# THE PHARMACEUTICAL INDEX

## 2014 Worldwide NCEs

A collection of drug information and preclinical research data
on worldwide approved NCEs in 2014

**Edited by Pharmacodia**

CHINA MEDICAL SCIENCE PRESS

**图书在版编目（CIP）数据**

世界新药概览. 2014 卷 / 药渡经纬信息科技（北京）有限公司主编.
—北京：中国医药科技出版社，2017.1
ISBN 978–7–5067–8744–4

Ⅰ. ①世… Ⅱ. ①药… Ⅲ. ①药品–介绍–世界 Ⅳ. ①R97

中国版本图书馆 CIP 数据核字（2016）第 266577 号

ISBN 978-7-5067-8744-4

The Pharmaceutical Index 2014 Worldwide NCEs

Compiled by Pharmacodia (Beijing) Co., LTD

Room 105, Haohai Building, No.7, 5th Street, Shangdi, Haidian District, Beijing, P.R. China, 100085

ISBN 978-7-5067-8744-4

Executive Editor: Yanyi Zhao    Yumeng Gao    Jin Ma
Cover Designer: Junqi Chen
Format Designer: Lu Zhang
Copyright © 2016 by China Medical Science Press
Published by China Medical Science Press, 2017.1
A-22 Northern Wenhuiyuan Road, Haidian District, Beijing, China, 100082

Printed in the People's Republic of China

# 编写委员会

# Editorial Board

| | |
|---|---|
| Liangren Zhang | Peking University, Beijing, P.R.China |
| Shu Liu | Pharmacodia, Beijing, P.R.China |
| Yi Cui | Pharmacodia, Beijing, P.R.China |
| Xiaomei Tang | Pharmacodia, Beijing, P.R.China |

## Editors

| | |
|---|---|
| Yuanwu Bao | BioDuro LLC (Shanghai), Shanghai, P.R.China |
| Haizhi Bu | 3D BioOptima, Suzhou, Jiangsu, P.R.China |
| Zengjiang Cheng | PharmaSea Beijing, P.R.China |
| Wenkui Fang | XuanZhu Pharma, Jinan, Shandong, P.R.China |
| Chun Guo | Shenyang Pharmaceutical University, Benxi, Liaoning, P.R.China |
| Zhenhua Huang | KBP BioSciences |
| Yunfeng Li | Institute of Pharmacology & Toxicology of AMMS, Beijing, P.R.China |
| Minyong Li | Shandong University, Jinan, Shandong, P.R.China |
| Zhenming Liu | Peking University, Beijing, P.R.China |
| Qianye Karen Liu | 3E Bioventures Capital |
| Chang Shi | Institute of Pharmacology & Toxicology of AMMS, Beijing, P.R.China |
| Wenjun Tang | Shanghai Institute of Organic Chemistry, Chinese Academy of Science, Shanghai, P.R.China |
| Qian Wan | Central China Normal University, Wuhan, Hubei, P.R.China |
| Lili Wang | Institute of Pharmacology & Toxicology of AMMS, Beijing, P.R.China |
| Peng Wu | The Scripps Research Institute, La Jolla, California, USA |
| Chunqi Wu | Institute of Pharmacology & Toxicology of AMMS, Beijing, P.R.China |
| Youjun Xu | Shenyang Pharmaceutical University, Benxi, Liaoning, P.R.China |

| Jianming Yu | Advantech Capital |
| Fuli Zhang | Shanghai Institute of Pharmaceutical Industry, Shanghai, P.R.China |
| Xumu Zhang | South University of Science and Technology of China, Shenzhen, Guangzhou, P.R.China |
| Linxiang Zhao | Shenyang Pharmaceutical University, Benxi, Liaoning, P.R.China |
| Bing Zhou | Shanghai Institute of Materia Medica, Chinese Academy of Science, Shanghai, P.R.China |

## Contributors in Pharmacodia

| | | | |
|---|---|---|---|
| Xinbi Cong | Xiaoduo Guan | Chunfang Huo | Rui Jiang |
| Zhi Jiang | Wenli Lan | Menghe Li | Dawei Li |
| Ai Mu | Wanying Qian | Ye Qiao | Yangyang Su |
| Jing Su | Jun Xu | Xiaoli Ye | Yongsheng Yu |
| Xiaowei Zhang | Man Zhang | | |

The Pharmaceutical Index
2014 Worldwide NCEs

# Acknowledgement

特别感谢药渡战略合作伙伴

尚珹资本和本草资本

对《世界新药概览》2014 年卷的大力支持

Special thanks to strategic partners of Pharmacodia,

Advantech Capital and 3E Bioventures Capital, for

*The Pharmaceutical Index 2014 Worldwide NCEs*

# Foreword

　　新药的发现是一个多学科协作的系统工程。药物化学家融合了化学、生物、医学、计算机和信息工程等学科的技术和进展，通过一系列细致的临床前和临床研究，才有可能开发出一个合格的临床用的上市药品。从发展的角度来看，新药的研究从经验的研究模式发展成现代的药物合理设计的模式。Aspirin 是从早期民间经验的基础上发展起来的，100 年后才研究清楚他解热镇痛和抗凝血的作用机制。后来发展的一系列基于动物的、细胞的、分子的药物筛选方法，开发出了大量新药，但大部分新药的作用机制是在药物上市后才进一步研究清楚。2001 年 Gleevec 的上市开创了新药研究历史上第一个针对疾病分子靶作用机制的新药。由于发现了慢性粒细胞白血病 chronic myeloid leukemia (CML)病人的第 9 和 22 位部分染色体的互换，形成了异常的 Bcr-Abl 酪氨酸蛋白激酶(Bcr-Abl tyrosine kinase)，以 Bcr-Abl 酪氨酸蛋白激酶为靶找到他的抑制剂 Gleevec。近年来，在研究了非小细胞肺癌的基因分类的基础上发现了 Iressa 对亚洲非小细胞肺癌病人群有比较好的治疗效果，从而开始了个体化精准医疗的年代，也开始了药物精准设计的年代。

Aspirin　　　　Gleevec　　　　Iressa

　　随着社会的发展和人类对疾病的深入了解，研究新药的难度也越来越大。根据这几年的资料，从 1996 至 2011 年，新药研发成功率逐年下降，2008～2011 年三年平均成功率 7.5%，是 1996～1999 三年平均成功率的一半不到(16.4%)。自 2011 年后开始反弹，2012～2014 年研究新药的成功率 11.6%。但小分子药物下降幅度还是巨大的(从 16%降到 5%)，而生物大分子则成功率相对平稳。因此小分子药物的研发需要新的疾病分子靶。

　　新的疾病分子靶的研究也有一个发现过程，如最近比较热门的 CDK4/6 抑制剂，其实已有 20 年的研发历史。第一个上市的 Palbociclib 早在 2001 年就由 Park-Davis 科学家合成，在辉瑞 2009 年开始 II 期临床之前大家都持观望态度，2007 年，UCLA 的科学家发现 Palbociclib 对乳腺癌(with estrogen-positive, HER2-negative)在体外十分有效，Palbociclib 2015 年首先上市，上市一年多，上季度销售额已达到 4.3 亿美元。同样的 CDK4/6 抑制剂，诺华的 Ribociclib (LEE011) III 期临床因疗效优异于今年 5 月被提前终止，有望今年上市。礼来的 Abemaciclib 则直接从 I 期跳进 III 期临床，紧随其后。

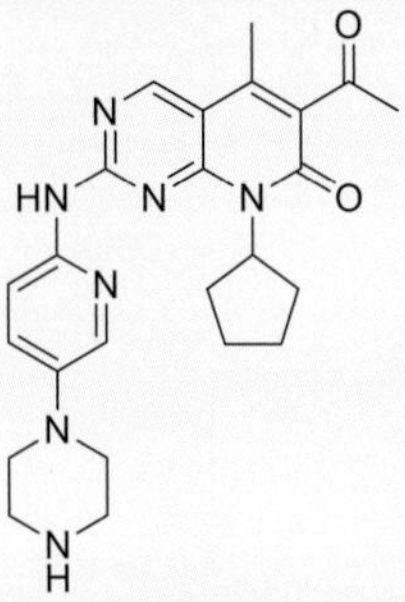

**Palbociclib** 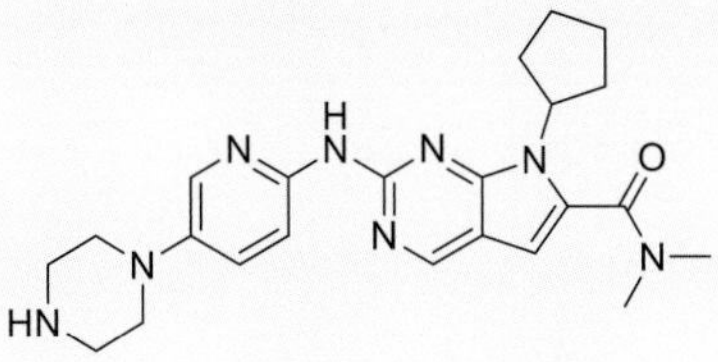          **Ribociclib (LEEO11)** 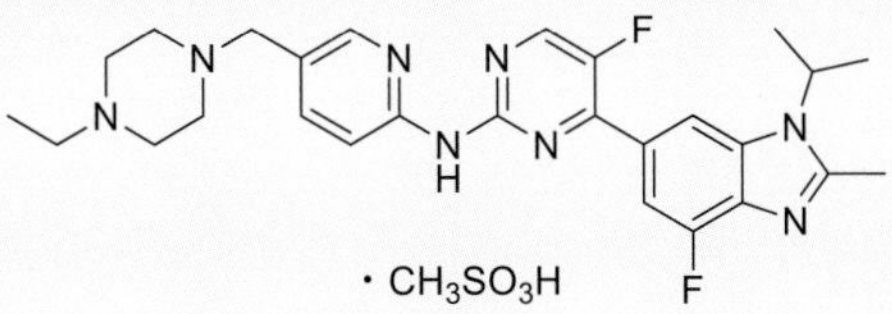          **Abemaciclib**

　　个体化精准医学需要生物、医学大数据的分析，从而也推动了信息科学以及相应的各类资料和数据的分析整理。我非常高兴的看到由"药渡"(Pharmacodia)主编的系列丛书《世界新药概览》(The Pharmaceutical Index)第一部(2013 年卷)已经出版，现在《世界新药概览》(The Pharmaceutical Index)第二部(2014 年卷)也将出版。这部丛书的 2014 年卷收集了当年世界各国上市的 31 个新药，书中详细整理了每个新药的临床前数据，包括合成路线、体内外的药理学实验数据、药物作用机制的研究、药物体内代谢和药物毒理数据，同时也给出了相关专利、文献和资料和数据的来源。这是我看到的第一部非常简明、非常实用又很方便查阅的药物工具书，我相信这部丛书对新药研究工作人员和临床研究工作人员都有很好的参考价值，在药学院校的教学工作中也是学生的一部很好的参考书。

张礼和

北京大学药学院

2016 年 7 月 12 日，北京

# Foreword

Every day brings fresh, tangible evidence of technology's impact on our lives. A couple years ago the internet streaked pass an astonishing landmark, the ability to level up and support ten million concurrent connections. Computer memory has increased a thousand-fold in the 21st Century. Why, then, has the number of small molecule drugs to come on the market only doubled in that same period of time?

Decades after Watson and Crick, most scientists still did not realize how profoundly complex is the living world. Medicinal chemists hoped logic would reduce the unpredictability of drug discovery, and that certainty would overtake serendipity. After a couple billion years on the defensive, however, nature rambled over a lot of territory and learned a lot of tricks.

Current pharmacological methods are more successful. Many of today's new drugs are found by optimizing small molecules using information from structures like proteins, or from hits found *via* high-throughput screening. Databases with the capacity to contain the big data generated by HTS are partnered with algorithms that facilitate delivering candidate compounds to targets. Nonetheless, rational drug design, to date, has not significantly shortened the time between a new therapeutics discovery and its becoming a commercial product.

There are other sources of fresh data to help advance the art of discovering useful biological activity, sources that haven't been systematically exploited yet. From 2001 through 2014, around 334 new chemical entities (NCEs) were approved, and each profile's documentation runs to thousands of pages. Data from this pool is cherry-picked by bioscientists, most of whom are looking to answer questions they've already framed. Until now, a universal methodology for organizing and presenting and evaluating all this data has not been attempted.

Now Pharmacodia, the publisher that maintains the most comprehensive body of information about the world's drugs, has created the Pharmaceutical Index. This first volume includes data for all the drugs approved in 2013; subsequently, the Pharmaceutical Index will be published annually, with each new volume presenting all the drugs receiving approval during the previous year. It assesses, and makes accessible, the most salient, significant and useful information about each of those NCEs. Every drug's data is summarized in twenty-or-so-pages of extensive chemistry, biology, pharmacokinetics, and medicinal chemistry data.

"The most fruitful basis for the discovery of a new drug," Nobel Laureate Sir James Whyte Black observed, "is to start with an old drug." A founding rational drug designer and iconic translational scientist, Sir James was an outstanding academician who was as good in the lab as he was in the board room. In a career full of accomplishments, the highlights were his team's discoveries of two entirely novel drug classes and the development of a unique, successful methodology that harnessed known agonists to search for specific new antagonists.

He created the beta blocker propranolol, the first reliable method for controlling blood pressure, and the world's best-selling drug until it was eclipsed by the H2 antagonist cimetidine (Tagamete®), also his discovery.  By eliminating the need for ulcer surgery, cimetidine changed the world practically over-night.

Though Sir James only had access to relatively 'small' data, he presciently looked for robust chemical/molecular tools.  Insights from propranolol's discovery became the starting point for developing cimetidine.  Likewise, this is the Pharmaceutical Index's philosophical starting point.

Unlike the data from optimized libraries and assays and high-throughput screens, the Index is a compendium of 'experiences' from hundreds of survivors of one of the most grueling events on Earth. There's no doubt a better understanding of the profiles of existing drug will assist in the design of future drugs.

Here are examples of the Pharmaceutical Index's utility:

1. Few pharma projects are pursued as much as the development of "me too drugs."  Good examples are the PDE5 inhibitors, used to treat erectile dysfunction, and proton pump inhibitors (PPIs) for

**Sildenafil**
**1998, Pfizer**

**Vardenafil**
**2003, Bayer, GSK**

**Udenafil**
**2005, Dong-A**

**Dexlansoprazole**
**2009, Takeda**

**Lansoprazole**
**1992, Takeda**

**Rabeprazole Sodium**
**1997, Eisai**

**Omeprazole**
**1988, AstraZeneca**

**Esomeprazole Magnesium Trihydrate**
**2000, AstraZeneca**

**Esomeprazole Sodium**
**2003, AstraZeneca**

**Esomeprazole Strontium**
**2013, Hanmi, Amneal**

**Pantoprazole Sodium Sesquihydrate**
**2000, Altana, Pfizer**

**Ilaprazole**
**2008, IL-Yang**

gastrointestinal disease. Knowing about their structure and pharmacology has been, and will continue to be, a well-traveled route to the designing of "me too drugs".

2. Information is data that's been organized, and effectively harvesting what's known about existing drugs will leverage the transformation of information into knowledge. Just an incremental increase in the odds that new candidate molecules survive clinical trials, and do so more rapidly, will save hundreds of millions. It is the help with their day-to-day challenges, however, that will be appreciated by researchers, like being able to access comprehensive knowledge bases for more strategic drug design selections. Absorption problems, for example, are often solved by a prodrug strategy. Used as a carboxylic acid promoiety, (5-methyl-2-oxo-1,3-dioxol-4-yl)methyl ester hydrolyzes *in vivo* in less than half an hour. While not a universal solution, it's quick and easy and gives useful feedback even if it's not successful.

**Olmesartan Medoxomil**
**2002, Daiichi-Sankyo**

**Ceftobiprole Medocaril Sodium**
**2008, Basilea & Janssen**

3. Collecting the 'nuggets' of historical medicinal chemistry gold can yield rich layers of treasure. A paradigm for exploiting the full texture of events is parecoxib, a salt form of valdecoxib whose approval in 2002 was a great accomplishment on multiple levels: not only was it the first injectable COX-2 inhibitor to reach the market, but the lessons from its discovery has had an impact on subsequent development programs. Clear, concise documentation of this and similar past practices will be useful to medicinal chemists and pharmaceutical scientists.

**Parecoxib Sodium**
**2002, Pfizer**

**Valdecoxib**
**2001, Pfizer**

This new series of *Pharmaceutical Indexes* will be a boon in academia and the pharmaceutical industry, and provide, as well, a significant addition to the therapeutics discovery arsenal. It should also find a wide audience in government, and the business community.

I am a chemist with a fundamental passion for making new molecular connectivity, and there is no measure by which I could be considered a representative member of the therapeutics community. While that group is unlikely to share my affinity for how Winston Churchill tackled his challenges, everyone should agree with what he thought was profoundly important. "Plans," he said, "are of little importance, but planning is essential."   The Pharmaceutical Index will make it easier to achieve the essential.

K. Barry Sharpless
*La Jolla, California, USA*
*December, 2015*

# Preface

Over the past decade, the process of drug discovery (from lead optimization to a clinical candidate) and development (from a clinical candidate to drug product approval) in the pharmaceutical industry has become an increasingly time-consuming and costly endeavor.[1]  On average, it takes approximately 10-15 years and $2.6 billion to develop a successful drug product.[2]  Major reasons preventing drugs from reaching the market are poor pharmacokinetic (PK) properties (20%), human toxicity (50%) and lack of efficacy (29%).[3]

As a result, a paradigm shift has occurred in the initial phases of drug discovery.  In addition to improving potency and selectivity towards the biological targets of interest, companies should also take into account the importance of PK and toxicity consideration at an early stage.  Hence, it is very important to design "drug-like" molecules, meaning molecules with functional groups that impart physical properties consistent with the majority of known drugs.

An ideal drug candidate should possess good pharmacological activity (potency and selectivity) as well as good ADME (absorption, distribution, metabolism, excretion) and toxicity (ADMET) properties.

Historically, there are 6000 drugs being used in humans.  There are currently around 3000 drugs still in clinical uses, not including herbal medicines.  These series of books focus on the profiles of the 500 pharmaceutical marketed products in the past two decades.  Underlying the basis of *The Pharmaceutical Index 2013 Worldwide NCEs* (1st volume), *The Pharmaceutical Index 2014 Worldwide NCEs* (2nd volume) improves the discription patterns of contents and styles.  "Patent Family" in text and "sales worldwide" as appendix have been added into the 2nd volume, which can provide more precise and detailed preclinical data, convenient for the new drug discovery.  The profile will include the following drug information:

1.  Sales
2.  Key patent information
3.  Mechanism of action
4.  Structural/physical chemistry
5.  Synthesis
6.  Target pharmacology
7.  *In vitro/in vivo* PK
8.  Drug-drug interaction
9.  Safety

The following paragraph will discuss the details covered in each category:

**1.  Sales:** The recent annual sales worldwide.  A summary table containing the drug worldwide sales in both 2014 and 2015 as an appendix.

**2.  Key Patent Information:** From the first matter of composition patent filing date and then adds 21 years as projected patent expiring date.   Besides, a summary of this part and the originator's international patent application list (patent family) are added, which is quite different from the 1$^{st}$ volume.

3. **Mechanism of Action:** Underlying mechanism of each drug.

4. **Structural/Physical Chemistry:** Lipinski's rule of five based drug-like properties.

Rule of five: Lipinski's Rule of Five is a rule of thumb to evaluate druglikeness, in other words, if a chemical compound with a certain pharmacological or biological activity has properties that would make it likely an orally active drug in humans. The rule was formulated by Christopher A. Lipinski in 1997, based on the observation that most drugs are relatively small and lipophilic molecules.[4] The rule describes molecular properties important for a drug's pharmacokinetics in the human body, including their absorption, distribution, metabolism, and excretion (ADME). However, the rule does not predict whether a compound will be pharmacologically active.

The Lipinski's rule is important for drug development since a pharmacologically active lead structure is optimized step-wise for not only increased activity and selectivity, but also drug-like properties before becoming a clinical candidate.[5]

Lipinski's rule states that, in general, an orally active drug has no more than one violation of the following criteria:

• Not more than 5 hydrogen bond donors (nitrogen or oxygen atoms with one or more hydrogen atoms)

• Not more than 10 hydrogen bond acceptors (nitrogen or oxygen atoms)

• A molecular mass not greater than 500 daltons

• An octanol-water partition coefficient[6] (log $P$) not greater than 5

Note that all numbers are five or multiples of five, which is the origin of the rule's name. As with many other rules of thumb, (such as Baldwin's guidelines for ring closure), there are many exceptions to Lipinski's rule.

5. **Synthesis**

Normally, for cost of goods reason, the synthetic steps involved for a given drug should not exceed 10 liner synthetic steps. The steps of synthesis in the drug table refer to the most scalable routes (process chemistry) based on author's judgment based on available publications and patents at the time of publication.

6. **Target Pharmacology**

6.1 $IC_{50}$: The half maximal inhibitory concentration ($IC_{50}$) is a measure of the effectiveness of a compound in inhibiting biological or biochemical function(s). This quantitative measure indicates how much of a particular drug or other substance (inhibitor) is needed to inhibit a given biological process (or component of a process, i.e. an enzyme, cell, cell receptor or microorganism) by half. In other words, it is the half maximal (50%) inhibitory concentration (IC) of a substance (50% IC, or $IC_{50}$). It is commonly used as a measure of antagonist drug potency in pharmacological research. Sometimes, it is also converted to the $pIC_{50}$ scale ($-\log IC_{50}$), in which higher values indicate exponentially greater potency. According to the FDA, $IC_{50}$ represents the concentration of a drug that is required for 50% inhibition *in vitro*. It is comparable to an $EC_{50}$ for agonist drugs. $EC_{50}$ also represents the plasma concentration required for obtaining 50% of a maximum effect *in vivo*.

6.2 Functional antagonist assay: The $IC_{50}$ of a drug can be determined by constructing a dose-response curve and examining the effect of different concentrations of antagonist on reversing agonist activity. $IC_{50}$ values can be calculated for a given antagonist by determining the concentration needed to inhibit half of the maximum biological response of the agonist. $IC_{50}$ values are very dependent on conditions under which they are measured. In general, the higher the concentration of inhibitor, the more agonist activity will be lowered. $IC_{50}$ value increases as enzyme concentration increases. Depending on the type of inhibition, furthermore, other factors may also influence $IC_{50}$ values. For ATP-dependent enzymes, $IC_{50}$ values have an interdependency with concentrations of ATP, especially so if the inhibition is competitive in nature. $IC_{50}$ values can be used to compare the potency of two antagonists.

6.3  Competition binding assays: In this type of assays, a single concentration of radioligand (usually an agonist) is used in every assay tube. The ligand is used at a low concentration, usually at or below its $K_d$ value. The level of specific binding of the radioligand is then determined in the presence of a range of concentrations of other competing non-radioactive compounds (usually antagonists), in order to measure the potency with which they compete for the binding of the radioligand. Competition curves may also be computer-fitted to a logistic function as described under direct fit. In this situation, the $IC_{50}$ is the concentration of competing ligand which displaces 50% of the specific binding of the radioligand. The $IC_{50}$ value is converted to an absolute inhibition constant $K_i$ using the Cheng-Prusoff equation (see $K_i$).[7]

6.4  Broad ligand profile screening: A concern with any given drug is that it selectively interacts with the target(s) of interest. It is quite common for projects to set up counter-screens to profile molecules *vs* related targets (isoforms that might have undesirable biological activity, other proteins from the same family with high sequence homology). For example, a CNS drug candidate may need to be profiled against other CNS targets (around 50) and may even be profiled further against more drug targets (around 250-300). One of the well-known companies in this field is CEREP. CEREP continues to expand and diversify the assay families, with an average of 100 assays added or updated each year. These assays are either integrated in the CEREP catalog, or are exclusively available to sponsor. The *in vitro* pharmacology and ADME-Tox & PK 2011 catalogs regroup about 1300 assays, of which 473 GPCRs, including 134 cellular functional targets (agonist and antagonist effects), 255 biochemical kinases and 32 cellular kinase assays (activator and inhibitor effects), 51 ion channels, 61 CYPs (phenotyping, inhibition, induction), 20 epigenetic and DNA-related enzymes, 14 PDEs, 24 phosphatases. Cerep's platforms cover a wide range of target classes including ADME-Tox related targets, GPCRs, various enzymes, transporters, nuclear receptors and ion channels, employing methods and assay types such as radioligand binding assays, calcium mobilization and cAMP measurement using TR-FRET, transporter/uptake assays, and bioluminescent and other fluorescent-based assays.

## 7.  Absorption and Bioavailability

7.1  While the gastrointestinal tract represents the first barrier to drug absorption after oral administration, it is the dynamic interplay between absorption, metabolism, distribution, and elimination that determines the amount of drug in the plasma. Two important pharmacokinetic parameters for understanding absorption following an extra-vascular dosing are area under the curve (AUC) and bioavailability (F). Rate-limiting steps to oral bioavailability may include: Dissolution, permeability, gut motility, and degree of ionization. Additional determination of bioavailability includes the first-pass effects. First-pass effects refer to the loss of drug, as it passes, for the first time, through sites of elimination following absorption through gastrointestinal tract and liver cell membranes. First-pass effects lower the amount of drug passing to the general circulation by extracting it through metabolic and transport mechanisms. Oral bioavailability may, therefore, be represented as the product of the fraction absorbed by gastrointestinal tract ($F_a$) and the fraction in the gastrointestinal tract ($F_g$), liver ($F_h$) and lung ($F_l$) which are not subjected to the first-pass effects: $F = F_a \cdot F_g \cdot F_h \cdot F_l$ or $F = F_a (1 - E_g)(1 - E_h)(1 - E_l)$ where E stands for extraction ratio of gut ($E_g$), Liver ($E_h$), and lung ($E_l$). When the molecule is mainly metabolized by the liver ($E_g \approx 0$ and $E_l \approx 0$), F can be expressed as following equation.

$$F = F_a (1 - E_h)$$

Where $E_h$ is the metabolic hepatic extraction ratio and $F_a$ the intestinal fraction absorption. In general, $E_h < 3$, ranked as low extraction, $3 < E_h < 7$, ranked as moderate extraction, and $E_h > 7$, ranked as high extraction.

7.2 Caco-2 and MDCK cells. Caco-2 cells, derived from a human colorectal carcinoma, are one of the most widely used *in vitro* models for understanding intestinal absorption and deciphering mechanism of transport. With respect to passively absorbed drugs, a correlation between Caco-2 cell permeability and human intestinal absorption has been established. In order to measure cell membrane permeability in an *in vitro* monolayer-based assay, test compounds are added onto the apical side (A) of a monolayer, and their appearance in the basolateral compartment (B) indicates membrane permeability. Permeability measurements for *in vitro* cellular models are generally described by an apparent permeability coefficient (Papp) and calculated according to the following equation:

$$Papp = dQ/dt \, (1/A)(C_0)$$

Where dQ/dt is the permeability rate (nmol/s), $C_0$ the initial substrate concentration in the donor compartment, and A the surface area of the monolayer (cm$^3$). Papp values (cm/s) of $<1 \times 10^{-6}$, $1 \times 10^{-6}$-$10 \times 10^{-6}$, and $>10 \times 10^{-6}$, may be associated with low, moderate and good absorption, respectively. It is important to note that the Papp ranges associated with absorption prediction can vary greatly from laboratory to laboratory. Despite the variability observed with Caco-2 cells, they are useful, not only for human absorption predictions but for the study of several transport systems. This is due to the fact that it expresses transporters for sugars, amino acids, bile acids, and thus, are a relevant system to assess transporters for many drugs. Most transporter-based studies focus on the use of Caco-2 for evaluating MDR1 (P-glycoprotein, P-gP) interactions. The significance of P-gP in limiting drug absorption and bioavailability is well established. Several factors are of concerns when assessing P-gP activity in Caco-2 cells. P-gP expression level may vary several-fold in both human intestine and Caco-2 cells. Caco-2 culture time and passage number appear to modulate P-gP expression. This means that culture conditions must be held constant to ensure consistent levels of P-gP when testing chemical compounds. Since Caco-2 cells express many transporters in addition to P-gP, they can also be used to assess drug-drug interactions with multiple transporters. For HTS screening purpose, the use of MDCK, derived from dog kidneys, has become increasingly popular. While Caco-2 cells require a three-week culture time to fully differentiate (i.e. establish tight junctions, cell polarity, and membrane transporter expression), MDCK cells form complete monolayer after 3 days of culture. In addition, human MDR1-transfected MDCK cells are available that significantly over-expressed human MDR1 when compared to endogenous transporters. Thus these cells offer superior resolution of transporter-specific efflux as compared to Caco-2 cells. While Caco-2 and MDCK cells are useful screening models to predict human absorption, both systems lack the expression of clinically significant drug metabolizing enzymes such as CYP3A4, an enzyme that is highly expressed in human intestine.[1] Cell monolayer permeability assay such as Caco-2 or MDCK can lead to over prediction of absorption potential if a compound is significantly metabolized by intestine CYP3A4. However, Caco-2 cells in combination with metabolic liability (hepatocytes or microsomal assays) may be used to predict bioavailability within a structural series of compounds.

### 8. Drug-Drug Interaction

8.1 A drug interaction is a situation in which a drug substance affects the activity of another drug, i.e. the effects are increased or decreased, or they produce a new effect that neither produces on its own. Hence the terminology is called drug-drug interaction. However, interactions may also exist between drugs & foods (drug-food interactions), as well as drugs & herbs (drug-herb interactions). These may occur out of accidental misuse, excessive use and mostly occur due to lack of knowledge of the active ingredients involved in the relevant herbs and food.

Generally speaking, drug interactions are to be avoided, due to the possibility of poor or unexpected outcomes in treatment. However, drug interactions have been deliberately used, such as co-administering probenecid with penicillin prior to mass production of penicillin. Probenecid retards the excretion of penicillin, so a dose of penicillin persists longer when taken with it, and it allowed patients to take less penicillin over a course of therapy. Because penicillin was difficult to manufacture, it was worthwhile to find a way to reduce the amount required.

A contemporary example of a drug interaction used as an advantage is the co-administration of carbidopa with levodopa (available as carbidopa/levodopa). Levodopa is used in the management of Parkinson's disease and must reach the brain in an un-metabolized state to be beneficial. When given by itself, levodopa is metabolized in the peripheral tissues outside the brain, which decreases the effectiveness of the drug and increases the risk of adverse effects. However, since carbidopa inhibits the peripheral metabolism of levodopa, the co-administration of carbidopa with levodopa allows more levodopa to reach the brain un-metabolized and also reduces the risk of side effects.

Drug interactions may be the result of various processes. These processes may include alterations in the pharmacokinetics of a drug, such as alterations in the ADME of the drug. Alternatively, drug interactions may be the result of the pharmacodynamic properties of the drug, e.g. the co-administration of a receptor antagonist and an agonist for the same receptor.

8.2 Metabolic drug interactions: Many drug interactions are due to alterations in drug metabolism. Further, human drug-metabolizing enzymes are typically activated through engagement of nuclear receptors.

One notable system involved in metabolic drug interactions is the enzyme system comprising the cytochrome P450 oxidases. This system may be affected by either enzyme induction or enzyme inhibition, as discussed in the examples below.

- Enzyme induction: Drug A induces the body to produce more of an enzyme which metabolizes drug B. This reduces the effective concentration of drug B, which may lead to loss of effectiveness of drug B. Drug A effectiveness is not altered.

- Enzyme inhibition: Drug A inhibits the production of the enzyme metabolizing drug B, thus an elevation of drug B occurs possibly leading to an overdose.

- Bioavailability: Drug A influences the absorption of drug B.

The examples described above may have different outcomes depending on the nature of the drugs. For example, if Drug B is a prodrug, then enzyme activation is required for the drug to reach its active form. Hence, enzyme induction by Drug A would increase the effectiveness of the drug B by increasing its metabolism to its active form. Enzyme inhibition by Drug A would decrease the effectiveness of Drug B. Additionally, Drug A and Drug B may affect each other's metabolism.

The phase I metabolic reactions commonly encountered in drug discovery are hydrolysis and oxidation. Hydrolysis is usually spontaneous enzymatic biotransformation of esters, amides, and epoxides to corresponding carboxylic acids, amines and alcohols in tissues and plasma. Thus these functional groups can be used as prodrug approaches for drug delivery to enhance the solubility and bioavailability. Enzymatic oxidation usually includes hydroxylation of aromatic and aliphatic carbons and heteroatoms (N-, S-, O-), as well as dealkylation and oxidations of carbons and direct oxidation of heteroatoms (N-, S-). The enzymes involved in these oxidations are mainly aldehyde oxidase (AO), xanthine oxidase (XO), monoamine oxidase (MAOs), flavin-containing monooxygenases (FMOs) and cytochrome P450s. Companies commonly set up routine assays to assess P450s activity, which includes CYP1A2, CYP3A4, CYP2D6, CYP2C19 and CYP2C9 isoforms. P450s constitute a superfamily of b-type heme-containing monooxygenases and are the most important drug metabolizing enzymes for numerous xenobiotics (drugs, pesticides, pollutants and dietary components) as well as some endogenous substrates (bile acids, steroids and cholesterol) in preclinical species and humans. Cytochrome P450 enzymes are present in many mammalian organs, such as kidneys, lungs and intestines with the majority residing in the liver.

Based on amino acid sequence homology, CYP superfamily members are divided into various subfamilies, which are further divided into various isoforms. More than 40 P450 subfamilies are currently identified and only four subfamilies (1, 2, 3, 4) are defined as drug metabolizing enzymes. Major isoforms involved in the biotransformation of drugs in humans are CYP1A2, CYP2C9, CYP2C19, CYP2D6 and CYP3A4. Among these isoforms, CYP3A4 is the most abundant isoform and account for approximately 30%-40% of the total content in the human liver and small intestine. CYP3A4 is estimated to metabolize 50%-70% of the currently used drugs. P450 isoforms exhibit significant substrate specificity during the biotransformation process, such as regio-and stereo selectivity. P450 enzymes can be inhibited, as well as induced by some xenobiotics, which possess the potential for drug-drug interaction. It is important to identify the polymorphically expressed isoforms (CYP2C9, CYP2C19, CYP2D6), which could cause inter-subject variability in human clinical PK.

### 9. Genetic Toxicity

Carcinogens, or cancer-inducing agents, can be divided into mutagenic and non-mutagenic in nature. Mutagenic carcinogens are agents that induce mutation or DNA sequence changes. The goal of genetic toxicity screening in drug discovery is to identify potential mutagenic and non-mutagenic carcinogens. Since the introduction of the Ames test, many *in vitro* tests have been proposed to identify mutagenic carcinogens.

The Ames test is a biological assay to assess the mutagenic potential of chemical compounds.[8] A positive test indicates that the chemical is mutagenic and therefore may act as a carcinogen, since cancer is often linked to mutation. However, a number of false-positives and false-negatives are known. The test serves as a quick and convenient assay to estimate the carcinogenic potential of a compound since standard carcinogen assays on rodents is time-consuming (taking around three years to complete) and expensive. The procedure is described in a series of papers from the early 1970s by Bruce Ames and his group at the University of California, Berkeley.

The test uses several strains of the bacterium *Salmonella typhimurium* that carry mutations in genes involved in histidine synthesis (i.e. an auxotrophic mutant) so that they require histidine for growth.

The method tests the capability of mutagen in creating mutations that can result in a reversion back to a non-auxotrophic state and thus the cells can grow on a histidine-free medium. The tester strains are specially constructed to detect either frameshift (e.g. strains TA-1537 and TA-1538) or point (e.g. strain TA-1531) mutations in the genes required to synthesize histidine, so that mutagens acting *via* different mechanisms may be identified. Some compounds are quite specific, causing reversions in just one or two strains.[9] The tester strains also carry mutations in the genes responsible for lipopolysaccharide synthesis, making the cell wall of the bacteria more permeable[10] and in the excision repair system to make the test more sensitive.[11] Rat liver extract is optionally added to simulate the effect of metabolism, as some compounds, like benzo[*a*]pyrene, are not mutagenic themselves but their metabolic products are.[12]

The bacteria are spread on an agar plate with a small amount of histidine. This small amount of histidine in the growth medium allows the bacteria to grow for an initial time and have the opportunity to mutate. When the histidine is depleted, only bacteria that have mutated to gain the ability to produce its own histidine will survive. The plate is incubated for 48 hours. The mutagenicity of a substance is proportional to the number of colonies observed.

Early studies by Ames showed that 90% of known carcinogens may be identified via this test.[13] Later studies, however, showed the identification of only 50%-70% of known carcinogens. The test was used to identify a number of compounds previously used in commercial products as potential carcinogens.[14] Examples include tris (2,3-dibromopropyl)phosphate which was used as a flame retardant in plastics and textiles, such as children's sleepware[15] and furylfuramide which was used as an antibacterial additive in food in Japan in 1960s and 1970s. Furylfuramide in fact had previously passed animal test, but more vigorous tests, after its identification in Ames test, showed it to be carcinogenic. The positive tests resulted in these chemicals being withdrawn from use in consumer product.

One interesting result from Ames test is that the dose response curve from Ames test using varying concentrations of chemical is almost always linear, indicating no threshold concentration for mutagenesis or in other words no safe threshold for mutagens or carcinogens. However, some researchers proposed that a low level of some mutagens may stimulate the DNA repair processes which can mitigate the effect of the mutagens and thus may not be harmful. Bruce Ames himself cautioned against the "hysteria over tiny traces of chemicals that may or may not cause cancer", that "completely drives out the major risks you should be aware of".[16]

Ames test is often used as one of the initial screens for potential drugs to weed out possible carcinogens and one of the eight tests required under Pesticide Act (USA) and one of six tests required under Toxic Substances Control Act (USA). *Salmonella typhimurium* is a prokaryote and not a perfect model for humans. Rat liver S9 fraction is used to mimic the mammalian metabolic conditions so that the mutagenic potential of metabolites formed from a parent molecule in the hepatic system can be assessed. As differences in metabolism and mutagenicity of chemicals exist between human and rat[17], the test may be improved by the use of human liver S9 fraction. The human liver S9 fraction was previously limited by its availability, but it is now commercially available. An adapted *in vitro* model has been made from eukaryotic cells, for example, yeast cells.

Mutagens identified in Ames test are not necessarily to be carcinogenic and further tests are required for any potential carcinogens identified in the test. Drugs that contain the nitrate moiety sometimes come back positive for Ames when they are indeed safe. The nitrate compounds may generate nitric oxide, an important signal molecule that can give a false positive. Nitroglycerin is an example that gives a positive Ames result yet is still used in treatment today. Long-term toxicology and outcome studies are needed with such compounds to disprove a positive Ames test.

### 10. Micronucleus Test

A micronucleus test is a test used in toxicological screening for potential genotoxic compounds. There are two major versions of this test, *in vivo* and *in vitro*. The *in vivo* test normally uses mouse bone marrow or mouse peripheral blood. Micronuclei were first used to quantify chromosomal damage, by H. J. Evans et al., in root tips of the Broad Bean, *Vicia faba*. Soon after, another *in vivo* assay was developed independently by W. Schmid and by J. A. Heddle and their colleagues. The assay is now recognized as one of the most successful and reliable assays for genotoxic carcinogens, i.e., carcinogens that act by causing genetic damage. The mouse peripheral blood assay was developed by J. T. Mac-Gregor and has now been adapted for measurement using flow cytometry by A. Tometsko and colleagues. The first use of micronuclei in cultured cells was developed by J. A. Heddle and colleagues using human lymphocytes. The assay has been improved by M. Fenech and colleagues for use in lymphocytes and other culture cells.

A micronucleus is the erratic (third) nucleus that is formed during the anaphase of mitosis or meiosis. Micronucleus, the name itself indicating small nucleus, are cytoplasmic bodies having a portion of acentric chromosome or the whole chromosome which is not carried during the anaphase to the opposite poles, finally resulting in missing of part or whole chromosome for the daughter cell. These chromosome fragments or whole chromosomes normally develop nuclear membranes and forms as micronuclei as a third nucleus. After cytokinesis, one daughter cell is with one nucleus and the other is with one large and one small nucleus, i.e. micronuclei. There is a chance of more than one micronuclei forming when more genetic damages happens. Micronucleus test is used as genotoxicity assessment of various chemicals and easy to conduct rather than chromosomal Aberration test because of its relative ease in conducting studies and evaluations. Using fluorescent in situ hybridization (FISH) with probes targeted to the centromere region, it can determine whether a whole chromosome or only a fragment is lost.

### 11. Acute Toxicity

Acute toxicity describes the adverse effects of a substance that result either from a single exposure or from multiple exposures in a short space of time (usually less than 24 hours). To be described as acute toxicity, the adverse effects should occur within 14 days of the administration of the substance.

Acute toxicity is distinguished from chronic toxicity, which describes the adverse health effects from repeated exposures, often at lower levels, to a substance over a longer time period (months or years).

It is widely considered unethical to use humans as test subjects for acute (or chronic) toxicity research. However, some information can be gained from investigating accidental human exposures (e.g., factory accidents). Otherwise, most acute toxicity data comes from animal testing or, more recently, *in vitro* testing methods and inference from data on similar substances.

### 12. Chronic Toxicity

Chronic toxicity is a property of a substance that has toxic effects on a living organism, when that organism is exposed to the substance continuously or repeatedly. Two distinct situations need to be considered:

- Prolonged exposure to a substance

For example if a person drinks too much alcohol on a regular basis then their health may suffer as a result. The alcohol does not have a long biological half-life but it is supplied on a regular basis to the body of the person.

- Prolonged internal exposure because a substance remains in the body for a long time

If a person was to ingest radium, for example, it would be absorbed into the bones where it would exert a harmful effect on a person's health. The radium might cause a disturbance in the blood cell-forming part of the bone (bone marrow).

Guidance on duration of chronic toxicity testing for tripartite development plan: Arising from the extensive analysis of non-rodents and based upon the achievements of ICH1 for testing in rodents, and so as to avoid duplication and follow a single development plan for chronic toxicity testing of new medicinal products, the following studies are considered acceptable for submission in the 3 regions:

1. Rodents

A study of 6 months duration.

2. Non-Rodents

A study of 9 months duration.

According to the limitation of editor's ability, the choices about the drug information and the aspect of editing might be somewhere inappropriate. It will be grateful for readers to provide your valuable comments and suggestions.

### References

[1]  Lin, J.; Sahakian, D. C.; de Morais, S. M., et al. *Curr. Top. Med. Chem.* **2003**, *3*, 1125-1154.

[2]  Tufts center for the study of drug development, 18 Nov, **2014**.

[3]  Cheng, A.; Diller, D. J.; Dixon, S. L., et al. *J. Comput. Chem.* **2002**, *23*, 172-183.

[4]  Lipinski, C. A.; Lombardo, F.; Dominy, B. W., et al. *Adv. Drug Deliv. Rev.* **2001**, *46*, 3-26.

[5]  Oprea, T. I.; Davis, A. M.; Teague, S. J., et al. *J. Chem. Inf. Comput. Sci.* **2001**, *41*, 1308-1315.

[6]  Leo, A.; Hansch, C.; Elkins, D. *Chem. Rev.* **1971**, *71*, 525-616.

[7]  Cheng, Y.; Prusoff, W. H. *Biochem. Pharmacol.* **1973**, *22*, 3099-3108.

[8]  Mortelmans, K.; Zeiger, E. *Mutat. Res.* **2000**, *455*, 29-60.

[9]  Ames, B. N.; Gurney, E. G.; Miller, J. A., et al. *Proc. Nat. Acad. Sci. U. S. A.* **1972**, *69*, 3128-3132.

[10]  Ames, B. N.; Lee, F. D.; Durston, W. E. *Proc. Natl. Acad. Sci. U. S. A.* **1973**, *70*, 782-786.

[11]  McCann, J.; Spingarn, N. E.; Kobori, J., et al. *Proc. Natl. Acad. Sci. U. S. A.* **1975**, *72*, 979-983.

[12]  Ames, B. N.; Durston, W. E.; Yamasaki, E., et al. *Proc. Natl. Acad. Sci. U. S. A.* **1973**, *70*, 2281-2285.

[13]  McCann, J.; Choi, E.; Yamasaki, E., et al. *Proc. Natl. Acad. Sci. U. S. A.* **1975**, *72*, 5135-5139.

[14]  Ames, B. N. *Science* **1979**, *204*, 587-593.

[15]  Prival, M. J.; McCoy, E. C.; Gutter, B., et al. *Science* **1977**, *195*, 76-78.

[16]  Twombly, R. *J. Natl. Cancer Inst.* **2001**, *93*, 1372.

[17]  Hakura, A.; Suzuki, S.; Satoh, T. *Mutat. Res., Genet. Toxicol. Environ. Mutagen.* **1999**, *438*, 29-36.

# Contents

This second volume of The Pharmaceutical Index includes thirty one NCEs instead of thirty two total approvals due to limited publications. The unprofiled NCE was Morinidazole (迈灵达®), which was developed by Hansoh Pharmaceutical and approved in Feb 2014 by CFDA.

The Pharmaceutical Index
2014 Worldwide NCEs

# Contents

## *NERVOUS SYSTEM*

## *OPHTHALMIC and ENT*

## *RESPIRATORY*

This second volume of The Pharmaceutical Index includes thirty one NCEs instead of thirty two total approvals due to limited publications.   The unprofiled NCE was Morinidazole (迈灵达®), which was developed by Hansoh Pharmaceutical and approved in Feb 2014 by CFDA.

# Executive Summary

## Alectinib Hydrochloride
## (Alecensa®)
AF-802; RG-7853; CH-5424802; RO-5424802
Capsule, oral, EQ 20 mg/40 mg Alectinib

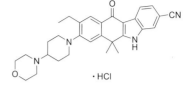
· HCl

❖ Alectinib hydrochloride is a small molecule inhibitor of ALK kinase, indicated for the treatment of patients with ALK fusion gene-positive unresectable, recurrent or advanced non-small cell lung cancer.   It was first approved in Jul 2014 by PMDA of Japan.
❖ Alectinib hydrochloride was discovered and marketed by Chugai (a subsidiary of Hoffmann-La Roche AG).
❖ *The recommended human starting dose* is 300 mg twice daily without food for adults.

| Worldwide Key Approvals | Global Sales ($Million) | | Key Substance Patent Expiration |
|---|---|---|---|
| Jul 04, 2014 (JP) | **2014** | 13.2 | May 29, 2031 (US9126931B2) (EP2441753A1: Examination) |
| Dec 11, 2015 (US) | **2015** | 71.3 | Mar 25, 2034 (JP4588121B1) Jun 09, 2030 (CN102459172B) |

## Mechanism of Action

As an ALK inhibitor, alectinib hydrochloride inhibits ALK and the downstream signals, thereby inhibiting tumor cells harboring ALK fusion, amplifications or activiating mutations.

**Target Binding Selectivity**
ALK: $IC_{50}$ = 1.9 nM
M4, ALK: $IC_{50}$ = 1.2 nM

**In Vitro Efficacy**
Human ALK fusion/amplification/mutation:
  $IC_{50}$ = 3.0-62 nM
Human ALK (fusion) nagetive cells:
  $IC_{50}$ = 400->1000 nM
Ba/F3 cells WT or EML-ALK mutation cells:
  $IC_{50}$ = 16-910 nM

**In Vivo Efficacy**
In NCI-H2228 models: TGI% = 59% at 0.8 mg/kg
In Karpas299 mouse models:
  TGI% = 94% at 6 mg/kg
In NB-1 mouse models:
  TGI% = 63% at 6 mg/kg
In crizotinib-resistant Ba/F3 models with L1196ALK-mutation:
  Tumor regression at 60 mg/kg/day

## Pharmacokinetics

| | Parameter | Rat | | Monkey | | Patient | | | | | |
|---|---|---|---|---|---|---|---|---|---|---|---|
| | Dose (mg/kg) | 1 (i.v.) | 1 (p.o.) | 0.5 (i.v.) | 0.5 (p.o.) | 20 (p.o.) | 40 (p.o.) | 80 (p.o.) | 160 (p.o.) | 240 (p.o.) | 300 (p.o.) |
| In Vivo | $C_{max}$ (ng/mL) | $C_0$: 175 | 60.9 | $C_0$: 283 | 55.8 | 4.52 | 12.3 | 41.4 | 60.3 | 58.6 | 84.1 |
| | $T_{max}$ (h) | NA | 8.0 | NA | 2.0 | 5.97 | 3.97 | 3.98 | 2.62 | 2.69 | 2.38 |
| | $AUC_{inf}$ (ng·h/mL) | 1580 | 1400 | 1380 | 696 | 206 | 288 | 696 | 1120 | 968 | 1640 |
| | $T_{1/2}$ (h) | 24.4 | 32.1 | 10.4 | 8.38 | 42.4 | 26.6 | 16.1 | 22.3 | 17.7 | 19.3 |
| | Cl (mL/min/kg) | 11.0 | NA | 6.04 | 13.0 | NA | NA | NA | NA | NA | NA |
| | $V_{ss}$ (L/kg) | 13.3 | NA | 5.28 | NA | NA | NA | NA | NA | NA | NA |
| | F (%) | - | 88.6 | - | 50.4 | NA | NA | NA | NA | NA | NA |
| | Most Abundant Drug-related Component in Plasma (%) | M0 (72.6) | | NA | | NA | | | | | |
| | Major Drug-related Metabolite in Plasma (%) | M1 (2.9) | | NA | | NA | | | | | |
| | Urine/Feces Excretion (%) | 0.5/95.7 | | NA | | <0.5/98 | | | | | |
| In Vitro | Caco-2 Permeability (%) | $Papp_{(A \to B)}$ = 1.88 ×$10^{-6}$ cm/s at 10 μM | | | | | | | | | |
| | Plasma Protein Binding (%Bound) | 99.1-99.6 | | 99.4-99.7 | | 99.1-99.5 | | | | | |
| | Hepatocytes Stability ($Cl_{int}$, mL/min/$10^6$ cells) | 0.0122 | | 0.0183 | | 0.0131 | | | | | |

## Drug-Drug Interaction

| | CYP Enzyme | Non-CYP Enzyme | Transporter |
|---|---|---|---|
| **Substrate** | CYP3A4 | NA | Not |
| **Inhibitor** | CYP2C8, 3A4, 1A2, 2B6, 2C9, 2D6, 2C19 | NA | P-gp, BCRP |
| **Inducer** | Not | NA | NA |

## Non-clinical Toxicology

| Single-Dose Toxicity | NA | Safety Pharmacology | • CVS: hERG $IC_{50}$ = 0.45 μM, Cav1.2 $IC_{50}$ = 0.461 μM<br>• No effects on respiratory, neurological effect or GI motor functions |
|---|---|---|---|
| **Repeated-Dose Toxicity (NOAEL)** | <3 mg/kg/day (rat, 13 weeks) <1.3 mg/kg/day (monkey, 13 weeks) | **Genotoxicity** | • Negative in the *in vitro* bacterial reverse mutation assay<br>• Positive in the *in vitro* mammalian cell chromosomal aberration assay and *in vivo* rat bone marrow micronucleus assay |
| | | **Reproductive and Developmental Toxicity** | • EFD in rats and rabbits: Increased fetal mortality, early embryonic mortality and total litter loss at 27 mg/kg; The NOAEL for maternal and fetal toxicity: 3 mg/kg/day in rats and 9 mg/kg/day in rabbits |
| | | **Carcinogenicity** | • NA |
| | | **Special Toxicology** | • Photo irritation factor: 94.8 |

## Apatinib Mesylate
(艾坦®)

YN-968D1

Tablet, oral, EQ 250 mg/375 mg/425 mg Apatinib

HENG RUI PHARMACEUTICALS

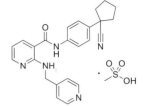

❖ Apatinib is a potent inhibitor of the vascular endothelial growth factor receptor-2 (VEGFR-2), indicated for the treatment of patients with progression and refractory advanced gastric cancer who have been treated with at least two prior lines of chemotherapy. It was first approved in Oct 2014 by CFDA.

❖ Apatinib was discovered and marketed by Hengrui Pharmaceuticals.

❖ ***The recommended human starting dose*** is 850 mg once daily, taken half an hour after a meal. For adverse reactions, considering dose interruption of treatments, dose reduces to 750 mg or 500 mg once daily.

| Worldwide Key Approvals | Global Sales ($Million) | Key Substance Patent Expiration |
|---|---|---|
| Oct 17, 2014 (CN) | Not available | Oct 08, 2024 (US7129252B2)<br>Jun 04, 2024 (EP1633712B1)<br>Jun 04, 2024 (JP5046643B2)<br>Nov 27, 2022 (CN1281590C) |

### Mechanism of Action

As a kinase inhibitor, apatinib suppresses the kinase activities of VEGFR-2 and inhibits cellular phosphorylation of VEGFR-2, c-kit and PDGFR.

| Target Binding and Inhibition | *In Vitro* Efficacy | *In Vivo* Efficacy |
|---|---|---|
| VEGFR-2: $IC_{50}$ = 1 nM<br>c-kit: $IC_{50}$ = 429 nM<br>Ret: $IC_{50}$ = 13 nM | Tube formation or transwell migration of HUVEC:<br>  Significant inhibition at 1 μM<br>Microvessel formation:<br>  Significantly inhibited at 0.1 μM | SGC-7901 human gastric tumor xenograft mouse model:<br>  Significant tumor growth inhibition at 100 mg/kg<br>  (T/C% = 33%) |

### Pharmacokinetics

| | Parameter | Rat | Human | | |
|---|---|---|---|---|---|
| | Dose (mg/kg, human: mg) | 20<br>(p.o.) | 500<br>(p.o.) | 750<br>(p.o.) | 850<br>(p.o.) |
| | $C_{max}$ (ng/mL) | 69.6 | 1521 | 2379 | 2833 |
| | $T_{max}$ (h) | 1.33 | NA | NA | NA |
| | $AUC_{0-t}$ (ng·h/mL) | 226 | 11295 | 18172 | 21975 |
| | $T_{1/2}$ (h) | 1.78 | 8 | 9 | 9 |
| *In Vivo* | Cl/F (L/h/kg) | 91.5 | NA | NA | NA |
| | $V_{ss}$/F (L/kg) | 300 | NA | NA | NA |
| | F (%) | NA | NA | NA | NA |
| | Most Abundant Drug-Related Component in Plasma (%) | NA | 4 h:M0 (41.4)/8 h:M9-2 (32.2) | | |
| | Major Drug-Related Metabolite in Plasma (%) | NA | M9-2 (19.6)/M9-2 (32.2) | | |
| | Urine/Feces Excretion (%) | NA | 7.02/69.8 | | |
| *In Vitro* | Caco-2 Permeability | NA | | | |
| | Plasma Protein Binding (%Bound) | NA | 92.4 | | |
| | LM/Hepatocytes Stability | NA | NA | | |

### Drug-Drug Interaction

| | CYP Enzyme | Non-CYP Enzyme | Transporter |
|---|---|---|---|
| Substrate | CYP3A4/5, 2D6, 2C9, 2E1 | UGT1A1/3/4/8/9, 2B4/7/17 | P-gp, BCRP |
| Inhibitor | NA | NA | P-gp, BCRP |
| Inducer | NA | NA | Not |

### Non-clinical Toxicology

| Single-Dose Toxicity (MTD) | 30 mg/kg (dog) | Safety Pharmacology | • NA |
|---|---|---|---|
| Repeated-Dose Toxicity (NOAEL) | NA | Genotoxicity | • NA |
| | | Reproductive and Developmental Toxicity | • NA |
| | | Carcinogenicity | • NA |

## Apremilast
## (Otezla®)
CC-10004
Tablet, oral, 10 mg/20 mg/30 mg Apremilast

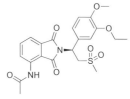

❖ Apremilast is a PDE4 inhibitor, indicated for the treatment of adults with active psoriatic arthritis. It was first approved in Mar 2014 by US FDA.
❖ Apremilast was discovered and marketed by Celgene.
❖ ***The recommended human dose*** is orally 30 mg of apremilast once daily until disease progression or unacceptable toxicity.

| Worldwide Key Approvals | Global Sales ($Million) | | Key Substance Patent Expiration |
|---|---|---|---|
| Mar 21, 2014 (US) | **2014** | 69.8 | Oct 30, 2018 (US6020358A) |
| Jan 15, 2015 (EU) | **2015** | 471.7 | Oct 19, 2019 (EP1752148B1) |
| | | | Oct 19, 2019 (JP4530543B2) |

## Mechanism of Action

As a phosphodiesterase 4 (PDE4) inhibitor, apremilast inhibits PDE4 and increases the intracellular cAMP levels, resulting in modulation of the expression of pro- and anti-inflammatory cytokines in inflammatory cells and attenuating the symptoms and course of psoriatic arthritis.

| Target Binding and Inhibition | *In Vitro* Efficacy | *In Vivo* Efficacy |
|---|---|---|
| PDE4: 95% inhibition at 10 µM | Pro-inflammatory cytokines in PBMCs: | Inhibited LPS-induced TNF-$\alpha$ in plasma: |
| PDE1-3: ≤30% inhibition | $IC_{50}$ = 46-440 nM | $ED_{50}$ = 0.018 mg/kg (rat) and 0.05 mg/kg (mouse) |
| PDE4 subtypes: $IC_{50}$ = 14-118 nM | Pro-inflammatory cytokines in T-cell: | In CIA mice: Reduced the severity of disease at 5 mg/kg/day |
| | $IC_{50}$ = 30-1000 nM | |

## Pharmacokinetics

| | Parameters | Healthy Human | | | | | | |
|---|---|---|---|---|---|---|---|---|
| | Dose (mg) | NA (i.v.) | 20 (p.o.) | 10 (p.o.) | 20 (p.o.) | 40 (p.o.) | 80 (p.o.) | 100 (p.o.) |
| | $T_{max}$ (h) | 0.25 | 2.29 | 1.0 | 1.75 | 2.05 | 2.25 | 3.0 |
| | $C_{max}$ (ng/mL) | 4.91 | 173 | 206 | 347 | 533 | 592 | 688 |
| | $AUC_{inf}$ (µg·h/mL) | 0.01 | 1.48 | 1.15 | 1.91 | 3.38 | 4.11 | 5.41 |
| *In Vivo* | $T_{1/2}$ (h) | 6.19 | 7.63 | 6.54 | 4.45 | 6.04 | 5.56 | 5.56 |
| | Cl (mL/min) | 169 | 230 | NA | NA | NA | NA | NA |
| | $V_{ss}$ (L) | 87.0 | NA | NA | NA | NA | NA | NA |
| | F (%) | - | 73.2 | NA | NA | NA | NA | NA |
| | Most Abundant Drug-related Component in Plasma (%) | M0 (44.8) | | | | | | |
| | Major Drug-related Metabolite in Plasma (%) | M12 (38.7) | | | | | | |
| | Urine/Feces Excretion (%) | 57.9/39.2 | | | | | | |
| *In Vitro* | LLC-PK1 Permeability | $P_{app}$ = 21 × $10^{-6}$ cm/s | | | | | | |
| | Plasma Protein Binding (%Bound) | 68.3 | | | | | | |
| | Human LM Stability (%Remining) | 80.2 | | | | | | |

## Drug-Drug Interaction

| | CYP Enzymes | Non-CYP Enzymes | Transporters |
|---|---|---|---|
| **Substrate** | CYP3A4, 1A2, 2A6 | NA | P-gp |
| **Inhibitor** | CYP2C8 | NA | Weak: OATP1B1/1B3, OAT1/3, OCT2, MRP1/2 |
| **Inducer** | Not | NA | NA |

## Non-clinical Toxicology

| | | | |
|---|---|---|---|
| **Single-Dose Toxicity (MLD)** | >2000 mg/kg (mouse, MNLD p.o.) 120/>120 mg/kg (mouse, male/female, i.v.) 2000/>300 mg/kg (rat, male/female, p.o.) >60 mg/kg (rat, i.v.) | **Safety Pharmacology** | • CVS: hERG $IC_{50}$ = 184 µM <br> • RS: A dose-related increase in peak inspiratory and expiratory flow at ≥0.5 mg/kg <br> • GI: No effects at doses up to 1000 mg/kg |
| **Repeated-Dose Toxicity (NOAEL)** | 10 mg/kg/day (mouse, 6 months) 600 mg/kg/day (monkey, 12 months) | **Genotoxicity** | • No genetic toxicity |
| | | **Reproductive Toxicity** | • FEED NOAEL: 50 mg/kg/day for males, 10 mg/kg/day for females <br> • EFD NOAEL: Not teratogenic, 20 mg/kg/day for mater in monkeys <br> • PPND NOAEL: 10 mg/kg/day for $F_0/F_1$ and male juvenile mice, 4 mg/kg/day for female juvenile mice |
| | | **Carcinogenicity** | • Not carcinogenic at doses up to 1000 mg/kg/day in mice, or up to 20 mg/kg/day in male rats and 3 mg/kg/day in female rats |

# Asunaprevir
## (Sunvepra®)
BMS-650032
Capsule, oral, 100 mg Asunaprevir

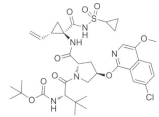

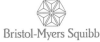

Bristol-Myers Squibb

- ❖ Asunaprevir is an inhibitor of NS3/4A protease, indicated for the treatment of patients with HCV infection.   It was approved in Jul 2014 by PMDA of Japan.
- ❖ Asunaprevir was discovered and marketed by Bristol-Myers Squibb.
- ❖ *The recommended human starting dose* is 100 mg orally twice daily until disease progression or unacceptable toxicity.

| Worldwide Key Approvals | Global Sales ($Million) | | Key Substance Patent Expiration |
| --- | --- | --- | --- |
| Jul 04, 2014 (JP) | **2014** | 55 | May 20, 2023 (US7915291B2) |
| | | | May 20, 2023 (EP1505963B1) |
| | **2015** | 288 | May 20, 2028 (JP4312710B2) |
| | | | May 20, 2023 (CN1974596B) |

## Mechanism of Action

As a selectively inhibitor of HCV NS3/4A protease, asunaprevir competitively binds to and inhibits the active site S1' and S4 of NS3/4A binding domain and prevents the proteolytic processing of HCV polyprotein, which is essential for HCV replication.

**Target Binding and Inhibition**

HCV NS3/4A from:
1a/1b/4a/5a/6a: $IC_{50}$ = 0.3-1.8 nM
2a/2b: $IC_{50}$ = 15/78 nM
3a: $IC_{50}$ = 320 nM

**In Vitro Efficacy**

Anti-HCV replicons:
1a/1b/4a: $EC_{50}$ = 1.2-4.0 nM; 2a/2b: $EC_{50}$ = 67-480 nM; 3a: $EC_{50}$ = 1162 nM
Resistant development: R155K, I170T and D168G in Genotype 1a; Q80R and D168 in Genotype 1b
Anti-HCV containing NS3/4A substitutions: V36/T54/Q80/I170: 0.4-6.5 folds increase in GT 1a/1b
R155/D168/double mutations: 14-713 folds $EC_{50}$ increase in GT 1a/1b

## Pharmacokinetics

| | Parameter | Mouse | | Rat | | Dog | | Monkey | | Human | |
| --- | --- | --- | --- | --- | --- | --- | --- | --- | --- | --- | --- |
| | Dose (mg/kg, human: mg) | 2 (i.v.) | 5 (p.o.) | 3 (i.v.) | 3 (p.o.) | 1 (i.v.) | 3 (p.o.) | 1 (i.v.) | 3 (p.o.) | 100 µg (i.v.) | 100 (p.o.) |
| | $C_{max}$ (µg/mL, human: ng/mL) | NA | 0.096 | 8.71 | 0.006 | 5.92 | 0.45 | 8.19 | 0.14 | 9.64 | 17.5 |
| | $T_{max}$ (h) | NA | 6 | 0.17 | 2.3 | NA | 3 | NA | 1.3 | 0.133 | 2.25 |
| | $AUC_{inf}$ (µg·h/mL, human: ng·h/mL) | 0.58 | 0.405 | 1.62 | 0.018 | 0.9 | 1.65 | 0.95 | 0.31 | 2.02 | 188 |
| | $T_{1/2}$ (h) | 4.6 | NA | 8.1 | ND | 1.0 | 2.0 | 1.3 | 1.1 | 13.7 | 19.7 |
| In Vivo | Cl (mL/min/kg, human: L/h) | 57.3 | NA | 38.9 | NA | 18.7 | NA | 18.3 | NA | 49.5 | NA |
| | $V_{ss}$ (L/kg, human: L) | 12.6 | NA | 7.4 | NA | 0.2 | NA | 0.5 | NA | 194 | NA |
| | F (%) | - | 28 | - | 1 | - | 42 | - | 10 | - | 9.3 |
| | Most Abundant Drug-related Component in Plasma (%) | M0 (40.3) | | M0 (79.0) | | M0 (74.3) | | M0 (16.0) | | M0 (54.9) | |
| | Major Drug-related Metabolite in Plasma (%) | M9 (9.0) | | M3 (2.3) | | M3 (5.4) | | M9 (10.2) | | M9 (4.6) | |
| | Urine/Feces Excretion (%) | 1.42/87.9 | | 0.29/86.9 | | 0.42/77.1 | | 0.40/55.6 | | 0.19/73.1 | |
| In Vitro | Caco-2 Permeability | $Papp_{(A→B)}$ = 1.1-5.4 × $10^{-6}$ cm/s | | | | | | | | | |
| | Plasma Protein Binding (%Bound) | 99.2 (serum) | | 98.8 (serum) | | 98.5 (serum) | | 97.2 (serum) | | 99.7-99.8 | |
| | Hepatocytes Stability (%Remaining) | 76.7 | | 63.3 | | 81.4 | | 65.5 | | 69.1 | |

## Drug-Drug Interaction

| | CYP Enzyme | Non-CYP Enzyme | Transporter |
| --- | --- | --- | --- |
| Substrate | CYP3A4, 3A5, 2A6, 2B6, 2C9, 2C19, 2D6 | NA | OATP1B1, OATP2B1, P-gp |
| Inhibitor | CYP3A4, 2C8, 1A2, 2B6, 2C9, 2C19, 2D6 | NA | OATP1B1, OATP2B1, OATP1B3, OAT1, P-gp |
| Inducer | CYP3A4, 2C9 | NA | NA |

## Non-clinical Toxicology

| Single-Dose Toxicity (MNLD) | 600 mg/kg (mouse) 2000 mg/kg (rat) 300 mg/kg (dog) | Safety Pharmacology | • CVS: hERG $IC_{50}$ >30 µM<br>• No effects on respiratory and CNS |
| --- | --- | --- | --- |
| | | Genotoxicity | • No genotoxicity |
| Repeated-Dose Toxicity (NOAEL) | 200 mg/kg/day (rat, 6 months) 100 mg/kg/day (dog, 9 months) | Reproductive and Developmental Toxicology | • FEED in rats: No anomalies<br>• EFD in mice and rabbits: No pronounced drug-related maternal toxicity or fetal malformation/variation<br>• PNND in rats: Maternal toxicity and decreased survival rate of $F_1$ fetus |
| | | Carcinogenicity | • No carcinogenicity |
| | | Special Toxicology | • Probably phototoxic |

# Ataluren
## (Translarna®)
PTC-124

Suspension, oral, 125 mg/250 mg/1000 mg Ataluren

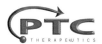

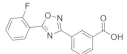

❖ Ataluren is an inhibitor of cystic fibrosis transmembrane conductance regulator (CFTR), indicated for the treatment of Duchenne muscular dystrophy (DMD) resulted from a nonsense mutation in the dystrophin gene, in ambulatory patients aged 5 years and older.   It was first approved in Jul 2014 by EMA.

❖ Ataluren was discovered and marketed by PTC Therapeutics.

❖ **_The recommended human starting dose_** is 10 mg/kg body weight in the morning and midday, 20 mg/kg body weight in the evening.

| Worldwide Key Approvals | Global Sales ($Million) | | Key Substance Patent Expiration |
|---|---|---|---|
| Jul 31, 2014 (EU) | **2014**<br>**2015** | 1.4<br>33.7 | May 17, 2024 (US7419991B2)<br>Apr 09, 2024 (EP1618098B1)<br>Apr 09, 2024 (JP4851933B2)<br>Apr 09, 2024 (CN1802360B) |

## Mechanism of Action

As an inhibitor of nonsense mutation in DNA, ataluren promotes read-through of premature translation termination codons, resulting in the formation of a full-length functional protein in patients with nonsense mutation genetic disorders.

### *In Vitro* Efficacy

Read-through of premature UGA codons in HEK 293 LUC-190 (UGA):
  Maximum ED = 3 µM
  Potenacy: UGA > UAG > UAA
Normal stop codons in HEK 293 cells:
  No effect at 10 or 100 µM

### *In Vivo* Efficacy

nmDMD *mdx* mouse model: Rescued functional dystrophin, reduced serum CK, and improved protection in muscles

The CF mouse model: Significantly increased hCFTR expression at 60 mg/kg

The Idua-W392X mouse model: Increased iduronidase activity at 0.1% (brain, spleen, heart and lungs) or 0.3% (liver)

The Idua-W402X mouse model: Read-through of premature stop codon in IDUA mRNA at 10 µg/mL

## Pharmacokinetics

| | Parameter | | Healthy Human | | | | | |
|---|---|---|---|---|---|---|---|---|
| *In Vivo* | Dose (mg/kg) | | 3 (p.o.) | 10 (p.o.) | 30 (p.o.) | 100 (p.o.) | 150 (p.o.) | 200 (p.o.) |
| | $C_{max}$ (µg/mL) | | 6 ± 0.5 | 27 ± 6 | 90 ± 22 | 210 ± 75 | 260 ± 33 | 314 ± 29 |
| | $T_{max}$ (h) | | 1.0 ± 1.0 | 0.7 ± 0.3 | 0.9 ± 0.2 | 2.2 ± 1.0 | 2.0 ± 1.3 | 2.7 ± 0.8 |
| | $AUC_{0-72}$ (µg·h/mL) | | 27 ± 6 | 110 ± 16 | 482 ± 95 | 2200 ± 1422 | 3001 ± 1214 | 2937 ± 436 |
| | $T_{1/2}$ (h) | | 3.1 ± 0.2 | 3.6 ± 0.2 | 4.7 ± 0.1 | 5.4 ± 1.1 | 5.1 ± 0.7 | 6.3 ± 2.0 |
| | Most Abundant Drug-related Component in Plasma (%) | | Ataluren (70-91) | | | | | |
| | Major Durg-related Metabolite in Plasma (%) | | NA | | | | | |
| | Urine/Feces Excretion (%) | | NA | | | | | |
| *In Vitro* | Permeability | | NA | | | | | |
| | Plasma Protein Binding (%Bound) | | NA | | | | | |
| | LM/Heptocytes Stability | | NA | | | | | |

## Drug-Drug Interaction

| | CYP Enzyme | Non-CYP Enzyme | Transporter |
|---|---|---|---|
| Substrate | Not | UGT1A9 | Not |
| Inhibitor | NA | NA | NA |
| Inducer | NA | NA | NA |

## Non-clinical Toxicology

| Single-Dose Toxicity | $LD_{50}$ >2000 mg/kg (rat)<br>Tolerated dose 1600 mg/kg (dog) | Safety Pharmacology | • No significant change on CNS, RS and CVS |
|---|---|---|---|
| Repeated-Dose Toxicity (NOAEL) | 120 mg/kg/day (rat, 26 weeks)<br><250 mg/kg/day (dog, 52 weeks) | Genotoxicity | • No genetic toxicity |
| | | Reproductive and Developmental Toxicity | • FEED NOAEL: 300 mg/kg/day fertility, 100 mg/kg/day for early embryo<br>• EFD NOAEL: 30 mg/kg/day for the maternal, 100 mg/kg/day (4 × RHD exposure) for fetuses in rats<br>• PPND: Maternal and neonatal toxicities at 150 mg/kg/day (5 × RHD exposure) |
| | | Carcinogenicity | • Endometrial hyperplasia and nephropathy in Tg.rasH2 mice and rats |

## Belinostat
### (Beleodaq®)
PX-105684; PXD-101

Lyophilized powder, intravenous, 500 mg Belinostat

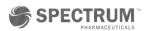

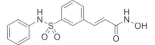

❖ Belinostat is a small molecule histone deacetylase (HDAC) inhibitor, indicated for the treatment of patients with relapsed or refractory peripheral T-cell lymphoma (PTCL).   It was first approved in Jul 2014 by US FDA.
❖ Belinostat was discovered by TopoTarget, developed and marketed by Spectrum pharmaceuticals.
❖ *The recommended human starting dose* is 1000 mg/m² administered over 30 minutes by intravenous infusion once daily on days 1-5 of a 21-day cycle.

| Worldwide Key Approvals | Global Sales ($Million) | | Key Substance Patent Expiration |
|---|---|---|---|
| Jul 03, 2014 (US) | **2014** | 4.9 | Sep 27, 2021 (US6888027B2) |
| | **2015** | 10.1 | Sep 27, 2021 (EP1328510B1) |
| | | | Sep 27, 2021 (JP4975941B2) |

## Mechanism of Action

As an HDAC inhibitor, belinostat inhibits the deacetylation of histone by HDACs and affects the access of transcription factors to the chromatin for gene transcription, which is an ongoing process that is required for normal cell growth and differentiation.

| Target Binding Selectivity | *In Vitro* Efficacy | *In Vivo* Efficacy |
|---|---|---|
| Class I HDAC: $EC_{50}$ = 30-125 nM | HeLa and bladder cancer cells growth: $IC_{50}$ = 1.0-10.0 μM | Mouse ascites model: |
| Class II HDAC: $EC_{50}$ = 67-128 nM | Multidrug-resistant cancer cell lines: $IC_{50}$ = 0.345-3.78 μM | H4 acetylation levels arise |
| Class III HDAC: $EC_{50}$ = 31.3-82 nM | In ovarian and HCT-116 cells: | In transgenic mice: |
| Class IV HDAC: $EC_{50}$ = 44.2 nM | Increased H3/4 acetylation and PARP cleavage, induced p21 expression | Reduced the weights of Ras-expressing bladders and decreased hematuria |
| | Increased the G1 proportion of tumor cells, not normal cells | |

## Pharmacokinetics

| | Parameter | Monkey | | | | | Human | | | | | |
|---|---|---|---|---|---|---|---|---|---|---|---|---|
| | Dose (i.v., mg/kg, human: mg/m²) | 10 | 25 | 35 | 50 | 60 | 150 | 300 | 600 | 900 | 1000 | 1200 |
| | $C_{max}$ (ng/mL) | NA | NA | NA | NA | NA | 6010 | 14777 | 28611 | 46278 | 32124 | 53793 |
| | $T_{max}$ (h) | NA | NA | NA | NA | NA | 0.02 | 0.00 | 0.00 | 0.00 | 0.00 | 0.02 |
| | $AUC_{inf}$ (ng·h/mL) | 13000 | 19200 | 43000 | 34700 | 27100 | 1220 | 3422 | 11008 | 15181 | 9990 | 19240 |
| | $T_{1/2}$ (h) | 0.47 | 1.23 | 1.58 | 0.89 | 0.89 | 0.45 | 0.54 | 0.52 | 0.90 | 0.69 | 0.79 |
| *In Vivo* | Cl (mL/min/m², human: L/h/m²) | 258 | 435 | 274 | 481 | 677 | 132 | 99.4 | 58.9 | 62.3 | 110 | 73.4 |
| | $V_{ss}$ (L/kg, human: L/m²) | 0.20 | 0.31 | 0.38 | 1.11 | 1.26 | 90.0 | 80.7 | 43.4 | 76.9 | 114 | 89.2 |
| | F (%) | - | - | - | - | - | - | - | - | - | - | - |
| | Most Abundant Drug-related Component in Plasma (%) | NA | | | | | M18 (16.2) | | | | | |
| | Major Drug-related Metabolite in Plasma (%) | NA | | | | | M18 (16.2) | | | | | |
| | Urine/Feces Excretion (%) | NA | | | | | NA | | | | | |
| | Caco-2 Permeability | NA | | | | | | | | | | |
| *In Vitro* | Plasma Protein Binding (%Bound) | NA | | | | | 92.9-95.8 | | | | | |
| | LM/Hepatocytes Stability | NA | | | | | NA | | | | | |

## Drug-Drug Interaction

| | CYP Enzyme | Non-CYP Enzyme | Transporter |
|---|---|---|---|
| **Substrate** | CYP2A6, 3A4, 2C9 | UGT1A1, 1A3, 1A8, 2B4, 2B7 | P-gp |
| **Inhibitor** | CYP2C9 | NA | Not |
| **Inducer** | CYP1A2 | NA | NA |

## Non-clinical Toxicology

| **Single-Dose Toxicity** | NA | **Safety Pharmacology** | • CVS: hERG $IC_{50}$ not reached<br>• No significant effects on RS and CNS |
|---|---|---|---|
| **Repeated-Dose Toxicity (NOEL)** | 10 mg/kg/day (dog, 4 weeks) | **Genotoxicity** | • Positive |
| | | **Reproductive and Developmental Toxicity** | • NA |
| | | **Carcinogenicity** | • NA |

## Ceritinib
## (Zykadia®)
LDK-378
Capsule, oral, 150 mg Ceritinib

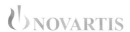

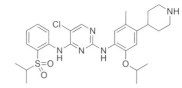

- ❖ Ceritinib is an anaplastic lymphoma kinase (ALK) inhibitor, indicated for the treatment of patients with ALK-positive metastatic non-small cell lung cancer (NSCLC) who have progressed on or are intolerant to crizotinib. It was first approved in Apr 2014 by US FDA.
- ❖ Ceritinib was discovered by IRM, developed and marketed by Novartis.
- ❖ *The recommended human starting dose* is 750 mg once daily without food.

| Worldwide Key Approvals | Global Sales ($Million) | | Key Substance Patent Expiration |
|---|---|---|---|
| Apr 29, 2014 (US) | | | Jun 29, 2030 (US8039479B2) |
| May 06, 2015 (EU) | **2014** | 31 | Nov 20, 2027 (EP2091918B1) |
| Mar 28, 2016 (JP) | **2015** | 79 | Nov 20, 2027 (JP5208123B2) |
| | | | (CN103641816A: Examination) |

## Mechanism of Action

As an ALK inhibitor, ceritinib inhibits autophosphorylation of ALK, ALK-mediated phosphorylation of the downstream signaling protein STAT3 and proliferation of ALK-dependent cancer cells.

**Target Inhibitory Selectivity**

ALK: $IC_{50}$ = 0.15 nM
IGF-1R: $IC_{50}$ = 8 nM
InsR: $IC_{50}$ = 7 nM
EML4-ALK: $IC_{50}$ = 31 nM

***In Vitro* Efficacy**

Anti-proliferation:
  NSCLC cell lines: $IC_{50}$ = 3.8-14.6 nM
  Ba/F3 cells_fusion ALK: $IC_{50}$ = 26-56 nM
  Ba/F3 cells_EMLA-ALK mutation: $IC_{50}$ = 37.6-940 nM
  Cells from crizotinib-resistant patients with ALK mutation:
    $IC_{50}$ = 25-230 nM

***In Vivo* Efficacy**

Human NSCLC model:
  Complete tumor regression at 25 mg/kg
In crizotinib-resistant H2228 cells model:
  T/C% = -100%-11.7% at 50 mg/kg
Karpas299 cell model:
  T/C% = -93%-74%

## Pharmacokinetics

| | Parameter | Mouse | | Rat | | Monkey | | Patient |
|---|---|---|---|---|---|---|---|---|
| | Dose (mg/kg, human: mg) | 5 (i.v.) | 20 (p.o.) | 10 (i.v.) | 25 (p.o.) | 5 (i.v.) | 30 (p.o.) | 750 (p.o.) |
| | $C_{max}$ (ng/mL, mouse: nM) | 1753 | 695 | 975 | 363 | 1410 | 881 | 186 |
| | $T_{max}$ (h) | - | 7 | 0.083 | 12.0 | 0.083 | 18.3 | 6.02 |
| | $AUC_{inf}$ (ng·h/mL, mouse: nM·h) | 5634 | 12296 | 6950 | 8390 | 6530 | 35800 | 7870 |
| | $T_{1/2}$ (h) | 6.2 | - | 9.7 | 13.2 | 29 | 12.1 | 40.6 |
| *In Vivo* | Cl (L/h/kg, mouse: mL/min/kg, human: L/h) | 26.6 | - | 1.49 | NA | 0.78 | - | 88.5 |
| | $V_{ss}$ (L/kg, human: L) | 9.7 | - | 19.9 | NA | 13.5 | - | 4230 |
| | F (%) | - | 54.6 | - | 48.3 | - | 43.0 | NA |
| | Most Abundant Drug-related Component in Plasma (%) | NA | | M0 (100) | | M0 (84.4) | | M0 (81.6) |
| | Major Drug-related Metabolite in Plasma (%) | - | | - | | M21.6 (3.6) | | M46.1 (2.3) |
| | Urine/Feces Excretion (%) | NA | | 0.18/101 | | 0.71/92.3 | | 1.2/91.0 |
| *In Vitro* | Permeability | Ceritinib was classified as a low passive permeability compound | | | | | | |
| | Plasma Protein Binding (%Bound) | NA | | 97.9-98.4 | | 94.4-95.2 | | 96.7-98.8 |
| | Hepatocytes Stability ($Cl_{int}$, μL/h/$10^6$ cells) | NA | | NC | | 38.5-98.7 | | 6.90-10.4 |

## Drug-Drug Interaction

| | CYP Enzyme | Non-CYP Enzyme | Transporter |
|---|---|---|---|
| **Substrate** | CYP3A, 2C19, 1A2, 2C8, 2D6, 2C9 | NA | P-gp, BCRP |
| **Inhibitor** | CYP3A4/5, 2A6, 2B6, 2C8/9/C19, 2D6 and 2E1 | NA | OATP1B1, OATP1B3, OAT1, OCT2 |
| **Inducer** | Not | NA | NA |

## Non-clinical Toxicology

| Single-Dose Toxicity (MNLD) | 250 mg/kg (monkey) | Safety Pharmacology | • CVS: hERG $IC_{50}$ = 0.4 μM<br>• No significant effects on respiratory or neurological function |
|---|---|---|---|
| **Repeated-Dose Toxicity (NOAEL)** | 10 mg/kg (monkey, 13 weeks) | Genotoxicity | • Positive in the *in vitro* micronucleus assay in TK6 cell<br>• Negative in other *in vitro* and *in vivo* genotoxicity studies |
| | | Reproductive and Developmental Toxicity | • EFD: No significant embryo lethality or fetotoxicity |
| | | Carcinogenicity | • NA |
| | | Special Toxicology | • Low phototoxicity in the *in vitro* 3T3 NRU assay |

## Chidamide
## (Epidaza®)
CS-055; HBI-8000
Tablet, oral, 5 mg Chidamide

微芯生物
CHIPSCREEN

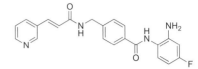

❖ Chidamide is a histone deacetylase (HDAC) inhibitor, indicated for the treatment of patients with relapsed or refractory peripheral T-cell lymphoma (PTCL).   It was first approved in Dec 2014 by CFDA.

❖ Chidamide was discovered and marketed by Chipscreen.

❖ *The recommended human starting dose* is 30 mg twice weekly for adult at least 30 min after eating breakfast and the minimum interval between doses is 3 days.

| Worldwide Key Approvals | Global Sales ($Million) | Key Substance Patent Expiration |
|---|---|---|
| Dec 23, 2014 (CN) | Not available | Feb 02, 2024 (US7550490B2) (EP2860174A2: Examination) Feb 09, 2024 (JP4637821B2) Jul 04, 2023 (CN1284772C) |

### Mechanism of Action

As an HDAC inhibitor, chidamide inhibits the enzymatic activity of histone deacetylases (HDAC) 1, 2, 3 and 10, thereby inhibiting tumor cell cycle and promoting apoptosis.

| Target Binding Selectivity | *In Vitro* Efficacy | *In Vivo* Efficacy |
|---|---|---|
| HDAC1: $IC_{50}$ = 95 nM<br>HDAC2: $IC_{50}$ = 160 nM<br>HDAC3: $IC_{50}$ = 67 nM<br>HDAC10: $IC_{50}$ = 78 nM | Transformed cell: $GI_{50}$ = 0.4-8.2 μM<br>Normal cell: $GI_{50}$ >100 μM<br>CAL-51 cell: $IC_{50}$ = 19.6 μM<br>A375 cell: $IC_{50}$ = 250 μM | In HL60 myelogenous leukaemia xenograft mouse model:<br>  Significantly decreased tumor weight at 50 mg/kg<br>  No gross body weight loss |

### Pharmacokinetics

| | Parameter | Rat | Human | | |
|---|---|---|---|---|---|
| *In Vivo* | Dose (p.o., mg/kg, human: mg) | 30 | 25 | 32.5 | 50 |
| | $C_{max}$ (ng/mL) | 4986 | 39.7 | 122 | 163 |
| | $T_{max}$ (h) | NA | 10.0 | 3.5 | 4.0 |
| | $AUC_{inf}$ (ng·h/mL) | 5013 | 867 | 875 | 1180 |
| | $T_{1/2}$ (h) | 11.9 | 16.8 | 17.5 | 18.3 |
| | Cl/F (L/h) | 6.8 | 35 | 59 | 50 |
| | $V_{ss}$/F (L/kg, human: L) | 118 | 790 | 1517 | 1285 |
| | F (%) | NA | NA | NA | NA |
| | Most Abundant Drug-related Component in Plasma (%) | NA | NA | | |
| | Major Drug-related Metabolite in Plasma (%) | NA | NA | | |
| | Urine/Feces Excretion (%) | 18.8/63.3 | NA | | |
| *In Vitro* | Caco-2 Permeability | NA | | | |
| | Plasma Protein Binding (%Bound) | NA | NA | | |
| | LM/Hepatocytes Stability | NA | NA | | |

### Drug-Drug Interaction

| | CYP Enzyme | Non-CYP Enzyme | Transporter |
|---|---|---|---|
| **Substrate** | NA | NA | NA |
| **Inhibitor** | NA | NA | NA |
| **Inducer** | NA | NA | NA |

### Non-clinical Toxicology

| | | | |
|---|---|---|---|
| **Single-Dose Toxicity** | NA | **Safety Pharmacology** | • NA |
| **Repeated-Dose Toxicity (NOAEL)** | NA | **Genotoxicity** | • NA |
| | | **Reproductive and Developmental Toxicity** | • NA |
| | | **Carcinogenicity** | • NA |

## Daclatasvir Dihydrochloride (Daklinza®)
BMS-790052
Tablet, oral, EQ 60 mg Daclatasvir

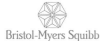

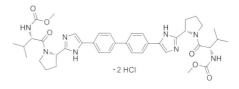

· 2 HCl

❖ Daclatasvir dihydrochloride is an inhibitor of NS5A, indicated for the treatment of patients with chronic HCV infection.　It was first approved in Jul 2014 by PMDA of Japan.
❖ Daclatasvir dihydrochloride was discovered and marketed by Bristol-Myers Squibb.
❖ **_The recommended human starting dose_** is 60 mg orally once daily.

| Worldwide Key Approvals | Global Sales ($Million) | | Key Substance Patent Expiration |
|---|---|---|---|
| Jul 04, 2014 (JP) | | | Apr 13, 2028 (US8329159B2) |
| Aug 22, 2014 (EU) | **2014** | 201 | Aug 09, 2027 (EP2049522B1) |
| Jul 24, 2015 (US) | **2015** | 1315 | Nov 06, 2028 (JP5235882B2) |
| | | | Aug 09, 2027 (CN101558059B) |

### Mechanism of Action

As an HCV NS5A inhibitor, daclatasvir dihydrochloride binds to the *N*-terminus of NS5A and inhibits both viral RNA replication and virion assembly.

**Mechanism of Action**

$S$-stereoisomer: $EC_{50}$ = 33 nM
$R$-stereoisomer: $EC_{50}$ >10 µM

***In Vitro* Efficacy**

Anti-HCV replicons in cell lines:
　Genotype 1a/1b/2a/4a/5a/6a:
　$EC_{50}$ = 1.2-54 pM
　Genotype 3a: $EC_{50}$ = 140-190 pM

Resistant NS5A substitution in HCV GT 1a replicon:
　L30, R30, L31, P32, Y93H: >340 folds
　Double and triple substitutions: >10000 folds (except T21I-L31M/M28T-Q30H/H58P-Y93H: 318-1205 folds)

### Pharmacokinetics

| | Parameter | Mouse | | Rat | | Dog | | Monkey | | Healthy Human | |
|---|---|---|---|---|---|---|---|---|---|---|---|
| | Dose (mg/kg, human: mg) | 3 (i.v.) | 3 (p.o.) | 5 (i.v.) | 5 (p.o.) | 1 (i.v.) | 3 (p.o.) | 1.13 (i.v.) | 2.83 (p.o.) | 100 (i.v., µg) | 60 (p.o.) |
| | $C_{max}$ (µg/mL, human: ng/mL) | NA | 2.3 | NA | 0.59 | NA | 0.85 | NA | 0.2 | 6.57 | 928 |
| | $T_{max}$ (h) | NA | 0.5 | NA | 2.7 | NA | 2.9 | NA | 2.0 | 0.133 | 1.38 |
| | $AUC_{inf}$ (µg·h/mL, human: ng·h/mL) | 5.4 | 6.6 | 5.66 | 3.6 | 1.31 | 5.66 | 1.63 | 1.45 | 23.6 | 9486 |
| | $T_{1/2}$ (h) | 1.1 | NA | 4.7 | NA | 3.9 | NA | 3.7 | NA | 9.51 | 11.9 |
| *In Vivo* | Cl (mL/min/kg, human: L/h) | 9.3 | NA | 14.8 | NA | 20.3 | NA | 12.4 | NA | 4.24 | NA |
| | $V_{ss}$ (L/kg, human: L) | NC | NA | 3.6 | NA | 5.4 | NA | 2.2 | NA | 47.1 | NA |
| | F (%) | - | 123 | - | 50.4 | - | 144 | - | 38 | - | 67.0 |
| | Most Abundant Drug-related Component in Plasma (%) | M0 (89.8) | | M0 (84.6) | | M0 (87.5) | | M0 (78.2) | | M0 (96.8) | |
| | Major Drug-related Metabolite in Plasma (%) | M4 (3.2) | | M28 (3.5) | | M15 (2.9) | | M2 (21.8) | | M2 (1.4) | |
| | Urine/Feces Excretion (%) | 1.4/87.4 | | 1.55/91.1 | | 8.75/54.2 | | 1.35/69.4 | | 6.60/87.6 | |
| | Caco-2 Permeability | $Papp_{(A→B)}$ <1.5 × $10^{-6}$ cm/s | | | | | | | | | |
| *In Vitro* | Serum Protein Binding (%Bound) | 98.2 | | 98.3 | | 96.5 | | 95.1 | | 95.6 | |
| | Hepatocytes Stability (pmol/min/$10^6$ cells) | 31.7 | | 5.6 | | 52.6 | | 43.8 | | 7.0 | |

### Drug-Drug Interaction

| | CYP Enzyme | Non-CYP Enzyme | Transporter |
|---|---|---|---|
| Substrate | CYP3A4 | Not | P-gp |
| Inhibitor | CYP3A4 | NA | OATP1B1,1B3,BCRP, OCT1, OCT2, P-gp, OAT1, OAT3 |
| Inducer | CYP3A4 | NA | NA |

### Non-clinical Toxicology

| Single-Dose Toxicity (MNLD) | 1000 mg/kg (mouse and rat) 150 mg/kg (dog and monkey) | Safety Pharmacology | • CVS: hERG $IC_{50}$ = 29.2 µM<br>• No respiratory or central nervous effect |
|---|---|---|---|
| Repeated-Dose Toxicity (NOAEL) | 25 mg/kg/day (rat, 6 months) 15 mg/kg/day (monkey, 9 months) 3 mg/kg/day (dog, 1 month) | Genotoxicity | • No genotoxicity |
| | | Reproductive and Developmental Toxicity | • FEED NOAEL: 50/200 mg/kg/day (male/female)<br>• EFD NOAEL: 50 mg/kg/day in rats, 40/20 mg/kg/day in rabbits (male/female)<br>• PPND/Juvenile NOAEL: 50 mg/kg/day |
| | | Carcinogenicity | • No drug-related tumor in Tg-rasH2 mouse or SD rats |

## Delamanid
### (Deltyba®)
OPC-67683
Tablet, oral, 50 mg Delamanid

 Otsuka

❖ Delamanid is a nitro-dihydro-imidazo-oxazole derivative, indicated for the treatment of multidrug-resistant tuberculosis (MDR-TB) in adult patients.   It was first approved in Apr 2014 by EMA.
❖ Delamanid was discovered and marketed by Otsuka.
❖ *The recommended human starting dose* is 100 mg twice daily.

| Worldwide Key Approvals | Global Sales ($Million) | Key Substance Patent Expiration |
|---|---|---|
| Apr 28, 2014 (EU) <br> Jul 04, 2014 (JP) | Not available | Feb 22, 2024 (US7262212B2) <br> Oct 10, 2023 (EP1555267B1) <br> Oct 14, 2028 (JP4186065B2) <br> Oct 10, 2023 (CN100366624C) |

### Mechanism of Action

As a nitro-dihydro-imidazo-oxazole derivative, delamanid inhibits the biosynthesis of methoxy- and keto-mycolic acid, which are mycobacterial cell wall components.

**Mechanism of Action**

Methoxy-mycolic acid:
$IC_{50}$ = 0.036 µg/mL
Keto-mycolic acid:
$IC_{50}$ = 0.021 µg/mL

***In Vitro* Efficacy**

TB/BCG strains: $MIC_{90}$ = 0.012-0.024 µg/mL
*M. tuberculosis*:
MIC ≤0.0005 µg/mL

***In Vivo* Efficacy**

In ICR mice model: ED = 0.52 mg/kg/day
Balb/c nude mice: Significantly reduced viable bacteria number at 0.625 mg/kg/day in lungs and spleen

### Pharmacokinetics

| | Parameter | Mouse | | Rat | | Dog | | | Healthy Chinese | | |
|---|---|---|---|---|---|---|---|---|---|---|---|
| | Dose (mg/kg, human: mg) | 3 (i.v.) | 1 (p.o.) | 3 (i.v.) | 3 (p.o.) | 3 (i.v.) | 3 (p.o.) | 30 (p.o.) | 100 (p.o.) | 200 (p.o.) | 400 (p.o.) |
| In Vivo | $C_{max}$ (ng/mL) | 1199 | 155 | 13923 | 494 | 1321 | 325 | 506 | 80.7 | 108 | 126 |
| | $T_{max}$ (h) | - | 2.0 | - | 6.0 | - | 9.5 | 14.0 | 3.00 | 2.00 | 3.00 |
| | $AUC_{inf}$ (ng·h/mL) | 13490 | 1818 | 21566 | 7529 | 14140 | 8488 | 14381 | 1130 | 1630 | 2010 |
| | $T_{1/2}$ (h) | 6.3 | 5.2 | 9.2 | 6.4 | 17.6 | 17.0 | 17.3 | 16.6 | 22.4 | 24.3 |
| | Cl (mL/h/kg) | 222 | 550 | 139 | 398 | 215 | 386 | 2168 | NA | NA | NA |
| | $V_{ss}$ (mL/kg) | 2026 | 4146 | 1841 | 3673 | 5388 | 9621 | 55435 | NA | NA | NA |
| | F (%) | - | NA | - | 34.9 | - | 60.0 | NA | NA | NA | NA |
| | Most Abundant Drug-Related Component in Plasma (%) | Parent (82.3) 3 mg/kg, p.o. | | Parent (85.9), 3 mg/kg, p.o. | | Parent (64.6), 10 mg/kg, p.o. | | | NA | | |
| | Major Drug-Related Metabolite in Plasma (%) | NA | | NA | | NA | | | NA | | |
| | Urine/Feces Excretion (%) | NA/NA | | 6.29/91.6 | | 3.0/89.8 | | | NA/NA | | |
| In Vitro | Permeability | NA | | | | | | | | | |
| | Plasma Protein Binding (%Bound) | NA | | 99.58-99.59 | | 99.34-99.45 | | | 99.54-99.57 | | |
| | S9 Stability (%Remaining) | 95.0 | | 93.2 | | 93.7 | | | 90.7 | | |

### Drug-Drug Interaction

| | CYP Enzyme | Non-CYP Enzyme | Transporter |
|---|---|---|---|
| **Substrate** | CYP3A4, 2D6, 1A1, 2E1 | NA | Not |
| **Inhibitor** | Not | NA | OAT1, OAT3, OATP1B1, OATP1B3, OCT1, OCT2, BSEP, P-gp, BCRP |
| **Inducer** | Not | NA | NA |

### Non-clinical Toxicology

| Single-Dose Toxicity (ALD) | >1000 mg/kg/day (rat) <br> >900 mg/kg/day (dog) | **Safety Pharmacology** | • CVS: hERG inhibition 35.4% at 1.6 µg/mL <br> • No *in vivo* effect on CNS, CVS or RS |
|---|---|---|---|
| **Repeated-Dose Toxicity (NOAEL)** | 30/300 mg/kg/day (rat, 26 weeks) <br> 1/3 mg/kg/day (dog, 39 weeks) | **Genotoxicity** | • No genetic toxicity |
| | | **Reproductive and Developmental Toxicity** | • FEED: No adverse effect <br> • EFD: Not teratogenic <br> • PPND: No adverse effect |
| | | **Carcinogenicity** | • No drug-related neoplasm |

# Eliglustat Tartrate
## (Cerdelga®)
Genz-112638
Capsule, oral, EQ 84 mg Eliglustat

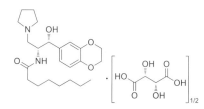

SANOFI GENZYME

- ❖ Eliglustat tartrate is a glucosylceramide synthase inhibitor, indicated for the treatment of adult patients with Gaucher disease type 1 (GD1) who are CYP2D6 extensive metabolizers (EMs), intermediate metabolizers (IMs), or poor metabolizers (PMs). It was first approved in Aug 2014 by US FDA.
- ❖ Eliglustat tartrate was discovered and marketed by Genzyme Corp (now a subsidiary of Sanofi).
- ❖ ***The recommended human starting dose*** is 84 mg taken orally twice daily in CYP2D6 EMs and IMs, and 84 mg once daily in CY2D6 PMs.

| Worldwide Key Approvals | Global Sales ($Million) | | Key Substance Patent Expiration |
|---|---|---|---|
| Aug 19, 2014 (US) | **2014** | 5.3 | Apr 29, 2022 (US7196205B2) |
| Jan 19, 2015 (EU) | **2015** | 73.3 | Jul 16, 2022 (EP1409467B1) |
| Mar 26, 2015 (JP) | | | Mar 28, 2025 (JP5038582B2) |

## Mechanism of Action

Eliglustat is a potent and selective inhibitor of glucosylceramide synthase, and acts as a substrate reduction therapy (SRT) for GD1.

### Target Inhibition and *In Vitro* Efficacy

Inhibition of glucosylceramide synthase in cells:
  $IC_{50}$ = 14-115 nM (GM1/3, GL-1 synthesis)
In both human microsomes and intact B16 cells (metabolites):
  GL-1 synthesis: $IC_{50}$ = 1.09->30 μM
  GM3 synthesis: $IC_{50}$ = 1.54->10 μM

### *In Vivo* Efficacy

In normal rats and dogs:
  Significantly decreased glucosylceramide levels in liver, kidneys and spleen
In Fabry mouse models:
  Significantly reduced GL-3 in the kidneys
In D490V/null Gaucher mouse models:
  Reduced GL-1 level in liver, lungs and spleen

## Pharmacokinetics

| | Parameter | Mouse | | Rat | | Rabbit | Dog | | Monkey | | Healthy Human (IMs) | |
|---|---|---|---|---|---|---|---|---|---|---|---|---|
| | Dose (mg/kg, human: mg) | 1 (i.v.) | 3 (p.o.) | 1 (i.v.) | 3 (p.o.) | 30 (p.o.) | 1 (i.v.) | 3 (p.o.) | 1.18 (i.v.) | 3.57 (p.o.) | 50 (i.v.) | 100 (p.o.) |
| | $C_{max}$ (ng/mL) | NA | 115 | NA | 109 | 88.5 | NA | 66.2 | NA | 4.66 | 93.2 | 25.4 |
| | $T_{max}$ (h) | NA | 0.0833 | NA | 0.292 | 0.708 | NA | 0.583 | NA | 0.250 | 1.08 | 3.5 |
| | $AUC_{inf}$ (ng·h/mL) | 146 | 20.5 | 436 | 114 | 128 | 459 | 171 | 222 | 4.74 | 653 | 253 |
| *In Vivo* | $T_{1/2}$ (h) | 0.546 | 0.214 | 0.266 | 0.407 | 3.90 | 1.03 | 1.39 | 1.43 | 0.737 | 6.87 | 6.99 |
| | Cl (mL/min/kg, human: L/h) | 96.0 | NA | 32.7 | NA | NA | 31.1 | NA | 77.8 | NA | 64.6 | NA |
| | $V_{ss}$ (L/kg, human: L) | 2.07 | NA | 0.556 | NA | NA | 2.38 | NA | 5.13 | NA | 641 | NA |
| | F (%) | - | 4.68 | - | 8.70 | NA | - | 12.3 | - | 0.803 | - | NA |
| | Most Abundant Drug-related Component in Plasma (%) | NA | | M0 (24.8) | | NA | M0 (22.2) | | NA | | NA | |
| | Major Drug-related Metabolite in Plasma (%) | NA | | M5 (7.08) | | NA | M17 (16.3) | | NA | | NA | |
| | Urine/Feces Excretion (%) | NA | | 11.4/82.1 | | NA | 25.6/63.9 | | NA | | 41.8/51.4 | |
| *In Vitro* | Caco-2 Permeability | $Papp_{(A-B)}$ = 22-23 × $10^{-6}$ cm/s | | | | | | | | | | |
| | Plasma Protein Binding (%Bound) | 95.3-98.9 | | 79.7-99.0 | | NA | 91.5-98.2 | | 80.7-92.2 | | 76.4-82.9 | |
| | LM Stability (%Remaining) | NA | | 33.1 | | NA | 8.13 | | - | | 44.0 | |

## Drug-Drug Interaction

| | CYP Enzyme | Non-CYP Enzyme | Transporter |
|---|---|---|---|
| **Substrate** | CYP2D6, CYP3A4 | NA | P-gp |
| **Inhibitor** | CYP2D6, CYP3A4 | NA | P-gp |
| **Inducer** | Not | NA | NA |

## Non-clinical Toxicology

| Single-Dose Toxicity (MNLD) | 200 mg/kg/day (rat, p.o.) 20 mg/kg (rat, i.v.) 100 mg/kg/day (dog, p.o.) | **Safety Pharmacology** | • CVS: hERG $IC_{50}$ = 0.35 μg/mL<br>• No statistically significant *in vivo* change in cardiovascular, respiratory, renal or GI function |
|---|---|---|---|
| | | **Genotoxicity** | • No genetic toxicity |
| **Repeated-Dose Toxicity (NOAEL)** | 50 mg/kg/day (rat) 10 mg/kg/day (dog) | **Reproductive and Developmental Toxicity** | • FEED NOAEL: 30 mg/kg/day in $F_0$ or 100 mg/kg/day in $F_1$<br>• Embryotoxic and teratogenic at 120 mg/kg/day in rats<br>• PPND: Maternal toxicity at 100 mg/kg/day in rats |
| | | **Carcinogenicity** | • No drug-related neoplasm in rats or mice |

## Empagliflozin
(Jardiance®)
BI-10773
Tablet, oral, 10 mg/25 mg Empagliflozin

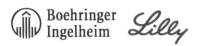

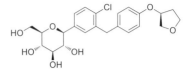

❖ Empagliflozin is an SGLT2 inhibitor, indicated for the treatment of type 2 diabetes. It was first approved in May 2014 by EMA.
❖ Empagliflozin was discovered by Boehringer Ingelheim, co-developed and co-marketed through a research collaboration with Eli-Lilly.
❖ *The human recommended starting dose* is 10 mg once a day before or after breakfast.

| Worldwide Key Approvals | Global Sales ($Million) | | Key Substance Patent Expiration |
|---|---|---|---|
| May 22, 2014 (EU)<br>Aug 01, 2014 (US)<br>Dec 26, 2014 (JP) | **2014**<br>**2015** | 10.1<br>Not available | Nov 05, 2025 (US7579449B2)<br>Mar 11, 2025 (EP1730131 B1)<br>Mar 11, 2030 (JP4181605B2)<br>Mar 11, 2025 (CN103450129B) |

### Mechanism of Action

As an SGLT2 inhibitor, empagliflozin selectively inhibits SGLT2, leading to inhibition of glucose reabsorption and increase of glucose excretion through urine, thereby reducing blood glucose.

**In Vitro Target Binding Selectivity**

hSGLT2: $IC_{50}$ = 1.3 nM
hSGLT1: $IC_{50}$ = 6278 nM
Selectivity SGLT2/SGLT1: >4800 folds

**In Vivo Efficacy**

Increased urinary glucose excretion:
  Significantly at ≥3 mg/kg (*db/db* mouse and ZDF rat)
  Beagle dog: $ED_{50}$ = 0.9 mg/kg

Decreased blood glucose:
  $ED_{50}$ = 0.6 mg/kg (*db/db* mouse and ZDF rat)
  Significantly decreased HbA1c from 7.93 to 6.84 at 3 mg/kg in ZDF rat

### Pharmacokinetics

| | Parameters | Mouse | | Rat | | Dog | | Healthy Human | | | |
|---|---|---|---|---|---|---|---|---|---|---|---|
| | Dose (mg/kg, human: mg) | 5 (i.v.) | 250 (p.o.) | 0.5 (i.v.) | 5 (p.o.) | 0.5 (i.v.) | 5 (p.o.) | 2.5 (p.o.) | 10 (p.o.) | 25 (p.o.) | 100 (p.o.) |
| *In Vivo* | $C_{max}$ (nM) | NA | 97700 | NA | 326 (ng/mL) | NA | 16100 | 53.2 | 226 | 505 | 2500 |
| | $T_{max}$ (h) | NA | 0.67 | NA | 1 | NA | 1 | 1.75 | 1.5 | 2.05 | 1.0 |
| | $AUC_{inf}$ (nM·h) | 4610 | 207000 | 595 (ng·h/mL) | 1798 (ng·h/mL) | 10200 | 101000 | 396 | 1730 | 3830 | 16500 |
| | $T_{1/2}$ (h) | 1.26 | 5.59 | 3.64 | 6.32 | 22.0 | 3.60 | 8.57 | 13.1 | 10.2 | 10.6 |
| | Cl (mL/min/kg) | 40.1 | 44.6 | 14.8 | 47.2 | 1.76 | 1.73 | NA | NA | NA | NA |
| | $V_{ss}$ (L/kg) | 1.17 | NA | 0.818 | NA | 0.836 | NA | NA | NA | NA | NA |
| | F (%) | - | 89.8 | - | 31.0 | - | 102 | NA | NA | NA | NA |
| | Most Abundant Drug-related Component in Plasma (%) | M0 (47.5) | | M0 (50.8) | | M0 (88.7) | | M0 (77.4) | | | |
| | Major Drug-related Metabolite in Plasma (%) | M482/1 (30.3) | | M482/1 (28.9) | | M482/1 (2.1) | | M626/3 (3.7) | | | |
| | Urine/Feces Excretion (%) | 15.4/81.7 | | 27.4/62.9 | | 29.6/61.4 | | 54.4/41.2 | | | |
| *In Vitro* | Caco-2 Permeability | $Papp_{(A \to B)}$ = 0.85 × $10^{-6}$ cm/s | | | | | | | | | |
| | Plasma Protein Binding (%Bound) | 87.5-88.5 | | 89.9-91.2 | | 88.2-89.3 | | 82.0-84.5 | | | |
| | Hepatocytes Stability ($Cl_{int}$, mL/min/kg) | NA | | 15.8 | | 7.70 | | <2.7 | | | |

### Drug-Drug Interaction

| | CYP Enzyme | Non-CYP Enzyme | Transporter |
|---|---|---|---|
| **Substrate** | Not | UGT2B7, 1A3, 1A8, 1A9 | hOAT3, hOATP1B1, hOATP1B3, P-gp, BCRP |
| **Inhibitor** | Not | Not | hOATP1B1, hOATP1B3, hOAT2B1 |
| **Inducer** | Not | NA | NA |

### Non-clinical Toxicology

| | | | |
|---|---|---|---|
| **Single-Dose Toxicity (NOAEL)** | 2000 mg/kg (mouse, p.o.)<br>300 mg/kg (mouse, i.p.)<br>2000 mg/kg (rat, p.o., i.p.) | **Safety Pharmacology** | • No cardiovascular, neurological, pulmonary, renal and GI effect |
| **Repeated-Dose Toxicity (NOAEL)** | 1000 mg/kg/day (mouse, 13 weeks)<br>700 mg/kg/day (rat, 26 weeks)<br>30 mg/kg/day (dog, 52 weeks) | **Genotoxicity** | • No genotoxicity |
| | | **Reproductive and Developmental Toxicity** | • FEED NOAEL: 700 mg/kg/day<br>• EFD NOAEL: 100 mg/kg/day for the maternal, 300 mg/kg/day for fetuses in rats; 300 mg/kg/day for the maternal, 700 mg/kg/day for fetuses in rabbits<br>• PPND NOAEL: 100 mg/kg/day for $F_0$, 30 mg/kg/day for $F_1$ |
| | | **Carcinogenicity** | • Mouse and rat: NOAEL = 100 mg/kg/day |

**Finafloxacin**
**(Xtoro®)**
AL-60371
Suspension, topical otic, 0.3% Finafloxacin

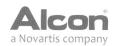
a Novartis company

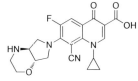

❖ Finafloxacin is a quinolone antimicrobial, indicated for the treatment of acute otitis externa (AOE) caused by susceptible strains of *Pseudomonas aeruginosa* and *Staphylococcus aureus*.   It was first approved in Dec 2014 by US FDA.
❖ Finafloxacin was discovered and marketed by Alcon Research.
❖ **_The recommended human starting dose_** is 4 drops in the affected ear(s) twice daily for 7 days.

| Worldwide Key Approvals | Global Sales($Million) | Key Substance Patent Expiration |
|---|---|---|
| Dec 17, 2014 (US) | Not available | Dec 04, 2017 (US6133260A)<br>Dec 04, 2017 (EP946176B1)<br>Dec 04, 2017 (JP3463939B2)<br>Dec 04, 2017 (CN100335054C) |

## Mechanism of Action

As a quinolone antimicrobial, finafloxacin involves the inhibition of bacterial type II topoisomerase enzymes, DNA gyrase and topoisomerase IV, which are required for bacterial DNA replication, transcription, repairation and recombination.

| Target Binding Selectivity | *In Vitro* Efficacy | *In Vivo* Efficacy |
|---|---|---|
| DNA gyrase: $CL_{50}$ = 25 ng/mL<br>DNA topoisomerase IV: $CL_{50}$ = 8 ng/mL | Antibacterial: $MIC_{50}$ = 0.008-32 µg/mL (pH 5.8)<br>Bactericidal: MBC = 0.03-2 µg/mL (pH 5.8)<br>MBC/MIC = 1-2 | Acute otitis externa model: 4-6 folds (at 24 h) or 0.5-1.5 folds (at 48 h) reduction in *P. aeruginosa* CFU at 0.3% finafloxacin |

## Pharmacokinetics

| | Parameter | Rat | | Dog | | Healthy Human | | | | | |
|---|---|---|---|---|---|---|---|---|---|---|---|
| | Dose (mg/kg, human: mg) | 2 (i.v.) | 2 (p.o.) | 1 (i.v.) | 2 (p.o.) | 25 (p.o.) | 50 (p.o.) | 100 (p.o.) | 200 (p.o.) | 400 (p.o.) | 800 (p.o.) |
| *In Vivo* | $C_{max}$ (µg eq./g, human: mg/L) | 2.19 | 0.38 | NA | NA | 0.24 | 0.44 | 1.32 | 1.90 | 5.06 | 11.1 |
| | $T_{max}$ (h) | - | 0.5 | NA | NA | 1.00 | 0.88 | 0.50 | 0.75 | 1.00 | 0.88 |
| | $AUC_{inf}$ (µg eq.·h/g, human: mg·h/L) | 1.69 | 0.986 | NA | NA | 0.42 | 1.26 | 2.80 | 4.08 | 14.2 | 29.2 |
| | $T_{1/2}$ (h) | 1.15 | 2.47 | 7.26 | 5.7 | 1.28 | 3.8 | 7.2 | 4.6 | 10.0 | 10.5 |
| | Cl (L/h) | NA | NA | NA | NA | 59.0 | 45.0 | 37.2 | 51.5 | 30.8 | 29.0 |
| | $V_z$/F (L) | NA | NA | NA | NA | 109 | 220 | 389 | 348 | 487 | 435 |
| | F (%) | - | 57.1 | - | 73 | NA | NA | NA | NA | NA | NA |
| | Most Abundant Drug-related Component in Plasma (%) | NA | | NA | | M0 | | | | | |
| | Major Drug-related Metabolite in Plasma (%) | AL-60317 | | AL-60317 | | AL-91591 | | | | | |
| | Urine/Feces Excretion (%) | 57.5/38.7 | | NA | | NA | | | | | |
| *In Vitro* | Permeability | | | | NA | | | | | | |
| | Plasma Protein Binding (%Bound) | 44.1-55.3 | | 70.4-79 | | 82.1-84.3 | | | | | |
| | LM/Hepatocytes Stability | NA | | NA | | NA | | | | | |

## Drug-Drug Interaction

| | CYP Enzyme | Non-CYP Enzyme | Transporter |
|---|---|---|---|
| Substrate | CYP3A4,1A2, 2D6, 2C19 | NA | NA |
| Inhibitor | Not | NA | NA |
| Inducer | NA | NA | NA |

## Non-clinical Toxicology

| Single-Dose Toxicity (MNLD) | NA | Safety Pharmacology | • NA |
|---|---|---|---|
| **Repeated-Dose Toxicity (NOAEL)** | 1.2%<br>(2.79 mg/animal/day, rabbit) | Genotoxicity | • Positive |
| | | Reproductive and Developmental Toxicity | • FEED NOAEL: 100 mg/kg<br>• EFD NOAEL: 9-100 mg/kg for mater |
| | | Carcinogenicity | • NA |
| | | Special Toxicdogy | • No phototoxicity |

## Idelalisib
## (Zydelig®)
CAL-101; GS-1101
Tablets, oral, 100 mg/150 mg Idelalisib

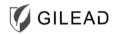

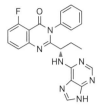

❖ Idelalisib is a small molecule PI3Kδ inhibitor, indicated for the treatment of patients with chronic lymphocytic leukemia (CLL) and indolent non-Hodgkin lymphoma (iNHL).　It was first approved in Jul 2014 by US FDA.
❖ Idelalisib was discovered by IWS Corp., then developed and marketed by Gilead Science.
❖ **_The recommended human starting dose_** is 150 mg orally twice daily.

| Worldwide Key Approvals | Global Sales ($Million) | | Key Substance Patent Expiration |
|---|---|---|---|
| Jul 23, 2014 (US) | **2014** | 23 | Aug 05, 2025 (US7932260B2) (EP2612862A2: Examination) |
| Sep 18, 2014 (EU) | **2015** | 132 | (JP2007537291A: Withdraw) May 12, 2025 (CN101031569B) |

## Mechanism of Action

As an inhibitor, idelalisib inhibits PI3Kδ kinase, a downstrearn signal molecule for several receptors involving in B-cell proliferation, motility, and in homing to and maintenance of the tumor microenvironment in B-cell malignancies.

**Target Inhibition Selectivity**
PI3Kδ: $IC_{50}$ = 19 nM
PI3Kα/β/γ: $IC_{50}$ = 2.1-8.6 μM

***In Vitro* Efficacy**
PI3Kδ activity in human basophil cell line: $EC_{50}$ = 8.9 nM (CD63 expression)
Anti-proliferation of WSU-FS-CCL and WSU-NHL cell lines: $IC_{50}$ = 30 nM (arrested in G1 phase)

## Pharmacokinetics

| | Parameter | Rat | | Dog | | | Human | | |
|---|---|---|---|---|---|---|---|---|---|
| | Dose (mg/kg, human: mg) | 3 (i.v.) | 3 (p.o.) | 1 (i.v.) | 1 (i.v. followed by p.o.) | 1 (p.o.) | 50 (p.o.) | 100 (p.o.) | 200 (p.o.) |
| *In Vivo* | $C_{max}$ (ng/mL) | 1437 | 129 | 977 | 510 | 209 | 598 | 1425 | 1769 |
| | $T_{max}$ (h) | 0.08 | 3.0 | 0.08 | 0.5 | 1.0 | NA | NA | NA |
| | $AUC_{inf}$ (ng·h/mL) | 1151 | 422 | 1432 | 1081 | 671 | 2301 | 4547 | 8110 |
| | $T_{1/2}$ (h) | 1.89 | 1.52 | 2.31 | 2.31 | 1.99 | 3.0 | 3.3 | 3.5 |
| | Cl (mL/min/kg) | 478 | NA | 0.76 | NA | NA | NA | NA | NA |
| | $V_{ss}$ (L/kg) | 2.49 | NA | 1.23 | NA | NA | NA | NA | NA |
| | F (%) | - | 39 | - | 79 | 48 | NA | NA | NA |
| | Most Abundant Drug-related Component in Plasma (%) | M0 (91-93) | | M0 (59) | | | M30A (62) | | |
| | Major Drug-related Metabolite in Plasma (%) | M30A (1.4) | | M30A (34) | | | M30A (62) | | |
| | Urine/Feces Excretion (%) | 3.04/83.9 | | 6.04/91.9 | | | 14/78 | | |
| *In Vitro* | Caco-2 Permeability | $Papp_{(A→B)}$ = 4.6-17 × $10^{-6}$ cm/s at 1-50 μM | | | | | | | |
| | Plasma Protein Binding (%Bound) | 81.3 | | 79.3 | | | 83.7 | | |
| | LM/Heptocytes Stability | NA | | NA | | | NA | | |

## Drug-Drug Interaction

| | CYP Enzyme | Non-CYP Enzyme | Transporter |
|---|---|---|---|
| **Substrate** | CYP3A4 | Aldehyde oxidase, UGT1A4 | P-gp, BCRP |
| **Inhibitor** | CYP3A, CYP2C8, CYP2C19 | NA | P-gp, OATP1B1, OATP1B3 |
| **Inducer** | CYP2B6, CYP2C8, CYP2C9, CYP3A4 | UGT1A1, UGT1A4 | NA |

## Non-clinical Toxicology

| **Single-Dose Toxicity (MTD)** | 25 mg/kg (dog) | **Safety Pharmacology** | • CVS: hERG $IC_{50}$ >50 μM<br>• No significant *in vivo* effect on neurological, cardiovascular or respiratory parameters |
|---|---|---|---|
| **Repeated-Dose Toxicity (NOAEL)** | NA | **Genotoxicity** | • Positive in *in vivo* chromosomal aberration assays at 2000 mg/kg<br>• Negative in the Ames assay and the *in vitro* HPBL chromosome aberration assay |
| | | **Reproductive and Developmental Toxicity** | • FEED: No effect on reproductive function<br>• EFD: Teratogenic, NOAEL was 25 mg/kg/day |
| | | **Carcinogenicity** | • NA |

# Ipragliflozin L-proline
## (Suglat®)
ASP-1941
Tablet, oral, EQ 25 mg/50 mg Ipragliflozin

   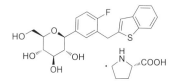

❖ Ipragliflozin is an SGLT2 (sodium-glucose cotransporter 2) inhibitor, indicated for the treatment of patients with type 2 diabetes. It was first approved by PMDA of Japan.
❖ Ipragliflozin was discovered by Kotobuki and Astellas, co-developed and co-marketed by Kotobuki, Merck and Astellas.
❖ **_The human recommended starting dose_** is 50 mg once daily, taken before or after breakfast.

| Worldwide Key Approvals | Global Sales ($Million) | | Key Substance Patent Expiration |
|---|---|---|---|
| Jan 17, 2014 (JP) | **2014** **2015** | 30.8 51.6 | May 27, 2024 (US7772407B2) Mar 12, 2024 (EP1980560B1) Mar 12, 2029 (JP4222450B2) Mar 12, 2024 (CN1802366B) |

## Mechanism of Action

Ipragliflozin reduces blood glucose levels by inhibiting the reuptake of glucose in kidneys *via* selectively inhibiting SGLT2.

**In Vitro Efficacy**
hSGLT2: $IC_{50}$ = 7.38 nM
hSGLT1: $IC_{50}$ = 1880 nM
Selectivity SGLT2/SGLT1: 254-fold

**In Vivo Efficacy**
Urinary glucose excretion (UGE): MED = 0.3 mg/kg in type 2 diabetic models
Blood glucose lower effect: MED = 0.1 mg/kg in type 2 diabetic and normal mice and rats
HbA1c lower effect: MED = 0.3 mg/kg in KK-A$^y$ mouse and 0.1 mg/kg in *db/db* mouse

## Pharmacokinetics

| | Parameters | Rat | | | | Monkey | | | | Healthy Human | |
|---|---|---|---|---|---|---|---|---|---|---|---|
| | Dose (mg/kg, human: mg) | 0.3 (i.v.) | 0.3 (p.o.) | 1 (p.o.) | 3 (p.o.) | 0.3 (i.v.) | 0.3 (p.o.) | 1 (p.o.) | 3 (p.o.) | 25 mg (i.v.) | 100 mg (p.o.) |
| | $C_{max}$ (ng/mL) | NA | 114 | 331 | 832 | NA | 133 | 444 | 1358 | 612 | 1406 |
| | $T_{max}$ (h) | NA | 0.5 | 1.0 | 0.5 | NA | 2.0 | 1.75 | 1.75 | 0.972 | 1.5 |
| | $T_{1/2}$ (h) | 3.85 | 4.43 | 3.61 | 3.93 | 9.45 | 8.65 | 10.1 | 9.56 | 16.8 | 16.3 |
| | $AUC_{inf}$ (ng·h/mL) | 692 | 541 | 1654 | 6277 | 1271 | 952 | 3231 | 9564 | 2374 | 8457 |
| In Vivo | $V_{ss}$ (L/kg, human: L) | 1.68 | NA | NA | NA | 2.32 | NA | NA | NA | 127 | NA |
| | Cl (L/h/kg, human: L/h) | 0.433 | NA | NA | NA | 0.252 | NA | NA | NA | 10.9 | 12.1 |
| | F (%) | - | 78.2 | 71.7 | 90.7 | - | 74.5 | 75.3 | 74.8 | - | 90.2 |
| | Mast Abundant Drug-related Component in Plasma (%) | M0 (82.2) | | | | M0 (47.6) | | | | M0 ($AUC_{inf}$ = 7326 ng·h/mL) | |
| | Major Drug-related Metabolite in Plasma (%) | M7 (1.9) | | | | M2 (6.3), M4 (6.3) | | | | M2 ($AUC_{inf}$ = 5065 ng·h/mL) | |
| | Urine/Feces Excretion (%) | 13.2/86.9 | | | | 44.7/48.4 | | | | 67.9/32.7 | |
| | MDCKII Permeability | $Papp_{(A-B)}$ = 5.98 ×10$^{-6}$ cm/s at 1 µM | | | | | | | | | |
| In Vitro | Plasma Protein Binding (%Bound) | 94.6-96.1 | | | | 93.2-95.3 | | | | 94.6-96.5 | |
| | LM Stability ($Cl_{int}$, mL/min/mg protein) | 0.0142 | | | | 0.0062 | | | | 0.0067 | |

## Drug-Drug Interaction

| | CYP Enzyme | Non-CYP Enzyme | Transporter |
|---|---|---|---|
| **Substrate** | NA | UGT2B7, 2B4, 1A9, 1A8 | P-gp |
| **Inhibitor** | CYP2B6 | Not | OATP1B1, OAT3, OCT1 |
| **Inducer** | Not | NA | NA |

## Non-clinical Toxicology

| **Single-Dose Toxicity (MTD)** | 2000/500 mg/kg (rat, male/female) 2000 mg/kg (monkey) | **Safety Pharmacology** | • CVS: 17.4% inhibition of hERG potassium current at 10 µM • No *in vivo* effetct on CNS, RS |
|---|---|---|---|
| | | **Genotoxicity** | • No genotoxic risk |
| **Repeated-Dose Toxicity (NOAEL)** | 0.1 mg/kg/day (rat, 26 weeks) 10/1 mg/kg/day (monkey, male/female, 52 weeks) | **Reproductive and Developmental Toxicity** | • FEED NOAEL: 300 mg/kg/day • EFD NOAEL: 100 mg/kg/day for mater and 300 mg/kg/day for fetus in rats/rabbits • PPND NOAEL: 100 mg/kg/day for $F_0/F_1$ • Placental barrier penetration and milk excretion |
| | | **Carcinogenicity** | • No significant malignant or benign neoplasia |

## Luseogliflozin Hydrate
## (Lusefi®)
TS-071
Tablet, oral, EQ 2.5 mg/5 mg Luseogliflozin

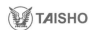 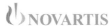

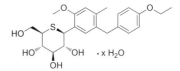

❖ Luseogliflozin hydrate is a sodium-glucose cotransporter 2 (SGLT2) inhibitor, indicated for the treatment of type 2 diabetes.   It was first approved in Mar 2014 by PMDA of Japan.

❖ Luseogliflozin hydrate was discovered by Taisho, co-developed and co-marketed by Taisho and Novartis.

❖ _**The recommended human starting dose**_ is 2.5 mg once daily, taken before or after breakfast.

| Worldwide Key Approvals | Global Sales ($Million) | | Key Substance Patent Expiration |
|---|---|---|---|
| Mar 24, 2014 (JP) | **2014** | 22.4 | Apr 04, 2028 (US7910619B2) |
| | **2015** | 5.7 | Jan 10, 2026 (EP1845095B1) |
| | | | Dec 17, 2029 (JP4492968B2) |
| | | | Jan 10, 2026 (CN101103013B) |

## Mechanism of Action

Luseogliflozin selectively inhibits SGLT2 which is responsible for glucose reabsorption, thereby increasing urine glucose excretion and reducing blood glucose concentration.

**_In Vitro_ Target Binding Selectivity**

hSGLT2: $IC_{50}$ = 2.26 nM
hSGLT1: $IC_{50}$ = 2900 nM
Selectivity hSGLT2/hSGLT1: 1283-fold

**_In Vivo_ Efficacy**

Urine glucose excretion: MED = 0.3-3 mg/kg in _db/db_ mice, ZDF and DIO rats
Blood glucose lower effect: MED = 0.3-3 mg/kg (blood glucose level, AUC and AUC in OGTT)

## Pharmacokinetics

| | Parameters | Rat | | | | Dog | | | | Healthy Human |
|---|---|---|---|---|---|---|---|---|---|---|
| | Dose (mg/kg, human: mg) | 1 (i.v.) | 0.3 (p.o.) | 1 (p.o.) | 3 (p.o.) | 1 (i.v.) | 0.3 (p.o.) | 1 (p.o.) | 3 (p.o.) | 2.5 (p.o.) |
| **In Vivo** | $C_{max}$ (ng/mL) | NA | 8.02 | 35.7 | 136 | NA | 301 | 914 | 2760 | 100 |
| | $T_{max}$ (h) | NA | 0.83 | 0.50 | 0.67 | NA | 0.67 | 0.67 | 1.33 | 1.11 |
| | $AUC_{inf}$ (ng·h/mL) | 462 | 42.0 | 163 | 524 | 5250 | 1480 | 4880 | 16000 | 1000 |
| | $T_{1/2}$ (h) | 4.92 | 3.17 | 2.93 | 2.52 | 3.89 | 3.84 | 4.07 | 4.25 | 11.2 |
| | Cl (L/h/kg, human: L/h) | 2.18 | NA | NA | NA | 0.19 | NA | NA | NA | NA |
| | $V_{ss}$ (L/kg, human: L) | 2.63 | NA | NA | NA | 0.80 | NA | NA | NA | NA |
| | F (%) | - | 30.3 | 35.3 | 37.8 | - | 94.0 | 92.7 | 101.6 | NA |
| | Most Abundant Drug-related Component in Plasma (%) | M8 (53.9) | | | | M0 (76.7) | | | | M0 |
| | Major Drug-Related Metabolite in Plasma (%) | M8 (53.9) | | | | M14,17 (7.2) | | | | M2 |
| | Urine/Feces Excretion (%) | 5.7/93.4 | | | | 35.2/65.1 | | | | 20/NA |
| **In Vitro** | Caco-2 Permeability | $Papp_{(A-B)}$ = 14 × $10^{-6}$ cm/s at 10 μM | | | | | | | | |
| | Plasma Protein Binding (%Bound) | 93.8-95.3 | | | | 91.7-95.6 | | | | 96.0-96.3 |
| | LM/Hepatocytes Stability | NA | | | | NA | | | | NA |

## Drug-Drug Interaction

| | CYP Enzyme | Non-CYP Enzyme | Transporter |
|---|---|---|---|
| **Substrate** | CYP3A, 4A11 | ADH, ALDH | P-gp |
| **Inhibitor** | CYP2C19 | NA | Not |
| **Inducer** | Not | NA | NA |

## Non-clinical Toxicology

| Single-Dose Toxicity (ALD) | >2000 mg/kg (rat) >1500 mg/kg (dog) | Safety Pharmacology | • Not much of special concern on CNS, CVS, RS and GI |
|---|---|---|---|
| | | Genotoxicity | • Negative overall |
| **Repeated-Dose Toxicity (NOAEL)** | 4 mg/kg/day (rat, 26 weeks) 2 mg/kg/day (dog, 52 weeks) 300 mg/kg/day (monkey, 13 weeks) | **Reproductive and Developmental Toxicity** | • FEED NOAEL: 300 mg/kg/day for males, 100 mg/kg/day for females<br>• EFD NOAEL: 150 mg/kg/day for the maternal, 50 mg/kg/day for fetuses in rats; 500 mg/kg/day for the maternal, 1000 mg/kg/day for fetuses in rabbits<br>• PPND NOAEL: 150 mg/kg/day for $F_0$, 50 mg/kg/day for $F_1$ |
| | | Carcinogenicity | • Adrenal pheochromocytoma, interstitial cell tumor in HD male rats |

## Naloxegol Oxalate
## (Movantik®/Moventig®)
NKTR-118
Tablets, oral, EQ 12.5 mg/25 mg Naloxegol

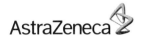

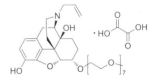

❖ Naloxegol is an opioid receptor antagonist, indicated for the treatment of opioid-induced constipation (OIC) in adult patients with chronic non-cancer pain. It was first approved in Sep 2014 by US FDA.
❖ Naloxegol was discovered by Nektar Therapeutics, developed and marketed by AstraZeneca.
❖ *The recommended human starting dose* is 25 mg once daily in the morning.

| Worldwide Key Approvals | Global Sales ($Million) | | Key Substance Patent Expiration |
|---|---|---|---|
| | | | Dec 19, 2027 (US7786133B2) |
| Sep 16, 2014 (US) | **2014** | Not available | Dec 16, 2024 (EP1694363B1) |
| Dec 08, 2014 (EU) | **2015** | 39 | Dec 16, 2024 (JP4991312B2) |
| | | | Dec 16, 2024 (CN101805343B) |

## Mechanism of Action

As a PEGylated derivative of naloxone, naloxegol binds to μ-opioid receptors in the gastrointestinal tract, thereby decreasing the constipating effects of opioids.

**Target Binding Selectivity**
μ-opioid receptor: $K_i$ = 7.42-77.3 nM
δ-opioid receptor: $K_i$ = 8.65-53.5 nM
κ-opioid receptor: $K_i$ = 186.5-230 nM

*In Vitro* **Efficacy**
μ-opioid receptor: $pIC_{50}$ = 6.64-7.25 (full antagonism)
δ-opioid receptor: $IC_{50}$ = 866 nM (antagonism)
κ-opioid receptor: $EC_{50}$ = 47 nM (partial agonism)

*In Vivo* **Efficacy**
Peripheral effects: $ED_{50}$ = 23.1 mg/kg
$ED_{50}$_analgesia/$ED_{50}$_GI = 2.4

## Pharmacokinetics

| | Parameter | Rat | Dog | | Monkey | | Healthy Human | | | |
|---|---|---|---|---|---|---|---|---|---|---|
| | Dose (mg/kg, human: mg) | 10, 30, 100 (i.v.) | 0.4 (i.v.) | 50 (p.o.) | 1.0 (i.v.) | 5 (p.o.) | 12.5 (p.o.) | 25 (p.o.) | 50 (p.o.) | 100 (p.o.) |
| | $C_{max}$ (ng/mL) | NA | NA | 1530 | NA | 41.6 | 19 | 46 | 152 | 375 |
| | $T_{max}$ (h) | NA | NA | 0.5 | NA | 0.69 | NA | NA | NA | NA |
| | $AUC_{inf}$ (ng·h/mL) | NA | NA | 3740 | NA | 78.1 | 86 | 158 | 371 | 847 |
| | $T_{1/2}$ (h) | 2.92 | 5.7 | 9.58 | 4.99 | 2.77 | 7.8 | 7.7 | 8.0 | 6.1 |
| *In Vivo* | Cl (L/h/kg, human: L/h) | 2.65 | 2.65 | NA | 1.46 | NA | 158 | 168 | 174 | 159 |
| | $V_{ss}$ (L/kg) | 3.14 | 4.66 | NA | 2.44 | NA | NA | NA | NA | NA |
| | F (%) | NA | NA | 20.6 | NA | 2.26 | NA | NA | NA | NA |
| | Most Abundant Drug-related Component in Plasma (%) | M0 (15.4) | M2 (62) | | NA | | M0 (64) | | | |
| | Major Drug-related Metabolite in Plasma (%) | M2 (5) | M2 (62) | | NA | | M10 (12) | | | |
| | Urine/Feces Excretion (%) | 18.8/78.9 | 25.2/63.4 | | NA | | <10/83 | | | |
| *In Vitro* | Caco-2 Permeability | $Papp_{(A \rightarrow B)}$ = 0.7 × $10^{-6}$ cm/s | | | | | | | | |
| | Plasma Protein Binding (%Bound) | 14.1 | 3.8-53.3 | | 9.7 | | 4.2 | | | |
| | Heptocytes Stability (%Remaining) | <12.4 | <16.9 | | <24.8 | | <29.9 | | | |

## Drug-Drug Interaction

| | CYP Enzyme | Non-CYP Enzyme | Transporter |
|---|---|---|---|
| **Substrate** | CYP3A4, 2D6 | NA | P-gp, BCRP, OATP1 B1, OATP1B3 |
| **Inhibitor** | CYP2D6 | NA | Not |
| **Inducer** | Not | NA | NA |

## Non-clinical Toxicology

| **Single-Dose Toxicity (MTD)** | 2000 mg/kg (mouse, rat, p.o.) 100 mg/kg (rat, i.v.) | **Safety Pharmacology** | • CVS: 13.3% hERG inhibition at 300 μM<br>• Gastrointestinal effect: Stomach weight increased by 28%-78%<br>• Renal effect: Urinary excretion of sodium, potassium, chloride and albumin increased |
|---|---|---|---|
| **Repeated-Dose Toxicity (NOAEL)** | 50 mg/kg/day (rat, 26 weeks) 200 mg/kg/day (dog, 39 weeks) | **Genotoxicity** | • Positive in Ames assay |
| | | **Reproductive and Developmental Toxicity** | • FEED NOAEL: 1000 mg/kg/day<br>• EFD NOAEL: 450 mg/kg/day (rabbit), 750 mg/kg/day (rat)<br>• PPND NOAEL: 500 mg/kg/day |
| | | **Carcinogenicity** | • Negative |

**Nintedanib Esylate**
**(Ofev®/Vargatef®)**
BIBF-1120
Capsule, oral, EQ 100 mg/150 mg Nintedanib

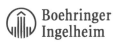 Boehringer
Ingelheim

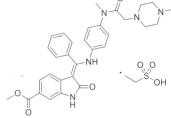

❖ Nintedanib is a tyrosine kinase inhibitor, indicated for the treatment of idiopathic pulmonary fibrosis (IPF) appoved by FDA, EMA and PMDA, non-small cell lung cancer approved by EMA. It was first approved in Oct 2014 by US FDA.
❖ Nintedanib was discovered and marketed by Boehringer Ingelheim.
❖ **_The recommended human starting dose_** is 150 mg twice daily for IPF or 200 mg twice daily for non-small cell lung cancer taken with food.

| Worldwide Key Approvals | Global Sales ($Million) | Key Substance Patent Expiration |
|---|---|---|
| Oct 15, 2014 (US)<br>Nov 21, 2014 (EU)<br>Jul 03, 2015 (JP) | Not available | Dec 10, 2020 (US6762180B1)<br>Oct 09, 2020 (EP1224170B1)<br>Oct 09, 2020 (JP4021664B2)<br>Oct 09, 2020 (CN100455568C) |

## Mechanism of Action

As a tyrosine kinase inhibitor, nintedanib competitively binds to the adenosine triphosphate (ATP) binding pocket of multiple receptor tyrosine kinases and blocks the intracellular signaling which is crucial for the proliferation, migration and transformation of fibroblasts.

**Target Inhibition**
PDGFR$\alpha/\beta$: $IC_{50}$ = 59/65 nM
FGFR 1-4: $IC_{50}$ = 37-610 nM
VEGFR 1-3: $IC_{50}$ = 13-34 nM

**_In Vitro_ Efficacy**
Auto-phosphorylation:
  PDGFR$\alpha/\beta$: $IC_{50}$ = 21.6-38.7 nM
Anti-proliferation: $IC_{50}$ = <1->4500 nM
Inhibition of migration: $IC_{50}$ = 19-228 nM
Transformation of IPF-HLF: $IC_{50}$ = 144 nM

**_In Vivo_ Efficacy**
Anti-tumour activities in Calu-6 xenograft mouse models:
  T/C% = 24% at 50 mg/kg, QD
Lung fibrosis in rats and mice:
  Decreased the severity of lung fibrosis

## Pharmacokinetics

| | Parameter | Mouse | Rat | | Cynomolgus Monkey | | Rhesus Monkey | | Healthy Human | |
|---|---|---|---|---|---|---|---|---|---|---|
| | Dose (mg/kg) | 50 (p.o.) | 2 (i.v.) | 50 (p.o.) | 5 (i.v.) | 40 (p.o.) | 5 (i.v.) | 40 (p.o.) | 0.078 (i.v.) | 1.29 (p.o.) |
| | $C_{max}$ (ng/mL) | 547 | 124 | 105 | 1300 | 175 | 1090 | 311 | 12.3 | 8.43 |
| | $T_{max}$ (h) | NA | NA | NA | NA | NA | NA | NA | NA | NA |
| | $AUC_{inf}$ (ng·h/mL) | 2720 | 181 | 375 | 2260 | 2390 | 2830 | 4440 | 71.9 | 56.2 |
| | $T_{1/2}$ (h) | 5.15 | 3.95 | - | 5.95 | - | 7.09 | - | 17.9 | 11.7 |
| _In Vivo_ | Cl (mL/min/kg) | - | 202 | - | 37.5 | - | 30.2 | - | 18 | - |
| | $V_d$ (L/kg) | - | 41.2 | - | 8.64 | - | 10.4 | - | 13.6 | - |
| | F (%) | NA | - | 11.9 | - | 13.2 | - | 23.8 | - | 4.7 |
| | Most Abundant Drug-related Component in Plasma (%) | M2 (31.4) M0 (31.3) | M2 (76.9) | | NA | | M2 (55.1) | | M1 (38.7) | |
| | Major Drug-related Metabolite in Plasma (%) | M2 (31.4)/ M2 (25.6) | M2 (76.9) | | NA | | M2 (55.1) | | M1 (38.7) | |
| | Urine/Feces Excretion (%) | 1.9/99.3 | 1.6/67.0 | | 1.2/87.7 | | | | 0.65/93.4 | |
| _In Vitro_ | Plasma Protein Binding (%Bound) | 97.2 | 95.8 | | 92.9 | | 91.4 | | 97.8 | |
| | LM/Hepatocytes Stability | NA | NA | | NA | | NA | | NA | |

## Drug-Drug Interaction

| | CYP Enzyme | Non-CYP Enzyme | Transporter |
|---|---|---|---|
| Substrate | CYP3A4 | Esterase, UGT1A1, 1A7, 1A8, 1A10 | P-gp, OCT1 |
| Inhibitor | Not | UGT1A1 | P-gp, BCRP, OCT1 |
| Inducer | Not | NA | NA |

## Non-clinical Toxicology

| Single-Dose Toxicity (ALD) | >2000 mg/kg (mouse, p.o.) >2000 mg/kg (rat, p.o.) | **Safety Pharmacology** | • CVS: hERG $IC_{50}$ = 4.0 μM<br>• No effect on neurobehavioral, respiratory or GI tract function |
|---|---|---|---|
| **Repeated-Dose Toxicity (NOAEL)** | 5 mg/kg/day (rat, 26 weeks). 10 mg/kg/day (monkey, 52 weeks) | **Genotoxicity** | • Negative |
| | | **Reproductive and Developmental Toxicology** | • FEED NOAEL: 100/20 mg/kg/day (male/female) for fertility; 3 mg/kg/day for embryo development<br>• EFD NOAEL: 10 mg/kg/day for mater and <2.5 mg/kg/day for fetus in rats; 60 mg/kg/day for mater and <15 mg/kg/day for fetus in rabbits<br>• PPND NOAEL: 5 mg/kg/day |
| | | **Carcinogenicity** | • No statistically significant pre- or neoplastic finding in mice or rats |

## Olaparib
### (Lynparza®)
AZD-2281; KU-0059436; KU-59436
Capsule, oral, 50 mg Olaparib

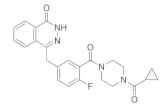

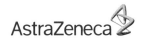

❖ Olaparib is a poly (ADP-ribose) polymerase (PARP) inhibitor, indicated for the treatment of patients with deleterious or suspected deleterious germline BRCA mutated advanced ovarian cancer. It was first approved in Dec 2014 by EMA.
❖ Olaparib was discovered and marketed by AstraZeneca.
❖ **_The recommended human starting dose_** is 400 mg orally twice daily.

| Worldwide Key Approvals | Global Sales ($Million) | | Key Substance Patent Expiration |
|---|---|---|---|
| | | | Oct 11, 2024 (US7449464B2) |
| Dec 16, 2014 (EU) | **2014** | Not available | Mar 12, 2024 (EP1633724B1) |
| Dec 19, 2014 (US) | **2015** | 94 | Mar 12, 2024 (JP4027406B2) |
| | | | Mar 12, 2024 (CN1788000B) |

## Mechanism of Action

Olaparib inhibits PARP1-3, which are required for the efficient repair of DNA single strand breaks, resulting in cancer cell death.

| Target Binding and Inhibition | *In Vitro* Efficacy | *In Vivo* Efficacy |
|---|---|---|
| PARP-1: $IC_{50}$ = 5 nM | Olaparib inhibited colony formation in cell lines: | Human derived tumor HBCx-10, 17 and Lu7433 models: |
| PARP-2: $IC_{50}$ = 1 nM | BRCA1/2 WT cell: $IC_{50}$ = 21-1463 nM | Tumor growth decreased at 50 mg/kg |
| PARP-3: $IC_{50}$ = 4 nM | BRCA1/2 mutation cell: $IC_{50}$ = 18-125 nM | |

## Pharmacokinetics

| | Parameter | Mouse (male) | | Rat (male) | | Dog (male) | | Healthy human | | | Patient | | |
|---|---|---|---|---|---|---|---|---|---|---|---|---|---|
| | Dose (mg/kg, human: mg) | 20 (i.v.) | 80 (p.o.) | 1 (i.v.) | 5 (p.o.) | 1 (i.v.) | 5 (p.o.) | 50 (p.o.) | 100 (p.o.) | 400 (p.o.) | 100 (p.o.) | 200 (p.o.) | 400 (p.o.) |
| | $C_{max}$ (μg/mL) | NA | 28.6 | 1.08 | 0.162 | 1.41 | 2.13 | 1.8 | 2.9 | 5.7 | 2.3 | 3.5 | 4.9 |
| | $T_{max}$ (h) | NA | 0.5 | 0.5 | 1.0 | 0.083 | 1.0 | 1.5 | 1.3 | 1.3 | 1.0 | 2.1 | 2.4 |
| | $AUC_{inf}$ (μg·h/mL) | 14.9 | 33.0 | 0.59 | 0.494 | 2.75 | 10.3 | 10 | 17 | 58 | 17 | 21 | 39 |
| | $T_{1/2}$ (h) | 0.648 | 1.74 | 0.8 | 2.5 | 1.71 | 4.61 | 7.9 | 8.4 | 12 | 7.8 | 6.9 | 11 |
| *In Vivo* | Cl (L/h/kg, human: L/h) | 1.34 | NA | NC | NC | 0.39 | NC | 5.4 | 6.2 | 8.6 | 9.3 | 10 | 12 |
| | $V_{ss}$ (L/kg) | 0.356 | NA | NC | NC | 0.93 | NC | 61 | 81 | 167 | 59 | 75 | 112 |
| | F (%) | - | 55.4 | - | 17.2 | - | 78.9 | NA | NA | NA | NA | NA | NA |
| | Most Abundant Drug-related Component in Plasma (%) | NA | | M0 (70.4) | | M0 (86.6-90.9) | | M0 (70.0) | | | NA | | |
| | Major Drug-related Metabolite in Plasma (%) | NA | | M12 (12.3) | | NI | | M18 (13.7) | | | NA | | |
| | Urine/Feces Excretion (%) | NA | | 7.8/88.7 | | 23.4/77.8 | | 44.1/41.8 | | | NA | | |
| | Permeability | | | | | NA | | | | | | | |
| *In Vitro* | Plasma Protein Binding (%Bound) | 69.4-71.6 | | 72.7-73.5 | | 54.7-61.9 | | 81.9-91.2 | | | NA | | |
| | LM/Heptocytes Stability | NA | | NA | | NA | | NA | | | NA | | |

## Drug-Drug Interaction

| | CYP Enzyme | Non-CYP Enzyme | Transporter |
|---|---|---|---|
| Substrate | CYP3A5, 2A6, 1A1 | NA | P-gp, OATs |
| Inhibitor | Not | NA | BCRP, OATP1B1, OCT1, OCT2, OAT1, OAT3, MATE1, MATE2K |
| Inducer | CYP2B6 | NA | NA |

## Non-clinical Toxicology

| Single-Dose Toxicity (MTD) | 300 mg/kg (mouse, p.o.) 70 mg/kg (mouse, i.v.) 240 mg/kg (rat, p.o.) 70 mg/kg (rat, i.v.) | Safety Pharmacology | • CVS: hERG $IC_{50}$ = 226 μM • No significant effect on CNS or RS |
|---|---|---|---|
| | | Genotoxicity | • Positive |
| Repeated-Dose Toxicity (NOAEL) | 30/5 mg/kg/day (rat, 26 weeks) 3 mg/kg/day (dog, 26 weeks) | Reproductive and Developmental Toxicity | • FEED NOEL: 0.5-40 mg/kg/day • EFD: Significantly embryotoxic and teratogenic |
| | | Carcinogenicity | • NA |

## Oritavancin Diphosphate
## (Orbactiv®)
LY-333328
Lyophilized powder, i.v., EQ 400 mg Oritavancin

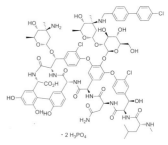

The
Medicines
Company

❖ Oritavancin diphosphate is a semi-synthetic, lipoglycopeptide antibacterial drug, indicated for the treatment of adult patients with acute bacterial skin and skin structure infections (ABSSSI) caused by susceptible isolates of designated Gram-positive microorganisms. It was first approved in Aug 2014 by US FDA.
❖ Oritavancin diphosphate was originally discovered by Eli Lilly, developed and marketed by The Medicines Company.
❖ *The recommended human starting dose* is 1200 mg as a single dose.

| Worldwide Key Approvals | Global Sales ($Million) | | Key Substance Patent Expiration |
|---|---|---|---|
| | | | Nov 24, 2016 (US5840684A) |
| Aug 06, 2014 (US) | **2014** | 0.8 | Jan 25, 2015 (EP0667353B1) |
| Mar 19, 2015 (EU) | **2015** | 9.1 | Jan 27, 2015 (JP3756539B2) |
| | | | Jan 27, 2015 (CN1071334C) |

## Mechanism of Action

As a semi-synthetic lipoglycopeptide antibacterial drug, oritavancin diphosphate inhibits bacterial cell wall biosynthesis and disrupts bacterial membrane integrity, leading to permeabilization and cell death.

| Target Binding and Inhibition | *In Vitro* Efficacy | *In Vivo* Efficacy |
|---|---|---|
| Increased proportion of D-Ala-D-Asp: | *Staphylococci/Enterococci/Streptococci*: MIC = 0.008-0.06 µg/mL | MSSA and MRSA infected endocarditis model: Reduced the bacterial burden by >4 $\log_{10}$ CFU |
| 13% at 25 µg/mL | *E. faecalis*/MRSA/MSSA: | *E. faecalis* infected model: |
| Increased proportion of tripeptides: | MIC = 0.008-0.5 µg/mL | Reduced the bacterial burden by 1.8-2.8 |
| 32% at 25 µg/mL | VISA/VRSA: MIC = 0.25-1 µg/mL | $\log_{10}$ CFU |

## Pharmacokinetics

| | Parameter | Rabbit | | | Human | | | |
|---|---|---|---|---|---|---|---|---|
| | | 10 (i.v.) | 15 (i.v.) | 20 (i.v.) | 0.5 (i.v.) | 1.0 (i.v.) | 2.0 (i.v.) | 3.0 (i.v.) |
| *In Vivo* | Dose (mg/kg) | | | | | | | |
| | $C_{max}$ (µg/mL) | 71.8 | 113 | 148 | 5.29 | 11.0 | 25.7 | 37.7 |
| | $T_{max}$ (h) | NA | NA | NA | 0.50 | 0.50 | 0.50 | 0.50 |
| | $AUC_{inf}$ (µg·h/mL, rabbit: $AUC_{0-24}$) | 450 | 786 | 966 | 101 | 179 | 448 | 650 |
| | $T_{1/2}$ (h) | NA | NA | NA | 240 | 178 | 285 | 322 |
| | Cl (mL/h/kg, human: L/h) | NA | NA | NA | 0.306 | 0.340 | 0.299 | 0.282 |
| | $V_{ss}$ (L) | NA | NA | NA | 78.8 | 53.7 | 66.7 | 61.4 |
| | F (%) | - | - | - | - | - | - | - |
| | Most Abundant Drug-related Component in Plasma (%) | NA | | | | | | |
| | Major Drug-related Metabolite in Plasma (%) | NA | | | | | | |
| | Urine/Feces Excretion (%) | NA | | | | | | |
| *In Vitro* | Permeability | NA | | | | | | |
| | Plasma Protein Binding (%Bound) | NA | | | 87.5 | | | |
| | LM/Heptocytes Stability | NA | | | NA | | | |

## Drug-Drug Interaction

| | CYP Enzyme | Non-CYP Enzyme | Transporter |
|---|---|---|---|
| **Substrate** | NA | NA | Not |
| **Inhibitor** | CYP3A4, 2D6, 2C9, 2C19, 2B6, 1A2 | NA | Not |
| **Inducer** | Not | NA | NA |

## Non-clinical Toxicology

| | | | |
|---|---|---|---|
| Single-Dose Toxicity (MNLD) | 40 mg/kg/day (rat) | Safety Pharmacology | • CVS: Ion channel current $IC_{50}$s ranged from 0.5 µM for $Na^+$ to 22 µM for $K^+$<br>• CNS: Slight prolonged hexobarbital sleep time and decrease of body temperature<br>• No significant change on GI and renal functions |
| Repeated-Dose Toxicity (NOAEL) | 5 mg/kg/day (rat, 4 weeks) 5 mg/kg/day (dog, 13 weeks) | Genotoxicity | • No genetic toxicity |
| | | Reproductive and Developmental Toxicology | • FEED NOAEL: 30 mg/kg/day<br>• EFD NOAEL: 30 mg/kg/day in rats and 15 mg/kg/day in rabbits<br>• PPND NOAEL: 30 mg/kg/day<br>• Juvenile NOAEL: 5 mg/kg/day in both rats and dogs |
| | | Carcinogenicity | • NA |

## Phenothrin (Sumithrin®)
KC-1001
Lotion, topical, 5% Phenothrin

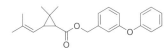

❖ Phenothrin, a synthetic type-I non-cyano pyrethroid insecticide, indicated for the treatment of keratinocytes type scabies and nail scabies. It was first approved in Mar 2014 by PMDA of Japan.

❖ Phenothrin was discovered by Sumitomo, developed and marketed by Kracie.

❖ *The recommended human starting dose* is 30 g of the lotion once weekly to the skin of neck below and plantar.

| Worldwide Key Approvals | Global Sales($Million) | Key Substance Patent Expiration |
|---|---|---|
| Mar 24, 2014 (JP) | Not available | May 29, 1989 (GB1243858A) |

### Mechanism of Action

As a pyrethroid insecticide, phenothrin kills insects by disrupting the transmission of nerve impulses along axons, the elongated parts of nerve cells.

#### *In Vitro* Efficacy

The $LD_{50}$ of farinae and tyrophagus:
  Farinae: $LD_{50}$ <0.01 µg/cm$^2$
  Tyrophagus: $LD_{50}$ = 0.46 µg/cm$^2$

Growth inhibition: 90.2% inhibition for ticks at 0.1% and 98.9% for tyrohagus at 0.001% on week 1
Insectticidal:
  Musca domestica: $LD_{50}$ = 0.022-0.056 µg/fly and $LC_{50}$ = 20.2-34.5 mg/100 mL
  Culex pipiens pallens: $LD_{50}$ = 0.0075 µg/insect

### Pharmacokinetics

| | Parameter | Rat (*Cis*-phenothrin/*Trans*-phenothrin) | | | Rabbit (Phenothrin) | Healthy Human (*Cis*-phenothrin/*Trans*-phenothrin) | |
|---|---|---|---|---|---|---|---|
| | Dose (mg/kg) | 50 (Topical) | 100 (Topical) | 200 (Topical) | 500 (p.o.) | *Cis*-phenothrin (Topical) | *Trans*-phenothrin (Topical) |
| **In Vivo** | $C_{max}$ (ng/mL) | 0.830/0.796 | 0.759/0.726 | 2.24/2.04 | 256 | 1.58 | 1.99 |
| | $T_{max}$ (h) | 4/4 | 12/8 | 48/48 | 3 | 24.0 | 14.3 |
| | $AUC_{0-t}$ (ng·h/mL) | 19.4/7.91 | 27.5/18.2 | 115/89.4 | 4877 | 42.4 | 50.2 |
| | $T_{1/2}$ (h) | NA | NA | NA | NA | NA | NA |
| | Cl (L/h/kg, human: L/h) | NA | NA | NA | NA | NA | NA |
| | $V_{ss}$ (L/kg) | NA | NA | NA | NA | NA | NA |
| | F (%) | NA | NA | NA | NA | NA | NA |
| | Most Abundant Drug-related Component in Plasma (%) | NA | | | NA | NA | |
| | Major Drug-related Metabolite in Plasma (%) | NA | | | NA | NA | |
| | Urine/Feces Excretion (%) | 4.5/12.3, 8.7/2.2 | | | NA | NA | |
| | Permeability | | | | NA | | |
| **In Vitro** | Plasma Protein Binding (%Bound) | NA | | | NA | >30.6-97.6/>27.5-98.6 | |
| | S9 Stability (%Remaining) | 76.2/73.4 | | | NA/67.0 | NA | |

### Drug-Drug Interaction

| | CYP Enzyme | Non-CYP Enzyme | Transporter |
|---|---|---|---|
| **Substrate** | NA | NA | NA |
| **Inhibitor** | Not | NA | NA |
| **Inducer** | Not | NA | NA |

### Non-clinical Toxicology

| Single-Dose Toxicity | No drug-related | Safety Pharmacology | • CNS NOAEL: 456 mg/kg/day for males and 1502 mg/kg/day for females |
|---|---|---|---|
| **Repeated-Dose Toxicity (NOAEL)** | 100-1000 mg/kg/day (rat, 21 days) | Genotoxicity | • No genotoxicity |
| | | Reproductive and Developmental Toxicity | • EFD NOAEL = 300 mg/kg/day<br>• Two generation reproductivity: 1000 ppm for $F_0$, 10000 ppm for $F_1$ |
| | | Carcinogenicity | • NOAEL: 51 mg/kg/day for males and 63 mg/kg/day for females |

## Ripasudil Hydrochloride Hydrate
### (Glanatec®ophthalmic solution 0.4%)
K-115

Ophthalmic solution, topical instillation, EQ 0.4% Ripasudil

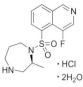

- ❖ Ripasudil hydrochloride hydrate is a Rho-associated coiled coil-containing protein kinase (ROCK) inhibitor, indicated for the treatment of the patients with glaucoma and ocular hypertension. It was approved in Sep 2014 by PMDA of Japan.
- ❖ Ripasudil hydrochloride hydrate was developed and marketed by Kowa Company.
- ❖ *The recommended human dose* is one drop in the affected eye, twice daily.

| Worldwide Key Approvals | Global Sales ($Million) | Key Substance Patent Expiration |
|---|---|---|
| Sep 26, 2014 (JP) | Not available | Oct 22, 2023 (JP4316794B2) |

### Mechanism of Action

As a ROCK inhibitor, ripasudil hydrochloride hydrate reduces intraocular pressure (IOP) by directly acting on the trabecular meshwork via increasing conventional outflow through the Schlemm's canal.

| Target Inhibition | In Vitro Efficacy | In Vivo Efficacy |
|---|---|---|
| Inhibition of ROCK: | In monkey TM cells: | IOP effects: |
| ROCK-1: $IC_{50}$ = 0.051 µM | Induced retraction and rounding | Dose-dependent reduction of IOP in rabbits and monkeys |
| ROCK-2: $IC_{50}$ = 0.019 µM | Reduced actin bundles | Significantly increased outflow facility by 2.2-fold, and reduced IOP in rabbits |

### Pharmacokinetics

| | Parameter | Rat | | | Rabbit | | | | Healthy Human | | | | |
|---|---|---|---|---|---|---|---|---|---|---|---|---|---|
| | Dose (mg/kg) | 1 (i.v.) | 1 (p.o) | 3 (p.o.) | 1.0% (o.s./o.d.) | 1 (i.v.) | 3 (i.v.) | 10 (i.v.) | 0.05% (o.u.) | 0.1% (o.u.) | 0.2% (o.u.) | 0.4% (o.u.) | 0.8% (o.u.) |
| In Vivo | $T_{max}$ (min, human: h) | NA | 14.9 | 15.0 | 6.26 | 6.00 | 5.02 | 5.29 | NC | 0.137 | 0.144 | 0.301 | 0.165 |
| | $C_{max}$ (µg/mL, human: ng/mL) | NA | 0.073 | 0.487 | 0.064 | NA | NA | NA | 0 | 0.115 | 0.456 | 0.656 | 0.880 |
| | $AUC_{0-t}$ (µg·h/mL, human: ng·h/mL) | NA | 3.01 | 24.5 | 2.08 | NA | NA | NA | 0 | 0.018 | 0.168 | 0.390 | 0.470 |
| | $T_{1/2}$ (min, human: h) | α: 10.4 β: 47.1 | 30.9 | 38.4 | 24.9 | α: 9.81 β: 32.2 | α: 15.4 β: 44.7 | α: 27.6 β: 88.5 | NC | NC | 0.730 | 0.620 | 0.495 |
| | Cl (mL/min/kg) | 35.0 | NA | NA | NA | 109 | 87.7 | 64.4 | NA | NA | NA | NA | NA |
| | $V_{ss}$ (mL/kg) | 1620 | NA | NA | NA | 3130 | 2800 | 2850 | NA | NA | NA | NA | NA |
| | F (%) | - | 11.7 | 29.2 | 95.8 | - | - | - | NA | NA | NA | NA | NA |
| | Most Abundant Drug-related Component in Plasma (%) | Parent (11.3) | | | NA | | | | NA | | | | |
| | Major Drug-related Metabolite in Plasma (%) | M5 (19.5) | | | NA | | | | M1 | | | | |
| | Urine/Feces Excretion (%) | 43.8/42.1 | | | NA | | | | Major/NA | | | | |
| In Vitro | Plasma Protein Binding (%Bound) | 35.3-36.7 | | | 41.2-41.9 | | | | 56.4-57.5 | | | | |
| | Hepatocytes Stability ($Cl_{int}$, µL/min/$10^6$ cells) | 5.86 | | | 46.7 | | | | 63.6/4.19/17.0 | | | | |

### Drug-Drug Interaction

| | CYP Enzyme | Non-CYP Enzyme | Transporter |
|---|---|---|---|
| Substrate | CYP3A4/5, 2C8 | Aldehyde oxidase | NA |
| Inhibitor | CYP3A4/5, CYP2D6 | Aldehyde oxidase | NA |
| Inducer | Not | NA | NA |

### Non-clinical Toxicology

| | | | |
|---|---|---|---|
| Single-Dose Toxicity (ALD) | 122 mg/kg (mouse, p.o.) ≥20.4 mg/kg (mouse, i.v.) 81.7 mg/kg (rat, p.o.) 20.4 mg/kg (rat, i.v.) | Safety Pharmacology | • CVS: hERG $IC_{50}$ = 39.5 µM, significant reduction on the maximum rate of repolarization • No effect on CNS or RS |
| | | Genotoxicity | • Negative |
| Repeated-Dose Toxicity (NOAEL) | 10/30 mg/kg/day (rat, 4 weeks) 2.0% (dog, 13 weeks) 1.0% (rabbit, 26 weeks) 2.0% (monkey, 52 weeks) | Reproductive Toxicity | • No FEED effects • EFD NOAEL: 10 mg/kg/day (rat/rabbit) • PPND NOAEL: 10 mg/kg/day, significant toxicity in $F_0$ and $F_1$ |
| | | Carcinogenicity | • Predicted no carcinogenic potential |
| | | Special toxicity | • Local irritation test: Conjunctival redness • No potential for skin sensitization and phototoxicity • Eye local toxicity: In rabbits, NOAEL: 2.0/1.0% BID In monkeys, NOAEL: 2.0% BID |

## Suvorexant
### (Belsomra®)
MK-4305
Tablet, oral, 5 mg/10 mg/15 mg/20 mg Suvorexant

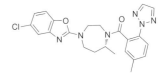

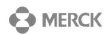

❖ Suvorexant is an orexin receptor antagonist, indicated for the treatment of insomnia, characterized by difficulties with sleep onset and/or sleep maintenance.   It was first approved in Aug 2014 by US FDA.
❖ Suvorexant was discovered and marketed by Merck & Co.
❖ ***The recommended human starting dose*** is 10 mg orally once daily.

| Worldwide Key Approvals | Global Sales ($Million) | Key Substance Patent Expiration |
|---|---|---|
| Aug 13, 2014 (US)<br>Sep 26, 2014 (JP) | Not available | Nov 20, 2029 (US7951797B2)<br>Nov 30, 2027 (EP2089382B1)<br>Jul 21, 2031 (JP4675427B2)<br>Nov 30, 2027 (CN101627028B) |

## Mechanism of Action

As an orexin receptor antagonist, suvorexant blocks the binding of wake-promoting neuropeptides orexin A and orexin B to receptors OX1R and OX2R, resulting in suppression of wake drive.

**Target Binding Selectivity**
OX1R: $IC_{50}$ = 49.9 nM, $K_i$ = 0.55 nM
OX2R: $IC_{50}$ = 54.8 nM, $K_i$ = 0.35 nM

***In Vivo* Efficacy**
Decreased locomotor activity in rats in a dose-dependent manner
Reduced the awake time and increased delta sleep, and REM sleep in rats, dogs and monkeys

## Pharmacokinetics

| | Parameter | Rat | | Dog | | Healthy Human | | | | | | | |
|---|---|---|---|---|---|---|---|---|---|---|---|---|---|
| | Dose (mg/kg, human: mg) | 3<br>(i.v.) | 10<br>(p.o.) | 2<br>(i.v.) | 5<br>(p.o.) | 5<br>(i.v.) | 10<br>(i.v.) | 20<br>(i.v.) | 30<br>(i.v.) | 10<br>(p.o.) | 20<br>(p.o.) | 40<br>(p.o.) | 80<br>(p.o.) |
| *In Vivo* | $C_{max}$ (µM, human $C_{eoi}$ or $C_{max}$) | NA | 2.3 | NA | 3.2 | 0.543 | 1.04 | 1.75 | 1.90 | 0.456 | 0.646 | 0.956 | 1.52 |
| | $T_{max}$ (h) | NA | 0.4 | NA | 0.7 | NA | NA | NA | NA | 1.5 | 1.0 | 2.0 | 2.0 |
| | $AUC_{inf}$ (µM·h) | 4.9 | 7.9 | 26.3 | 22.3 | 3.46 | 6.92 | 15.1 | 13.7 | 5.32 | 9.51 | 16.2 | 27.3 |
| | $T_{1/2}$ (h) | 0.8 | NA | 3.8 | NA | 9.2 | 9.9 | 13.5 | 8.9 | 12.1 | 12.5 | 12.6 | 13.6 |
| | Cl (mL/min/kg, human: mL/min) | 35.3 | NA | 3.5 | NA | 52.3 | 52.7 | 48.6 | 80.6 | NA | NA | NA | NA |
| | $V_{ss}$ (L/kg) | 1.9 | NA | 1.3 | NA | 36.5 | 42.5 | 57.1 | 57.3 | NA | NA | NA | NA |
| | F (%) | - | 48.2 | - | 33.9 | NA | NA | NA | NA | NA | NA | NA | NA |
| | Most Abundant Drug-related Component or Metabolite in Plasma (%) | NA | | NA | | M0 (30.1), M9 (36.1) | | | | | | | |
| | Major Durg-related Metabolite in Plasma (%) | NA | | NA | | M9 (36.1) | | | | | | | |
| | Urine/Feces Excretion (%) | 1.8/92.1 | | 10.2/74.5 | | 23.0/66.4 | | | | | | | |
| *In Vitro* | LLC-PK1 Permeability | $Papp_{(A-B)}$ = 22.8-25.9 × $10^{-6}$ cm/s at 0.5-5 µM | | | | | | | | | | | |
| | Plasma Protein Binding (%unbound) | 1.1-1.7 | | 0.9-1.9 | | 0.3-0.5 | | | | | | | |
| | Hepatocytes Stability (%Romaining) | NA | | NA | | 48 | | | | | | | |

## Drug-Drug Interaction

| | CYP Enzyme | Non-CYP Enzyme | Transporter |
|---|---|---|---|
| Substrate | CYP3A, 2C19 | NA | Not |
| Inhibitor | CYP3A4, 2C19, 2C8, 2C9, 2D6 | NA | P-gp, OCT2, BCRP, OATP1B1 |
| Inducer | CYP3A4, 1A2, 2B6 | NA | NA |

## Non-clinical Toxicology

| | | | |
|---|---|---|---|
| **Single-Dose Toxicity (NOAEL)** | NA | **Safety Pharmacology** | • CVS: hERG $IC_{50}$ = 2.6 µM<br>• No significant *in vivo* effects on cardiovascular, central nervous and respiratory system |
| **Repeated-Dose Toxicity (NOAEL)** | 100/25 mg/kg/day (rat, TPGS, 6 months)<br>160/80 mg/kg/day (rat, SDF, 6 months)<br>25 mg/kg/day (dog, TPGS, 9 months)<br>50 mg/kg/day (dog, SDF, 9 months) | **Genotoxicity** | • Negative in genotoxicity |
| | | **Reproductive and Developmental Toxicology** | • FEED NOAEL: 75->1200 mg/kg/day<br>• EFD NOAEL: 30-300 mg/kg/day<br>• PPND NOAEL: 80 mg/kg/day |
| | | **Carcinogenicity** | • Thyroid follicular cell adenomas, combined adenomas and carcinomas was significantly increased in rat at 325 mg/kg/day |
| | | **Special Toxicology** | • The NOEL for phototoxicity was greater than 325 mg/kg/day |

## Tasimelteon
## (Hetlioz®)
VEC-162
Capsule, oral, 20 mg Tasimelteon

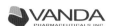 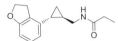

❖ Tasimelteon is a melatonin receptor agonist, indicated for the treatment of Non-24-Hour Sleep-Wake Disorder. It was first approved in Jan 2014 by US FDA.
❖ Tasimelteon was discovered by Bristol-Myers Squibb, developed and marketed by Vanda.
❖ *The recommended human starting dose* is 20 mg orally once daily prior to bedtime without food.

| Worldwide Key Approvals | Global Sales ($Million) | | Key Substance Patent Expiration |
|---|---|---|---|
| Jan 31, 2014 (US) | **2014** | 12.8 | Dec 09, 2017 (US5856529A) |
| | | | Dec 09, 2017 (EP1027043B1) |
| Jul 03, 2015 (EU) | **2015** | 44.3 | Dec 09, 2017 (JP4290765B2) |
| | | | Dec 09, 2017 (CN1152679C) |

## Mechanism of Action

Tasimelteon is a full agonist at melatonin receptors $MT_1$ and $MT_2$, believed to contribute to its sleep-promoting properties.

**Target Binding Selectivity**

$MT_1$: $IC_{50}$ = 0.586 nM; $K_i$ = 0.304 nM
$MT_2$: $IC_{50}$ = 0.133 nM; $K_i$ = 0.0692 nM

***In Vitro* Efficacy**

NIH-3T3 cell lines:
$MT_1$: $K_i$ = 0.35 nM, $EC_{50}$ = 0.74 nM
$MT_2$: $K_i$ = 0.17 nM, $EC_{50}$ = 0.1 nM

***In Vivo* Efficacy**

SCN electrical activity rhythms shifted significantly faster in the brain slices taken from treated rats
Entrainment of "free-running" activity rhythms model: $ED_{50}$ = 0.21 mg/kg

## Pharmacokinetics

| | Parameter | Rat | | Monkey | | Healthy Human | |
|---|---|---|---|---|---|---|---|
| | Dose (mg/kg, human: mg) | 1.0 (i.v.) | 1.0 (p.o.) | 1.0 (i.v.) | 1.0 (p.o.) | 2 (i.v.) | 20 (p.o.) |
| ***In Vivo*** | $C_{max}$ (ng/mL) | NA | 51 | NA | 54.2 | 82.2 | 260 |
| | $T_{max}$ (h) | NA | 0.25 | NA | 0.67 | 0.28 | 0.50 |
| | $AUC_{inf}$ (ng·h/mL) | NA | NA | NA | NA | 71.6 | 358 |
| | $T_{1/2}$ (h) | 2.1 | NA | 2.1 | NA | 1.02 | 1.06 |
| | Cl (L/h/kg, human: mL/min) | 5.3 | NA | 1.6 | NA | 505 | 2241 |
| | $V_{ss}$ (L/kg, human: L) | 3.8 | NA | 1.4 | NA | 42.7 | 178 |
| | F (%) | - | 58.5 | - | 11.7 | - | 50 |
| | Most Abundant Drug-related Component in Plasma (%) | M12 (48.4) | | M9 (10.3)/ M0 (17.7) | | M9 (19.8) | |
| | Major Drug-related Metabolite in Plasma (%) | M12 (48.4) | | M9 (10.3)/ M12 (10) | | M9 (19.8) | |
| | Urine/Feces Excretion (%) | NA | | 80/5 | | 80.4/3.72 | |
| ***In Vitro*** | Caco-2 Permeability | $Papp_{(A \rightarrow B)}$ = 19.4-63.9 × $10^{-6}$ cm/s | | | | | |
| | Plasma Protein Binding (%Bound) | 76.8-84.8 | | 69.0-79.7 | | 85.8-90.3 | |
| | LM/Hepatocytes Stability | NA | | NA | | NA | |

## Drug-Drug Interaction

| | CYP Enzyme | Non-CYP Enzyme | Transporter |
|---|---|---|---|
| Substrate | CYP1A2, 3A4, 1A1, 2C9/19, 2D6 | NA | Not |
| Inhibitor | CYP3A4, 2C19 | NA | OCT2, OAT3 |
| Inducer | CYP2C8, CYP3A4 | NA | NA |

## Non-clinical Toxicology

| | | | |
|---|---|---|---|
| **Single-Dose Toxicity (MNLD)** | 400 mg/kg (mouse) 1750 mg/kg (rat) 200 mg/kg (monkey) | **Safety Pharmacology** | • CVS: hERG: 14% inhibition at 100 μM, *in vivo* reductions on BP and HR, and shortened APD in anesthetized dogs <br> • Besides, tasimelteon seemed vasoconstrictive |
| **Repeated-Dose Toxicity (NOAEL)** | 100 mg/kg/day (mouse, 13 weeks) 5 mg/kg/day (rat, 26 weeks) 3 mg/kg/day (monkey, 12 months) | **Genotoxicity** | • Negative in an Ames assay and in *in vivo* rat micronucleus assay <br> • Metabolite M11 was clastogenic in an *in vitro* chromosomal aberration assay |
| | | **Reproductive and Developmental Toxicity** | • FEED: ↑ Irregular estrus cycles in MDF and HDF <br> • EFD: No malformations in any groups in rats <br> • PPND: Slight ↓ BW at MD and/or HD during gestation and in all dams during lactation |
| | | **Carcinogenicity** | • Drug-related neoplasms in liver, uterus and cervix in rats, but not identified in mice |

**Tavaborole
(Kerydin®)**
AN-2690
Topical solution, topical, 5% Tavaborole

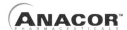

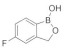

❖ Tavaborole is an oxaborole antifungal drug, indicated for the treatment of onychomycosis of the toenails due to *Trichophyton rubrum* or *Trichophyton mentagrophytes* infection.   It was first approved in Jul 2014 by US FDA.
❖ Tavaborole was discovered and marketed by Anacor Pharmaceuticals.
❖ **The recommended human starting dose** is once daily for 48 weeks.

| Worldwide Key Approvals | Global Sales ($Million) | Key Substance Patent Expiration |
|---|---|---|
| Jul 07, 2014 (FDA) | Not available | NA |

## Mechanism of Action

Tavaborole inhibits fungal protein synthesis by inhibition of aminoacyl-transfer ribonucleic acid (tRNA) synthetase (AARS).

| **Target Efficacy** | *In Vitro* **Efficacy** | *In Vivo* **Efficacy** |
|---|---|---|
| Aminoacylation inhibition: $IC_{50}$ = 2.1 µM  tRNA: $K_i$ = 1.85-31.4 µM | Antifungal spectrum of tavaborole:  MIC = 0.25-2 µg/mL  Antifungal against *Trichophyton* from clinical:  MIC = 1.0-8.0 µg/mL and $MIC_{90}$ = 8.0 µg/mL  MFC = 8.0->128 µg/mL and $MFC_{90}$ = 64 µg/mL | In systemic candidiasis infection mouse model:  No significant effect on mortality |

## Pharmacokinetics

| | Parameters | Patient |
|---|---|---|
| *In Vivo* | Dose (µL) | 200 |
| | $C_{max}$ (ng/mL) | 3.54 ± 2.26 |
| | $T_{max}$ (h) | 12.0 (4.03-23.9) |
| | $AUC_{last}$ (ng·h/mL) | 44.4 ± 25.5 |
| | $T_{1/2}$ (h) | 7.68 |
| | Most Abundant/Major Drug-related Metabolite in Plasma (%) | NA |
| | Urine/Feces Excretion (%) | NA |
| *In Vitro* | Permeability | NA |
| | Plasma Protein Binding (%Bound) | 45.8-76.9 |
| | LM/Hepatocytes Stability | NA |

## Drug-Drug Interaction

| | CYP Enzymes | Non-CYP Enzymes | Transporters |
|---|---|---|---|
| **Substrate** | CYP3A5, 2C18, 2C19, 3A4 | FMO3 and FMO5 | NA |
| **Inhibitor** | CYP2A6, CYP2E1 | NA | NA |
| **Inducer** | Not | NA | NA |

## Non-clinical Toxicology

| **Single-Dose Toxicity (MTD)** | NA | **Safety Pharmacology** | • CVS: Low-potency hERG-channel blocker (<25% inhibition)  • No effect on CNS |
|---|---|---|---|
| **Repeated-Dose Toxicity (NOAEL)** | 30 mg/kg/day (rat, 6 months)  3% (minipig, systemic, 9 months) | **Genotoxicity** | • No genotoxicity |
| | | **Reproductive and Developmental Toxicity** | • FEED NOAEL: 300 mg/kg/day  • EFD NOAEL: 100 mg/kg/day in rats, 5% (dermal) and 50 mg/kg/day (p.o.) for fetuses in rabbits  • PNND NOAEL: 60 mg/kg/day for $F_0$, 100 mg/kg/day for $F_1$ |
| | | **Carcinogenicity** | • Rat NOAEL: 50 mg/kg/day  • Mouse NOAEL: 15% |

## Tedizolid Phosphate
### (Sivextro®)
TR-701FA; TR-701; DA-7218
Table or powder, oral or i.v., 200 mg tedizolid phosphate

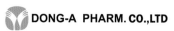   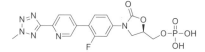

❖ Tedizolid phosphate belongs to the oxazolidinone class of antibacterial drugs, indicated for the treatment of acute bacterial skin and skin structure infections (ABSSSI) caused by designated susceptible bacteria. It was first approved in Jun 2014 by US FDA.
❖ Tedizolid phosphate was discovered by Dong-A, developed and marketed by Cubist.
❖ **_The recommended human starting dose_** is 200 mg orally once daily or as an intravenous (i.v.) infusion over 1 h for six days.

| Worldwide Key Approvals | Global Sales ($Million) | Key Substance Patent Expiration |
|---|---|---|
| Jun 20, 2014 (US)<br>Mar 23, 2015 (EU) | Not available | Feb 23, 2028 (US8420676B2)<br>Dec 17, 2024 (EP1699784B1)<br>Dec 17, 2024 (JP4739229B2)<br>Dec 17, 2024 (CN101982468B) |

### Mechanism of Action

Tedizolid phosphate is an oxazolidinone prodrug antibiotic that is converted *in vivo* to tedizolid, which is a protein synthesis inhibitor that interacts with bacterial ribosome and prevents translation.

| Target Binding Selectivity | *In Vitro* Efficacy | *In Vivo* Efficacy |
|---|---|---|
| Tedizolid:<br>$IC_{50}$ = 956.7 nM<br>Tedizolid phosphate:<br>$IC_{50}$ = 3495.7 nM | Antibacterial spectrum of tedizolid phosphate:<br>*Staphylococci*: $MIC_{50}$ = 0.25-0.5 µg/mL<br>*Enterococci*: $MIC_{50}$ = 0.25-0.5 µg/mL<br>*Streptococci*: $MIC_{50}$ = 0.12-0.25 µg/mL | Systematic infection in mice: $ED_{50}$ = 0.46->40 mg/kg<br>Skin and soft tissue infection (MRSA) in mice:<br>3.16-5.42 $log_{10}$/mL CFU in thigh<br>2.33-9.07 $log_{10}$/mL CFU in air pouch |

### Pharmacokinetics

| | Parameter | Mouse | | Rat | | Long-Evans Rat | | | Dog | | | | Healthy Human | |
|---|---|---|---|---|---|---|---|---|---|---|---|---|---|---|
| | Dose (mg/kg, human: mg) | 10 (i.v.) | 10 (p.o.) | 10 (i.v.) | 10 (p.o.) | 10 (p.o.) | 30 (p.o.) | 100 (p.o.) | 10 (i.v.) | 30 (i.v.) | 10 (p.o.) | 30 (p.o.) | 200 (i.v.) | 200 (p.o.) |
| *In Vivo* | $C_{max}$ (µg/mL) | 8.81 | 8.37 | NA | 1.87 | 6.18 | 15.7 | 35.3 | 5.37 | 17.43 | 1.38 | 5.85 | 2.3 | 2.0 |
| | $T_{max}$ (h) | 0.0167 | 0.5 | NA | 5.00 | 1 | 1 | 8 | 0.08 | 0.19 | 1.67 | 0.83 | 1.1 | 2.5 |
| | $AUC_{inf}$ (µg·h/mL) | 53.6 | 49.8 | 53.1 | 15.8 | 24.6 | 134 | 500 | 4.42 | 18.6 | 2.78 | 14.2 | 26.6 | 23.8 |
| | $T_{1/2}$ (h) | 3.42 | 3.82 | 2.15 | 3.59 | 3.3 | 2.1 | 2.8 | 0.58 | 0.90 | 0.64 | 0.94 | NA | NA |
| | Cl (mL/min/kg, human: L/h) | 3.11 | NA | 3.15 | NA | NA | NA | NA | 39.2 | 26.9 | NA | NA | 6.4 | 6.9 |
| | $V_{ss}$ (L/kg, human: L) | 0.918 | NA | 0.274 | NA | NA | NA | NA | 1.66 | 1.93 | NA | NA | NA | NA |
| | F (%) | - | 92.9 | - | 29.8 | NA | NA | NA | - | - | NA | NA | - | NA |
| | Most Abundant/major Drug-related Metabolite in Plasma (%) | M5 (100) | | M5 (100) | | | | | M5 (100) | | | | M5 (94.5-98.2) | |
| | Urine/Feces Excretion (%) | NA/NA | | 11.3/87.8 | | | | | 10.1/81.4 | | | | 18.0/81.5 | |
| *In Vitro* | Caco-2 Permeability | $Papp_{(A-B)}$ = 18.5-29.1 × $10^{-6}$ cm/s | | | | | | | | | | | | |
| | Plasma Protein Binding (%Bound) | 74.8 | | 97.2 | | | | | 85.1 | | | | 86.6 | |
| | LM Stability (%Remaining) | NA | | 87.1 | | | | | 92.7 | | | | 88.7 | |

### Drug-Drug Interaction

| | CYP Enzyme | Non-CYP Enzyme | Transporter |
|---|---|---|---|
| Substrate | Not | Phosphatase | Not |
| Inhibitor | Not | Not | BCRP |
| Inducer | Not | NA | NA |

### Non-clinical Toxicology

| Single-Dose Toxicity (NOAEL) | 500 mg/kg/day (mouse)<br>62 mg/kg/day (rat) | Safety Pharmacology | • No toxic potential for neurological, cardiovascular, and pulmonary, renal and GI function |
|---|---|---|---|
| | | Genotoxicity | • Negative |
| Repeated-Dose Toxicity (NOAEL) | 30/10 mg/kg/day (rat, 9 months)<br>400 mg/kg/day (dog, 3 months) | Reproductive and Developmental Toxicity | • FEED NOAEL: 50/15 mg/kg/day (male/female)<br>• EFD NOAEL: 2.5 mg/kg/day in rats; 25 mg/kg/day for mater and 5 mg/kg/day for fetus in mice; 1.0 mg/kg/day in rabbits<br>• PPND NOAEL: 3.75 mg/kg/day |
| | | Carcinogenicity | • NA |

## Tofogliflozin Hydrate
## (Deberza®)
CSG-452
Tablet, oral, EQ 20 mg Tofogliflozin

Roche Group

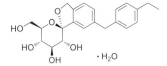

- ❖ An SGLT2 (sodium-glucose cotransporter 2) inhibitor, indicated for the treatment of type 2 diabetes. It was first approved in Mar 2014 by PMDA of Japan.
- ❖ It was discovered by Chugai (Roche), co-developed and co-marketed by Chugai, Sanofi and Kowa.
- ❖ *The recommended human starting dose* for adults is 20 mg once daily, taken before or after breakfast.

| Worldwide Key Approvals | Global Sales ($Million) | Key Substance Patent Expiration |
|---|---|---|
| Mar 24, 2014 (JP) | Not available | Jan 31, 2027 (US7767651B2)<br>(EP1852439A1: Examination )<br>Jan 27, 2026 (JP4093587B2)<br>Jan 27, 2026 (CN101111508B) |

## Mechanism of Action

As an SGLT2 inhibitor, tofogliflozin inhibits the reuptake of glucose and urine glucose excretion in kidneys, thereby reducing blood glucose levels.

### *In Vitro* Target Binding Selectivity
hSGLT2: $K_i$ = 2.9 nM, $IC_{50}$ = 2.9 nM
hSGLT1: $K_i$ = 6000 nM
Selectivity: 2069-fold for $K_i$

### *In Vivo* Efficacy
Blood glucose reduction: Decreased blood glucose at 0.1-3 mg/kg
Glucosuria renal clearance:
    Increased UGE: 3 mg/kg in ZDF rats and 0.005% in *db/db* mice,
    0.05% in DIO rats and 1 mg/kg of $AUC_{0-6}$ in normal rats

## Pharmacokinetics

| | Parameters | Rat | | Monkey | | Healthy Human | |
|---|---|---|---|---|---|---|---|
| | Dose (mg/kg, Human: mg) | 1 (i.v.) | 1 (p.o.) | 1 (i.v.) | 1 (p.o.) | 0.1 (i.v.) | 20 (p.o.) |
| | $C_{max}$ (ng/mL) | 1060 | 221 | 2170 | 550 | 4.47 | 489 |
| | $T_{max}$ (h) | 0.083 | 1 | 0.083 | 1 | 0.25 | 0.75 |
| | $AUC_{inf}$ (ng·h/mL) | 869 | 807 | 4690 | 2750 | 9.57 | 1970 |
| | $T_{1/2}$ (h) | 1.15 | 2.56 | 5.02 | 10.5 | 4.65 | 6.33 |
| *In Vivo* | Cl (mL/min/kg, Human: L/h) | 19.4 | NA | 3.65 | NA | 9.96 | 10.4 |
| | $V_{ss}$ (L/kg, Human: L) | 1.15 | NA | 0.919 | NA | 50.6 | 92.6 |
| | F (%) | - | 75.0 | - | 58.6 | - | 97.5 |
| | Most Abundant Drug-related Component in Plasma (%) | M0 (38.7) | | M0 (64.4) | | M1 (52) | |
| | Major Drug-related Metabolites in Plasma (%) | M2,M3 (33.4) | | M2, M3-GA (10.9) | | M1 (52) | |
| | Urine/Feces Excretion (%) | 54.9/NA | 44.6/52.7 | 42.9/44.7 | NA | NA | 77/21.7 |
| *In vitro* | Permeability | NA | | | | | |
| | Plasma Protein Binding (%Bound) | 83.0-83.8 | | 76.2-76.9 | | 82.3-82.6 | |
| | Hepatocytes Stability (%Remaining) | 55.2 | | 65.1 | | 89.3 | |

## Drug-Drug Interaction

| | CYP Enzyme | Non-CYP Enzyme | Transporter |
|---|---|---|---|
| Substrate | CYP4A11, 4F3B, 3A4/5, 2C18 | ADH | P-gp |
| Inhibitor | Not | NA | Not |
| Inducer | Not | NA | NA |

## Non-clinical Toxicology

| Single-Dose Toxicity (ALD) | 1000 mg/kg (rat) | Safety Pharmacology | • No effects on CNS, CVS and RS |
|---|---|---|---|
| **Repeated-Dose Toxicity (NOAEL)** | 20 mg/kg/day (mouse, 3 months)<br>5 mg/kg/day (rat, 6 months)<br>30 mg/kg/day (monkey, 12 months) | **Genotoxicity** | • Negative |
| | | **Reproductive and Developmental Toxicity** | • NOAEL was 80-320 mg/kg/day for rats<br>• NOAEL was 60 mg/kg/day for rabbits in EFD assay |
| | | **Carcinogenicity** | • NOAEL for mice: 30/125 mg/kg/day (male/female)<br>• NOAEL for rats: 100 mg/kg/day |

## Umeclidinium Bromide
## (Incruse®/Incruse Ellipta®/Encruse®)
GSK-573719
Powder, inhalation, 65 µg Umeclidimium

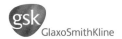 GlaxoSmithKline

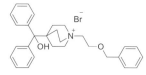

❖ Umeclidinium bromide is an inhaled long-acting muscarinic antagonist (LAMA), indicated for the treatment of patients with chronic obstructive pulmonary disease (COPD).   It was first approved in Apr 2014 by EMA.
❖ Umeclidinium bromide was discovered and marketed by GlaxoSmithKline Plc.
❖ ***The recommended human starting dose*** is 62.5 µg once daily.

| Worldwide Key Approvals | Global Sales ($Million) | | Key Substance Patent Expiration |
|---|---|---|---|
| Apr 28, 2014 (EU) Apr 30, 2014 (US) Mar 26, 2015 (JP) | **2014** **2015** | Not available 21.4 | Apr 27, 2025 (US7488827B2) Apr 27, 2025 (EP1740177B1) Feb 06, 2028 (JP5014121B2) (CN102040602A: Examination) |

## Mechanism of Action

As an inhaled LAMA, umeclidinium bromide competitively inhibits the binding of acetylcholine with muscarinic cholinergic receptors on airway smooth muscle leading to brochodilation.

| Target Inhibition | *In Vitro* Efficacy | *In Vivo* Efficacy |
|---|---|---|
| M1-5 mAChRs: $K_i$ = 0.05-0.16 nM | Antagonist at hM1-3 AChRs: $pA_2$ = 9.6-10.6 Reversibility of antagonism at the M3 receptor in CHO cells: $EC_{50}$_ Washout < $EC_{50}$_ No washout | In Balb/c mouse models: $ED_{50}$ = 0.02 µg/mouse In Dunkin-Hartley guinea pig models: Significant inhibition (74.4%), 4 h post instillation |

## Pharmacokinetics

| | Parameter | Rat | Dog | Healthy human/Male | | | | | | |
|---|---|---|---|---|---|---|---|---|---|---|
| | Dose (mg/kg, human: µg) | 0.5 (i.v.) | 1 (i.v.) | 65 (i.v.) | 65 (i.v.) | 1000 (p.o.) | 20 (i.v.) | 50 (i.v.) | 65 (i.v.) | 1000 (i.h.) |
| | $C_{max}$ (ng/mL) | 30.3 | 651 | 0.906 | 1.39 | 0.07 | 0.376 | 1.14 | 1.55 | 1.66 |
| | $T_{max}$ (h) | 0.33-0.67 | 0.75-1.0 | 0.53 | 0.5 | 4 | 0.483 | 0.483 | 0.483 | 0.083 |
| | $AUC_{inf}$ (ng·h/mL) | 25.2 | 502 | 0.268 | 1.04 | 0.796 | 0.132 | 0.525 | 0.543 | 1.33 |
| | $T_{1/2}$ (h) | 3.35 | 11.6 | NA | NA | NA | NA | NA | NA | NA |
| *In Vivo* | Cl (mL/min/kg, human: L/h) | 328 | 32.5 | 151 | 46.5 | 988 | 108 | 95.3 | 90.9 | 752 |
| | $V_{ss}$ (L/kg, human: L) | 14.6 | 4.67 | 86.2 | 1801 | 66958 | 12.8 | 16.2 | 14.5 | 2717 |
| | F (%) | - | - | - | - | 5.4 | - | - | - | 12.8 |
| | Most Abundant Drug-related Component in Plasma (%) | M0 (98) | M0 (94.7) | NA | | | | | | |
| | Major Drug-related Metabolite in Plasma (%) | NA | NA | M14 (4, 10) | | | | | | |
| | Urine/Feces Excretion (%) | 16.9/65.3 | 11.9/61.8 | 22/58 (i.v., 65 µg) | | | | | | |
| | MDCK Permeability | | | Low | | | | | | |
| *In Vitro* | Plasma Protein Binding (%Bound) | 84.3-86.9 | 77.2-83.0 | 87.1-88.9 | | | | | | |
| | Heptocytes Stability (%Remaining) | 74 | 72 | 57 | | | | | | |

## Drug-Drug Interaction

| | CYP Enzyme | Non-CYP Enzyme | Transporter |
|---|---|---|---|
| **Substrate** | CYP2D6, 3A4, 1A1 | NA | P-gp, OCT1, OCT2 |
| **Inhibitor** | CYP3A4, CYP2D6 | NA | OCT2 |
| **Inducer** | Not | NA | NA |

## Non-clinical Toxicology

| Single-Dose Toxicity (ALD) | NA | Safety Pharmacology | • CVS: hERG $IC_{50}$ = 9.41 µM, minimal *in vivo* effect • CNS: No significant effect • RS: Only minimal effects |
|---|---|---|---|
| **Repeated-Dose Toxicity (NOAEL)** | 87.1 µg/kg/day (rat, 26 weeks) 109 µg/kg/day (dog, 39 weeks) | Genotoxicity | • No genetic toxicity |
| | | Reproductive and Developmental Toxicity | • FEED: No effect • EFD: No effect • PPND: No effect |
| | | Carcinogenicity | • No drug-related neoplastic or non-neoplastic finding |

**Vaniprevir**
**(Vanihep®)**
MK-7009
Capsule, oral, EQ 150 mg Vaniprevir

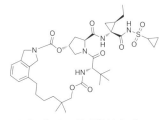

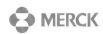 MERCK

❖ Vaniprevir is a hepatitis C virus (HCV) non-structural 3/4A protease inhibitor, indicated for the treatment of patients with HCV infection. It was first approved in 2014 by PMDA of Japan.
❖ Vaniprevir was discovered and marketed by Merck & Co.
❖ *The recommended human starting dose* is 300 mg twice daily with or without food last for 12 weeks.

| Worldwide Key Approvals | Global Sales($Million) | Key Substance Patent Expiration |
|---|---|---|
| Sep 26, 2014 (JP) | Not available | Jan 26, 2027 (US7470664B2) <br> Jul 14, 2026 (EP1910404B1) <br> Jun 03, 2030 (JP4621282B2) <br> Jul 14, 2026 (CN101228181B) |

## Mechanism of Action

As a macrocyclic HCV NS3/4A protease inhibitor, vaniprevir reversible inhibits HCV NS3/4A protease and prevents the proteolytic processing of the HCV polyprotein, which is essential for viral replication.

**Target Inhibition**
GT 1a/b, 2a/4a/5a/6a/2b:
  $IC_{50}$ = 0.016-1.4 nM
GT 3a: $IC_{50}$ = 53 nM

**In Vitro Efficacy**
Anti-HCV replicons: WT $EC_{50}$ = 1-7 nM
Anti-NS3/4A mutant HCV 1a/1b replicons ($EC_{50}$ increase):
  V36/Q41/T54/V55/Q80/V107: 0.4-7.7 folds
  R155/A156/D168: 15.3->1000 folds
  A156S/D168N: 2.6-7 folds

**In Vivo Efficacy**
HCV genotype 1a infection in Chimpanzee:
  Decreased 5 Log IU/mL in plasma viral load at 5 mg/kg
  Decreased 2-3 Log IU/mL in plasma viral load at 1 mg/kg
HCV genotype 1b infected model:
  Decreased 2-3 Log IU/mL in plasma at 1 mg/kg

## Pharmacokinetics

| | Parameter | Rat | | Dog | | Monkey | | Chrimpanzee | Rabbit | Human | |
|---|---|---|---|---|---|---|---|---|---|---|---|
| | Dose (mg/kg, human: mg) | 2 (i.v.) | 5 (p.o.) | 2 (i.v.) | 10 (p.o.) | 2 (i.v.) | 50 (p.o.) | 10 (p.o.) | 240 (p.o.) | 200 (p.o.) | 1000 (p.o.) |
| *In Vivo* | $C_{max}$ (µM) | NA | 0-0.1 | NA | 0.7 | NA | 0.8 | 0.7, 1.1 | 1.7 | 0.319 | 9.44 |
| | $T_{max}$ (h) | NA | 0.5 | NA | 1 | NA | 4 | 2, 4 | 1.3 | 1.75 | 4.00 |
| | $AUC_{0-24}$ (µM·h) | 0.6 | 0-0.1 | 4.1 | 1.5 | 2.5 | 3.1 | 3.8, 6.5 | 7.5 | 0.918 | 30.2 |
| | $T_{1/2}$ (h) | 0.9 | NA | 1.2 | NA | 1.3 | NA | NA | NA | 5.96 | 4.27 |
| | Cl (mL/min/kg, human: L/h) | 74 | NA | 11 | NA | 18 | NA | NA | NA | NA | NA |
| | $V_{ss}$ (L/kg) | 1.9 | NA | 0.3 | NA | 0.4 | NA | NA | NA | NA | NA |
| | F (%) | - | 0-5 | - | NA | - | NA | NA | NA | NA | NA |
| | Most Abundant Drug-related Component in Plasma (%) | NA | | NA | | NA | | NA | NA | NA | |
| | Urine/Feces Excretion (%) | 0.5/81.3 | | 0.78/87.3 | | NA | | NA | 0.5/66.9 | 0.4/95.5 | |
| *In Vitro* | Caco-2 Permeability | NA | | | | | | | | | |
| | Plasma Protein Binding (%Bound) | 99.5 | | 99.3 | | 98.2-98.7 | | 98.9 | 99.0 | 97.7-98.8 | |
| | LM/Hepatocytes Stability | NA | | NA | | NA | | NA | NA | NA | |

## Drug-Drug Interaction

| | CYP Enzyme | Non-CYP Enzyme | Transporter |
|---|---|---|---|
| Substrate | CYP3A | NA | P-gp, OATP1B1, OATP1B3 |
| Inhibitor | CYP3A | UGT1A1 | P-gp, OATP1B1, OATP1B3, BESP, BCRP, MRP2, MRP3, MRP4 |
| Inducer | Not | NA | NA |

## Non-clinical Toxicology

| | | | |
|---|---|---|---|
| Single-Dose Toxicity (MTD) | 2000 mg/kg (mouse) | Safety Pharmacology | • CVS: 36% inhibition of hERG tail current at 30 µM <br> • No significan *in vivo* effects on respiratory, cardiovascular or neurological function |
| Repeated-Dose Toxicity (NOAEL) | 120 mg/kg/day (rat, 6 months) 15 mg/kg/day (dog, 9 months) | Genotoxicity | • Negative |
| | | Reproductive and Developmental Toxicity | • FEED NOAEL: 250 mg/kg/day <br> • EFD NOAEL: 120 mg/kg/day (3.8 × MRHD) in rats; 120 mg/kg/day (0.37 × MRHD) for mater and 240 mg/kg/day (2.0 × MRHD) for fetus in rabbits <br> • PPND NOAEL: 120 and 180 mg/kg/day for $F_0$ and $F_1$ |
| | | Carcinogenicity | • No carcinogenicity |
| | | Special Toxicology | • No significant phototoxicity |

## Vonoprazan Fumarate
### (Takecab®)
TAK-438

Tablet, oral, EQ 10 mg/20 mg Vonoprazan

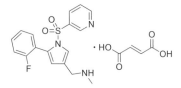

  Otsuka

- ❖ Vonoprazan fumarate is a proton pump inhibitor (PPI), indicated for gastric ulcer, duodenal ulcer, and reflux esophagitis.  It was first approved in Dec 2014 by PMDA of Japan.
- ❖ Vonoprazan fumarate was discovered by Takeda, co-developed and co-marketed by Takeda and Otsuka.
- ❖ *The recommended human starting dose* is 20 mg once daily.

| Worldwide Key Approvals | Global Sales ($Million) | Key Substance Patent Expiration |
|---|---|---|
| Dec 26, 2014 (JP) | Not available | Aug 11, 2028 (US7977488B2) <br> Aug 29, 2026 (EP1919865B1) <br> Aug 29, 2031 (JP4035559B1) <br> Aug 29, 2026 (CN101300229B) |

## Mechanism of Action

Vonoprazan fumarate belongs to potassium-competitive acid blockers (P-CAB), inhibiting $H^+$, $K^+$-ATPase (proton pump) which is the final step of acid secretion in the gastric parietal cells.

### Target Binding Selectivity

$H^+$, $K^+$-ATPase: $IC_{50}$ = 19.3 nM, pH = 6.5
Acid secretion in gastric parietal cells: $IC_{50}$ = 300 nM

### *In Vivo* Efficacy

Upper gastrointestinal tract lesion formation: $ID_{50}$ = 0.73-1.65 mg/kg
Gastric acid secretion: $ID_{50}$ = 0.21-1.26 mg/kg

## Pharmacokinetics

| | Parameter | Rat | | | | | Dog | | | | | Healthy Human | | | |
|---|---|---|---|---|---|---|---|---|---|---|---|---|---|---|---|
| | Dose (mg/kg, human: mg) | 0.75 (i.v.) | 2.25 (i.v.) | 2 (p.o.) | 6 (p.o.) | 18 (p.o.) | 0.1 (i.v.) | 0.3 (p.o.) | 0.1 (p.o.) | 0.3 (p.o.) | 1 (p.o.) | 1 (p.o.) | 10 (p.o.) | 40 (p.o.) | 120 (p.o.) |
| | $C_{max}$ (ng/mL) | NA | NA | 17.4 | 195 | 953 | - | 29.5 | 5.3 | 29.9 | 149 | 0.692 | 9.69 | 71.9 | 304 |
| | $T_{max}$ (h) | NA | NA | 0.3 | 0.4 | 0.5 | - | 1.0 | 0.8 | 0.6 | 0.6 | 1.5 | 1.75 | 1.5 | 1.0 |
| | $AUC_{inf}$ (ng·h/mL) | 99.2 | 384 | 27.2 | 417 | 2629 | 44 | 68 | 13.9 | 80.4 | 601 | 4.27 | 60.8 | 475 | 1985 |
| | $T_{1/2}$ (h) | 1.2 | 1.3 | 1.3 | 1.3 | 1.8 | 1.2 | 1.1 | 1.1 | 1.3 | 1.9 | 5.11 | 6.95 | 7.09 | 6.58 |
| *In Vivo* | Cl (mL/min/kg) | NA | NA | NA | NA | NA | NA | NA | NA | NA | NA | NA | NA | NA | NA |
| | $V_{ss}$ (L/kg) | NA | NA | NA | NA | NA | NA | NA | NA | NA | NA | NA | NA | NA | NA |
| | F (%) | - | - | 10.3 | NA | NA | - | 52.4 | NA | NA | NA | NA | NA | NA | NA |
| | Most Abundant Drug-related Component in Plasma (%) | M-I (51.9) | | | | | M-II-G (39.4) | | | | | M-I-G (19.2) | | | |
| | Most Metabolite Drug-related in Plasma (%) | M-I (51.9) | | | | | M-II-G (39.4) | | | | | M-I-G (19.2) | | | |
| | Urine/Feces Excretion (%) | 16.8/80.3 | | | | | 64.4/34.3 | | | | | NA | | | |
| | Caco-2 Permeability | $Papp_{(A-B)}$ = 17.8 × $10^{-6}$ cm/s at concentration of 3 µM | | | | | | | | | | | | | |
| *In Vitro* | Plasma Protein Binding (%Bound) | 67.3-69.5 | | | | | 71.7-83.3 | | | | | 85.2-88.0 | | | |
| | Hepatocytes Stability (Remaining) | 3180 nM | | | | | 1324 nM | | | | | 1593/1496 nM | | | |

## Drug-Drug Interaction

| | CYP Enzyme | Non-CYP Enzyme | Transporter |
|---|---|---|---|
| Substrate | CYP3A4, 2B6, 2C19, 2D6 | NA | Not |
| Inhibitor | CYP3A4/5, 2B6 | NA | P-gp, OAT3, OCT2 |
| Inducer | Not | NA | NA |

## Non-clinical Toxicology

| Single-Dose Toxicity (MNLD) | 200 mg/kg (rat) <br> 10 mg/kg (dog) | Safety Pharmacology | • NA |
|---|---|---|---|
| | | Genotoxicity | • Negative |
| Repeated-Dose Toxicity (NOAEL) | 5/10 mg/kg/day (rat, 26 weeks) <br> 0.6 mg/kg/day (dog, 39 weeks) | Reproductive and Developmental Toxicology | • FED NOAEL: ≥300 mg/kg/day for both male and female rats <br> • EFD NOAEL: 30 mg/kg/day in rats and 3 mg/kg/day in rabbits for the maternal; 100 mg/kg/day in rats and >30 mg/kg/day in rabbits for fetuses <br> • PNND NOAEL: 10 mg/kg/day for $F_0$ and $F_1$ in rats |
| | | Carcinogenicity | • Increased incidence of tumor in liver and stomach in mice and rats |
| | | Special Toxicology | • Only minor irritation function in paravenous tolerance study |

## Vorapaxar Sulfate
## (Zontivity®)
SCH-530348
Table, oral, EQ 2.08 mg Vorapaxar

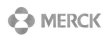 MERCK

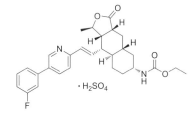

❖ Vorapaxar sulfate is a PAR-1 antagonist, indicated for the treatment of reduction of thrombotic cardiovascular events in patients with a history of myocardial infarction (MI) or with peripheral arterial disease (PAD). It was first approved in May 2014 by US FDA.
❖ Vorapaxar sulfate was discovered and marketed by Merck & Co.
❖ *The recommended human starting dose* is 2.08 mg once daily.

| Worldwide Key Approvals | Global Sales ($Million) | Key Substance Patent Expiration |
|---|---|---|
| May 08, 2014 (US) <br> Jan 19, 2014 (EU) | Not available | Apr 06, 2024 (US7304078B2) <br> Apr 14, 2023 (EP1495018B1) <br> Apr 14, 2023 (JP4558331B2) <br> Apr 14, 2023 (CN1659162B) |

## Mechanism of Action

As an antagonist of protease-activated receptor-1 (PAR-1), vorapaxar sulfate inhibits thrombin-induced and thrombin receptor agonist peptide (TRAP)-induced platelet aggregation.

**Target Binding Affinity and *In Vitro* Efficacy**

Binding Affinity: PAR-1: $K_d$ = 1.2 nM (M20: $K_d$ = 1.6 nM)
Washed human platelet: $K_d$ = 1.08-1.2 nM (M20: $K_d$ = 1.14-1.6 nM)
Thrombin/TRAP-induced platelet aggregation: $IC_{50}$ = 15-76 nM
Human CASMC: TK agonist-induced $Ca^{2+}$ efflux transients: $EC_{50}$ = 4.5 nM and $K_b$ = 0.63 nM
Rat ASMC: TK agonist- or thrombin-induced $Ca^{2+}$ transients: $K_b$ = 1.3-2.9 nM

**Ex Vivo Efficacy**

Inhibition of aggregation in whole blood derived from monkeys:
  Minimum Effective dose: 0.05 mg/kg
  Complete inhibition at 0.1 mg/kg

## Pharmacokinetics

| | Parameter | Rat | | Monkey | | Human | |
|---|---|---|---|---|---|---|---|
| | Dose (mg/kg) | 10 (i.v.) | 10 (p.o.) | 1 (i.v.) | 1 (p.o.) | 73.7 µg (i.v.) | 2.5 mg (p.o.) |
| *In Vivo* | $C_{max}$ (µg/mL, human: ng/mL) | NA | 0.33 | NA | 0.65 | 1.17 | 27.0 |
| | $T_{max}$ (h) | NA | 3.3 | NA | 1.0 | 0.30 | 1.25 |
| | $AUC_{0-48}$ (µg·h/mL, human: ng·h/mL) | 7.9 | 2.6 | 5.6 | 4.8 | 43.2 | 1300 |
| | $T_{1/2}$ (h) | 5.1 | NA | 13 | NA | 159 | 196 |
| | Cl (mL/min/kg, human: L/h) | 21 | NA | 3.0 | NA | NA | NA |
| | $V_{ss}$ (L/kg, human: L) | 4.6 | NA | 2.2 | NA | NA | NA |
| | F (%) | - | 33 | - | 86 | - | 88.7 |
| | Most Abundant Drug-related Component in Plasma (%) | M0 (67.7/73.4) | | M0 (53.5/46.5) | | M0 ($AUC_{0-24}$ = 181 ng·h/mL) | |
| | Major Drug-related Metabolite in Plasma (%) | M19 (23.5/10.6) | | M20 (38.2/43.2) | | M20 ($AUC_{0-24}$ = 32.2 ng·h/mL) | |
| | Urine/Feces Excretion (%) | <1/>82 | | 5.0/NA | | 4.23/42.2 | |
| *In Vitro* | Caco-2 Permeability | $Papp_{(A-B)}$ = 27.9-34.0 × $10^{-6}$ cm/s | | | | | |
| | Plasma Protein Binding (%Bound) | 99.6-99.7 | | 99.8 | | 99.82-99.84 | |
| | Heptocytes Stability (%Remaining) | NA | | NA | | NA | |

## Drug-Drug Interaction

| | CYP Enzyme | Non-CYP Enzyme | Transporter |
|---|---|---|---|
| Substrate | CYP3A4, 2C19, 1A1, 1A2 | NA | Not |
| Inhibitor | CYP2C8 | NA | P-gp, OAT3, BCRP |
| Inducer | CYP1A2, 2B6 | NA | NA |

## Non-clinical Toxicology

| | | | |
|---|---|---|---|
| **Single-Dose Toxicity ($LD_{50}$)** | >2000 mg/kg (rat) <br> >800 mg/kg (monkey) | **Safety Pharmacology** | • CVS: hERG inhibition: $IC_{50}$ = 341 nM <br> • No effect on CNS, respiratory gastrointestinal and renal function |
| **Repeated-Dose Toxicity (NOAEL)** | 3/10 mg/kg/day (rat, 6 months) <br> 5 mg/kg/day (monkey, 12 months) | **Genotoxicity** | • No genetic toxicity |
| | | **Reproductive and Developmental Toxicity** | • FEED NOAEL: 50 mg/kg/day <br> • EFD NOAEL: 25 mg/kg/day in rats; 20 mg/kg/day for the maternal and 10 mg/kgy/day for fetuses in rabbits <br> • PPND NOAEL: 50 mg/kg/day for $F_0$, 5 mg/kg/day for $F_1$, 25 mg/kg/day for $F_2$ |
| | | **Carcinogenicity** | • No drug-related tumor |
| | | **Special toxicity** | • No drug-related photoallergy |

# CHAPTER

# 1

## Alectinib Hydrochloride

# Alectinib Hydrochloride

## (Alecensa®)

Research code: AF-802; RG-7853; CH-5424802; RO-5424802

## 1 General Information

❖ Alectinib hydrochloride is a small molecule inhibitor of anaplastic lymphoma kinase (ALK) and RET kinase, which was first approved in Jul 2014 by PMDA of Japan.

❖ Alectinib hydrochloride was discovered and marketed by Chugai (now a subsidiary of Hoffmann-La Roche AG).

❖ Alectinib hydrochloride inhibits ALK and its downstream signaling protein, thereby inhibiting cancer cells harboring ALK fusion, amplifications, or activating mutations.

❖ Alectinib hydrochloride is indicated for the treatment of patients with ALK fusion gene-positive unresectable, recurrent or advanced non-small cell lung cancer.

❖ Available as capsules, with each containing 20 mg or 40 mg (Japan) and 150 mg (US) of alectinib hydrochloride, and the recommended dose is 300 mg (Japan) and 600 mg (US) orally twice daily.

❖ The 2014 and 2015 sales of Alecensa® were 13.2 and 71.3 million US$, respectively, referring to the financial reports of Chugai and Roche.

## Key Approvals around the World*

|  | Japan (PMDA) | USA (FDA) |
|---|---|---|
| First approval date | 07/04/2014 | 12/11/2015 |
| Application or approval No. | 22600AMX00760; 22600AMX00761 | NDA 208434 |
| Brand name | Alecensa® | Alecensa® |
| Indication | NSCLC | NSCLC |
| Authorisation holder | Chugai | Hoffmann-LA Roche |

* Till Mar 2016, it had not been approved by EMA (Europe) and CFDA (China).

## Active Ingredient

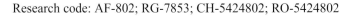

*Molecular formula*: $C_{30}H_{34}N_4O_2 \cdot HCl$
*Molecular weight*: 519.08
*CAS No.*: 1256580-46-7 (Alectinib)
1256589-74-8 (Alectinib hydrochloride)
*Chemical name*: 9-Ethyl-6,6-dimethyl-8-[4-(morpholin-4-yl)piperidin-1-yl]-11-oxo-6,11-dihydro-5H-benzo[b]carbazole-3-carbonitrile hydrochloride

*Parameters of Lipinski's "Rule of 5"*

| MW[a] | H$_D$ | H$_A$ | FRB[b] | PSA[b] | cLogP[b] |
|---|---|---|---|---|---|
| 482.62 | 1 | 6 | 3 | 72.4Å$^2$ | 5.88 ± 1.12 |

[a] Molecular weight of alectinib.  [b] Calculated by ACD/Labs software V11.02.

## Drug Product*

*Dosage route*: Oral
*Strength*: 20 mg/40 mg in Japan (Alectinib)
150 mg in US (Alectinib)
*Dosage form*: Capsule
*Inactive ingredient*: Lactose hydrate, crystal cellulose, sodium starch glycolate, hydroxypropyl cellulose, sodium lauryl sulfate, magnesium stearate, hypromellose, carrageenan, potassium chloride, titanium oxide, yellow iron oxide (20 mg), iron oxide (40 mg) and carnauba wax.
*Recommended dose*: The recommended starting dose is 300 mg twice daily without food for adults.
Fasting 1 h or more prior to the administration and more than 2 h after the administration.
600 mg twice daily with food in US.

* Sourced from Japan PMDA drug label information

## 2   Key Patents Information

### Summary

❖ Alecensa® (Alectinib hydrochloride) was initially approved by PMDA of Japan on Jul 04, 2014.

❖ Alectinib was originally developed by Chugai, and its compound patent application was filed as PCT application by Chugai in 2010.

❖ The compound patent will expire in 2030 foremost, which has been granted in China, the United States and Japan successively.

Table 1   Alectinib's Compound Patent Protection in Drug-Mainstream Country

| Country | Publication/Patent NO. | Application Date | Granted Date | Estimated Expiry Date |
|---------|------------------------|------------------|--------------|-----------------------|
| WO | WO2010143664A1 | 06/09/2010 | / | / |
| US | US9126931B2 | 06/09/2010 | 09/08/2015 | 05/29/2031[a] |
| EP | EP2441753A1 | 06/09/2010 | / | / |
| JP | JP4588121B1 | 06/09/2010 | 11/24/2010 | 03/25/2034[b] |
| CN | CN102459172B | 06/09/2010 | 06/24/2015 | 06/09/2030 |

[a] The term of this patent is extended by 354 days.   [b] The term of this patent is extended by 1385 days.

Table 2   Originator's International Patent Application List (Patent Family)

| Publication NO. | Title | Applicant/Assignee/Owner | Publication Date |
|-----------------|-------|--------------------------|------------------|
| **Technical Subjects** | **Active Ingredient (Free Base)'s Formula or Structure and Preparation** | | |
| WO2010143664A1 | Tetracyclic compound | Chugai | 12/16/2010 |
| **Technical Subjects** | **Salt, Crystal, Polymorphic, Solvate (Hydrate), Isomer, Derivative Etc. and Preparation** | | |
| WO2015163447A1 | Novel crystal of tetracyclic compound | Chugai | 10/29/2015 |
| **Technical Subjects** | **Formulation and Preparation** | | |
| WO2012023597A1 | Composition containing tetracyclic compound | Chugai | 02/23/2012 |
| WO2015163448A1 | Preparation containing tetracyclic compound at high dose | Chugai | 10/29/2015 |
| WO2015193309A1 | New pharmaceutical composition comprising non-ionic surfactants | Chugai | 12/23/2015 |
| **Technical Subjects** | **Indication or Methods for Medical Needs** | | |
| WO2014050781A | RET inhibitor | Chugai | 04/03/2014 |

The data was updated until Jan 2016.

# 3 Chemistry

## Route 1: Original Discovery Route

*Synthetic Route*: The original synthetic route to alectinib began with commercially ready 7-methoxy-2-tetralone **1**. Bis-methylation of **1** with MeI in TBAHS/*aqueous* KOH, followed by bromination with NBS provided the 1,1-dimethyl bromo-tetralone **3** in 67% yield over two steps. Further transformation of **3** with 3-hydrazinobenzonitrile **4** in TFA at 100 °C led to the desired Fischer indole product **5**, which was carried forward to oxidation with DDQ to yield ketone **6**, which was isolated as a single isomer *via* precipitation from the crude reaction mixture. Installation of the 4-morpholinopiperidine moiety took place *via* three transformations from **6**: Initiating the demethylation with 1-dodecanethiol/NMP/NaOMe; then, the corresponding phenol **7** was readily converted into the triflate intermediate **8** and displaced with 4-(piperidin-4-yl)morpholine **9** at an elevated temperature, providing intermediate **10**; thirdly, Pd-catalyzed cross-coupling of the bromide **10** with ethynyl triiso-propylsilane **11** followed by cleavage of the resulting alkylsilane with TBAF yielded the key ethynyl precursor **12** to alectinib. Finally, hydrogenation of this unsaturated precursor furnished the final target alectinib, which was transferred to its HCl salt as active pharmaceutical ingredient (API).[1-5]

[1]  Kazutomo, K.; Kohsuke, A.; Noriyuki, F. US2012083488A1, **2012**.
[2]  Furumoto, K.; Shiraki, K.; Hirayama, T. WO2012023597A1, **2012**.
[3]  Furumoto, K.; Shiraki, K.; Hirayama, T. US2013143877A1, **2013**.
[4]  Kinoshita, K.; Kobayashi, T.; Asoh, K., et al. *J. Med. Chem.* **2011**, *54*, 6286-6294.
[5]  Kinoshita, K.; Asoh, K.; Furuichi, N., et al. *Bioorg. Med. Chem.* **2012**, *20*, 1271-1280.

## Route 2

*Synthetic Route*: Chugai also reported a scale-up procedure for preparing alectinib hydrochloride which was involved in the same patent as referred to route 1. Palladium-catalyzed coupling of 2-(4-bromophenyl)-2-methylpropanoic acid **1** with potassium trifluoro(vinyl)borate **2** afforded propanoic acid **3** in 93% yield, which was subjected to the hydrogenation and future iodation to yield iodobenzene **5** with the yield of 94% from acid **3**. CDI-activated condensation of **5** with 3-(*tert*-butoxy)-3-oxopropanoic acid **6** in the presence of TEA and MgCl$_2$ provided *tert*-butyl 3-oxopentanoate **7**, which was further condensed with 3-nitrobenzonitrile **8** under basic and reductive conditions to provide *tert*-butyl indole-3-carboxylate **9** in 64% yield from **5**. Buchwald-Hartwig type amination of the carboxylate **9** with 4-(piperidin-4-yl)morpholine **10**, and further two-step saltifications finally led to hydrochloride salt of 4-(morpholin-4-yl)piperidine derivative **11** in 83% yield, which upon deprotection with TMSCl produced indole-3-carboxylic acid **12** in excellent yield. As the precursor to the alectinib, **12** underwent the annulation to provide the free base of alectinib. The preparation was completed in 32% overall yield while alectinib hydrochloride was achieved in 83% yield by treatment of alectinib with diluted HCl.[1]

[1] Kazutomo, K.; Kohsuke, A.; Noriyuki, F. US2012083488A1, **2012**.

## Route 3

*Synthetic Route*:　This synthesis of alectinib using 1-(3-bromo-4-ethyl-phenyl)ethanone **1** and 4-(piperidin-4-yl)morpholine **2** as starting materials was described.　Initial condensation of 4-(piperidin-4-yl)morpholine **2** with 1-(3-bromo-4-ethylphenyl) ethanone **1** in the presence of *t*-BuOK in DMSO under microwave irradiation gave phenylethanone **3** in 95% yield, which upon Grignard reaction with methyl magnesium bromide produced tertiary alcohol **4** with the yield of 87%.　Catalyzed by TFA, a Fridel-Craft alkylation of methyl 6-cyanoindole-3-carboxylate **5** with tertiary alcohol **4** afforded the corresponding intermediate **6** in 80% yield, which was then subjected to ester hydrolysis with TMSCl in trifluoroethanol to yield carboxylic acid **7** in 94% yield.　Finally, alectinib was obtained upon cyclization of **7** mediated by Ac₂O/DIPEA in DMA with the yield of 87% and the overall yield of 54%.[6]

## 4　Pharmacology

### Summary

Mechanism of Action

❖ Alectinib hydrochloride is an ALK kinase inhibitor, which inhibits ALK phosphorylation and ALK-mediated activation of the downstream signaling proteins STAT3 and AKT, and decreases tumor cell viability in multiple cell lines harboring ALK fusions, amplifications, or activating mutations in nonclinical studies.

❖ Alectinib hydrochloride, bound to the ATP binding site of ALK as an ATP competitor showed in X-ray structure analysis, inhibited ALK ($IC_{50}$ = 1.9 nM), RET ($IC_{50}$ = 4.8 nM), and mutant ALK ($IC_{50}$ = 0.93-41 nM), mutant RET ($IC_{50}$ = 5.7-53 nM) as well.

❖ The main metabolite M4 of alectinib hydrochloride in humans also inhibited ALK ($IC_{50}$ = 1.2 nM).

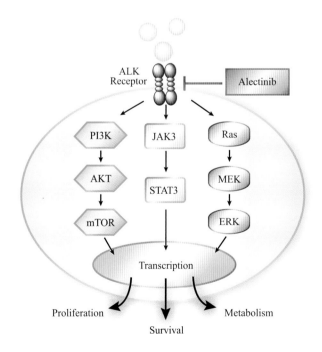

[6]　Xu, X. CN104402862A, **2015**.

❖ Alectinib hydrochloride showed no off-target effects (inhibition >50%) on a panel of 109 receptors, ion channels and 42 enzymes at 1 or 10 μM, except 5-HT$_{2B}$ (IC$_{50}$ = 100 nM), NE (IC$_{50}$ = 330 nM), DA (IC$_{50}$ = 260 nM), CaMK2$\alpha$, Ca$^{2+}$-L.

*In Vitro* Efficacy
❖ Anti-proliferation in cancer cell lines:
  • Human ALK fusion positive, gene amplification and mutant ALK cell lines: IC$_{50}$ = 3.0-62 nM.
  • Human ALK fusion gene negative cell lines: IC$_{50}$ = 400->1000 nM.
  • Ba/F3 cells WT or EML-ALK mutation cells: IC$_{50}$ = 16-240 nM.

*In Vivo* Efficacy
❖ Human NSCLC xenograft models in SCID mice:
  • In NCI-H2228 models:
    ◆ Significant tumor inhibition at 0.8 mg/kg (TGI% = 59%).
    ◆ Tumor regression at 4 mg/kg/day on Day 31.
  • In A549 models: No significant tumor growth inhibition.
❖ In Karpas299 and NB-1 models:
  • Significant tumor growth inhibition at 6 mg/kg (TGI% = 94% or 63%).
  • Tumor regression at 20 mg/kg/day on Day 20.
❖ In crizotinib-resistant Ba/F3 models with L1196M ALK-mutation:
  • Tumor regression at 60 mg/kg/day on Day 16.
  • No tumor growth inhibition with crizotinib.

## Mechanism of Action

Table 3   Inhibitory Activity of Alectinib Hydrochloride on Human Protein Kinases[7, 8]

| Kinase | Type | IC$_{50}$ (nM) Alectinib Hydrochloride | M4 | Kinase | Type | IC$_{50}$ (nM) Alectinib Hydrochloride | M4 |
|---|---|---|---|---|---|---|---|
| ALK | TK | 1.9 | 1.2 | RET | RET kinase | 4.8 | 3.0 |
| ALK (C1156Y) | TK | 0.93 | 0.62 | RET (G691S) | RET kinase | 9.5 | 3.3 |
| ALK (F1174L) | TK | 1.0 | 1.1 | RET (M918T) | RET kinase | 5.7 | 2.3 |
| ALK (L1196M) | TK | 2.1 | 0.87 | RET (S891A) | RET kinase | 8.3 | 2.1 |
| ALK (R1275Q) | TK | 3.5 | 3.4 | RET (V791F) | RET kinase | 14 | 3.1 |
| ALK (T1151_L1152insT) | TK | 4.7 | 1.1 | RET (V804L) | RET kinase | 32 | 9.1 |
| ALK (L1152R) | TK | 4.8 | 0.83 | RET (V804M) | RET kinase | 53 | 8.1 |
| ALK (G1202R) | TK | 41 | 34 | AKT1 | S/T kinase | >5000 | >5000 |
| ALK (G1269A) | TK | 17 | 2.6 | PKC$\beta$1 | S/T kinase | >5000 | >5000 |

The inhibitory activities of kinases were studied by time-resolved fluorescence resonance energy transfer method or fluorescence polarization method.   RET: Rearranged during transfection.   TK: Tyrosine kinase.   S/T: Serine/threonine kinase.   ALK: Anaplastic lymphoma kinase.

Table 4   *In Vitro* Off-Target Activity of Alectinib Hydrochloride[8]

| Screening Assay[a] | | | Binding Test[b] | | | |
|---|---|---|---|---|---|---|
| Target | Conc. (μM) | %Inhibition | Target | IC$_{50}$ (nM) | Conc. (μM) | %Inhibition |
| Dopamine receptor | 10 | >50 | Norepinephrine | 330 | 1 | >50 |
| Ca$^{2+}$-L | 10 | >50 | Dopamine | 260 | 1 | >50 |
| CaMK2$\alpha$ | 10 | >50 | 5-HT$_{2B}$ | 100 | 10 | >50 |

[a] In the screening assay, the ligand-binding and effects of 109 receptors, ion channels or transporters, and 42 enzymes were tested in a concentration (10 μM, 4826 ng/mL) of alectinib hydrochloride.   [b] The binding test was conducted with twenty receptors and two monoamines (norepinephrine and dopamine) which expressed on the cells from rat synaptosomes, and the test was evaluated at two concentrations (1 and 10 μM, 482.6 and 4826 ng/mL) of alectinib hydrochloride.

[7]  U.S. Food and Drug Administration (FDA) Database.   http://www.accessdata.fda.gov/drugsatfda_docs/nda/2015/208434Orig1s000PharmR.pdf (accessed Mar 2016).
[8]  Japan Pharmaceuticals and Medical Devices Agency (PMDA) Database.   http://www.pmda.go.jp/drugs/2014/P201400094/index.html (accessed Mar 2016).

## *In Vitro* Efficacy

Table 5    *In Vitro* Inhibitory Activity of Alectinib Hydrochloride in Cancer Cell Lines[7, 8]

| Cell Type | Cell Line | ALK Status | IC$_{50}$ (nM) |
|---|---|---|---|
| NCI-H2228 | Human NSCLC | EML4-ALK-positive | 12 |
| Karpas299 | Human ALCL | NPM-ALK-positive | 14/3.0[a] |
| SR | Human ALCL | NPM-ALK-positive | 14/6.9[a] |
| NB-1 | Human neuroblastoma | Gene amplification | 4.5 |
| KELLY | Human neuroblastoma | F1174L | 62 |
| SK-N-FI | Human neuroblastoma | Wild type | >10000 |
| PC-9[b] | Human NSCLC | EML4-ALK-negative | 400 |
| A549[c] | Human NSCLC | EML4-ALK-negative | >1000[c] |
| NCI-H1993[d] | Human NSCLC | EML4-ALK-negative | >1000 |
| U-937 | Human ALCL | ALK-negative | >1000 |
| Ba/F3 | Mouse primary B cell | Wild type | 910 |
| | | EML4-ALK | 19 |
| | | EML4-ALK (1151Tins) | 110 |
| | | EML4-ALK C1156Y | 38 |
| | | EML4-ALK F1174L | 34 |
| | | EML4-ALK L1196M | 75 |
| | | EML4-ALK G1202R | 240 |
| | | EML4-ALK S1206Y | 16 |
| | | EML4-ALK G1268A | 40 |

NSCLC: Non-small cell lung cancer.    ALCL: Anaplastic large-cell lymphoma.    Each human cancer cell lines (2.0 × 10$^3$ cells/well) were seeded in 96-well plates, treated with 0 or 1-1000 nM of alectinib hydrochloride, 96-120 h post-treatment in the next day, and the number of viable cells was studied by quantifying the amount of ATP.    [a] In two separated experiments.    [b] PC-9 is a cell line with Exon19 deficient mutations of EGFR.    [c] A549 is a cell line with activating mutations of KRAS gene. [d] NCI-H1993 is a cell line with c-MET gene amplified.

[7]  FDA Database.    http://www.accessdata.fda.gov/drugsatfda_docs/nda/2015/208434Orig1s000PharmR.pdf (accessed Mar 2016).
[8]  PMDA Database.    http://www.pmda.go.jp/drugs/2014/P201400094/index.html (accessed Mar 2016).

## *In Vivo* **Efficacy**

Table 6    *In Vivo* Efficacy of Alectinib Hydrochloride in Xenograft Models[7, 8]

| Source | Cell Line | ALK Status | Animal | Dose (mg/kg/day, p.o.) | Duration (Day) | TGI (%) | P | Finding |
|---|---|---|---|---|---|---|---|---|
| Human NSCLC | NCI-H2228 | ALK-positive (Wild type) | SCID mouse | 0.8 | QD × 14 | 59 | 0.0006 | Tumor regression at 4 mg/kg on Day 31. |
| | | | | 4 | QD × 14 | 129 | <0.0001 | |
| | | | | 20 | QD × 14 | 137 | <0.0001 | |
| | | | | Alectinib: 60 mg/kg Crizotinib: 100 mg/kg | QD × 26 | - | - | Survival time: 39 days (control); 102.5 days (alectinib hydrochloride); 57 days (crizotinib). |
| | A549 | ALK-negative (Wild type) | SCID mouse | 0.8 | QD × 14 | -6 | 0.6427 | No tumor growth inhibition. |
| | | | | 4 | QD × 14 | -2 | 0.9765 | |
| | | | | 20 | QD × 14 | 0 | 0.9981 | |
| | | | | 2 | QD × 11 | -1 | 1.0000 | 31% inhibition at 20 mg/kg/day. Rarely effect on tumor growth. |
| | | | | 6 | QD × 11 | 22 | 0.5448 | |
| | | | | 20 | QD × 11 | 31 | 0.2874 | |
| Human ALCL | Karpas299 | ALK-positive (Wild type) | SCID mouse | 6 | QD × 11 | 94 | <0.0001 | Tumor regression at 20 mg/kg on Day 20. |
| | | | | 20 | QD × 11 | 119 | <0.0001 | |
| Human neuroblastoma cells | NB-1 | ALK-positive (Wild type) | SCID mouse | 6 | QD × 11 | 63 | 0.0003 | Tumor regression at 20 mg/kg on Day 20. |
| | | | | 20 | QD × 11 | 104 | <0.0001 | |
| Murine pro-B lymphoma cells | Ba/F3 | Crizotinib-resistant (L1196M) | SCID mouse | 60 | QD × 7 | 123 | <0.0001 | Tumor regression at 60 mg/kg. |
| | | | | Crizotinib: 100 | QD × 7 | 1 | 0.8811 | Tumor growth inhibition at crizotinib 100 mg/kg on Day 16. |

NSCLC: Non-small cell lung cancer.    ALCL: Anaplastic large-cell lymphoma.    SCID: Severe combined immunodeficient.    TGI: Tumor growth inhibition.    TGI (%) = [1- (the average value of the tumor volume change in treatment group)/(the average value of the tumor volume change in control group)] × 100.    Δtumor volumes = (tumor volume of the final measurement date) - (tumor volume of the administration start date).

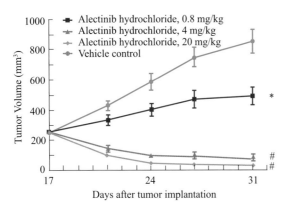

**Study:** Anti-tumor activities in NCI-H2228 xenograft mouse models.

**Animal:** SCID beige mouse.

**Model:** $1 × 10^7$ NCI-H2228 cells/mouse were implanted s.c. into SCID mice.

**Administration:** Treated daily, p.o. for 14 days, alectinib hydrochloride 0.8, 4, 20 mg/kg; Vehicle control: NA.

**Starting:** Established tumors in mice (Day 18).

**Test:** Tumor volumes, twice weekly.

**Result:** Treatment with 4 mg/kg alectinib hydrochloride resulted in complete tumor regression after 31 days of treatment.    $^*P = 0.0006$; $^\#P < 0.0001$.

Figure A    Effect of Alectinib Hydrochloride on Human NCI-H2228 NSCLC Xenograft in SCID Mouse Models[8]

[7]  FDA Database.    http://www.accessdata.fda.gov/drugsatfda_docs/nda/2015/208434Orig1s000PharmR.pdf (accessed Mar 2016).
[8]  PMDA Database.    http://www.pmda.go.jp/drugs/2014/P201400094/index.html (accessed Mar 2016).

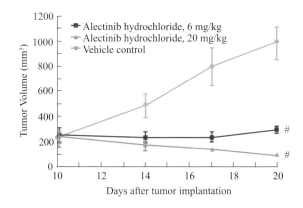

**Study:** Anti-tumor activities in Karpas299 ALCL xenograft mouse model.

**Animal:** SCID beige mouse.

**Model:** $4.9 \times 10^6$ Karpas299 cells/mouse were implanted s.c. into SCID mice.

**Administration:** Treated daily, p.o. for 11 days, alectinib hydrochloride 6 and 20 mg/kg; Vehicle control: NA.

**Starting:** Mice bearing established tumors (Day 10).

**Test:** Tumor volumes, twice weekly.

**Result:** Treatment with 20 mg/kg alectinib hydrochloride resulted in tumor regression after 20 days of treatment. [#] $P < 0.0001$.

Figure B    Effect of Alectinib Hydrochloride on Human Karpas299 ALCL Xenografts in SCID mouse Models[7]

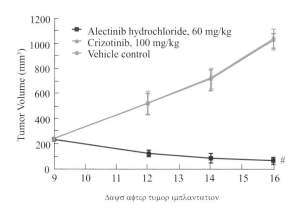

**Study:** Anti-tumor activities in crizotinib-resistant Ba/F3 with ALK-L1196M-mutations xenograft mouse models.

**Animal:** SCID beige mouse.

**Model:** $5.0 \times 10^6$ Ba/F3 cells with ALK-L1196-mutations were implanted s.c. into SCID mice.

**Administration:** Treated daily, p.o. for 7 days, alectinib hydrochloride 60 mg/kg, crizotinib 100 mg/kg/day; Vehicle control: NA.

**Starting:** Mice bearing established tumors (Day 9).

**Test:** Tumor volumes, twice weekly.

**Result**: Treatment with 60 mg/kg alectinib hydrochloride, significant tumor growth inhibitory effects and tumor regression were observed. [#]$P < 0.0001$.

Figure C    Effect of Alectinib Hydrochloride on Crizotinib-resistant Ba/F3 Cells with ALK-L1196M-Mutations Xenograft in SCID Mouse Models[8]

# 5    ADME & Drug-Drug Interaction

## Summary

### Absorption of Alectinib

❖ Exhibited a non-linear pharmacokinetics in humans following oral dosing.    The increases in $C_{max}$ and AUC did not appear to be dose-proportional in the dose range of 20 to 300 mg of alectinib.

❖ Had high oral bioavailability in rats (88.6%) and monkeys (50.4%).

❖ Was absorbed slowly in rats ($T_{max} = 8$ h) and humans (3.97-5.97 h) at 20-80 mg/kg, but moderately in monkeys (2 h).

❖ Showed a half-life ranging between 16.1-42.4 h in humans, 32.1 h in rats and 8.38 h in monkeys, after oral administrations.

❖ Had low clearance in rats (11 mL/min/kg) and monkeys (6.04 mL/min/kg), in contrast to liver blood flow, after intravenous administrations.

❖ Exhibited an extensive tissue distribution in rats and monkeys, with apparent volumes of distribution at 13.3 and 5.28 L/kg, after intravenous administrations.

❖ Showed a moderate permeability with $Papp_{(A \to B)}$ of $1.88 \times 10^{-6}$ cm/s in Caco-2 cell monolayer model.

### Distribution of Alectinib

❖ Exhibited high plasma protein binding in humans, rats, mice and monkeys (99.1%-99.7%).    Note that the drug was mainly bound to HSA.

❖ Had a $C_b:C_p$ ratio of 1.29 to 2.92 in humans, suggesting more penetration into red blood cells.

[7]  FDA Database.    http://www.accessdata.fda.gov/drugsatfda_docs/nda/2015/208434Orig1s000PharmR.pdf (accessed Mar 2016).
[8]  PMDA Database.    http://www.pmda.go.jp/drugs/2014/P201400094/index.html (accessed Mar 2016).

❖ In WIST and Long-Evans rats after single oral administration:
  - [14C]Alectinib was extensively distributed into most tissues in rats including the central nervous system, with the concentration in cerebrum close to that in plasma.
  - Relatively higher concentration levels were observed in adrenal gland, spleen, liver, lungs, kidneys, pancreas, small intestine and stomach.
  - Elimination was not complete at 168 h post-dose from high concentration tissues.
  - Radioactivity was detected in pigmented skin, suggesting [14C]alectinib was bound to melanin.

## Metabolism of Alectinib

❖ Was stable in mouse and dog hepatocytes comparing to other species hepatocytes.   10 metabolites could be detected in human liver microsomes, rhCYPs and hepatocytes.

❖ The major metabolizing enzyme was CYP3A4.

❖ The major metabolites in hepatocytes were M1, M4 (CH5468924-000) and M6 (CH5507197-000).   No human specific metabolite of alectinib was identified.

❖ Overall, the parent drug was the most abundant component in rat plasma, with M1 as the major metabolite in rat plasma.

## Excretion of Alectinib

❖ Was predominantly excreted in bile, with M5 as the most significant component in rat bile.

## Drug-Drug Interaction

❖ Alectinib had moderate time-dependent inhibition for CYP2C8 ($IC_{50}$ = 3.87-6.81 μM) and CYP3A4 ($IC_{50}$ = 6.07-7.46 μM), but weak inhibitions for other CYPs.

❖ Alectinib had no induction for CYP1A2, 2B6 or 3A4.

❖ Alectinib was not a substrate of P-gp or BCRP, but had inhibitions for P-gp ($IC_{50}$ = 1.13 μM) and BCRP ($IC_{50}$ = 0.103 μM).

❖ Alectinib had no inhibition for OATP1B1, OAT1, OAT3 or OCT2.

# Absorption

Table 7   *In Vivo* Pharmacokinetic Parameters of Alectinib in Rats and Monkeys after Single Oral and Intravenous Dose of Alectinib[7, 8]

| Species | Route | Dose (mg/kg) | $T_{max}$ (h) | $C_{max}$ (ng/mL) | $AUC_{inf}$ (ng·h/mL) | $T_{1/2}$ (h) | Cl or Cl/F (mL/min/kg) | $V_{ss}$ (L/kg) | F (%) |
|---------|-------|------|------|------|------|------|------|------|------|
| WIST rat (fasted male) | i.v. | 1 | NA | $C_0$: 175 ± 59 | 1580 ± 450 | 24.4 ± 10.9 | 11.0 ± 2.8 | 13.3 ± 4.3 | - |
| | p.o. | 1 | 8.0 ± 0.0 | 60.9 ± 14.0 | 1400 ± 320 | 32.1 ± 4.9 | NA | NA | 88.6 |
| Monkey | i.v. | 0.5 | NA | $C_0$: 283 | 1380 | 10.4 | 6.04 | 5.28 | - |
| | p.o. | 0.5 | 2.0 | 55.8 | 696 | 8.38 | 13.0 | NA | 50.4 |

Mean ± SD.   $C_0$: Extrapolated plasma concentration at time 0 after administration.

Table 8   *In Vivo* Pharmacokinetic Parameters of Alectinib in Humans after Single Oral Dose of Alectinib[8]

| Species | Route | Dose (mg) | $AUC_{0-72}$ (ng·h/mL) | $AUC_{inf}$ (ng·h/mL) | $C_{max}$ (ng/mL) | $T_{1/2}$ (h) | $T_{max}$ (h) |
|---------|-------|------|------|------|------|------|------|
| Patient (male & female) | p.o. | 20 | 143 | 206 | 4.52 | 42.4 | 5.97 |
| | p.o. | 40 | 248 | 288 | 12.3 | 26.6 | 3.97 |
| | p.o. | 80 | 670 | 696 | 41.4 | 16.1 | 3.98 |
| | p.o. | 160 | 1030 | 1120 | 60.3 | 22.3 | 2.62 |
| | p.o. | 240 | 920 | 968 | 58.6 | 17.7 | 2.69 |
| | p.o. | 300 | 1540 | 1640 | 84.1 | 19.3 | 2.38 |

[7] FDA Database.   http://www.accessdata.fda.gov/drugsatfda_docs/nda/2015/208434Orig1s000PharmR.pdf (accessed Mar 2016).
[8] PMDA Database.   http://www.pmda.go.jp/drugs/2014/P201400094/index.html (accessed Mar 2016).

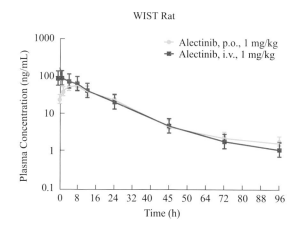
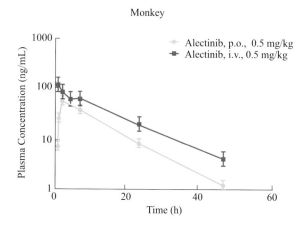

Figure D  *In Vivo* Plasma Concentration-Time Profiles of Alectinib in Rats and Monkeys
after Single Intravenous and Oral Dose of Alectinib[7, 8]

Table 9  *In Vitro* Permeability of Alectinib in Caco-2 Cell Monolayer Model[8]

| Compound | Conc. | $Papp_{(A \to B)}$ ($1 \times 10^{-6}$ cm/s) | Permeability Class |
|---|---|---|---|
| Alectinib | 10 μM | 1.88 ± 0.23 | Moderate |
| Lucifer yellow | 0.5 mg/mL | 0.15 ± 0.03 | Low |

## Distribution

Table 10  *In Vitro* Plasma Protein Binding and Blood Partitioning of Alectinib in Several Species[8]

| Study | Plasma Protein Binding (%) | | | Isolated Human Plasma Protein Binding (%) | | | | Blood Partitioning ($C_b$:$C_p$) | | | |
|---|---|---|---|---|---|---|---|---|---|---|---|
| Conc. (ng/mL) | 100 | 1000 | 10000 | Conc. (ng/mL) | 100 | 300 | 1000 | Conc. (ng/mL) | 100 | 1000 | 10000 |
| Mouse | ND | 99.4 ± 0.1 | ND | HSA | 97.0 | 97.0 | 96.9 | Mouse | ND | 1.11 | ND |
| Rat | 99.5 ± 0.1 | 99.5 ± 0.1 | 99.6 ± 0.0 | $\alpha_1$-AGP | 4.9 | 2.5 | ND | Rat | 2.06 | 2.06 | 1.40 |
| Monkey | 99.6 ± 0.0 | 99.6 ± 0.0 | 99.6 ± 0.0 | | | | | Monkey | 3.95 | 3.52 | 1.68 |
| Human | 99.6 ± 0.1 | 99.7 ± 0.0 | 99.7 ± 0.0 | | | | | Human | 2.92 | 2.64 | 1.29 |

Each value represented mean ± SD of 3 samples.   ND: Not detected.   HSA: Human serum albumin.   $\alpha_1$-AGP: $\alpha_1$-acid glycoprotein.

Table 11  *In Vitro* Plasma Protein Binding and Blood Partitioning of M4 (CH5468924-000) in Several Species[7]

| | Plasma Protein Binding (%) | | | Blood Partitioning | | |
|---|---|---|---|---|---|---|
| Species | Conc. (μg/mL) | %Bound | Species | Conc. (μg/mL) | %Partition | $C_b$:$C_p$ |
| Rat | 0.3 | 99.1 ± 0.1 | Rat | 0.3 | 77.7 ± 1.3 | 2.52 ± 0.14 |
| | 1 | 99.5 ± 0.0 | | 1 | 79.2 ± 1.5 | 2.70 ± 0.19 |
| | 2 | 99.6 ± 0.0 | | 2 | 77.2 ± 0.2 | 2.45 ± 0.02 |
| Monkey | 0.3 | 99.4 ± 0.2 | Monkey | 0.3 | 76.5 ± 1.2 | 2.26 ± 0.12 |
| | 1 | 99.6 ± 0.0 | | 1 | 75.8 ± 0.7 | 2.19 ± 0.06 |
| | 2 | 99.7 ± 0.1 | | 2 | 75.6 ± 1.4 | 2.18 ± 0.13 |
| Human | 0.3 | 99.1 ± 0.1 | Human | 0.3 | 79.8 ± 0.6 | 2.58 ± 0.08 |
| | 1 | 99.5 ± 0.0 | | 1 | 79.2 ± 0.5 | 2.50 ± 0.07 |
| | 2 | 99.5 ± 0.1 | | 2 | 79.2 ± 0.4 | 2.50 ± 0.05 |

[7]  FDA Database.   http://www.accessdata.fda.gov/drugsatfda_docs/nda/2015/208434Orig1s000PharmR.pdf (accessed Mar 2016).
[8]  PMDA Database.   http://www.pmda.go.jp/drugs/2014/P201400094/index.html (accessed Mar 2016).

Table 12   *In Vivo* Tissue Distribution of Alectinib in WIST and Long-Evans Rats
after Single Oral Dose of [$^{14}$C]Alectinib[8]

| Species | WIST Rat (male) | | | | | Long-Evans Rat (male) | | | | | |
|---|---|---|---|---|---|---|---|---|---|---|---|
| Method | 1 mg/4.5 MBq/kg | | | | | 10 mg/4.48 MBq/kg | | | | | |
| Tissue | Radioactivity Conc. (ng eq./g) | | | | Tissue/Plasma AUC$_{0-168}$ Ratio | Radioactivity Conc.(ng eq./g) | | | | | Tissue/Plasma AUC$_{0-504}$ Ratio |
| | 8 h | 24 h | 168 h | T$_{1/2}$ (h) | | 12 h | 48 h | 168 h | 504 h | T$_{1/2}$ (h) | |
| Plasma | 50.0 | 13.9 | 0.923 | 41.6 | 1.0 | 503 | 52.3 | 10.1 | ND | 49.5 | 1.0 |
| Blood | 139 | 55.2 | ND | 56.0 | 2.9 | 1360 | 150 | BLQ | BLQ | 16.6 | 2.3 |
| Cerebrum | 46.9 | 21.4 | ND | 23.1 | 0.9 | 498 | BLQ | BLQ | BLQ | 29.0 | 1.2 |
| Lungs | 2820 | 841 | ND | 41.6 | 47.4 | 23600 | 2680 | 1030 | 600 | 401 | 50.3 |
| Liver | 2100 | 817 | 120 | 38.0 | 42.8 | 15900 | 2450 | 717 | 196 | 180 | 38.4 |
| Kidneys | 1440 | 851 | 55.7 | 51.1 | 34.0 | 8170 | 1340 | 469 | 134 | 189 | 21.2 |
| Adrenal gland | 8960 | 5370 | 275 | 42.9 | 193.4 | 16300 | 6040 | 1520 | 1950 | NC | 63.3 |
| Spleen | 1780 | 841 | ND | 39.1 | 44.4 | 9740 | 2650 | 1930 | 1320 | NC | 39.0 |
| Pancreas | 1550 | 610 | ND | 28.8 | 28.1 | 10600 | 1410 | 420 | 132 | 202 | 24.1 |
| Skin (non-pigmented) | 314 | 595 | ND | 48.6 | 19.9 | 2310 | 636 | 233 | BLQ | 133 | 8.6 |
| Skin (pigmented) | - | - | - | - | - | 2870 | 1260 | 524 | 157 | 193 | 11.5 |
| Small intestine (content) | 5040 | 2010 | ND | NA | 9.4 | 7190 | 1470 | 334 | 243 | NC | 17.5 |
| Stomach (content) | 7400 | 299 | ND | NA | 9.8 | 4300 | 802 | 411 | 200 | NC | 12.2 |

Sample times: 4, 8, 12, 24, 48, 72, 120 and 168 h post-dose for WIST Rats.   12, 24, 48, 72, 120, 168, 336 and 504 h post-dose for Long-Evans rats.   BLQ: Below the lower limit of quantification.   ND: Not detected.   NC: Not calculated.

## Metabolism

Table 13   *In Vitro* Metabolic Phenotype of Alectinib in Hepatocytes and Liver Microsomes[8]

| %Inhibition | Hepatocytes | | | | Liver Microsomes | |
|---|---|---|---|---|---|---|
| | Benzylimidazole | Ketoconazole | | | Benzylimidazole | Ketoconazole |
| | 1000 µM | 1 µM | 10 µM | 1000 µM | 1000 µM | 1 µM |
| Alectinib | 99 | 43 | 47 | 85 | 93 | 78 |
| Testosterone | NA | NA | 97 | NA | NA | 83 |

Testosterone: Typical substrate for CYP3A (concentration: 100 µM).   Ketoconazole: Inhibitor of CYP3A.   Benzylimidazole: Inhibitor of Pan-CYP.   NA: Not available.

Table 14   *In Vitro* the Intrinsic Clearance of [$^{14}$C]Alectinib in Mouse, Rat, Dog, Monkey and Human Hepatocytes[7]

| Species | Mouse | | | Rat | | | Dog | | | Monkey | | | Human | | |
|---|---|---|---|---|---|---|---|---|---|---|---|---|---|---|---|
| Incubation time (h) | 0 | 1 | 4 | 0 | 1 | 4 | 0 | 1 | 4 | 0 | 1 | 4 | 0 | 1 | 4 |
| Alectinib (µM) | 9.80 | 9.38 | 8.81 | 9.69 | 8.38 | 6.59 | 9.78 | 9.30 | 8.40 | 9.74 | 6.15 | 4.63 | 9.75 | 8.59 | 6.51 |
| Cl$_{int}$ (mL/min/10$^6$ cells) | 0.00390 | | | 0.0122 | | | 0.00558 | | | 0.0183 | | | 0.0131 | | |

[7]   FDA Database.   http://www.accessdata.fda.gov/drugsatfda_docs/nda/2015/208434Orig1s000PharmR.pdf (accessed Mar 2016).
[8]   PMDA Database.   http://www.pmda.go.jp/drugs/2014/P201400094/index.html (accessed Mar 2016).

Table 15  *In Vitro* Metabolic Stability of [$^{14}$C]Alectinib in Recombinant CYP Enzymes[7]

| CYPs | Control-1 | Control-2 | 1A1 | 1A2 | 2A6 | 2B6 | 2C8 | 2C9 | 2C18 | 2C19 | 2D6 | 2E1 | 3A4 | 3A5 | 4A11 |
|---|---|---|---|---|---|---|---|---|---|---|---|---|---|---|---|
| Remaining conc. of [$^{14}$C] alectinib ($\mu$M) | 9.61 | 9.63 | 9.40 | 9.55 | 9.54 | 9.52 | 9.21 | 9.52 | 9.59 | 9.57 | 9.47 | 9.62 | 4.66 | 9.28 | 9.26 |
| % of control | 100 | 100 | 97.8[a] | 99.4[a] | 99.1[b] | 98.9[b] | 95.6[b] | 98.9[b] | 99.8[a] | 99.4[b] | 98.5[a] | 99.9[b] | 48.4[b] | 96.4[b] | 96.4[a] |

[a] % of control = (Conc. of [$^{14}$C]alectinib in CYPs/conc. of [$^{14}$C]alectinib in control-1) × 100.    [b] % of control = (Conc. of [$^{14}$C]alectinib in CYPs/conc. of [$^{14}$C]alectinib in control-2) × 100.

Table 16  *In Vitro* Metabolism of Alectinib in Cryopreserved Hepatocytes[8]

| Species | Incubated Time (h) | Composition of Drug-Related Material in Reaction Mixture (% of initial parent content) | | | | | | | | | |
|---|---|---|---|---|---|---|---|---|---|---|---|
| | | Parent | M1 | M3 | M4 | M5 | M6 | M7 | M8 | M9 | M10 |
| Mouse | 1 | 95.7 | 2.0 | 0.3 | 2.1 | 0.3 | 0.6 | 0.6 | 0.1 | 0.1 | ND |
| | 4 | 89.9 | 4.2 | 0.4 | 4.5 | 0.2 | 1.4 | 0.4 | 0.1 | 0.4 | 0.0 |
| Rat | 1 | 86.5 | 2.2 | 0.2 | 7.5 | 0.6 | 0.5 | 1.2 | 1.0 | 1.8 | 0.2 |
| | 4 | 68.0 | 7.4 | 0.4 | 20.0 | 0.7 | 0.9 | 0.5 | 1.2 | 1.8 | 0.6 |
| Dog | 1 | 95.1 | 1.1 | 0.2 | 4.2 | 1.0 | 0.1 | 0.2 | 0.1 | 0.1 | 0.1 |
| | 4 | 85.9 | 3.7 | ND | 10.8 | 0.9 | 0.2 | 0.1 | 0.0 | 0.1 | 0.1 |
| Monkey | 1 | 63.1 | 5.5 | 2.2 | 8.9 | 1.0 | 6.2 | 1.3 | 3.9 | 7.1 | 1.1 |
| | 4 | 47.5 | 10.9 | 2.7 | 18.8 | 1.0 | 8.5 | 0.9 | 3.7 | 4.8 | 1.3 |
| Human | 1 | 88.1 | 2.5 | 0.9 | 4.5 | 0.9 | 1.9 | 0.5 | 0.6 | 1.5 | 0.4 |
| | 4 | 66.8 | 8.6 | 1.9 | 13.5 | 1.3 | 4.3 | 0.4 | 1.7 | 2.6 | 0.8 |

M4 (CH5468924-000).   M6 (CH5507197-000).   Cryopreserved hepatocytes suspension (1 × 10$^6$ cells/mL) containing 10 $\mu$M [$^{14}$C]alectinib were incubated at 37 °C for 1 or 4 h in CO$_2$ incubator.

Table 17  *In Vitro* Metabolism of Alectinib in Recombinant Human CYP (rhCYP) Microsomes[8]

| rhCYP | Composition of Drug-Related Material in Reaction Mixture (% of initial parent content) | | | | | | | | |
|---|---|---|---|---|---|---|---|---|---|
| | Parent | M1 | M2 | M3 | M4 | M5 | M6 | M9 | M10 |
| 1A1 | 95.6 | 0.5 | ND | 0.9 | 1.7 | 0.4 | 0.4 | 0.2 | 0.1 |
| 1A2 | 95.6 | 0.4 | ND | 0.7 | ND | ND | ND | 0.1 | ND |
| 2A6 | 94.0 | ND | ND | 0.6 | 1.5 | ND | 0.2 | ND | ND |
| 2B6 | 93.8 | 0.3 | ND | 0.7 | 1.5 | 0.2 | ND | ND | 0.0 |
| 2C8 | 91.2 | ND | ND | 1.4 | 2.6 | 1.8 | 0.3 | 0.1 | 0.1 |
| 2C9 | 95.1 | ND | ND | 0.8 | 1.4 | ND | ND | ND | ND |
| 2C18 | 94.5 | ND | ND | 0.6 | ND | 0.4 | ND | 0.1 | ND |
| 2C19 | 94.3 | ND | ND | ND | 1.4 | 0.1 | 0.2 | ND | ND |
| 2D6 | 95.9 | 0.4 | ND | 0.8 | 1.7 | 0.4 | ND | 0.2 | 0.0 |
| 2E1 | 95.7 | ND | ND | ND | ND | 0.2 | ND | ND | ND |
| 3A4 | 46.7 | 2.8 | 1.6 | 3.6 | 28.1 | 3.2 | 5.2 | 1.5 | 1.8 |
| 3A5 | 91.0 | 0.3 | ND | 1.2 | 2.8 | 0.5 | 0.3 | 0.2 | 0.1 |
| 4A11 | 94.5 | ND | ND | 0.6 | 1.7 | 3.0 | ND | ND | 0.1 |

M4 (CH5468924-000).   M6 (CH5507197-000).   ND: Not detected.   rhCYP suspension (100 nM CYP and 1.4 mg protein/mL) containing 10 $\mu$M [$^{14}$C]alectinib and NADPH generating system were incubated at 37 °C for 60 min.

[7]  FDA Database.   http://www.accessdata.fda.gov/drugsatfda_docs/nda/2015/208434Orig1s000PharmR.pdf (accessed Mar 2016).
[8]  PMDA Database.   http://www.pmda.go.jp/drugs/2014/P201400094/index.html (accessed Mar 2016).

Table 18   *In Vitro* Metabolism of Alectinib in Human Liver Microsomes[8]

| System | Condition | | Composition of Drug-Related Material in Reaction Mixture (% of peak area) | | | | | | | | | | |
|---|---|---|---|---|---|---|---|---|---|---|---|---|---|
| | | | Parent | M1 | M2 | M3 | M4 | M5 | M6 | M7 | M8 | M9 | M10 |
| NADPH dependent metabolism | Without NADPH | | 98.8 | 0.0 | 0.0 | 0.1 | 0.2 | 0.0 | 0.0 | 0.0 | 0.0 | 0.0 | 0.0 |
| | With NADPH | | 86.5 | 0.4 | 0.1 | 1.3 | 4.1 | 1.4 | 1.4 | 0.1 | 1.4 | 2.2 | 0.2 |
| Metabolism in the specific inhibitor for CYP isoform | Without inhibitor | 0 min | 97.9 | 0.2 | ND | 0.2 | 0.3 | 0.1 | 0.1 | 0.0 | 0.1 | 0.1 | 0.0 |
| | | 15 min | 88.2 | 0.7 | 0.0 | 1.6 | 4.5 | 1.3 | 1.5 | 0.0 | 0.6 | 0.5 | 0.1 |
| | With inhibitor | CYP1A2 | 88.0 | 0.4 | 0.1 | 1.6 | 4.6 | 1.4 | 1.4 | 0.1 | 0.7 | 0.4 | 0.1 |
| | | CYP2C9 | 89.1 | 0.4 | 0.1 | 1.4 | 4.3 | 1.3 | 1.1 | 0.0 | 0.6 | 0.1 | 0.0 |
| | | CYP2C19 | 89.0 | 0.3 | 0.1 | 1.5 | 4.3 | 1.2 | 1.2 | 0.0 | 0.7 | 0.3 | 0.0 |
| | | CYP2D6 | 88.9 | 0..3 | 0.1 | 1.8 | 4.1 | 1.4 | 1.1 | 0.1 | 0.7 | 0.4 | 0.0 |
| | | CYP3A4/5 | 97.6 | 0.2 | 0.0 | 0.2 | 0.4 | 0.3 | 0.0 | 0.0 | 0.1 | 0.0 | ND |

M4 (CH5468924-000).   M6 (CH5507197-000).   NADPH dependent metabolism: Human liver microsomes suspension (0.5 mg protein/mL) containing 10 μM [$^{14}$C]alectinib was incubated with or without NADPH generating system at 37 °C for 15 min.   Metabolism in the specific inhibitor for CYP isoform: Human liver microsomes suspension (0.5 mg protein/mL) containing 10 μM [$^{14}$C]alectinib and NADPH generating system was incubated with or without specific inhibitor for each CYP isoform at 37 °C for 15 min.

Table 19   Metabolites in Plasma, Urine and Feces in Rats after Single Oral Dose of [$^{14}$C]Alectinib[8, 9]

| Matrix | Species | Dose (mg/kg) | Time (h) | % of Radioactivity | | | | | | | | | |
|---|---|---|---|---|---|---|---|---|---|---|---|---|---|
| | | | | M0 | M1 | M2 | M3 | M4 | M5 | M6 | M7 | M8 | Others |
| Plasma | Rat | 1 | 24 | 72.6 | 2.9 | 1.0 | 1.0 | 1.5 | 1.5 | 1.0 | ND | 1.0 | 4.1 |
| Urine | Rat | 1 | 0-24 | 8.1 | 40.0 | 48.1 | - | - | - | - | - | - | 1.2 |
| | | | 24-48 | 6.5 | 22.7 | 63.3 | - | - | - | - | - | - | 2.3 |
| Bile | Rat | 1 | 0-24 | 4.0 | 5.7 | 19.2 | 21.4 | 2.0 | 40.6 | 2.4 | - | - | 4.7 |
| Feces | Rat | 1 | 0-24 | 51.8 | 12.6 | 2.0 | 22.1 | 1.3 | ND | - | - | - | 2.6 |
| | | | 24-48 | 30.2 | 13.6 | 1.4 | 39.3 | 1.9 | 1.4 | - | - | - | 1.9 |
| | Human[a] | NA | NA | 84 | NA | NA | NA | 6 | NA | NA | NA | NA | NA |

[a] % of dose.

[8] PMDA Database.   http://www.pmda.go.jp/drugs/2014/P201400094/index.html (accessed Mar 2016).
[9] FDA Database.   http://www.accessdata.fda.gov/drugsatfda_docs/label/2015/208434s000lbl.pdf (accessed May 2016).

Figure E    Proposed Pathway for *In Vitro* Biotransformation of Alectinib in Human Liver Microsomes or Hepatocytes[8]

## Excretion

Table 20    Excretion Profiles of [$^{14}$C]Alectinib in Rats and Humans after Single Oral Dose of [$^{14}$C]Alectinib[8, 9]

| Species | State | Dose (mg/kg) | Route | Time (h) | Bile (% of dose) | Urine (% of dose) | Feces (% of dose) | Cage Washing (% of dose) | Recovery (% of dose) |
|---|---|---|---|---|---|---|---|---|---|
| Rat (male) | Intact | 1 | p.o. | 0-168 | - | $0.5 \pm 0.1$ | $95.7 \pm 0.7$ | $0.3 \pm 0.2$ | $96.4 \pm 0.6$ |
| Rat (male) | BDC | 1 | p.o. | 0-48 | $42.5 \pm 7.1$ | $2.0 \pm 0.1$ | $10.3 \pm 4.3$ | $0.1 \pm 0.1$ | $54.9 \pm 8.8$ |
| Human | Intact | NA | p.o. | NA | - | <0.5 | 98 | - | NA |

[8]  PMDA Database.   http://www.pmda.go.jp/drugs/2014/P201400094/index.html (accessed Mar 2016).
[9]  FDA Database.   http://www.accessdata.fda.gov/drugsatfda_docs/label/2015/208434s000lbl.pdf (accessed May 2016).

## Drug-Drug Interaction

Table 21　*In Vitro* Evaluation of Alectinib as an Inhibitor and an Inducer of CYP Enzymes[8]

| | Alectinib as an Inhibitor | | | Alectinib as an Inducer | | | | Enzyme Activity | | mRNA | |
|---|---|---|---|---|---|---|---|---|---|---|---|
| CYPs | Pre-incubation (min) | IC$_{50}$ (µM) | %Inhibition (10 µM) | CYPs | Hepatocyte | Conc. (µM) | | Fold Induction | % of Positive | Fold Induction | % of Positive |
| 1A2 | 0/30 | >10/>10 | 13.0/11.4 | | Hu1319 | 0.01-1 | | 1.5-1.7 | 2.1-2.9 | 0.9-1.1 | -0.1-0.2 |
| 2B6 | 0/30 | >10/>10 | 30.8/31.3 | 1A2 | Hu4197 | 0.01-1 | | 1.0-1.2 | 0.2-4.3 | 1.0-1.9 | 0.1-2.6 |
| 2C8 | 0/30 | 3.87/6.81 | 71.3/59.7 | | Hu8084 | 0.01-1 | | 1.1-2.0 | 0.6-5.8 | 1.1-2.0 | 0.1-1.8 |
| 2C9 | 0/30 | >10/>10 | 23.8/27.3 | | Hu1319 | 0.01-1 | | 1.4-1.7 | 9.1-14.6 | 0.9-1.5 | -0.4-3.3 |
| 2C19 | 0/30 | >10/>10 | 28.9/29.8 | 2B6 | Hu4197 | 0.01-1 | | 1.1-1.5 | 3.9-19.8 | 1.1-3.1 | 0.7-25.8 |
| 2D6 | 0/30 | >10/>10 | 12.7/5.4 | | Hu8084 | 0.01-1 | | 1.2-1.9 | 1.3-6.6 | 1.0-1.7 | -0.1-2.2 |
| 3A4[a] | 0/30 | >10/6.07 | 37.0/62.4 | | Hu1319 | 0.01-1 | | 1.3-1.7 | 6.5-16.5 | 0.9-2.5 | -0.3-5.1 |
| 3A4[b] | 0/30 | >10/7.46 | 29.5/57.1 | 3A4 | Hu4197 | 0.01-1 | | 1.2-1.8 | 3.2-11.4 | 0.9-3.8 | -0.4-11.5 |
| | | | | | Hu8084 | 0.01-1 | | 1.1-2.1 | 1.3-13.0 | 1.1-3.9 | 0.2-4.9 |

[a] Midazolam was substrate.　[b] Testosterone was substrate.

Table 22　*In Vitro* Evaluation of Alectinib as an Inhibitor of CYP2C8 and CYP3A4[8]

| | CYP2C8 | | | | CYP3A4 | | | | | |
|---|---|---|---|---|---|---|---|---|---|---|
| Parameter | $V_{max}$ (nmol/min /mg protein) | $K_m$ (µM) | $K_i$ (µM) | Inhibition Model | Conc. (µM) | $K_{obs}$ (min$^{-1}$) | $K_{inact}$ (min$^{-1}$) | $K_I$ (µM) | $K_{inact}/K_i$ Ratio (min$^{-1}$·µM$^{-1}$) | % Loss of Initial Enzyme Activity with Pre-Incubation (30-min) |
| Alectinib | 2.18 | 1.74 | 1.98 | Competitive | 3.75-60 | 0.000892-0.0102 | 0.0624 | ≥60 | ≤0.00104 | 5.9-35.6 |

$K_I$: Inhibitor concentration producing $K_{obs} = K_{inact}/2$.　$K_{obs} = K_{inact} \times [I]/(K_i + [I])$.　$K_{obs}$: Apparent inactivation rate constant.　$K_{inact}$: Maximum inactivation rate constant. $K_i$: Inhibition constant.

Table 23　*In Vitro* Evaluation of Alectinib as a Substrate and an Inhibitor of P-gp in Caco-2 Cells[8]

| | Alectinib as a P-gp Substrate | | | | Alectinib as a P-gp Inhibitor | | | | |
|---|---|---|---|---|---|---|---|---|---|
| Conc. (µM) | Papp of [$^{14}$C]Alectinib | | | Conc. (µM) | Papp of [$^3$H]Digoxin | | | | IC$_{50}$ (µM) |
| | Papp$_{(A \to B)}$ (1 × 10$^{-6}$ cm/s) | Papp$_{(B \to A)}$ (1 × 10$^{-6}$ cm/s) | Efflux Ratio | | Papp$_{(A \to B)}$ (1 × 10$^{-6}$ cm/s) | Papp$_{(B \to A)}$ (1 × 10$^{-6}$ cm/s) | Efflux Ratio | % of Control | |
| 0.3 | 4.48 (n = 2) | 4.14 ± 0.28 | 0.924 | 0.03-0.3 | 1.74-1.91 | 12.5-13.9 | 6.56-7.76 | 83.3-102 | 1.13 |
| 1 | 3.80 ± 0.55 | 5.0 ± 0.69 | 1.32 | 1-3 | 2.58-3.31 | 8.9-12.4 | 2.70-4.82 | 22.7-56.0 | |

% of control = (ER of Alectinib - ER of positive inhibitor)/(ER of vehicle - ER of positive inhibitor) × 100.　Digoxin was a positive substrate.

Table 24　*In Vitro* Evaluation of Alectinib as a Substrate and an Inhibitor of BCRP[8]

| | Alectinib as a BCRP Substrate | | | | Alectinib as a BCRP Inhibitor | | | | |
|---|---|---|---|---|---|---|---|---|---|
| Conc. (µM) | [$^{14}$C]Alectinib | | | Conc. (µM) | [$^3$H]Prazosin | | | | IC$_{50}$ (µM) |
| | Papp$_{(A \to B)}$ (1 × 10$^{-6}$ cm/s) | Papp$_{(B \to A)}$ (1 × 10$^{-6}$ cm/s) | Corrected ER | | Papp$_{(A \to B)}$ (1 × 10$^{-6}$ cm/s) | Papp$_{(B \to A)}$ (1 × 10$^{-6}$ cm/s) | Corrected ER | % of Control | |
| 0.3 | 2.86 (n = 2) | 5.41 ± 0.83 | 1.20 | 0.01-0.03 | 5.83-6.36 | 26.4-26.9 | 3.50-3.94 | 78.5-92.4 | |
| 1 | 3.22 ± 0.41 | 5.63 ± 0.55 | 1.62 | 0.1-0.3 | 8.51-10.9 | 23.6-25.0 | 1.79-2.43 | 24.4-44.6 | 0.103 |
| 3 | 3.59 ± 0.38 | 4.20 ± 0.23 | 1.13 | 1-3 | 12.8-13.9 | 12.7-16.6 | 0.914-1.19 | -3.4-5.4 | |

Corrected ER: ER in human BCRP expressing cells/ER in control cells (host cells).　% of control = (Corrected ER of inhibitor - Corrected ER of positive inhibitor)/ (Corrected ER of vehicle - Corrected ER of positive inhibitor) × 100 .　Prazosin was a positive substrate.

[8]　PMDA Database.　http://www.pmda.go.jp/drugs/2014/P201400094/index.html (accessed Mar 2016).

Table 25   *In Vitro* Evaluation of Alectinib as an Inhibitor of Uptake Transporters[8]

| Inhibitor | %Uptake Activity | | | |
| --- | --- | --- | --- | --- |
| | OATP1B1 | OAT1 | OAT3 | OCT2 |
| Vehicle (control) | 100 | 100 | 100 | 100 |
| Rifampicin, probenecid or quinidine | 16.3 | 1.5 | 6.9 | 1.1 |
| Alectinib (3 µM) | 96.7 | 106.2 | 92.3 | 106.3 |

Rifampicin, probenecid or quinidine were positive inhibitors of OATP1B1, OAT1, OAT3 and OCT2.

# 6   Non-Clinical Toxicology

## Summary

### Single-Dose Toxicity
❖ Not conducted.

### Repeated-Dose Toxicity
❖ Repeated-dose toxicity of alectinib in rats and monkeys by oral administration for up to 13 weeks:
  • The predominant targets of toxicity in both species consistently included GI tract, adrenal gland, liver, reproductive organs, and respiratory system.   Meanwhile, all lesions were considered reversible.
  • Toxicities only observed in rats focused on trachea, lungs, bone and incisor, as well as extension of blood clotting time and hemorrhagic transformation of the ileum.   However, since trachea and lungs lesions were reversible and not accompanied with hyperplasia or fibrosis, respiratory disorder was not considered a clinical problem.   Likewise, certainty was limited for extrapolation of bone and incisor abnormalities to adult patients, due to rare occurrence in primates and developmental differences from human, but effects on infants and juveniles were not deniable.

### Safety Pharmacology
❖ Both *in vitro* and *in vivo* safety pharmacology studies to assess the risk on neurological, cardiovascular, respiratory and gastrointestinal system:
  • No effects on CNS, respiratory, or gastrointestinal motor functions.
  • Cardiovascular effects: The $IC_{50}$ of hERG currents was 0.45 µM, suggesting some potential for QTc prolongation, yet not reported clinically.   However, slight hypotension was observed in monkeys, likely due to the inhibitory effects on Cav1.2 currents with a low $IC_{50}$ of 0.461 µM.

### Genotoxicity
❖ A standard battery of genotoxicity studies on alectinib:
  • It was negative in the *in vitro* reverse mutation (Ames) assays, but positive for clastogenicity in the *in vivo* micronucleus assay.   In addition, the observed chromosomal effects were more numerical rather than structural.

### Reproductive and Developmental Toxicity
❖ Male and female fertility and pre- and postnatal developmental toxicity studies were not conducted.
❖ Embryo-fetal development in rats and rabbits:
  • Alectinib administration during organogenesis resulted in abortion, embryo-fetal lethality and structural teratogenicity (visceral and skeletal) at maternally toxic doses in both species.
  • The NOAEL for maternal and fetal toxicity was 3 mg/kg/day in rats and 9 mg/kg/day in rabbits, approximately 0.9- and 0.4-fold the estimated human exposure, respectively.

### Carcinogenicity
❖ No carcinogenicity evaluation was conducted or required for the indicated patients with advanced cancer.

### Special Toxicology
❖ There appeared to be a potential for phototoxic response, based on the calculated photo irritation factor.

[8]  PMDA Database.   http://www.pmda.go.jp/drugs/2014/P201400094/index.html (accessed Mar 2016).

## Repeated-Dose Toxicity

Table 26    Repeated-Dose Toxicity Studies of Alectinib by Oral (Gavage) Administration[8]

| Species | Duration (Week) | Dose (mg/kg/day) | NOAEL | | Finding |
|---|---|---|---|---|---|
| | | | Dose (mg/kg/day) | $AUC_{0-24}^{a}$ (ng·h/mL) | |
| Wistar rat | 4 | 0, 6, 20, 60 | <6 | 9340/13900 | 6 mg/kg: Abnormality of RBCs, ↑ ALP, giant PLTs, infiltration of alveoli macrophage. <br> 20 mg/kg: ↓ BWG, ↑ mature megakaryocytes of spleen, swelling hepatocytes, vacuolation of the bile duct epithelium, high adrenal gland weight, hypertrophy of adrenal cortex, degeneration of stomach glandular epithelium, inflammatory cells invaded into gastrointestinal mucosa, extension of growth zone. <br> 60 mg/kg: ↑ Activated osteoclasts, ↓ trabecular bone, ↑ γ-GT in neutrophils in males and females. |
| | 13 | 0, 3, 9, 27 | <3 | 5100/8450 | 3 mg/kg: ↓ BWG, ↑ AST, unicellular/localized necrosis of liver cells, ↑ hematopoiesis of the spleen. <br> 9 mg/kg: Large PLTs, abnormality of RBCs. <br> 27 mg/kg: ↑ Mature megakaryocytes in the spleen, vacuolation, degeneration or necrosis of bile duct epithelium, ↑ neutrophils and megakaryocytes in bone marrow, infiltration of megakaryocytes, polynuclear giant cells and inflammatory cells in tracheal mucosa lamina propria, disarrangement or peeling of the small intestine mucosal epithelium, bleeding of ileal mucosa. |
| Cynomolgus monkey | 4 | 0, 1.7, 5, 15 | <1.7 | 1160/1300 | 15 mg/kg: Colon expansion, growth zone extension of the small intestine mucosa, ↑ direct bilirubin, ↑ liver weight, hepatocyte enlargement. |
| | 13 | 0, 1.3, 4, 12 | <1.3 | 894/1030 | 12 mg/kg: Bowel dilatation and hepatocyte enlargement, inflammatory cell infiltration of grisons sheath (female), ↓ RBCs, hypertrophy of adrenal cortical (male). |

[a] Male/Female.

## Safety Pharmacology

Table 27    Safety Pharmacology Studies of Alectinib[8]

| Study | System | Dose | Finding |
|---|---|---|---|
| Cardiovascular effect | hERG current/Transfected HEK293 cell | 0.141, 0.246, 0.470 μM | The $IC_{50}$ of hERG tail current: 0.45 μM. |
| | Cynomolgus monkey | 20, 60 mg/kg, p.o. | Decrease of BP at 20 and 60 mg/kg. |
| | | 1.7, 5, 15 mg/kg, p.o. | No effects on HR, BP, ECG or body temperature. |
| | Cav 1.2 calcium current/CHO cell | 0.189, 0.339, 0.764 μM | The $IC_{50}$ of $Ca^{2+}$ current: 0.461 μM. |
| | Vasomotion/Isolated rat aorta | 0.0160, 0.0723, 0.247, 0.860, 3.38 μM | The $IC_{50}$ of vasomotion: 0.168 μM. |
| Respiratory effect | Male Wistar rat | 3, 30, 300 mg/kg, p.o. | No effects on respiratory rate, tidal volume or min volume. |
| Neurological effect | Male Wistar rat | 3, 30, 300 mg/kg, p.o. | No effects on general condition or behavior. |

[8]    PMDA Database.    http://www.pmda.go.jp/drugs/2014/P201400094/index.html (accessed Mar 2016).

# Genotoxicity

Table 28　Genotoxicity Studies of Alectinib[8]

| Assay | Species/System | Metabolism Activity | Dose | Finding |
|---|---|---|---|---|
| *In vitro* bacterial reverse mutation assay (Ames) | *S. typhimurium* TA100, TA1535, TA98, TA1537; *E. coli* WP2 *uvr*A | ±S9 | 31.3-1000 μg/plate | Negative. |
| *In vitro* mammalian cell chromosomal aberration assay | CHL | ±S9 | 0, 4, 5, 6 μg/mL (6 h, -S9) 0, 3, 4, 5 μg/mL (24 h, -S9) 0, 7, 8, 9, 10 μg/mL (6 h, +S9) | Slightly ↑ polyploidy at 10 μg/mL in the short-term treatment assay with S9 mix. |
| | TK6 | -S9 | 0.4-6.3 μg/mL (-S9) | Cytotoxicity: 6.3 μg/mL. Significant ↑ CMN. |
| *In vivo rat* bone marrow micronucleus assay | Male Wistar rat | + | 6-2000 mg/kg/day, p.o. | Toxic/Cytotoxic effects: None. ≥500 mg/kg: statistically significant ↑ incidence of MN-PCEs. |
| | Wistar rat | + | 100-1000 mg/kg/day, p.o. | ≥500 mg/kg: statistically significant ↑ number of Fish-signal positive MNPCEs. |

Vehicle: DMSO for *in vitro* assays.

# Reproductive and Developmental Toxicity

Table 29　Reproductive and Developmental Toxicology Studies of Alectinib by Oral (Gavage) Administration[7, 8]

| Study | Species | Dose (mg/kg/day) | NOAEL Endpoint | NOAEL Dose (mg/kg/day) | NOAEL AUC$_{0-24}$ (ng·h/mL) | NOAEL Safety Margin (× MRHD) | Finding |
|---|---|---|---|---|---|---|---|
| Embryo-fetal development | Wistar rat | 0, 3, 9, 27 | Maternal | 3 | 13900 | 0.9 | >9 mg/kg: ↓ BWG and food consumption. 27 mg/kg: Red focus of the glandular stomach, dark-red discoloration in the mesenteric LNs, diminished size and black-brown discoloration in the adrenal gland. |
| | | | Fetal development | 3 | 13900 | 0.9 | 9 mg/kg: Low BW, delayed ossification (reduction of sacral and caudal vertebrae number), ↑ incidence of visceral abnormalities (ureter expansion, thymus cord, small ventricle, wall thinning ventricle). 27 mg/kg: ↑ Fetal mortality, early embryonic mortality and total litter loss. |
| | NZW rabbit | 0, 3, 9, 27 | Maternal | 9 | 6650 | 0.4 | >9 mg/kg: Morphological abnormality of RBCs. 27 mg/kg: Abortion, decrease in stool volume/no-stool, significant ↓ food consumption, low BW, anemia, deterioration and changes of nutritional status associated with inflammation or stress. |
| | | | Fetal development | 9 | 6650 | 0.4 | 27 mg/kg: Whole embryo lethality, ↑ resorption of post-implantation, ↑ number of embryo-fetal death, ↓ number of viable fetuses, low fetal weight and placental weight, abnormality of appearance, visceral and skeleton, ↑ skeletal variation. |

The AUC$_{ss,24}$ for the MRHD of 600 mg BID was 14900 ng·h/mL.

[7] FDA Database.　http://www.accessdata.fda.gov/drugsatfda_docs/nda/2015/208434Orig1s000PharmR.pdf (accessed Mar 2016).
[8] PMDA Database.　http://www.pmda.go.jp/drugs/2014/P201400094/index.html (accessed Mar 2016).

## Special Toxicology

Table 30    Special Toxicology Studies of Alectinib[8]

| Study | Species | Dose | Finding |
|-------|---------|------|---------|
| Neutral red uptake phototoxicity assay | Murine (Balb/c 3T3) fibroblast | 0, 0.02-50 µg/mL | Photo irritation factor: 94.8. |

Vehicle: PBS/1% DMSO.    The photo irritation factor (PIF): 94.8 (Calculated based on $IC_{50}$ (dark)/$IC_{50}$ (UVA) with the Photox version 2.0.

[8]  PMDA Database.    http://www.pmda.go.jp/drugs/2014/P201400094/index.html (accessed Mar 2016).

# CHAPTER

## 2

## Apatinib Mesylate

# Apatinib Mesylate

## (艾坦®)

Research code: YN-968D1

## 1 General Information

❖ Apatinib mesylate is a selective vascular endothelial growth factor receptor-2 (VEGFR-2) inhibitor, which was approved in Oct 2014 by CFDA.

❖ Apatinib mesylate was developed and marketed by Hengrui Pharmaceuticals.

❖ Apatinib mesylate inhibits VEGFR-2 and its related downstream signaling pathway, leading to inhibition of angiogenesis, which plays an important role in the growth and metastasis of malignant tumors.

❖ Apatinib mesylate is indicated for the treatment of patients with progression and refractory advanced gastric cancer who have been treated with at least two prior lines of chemotherapy.

❖ Available as tablet, with each containing 250 mg, 375 mg, or 425 mg of apatinib and the recommended starting dose is 850 mg once daily.

❖ The sale of 艾坦® was not available up to Mar 2016.

### Key Approvals around the World*

|  | China (CFDA) |
| --- | --- |
| First approval date | 10/17/2014 |
| Application or approval No. | 国药准字 H20140103 国药准字 H20140104 国药准字 H20140105 |
| Brand name | 艾坦® |
| Indication | Advanced gastric cancer |
| Authorisation holder | Hengrui Pharmaceuticals |

* Till Mar 2016, it had not been approved by FDA (US), EMA (EU) and PMDA (Japan).

## Active Ingredient

*Molecular formula*: $C_{24}H_{23}N_5O \cdot CH_4SO_3$
*Molecular weight*: 493.58
*CAS No.*: 811803-05-1 (Apatinib)
1218779-75-9 (Apatinib mesylate)
*Chemical name*: *N*-[4-(cyanocyclopentyl)-phenyl] {2-[(4-pyridylmethyl)amino](3-pyridyl)}carboxamide mesylate

*Parameters of Lipinski's "Rule of 5"*

| MW[a] | H$_D$ | H$_A$ | FRB[b] | PSA[b] | cLogP[b] |
| --- | --- | --- | --- | --- | --- |
| 397.47 | 2 | 6 | 5 | 90.7Å$^2$ | 3.66 ± 0.69 |

[a] Molecular weight of apatinib.  [b] Calculated by ACD/Labs software V11.02.

## Drug Product*

*Dosage route*: Oral
*Strength*: 250 mg/375 mg/425 mg (Apatinib)
*Dosage form*: Tablet
*Inactive ingredient*: Unknown
*Recommended dose*: The recommended dose is 850 mg once daily, taken half an hour after a meal.

* Sourced from CFDA drug label information

# 2 Key Patents Information

## Summary

❖ 艾坦® (Apatinib mesylate) was approved by CFDA on Oct 17, 2014.

❖ Apatinib was originally discovered by Chen guoqing (Paul), and then developed by Hengrui (Jiangsu Hengrui Medicine Co., Ltd.), and its compound patent application was filed as PCT application by Chen guoqing in 2004.

❖ The compound patent will expire in 2022 foremost, which has been granted in China, United States, Japan and Europe successively.

Table 1　Apatinib mesylate's Compound Patent Protection in Drug-Mainstream Country

| Country | Publication/Patent NO. | Application Date | Granted Date | Estimated Expiry Date |
| --- | --- | --- | --- | --- |
| WO | WO2005000232A2 | 06/04/2004 | / | / |
| US | US7129252B2 | 06/02/2004 | 10/31/2006 | 10/08/2024 |
| EP | EP1633712B1 | 06/04/2004 | 06/25/2014 | 06/04/2024 |
| JP | JP5046643B2 | 06/04/2004 | 10/10/2012 | 06/04/2024 |
| CN | CN1281590C | 11/27/2002 | 10/25/2006 | 11/27/2022 |

Table 2　Originator's International Patent Application List (Patent Family)

| Publication NO. | Title | Applicant/Assignee/Owner | Publication Date |
| --- | --- | --- | --- |
| **Technical Subjects** | **Active Ingredient (Free Base)'s Formula or Structure and Preparation** | | |
| WO2005000232A2 | Six membered amino-amide derivatives as angiogenesis inhibitors | Chen Guoqing (Paul) | 01/06/2005 |
| **Technical Subjects** | **Salt, Crystal, Polymorphic, Solvate (Hydrate), Isomer, Derivative Etc. and Preparation** | | |
| WO2010031266A1 | The salts of N-[4-(1-cyanocyclopentyl)phenyl]-2-(4-pyridylmethyl)amino-3-pyridine carboxamide | Hengrui | 03/25/2010 |
| **Technical Subjects** | **Indication or Methods for Medical Needs** | | |
| WO2010031265A1 | Pharmaceutical composition for the treatment of proliferative diseases | Hengrui | 03/25/2010 |
| **Technical Subjects** | **Combination Including at Least Two Active Ingredients** | | |
| WO2011050684A1 | Pharmaceutical composition for treating tumor | Hengrui | 05/05/2011 |

The data was updated until Jan 2016.

# 3 Chemistry

## Route 1: Original Discovery Route

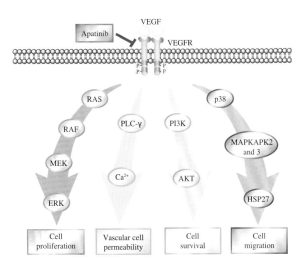

*Synthetic Route*: The synthetic route of apatinib mesylate based on a patent disclosure outlined preparation of the active pharmaceutical ingredient (API). The synthesis started from commercially available 1-phenyl cyclopentane carbonitrile **1**, which was regioselectively nitrated to provide nitrobenzene **2**. Subsequent reduction of **2** *via* catalytic hydrogenation gave the corresponding aniline **3**, which was subsequently coupled with 2-chloronicotinoyl chloride **4** to afford aryl amide **5**. No yield was reported for the preparation of aryl amide **5** from starting material **1**. Amination of the 2-pyridyl chloride **5** with pyridin-4-ylmethanamine **6** in hot pentanol followed by salt formation with methylsulfonic acid afforded apatinib mesylate in 77% yield.[1-5]

# 4 Pharmacology

## Summary

Mechanism of Action

❖ Apatinib is an oral tyrosine kinase inhibitor targeting VEGFR-2 (IC$_{50}$ = 1 nM), thereby inhibiting angiogenesis, which plays an important role in the growth and metastasis of malignant tumors.

❖ Apatinib inhibited VEGFR-2, resulting in inhibition of angiogenesis, migration, and stimulated cell proliferation *in vitro* studies.

❖ M1-1, a metabolite of apatinib, showed significant inhibition to VEGFR-2 (IC$_{50}$ = 19.2 nM), c-kit (IC$_{50}$ = 125 nM) and PDGFR-$\beta$ (IC$_{50}$ = 46.9 nM).

❖ Apatinib inhibited the growth in a broad range of xenografted human tumors *in vivo* in a dose-dependent manner, but did not inhibit the growth of these cancer cell lines *in vitro*, suggesting that the antitumor activity was *via* an anti-angiogenic mechanism rather than due to a direct inhibition of cell proliferation.

[1] Chen, G. P. US20040259916A1, **2004**.
[2] Yuan, K.; Sun, P.; Zhou, Y., et al. WO2010031266A1, **2010**.
[3] Yuan, K.; Sun, P.; Zhou, Y., et al. US8362256B2, **2013**.
[4] Yuan, K.; Sun, P. WO2010031265A1, **2010**.
[5] Sun, Z.; Tao, H. CN1502608A, **2004**.

*In Vitro* Efficacy

❖ Apatinib inhibited phosphorylation of RTKs and its related downstream molecules in cells:
  • VEGFR and ERK1/2: Completely blocked at 10 μM.
  • c-kit and PDGFR: Completely blocked at 1 μM.
  • HER2 and EGFR: No effect.
❖ Inhibited proliferation of HUVEC cells:
  • In 20% FBS condition: $IC_{50}$ = 23.4 μM.
  • Activated by VEGF: $IC_{50}$ = 0.17 μM.
❖ Inhibited *in vitro* angiogenesis and migration:
  • In HUVEC tube formation assay: Significant inhibition at 1 μM.
  • In HUVEC transwell migration assay: Significant inhibition at 1 μM.
  • In microvessel growth from rat aortic ring: Significant inhibition at 0.1 μM.

*In Vivo* Efficacy

❖ Tumor growth inhibition in human lung carcinoma xenograft mice models:
  • Significant inhibition at 100 mg/kg/day in both NCI-H460 (T/C% = 57%) and A549 (T/C% = 41%) models.
  • Apatinib was enhanced by the combination with docetaxel or doxorubicin ($P$ <0.05) in NCI-H460 model.
❖ Tumor growth inhibition in human colon carcinoma xenograft mice models:
  • Significant inhibition at 50 mg/kg/day in both HCT-116 (T/C% = 63%), HT-29 (T/C% = 59%) and Ls174t (T/C% = 72%) models.
  • Apatinib was enhanced by the combination with oxaliplatin or 5-FU ($P$ <0.05) in Ls174t model.
❖ Tumor growth inhibition in human stomach carcinoma SGC-7901 xenograft mice models:
  • Significant at 100 mg/kg/day (T/C% = 33%).

# Mechanism of Action

Table 3　*In Vitro* Kinase Activity of Apatinib[6]

| Kinase | $IC_{50}$ (nM) | | Kinase | $IC_{50}$ (nM) | |
| --- | --- | --- | --- | --- | --- |
| | Apatinib | Sunitinib | | Apatinib | Sunitinib |
| VEGFR-2 | 1 | 5 | c-src | 530 | 2200 |
| c-kit | 429 | 1 | EGFR | >10000 | >10000 |
| PDGFR-$\alpha$ | >1000 | 13 | HER2 | >10000 | >10000 |
| Ret | 13 | 72 | FGFR1 | >10000 | 510 |

The inhibitory activity of apatinib against tyrosine kinases was determined using ELISA methodology.　In US2011/0184023A1, the $IC_{50}$ value of c-src was >10000 nM.

Table 4　Binding of Apatinib and Its Metabolite to Human Plasma Proteins and *In Vitro* Pharmacological Studies[7]

| Compound | $IC_{50}$ (nM) | | | PAI (%) | | |
| --- | --- | --- | --- | --- | --- | --- |
| | VEGFR-2 | PDGFR-$\beta$ | c-kit | VEGFR-2 | PDGFR-$\beta$ | c-kit |
| Apatinib | 1.90 | 16.5 | 12.9 | 100 | 100 | 100 |
| M1-1 | 19.2 | 46.9 | 125 | 5.42 | 19.3 | 5.66 |
| M1-2 | 179 | 1352 | 2511 | 0.22 | 0.25 | 0.11 |
| M1-6 | 265 | 369 | 981 | 0.32 | 0.80 | 0.77 |
| M9-2 | Inactive | Inactive | Inactive | Inactive | Inactive | Inactive |

Percent of protein binding was measured by ultracentrifugation.　PAI = (metabolite AUC at steady state × percent of protein binding of metabolite × $IC_{50}$ of parent)/(parent AUC at steady state × parent percent of protein binding × $IC_{50}$ of metabolite) × 100.　PAI: Pharmacological activity index.

[6]　Tian, S.; Quan, H.; Xie, C., et al. *Cancer Sci.* **2011**, *102*, 1374-1380.
[7]　Ding, J.; Chen, X.; Gao, Z., et al. *Drug Metab. Dispos.* **2013**, *41*, 1195-1210.

## *In Vitro* Efficacy

Table 5　*In Vitro* Efficacy of Apatinib[6]

| Study | | Cell Line | Stimulator/Condition | Effect | |
|---|---|---|---|---|---|
| **Test** | **Target** | | | **Effect Dose (μM)[a]** | **Finding** |
| Phosphorylation | VEGFR-2 | HUVEC | VEGF | 10 | Completely blocked |
| | ERK1/2 | HUVEC | VEGF | 10 | Completely blocked |
| | c-kit | Mo7e | Stem cell factor | 1 | Completely blocked |
| | PDGFR | NIH-3T3 | PDGF | 1 | Completely blocked |
| | EGFR | NA | EGF | No effect | Up to 10 μM |
| | HER2 | NA | NA | No effect | Up to 10 μM |
| Cell proliferation[b] | | HUVEC | 20% FBS | $IC_{50} = 23.4$ μM | Sunitinib: $IC_{50} = 7.4$ μM |
| | | HUVEC | VEGF | $IC_{50} = 0.17$ μM | Sunitinib: $IC_{50} = 0.034$ μM |
| Tube formation[c] | | HUVEC | 20% FBS | 1 | - |
| Transwell migration[d] | | HUVEC | 20% FBS | 1 | - |
| Microvessel formation[e] | | Rat aortic ring | FBS | 0.1 | - |

HUVEC: Human umbilical vein endothelial cells.　VEGF: Vascular endothelial growth factor.　VEGFR: Vascular endothelial growth factor receptor.　ERK: A downstream of VEGF signaling.　PDGF: Platelet derived growth factor.　PDGFR: Platelet derived growth factor receptor.　EGF: Endothelial growth factor.　EGFR: Endothelial growth factor receptor.　Sunitinib is an oral multikinase inhibitor with antiangiogenic and antitumor properties that targets VEGFR, c-kit, platelet derived growth factor receptors (PDGFR), FLT-3, CSF-1R and Ret.　[a] $P <0.05$ versus vehicle control.　[b] HUVEC were incubated with test agent together with 20% FBS or 20 ng/mL VEGF.　[c] HUVEC suspended in M199 medium with 20% FBS were added into solidified matrigel, with different test agents for 8 h, and the cells were imaged using a high magnificent field.　[d] Transwell migration assays using the corning chamber showed that the migration of HUVEC induced by 20% FBS.　[e] The aortic rings were embedded in matrigel and incubated in supplemented media at 37 °C, 5% $CO_2$ for 6 days.

## *In Vivo* Efficacy

Table 6　Anti-tumor Efficacy in Xenograft Tumor Models[6, 8]

| Tumor Xenograft Model | | | Administration | | Effect | |
|---|---|---|---|---|---|---|
| **Model** | **Origin** | **Animal** | **Dose (mg/kg)** | **Route & Schedule (day)** | **T/C (%)[a]** | ***P*-value** |
| NCI-H460 | Lung | Balb/cA nude mouse | 100 | p.o., QD × 14 | 57 | 0.017 |
| | | | 200 | p.o., QD × 14 | 17 | <0.001 |
| | | | 150 | p.o., QD × 14 | 46 | - |
| | | | Docetaxel: 12 | i.v., Q4D × 3 | 37 | - |
| | | | Apatinib: 150 Docetaxel: 12 | Apatinib: p.o., QD × 14 Docetaxel: i.v., Q4D × 3 | 7 | <0.05[b] |
| | | | Doxorubicin: 10 | i.v., single dose | 35 | - |
| | | | Apatinib: 150 Doxorubicin: 10 | Apatinib: p.o., QD × 14 Doxorubicin: i.v., single dose | 14 | <0.05[b] |
| A549 | Lung | Balb/cA nude mouse | 50 | p.o., QD × 14 | 73 | 0.198 |
| | | | 100 | p.o., QD × 14 | 41 | 0.012 |
| | | | 200 | p.o., QD × 14 | 17 | 0.001 |
| HCT 116 | Colon | Balb/cA nude mouse | 50 | p.o., QD × 21 | 63 | 0.009 |
| | | | 100 | p.o., QD × 21 | 40 | <0.001 |
| | | | 200 | p.o., QD × 21 | 14 | <0.001 |

[6]　Tian, S.; Quan, H.; Xie, C., et al. *Cancer Sci.* **2011**, *102*, 1374-1380.
[8]　Yuan, K., Sun, P. Y. US2011/0184023A1, **2011**.

*Continued*

| Tumor Xenograft Model | | | Administration | | Effect | |
|---|---|---|---|---|---|---|
| **Model** | **Origin** | **Animal** | **Dose (mg/kg)** | **Route & Schedule (Day)** | **T/C (%)[a]** | **P-value** |
| HT-29 | Colon | Balb/cA nude mouse | 50 | p.o., QD × 21 | 59 | 0.005 |
| | | | 100 | p.o., QD × 21 | 42 | <0.001 |
| | | | 200 | p.o., QD × 21 | 18 | <0.001 |
| Ls174t | Colon | Balb/cA nude mouse | 50 | p.o., QD × 14 | 72 | 0.014 |
| | | | 100 | p.o., QD × 14 | 43 | <0.001 |
| | | | 200 | p.o., QD × 14 | 8 | <0.001 |
| | | | 150 | p.o., QD × 14 | 28 | - |
| | | | Oxaliplatin: 6 | i.v., QD × 3 | 54 | - |
| | | | Apatinib: 150 Oxaliplatin: 6 | Apatinib: p.o., QD × 14 Oxaliplatin: i.v., QD × 3 | 5 | <0.05[b] |
| | | | 75 | p.o., QD × 14 | 60 | - |
| | | | 5-FU: 50 | i.v., QD × 3 | 60 | - |
| | | | Apatinib: 75 5-FU: 50 | Apatinib: p.o., QD × 14 5-FU: i.v., QD × 3 | 40 | <0.05[b] |
| SGC-7901 | Stomach | Balb/cA nude mouse | 50 | p.o., QD × 18 | 58 | 0.067 |
| | | | 100 | p.o., QD × 18 | 33 | 0.006 |
| | | | 200 | p.o., QD × 18 | 12 | 0.001 |

Q4D: Once daily for four days.   [a] T/C (%) = Mean increase of tumor volumes of treated groups/mean increase of tumor volumes of control groups × 100%.   [b] $P$ <0.05 versus apatinib alone or cytotoxic drugs alone (n = 6).

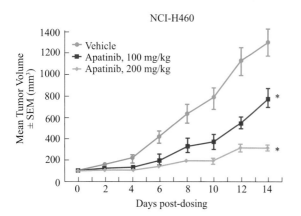

**Study:** Anti-tumor activities in NCI-H460 xenograft model.

**Animal:** Balb/cA nude mouse.

**Model:** NCI-H460 cells s.c. injected in Balb/cA nude mice.

**Administration:** Oral, once daily for 14 days.   Apatinib: 100, 200 mg/kg; Vehicle: NA.

**Starting:** Tumors were established (100-300 mm³).

**Test:** Tumor volume, formula: (a × b²)/2.

**Results:** Significantly inhibited tumor growth at 100 mg/kg (T/C% = 57%) or 200 mg/kg (T/C% = 17%).   * $P$ <0.05 versus control.

Figure A   Anti-tumor Activities of Apatinib in Human Lung Carcinoma NCI-H460 Xenograft Model[6]

[6]   Tian, S.; Quan, H.; Xie, C., et al. *Cancer Sci.* **2011**, *102*, 1374-1380.

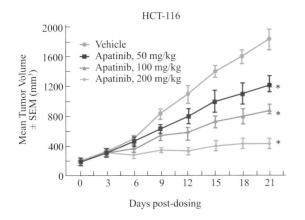

**Study:** Anti-tumor activities in HCT-116 xenograft model.

**Animal:** Balb/cA nude mouse.

**Model:** HCT-116 cells s.c. injected in Balb/cA nude mice.

**Administration:** Oral, once daily for 21 days.    Apatinib: 50, 100, 200 mg/kg; Vehicle: NA.

**Starting:** Tumors were established (100-300 mm$^3$).

**Test:** Tumor volume, formula: $(a \times b^2)/2$.

**Results**: Significantly inhibited tumor growth at 50 mg/kg (T/C% = 63%), 100 mg/kg (T/C% = 40%) and 200 mg/kg (T/C% = 14%).   * $P$ <0.05 versus control.

Figure B    Anti-tumor Activities of Apatinib in Human Colon Carcinoma HCT-116 Xenograft Model[6]

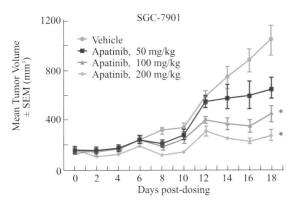

**Study:** Anti-tumor activities in SGC-7901 xenograft model.

**Animal:** Balb/cA nude mouse.

**Model:** SGC-7901 cells s.c. injected in Balb/cA nude mice.

**Administration:** Oral, once daily for 18 days.    Apatinib: 50, 100, 200 mg/kg; Vehicle: NA.

**Starting:** Tumors were established (100-300 mm$^3$).

**Test:** Tumor volume, formula: $(a \times b^2)/2$.

**Results**: Significantly inhibited tumor growth at 100 mg/kg (T/C% = 33%) or 200 mg/kg (T/C% = 12%).   * $P$ <0.05 versus control.

Figure C    Anti-tumor Activities of Apatinib in Human Stomach Carcinoma SGC-7901 Xenograft Model[6]

# 5   ADME & Drug-Drug Interaction

## Summary

### Absorption of Apatinib
❖ Had low oral bioavailability in male dogs (9.24%) and female dogs (15.4%) after single oral administration of apatinib mesylate.
❖ Was absorbed moderately in humans ($T_{max}$ = 2.9 h) and in rats (1.33 h).
❖ Showed a half-life ranging between 8-9 h in humans after oral administration, longer than that in rats (1.78 h).

### Distribution of Apatinib
❖ Apatinib and M1-1 exhibited high plasma protein binding in humans (92.4% and 90.1%), M1-2 and M1-6 exhibited moderate plasma protein binding (88% and 75.8%).

### Metabolism of Apatinib
❖ Was extensively metabolized in human liver microsomes and recombinant enzymes.
❖ Was metabolized primarily by CYP3A4/5, to a lesser extent, by CYP2D6, 2C9 and 2E1.
❖ UGT2B7 was the main enzyme responsible for the formation of M9-2.    Both UGT1A4 and UGT2B7 were responsible for the formation of *Z*-3-hydroxy-apatinib-*O*-glucuronide (M9-1).
❖ Overall, the parent drug represented the most abundant component in human plasma, with M9-2 (*O*-glucuronide) as the major metabolite.
❖ The steady-state exposures of *E*-3-hydroxy-apatinib (M1-1), *Z*-3-hydroxy-apatinib (M1-2), and apatinib-25-*N*-oxide (M1-6) were 56%, 22% and 32% of parent drug exposure, respectively.
❖ M1-1, M1-2 and M1-6 were pharmacologically active in inhibiting VEGFR-2 and VEGFR-*β*, but the major circulating metabolite (M9-2) was inactive.

[6]   Tian, S.; Quan, H.; Xie, C., et al. *Cancer Sci.* **2011**, *102*, 1374-1380.

Excretion of Apatinib

❖ Was predominantly excreted in feces with the parent drug as the most significant component in human feces.

❖ Unchanged apatinib was detected in negligible quantities in urine, indicating that systemically available apatinib was extensively metabolized.

Drug-Drug Interaction

❖ Apatinib had a higher affinity for BCRP compared with P-gp and it was likely a substrate for both BCRP and P-gp.

❖ Apatinib significantly inhibited P-gp ($IC_{50} = 2.9$ µM) and BCRP-mediated ($IC_{50} = 11$ µM) transport in MDR cells.

❖ Apatinib did not significantly alter the mRNA or protein levels of P-gp and BCRP.

## Absorption

Table 7    *In Vivo* Pharmacokinetic Parameters of Apatinib in SD Rats after Single Oral Dose of Apatinib[8]

| Species | Dose (mg/kg) | Compound | $T_{max}$ (h) | $C_{max}$ (ng/mL) | $AUC_{0-8}$ (ng·h/mL) | $T_{1/2}$ (h) | Cl/F (L/h/kg) | $V_d$/F (L/kg) |
|---|---|---|---|---|---|---|---|---|
| SD rat | 20 | Apatinib | 1.33 ± 0.29 | 69.6 ± 9.2 | 226 ± 63 | 1.78 ± 0.57 | 91.5 ± 23.6 | 300 ± 69.4 |
| | 20 | Hydrochloride | 0.92 ± 0.95 | 463 ± 334 | 814 ± 149 | 1.96 ± 1.25 | 22.6 ± 6.7 | 67.9 ± 37.9 |
| | 20 | Phosphate | 0.33 ± 0.14 | 237 ± 131 | 366 ± 254 | 1.02 ± 0.43 | 65.6 ± 31.1 | 109 ± 65.1 |
| | 20 | Maleate | 0.92 ± 0.94 | 156 ± 86 | 456 ± 343 | 0.77 ± 0.04 | 69.1 ± 56 | 154 ± 118 |
| | 20 | Mesylate | 0.33 ± 0.14 | 489 ± 296 | 697 ± 283 | 0.87 ± 0.39 | 32.4 ± 15.5 | 57.3 ± 43.2 |

Table 8    *In Vivo* Pharmacokinetic Parameters of Apatinib in Humans after Single Oral Dose of Apatinib[9]

| Species | Dose (mg) | $C_{max}$ (ng/mL) | $AUC_{0-24}$ (ng·h/mL) | $T_{1/2}$ (h) |
|---|---|---|---|---|
| Human | 500 | 1521 | 11295 | 8 |
| | 750 | 2379 | 18172 | 9 |
| | 850 | 2833 | 21975 | 9 |

Table 9    *In Vivo* Pharmacokinetic Parameters of Apatinib and Metabolites in Humans with Advanced Colorectal Cancer after Single Oral Dose of 750 mg Apatinib Mesylate (n =12)[7]

| Parameter | Apatinib | M1-1 | M1-2 | M1-6 | M9-1 | M9-2 |
|---|---|---|---|---|---|---|
| $T_{max}$ (h) | 2.9 ± 1.4 | 5.2 ± 4.8 | 5.0 ± 4.8 | 7.7 ± 6.3 | 7.1 ± 4.5 | 10.2 ± 3.7 |
| $C_{max}$ (nM) | 3819 ± 2204 | 849 ± 268 | 339 ± 131 | 375 ± 172 | 36.5 ± 22.0 | 1543 ± 819 |
| $AUC_{0-24}$ (nM·h) | 30941 ± 18794 | 12458 ± 4380 | 4796 ± 2049 | 6605 ± 2806 | 555 ± 322 | 27276 ± 14147 |

The values were mean ± SD, n = 20.

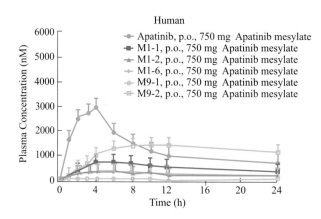

Human
- Apatinib, p.o., 750 mg  Apatinib mesylate
- M1-1, p.o., 750 mg  Apatinib mesylate
- M1-2, p.o., 750 mg  Apatinib mesylate
- M1-6, p.o., 750 mg  Apatinib mesylate
- M9-1, p.o., 750 mg  Apatinib mesylate
- M9-2, p.o., 750 mg  Apatinib mesylate

Figure D    *In Vivo* Plasma Concentration-Time Profiles of Apatinib and Metabolites in Humans after Single Oral Dose of Apatinib Mesylate (n = 12)[7]

[7]  Ding, J.; Chen, X.; Gao, Z., et al. *Drug Metab. Dispos.* **2013**, *41*, 1195-1210.

[8]  Yuan, K., Sun, P. Y. US2011/0184023A1, **2011**.

[9]  Li, J.; Zhao, X.; Chen, L., et al. *BMC Cancer* **2010**, *10*, 529.

**Key Findings:**[7]

❖ Apatinib exhibited low oral bioavailability in male dogs (9.24%) and female dogs (15.4%) after single oral administration of apatinib mesylate.

❖ The systemic clearances for all the metabolites quantified were slightly slower than that for the parent drug.

❖ The accumulation degrees of apatinib and its metabolites seemed moderate, with mean $AUC_{0-24}$ accumulation ratios ranging from 1.77 to 3.69.

## Distribution

Table 10    *In Vitro* Plasma Protein Binding of Apatinib and Metabolites[7]

| Species | Compound | Apatinib | M1-1 | M1-2 | M1-6 |
|---------|----------|----------|------|------|------|
| Human | %Bound | 92.4 ± 3.2 | 90.1 ± 2.2 | 88.0 ± 3.2 | 75.8 ± 3.7 |

**Key Findings:**[10]

❖ The binding efficiencies of apatinib to multiple plasma protein in rats, canines, monkeys and humans were in the range of 86%-93%.

## Metabolism

Table 11    *In Vitro* Metabolic Stability of Apatinib in Human Liver Microsomes and Recombinant CYP Enzymes[7]

| Formation of Metabolite | Kinetic Parameter | HLM | Recombinant CYP Enzyme | | |
|---|---|---|---|---|---|
| | | | CYP3A4 | CYP3A5 | CYP2D6 |
| M1-1 | $K_m$ (μM) | 1.93 ± 0.33 | 0.57 ± 0.13 | 0.28 ± 0.05 | 0.69 ± 0.15 |
| | $V_{max}$ | 3.28 ± 0.19 | 0.05 ± 0.003 | 0.02 ± 0.0007 | 1.07 ± 0.06 |
| | $Cl_{int}$ | 1.70 ± 0.21 | 0.09 ± 0.02 | 0.07 ± 0.01 | 1.56 ± 0.29 |
| | $R^2$ | 0.973 | 0.912 | 0.932 | 0.946 |
| M1-2 | $K_m$ (μM) | 2.18 ± 0.29 | 0.90 ± 0.15 | 0.26 ± 0.03 | NA |
| | $V_{max}$ | 39.1 ± 1.79 | 1.29 ± 0.06 | 0.88 ± 0.02 | NA |
| | $Cl_{int}$ | 17.9 ± 1.74 | 1.44 ± 0.20 | 3.38 ± 0.35 | NA |
| | $R^2$ | 0.985 | 0.964 | 0.975 | NA |
| M1-6 | $K_m$ (μM) | 1.41 ± 0.22 | 1.02 ± 0.17 | 0.30 ± 0.03 | 0.53 ± 0.12 |
| | $V_{max}$ | 9.82 ± 0.46 | 0.31 ± 0.01 | 0.16 ± 0.004 | 4.60 ± 0.24 |
| | $Cl_{int}$ | 7.01 ± 0.83 | 0.30 ± 0.04 | 0.52 ± 0.05 | 8.68 ± 1.61 |
| | $R^2$ | 0.976 | 0.969 | 0.979 | 0.939 |

The values were mean ± SD.    The unit for $V_{max}$ was pmol/min/mg protein for HLM and pmol/min/pmol P450 for CYP3A4, 3A5 and 2D6.    The unit for $Cl_{int}$ was μL/min/mg protein for HLM and μL/min/pmol P450 for CYP3A4, 3A5 and 2D6.    $Cl_{int}$: Intrinsic clearance.    HLM: Human liver microsomes.    $K_m$: Michaelis constant. $R^2$: Calculated correlation coefficient.

[7]    Ding, J.; Chen, X.; Gao, Z., et al. *Drug Metab. Dispos.* **2013**, *41*, 1195-1210.
[10]   Geng, R. X.; Li, J. *Expert. Opin. Pharmacother.* **2015**, *16*, 117-122.

## Key Findings:[7]

❖ Apatinib was incubated in human microsomes and cytochrome enzymes for 1 h:
  • More than 95% of the parent drug was consumed in CYP2D6, 3A4 and 3A5 incubations.
  • About 30% to 50% of the parent drug was consumed in CYP2C9 and 2E1 incubations.
  • About 5% to 15% of the parent drug was consumed in CYP1B1, 2C8 and 2C19 incubations.
  • Less than 5% of the parent drug was consumed in CYP1A2, 2A6, 2B6, 4A11, FMO1, 3 and 5 incubations, indicating that these cytochromes and FMO enzymes contributed minimally to the metabolism of apatinib.
  • M1-1, M1-2 and M1-6 had pharmacological activity to inhibit VEGFR-2 ($IC_{50}$ = 19, 179 and 265 nM, respectively), VEGFR-$\beta$ ($IC_{50}$ = 47, 1352 and 369 nM, respectively) and c-kit ($IC_{50}$ = 125, 2511 and 981 nM, respectively).
  • Apatinib was metabolized primarily by CYP3A4/5, to a lesser extent, by CYP2D6, CYP2C9 and CYP2E1.   UGT2B7 was the main enzyme responsible for M9-2 formation.   Both UGT1A4 and UGT2B7 were responsible for Z-3-hydroxy-apatinib-O-glucuronide (M9-1) formation.

Table 12   Metabolites in Plasma, Urine and Feces of Humans after Oral Dose of Apatinib Mesylate[7]

| Matrix | Dose (mg) | Time (h) | %Relative Peak Area | | | | | | | | | | | |
|---|---|---|---|---|---|---|---|---|---|---|---|---|---|---|
| | | | M0 | M1-1 | M1-2 | M1-3 | M1-6 | M2 | M3-1 | M3-2 | M3-3 | M8-2 | M9-1 | M9-2 |
| Plasma | 750 | 4 | 41.4 | 19.2 | 7.43 | 1.61 | 1.70 | 2.67 | 1.51 | 1.65 | 0.40 | 0.52 | 0.69 | 19.6 |
| | | 8 | 27.8 | 17.8 | 6.31 | 1.41 | 2.28 | 3.55 | 2.85 | 1.73 | 0.74 | 0.82 | 0.53 | 32.2 |
| Urine | 750 | 0-24 | ND | 14.6 | 12.0 | 1.71 | 2.35 | ND | 2.26 | 0.52 | 0.17 | 10.3 | 1.07 | 27.9 |
| Feces | 750 | 34-48 | 76.7 | 7.43 | 2.92 | 0.47 | 0.12 | 1.05 | ND | ND | ND | ND | ND | ND |
| | | 0-96 | 59[a] | 2.76[a] | 1.20[a] | NA | 0.02[a] | NA | NA | NA | NA | NA | NA | NA |

M0: Parent.   M1-1: E-3-hydroxylation.   M1-2: Z-3-hydroxylation.   M1-3: Mono-oxygenation.   M1-6: 25-N-oxidation.   M2: N-dealkylation.   M3-1: Z-3-hydroxylation and N-dealkylation.   M3-2: E-3-hydroxylation and N-dealkylation.   M3-3: Mono-oxygenation and N-dealkylation.   M8-2: E-3-hydroxylation, N-dealkylation and O-glucuronidation.   M9-1: Z-3-hydroxylation and O-glucuronidation.   M9-2: E-3-hydroxylation and O-glucuronidation.   [a] % of dose.

## Key Findings:[7]

❖ Systemically available apatinib was extensively metabolized.
❖ The major circulating metabolite, M9-2 (E-3-hydroxy-apatinib-O-glucuronide), was pharmacologically inactive, the steady-state exposure of which was 125% of the parent drug at steady state.   The systemic exposure of M1-1, M1-2, and M1-6 was 56%, 22% and 32% of the parent drug, respectively.
❖ Calculated as pharmacological activity index values, the contribution of M1-1 to the pharmacology of the drug was 5.42%-19.3% of the parent drug.   The contribution of M1-2 and M1-6 to the drug's pharmacology was less than 1%.

[7]   Ding, J.; Chen, X.; Gao, Z., et al. *Drug Metab. Dispos.* **2013**, *41*, 1195-1210.

Figure E    Proposed Pathways for *In Vivo* Biotransformation of Apatinib in Humans[7]
The red labels represent the main components in the matrices.    P = Plasma, U = Urine and F = Feces.

## Metabolic Phenotyping:[7]

❖ *In vitro* metabolism studies on recombinant human isozymes and inhibition studies on selective chemical inhibitors of human P450 enzymes demonstrated that the oxidative metabolism of apatinib was mediated by CYP3A4/5 and, to a lesser extent, by CYP2D6, 2C9 and 2E1.    All tested cytochrome isoforms were capable of the formation of M1-1 and M1-2.

❖ M1-1 was produced to the greatest extent by CYP2D6 and to a lesser extent by CYP3A4 and 3A5.    M1-2 was produced to the greatest extent by CYP3A4 and 3A5.    M1-6 was predominantly formed by CYP2D6 and to a lesser extent by CYP3A4 and 3A5.    *N*-dealkylation of apatinib was mediated predominantly by CYP3A4/5.

[7]    Ding, J.; Chen, X.; Gao, Z., et al. *Drug Metab. Dispos.* **2013**, *41*, 1195-1210.

❖ UGT1A1, 1A3, 1A4, 1A8, 1A9, 2B4, 2B7 and 2B17 all catalyzed the formation of M9-2, with UGT2B7 having the highest activity.

❖ UGT1A1, 1A3, 1A4, 1A8, 2B4, and 2B7 all catalyzed the formation of M9-1, with UGT1A4 having the highest activity, followed by UGT2B7.

## Excretion

Table 13    Excretion Profiles of Apatinib-Related Compounds after Single Oral Dose of Apatinib Mesylate in Healthy Subjects[7]

| Species | Gender | Route | Dose (mg) | Time (h) | Urine (% of dose) | Feces (% of dose) | Recovery (% of dose) |
|---------|--------|-------|-----------|----------|-------------------|-------------------|----------------------|
| Human | Male & Female | p.o. | 750 | 0-96 | 7.02 ± 1.77 | 69.8 ± 16.1 | 76.8 ± 14.9 |

Mean ± SD, n = 12.

## Drug-Drug Interaction[11]

❖ Apatinib had a higher affinity with BCRP compared with P-gp and that was likely a substrate for both BCRP and P-gp.

❖ Apatinib significantly inhibited P-gp ($IC_{50}$ = 2.9 μM) and BCRP-mediated ($IC_{50}$ = 11 μM) transport in MDR cells.

❖ Apatinib did not significantly alter the mRNA or protein levels of P-gp and BCRP.    Apatinib reversed ABCB1- and ABCG2-mediated MDR by directly inhibiting ABCB1 and ABCG2 function, resulting in elevated intracellular concentrations of substrate chemotherapeutic drugs.

# 6    Non-Clinical Toxicology

## Summary

Single-Dose Toxicity
❖ Dog MTD: 30 mg/kg.[9]

Repeated-Dose Toxicity
❖ NA.

Safety Pharmacology
❖ NA.

Genotoxicity
❖ NA.

Reproductive and Developmental Toxicity
❖ NA.

Carcinogenicity
❖ NA.

[7]  Ding, J.; Chen, X.; Gao, Z., et al. *Drug Metab. Dispos.* **2013**, *41*, 1195-1210.

[9]  Li, J.; Zhao, X.; Chen, L., et al. *BMC Cancer* **2010**, *10*, 529.

[11]  Mi, Y. J.; Liang, Y. J.; Huang, H. B., et al. *Cancer Res.* **2010**, *70*, 7981-7991.

# CHAPTER

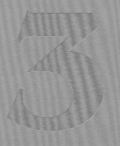

## Apremilast

# Apremilast

(Otezla®)

Research code: CC-10004

## 1  General Information

- ❖ Apremilast is an inhibitor of phosphodiesterase 4 (PDE4), which was first approved in Mar 2014 by US FDA.

- ❖ Apremilast was originally discovered, developed and marketed by Celgene.

- ❖ Apremilast inhibits PDE4 and elevates intracellular cyclic adenosine monophosphate (cAMP) levels, which works intracellularly to modulate a network of pro- and anti-inflammatory mediators in psoriasis and psoriatic arthritis (PsA).

- ❖ Apremilast is indicated for the treatment of adult patients with active psoriatic arthritis.

- ❖ Available as tablet, with each containing 10 mg, 20 mg or 30 mg of apremilast and the recommended dose is 30 mg orally once daily until disease progression or unacceptable toxicity.

- ❖ The 2014 and 2015 worldwide sales of Otezla® were 69.8 and 471.7 million US$, respectively, referring to the financial reports of Celgene.

### Key Approvals around the World*

|  | US (FDA) | EU (EMA) |
|---|---|---|
| First approval date | 03/21/2014 | 01/15/2015 |
| Application or approval No. | NDA 205437 | EMEA/H/C/003746 |
| Brand name | Otezla® | Otezla® |
| Indication | Active psoriatic arthritis | Active psoriatic arthritis |
| Authorisation holder | Celgene | Celgene |

* Till Mar 2016, it had not been approved by PMDA (Japan) and CFDA (China).

## Active Ingredient

*Molecular formula*:  $C_{22}H_{24}N_2O_7S$
*Molecular weight*:  460.50
*CAS No.*:  608141-41-9 (Apremilast)
*Chemical name*:  $N$-[2-[(1$S$)-1-(3-ethoxy-4-methoxy-phenyl)-2-(methylsulfonyl)ethyl]-2,3-dihydro-1,3-dioxo-1$H$-isoindol-4-yl]acetamide

*Parameters of Lipinski's "Rule of 5"*

| MW | $H_D$ | $H_A$ | FRB[a] | PSA[a] | cLogP[a] |
|---|---|---|---|---|---|
| 460.50 | 1 | 9 | 8 | 127Å² | 0.48 ± 0.82 |

[a] Calculated by ACD/Labs software V11.02.

## Drug Product*

*Dosage route*:  Oral
*Strength*:  10 mg/20 mg/30 mg (Apremilast)
*Dosage form*:  Tablet
*Inactive ingredient*:  Lactose monohydrate, microcrystalline cellulose, croscarmellose sodium, magnesium stearate, polyvinyl alcohol, titanium dioxide, polyethylene glycol, talc, iron oxide red, iron oxide yellow (20 and 30 mg only) and iron oxide black (30 mg only).
*Recommended dose*: The recommended dose is 30 mg once daily.
  To reduce risk of gastrointestinal symptoms, titrate to recommended dose of 30 mg twice daily according to the following schedule:
  Day 1: 10 mg in morning.
  Day 2: 10 mg in morning and 10 mg in evening.
  Day 3: 10 mg in morning and 20 mg in evening.
  Day 4: 20 mg in morning and 20 mg in evening.
  Day 5: 20 mg in morning and 30 mg in evening.
  Day 6 and thereafter: 30 mg twice daily.

* Sourced from US FDA drug label information

## 2 Key Patents Information

### Summary

❖ Otezla® (Apremilast) has got five-year NCE market exclusivity protection after it was initially approved by US FDA on Mar 21, 2014.

❖ Apremilast was originally discovered by Celgene, and its compound patent application was filed as PCT application by Celgene in 1999.

❖ The compound patent will expire in 2018 foremost, which has been granted in the United States, Europe and Japan successively.

❖ The compound patent has not been filed in China yet.

Table 1    Apremilast's Compound Patent Protection in Drug-Mainstream Country

| Country | Publication/Patent NO. | Application Date | Granted Date | Estimated Expiry Date |
|---------|------------------------|------------------|--------------|-----------------------|
| WO | WO0025777A1 | 10/19/1999 | / | / |
| US | US6020358A | 10/30/1998 | 02/01/2000 | 10/30/2018 |
| EP | EP1752148B1 | 10/19/1999 | 06/23/2010 | 10/19/2019 |
| | EP1126839B1 | 10/19/1999 | 01/03/2007 | 10/19/2019 |
| JP | JP4530543B2 | 10/19/1999 | 08/25/2010 | 10/19/2019 |
| CN | NA | / | / | / |

Table 2    Originator's International Patent Application List (Patent Family)

| Publication NO. | Title | Applicant/Assignee/Owner | Publication Date |
|-----------------|-------|--------------------------|------------------|
| **Technical Subjects** | **Active Ingredient (Free Base)'s Formula or Structure and Preparation** | | |
| WO0025777A1 | Substituted phenethylsulfones and method of reducing TNF α levels | Celgene | 05/11/2000 |
| **Technical Subjects** | **Salt, Crystal, Polymorphic, Solvate (Hydrate), Isomer, Derivative Etc. and Preparation** | | |
| WO2009120167A1 | Solid forms comprising (+)-2-[1-(3-ethoxy-4-methoxyphenyl)-2-methylsulfonylethyl]-4-acetylaminoisoindoline-1,3-dione, compositions thereof, and uses thereof | Celgene | 10/01/2009 |
| WO2013126360A3 | Processes for the preparation of (S)-1-(3-ethoxy-4-methoxyphenyl)-2-methanesulfonylethylamine | Celgene | 10/31/2013 |
| **Technical Subjects** | **Formulation and Preparation** | | |
| WO2013101810A1 | Formulations of (+)-2-[1-(3-ethoxy-4-methoxyphenyl)-2-methanesul-fonylethyl]-4-acetyl aminoisoindoline-1,3-dione | Celgene | 07/04/2013 |
| WO2014204825A1 | Tablet formulations of (+)-2-[1-(3-ethoxy-4-methoxyphenyl)-2-methyl-sulfonylethyl]-4-acetylaminoisoindoline-1,3-dione | Celgene | 12/24/2014 |
| WO2013119607A2 | Modified release formulations of (+)-2-[1-(3-ethoxy-4-methoxy-phenyl)-2-methanesulfonylethyl]-4-acetyl aminoisoindoline-1,3-dione | Celgene | 08/15/2013 |
| WO2011059931A2 | Nanosuspension of a poorly soluble drug via microfluidization process | Celgene | 05/19/2011 |
| WO2012083017A2 | Controlled release oral dosage forms of poorly soluble drugs and uses thereof | Celgene | 06/21/2012 |
| **Technical Subjects** | **Indication or Methods for Medical Needs** | | |
| WO2014025958A2 | Treatment of immune-related and inflammatory diseases | Celgene | 02/13/2014 |
| WO2005044269A1 | Cytokine inhibitory drugs for treatment of macular degeneration | Celgene | 05/19/2005 |
| WO2007079182A1 | Methods for treating cutaneous lupus using aminoisoindoline compounds | Celgene | 07/12/2007 |
| WO2014074846A1 | Methods for the treatment of bone loss | Celgene | 05/15/2014 |
| WO03080048A1 | (-)-2-[1-(3-Ethoxy-4-methoxyphenyl)-2-methylsulfonylethyl]-4-acetylamino-isoindoline-1,3-dione: methods of using and compositions thereof | Celgene | 10/02/2003 |
| WO2011063102A1 | Apremilast for the treatment of sarcoidosis | Celgene | 05/26/2011 |
| WO03097052A3 | Methods and compositions using immunomodulatory compounds for treatment and management of cancers and other diseases | Celgene | 12/18/2003 |

*Continued*

| Publication NO. | Title | Applicant/Assignee/Owner | Publication Date |
|---|---|---|---|
| WO2012121988A2 | Methods for treating diseases using isoindoline compounds | Celgene | 09/13/2012 |
| WO2006065814A1 | Compositions comprising PDE4 modulators and their use for the treatment or prevention of airway inflammation | Celgene | 06/22/2006 |
| WO03080049A1 | (+)-2-[1-(3-Ethoxy-4-methoxyphenyl)-2-methylsulfonylethyl]-4-acetylaminoisoindoline-1,3-dione: methods of using and compositions thereof | Celgene | 10/02/2003 |
| WO2014151180A1 | Treatment of psoriatic arthritis using apremilast | Celgene | 09/25/2014 |
| WO2010093588A1 | Methods of using and compositions comprising PDE4 modulators for treatment, prevention and management of tuberculosis | Celgene | 08/19/2010 |
| WO2015175956A1 | Compositions and methods for the treatment of atherosclerotic cardiovascular diseases with PDE4 modulators | Celgene | 11/19/2015 |
| WO2015200177A1 | Apremilast for the treatment of a liver disease or a liver function abnormality | Celgene | 12/30/2015 |
| WO2015112568A1 | Methods for the treatment of obesity using apremilast | Celgene | 07/30/2015 |
| **Technical Subjects** | **Combination Including at Least Two Active Ingredients** | | |
| WO2012149251A1 | Methods and compositions using PDE4 inhibitors for the treatment and management of autoimmune and inflammatory diseases | Celgene | 11/01/2012 |
| WO2012096884A1 | Phenethylsulfone isoindoline derivatives as inhibitors of PDE4 and/or cytokines | Celgene | 07/19/2012 |
| **Technical Subjects** | **Others** | | |
| WO2011159750A1 | Biomarkers for the treatment of psoriasis | Celgene | 12/22/2011 |

The data was updated until Jan 2016.

# 3 Chemistry

## Route 1: Original Discovery Route

*Synthetic Route*: The original discovery route was initiated with the preparation of $\beta$-aminosulfone **2** derived from the addition to the *in situ* generated imine of 3-ethoxy-4-methoxybenzaldehyde **1** by LiHMDS with dimethylsulfone lithium, catalyzed by BF$_3$·Et$_2$O in 41% yield. Resolution of racemic $\beta$-aminosulfone **2** with *N*-acetyl-L-leucine **3** gave the *S*-isomer **4** in 90% yield and with 98% *ee*. Condensation of **4** with 3-*N*-acetylamidophthalic anhydride **5** in refluxing acetic acid provided the titled compound in 75% yield with 98% *ee*.　The overall yield was 14%.[1-3]

3-*N*-acetylaminophthalic anhydride **5** was prepared upon catalytic hydrogenation of 3-nitrophthalic acid **6**, followed by acetylation of **7** in refluxing acetic anhydride in 51% yield over two steps.[1-3]

## Route 2

*Synthetic Route*:　This route presented a process of asymmetric synthesis of apremilast.　3-Ethoxy-4-methoxybenzaldehyde **1** as starting material was condensed with chiral auxiliary (*R*)-1-(*α*-aminobenzyl)-2-naphthol **2** in basic conditions, generating chiral oxazine **3** in 90% yield, which underwent ring-opening addition with dimethyl sulfone lithium **4** to furnish the corresponding aminosulfone **5** in 87% yield.　Hydrogenation of **5** and subsequent condensation of **6** with 3-*N*-acetylamidophthalic anhydride **7** produced apremilast with the yield of 88% and 73%, respectively.　The overall yield was 50%.[4]

## Route 3

Rh(COD)$_2$OTf: Bis(1,5-cyclooctadiene)rhodium(I) trifluoromethanesulfonate
(*S*,*R*)-*t*-Bu-Josiphos: (*S*)-1-[(*R*)-2-(Diphenylphosphino)ferrocenyl]ethyldi-*tert*-butylphosphine

[1]　Schafer, P. H.; Muller, G. W.; Man, H. W., et al. WO2003080049A1, **2003**.
[2]　Muller, G. W.; Schafer, P. H.; Man, H. W., et al. US6962940B2, **2005**.
[3]　Man, H. W.; Schafer, P.; Wong, L. M., et al. *J. Med. Chem.* **2009**, *52*, 1522-1524.
[4]　Xu, X. CN103864670A, **2014**.

*Synthetic Route*:    Dimethyl sulfone was first subjected to *n*-butyllithium in THF prior to exposure to commercially available 3-ethoxy-4-methoxybenzonitrile **1** at low temperature to afford enamine **2** in 83% yield.    The enamine **2** was submitted to asymmetric hydrogenation, catalyzed by [Rh(COD)₂]OTf and (*S,R*)-*t*-Bu-Josiphos in trifluoroethanol (TFE) to afford the corresponding optically active amine **3** in 70% yield with 95% *ee*.    Finally, **3** was condensed with commercially available 3-*N*-acetylamidophthalic anhydride **4** in refluxing acetic acid to provide desired apremilast.[5]

## Route 4

*Synthetic Route*:    In this process route, 1-(3-ethoxy-4-methoxyphenyl)-2-methanesulfonyl ethanone **3** was obtained from 3-ethoxy-4-methoxybenzonitrile **1** *via* coupling with dimethylsulfone in the presence of *n*-butyllithium, and followed by *in situ* hydrolysis with 2N HCl with the yield of 88%-93% over two steps.    Then compound **3** was treated with chiral auxiliary (*S*)-(-)-1-phenylethylamine **4** and reduced with sodium borohydride in acidic conditions to yield chiral *N*-benzylated derivative of aminosulfone **5** as a hydrochloride salt with the yield of 79%-81% and an *ee* of >99%.    Finally, **5** was hydrogenated with 5% Pd/C in methanol to afford the key intermediate *β*-aminosulfone **6** in the yield of 86%-94% and with an *ee* of >99%.[6]

In an alternative process route, condensation of commercially available (*R*)-*tert*-butylsulfinamide **8** with 3-ethoxy-4-methoxy-benzaldehyde **7** under mild conditions provided *tert*-butanesulfinyl imine **9**.    Then nucleophile addition of dimethylsulfone to imine **9** in the presence of *n*-butylliuthium and aluminium methide yielded sulfinamide **10**, which upon *in situ* removal of the *tert*-butylsulfinyl group under acid conditions provided the key intermediate *β*-aminosulfone **6** with 80% *ee*.[6]

[5]   Connolly, T. J.; Ruchelman, A. L.; Yong, K. H. Y., et al. US20140081032A1, **2014**.
[6]   Venkateswaralu, J.; Rajendiran, C.; Reddy, N. R., et al. US20130217918A1, **2013**.

## Route 5

RuCl(p-cymene)[(S,S)-Ts-DPEN]: [N-[(1S,2S)-2-(amino-κN)-1,2-diphenylethyl]-4-methylbenzenesulfonamidato-κN]chloro[(1,2,3,4,5,6-η)-1-methyl-4-(1-methylethyl)benzene]-ruthenium

*Synthetic Route*: Catalyzed by RuCl(p-cymene)[(S,S)-Ts-DPEN], Noyori's asymmetric transfer hydrogenation of ketone **1** generated optical active alcohol **2** in 87% yield and with 99% *ee*. Subsequent conversion of β-hydroxysulfone **2** into azide **3** was achieved upon the Mitsunobu reaction in 81% yield and with 36.3% *ee*. Reduction of azide **3** to the free amine, then followed by resolution of its *N*-Ac-Leu salt **5** was completed in 44% yield with 94.4% *ee*. The overall yield was 31%.[7]

## 4 Pharmacology

### Summary

Mechanism of Action

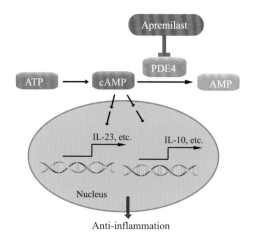

- ❖ Apremilast is a novel oral small molecule inhibitor of PDE4 (IC$_{50}$ = 74 nM), a cAMP-specific PDE as a dominant PDE in inflammatory cells.
- ❖ Apremilast inhibits PDE4 and elevates intracellular cAMP levels, which in turn downregulates the inflammatory response by modulating the expression of pro- and anti-inflammatory cytokines, such as tumor necrosis factor alpha (TNF-α), interleukin (IL)-23, IL-17, and anti-inflammatory cytokines.
- ❖ The metabolites of apremilast had no significant inhibition of PDE4, but the apremilast *S*-isomer metabolite M17 significantly inhibited PDE4 (IC$_{50}$ = 94 nM) and TNF-α (IC$_{50}$ = 21 nM).
- ❖ Apremilast (10 μM) had no significant activity on a panel of 68 cell surface receptors or 17 enzymes, except for *L*-calcium channel receptor. It did not significantly inhibit any of the 255 kinases in Invitrogen's Select Screen profile either.[8, 9]

[7] Ruchelman, A. L.; Connolly, T. J. *Tetrahedron Asymmetr.* **2015**, *26*, 553-559.

[8] U.S. Food and Drug Administration (FDA) Database. http://www.accessdata.fda.gov/drugsatfda_docs/nda/2014/206088Orig1s000PharmR.pdf (accessed Mar 2016).

[9] European Medicines Agency (EMA) Database. http://www.ema.europa.eu/docs/en_GB/document_library/EPAR_-_Public_assessment_report/human/003746/WC500182629.pdf (accessed Mar 2016).

*In Vitro* Efficacy

❖ Effects on cytokines and anti-inflammation by apremilast in cell lines:
- In LPS-stimulated PBMCs:
  - Decreased TNF-$\alpha$, MIP-$1\alpha$ and IL-12: $IC_{50}$ = 110-440 nM.
  - Increased IL-10: $EC_{50}$ = 80 nM.
- In LPS-stimulated human cutaneous lupus PBMCs:
  - TNF-$\alpha$: $IC_{50}$ = 77 nM.
  - IL-12: $IC_{50}$ = 140 nM.
  - IL-10: $EC_{50}$ = 2300 nM.
- In TLR9 agonist CpG-A stimulated human cutaneous lupus PBMCs:
  - Significantly inhibited gene expression of CXCL9, CXCL10, and CXCL11.
- IL-$1\beta$-stimulated human cutaneous lupus PBMC model:
  - TNF-$\alpha$: $IC_{50}$ = 83 nM.
- In anti-CD3 mAb stimulated T-cell line:
  - Decreased TNF-$\alpha$, IL-5, IL-10, IL-13 and IL-17: $IC_{50}$ = 30-930 nM.
- In CIA synovial membrane tissue:
  - TNF-$\alpha$: $IC_{50}$ = 100 nM.
- In pDC/HEKa co-culture cells:
  - Inhibited the production of IFN-$\alpha$ and TNF-$\alpha$ protein, and expression of HEKa intracellular MxA protein.

*In Vivo* Efficacy

❖ In rat models:
- Plasma TNF-$\alpha$ in LPS-stimulated CD rats: $ED_{50}$ = 0.018 mg/kg.
- Air pouch TNF-$\alpha$ in carrageenan-stimulated CD rats: 82% inhibition at 10 mg/kg.
- Lung neutrophilia in LPS-stimulated CD rat lung models: $ED_{50}$ = 0.25 mg/kg.

❖ In mouse models:
- Serum TNF-$\alpha$ in LPS-stimulated Balb/c mice: $ED_{50}$ = 0.05 mg/kg.
- Type II CIA: 49% reduction of mean severity score on day 14.
- Mab/LPS-induced: Reduced paw thickness and hind-paw arthritic reactions in dose-dependent manner at 5 and 25 mg/kg/day.

## Mechanism of Action

Table 3   *In Vitro* Inhibition of Apremilast against PDE and PDE4 Subtypes[8, 9]

| PDE4 Subtype | $IC_{50}$ (nM) | | PDE | Conc. ($\mu$M) | %Inhibition |
| --- | --- | --- | --- | --- | --- |
| | Apremilast | Rolipram[a] | | | |
| PDE4-A1A | 14 | 188 | PDE1 | 10 | 12 |
| PDE4-B1 | 43 | 418 | | | |
| PDE4-B2 | 27 | 135 | PDE2 | 10 | 30 |
| PDE4-C1 | 118 | 847 | | | |
| PDE4-D2 | 33 | 858 | PDE3 | 10 | 26 |
| PDE4-D3 | 28 | 825 | | | |
| PDE4-D7 | 30 | 913 | PDE4 | 10 | 95 |

[a] Rolipram was used as a positive control.

[8] FDA Database.   http://www.accessdata.fda.gov/drugsatfda_docs/nda/2014/206088Orig1s000PharmR.pdf (accessed Mar 2016).
[9] EMA Database.   http://www.ema.europa.eu/docs/en_GB/document_library/EPAR_-_Public_assessment_report/human/003746/WC500182629.pdf (accessed Mar 2016).

Table 4  *In Vitro* Inhibition of PDE4 and Expression of TNF-$\alpha$ by Apremilast and Its Metabolites[8, 10]

| Compounds | Source | Type | IC$_{50}$ (nM) | |
|---|---|---|---|---|
| | | | PDE4 | TNF-$\alpha$ |
| Apremilast | NA | Parent | 74[a] | NA |
| Apremilast | Synthesize | Parent | 80/47[b] | 11/36[b] |
| M12 | Urine (*S*-isomer) | Metabolite | 5500 | IC$_{40}$ = 10000 |
| M12 | Synthesize (*S*-isomer) | Metabolite | >10000 | IC$_{24}$ = 10000 |
| M3 | Synthesize (*S*-isomer) | Metabolite | 8300 | 5600 |
| M16 | Synthesize (*S*-isomer) | Metabolite | 6500 | IC$_{24}$ = 10000 |
| M17 | Synthesize (*S*-isomer) | Metabolite | 94 | 21 |

Apremilast was used as a comparative positive control in metabolite and *S*-isomer studies.   The M12 metabolite of apremilast was tested for PDE4 enzyme activity and for bioactivity by quantifying TNF-$\alpha$ release from lipopolysaccharide (LPS)-stimulated peripheral blood mononuclear cells.   [a] PDE4 was isolated from U937 human monocytic cells.   [b] Data from two independent experiments, prior to testing with M12, and following with M3, M16 and M17.   M3: Apremilast-*O*-desmethyl.   M12: Apremilast-*O*-desmethyl glucuronide.   M16: Acetamide hydroxyl-glucuronide.   M17: Acetamide-hydroxy.

## *In Vitro* Efficacy

Table 5  *In Vitro* Effects on Cytokines and Anti-Inflammatory by Apremilast[8-10]

| Line/Tissue | Source/Type Cell | Stimulus | Cytokine | IC$_{50}$ (nM) |
|---|---|---|---|---|
| PBMC[a] | Human | LPS | TNF-$\alpha$ | 110 |
| | | | IL-12 | 120 |
| | | | MIP-1$\alpha$ | 440 |
| | | | IL-10 | EC$_{50}$ = 80 |
| | Human cutaneous lupus | LPS | TNF-$\alpha$ | 77 |
| | | | IL-12 | 140 |
| | | | IL-10 | EC$_{50}$ = 2300 |
| | | TLR9 agonist CpG-A | CXCL9 | Significant inhibition of CXCL9, CXCL10, and CXCL11 gene expression. |
| | | | CXCL10 | |
| | | | CXCL11 | |
| | | SEB | IL-2 | 291 |
| | | | IFN-$\gamma$ | 46 |
| | | IL-1$\beta$ | TNF-$\alpha$ | 83 |
| | | PGE$_2$ | cAMP | EC$_{50}$ = 1510 |
| T Cell[b] | Human | Anti-CD3 mAb | TNF-$\alpha$ | 930 |
| | | | IL-5 | 30 |
| | | | IL-10 | 190 |
| | | | IL-13 | 280 |
| | | | IL-17 | 90 |
| | | | GM-CSF | 1000 |
| pDC/HEKa co-cultures | Cutaneous lupus | TLR9 agonist CpG-A | IFN-$\alpha$ | Inhibited the production of IFN-$\alpha$ and TNF-$\alpha$ protein, as well as the expression of HEKa intracellular MxA protein. |
| | | | TNF-$\alpha$ | |
| | | | MxA | |
| Synovial membrane tissue[c] | Human | CIA | TNF-$\alpha$ | 100 |

LPS: Lipopolysaccharide.   CIA: Collagen-induced arthritis.   mAb: Monoclonal antibody.   [a] PBMC: Peripheral blood mononuclear cell.   Luminex technology was used to determine the 50% inhibitory or enhancement concentration, IC$_{50}$ or EC$_{50}$, for apremilast effects on pro-inflammatory cytokines and IL-10 (anti-inflammatory cytokine).   [b] Anti-CD3 mAb was used to stimulate primary human T cells in an *in vitro* plate-bound antibody assay.   [c] Cytokine levels in the supernatant were measured by ELISA.   There was no effect on cell viability.

[8]  FDA Database.   http://www.accessdata.fda.gov/drugsatfda_docs/nda/2014/206088Orig1s000PharmR.pdf (accessed Mar 2016).
[9]  EMA Database.   http://www.ema.europa.eu/docs/en_GB/document_library/EPAR_-_Public_assessment_report/human/003746/WC500182629.pdf (accessed Mar 2016).
[10]  Perez-Aso, M.; Montesinos, M. C.; Mediero, A., et al. *Arthritis Res. Ther.* **2015**, *17*, 249-262.

## *In Vivo* **Efficacy**

Table 6 *In Vivo* and *Ex Vivo* Anti-Arthritic and Anti-Inflammatory Activity of Apremilast[8, 9, 11]

| Study | Animal Model Modeling | Animal | Dose (mg/kg) | Route & Duration | Effect ED (mg/kg/day) | Finding |
|---|---|---|---|---|---|---|
| Anti-inflammatory activity | LPS | Balb/c mouse (female) | 0.01-1 | p.o., 3.5 h | $ED_{50} = 0.05$ | Inhibited LPS-induced serum TNF-$\alpha$ levels. |
| | | CD rat (female) | 0.01-10 | p.o., 2.5 h | $ED_{50} = 0.018$ | Inhibited LPS-induced plasma TNF-$\alpha$ levels >80%. |
| | Carrageenan | CD rat (female) | 10 | p.o., 5 h | 10 | Pretreatment reduced air pouch TNF-$\alpha$ levels by 82%. |
| | | SD rat (male) | 50 | i.p., 3 days | 50 | Significantly reduced paw edema and biologically relevant increased in 3 h post-dose threshold for both mechanical and thermal hyperalgesia. |
| | | CD rat (female) | 10 | p.o., 4 h | NA | No effect c    edema following carrageenan injection. |
| Anti-arthritic activity | Type II CIA + LPS | DBA/1LacJ mouse (female) | 1 or 10 | p.o., QD × 14 days | NA | Reduced mean severity score of 49% at 1 mg/kg, 32% at 10 mg/kg. |
| | Nonresponding control (CIA + LPS) | DBA/1LacJ mouse (female) | 1 or 25 | p.o., QD × 17 days | 5 | Inhibited the severity of disease only on Day 17. |
| | Type II CIA + LPS | DBA/1Ols-Hsd mouse (female) | 5 or 25 | i.p., QD × 10 days | NA | Reduced the clinical severity scores and reduced histological evidence of arthritic severity. |
| | Collagen mAb + LPS | BALB/c mouse (male) | 1, 5, or 25 | p.o., QD × 5 days | 5 (paw thickness) 25 (clinical score) | Significantly reduced paw thickness at 5 mg/kg/day and clinical score at 25 mg/kg/day. |
| Amyloid lateral Sclerosis (ALS) | NA | B6S JL-TgN (SOD1-G93A) dl 1 Gur mouse | 4-8 | NA, QD × 130 days | NA | High dose delayed onset of ALS clinical symptoms, non-significant increased survival.    Plasma concentrations in fed mice were higher in females than in males. There was a weak correlation between survival and plasma apremilast concentration. |
| Lung models of inflammation and asthma | LPS | CD rat (female) | 0.1, 0.3, 1, 3 | p.o., pre- and post-LPS injection | $ED_{50} = 0.25$ | Inhibited lung neutrophilia after LPS stimulation. |
| | | | 0.003-0.1 | i.t., pre- and post-LPS injection | $ED_{50} = 0.003$ | Inhibited lung neutrophilia intratracheally, ~100-fold more potent than oral administration. |
| | | Ferret (male) | 0.1-30 | p.o., pre- and post-LPS exposure | $ED_{50} = 0.8$ | The threshold emetic dose = 10 mg/kg (average 0.5 emetic events (retches only) per ferret).   $ED_{50}$ lung neutrophilia = 0.8 mg/kg (therapeutic index = 12). |
| | OVA | Balb/c mouse (male) | 1-25 | p.o., 1 h prior to LPS, QD × 5 days | NA | Inhibited AHR by 59% at 1 mg/kg and by 91% at 25 mg/kg. |
| | | | 10 | p.o., 1 h prior to LPS, QD × 9 days | 10 | Inhibited AHR by more than 96% at 24 and 48 h, and by 83% at 72 h post-OVA (day 22) challenge. Reduced lung levels of macrophages, neutrophils, lymphocytes, eosinophils, IL-4, RANTES, and eotaxin, as well as plasma IgE levels. |
| *Ex vivo* of lung model | NA | Tissue bath of guinea pig, trachea | 0.0001-1 μM (incubation) | NA | $EC_{50} = 310$ nM | Produced a significant relaxation of guinea pig trachea under spontaneous tone contraction. |

LPS: Lipopolysaccharide.   TNF-$\alpha$: Tumor necrosis factor alpha.   CIA: Collagen-induced arthritis.   mAb: Monoclonal antibody.   i.t.: Administered intratracheally.

[8]  FDA Database.   http://www.accessdata.fda.gov/drugsatfda_docs/nda/2014/206088Orig1s000PharmR.pdf (accessed Mar 2016).
[9]  EMA Database.   http://www.ema.europa.eu/docs/en_GB/document_library/EPAR_-_Public_assessment_report/human/003746/WC500182629.pdf (accessed Mar 2016).
[11]  McCann, F. E.; Palfreeman, A. C.; Andrews, M., et al. *Arthritis Res. Ther.* **2010**, *12*, R107-R118.

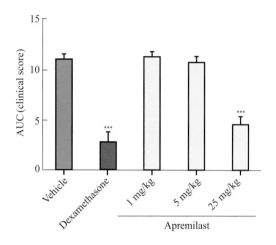 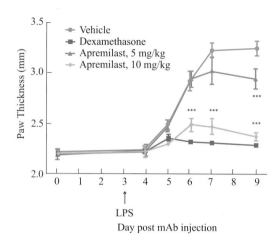

Figure A    Apremilast Reduced Severity of mAb-Induced Arthritis in Balb/c Mice[11]

**Study:** Efficacy of apremilast in collagen mAb-induced arthritis mouse models.

**Animal:** Balb/c mouse (male).

**Model:** Initial injection of a four-component arthritogenetic mAb cocktail (i.v. 100 mg/kg mAb cocktail on Day 0) and the subsequent administration of LPS (i.p. 2.5 mg/kg LPS, 3 days later).

**Administration:** 1 h prior to administration of LPS orally (Day 3) and then daily for 4 days until Day 7.   Apremilast: p.o., 1, 5 or 25 mg/kg.   Vehicle: 0.5% carboxymethyl cellulose, 0.25% Tween 80.

**Test:** Paw thickness and clinical score.   0, normal; 1, mild swelling and redness restricted to digits; 2, moderate swelling and redness of ankle; 3, severe redness and swelling of the entire paw including digits; 4, maximally inflamed limb with involvement of multiple joints.

**Result:** Significantly reduced paw thickness at 5 mg/kg on Day 9 (*** $P < 0.001$), and clinical score at 25 mg/kg (*** $P < 0.001$).

# 5    ADME & Drug-Drug Interaction

## Summary

Absorption of Apremilast

❖ Exhibited a non-linear pharmacokinetics in humans following oral dosing.   The increases in $C_{max}$ and AUC appeared to be less than dose-proportional in the dose range of 10 to 100 mg apremilast.

❖ Had high oral bioavailability in humans (73.2%), monkeys (78%) and female rats (63%), but moderate in mice (27%) and low in male rats (11.5%).

❖ Was absorbed moderately with the $T_{max}$ occurring 1-3 h in humans.

❖ Showed a half-life ranging between of 4.5-7.6 h in humans, much longer than that in mice (1.7 h for males and 2.3 h for females).

❖ Had low clearance in humans (169 mL/min) and rabbits (2039 mL/h/kg), in contrast to liver blood flow, after intravenous administrations.

❖ Exhibited an extensive tissue distribution in humans but moderate in rabbits, with apparent volumes of distribution at 87 L and 1843 mL/kg, respectively, after intravenous administrations.

❖ Showed a low permeability, with a $Papp_{(A \to B)}$ of $21 \times 10^{-6}$ cm/s in LLC-PK1 cell monolayer model.

Distribution of Apremilast

❖ Exhibited moderate plasma protein binding in humans (68.3%), mice (88.6%), rabbits (80.9%) and monkeys (84.3%), but high in rats (90.6%).

[11]   McCann, F. E.; Palfreeman, A. C.; Andrews, M., et al. *Arthritis Res. Ther.* **2010**, *12*, R107-R118.

❖ Albino mice following single oral administration:
   • Absorbed radioactivity was rapidly distributed into tissues.
   • Relatively higher concentration levels were observed in these tissues generally associated with the principal of biotransformation and excretion (i.e liver and kidneys), the pancreas, and gall bladder (biliary elimination).
   • Concentrations measured in the central nervous system were consistently low, indicating that penetration of the blood-brain barrier was limited.
   • Males and females had similar patterns of tissue distribution.
   • Radioactivity was not associated with melanin-containing tissues (i.e uveal tract and pigmented skin) in pigmented male mice.
   • By the 72 h post-dose, levels were below the lower limit of quantification of 0.71 μg eq./g, except for the liver for males only, kidneys (cortex and medulla), skin, uveal tract, nasal mucosa and gastrointestinal mucosa.
   • Radioactivity was not detected in any tissues at 168 h after dosing or even later.

## Metabolism of Apremilast

❖ Could be metabolized in human and animal liver microsomes and hepatocytes with different extents.
❖ *In vitro*, oxidative metabolism of apremilast was mediated by CYP3A4 to a large extent, with minor contributions from CYP1A2 and CYP2A6.
❖ Overall, the parent drug represented the most abundant component, with M12 (glucuronide conjugate of *O*-demethylated apremilast) as the major metabolite in human plasma.   The major component in mice was M1/2.
❖ The major circulating M12 was not pharmacologically active.

## Excretion of Apremilast

❖ Was predominantly excreted in urine, with M12 as the major component in human urine.
❖ Was predominantly excreted in feces in rats and monkeys, and M3 as the major component in rat and monkey feces.
❖ About 59% (i.v.) and 54% (p.o.) of apremilast was recovered *via* biliary excretion in bile duct-cannulated (BDC) female mice.

## Drug-Drug Interaction

❖ Apremilast did not inhibit CYP1A2, 2A6, 2B6, 2C9, 2C19, 2D6, 2E1 or 3A4, but had a weak inhibition for CYP2C8 ($IC_{50}$ = 56.1 μM).
❖ Apremilast had no effect on CYP3A4, 1A2 or 2C9 at 1 μM.   A 3.7-fold induction of CYP3A4 was observed at 100 μM. Treatment at higher concentrations caused 35% (10 μM) and up to 70% (100 μM) decreases in CYP1A2 and CYP2C9 activities.
❖ Apremilast was a substrate of P-gp, but not of BCRP.
❖ Apremilast had no inhibition for P-gp or BCRP, but had weak inhibition for MRP1 and MRP2 ($IC_{50}$ >10 μM).
❖ Apremilast was not a substrate of OATP1B1, OATP1B3, OAT1, OAT3 or OCT2, and had weak inhibition for them ($IC_{50}$ >10 μM).

# Absorption

**Key Findings:**[8, 9]
❖ In mice:
   • Following intravenous dosing of 10 mg/kg, [$^{14}$C]apremilast had a shorter elimination time, 1.7 h in males and 2.3 h in females, compared to total radioactivity in plasma approximately 19 h in males and 30 h in females.   AUC and $T_{1/2}$ values indicated total radioactivity persisted, indicating persistent metabolism.
   • Following oral dosing of 500 mg/kg, the terminal elimination half-life of [$^{14}$C]apremilast was approximately 15 h in males and 22 h in females with similar values for plasma and blood.   No significant sex-related differences were observed.
   • Oral bioavailability ranged from approximately 20% to 33% (average 27%).
   • The exposure to parent-derived radioactivity (i.e., metabolites) was about 2-fold higher than that of the parent.
   • For both dose routes, concentrations of radioactivity in blood were consistently lower than those in plasma at the same time point, indicating that there was no specific association of apremilast or its metabolites with blood cells.
❖ In monkeys:
   • Bioavailability of total administered radioactivity was approximately 78% in plasma for a 10 mg/kg oral dose.   However, it was not possible to calculate the bioavailability of [$^{14}$C]apremilast due to the lack of detection of [$^{14}$C]apremilast from the low dose after intravenous dosing.

[8] FDA Database.   http://www.accessdata.fda.gov/drugsatfda_docs/nda/2014/206088Orig1s000PharmR.pdf (accessed Mar 2016).
[9] EMA Database.   http://www.ema.europa.eu/docs/en_GB/document_library/EPAR_-_Public_assessment_report/human/003746/WC500182629.pdf (accessed Mar 2016).

- In multiple-dose toxicity studies with monkeys, there was a dose-related increase in exposure, which was less than dose proportional in range of 200 mg/kg/day to 2000 mg/kg/day.
- There were no sex-related differences in pharmacokinetics parameters.

❖ In rats:
  - Following intravenous dosing, plasma concentrations declined steadily in both males and females, however, concentrations were below the limit of quantification by 8 h post-dose in male animals but still detected at 24 h in females. Sex differences in exposure were also reflected in the lower AUC and shorter $T_{1/2}$ in males compared with females and systemic clearance was high in males but low in females.
  - Following oral dosing at 50 mg/kg in males and 10 mg/kg in females, exposure was 6-fold greater in females.
  - In males, plasma total radioactivity AUC was 25-96 times greater than those for [$^{14}$C]apremilast, but in females total radioactivity AUC was 2-3 times greater than those for the [$^{14}$C]apremilast, suggesting that the metabolism was more extensive in males than that in females.
  - The bioavailability following oral dosing of apremilast was approximately 11.5% in males and 63% in females.

❖ In rabbits:
  - For female New Zealand White rabbits, following a single 1000 mg/kg oral dose, apremilast was rapidly absorbed.
  - Following a 250 mg/kg oral dose, exposure was negligible, with a mean $C_{max}$ of 2.62 ng/mL and an absolute oral bioavailability of less than 0.02%. The AUC ratio of CC-10007 (*R*-enantiomer) to apremilast was approximately 0.02, which was similar to the level in the administered dose.
  - In pregnant female New Zealand White rabbits infused 10 mg/kg apremilast, following termination of infusion apremilast concentrations declined rapidly with a mean half-life of 1.2 h.
  - The mean plasma clearance was high (2039 mL/h/kg), which was greater than 50% of the hepatic blood flow in rabbits, after intravenous administration.
  - The volume of distribution was moderate (1843 mL/kg) and was approximately 2.5 times of the total body water volume.

Table 7   *In Vivo* Pharmacokinetic Parameters of Apremilast in Humans after Single Intravenous and Oral Dose of Apremilast[12]

| Species | Route | Dose (mg) | $T_{max}$ (h) | $C_{max}$ (ng/mL) | $AUC_{inf}$ (ng·h/mL) | $T_{1/2}$ (h) | Cl/F (mL/min) | $V_{ss}$ (L) | F (%) |
|---|---|---|---|---|---|---|---|---|---|
| | i.v. | NA | 0.25 (0.25-0.33) | 4.91 (27.2) | 10.1 (22.8) | 6.19 (1.21) | 169 (41.6) | 87.0 | - |
| | p.o. | 20 | 2.29 (1.0-4.0) | 173 (27.2) | 1480 (21.8) | 7.63 (1.14) | 230 (46.4) | NA | 73.2 (12.5) |
| | p.o. | 10 | 1.0 (0.5-2.0) | 206 (32.3) | 1153 (18.0) | 6.54 (19.9) | NA | NA | NA |
| Healthy human (male & female) | p.o. | 20 | 1.75 (1.0-4.0) | 347 (36.6) | 1908 (40.8) | 4.45 (33.2) | NA | NA | NA |
| | p.o. | 40 | 2.05 (1.5-3.0) | 533 (35.9) | 3379 (47.1) | 6.04 (31.0) | NA | NA | NA |
| | p.o. | 80 | 2.25 (1.0-3.0) | 592 (49.0) | 4106 (42.0) | 5.56 (23.5) | NA | NA | NA |
| | p.o. | 100 | 3.0 (1.5-6.0) | 688 (43.4) | 5407 (32.4) | 5.56 (20.7) | NA | NA | NA |

Median (range) for $T_{max}$, Mean (CV%) for other parameters.

Table 8   *In Vivo* Plasma Pharmacokinetic Parameters for Apremilast and Metabolites in Humans after Single Oral Dose of 20 mg [$^{14}$C]Apremilast[13]

| Analyte | $T_{max}$ (h) | $C_{max}$ (ng eq./mL) | $AUC_{inf}$ (ng eq.·h/mL) | $T_{1/2}$ (h) |
|---|---|---|---|---|
| Total radioactivity | 1.5 (1.0-3.0) | 527 ± 127 | 6632 ± 653 | 50.4 ± 8.7 |
| Apremilast[a] | 1.5 (1.0-3.0) | 333 ± 76 | 1970 ± 343 | 6.8 ± 2.6 |
| Apremilast[b] | 1.8 (1.0-2.5) | 321 ± 134 | 2636 ± 705 | 7.1 ± 2.7 |
| M11 | 1.0 (0.5-2.5) | 20.2 ± 7.6 | 232 ± 151 | 10.7 ± 10.2 |
| M12 | 2.5 (1.0-2.5) | 111 ± 36 | 2446 ± 416 | 15.8 ± 3.9 |
| M13 | 2.5 (1.0-24) | 7.5 ± 6.8 | NC | NC |
| M14 | 2.5 (1.0-24) | 9.4 ± 4.3 | NC | NC |
| M16 | 5.3 (1.0-8.0) | 27.6 ± 26.0 | 389 ± 91 | 11.0 ± 2.4 |

[a] Apremilast concentrations in plasma were determined by using a Chiral LC/MS/MS assay.   [b] Apremilast and metabolite concentrations in plasma were calculated by using plasma radioactivity concentrations and radiochromatography.   NC: Not calculated.

[12]  FDA Database.   http://www.accessdata.fda.gov/drugsatfda_docs/nda/2014/205437Orig1s000ClinPharmR.pdf (accessed Mar 2016).
[13]  Hoffmann, M.; Kumar, G.; Schafer, P., et al. *Xenobiotica.* **2011**, *41*, 1063-1075.

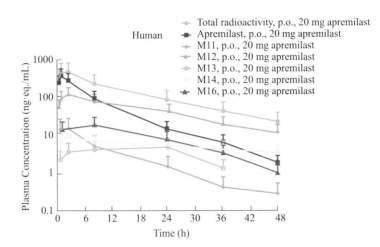

Figure B    *In Vivo* Plasma Concentration-Time Profiles of Total Radioactivity, Apremilast and Metabolites in Healthy Male Subjects after Single Oral Dose of 20 mg [$^{14}$C]Apremilast[13]

## Permeability:[9]

❖ The determined intrinsic apparent permeability (Papp) value was $21 \times 10^{-6}$ cm across native LLC-PK1 cell monolayer following a 120-min incubation.

## Distribution

Table 9    *In Vitro* Plasma Protein Binding of Apremilast in All Tested Species[8, 9, 12]

| Species | Conc. (µg/mL) | Human | Mouse | Rat | Rabbit | Monkey |
|---|---|---|---|---|---|---|
| %Bound | 0.25, 0.75, 2.5 | 68.3 ± 0.9 | 88.6 ± 2.3 | 90.6 ± 0.9 | 80.9 ± 1.2 | 84.3 ± 1.5 |

## Key Findings:[8, 9]

❖ Albino mouse tissue distribution of [$^{14}$C]apremilast:
- Absorbed radioactivity was rapidly distributed into tissues in mice after oral administration of 500 mg/kg, although the concentrations measured were generally low.
- The highest levels of radioactivity were generally associated with the principal of biotransformation and excretion (i.e liver and kidneys), pancreas, and gall bladder (biliary elimination).
- Concentrations measured in the central nervous system were consistently low, indicating that penetration of the blood-brain barrier was limited.
- In albino mice, at 72 h post-dose, levels had fallen below the lower limit of quantification (0.71 µg eq./g) except for liver and, in males only, kidneys (cortex and medulla), skin, uveal tract, nasal mucosa, and gastrointestinal mucosa.
- Males and females had similar patterns of tissue distribution.
- Radioactivity was not associated with melanin-containing tissues (i.e uveal tract and pigmented skin) in pigmented male mice.
- Radioactivity was not detected in any tissues at 168 h post-dose or later.
- In pigmented mice, levels of radioactivity were elevated in the uveal tracts of the eyes compared to albino mice at 1 and 3 days post-dose.

[8]  FDA Database.   http://www.accessdata.fda.gov/drugsatfda_docs/nda/2014/206088Orig1s000PharmR.pdf (accessed Mar 2016).
[9]  EMA Database.   http://www.ema.europa.eu/docs/en_GB/document_library/EPAR_-_Public_assessment_report/human/003746/WC500182629.pdf (accessed Mar 2016).
[12]  FDA Database.   http://www.accessdata.fda.gov/drugsatfda_docs/nda/2014/205437Orig1s000ClinPharmR.pdf (accessed Mar 2016).
[13]  Hoffmann, M.; Kumar, G.; Schafer, P., et al. *Xenobiotica.* **2011**, *41*, 1063-1075.

## Metabolism

Table 10   *In Vitro* Metabolism of Apremilast in Liver Microsomes after 120-min Incubation with 10 μM Apremilast[8]

| Species | Condition | Gender | % of Radioactivity | | | | | | | | |
|---|---|---|---|---|---|---|---|---|---|---|---|
| | | | M1 | M2 | M3 | M4 | M5 | M7 | M8 | M9 | M10 |
| Mouse | With NADPH | Male | 10.3 | 9.2 | 4.9 | - | 4.6 | 0.8 | - | - | - |
| | | Female | 6.9 | 5.4 | 1.5 | - | 0.7 | 2.5 | - | - | - |
| | Without NADPH | Male | 8.2 | 7.9 | - | - | - | 2.1 | - | - | - |
| | | Female | 7.0 | 5.3 | - | - | - | 3.1 | - | - | - |
| Rat | With NADPH | Male | 7.4 | 5.6 | 9.4 | - | - | - | - | - | - |
| | | Female | 6.4 | 5.0 | - | - | - | - | - | - | - |
| | Without NADPH | Male | 8.2 | 6.5 | - | - | - | - | - | - | - |
| | | Female | 7.5 | 5.9 | - | - | - | - | - | - | - |
| Rabbit | With NADPH | Male | 4.8 | 2.1 | 36.2 | 21.2 | - | 4.8 | 4.1 | 4.1 | 4.2 |
| | | Female | 4.0 | 3.1 | 28.5 | 12.0 | - | 13.4 | - | 2.1 | 1.9 |
| | Without NADPH | Male | 5.8 | 4.2 | - | - | - | 51.4 | - | - | - |
| | | Female | 4.8 | 4.3 | - | - | - | 32.6 | - | - | - |
| Dog | With NADPH | Male | 4.1 | 3.0 | 2.8 | - | - | 3.0 | - | - | - |
| | | Female | 3.1 | 2.6 | 4.0 | - | - | 2.8 | - | - | - |
| | Without NADPH | Male | 3.9 | 2.9 | - | - | - | 3.0 | - | - | - |
| | | Female | 4.2 | 3.5 | - | - | - | 3.9 | - | - | - |
| Monkey | With NADPH | Male | 7.0 | 5.4 | 11.2 | - | 1.9 | - | - | - | - |
| | | Female | 7.0 | 5.9 | 12.8 | - | 2.7 | - | - | - | - |
| | Without NADPH | Male | 7.4 | 6.2 | - | - | - | - | - | - | - |
| | | Female | 7.3 | 5.8 | - | - | - | - | - | - | - |
| Human | With NADPH | Male | 8.7 | 6.6 | 3.5 | - | - | 1.0 | - | - | - |
| | | Female | 9.4 | 7.1 | 8.4 | - | - | 1.0 | - | - | - |
| | Without NADPH | Male | 12.1 | 11.3 | - | - | - | 1.1 | - | - | - |
| | | Female | 9.4 | 8.1 | - | - | - | 1.1 | - | - | - |

M1/M2: Hydrolysis products.   M3: *O*-Demethylated.   M4: *O*-Demethylated *N*-deacetylated.   M5: *O*-Demethylated.   M7: *N*-Demethylated.   M8: Hydroxylated *O*-demethylated *N*-Demethylated.   M9: Hydrolysis products of M3.   M10: *O*-Demethylated hydroxylated acetamide.

### Key Findings:[8, 9]

❖ Metabolism in liver microsomes:
- All the metabolites formed by human liver microsomes were formed by microsomes of one or more animal species.
- The order of the extent of metabolism from the greatest to the least was rabbit >> monkey > mouse = male rat > human > dog > female rat.
- The rat was the only species with sex differences in the metabolism of apremilast.
- Incubation of [14C]apremilast with liver microsomes resulted in both enzymatic (CYP mediated) and non-enzymatic means (hydrolysis, forming M1/M2 and M7).
- The major metabolite, M3, was formed in all species except for the female rat liver microsomes.   M5 was formed in the mouse and monkey liver microsomes.
- The *N*-deacetylated product (M7) was formed to a minor extent in the absence of NADPH in mouse, dog and human liver microsomes, but to a greater extent in the presence of rabbit liver microsomes.

[8]   FDA Database.   http://www.accessdata.fda.gov/drugsatfda_docs/nda/2014/206088Orig1s000PharmR.pdf (accessed Mar 2016).
[9]   EMA Database.   http://www.ema.europa.eu/docs/en_GB/document_library/EPAR_-_Public_assessment_report/human/003746/WC500182629.pdf (accessed Mar 2016).

❖ Metabolism in hepatocytes:
- [$^{14}$C]Apremilast was metabolized most extensively by rabbit hepatocytes, moderately by rat hepatocytes, and to a limited extent by hepatocytes from mice, dogs, monkeys and humans.
- Twelve metabolites (M1/M2, M3, M4, M7, M11, M12, M14, M15, M16, M17, M18 and M23) were characterized or identified.
- Significant hydrolysis products M1/M2 and M18 were observed, accounting for 13.3%-13.9% and 11.6%-13.0%, respectively.
- All metabolites formed *in vitro* by human hepatocytes were formed by hepatocytes from one or more animal species, although the amounts differed among the species.
- A much lower amount of M14 was observed, ranging from 0.8%-2.6% of the total radioactivity in the hepatocyte incubations of the other five species. M3, M7 and M12 were observed in the hepatocyte incubations of all species.

❖ Metabolizing enzyme identification:
- *In vitro*, oxidative metabolism of apremilast was mediated by CYP3A4 to a large extent, with minor contributions from CYP1A2 and CYP2A6.
- Following incubations with cDNA expressed human P450 isoforms, CYP3A4 was found to be capable of efficiently metabolizing apremilast to M3, CYP2C8 and CYP2D6 to a small extent. Apremilast was metabolized to M5 predominantly by CYP3A4, CYP2A6 and to some extent by CYP1A2.

Table 11 Metabolites in Plasma, Urine, Bile and Feces in Humans and Non-clinical Test Species after Single Oral Dose of Apremilast[8, 12]

| Matrix | Species | Dose (mg/kg) | Time (h) | % of Dose | | | | | | | | | | |
| --- | --- | --- | --- | --- | --- | --- | --- | --- | --- | --- | --- | --- | --- | --- |
| | | | | M0 | M1/M2 | M3 | M4 | M7 | M8 | M9 | M10 | M11 | M12 | M13 |
| Plasma | Mouse | 500 | 0-48 | NA | Major | NA | NA | Trace | NA | NA | NA | NA | √ | Trace |
| | Rat | 10 | NA | NA | √ | NA | NA | NA | NA | NA | NA | NA | √ | - |
| | Monkey | 10 | NA | NA | √ | NA | NA | NA | NA | NA | NA | NA | √ | NA |
| | Human | 20 mg | NA | 44.8 | √ | √ | - | √ | - | - | - | 2.5 | 38.7 | 2.4 |
| Urine | Mouse | 500 | 0-48 | NA | √ | √ | - | - | - | √ | - | - | 4.01 | 7.14 |
| | Rat | 10 | - | NA | - | - | - | - | - | - | - | Major | - | |
| | Monkey | 10 | NA | NA | √ | √ | - | - | - | √ | - | - | Major | √ |
| | Human | 20 mg | NA | 2.82 | 0.92 | √ | - | √ | - | - | - | - | 33.7 | 2.04 |
| Bile | Mouse | 10 | 0-48 | NA | NA | NA | NA | NA | NA | NA | NA | NA | 30 | 10 |
| Feces | Mouse | 500 | NA | NA | √ | √ | - | - | - | √ | - | - | √ | - |
| | Rat | 10 | NA | NA | NA | Major | - | - | - | - | - | - | - | - |
| | Monkey | 10 | NA | NA | - | Major | - | - | - | - | √ | - | - | - |
| | Human | 20 mg | NA | 4.06 | 0.53 | 4.55 | 2.36 | 0.11 | 0.97 | 7.67 | 1.34 | 1.41 | - | - |

√: Be observed.   BDC: Bile duct-cannulated.

## Key Findings:[12]
❖ The major metabolic route of apremilast in humans was *O*-demethylation, with approximately 50% of the dose metabolized via this pathway.
❖ Other minor metabolic routes included *O*-deethylation, *N*-deacetylation, hydroxylation (oxidative), hydrolysis of the imide ring, and a combination of these pathways.

[8]  FDA Database.   http://www.accessdata.fda.gov/drugsatfda_docs/nda/2014/206088Orig1s000PharmR.pdf (accessed Mar 2016).
[12]  FDA Database.   http://www.accessdata.fda.gov/drugsatfda_docs/nda/2014/205437Orig1s000ClinPharmR.pdf (accessed Mar 2016).

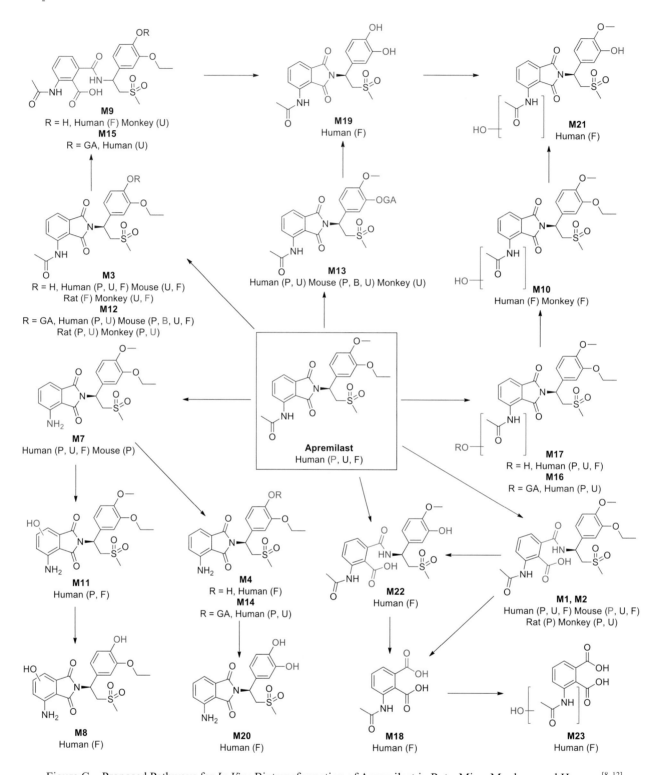

Figure C    Proposed Pathways for *In Vivo* Biotransformation of Apremilast in Rats, Mice, Monkeys and Humans[8, 12]
The red labels represent the main components in matrices.    P = Plasma, U = Urine, F = Feces, B = Bile and GA = Glucuronic acid.

[8]   FDA Database.   http://www.accessdata.fda.gov/drugsatfda_docs/nda/2014/206088Orig1s000PharmR.pdf (accessed Mar 2016).
[12]   FDA Database.   http://www.accessdata.fda.gov/drugsatfda_docs/nda/2014/205437Orig1s000ClinPharmR.pdf (accessed Mar 2016).

# Excretion

Table 12    Excretion Profiles of [$^{14}$C]Apremilast in Various Species after Single Intravenous and Oral Dose of Apremilast[8, 12]

| Species | State | Route | Dose (mg/kg) | Time (h) | Bile (% of dose) | Urine (% of dose) | Feces (% of dose) | Recovery (% of dose) |
|---|---|---|---|---|---|---|---|---|
| Mouse (male) | Intact | i.v. | 10 | 0-48 | - | 7.8 | 66.2 | 90.6 |
| | | p.o. | 500 | 0-48 | - | 4.1 | 71.5 | 97.7 |
| Mouse (female) | | i.v. | 10 | 0-48 | - | 8.7 | 71.3 | 91.1 |
| | | p.o. | 500 | 0-48 | - | 3.0 | 73.1 | 92.8 |
| Mouse (male) | BDC | i.v. | 5 | 0-48 | 59.1 | 17.8 | 10.5 | 90.2 |
| | | p.o. | 10 | 0-48 | 53.9 | 15.1 | 15.6 | 91.0 |
| Rat (male) | Intact | p.o. | 10 | 0-24 | - | 8.5 | 33.4 | 45.4 |
| | | p.o. | 10 | 0-24 | - | 15.7 | 57.9 | 74.5 |
| Rat (female) | | p.o. | 10 | 0-24 | - | 12.1 | 44.5 | 60.8 |
| | | p.o. | 10 | 0-24 | - | 29.6 | 28.2 | 52.6 |
| Monkey (male) | Intact | i.v. | 1 | 0-168 | - | 15.7 | 56.6 | 79.6 |
| | | i.v. | 10 | 0-168 | - | 17.2 | 69.3 | 93.5 |
| Monkey (female) | | p.o. | 1 | 0-168 | - | 16.2 | 56.0 | 81.1 |
| | | p.o. | 10 | 0-168 | - | 20.3 | 68.2 | 95.8 |
| Human (male) | Intact | p.o. | 20 mg | NA | - | 57.9 | 39.2 | 97.1 |

BDC: Bile duct-cannulated.

# Drug-Drug Interaction

## CYP-Based DDI:[9]

❖ Apremilast did not significantly inhibit marker enzyme activities for CYP1A2, CYP2A6, CYP2B6, CYP2C9, CYP2C19, CYP2D6, CYP2E1, or CYP3A4 at any concentration evaluated.    Apremilast was a weak direct inhibitor of CYP2C8, estimated half-maximal inhibition (IC$_{50}$) of 56.1 μM.

❖ There was no effect on CYP3A4 activities at 1 and 10 μM apremilast.    A 3.7-fold induction of CYP3A4 (roughly half the extent induced by rifampin) was observed at 100 μM.

❖ Apremilast had no effects on CYP1A2 or CYP2C9 at 1 μM.    Treatment at higher concentrations caused 35% (10 μM) and up to 70% (100 μM) decreases in CYP1A2 and CYP2C9 activities.

Table 13    *In Vitro* Evaluation of Apremilast as an Inhibitor and a Substrate of Transporters[9, 12]

| Transporter | ABC | | | | SLC | | | | |
|---|---|---|---|---|---|---|---|---|---|
| | BCRP | P-gp | MRP2 | MRP1 | OATP1B1 | OATP1B3 | OAT1 | OAT3 | OCT2 |
| Substrate (efflux ratio) | No | 24-30 | NA | NA | No | No | No | No | No |
| Inhibitor (IC$_{50}$, μM) | No | No | >10 | >10 | >20 | >10 | >10 | >10 | >10 |

MDR1-LLC-PK1 cells for P-gp substrate study *in vitro*.

[8]   FDA Database.    http://www.accessdata.fda.gov/drugsatfda_docs/nda/2014/206088Orig1s000PharmR.pdf (accessed Mar 2016).
[9]   EMA Database.    http://www.ema.europa.eu/docs/en_GB/document_library/EPAR_-_Public_assessment_report/human/003746/WC500182629.pdf (accessed Mar 2016).
[12]   FDA Database.    http://www.accessdata.fda.gov/drugsatfda_docs/nda/2014/205437Orig1s000ClinPharmR.pdf (accessed Mar 2016).

# 6 Non-Clinical Toxicology

## Summary

### Single-Dose Toxicity

❖ Acute toxicity by the i.v. and p.o. route in two rodent species, and the observed MNLDs/MLDs were concluded:
- For mice: The oral MNLD was >2000 mg/kg, and the intravenous MLD was ≥120 mg/kg.
- For rats: The oral MLD was 2000 mg/kg in males and >300 mg/kg in females, and the intravenous MLD was >60 mg/kg.

### Repeated-Dose Toxicity

❖ Sub- and chronic toxicity by the oral route in mice (up to 6 months) and monkeys (up to 12 months):
- In mice:
  - The major apremilast-related finding was arteritis within the thoracic organs, particularly prominent at the junction of the aortic root and the heart, but non-prevalent in the thymus. Perivascular inflammation of the lungs was also observed.
  - Other findings included centrilobular hepatocyte hypertrophy and gastrointestinal effects at high doses such as histopathological changes in the stomach (distension, thickening, irregular surface and raised foci) and associated reduction in food consumption and weight loss.
- In monkeys:
  - Arteritis was observed in a shorter duration and higher doses studies. Arteritis was generally found in the myocardium and other locations that included connective tissues of the sciatic nerve and kidneys.
  - Other findings at higher doses included emesis, retching or excessive salivation, and thin body condition.

### Safety Pharmacology

❖ Both *in vitro* and *in vivo* safety pharmacology studies were conducted to assess the effects of apremilast on neurological, cardiovascular, respiratory system and gastrointestinal effects.
- Neurological effects: Apremilast produced sympathetic activation responses, and one death at HD (2000 mg/kg) the day after neurological testing.
- Cardiovascular effects: The $IC_{50}$ of 184 μM for $I_{Kr}$ would be >100-fold the human $C_{max}$ at 30 mg BID dose, suggesting rare potential for QT prolongation, which was confirmed by an *in vivo* dog study.
- No finding of initial concern in studies of respiratory function or gastrointestinal transport.

### Genotoxicity

❖ Apremilast was considered neither mutagenic nor clastogenic, based on the whole battery of genotoxicological assays employed.

### Reproductive and Developmental Toxicity

❖ Fertility and early embryonic development in mice:
- Prolonged the estrus cycle and increased the interval to mating in female mice.

❖ Embryo-fetal developmental in mice and monkeys:
- Dystocia reduced viability, fetal weight and litter size, and increased abortion and embryo-fetal death.
- Not teratogenic in mice or monkeys.

❖ Pre- and postnatal development in mice:
- Premature delivery, dystocia, reduced viability and birth weights at doses ≥10 mg/kg.

❖ Repeated-dose toxicity in juvenile mice:
- Apremilast was considered to be well tolerated in male and female juvenile mice.

### Carcinogenicity

❖ Two 2-year oral carcinogenicity studies with apremilast assays were conducted in mice and rats:
- Not carcinogenic in mice at doses up to 1000 mg/kg/day or in rats at doses up to 20 mg/kg/day in males and 3 mg/kg/day in females.

### Special Toxicology

❖ Phototoxicity: Negative.

# Single-Dose Toxicity

Table 14　Single-Dose Toxicity Studies of Apremilast[9]

| Species | Dosage (mg/kg) | | MLD (mg/kg) | Finding |
|---|---|---|---|---|
| | Preliminary | Main | | |
| ICR mouse | 2000, p.o. | 2000, p.o. | MNLD: >2000 | No body weight effect or gross macroscopic necropsy findings.　Isolated palpebral closure. |
| | 50, 75, 100, 150, 200, i.v. | 120, i.v. | 120 (male) >120 (female) | Preliminary: Mortality at 150 and 200 mg/kg. Clinical signs at dose ≥50 mg/kg included tachypnea, lethargy and palpebral closure. Main: 1 mortality (male) at 120 mg/kg, tachypnea, palpebral closure (male). |
| Wistar rat | 200, 400, 700, 1000, 1500, 2000, p.o. | 300 (female) 2000 (male) p.o. | 2000 (male) >300 (female) | Preliminary: Mortality (female) at ≥400 mg/kg. Main: Mortality (male) at 2000 mg/kg, weight loss, vasodilatation, diarrhea, staining of the snout, soiling of the anogenital region, palpebral closure, lethargy, a hunched posture, chromodacryorrhea, dyspnea, a wasted appearance GI macroscopic changes. |
| | 50, 60, 75, 100, i.v. | 60, i.v. | >60 | Preliminary: Mortality (female) at ≥75 mg/kg, tachypnea, lethargy, haematuria, salivation, palpebral closure, pilo-erection and rales, tremors, stained snout, chromodacryorrhea. Main: No mortality at 60 mg/kg, tachypnea, lethargy, lachrymation and palpebral closure within 2 h of dosing and pilo-erection and stained snouts (female). |

# Repeated-Dose Toxicity

Table 15　Repeated-Dose Toxicity Studies of Ameprilast by Oral Administration[8, 9]

| Species | Duration | Dose (mg/kg/day) | NOAEL | | | Finding |
|---|---|---|---|---|---|---|
| | | | Dose (mg/kg/day) | AUC$_{0-24}$[a] (ng·h/mL) | Safety Margin[a] (× MRHD) | |
| ICR mouse | 2 weeks | 500, 1000, 2000 | 500 | 146245/158868 | 20.0/21.7 | ↓ Body weight and ↓ food consumption. GI tract: Distension, thickening, irregular surface and raised foci in the stomach. Clinical pathology included increased neutrophils, total protein and globulin, and reduced albumin, AST and ALT. |
| | 4 weeks | 1, 2, 4, 5, 25, 75, 150 | 4 | 3810/3992 | 0.5/0.5 | Arteritis at ≥5 mg/kg. Essentially no toxicity ≤4 mg/kg. |
| | 13 weeks | 2, 4, 8, 16 | 8 | 9608/8988 | 1.3/1.2 | Arteritis at 16 mg/kg/day in a few animals, at the root of the aorta and in 1 female also the thymus. |
| | 3 months | 100, 300, 1000 | 100 | 24318/25478 | 3.3/3.5 | No mortality at all doses. Inflammatory lesions associated with organs in the thoracic cavity (heart, aortic root and lungs). |
| | 6 months | 0, 10, 100, 1000, QD | 10 | 5614/5842 | 0.8/0.8 | Mortalities at 100 and 1000 mg/kg/day. Arteritis of the aortic root and other cardiac arteries and myocardium, inflammation and vascular lesions in abdominal organs. |
| Cynomolgus monkey | 4 weeks | 0, 50, 180, 650 | 50 | 15079/9666 | 2.1/1.3 | A dose-dependent increase in white blood cells and a reduction in lymphocytes, vasculitis in 1 male at 180 mg/kg/day and 2 females at 650 mg/kg/day. |
| | 13 weeks | 0, 25, 85, 300 | 300 | 32523/23307 | 4.5/3.2 | Excessive salivation, occasional emesis or retching at high doses. |
| | 12 months | 0, 60, 180, 600 | 600 | 42608/26936 | 5.8/3.7 | Increase in total white blood cells due to an increase in neutrophils, a reduction in lymphocytes and an elevated fibrinogen. |

[a] Male/Female.　The AUC$_{0-24}$ for the maximum recommended human dose of 30 mg BID was 7440 ng·h/mL.

[8] FDA Database.　http://www.accessdata.fda.gov/drugsatfda_docs/nda/2014/206088Orig1s000PharmR.pdf (accessed Mar 2016).
[9] EMA Database.　http://www.ema.europa.eu/docs/en_GB/document_library/EPAR_-_Public_assessment_report/human/003746/WC500182629.pdf (accessed Mar 2016).

## Safety Pharmacology

Table 16    Safety Pharmacological Studies of Apremilast[8]

| Study | System | Dose | Finding |
|---|---|---|---|
| Cardiovascular effect | hERG channel transfected HEK293 cell | 16.8, 49.7, 87.5, 249.7 μM | $IC_{50}$ of hERG tail current: 184 μM. |
| | Beagle dog | 0.5, 1, 5 mg/kg, i.v. | Dose-related increases in dP/dtmax and heart rate were observed at doses ≥0.5 mg/kg, but QT prolongation was not observed. |
| Respiratory effect | Beagle dog | 0.5, 1, 5 mg/kg, i.v. | Dose-related increases in peak inspiratory and expiratory flow were observed at doses ≥0.5 mg/kg. |
| Central nervous effect | ICR mouse | 500, 1000, 2000 mg/kg, p.o. | At doses ≥1000 mg/kg: Lacrimation and ptosis were observed. At 2000 mg/kg: Apathy (sluggish movement) and death of one animal. |
| Gastrointestinal tract | ICR mouse | 10, 100, 1000 mg/kg, p.o. | No effect at doses up to 1000 mg/kg. |

## Genotoxicity

Table 17    Genotoxicity Studies of Apremilast[8, 9]

| Assay | Species/System | Metabolism Activity | Dose | Finding |
|---|---|---|---|---|
| In vitro reverse mutation assay in bacterial cells (Ames) | S. typhimurium TA98, TA100, TA1535, TA1537, TA102; E. coli WP2 uvrA | ±S9 | Up to 5000 μg/plate | Negative. |
| In vitro chromosomal aberrations assays in mammalian cells | HPBL | ±S9 | Up to 448 μg/mL (-S9) Up to 700 μg/mL (+S9) | Negative. |
| In vivo bone marrow micronucleus assay | Mouse | + | Single, p.o., 0, 500, 1000, 2000 mg/kg/day | Negative. |

## Reproductive and Developmental Toxicity

Table 18    Reproductive and Developmental Toxicology Studies of Apremilast by Oral Administration[8, 9]

| Studies | Species | Dose (mg/kg/day) | NOAEL Endpoint | NOAEL Dose (mg/kg/day) | NOAEL $AUC_{0-24}$ (ng·h/mL) | NOAEL Safety Margin[a] (× MRHD) | Finding |
|---|---|---|---|---|---|---|---|
| Fertility and early embryonic development | ICR mouse | 1, 10, 25, 50 | Male fertility | 50 | 21040 | 2.8 | No effect on fertility. |
| | ICR mouse | 10, 20, 40, 80 | Female fertility | 10 | 29215 | 3.9 | ↓ Number of estrus cycles, ↑ extended cycles at 20 & 80 mg/kg/day. ↑ #days of cohabit ≥20 mg/kg/day. ↑ Post-implant losses, total/early resorption ≥20 mg/kg/day, ↓ litter sizes, number of live fetuses and fetal BW at ≥40 mg/kg. ↓ Ossified tarsals ≥20 mg/kg/day, ↑ incompletely ossified supraoccipitals at ≥40 mg/kg/day. |
| Embryo-fetal development | ICR mouse | 250, 500, 750 | EFD | 750 | NA | NA | Pregnancy rate unaffected, ↑ embryo-fetal loss, ↑ intrauterine deaths & post-implantation losses. ↓ Litter weight and fetal weight at all doses, ↓ placental weight ≥500 mg/kg/day. ↑ Rate incomplete ossification and/or sternabrae development. |

[8] FDA Database. http://www.accessdata.fda.gov/drugsatfda_docs/nda/2014/206088Orig1s000PharmR.pdf (accessed Mar 2016).
[9] EMA Database. http://www.ema.europa.eu/docs/en_GB/document_library/EPAR_-_Public_assessment_report/human/003746/WC500182629.pdf (accessed Mar 2016).

*Continued*

| Studies | Species | Dose (mg/kg/day) | NOAEL | | | | Finding |
|---------|---------|------------------|-------|---|---|---|---------|
| | | | Endpoint | Dose (mg/kg/day) | $AUC_{0-24}$ (ng·h/mL) | Safety Margin[a] (× MRHD) | |
| Embryo-fetal development | Cynomolgus monkey | 20, 50, 200, 1000 | Maternal | 20 | 10100 | 1.4 | ↓ BW in animals that aborted. ↑ Dose-dependent in embryo/fetal loss. External fetal findings not considered treatment-related due to absence of dose response. Ossification or misaligned vertebrae, used ribs, scoliosis, all considered not related to treatment. |
| | | | EFD | 1000 | 62400 | 8.4 | |
| Pre- and postnatal development | ICR mouse | 10, 80, 300 | Maternal | 10 | NA | NA | $F_0$: One death at HD, ↓ maternal BW on DL 4 & 14, ↓ BWG GD 12-18, DL 1-14 at 300 mg/kg/day. PPN: ↑ Stillborn pups at ≥80 mg/kg/day and dams with no surviving pups (300 mg/kg/day). ↓ Litter sizes and average litter weight, and pup weight ≥80 mg/kg/day. ↑ 80 mg/kg/day dead, sacrificed due to adverse signs or missing and presumed cannibalize. $F_1$: No treatment-related effect on clinical signs, body weights, sexual maturation, passive avoidance, motor activity, mating, fertility, or C-section parameters. |
| | | | $F_1$ | 10 | NA | NA | |
| Juvenile | ICR mouse | 1, 4, 10 | Male | 10 | 7470[b] | 1.0 | Well-tolerated in juvenile mice. Mortalities at all doses. Mild/moderate dyhydration decreased activity and body weights, delayed sexual maturation, and increased lymphocytes. |
| | | | Female | 4 | 13600[b] | 1.8 | |

\#: The number of days.  [a] Calculated based on the $AUC_{0-24}$ for the MRHD of 30 mg BID (7440 ng·h/mL).  [b] The highest data obtained, which was on PND 7.

# Carcinogenicity

Table 19    Carcinogenicity Studies of Apremilast by Oral Administration for 104 Weeks[8, 9]

| Species | Dose (mg/kg/day) | NOAEL | | | Finding |
|---------|------------------|-------|---|---|---------|
| | | Dose (mg/kg/day) | $AUC_{0-24}$ (ng·h/mL) | Safety Margin[a] (× MRHD) | |
| ICR mouse | 100, 300 (200), 1000 (500 female) | 1000 | 63952 | 8.6 | No treatment-related neoplastic change up to 1000/500 mg/kg/day. |
| SD rat | Male, 3, 10/6, 20 | 20 | 608 | 0.08 | No treatment-related neoplastic change up to 20 or 3 mg/kg/day in males and females, respectively. |
| | Female, 0.3, 1, 3 | 3 | 7721 | 1.1 | |

Vehicle: 1% CMC-Na for the mouse study, 1% MC for the rat study.    [a] Calculated based on the $AUC_{0-24}$ for the MRHD of 30 mg BID (7440 ng·h/mL).

[8]  FDA Database.    http://www.accessdata.fda.gov/drugsatfda_docs/nda/2014/206088Orig1s000PharmR.pdf (accessed Mar 2016).
[9]  EMA Database.    http://www.ema.europa.eu/docs/en_GB/document_library/EPAR_-_Public_assessment_report/human/003746/WC500182629.pdf (accessed Mar 2016).

## Special Toxicology

Table 20    Special Toxicology Studies of Apremilast[8]

| Study | Species | Finding |
|---|---|---|
| Neutral red uptake phototoxicity assay | Murine (Balb/c 3T3) fibroblast | Not phototoxic at doses up to 101.8 mg/L. |

[8]  FDA Database.   http://www.accessdata.fda.gov/drugsatfda_docs/nda/2014/206088Orig1s000PharmR.pdf (accessed Mar 2016).

# CHAPTER

## 4

## Asunaprevir

# Asunaprevir

## (Sunvepra®)

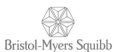

Bristol-Myers Squibb

## 1  General Information

❖ Asunaprevir is an inhibitor of NS3/4A protease, which was first approved in Jul 2014 by PMDA of Japan.

❖ Asunaprevir was discovered, developed and marketed by Bristol-Myers Squibb.

❖ Asunaprevir is a selectively inhibitor of NS3/4A protease which is essential for HCV replication.  Asunaprevir competitively binds to and inhibits the active site S1' and S4 of NS3/4A binding domain, resulting in preventing the proteolytic process of the HCV nonstructural polyprotein.

❖ Asunaprevir is indicated for the treatment of patients with HCV infection.

❖ Available as capsule, with each containing 100 mg of asunaprevir and the recommended dose is 100 mg orally twice daily until disease progression or unacceptable toxicity.

❖ Sales of Sunvepra® were 55 and 288 million US$ in 2014 and 2015, respectively, referring to the financial reports of Bristol-Myers Squibb.

## Key Approvals around the World*

|  | Japan (PMDA) |
| --- | --- |
| First approval date | 07/04/2014 |
| Application or approval No. | 22600AMX00765000 |
| Brand name | Sunvepra® |
| Indication | HCV infection |
| Authorisation holder | Bristol-Myers Squibb |

* Till Mar 2016, it has not been approved by FDA (US), EMA (EU) and CFDA (China).

## Active Ingredient

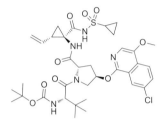

*Molecular formula*:  $C_{35}H_{46}ClN_5O_9S$
*Molecular weight*:  748.29
*CAS No.*:  630420-16-5 (Asunaprevir)
*Chemical name*:  1,1-Dimethylethyl{(2S)-1-[(2S,4R)-4-({7-chloro-4-methoxyisoquinolin-1-yl}oxy)-2-({{(1R,2S)-1-[(cyclopropanesulfonyl)carbamoyl]-2-ethenylcyclopropyl}carbamoyl)pyrrolidin-1-yl]-3,3-dimethyl-1-oxobutan-2-yl} carbamate

*Parameters of Lipinski's "Rule of 5"*

| MW | $H_D$ | $H_A$ | FRB[a] | PSA[a] | cLogP[a] |
| --- | --- | --- | --- | --- | --- |
| 748.29 | 3 | 14 | 13 | 191Å² | 4.25 ± 1.46 |

[a] Calculated by ACD/Labs software V11.02.

## Drug Product*

*Dosage route*:  Oral
*Strength*:  100 mg (Asunaprevir)
*Dosage form*:  Capsule
*Inactive ingredient*:  Medium chain fatty acid triglycerides, monoglycerides capric caprylic acid, polysorbate 80, dibutyl hydroxy toluene, gelatin, corn starch, glycerin and titanium oxide.
*Recommended dose*:  The recommended dose is 100 mg orally twice daily for adults.
  Asunaprevir is used in combination with daclatasvir dihydrochloride, administration period for 24 weeks.

* Sourced from Japan PMDA drug label information

## 2  Key Patents Information

### Summary

❖ Sunvepra® (Asunaprevir) was approved by PMDA of Japan on Jul 04, 2014.

❖ Asunaprevir was originally discovered by Bristol-Myers Squibb, and its compound patent application was filed as PCT application by Bristol-Myers Squibb in 2003.

❖ The compound patent will expire in 2023 foremost, which has been granted in the United States, China, Japan and Europe successively.

Table 1  Asunaprevir's Compound Patent Protection in Drug-Mainstream Country

| Country | Publication/Patent NO. | Application Date | Granted Date | Estimated Expiry Date |
|---|---|---|---|---|
| WO | WO03099274A1 | 05/20/2003 | / | / |
| US | US6995174B2 | 05/20/2003 | 02/07/2006 | 05/20/2023 |
| | US7915291B2 | 05/20/2003 | 03/29/2011 | 05/20/2023 |
| EP | EP1505963B1 | 05/20/2003 | 04/20/2011 | 05/20/2023 |
| JP | JP4312710B2 | 05/20/2003 | 08/12/2009 | 05/20/2028[a] |
| CN | CN1299677C | 05/20/2003 | 02/14/2007 | 05/20/2023 |
| | CN1974596B | 05/20/2003 | 07/28/2010 | 05/20/2023 |

[a] The term of this patent is extended by 5 years.

Table 2  Originator's International Patent Application List (Patent Family)

| Publication NO. | Title | Applicant/Assignee/Owner | Publication Date |
|---|---|---|---|
| **Technical Subjects** | **Active Ingredient (Free Base)'s Formula or Structure and Preparation** | | |
| WO03099274A1 | Hepatitis C virus inhibitors | Bristol-Myers Squibb | 12/04/2003 |
| **Technical Subjects** | **Salt, Crystal, Polymorphic, Solvate (Hydrate), Isomer, Derivative Etc. and Preparation** | | |
| WO2009085659A1 | Crystalline forms of N-(tert-butoxycarbonyl)-3-methyl-l-valyl-(4R)-4-((7-chloro-4-methoxy-1-isoquinolinyl)oxy)-N-((1R,2S)-1-((cyclopropylsulfonyl)carbamoyl)-2-vinylcyclo-propyl)-l-prolinamide | Bristol-Myers Squibb | 07/09/2009 |
| WO2009129109A1 | Hepatitis C virus inhibitors | Bristol-Myers Squibb | 10/22/2009 |
| WO2012166459A1 | Tripeptides incorporating deuterium as inhibitors of hepatitis C virus | Bristol-Myers Squibb | 12/06/2012 |
| **Technical Subjects** | **Formulation and Preparation** | | |
| WO2013169520A1 | Solubilized capsule formulation of 1,1-dimethylethyl[(1S)-1-{[(2S,4R)-4-(7-chloro-4-methoxyisoquinolin-1-yloxy)-2-({(1R,2S)-1-[(cyclopropysulfonyl)carbamoyl]-2-ethenylcyclopropyl}carbamoyl)pyrrolidin-1-yl]carbonyl}-2,2-dimethylpropyl]carbamate | Bristol-Myers Squibb | 11/14/2013 |
| WO2013169577A1 | Oral solid dosage formulation of 1,1-dimethylethyl[(1S)-1-{[(2S,4R)-4-(7-chloro-4-methoxyisoquinolin-1-yloxy)-2-({(1R,2S)-1-[(cyclopropysulfonyl)carbamoyl]-2-ethenylcyclopropyl}carbamoyl)pyrrolidin-1-yl]carbonyl}-2,2-dimethylpropyl]carbamate | Bristol-Myers Squibb | 11/14/2013 |

The data was updated until Jan 2016.

# 3 Chemistry

## Route 1: Original Discovery Route

*Synthetic Route*: The synthesis of enantioenriched cyclopropylamine **10** commenced with condensation of commercially available glycine ethyl ester hydrochloride **2** and benzaldehyde **1** to afford imine **3**. A subsequent four-step sequence in which base-promoted cyclization was followed by Boc-protection to afford **5** in 53% from **2**, as a 1:1 mixture of (1*R*,2*S*) : (1*S*,2*R*) cyclopropanes, and then treated **5** with alcalase in a buffered solution in a mix solution of aqueous NaOH and DMSO to seperate enantiomer **6** in 52% isolated yield (>98% expected recovery) and with 100% *ee*. Saponification with LiOH afforded acid **7**, and this was followed by a CDI-promoted amide bond formation to give **9** in excellent yield (92%). Deprotection with TFA followed by an ion swap gave rise to the key enantiopure intermediate **10** in 92% yield. Three conventional peptide coupling steps achieved tripeptide **15** in 98% yield within three steps, which was then condensed with 1,7-dichloro-4-methoxyisoquinoline **16** in the presence of LaCl₃ under basic conditions to complete the synthesis of the titled compound in 31% yield and 6% overall yield.[1-4]

[1] Wang, X. A.; Sun, L.; Sit, S., et al. WO2003099274A1, **2003**.
[2] Wang, X. A.; Sun, L.; Sit, S., et al. US6995174B2, **2006**.
[3] Sin, N.; Venables, B. L.; Scola, P. M., et al. WO2009129109A1, **2009**.
[4] Sin, N.; Venables, B. L.; Scola, P. M., et al. US8163921B2, **2012**.

## Route 2

*Synthetic Route*:   Preparation of asunaprevir was initiated with commercially available *p*-chlorocinnamic acid **1** which was treated with diphenylphosphoryl azide (DPPA) to effect a Curtius rearrangement followed by ring closure to give isoquinoline **2** in 53% yield.   Regioselective bromination of **2** followed by conversion of the hydroxyl group within **3** to C1-chloroiso-quinoline **4** with the yield of 90% and 73%, respectively.   Next, oxygenation of the isoquinoline C4 position in isoquinoline **4** was accomplished in a single operation by a lithium-halogen exchange, which selectively engaged the C4-bromo group in the presence of both the C1 and C7 chloro substituents.   The intermediate aryl-lithium species was quenched by the addition of isopropylboronic acid ester which gave rise to the isoquinoline-4-boronate derivative.   The crude boronate derivative was directly converted to 4-hydroxy-1,7-dicholoroisoquinoline **5** by oxidizing condition of aqueous H$_2$O$_2$ in good overall yield (82%), which was smoothly converted to methyl ether **6** in 97% yield.   Thus, S$_N$Ar involving *N*-Boc-3-(*R*)-hydroxy-L-pro-line **7** and chloriquinoline **6** under basic conditions furnished aryl pyrrolidino ether **8** which was carried forward as crude for the subsequent transformation.   Proline-derived acid **8** was activated prior to the subjection to **9** in the presence of base to afford amide **10** in 88% yield over two steps, which upon quantitative acidic Boc-removal and successive HATU-mediated coupling with *N*-Boc-L-*tert*-Leucine **12** completed the synthesis of asunaprevir in 94% yield and the overall yield of 23%.[5-9]

[5]   Scola, P. M.; Sun, L.; Wang A. X., et al. *J. Med. Chem.* **2014**, *57*, 1730-1752.
[6]   Perrone, R. K.; Wang, C.; Ying, W., et al. WO2009085659A1, **2009**.
[7]   Perrone, R. K.; Song, A. I.; Wang, C., et al. US8202996B2, **2012**.
[8]   Sun, L.; Scola, P. M. WO2012166459A1, **2012**.
[9]   Sun, L.; Scola, P. M. US20130129671A1, **2013**.

# 4   Pharmacology

## Summary

### Mechanism of Action

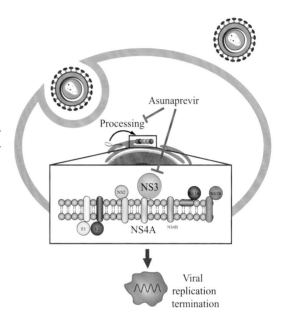

❖ Asunaprevir is a small molecule inhibitor of HCV NS3/4A protease, which is required for cleavage of the HCV polyprotein and viral replication.

❖ In a biochemistry assay, asunaprevir competitively bound to and inhibited the active site S1' and S4 of NS3/4A binding domain, resulting in preventing the proteolytic process of the HCV nonstructural polyprotein (Genotype 1: $K_i$ = 0.24-1.0 nM).[10]

❖ The inhibitions were exhibited as:
  • Genotype 1a/1b/4a/5a/6a: $IC_{50}$ = 0.3-1.8 nM.
  • Genotype 2a/2b: $IC_{50}$ = 15/78 nM.
  • Genotype 3a: $IC_{50}$ = 320 nM.

❖ Asunaprevir had no significant inhibition of ligand binding in a panel of all other serine/cysteine proteases ($IC_{50} \geq$ 5000 nM), or a panel of 37 targets including receptors, enzymes, or ion channels at 10 μM.[10]

### *In Vitro* Efficacy

❖ Anti-HCV potency in HCV replicon cells:
  • 1a/1b/4a: $EC_{50}$ = 1.2-4.0 nM.
  • 2a/2b: $EC_{50}$ = 67-480 nM.
  • 3a: $EC_{50}$ = 1162 nM.

❖ Resistant development in cells containing genotype 1a/1b HCV replicons:
  • GT 1a: R155K, I170T and D168G, with 49 folds increase for $EC_{50}$ at 30 × $EC_{50}$_wild type.
  • GT 1b: Q80R and D168V/G/A/Y with 170-400 folds increase for $EC_{50}$ at 30 × $EC_{50}$_wild type.

❖ Anti-HCV potency against HCV replicons containing NS3/4A substitutions:
  • 1a containing V36/T54/Q80K/I170T: $EC_{50}$ = 0.33-3.6 nM (0.4-5 folds increase).

❖ 1a containing R155K, D168 and double site mutations: $EC_{50}$ = 11-542 nM (14-713 folds increase).
  • 1b containing V36/T54A/Q80/V170A: $EC_{50}$ = 0.35-5.6 nM (0.4-6.5 folds).
  • 1b containing A156S/T/V: $EC_{50}$ = 5.4-17 nM (6-20 folds).
  • 1b containing D168: $EC_{50}$ = 13-241 nM (16-280 folds).

❖ Substitutions in (Daclatasvir + Asunaprevir)-resistant HCV replicons from clinical patients:
  • GT1b (Con1) replicon: $EC_{50}$ = 2 nM.
  • GT 1b NS3-D168V/NS5A-L31M-Y93H: $EC_{50}$ = 401 nM.

❖ Effect on NS3 protease and NS5A amino acid in genotype 1a replicon in clinical patients:
  • NS3/NS5 WT: $EC_{50}$ = 10.1/4.5 nM.
  • From patients (NS3/NS5 mutation): $EC_{50}$ = 5.3-1883 nM, 1-418 folds.

[10]   Japan Pharmaceuticals and Medical Devices Agency (PMDA) Database.   http://www.pmda.go.jp/drugs/2014/P201400113/index.html (accessed Mar 2016).

## Mechanism of Action

Table 3    The Activity of Asunaprevir against Recombinant HCV NS3/4A Protease in Major HCV Genotype[10, 11]

| Genotype (strain) | IC$_{50}$ (nM) | | Genotype (strain) | IC$_{50}$ (nM) | |
| --- | --- | --- | --- | --- | --- |
| | Asunaprevir | Telaprevir | | Asunaprevir | Telaprevir |
| 1a (BMS) | 1.8 ± 0.2 | 12 ± 2 | 3a (S52) | 320 ± 13 | 537 ± 4 |
| 1a (H77) | 0.7 ± 0.06 | 33 ± 7 | 4a (ED43) | 1.6 ± 0.1 | 12 ± 1 |
| 1b (J4L6S) | 0.3 ± 0.02 | 22 ± 6 | 5a (SA13) | 1.7 ± 0.2 | 38 ± 3 |
| 2a (HC-J6) | 15 ± 1.2 | 95 ± 17 | 6a (HK-6A) | 0.9 ± 0.09 | 86 ± 2 |
| 2b (HC-J8) | 78 ± 2 | 12 ± 1 | | | |

BMS: Bristol-Myers Squibb.    Data were means ± SD from at least three independent experiments.

Table 4    *In Vitro* Potency of Asunaprevir against Serine and Cysteine Proteases[11]

| Protease | IC$_{50}$ (nM) | |
| --- | --- | --- |
| | Asunaprevir | Telaprevir |
| HCV 1a NS3/4A (BMS) | 0.7 ± 0.1 | 12 ± 2 |
| GBV-B NS3/4A | 21000 ± 6000 | 7700 ± 0 |
| Human leukocyte elastase | >50000 | 3200 ± 100 |
| PPE | >50000 | 5600 ± 300 |
| Human chymotrypsin | >50000 | 45000 ± 8000 |
| Human cathepsin B | >50000 | 1700 ± 200 |
| Human cathepsin A | >5000[a] | 330 ± 20 |
| Trypsin | >30000 | ND |
| Thrombin | >30000 | ND |
| Factor VIIa | >30000 | ND |
| Factor Xa | >30000 | ND |
| Factor XIa | >30000 | ND |
| Kallikrein | >30000 | ND |

BMS: Bristol-Myers Squibb.    PPE: Porcine pancreas elastase.    ND: Not determined.    [a] Assay interference was observed at 20 μM.

## *In Vitro* Efficacy

Table 5    Anti-HCV Potency of Asunaprevir on Different Genotype HCV Replicon in Cell Lines[10, 11]

| Genotype | Strain | System | Method | EC$_{50}$ (nM) | |
| --- | --- | --- | --- | --- | --- |
| | | | | Asunaprevir | Telaprevir |
| 1a | H77 | Stable cell line | Luciferase | 4.0 ± 0.3 | 995 ± 11 |
| 1b | Con1 | Stable cell line | Luciferase | 1.2 ± 0.3 | 427 ± 3 |
| | | | FRET | 2.9 ± 0.5 | 573 ± 21 |
| | | Transient | Luciferase | 1.3 ± 0.1 | 266 ± 77 |
| 2a | JFH-1 | Stable cell line | FRET | 230 ± 74 | 229 ± 32 |
| | | Transient | Luciferase | 67 ± 23 | 108 ± 12 |
| 2b | HC-J8 | Transient | Luciferase | 480 ± 104 | 1236 ± 96 |
| 3a | S52 | Stable cell line | Luciferase | 1162 ± 274 | 2731 ± 188 |
| 4a | ED43 | Transient | Luciferase | 1.8 ± 0.2 | 1137 ± 223 |

Therapeutic index: Asunaprevir = 9300, Telaprevir >175.    Therapeutic index = Genotype 1b (Con1) in replicon cells CC$_{50}$/EC$_{50}$ (FRET), CC$_{50}$ = 50% cytotoxic concentration, EC$_{50}$ = 50% effective concentration.    1b (Con 1), CC$_{50}$ = 27000 ± 2000 nM (asunaprevir) or >100000 nM (telaprevir).    Telaprevir was preincubated with each of the respective NS3/4A protease complexes for 30 min before the addition of substrate to obtain optimum potency.    Data were means ± SD from at least three independent experiments.    FRET: Fluorescent resonance energy transfer.

[10]  PMDA Database.    http://www.pmda.go.jp/drugs/2014/P201400113/index.html (accessed Mar 2016).
[11]  McPhee, F.; Sheaffer, A. K.; Friborg, J., et al. *Antimicrob. Agents Chemother.* **2012**, *56*, 5387-5396.

Table 6 *In Vitro* Cytotoxicity of Asunaprevir in Human Tissue-Derived Cell Lines[10, 11]

| Cell Line | Tissue | Virus | $CC_{50}$ (μM) | $EC_{50}$ (μM) | $CC_{50}/EC_{50}$ Rate |
|-----------|--------|-------|----------------|----------------|------------------------|
| HuH-7 | Liver | HCV-1a[a] | 25 ± 5.2 | 0.004 ± 0.0003 | 6250 |
| HepG2 | Liver | BVDV[b] | 38 ± 4.6 | NA | NA |
| MT2 | T lymphocytes | HIV | 34 ± 2.8 | 13 ± 2 | 2.6 |
| MRC5 | Lung | HCoVOC43, HRV2 | 32 ± 5.0 | >32 | <1 |
| HeLa | Uterine cervix | NA | 19 ± 0.5 | NA | NA |
| HEK-293 | Embryonic kidney | NA | 11 ± 2.1 | NA | NA |

Data were means ± SD from at least three independent experiments. [a] Subgenomic replicon. [b] Full-length replicon.

Table 7 *In Vitro* Resistant Development of Asunaprevir Selection in HCV Genotype 1a and 1b[10]

| Genotype | Conc. | Effect | | Major NS3 Protease Replacement | NS3 Mutation Frequency |
|----------|-------|--------|--|--------------------------------|------------------------|
| | | $EC_{50}$ (nM) | Fold of $EC_{50}$ | | |
| 1a (H77) | 0 | 6.5 ± 2.2 | 1 | Wild type | - |
| 1a Mutation | $10 \times EC_{50\_WT}$[a] | 91 ± 39 | 13 | V51A, D79E | 1/9 |
| | | | | T95A, I170T | 1/9 |
| | | | | R155K | 8/9 |
| 1a Mutation | $10 \times EC_{50\_WT}$[a] | 77 ± 26 | 11 | Q41E, R62K | 1/9 |
| | | | | I114V, N174Y | 1/9 |
| | | | | D168G | 3/9 |
| | | | | I170T | 4/9 |
| 1a Mutation | $30 \times EC_{50\_WT}$[a] | 315 ± 72 | 49 | T40A, R123G | 1/10 |
| | | | | R155K | 4/10 |
| | | | | I170T | 5/10 |
| | | | | L175P, G176E | 1/10 |
| 1b (Con 1) | 0 | 3 | 1 | Q41R | - |
| | | | | Q86R | - |
| 1b Mutation | $10 \times EC_{50\_WT}$[b] | 590-1100 | 197-367 | Q41R | 6/10 |
| | | | | Q86R | 10/10 |
| | | | | D168G/A/H | 5/10; 1/10; 1/10 |
| | | | | E173G, E176G | 1/10 |
| 1b Mutation | $30 \times EC_{50\_WT}$[b] | 510-1200 | 170-400 | Q41R | 7/12 |
| | | | | Q80R | 1/12 |
| | | | | Q86R | 10/12 |
| | | | | P89L, Y105C | 1/12 |
| | | | | D168V/G/A/Y | 7/12; 3/12; 1/12; 1/12 |

R155K, I170T, D168V/G/A/Y, and Q80R were the substitutions around the binding sites of asunaprevir. [a] $EC_{50\_WT}$ = 1a (H77) $EC_{50}$ (6.5 ± 2.2 nM). [b] $EC_{50\_WT}$ = 1b (Con 1) $EC_{50}$ (3nM).

[10] PMDA Database. http://www.pmda.go.jp/drugs/2014/P201400113/index.html (accessed Mar 2016).
[11] McPhee, F.; Sheaffer, A. K.; Friborg, J., et al. *Antimicrob. Agents Chemother.* **2012**, *56*, 5387-5396.

Table 8    Anti-HCV of Asunaprevir against HCV Replicon Containing NS3/4A Substitutions in Cells[10, 12]

| Type | Amino Acid Substitution | Replication Ability (%) | Asunaprevir Effect | | Telaprevir | |
|---|---|---|---|---|---|---|
| | | | EC$_{50}$ (nM) | Fold Increase of the EC$_{50}$ Values | EC$_{50}$ (nM) | Fold Increase of the EC$_{50}$ Values |
| Genotype 1a | Wild type | 100 | 0.76 ± 0.3 | 1 | 181 ± 87 | 1 |
| | V36A | 89 | 2.3 ± 0.7 | 3 | 2689 ± 241 | 15 |
| | V36L | 137 | 1.8 ± 0.6 | 2 | 1248 ± 427 | 7 |
| | V36M | 171 | 1.5 ± 0.5 | 2 | 2989 ± 1813 | 17 |
| | T54A | 39 | 0.33 ± 0.1 | 0.4 | 847 ± 209 | 5 |
| | T54S | 36 | 0.74 ± 0.2 | 1 | 664 ± 150 | 4 |
| | Q80K | 119 | 2.5 ± 1.0 | 3 | 152 ± 75 | 1 |
| | R155K | 7 | 16 ± 3 | 21 | 860 ± 256 | 5 |
| | V36M + R155K | 5 | 42 ± 19 | 55 | >10000 | >55 |
| | **D168G** | 2 | 11 ± 4 | 14 | 133 ± 76 | 1 |
| | D168V | 33 | 283 ± 4 | 373 | 162 ± 10 | 1 |
| | Q80K + D168V | 46 | 542 ± 111 | 713 | 130 ± 37 | 1 |
| | **I170T** | 12 | 3.6 ± 1.6 | 5 | 647 ± 202 | 4 |
| Genotype 1b | Wild Type | 100 | 0.86 ± 0.3 | 1 | 176 ± 41 | 1 |
| | V36A | 124 | 1.6 ± 0.6 | 2 | 933 ± 281 | 5 |
| | V36L | 77 | 0.65 ± 0.1 | 1 | 395 ± 19 | 2 |
| | T54A | 101 | 0.35 ± 0.1 | 0.4 | 718 ± 31 | 4 |
| | D168E | 25 | 67 ± 11 | 78 | 129 ± 7 | 1 |
| | Q80K | 139 | 5.6 ± 1 | 6.5 | ND | ND |
| | Q80L | 98 | 0.86 ± 0.1 | 1 | 167 ± 14 | 1 |
| | **Q80R** | 102 | 3.5 ± 0.9 | 4 | ND | ND |
| | A156S | 120 | 5.9 ± 0.9 | 7 | 2515 ± 624 | 15 |
| | A156T | 17 | 5.4 ± 1 | 6 | >10000 | >57 |
| | A156V | 3 | 17 ± 2 | 20 | >10000 | >57 |
| | **D168A** | 37 | 109 ± 19 | 127 | 21 ± 4 | 0.1 |
| | **D168G** | 29 | 13 ± 4 | 16 | 56 ± 12 | 0.3 |
| | **D168V** | 29 | 241 ± 17 | 280 | 42 ± 7 | 0.2 |
| | **D168Y** | 2 | 205 ± 29 | 238 | 71 ± 43 | 0.4 |
| | V170A | 96 | 1.6 ± 0.4 | 2 | 699 ± 237 | 4 |

Substitutions associated with asunaprevir resistance selection in genotype 1a and 1b replicons were in bold.    Values were means ± SD from ≥3 independent experiments.    ND: Not determined.

[10]  PMDA Database.    http://www.pmda.go.jp/drugs/2014/P201400113/index.html (accessed Mar 2016).
[12]  McPhee, F.; Friborg, J.; Levine, S., et al. *Antimicrob. Agents Chemother.* **2012**, *56*, 3670-3681.

Table 9 Cell Potency of Compounds against Genotype 1b Wild Type and (Daclatasvir + Asunaprevir)-resistant Replicons and $C_{trough}$ Concentration Observed in Clinical Settings[13]

| Agent | EC$_{50}$ (nM) | | | $C_{trough}$ (nM) |
| | GT 1b (Con1) Replicon | GT 1b NS3-D168V, NS5A-L31M-Y93H | Fold | |
| --- | --- | --- | --- | --- |
| Asunaprevir | 2.0 ± 0.4 | 401 ± 102 | 201 | 40 |
| Daclatasvir | 0.002 ± 0.001 | 49 ± 9 | 24500 | 250 |
| Beclabuvir | 3.4 ± 0.2 | 4.0 ± 0.7 | 1 | 500 |
| Ledipasvir | 0.002 ± 0.0004 | 131 ± 40 | 65500 | 120 |
| Sofosbuvir | 147 ± 27 | 102 ± 12 | 1 | 1100 |
| Simeprevir | 1.9 ± 0.1 | 6296 ± 203 | 3313 | 2200 |
| Next-gen NS5A (BMS-1) | 0.010 ± 0.002 | 0.354 ± 0.05 | 39 | - |
| Next-gen NS3 PI (BMS-2) | 0.7 ± 0.1 | 4.1 ± 0.6 | 6 | 100 |
| Ribavirin | 8.1 ± 1.2 | 7.8 ± 5.7 | 1 | 2.5 |
| Peginterferon alfa | 1.2 ± 0.2 | 2.6 ± 0.6 | 2 | 15 |

Data were means ± SD.

Table 10 Effect of NS3 Protease and NS5A Amino Acid Substitutions on Asunaprevir and Daclatasvir Potency in Genotype 1a Replicon Assays in Clinical Patients[14]

| | Variant | | Asunaprevir | | Daclatasvir | |
| | NS3 | NS5A | EC$_{50}$ (nM) | Fold Resistance | EC$_{90}$ (nM) | Fold Resistance |
| --- | --- | --- | --- | --- | --- | --- |
| Cell line | WT | WT | 10.1 ± 5.5 | 1 | 0.060 ± 0.003 | 1 |
| Transient | WT[a] | WT[a] | 4.5 ± 1.7 | 1 | 0.020 ± 0.006 | 1 |
| | D168Y | WT | 938 | 93 | 0.030 ± 0.006 | 1 |
| | D168A | WT | 132 | 29 | ND | ND |
| Patient 1 | D168T[a] | WT[a] | 924 ± 3 | 205 | 0.020 ± 0.001 | 1 |
| | WT | Y93N | 7.7 ± 0.8 | 1 | 1156 ± 53 | 19267 |
| | D168Y | Y93N | ND | ND | ND | ND |
| | D168T | Y93N | 934 ± 75 | 92 | 708 ± 104 | 11800 |
| | Q80K + R155K[a] | WT[a] | 292 ± 114 | 65 | 0.020 ± 0.003 | 1 |
| | Q80K + D168Y | WT | >1000 | >99 | 0.050 ± 0.009 | 1 |
| Patient 2 | WT | L31V + H58P | 5.3 ± 0.0 | 1 | 144 ± 29 | 2400 |
| | Q80K + R155K | L31V + H58P | 639 ± 138 | 63 | 272 ± 21 | 4533 |
| | Q80K + D168Y | L31V + H58P | >1000 | >99 | 312 ± 106 | 5200 |
| | D168Y | WT | 938 | 93 | 0.030 ± 0.006 | 1 |
| Patient 3 | WT | Q30R + L31M | 6.1 ± 0.4 | 1 | 564 ± 6 | 9400 |
| | D168Y[a] | Q30R + L31M[a] | 1883 ± 156 | 418 | >2000 | >100000 |
| | Q80K+D168E[a] | WT[a] | 209 ± 8 | 46 | 0.010 ± 0.002 | 1 |
| | WT | Q30R + L31V | 6.1 ± 0.6 | 1 | >2000 | 33333 |
| | WT[a] | L31V[a] | ND | ND | 42 ± 12 | 2100 |
| Patient 4 | WT | L31V + Y93C | 7.2 ± 0.5 | 1 | >2000 | 33333 |
| | Q80K + D168E | Q30R + L31V | 374 ± 29 | 37 | >2000 | 33333 |
| | Q80K + D168E | L13V + Y93C | 446 ± 88 | 44 | >2000 | 33333 |
| | Q80K + D168E[a] | L31V[a] | 223 ± 4 | 50 | 70 ± 14 | 3500 |

[13] Friborg, J.; Zhou, N.; Han, Z., et al. *Infect. Dis. Ther.* **2014**, *4*, 137-144.
[14] McPhee, F.; Hernandez, D.; Yu, F., et al. *Hepatology (Hoboken, NJ, U. S.).* **2013**, *58*, 902-911.

*Continued*

| Variant | | Asunaprevir | | Daclatasvir | |
|---|---|---|---|---|---|
| NS3 | NS5A | $EC_{50}$ (nM) | Fold Resistance | $EC_{90}$ (nM) | Fold Resistance |
| Q80L + R155K | WT | 485 ± 30 | 48 | 0.050 ± 0.007 | 1 |
| WT | Y93N | 7.7 ± 0.8 | 1 | 1156 ± 53 | 19267 |
| WT | Q30R + L31V | 6.1 ± 0.6 | 1 | >2000 | 33333 |
| WT | L31V + H58P | 5.3 ± 0.0 | 1 | 144 ± 29 | 2400 |
| Q80L + R155K | Y93N | 348 ± 197 | 34 | 637 ± 129 | 10617 |
| Q80L + R155K[a] | Q30R + L31V[a] | 97 ± 37 | 22 | >1000 | >50000 |
| Q80L + R155K[a] | L31V + H58P[a] | 101 ± 33 | 22 | 161 ± 43 | 8050 |
| R155K | WT | 270 ± 7 | 27 | 0.04 ± 0.01 | 1 |
| WT | Q30E | 12 ± 2 | 1 | 373 ± 4 | 6217 |
| Q80L-R155K | Q30E | 438 ± 6 | 43 | 350 ± 17 | 5833 |

Patient 5 (rows 1–7); Patient 7 (rows 8–10).

Predominant resistance variants, as determined by clonal analysis (≥10% of clones) were shown.    In general, $EC_{90}$ values represented the average of at least three independent experiments (standard deviation provided).    For variants where a standard deviation was not provided, $EC_{90}$ values represented the average of two independent experiments.    WT referred to the parental HCV genotype 1a (H77c) replicon used to compare the impact of NS3 and NS5A resistance substitutions on asunaprevir and daclatasvir antiviral activity.    [a] Transient HCV replication assay.    ND: Not determined because the variant did not replicate.    WT: Wild type.

# 5   ADME & Drug-Drug Interaction

## Summary

### Absorption of Asunaprevir

❖ Exhibited a non-linear pharmacokinetics in rats and humans following oral dosing.    The increases in $C_{max}$ and AUC appeared not to be proportional in the dose range of 10 to 90 mg/kg in rats and 200 to 1200 mg in humans, respectively.

❖ Showed high and moderate oral bioavailability in dogs (100% at 6 mg/kg, 42% at 3 mg/kg), and moderate in mice (28%), but low in rats (1%-14%) and monkeys (10%).

❖ Was absorbed rapidly in monkeys ($T_{max}$ = 1.3 h), moderately in dogs ($T_{max}$ = 1.7-3 h), rapidly to slowly in rats ($T_{max}$ = 1.8-9.6 h) and humans ($T_{max}$ = 2.8-4.0 h), but slowly in mice ($T_{max}$ = 6 h).

❖ Showed a half-life of 13.7 h in humans, longer than that in mice (4.6 h), rats (4.2-8.1 h) and monkeys (1.3 h), after intravenous administrations.

❖ Had moderate clearance in mice (57.3 mL/min/kg), rats (38.4-38.9 mL/min/kg), dogs (15.4-18.7 mL/min/kg), monkeys (18.3 mL/min/kg) and humans (49.5 L/h), after intravenous administrations.

❖ Exhibited a moderate tissue distribution in dogs and monkeys, with apparent volumes of distribution at 0.2-0.6 L/kg and 0.5 L/kg, respectively, but an extensive tissue distributions in mice, rats and humans, with apparent volumes of distribution at 12.6, 7.4-7.9 L/kg and 194 L, respectively, after intravenous administrations.

❖ Showed a high permeability in PAMPA model with Pe = 473-1012 nm/s and Pe = 492-610 nm/s at pH 5.5 and 7.4 separately, but moderate in Caco-2 cell monolayer model with $Papp_{(A \to B)}$ of 1.1-5.4 × $10^{-6}$ cm/s.

### Distribution of Asunaprevir

❖ Exhibited high serum protein binding in mice (99.2%), rats (98.8%), dogs (98.5%), monkeys (97.2%) and humans (98.8%).

❖ Had a $C_b:C_p$ ratio of 0.55 in humans, indicating low distribution into blood cells.

❖ Male rats after oral administration:
  • The drug was rapidly distributed into most tissues except for central nervous system.
  • Relatively higher concentration levels were observed in liver, bile, esophagus, stomach and small intestine, while the radioactivity in eyes was below limit of quantitation.
  • By 96 h post-dose, the remaining trace of radioactivity was detectable in liver and intestine.
  • Radioactivity was almost completely cleared at 168 h post-dose.

### Metabolism of Asunaprevir

❖ The metabolism of asunaprevir was relatively stable in liver microsomes and hepatocytes of humans, mice, rats, dogs and monkeys.

❖ Overall, the parent drug represented the most abundant component in human plasma, with M9 (BMS558364) as the major metabolite.

❖ The most abundant metabolites were similar among mice, rats, dogs, monkeys and humans.
❖ CYP3A4 and CYP3A5 were the major metabolizing enzymes, with minor contribution of CYP2A6, CYP2B6, CYP2C9, CYP2C19 and CYP2D6.[10]

## Excretion of Asunaprevir

❖ Was predominantly excreted in feces in humans and tested animals, with the parent drug as the most significant component in feces of mice, rats, dogs and rabbits.

## Drug-Drug Interaction

❖ Asunaprevir had reversible inhibition for CYP3A4 ($IC_{50}$ = 27.3->45 μM), 2C8 ($IC_{50}$ = 30.9 μM), 1A2, 2B6, 2C9, 2C19 and 2D6 ($IC_{50}$ >40 μM).
❖ Asunaprevir had induction for CYP3A4 and CYP2C9, but had no induction for CYP1A2.
❖ Asunaprevir was a substrate of P-gp, and had a low potential inhibition for P-gp.
❖ Asunaprevir was a substrate of OATP1B1 and OATP2B1, and had inhibition for OATP1B1 ($IC_{50}$ = 0.3 μM), OATP2B1 ($IC_{50}$ = 1.2 μM), OATP1B3 ($IC_{50}$ = 3.0 μM) and OAT1 ($IC_{50}$ = 11.8 μM).

# Absorption

Table 11   *In Vivo* Pharmacokinetic Parameters of Asunaprevir in Mice, Rats, Dogs and Monkeys after Single Dose of Asunaprevir (n = 3)[10]

| Species | Route | Dose (mg/kg) | $T_{max}$ (h) | $C_{max}$ (μg/mL) | $AUC_{inf}$ (μg·h/mL) | $T_{1/2}$ (h) | $V_{ss}$ (L/kg) | Cl (mL/min/kg) | F (%) |
|---|---|---|---|---|---|---|---|---|---|
| Mouse (male) | i.v. (PEG-400/ethanol) | 2[a] | NA | NA | 0.58 | 4.6 | 12.6 | 57.3 | - |
| | p.o. (PEG-400/ethanol) | 5[a] | 6 | 0.096 ± 0.059 | 0.405 | NA | NA | NA | 28 |
| | i.v. (PEG-400/ethanol) | 2[b] | NA | NA | 0.37 | 9.7 | 57.8 | 90.3 | - |
| | p.o. (PEG-400/ethanol) | 5[b] | 8 | 0.37 ± 0.07 | 2.38 | NA | NA | NA | 258 |
| Rat (male, fasted) | i.v. (PEG-400/ethanol) | 1 | 0.17 | 2.49 ± 0.68 | 0.53 ± 0.26 | ND | ND | ND | - |
| | | 3 | 0.17 | 8.71 ± 2.31 | 1.62 ± 0.56 | 8.1[g] | 7.4[g] | 38.9[g] | - |
| | | 5 | 0.17 | 11.5 ± 5.19 | 2.27 ± 0.55 | 4.2 ± 0.6 | 7.9 ± 7.2 | 38.4 ± 10.3 | - |
| | IPT[c] (PEG-400/ethanol) | 5 | 0.5 | 5.50 | 2.44 | 3.9 | 9.0 | 34.6 | - |
| | p.o. (PEG-400/ethanol) | 3 | 2.3 ± 1.5 | 0.006 ± 0.003 | 0.018 ± 0.006 | ND | NA | NA | 1 |
| | | 5 | 1.8 ± 1.9 | 0.032 ± 0.020 | 0.227 ± 0.173 | 4.5[g] | NA | NA | 10 |
| | | 10 | 9.6 ± 12.6 | 0.031 ± 0.009 | 0.317 ± 0.203 | 6.1[g] | NA | NA | 7 |
| | | 15 | 4.0 ± 0.0 | 0.137 ± 0.063 | 0.945 ± 0.220 | 8.3 ± 2.2 | NA | NA | 14 |
| | p.o.[d] (Water/povidone K-30/docusate sodium) | 10 | 1.2 ± 0.8 | 0.122 ± 0.112 | 0.300 ± 0.053 | 2.8[g] | NA | NA | 7 |
| | | 30 | 6.0 ± 0 | 1.44 ± 0.820 | 4.03 ± 2.63 | 3.7 ± 1.4 | NA | NA | 30 |
| | | 60 | 6.0 ± 2.0 | 3.98 ± 0.750 | 17.0 ± 1.28 | 2.2 ± 0.2 | NA | NA | 63 |
| | | 90 | 4.7 ± 1.2 | 4.59 ± 2.59 | 16.8 ± 4.90 | 2.5 ± 0.1 | NA | NA | 41 |
| | p.o.[e] (Water/povidone K-30/docusate sodium) | 10 | 1.9 ± 1.8 | 0.038 ± 0.036 | 0.201 ± 0.043 | 9.1[g] | NA | NA | 4 |
| | | 30 | 4.7 ± 2.3 | 1.59 ± 0.859 | 4.28 ± 0.882 | 1.8[g] | NA | NA | 32 |
| | | 60 | 6 ± 0 | 4.66 ± 1.07 | 27.6 ± 2.79 | 1.9 ± 0.1 | NA | NA | >100 |
| | | 90 | 4.7 ± 2.3 | 4.75 ± 3.46 | 24.3 ± 16.8 | 2.2 ± 0.4 | NA | NA | 60 |

[10]   PMDA Database. http://www.pmda.go.jp/drugs/2014/P201400113/index.html (accessed Mar 2016).

*Continued*

| Species | Route | Dose (mg/kg) | $T_{max}$ (h) | $C_{max}$ (µg/mL) | $AUC_{inf}$ (µg·h/mL) | $T_{1/2}$ (h) | $V_{ss}$ (L/kg) | Cl (mL/min/kg) | F (%) |
|---|---|---|---|---|---|---|---|---|---|
| Beagle dog (male, fasted) | i.v. (PEG-400/water) | 1[g] | NA | 5.92 | 0.9 | 1.0 | 0.2 | 18.7 | - |
| | | 2 | NA | 10.3 ± 4.06 | 2.62 ± 0.86 | 0.3 ± 0.2 | 0.6 ± 0.2 | 15.4 ± 5.6 | - |
| | p.o. (PEG-400/water) | 3[g] | 3 | 0.45 | 1.65 | 2.0 | NA | NA | 42 |
| | | 6 | 1.7 ± 0.6 | 5.60 ± 2.60 | 16.4 ± 4.83 | 2.4 ± 0.2 | NA | NA | >100 |
| | p.o.[e] (Croscamellose sodium/avicel 101) | 4[h] | 2.3 ± 0.5 | 0.35 ± 0.16 | 0.80 ± 0.37 | 0.7 ± 0.1 | NA | NA | 15 |
| | | 10 | 2.3 ± 1.5 | 4.32 ± 2.26 | 12.2 ± 7.19 | 2.8 ± 0.1 | NA | NA | 93 |
| Monkey[f] | i.v. (PEG-400/water) | 1 | NA | 8.19 ± 1.88 | 0.95 ± 0.26 | 1.3 ± 0.3 | 0.5 ± 0.2 | 18.3 ± 5.1 | - |
| | p.o. (PEG-400/water) | 3 | 1.3 ± 0.6 | 0.14 ± 0.13 | 0.31 ± 0.21 | 1.1 ± 0.3 | NA | NA | 10 |

[a] Wild type (FVB) mouse.  [b] P-gp knock-out (*mdr1a/1b*) mouse.  [c] 30-minute IPT (intraportal) infusion.  [d] The test article was asunaprevir amorphous free acid.
[e] The test article was asunaprevir potassium salt.  [f] This was a cross-over study with 2 weeks wash-out between doses.  [g] n = 2.  [h] n = 4.

Table 12    *In Vivo* Pharmacokinetic Parameters of Asunaprevir in Humans after Single Dose of Asunaprevir[10]

| Species | Route | Dose (mg) | $T_{max}$ (h)[a] | $C_{max}$ (ng/mL)[b] | $AUC_{0-t}$ (ng·h/mL)[b] | $AUC_{inf}$ (ng·h/mL)[b] | $T_{1/2}$ (h)[c] | Cl or Cl/F (L/h)[b] | $V_{ss}$ (L)[c] | F (%)[b] |
|---|---|---|---|---|---|---|---|---|---|---|
| Healthy Human | i.v.[d] | 100 µg [14C]asunaprevir | 0.133 (0.133-0.150) | 9.64 (25) | 1.98 (21) | 2.02 (21) | 13.7 (9.81) | 49.5 (24) | 194 (140) | - |
| | p.o.[d] | 100 mg softgel capsule | 2.25 (1.00-4.00) | 17.5 (74) | 175 (53) | 188 (52) | 19.7 (3.29) | NA | NA | 9.3 (45) |
| | p.o.[e] | 200 | 4.0 (4.0-6.0) | 68.3 (81) | 540 (65) | 571 (67) | 19.6 (8.01) | 351 (67) | NA | NA |
| | | 400 | 3.5 (3.0-4.0) | 812 (47) | 2477 (43) | 2492 (43) | 15.4 (2.19) | 161 (78) | NA | NA |
| | | 600 | 4.0 (2.5-4.0) | 448 (153) | 1844 (103) | 1871 (102) | 17.1 (3.00) | 321 (58) | NA | NA |
| | | 900 | 4.0 (3.0-6.0) | 704 (110) | 2745 (90) | 2794 (89) | 21.2 (11.6) | 322 (90) | NA | NA |
| | | 1200 | 2.8 (1.5-4.0) | 728 (147) | 2693 (137) | 2726 (137) | 15.7 (7.75) | 440 (147) | NA | NA |

[a] Median (minimum-maximum).  [b] Mean (CV%).  [c] Mean (SD).  [d] n = 10.  [e] n = 6.

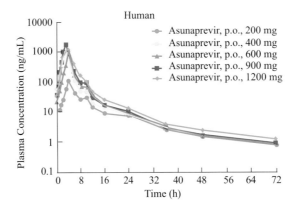

Figure A    *In Vivo* Plasma Concentration-Time Profiles of Asunaprevir in Humans after Single Oral Dose of Asunaprevir[10]

[10]  PMDA Database. http://www.pmda.go.jp/drugs/2014/P201400113/index.html (accessed Mar 2016).

Table 13   *In Vitro* Permeability of Asunaprevir in Caco-2 Cell and PAMPA Monolayer Model[10]

| Compound | Conc. (μM) | Papp(A−B) (1 × 10^{-6} cm/s) | Permeability Class | Donor pH | Conc. (μM) | Pe (nm/s) | Permeability Class |
|---|---|---|---|---|---|---|---|
| | | **Caco-2 Cell Model**[a] | | | | **PAMPA Monolayer Model**[b] | |
| Asunaprevir | 5 | 1.1 | Moderate | 5.5 | 100 | 473 ± 43 | High |
| | | | | | 100 | 812 ± 99 | High |
| Asunaprevir | 25 | 5.4 | Moderate | | 100 | 1012 ± 161 | High |
| | | | | | 100 | 570 ± 90 | High |
| Asunaprevir | 100 | NA | - | 7.4 | 100 | 492 ± 140 | High |
| | | | | | 100 | 610 ± 80 | High |

Values were mean ± SD (n = 3).   PAMPA: Parallel artificial membrane permeability assay.   [a] Incubation of asunaprevir with Caco-2 cells and measurement of permeability across the Caco-2 cell monolayers (pH 7.4 on both sides).   [b] Incubation of asunaprevir in 96-well PAMPA model followed by sample analysis using a UV plate reader.   The study was conducted at 100 μM with 4 h incubation at room temperature.

## Distribution

Table 14   *In Vitro* Plasma Protein Binding and Blood Partitioning of Asunaprevir in Several Species[10]

| Species | Matrix | Conc. (μM) | %Bound | Species | Conc. (μM) | Time (h) | C_b:C_p |
|---|---|---|---|---|---|---|---|
| | **Protein Binding**[a] | | | | **Blood Cell Partitioning**[b] | | |
| Mouse | Serum | 10 | 99.2 | Rat | 1 | 1 | 0.41 |
| Rat | Serum | 10 | 98.8 ± 0.55 | | 1 | 2 | 0.49 |
| Dog | Serum | 10 | 98.5 ± 0.77 | Dog | 1 | 1 | 0.79 |
| Monkey | Serum | 10 | 97.2 ± 1.4 | | 1 | 2 | 0.82 |
| Human | Serum | 10 | 98.8 ± 0.54 | Monkey | 1 | 1 | 0.34 |
| | Plasma | 0.1 | 99.8 ± 0.02 | | 1 | 2 | 0.37 |
| | Plasma | 1.0 | 99.7 ± 0.03 | Human | 1 | 1 | 0.55 |
| | Plasma | 10 | 99.8 ± 0.02 | | 1 | 2 | 0.55 |

Values were mean ± SD.   [a] n = 2 for mouse; n = 3 for rat, dog and monkey; n = 9 for human serum; n = 6 for human plasma.   [b] n = 2.

Table 15   *In Vivo* Tissue Distribution of [^{14}C]Asunaprevir in Male Rats after Oral Dose of 80 mg/kg[10]

| Tissue | 0.5 h | 2 h | 4 h | 8 h | 24 h | 48 h | 96 h | 168 h | 1 h | 8 h | 24 h |
|---|---|---|---|---|---|---|---|---|---|---|---|
| | **Radioactivity Concentration (μg eq./g)** | | | | | | | | | | |
| | **Pigmented Long-Evans Rat**[a] | | | | | | | | **Albino Sprague-Dawley Rat**[b] | | |
| Adipose (brown) | BLQ | BLQ | BLQ | BLQ | BLQ | BLQ | BLQ | BLQ | 0.088 | 0.250 | BLQ |
| Adrenal gland | BLQ | BLQ | BLQ | BLQ | BLQ | BLQ | BLQ | BLQ | 0.230 | 0.076 | BLQ |
| Bile | 12.1 | 30.0 | 15.1 | 12.8 | 5.55 | 2.13 | BLQ | BLQ | 15.0 | 15.7 | 1.69 |
| Blood (cardiac) | 0.108 | NS | BLQ | BLQ | BLQ | BLQ | BLQ | BLQ | 0.321 | BLQ | BLQ |
| Brain (entire) | BLQ | BLQ | BLQ | BLQ | BLQ | BLQ | BLQ | BLQ | BLQ | BLQ | BLQ |
| Cecum | BLQ | 13.3 | 14.6 | 10.9 | 2.85 | 0.166 | BLQ | BLQ | 2.22 | 53.6 | 6.86 |
| Esophagus | 1.66 | BLQ | BLQ | BLQ | BLQ | BLQ | BLQ | BLQ | BLQ | BLQ | BLQ |
| Eyes (entire) | BLQ | BLQ | BLQ | BLQ | BLQ | BLQ | BLQ | BLQ | BLQ | BLQ | BLQ |
| Heart (myocardium) | 0.078 | BLQ | BLQ | BLQ | BLQ | BLQ | BLQ | BLQ | 0.333 | BLQ | BLQ |
| Kidneys (entire) | BLQ | 0.100 | 0.081 | BLQ | BLQ | BLQ | BLQ | BLQ | 0.188 | BLQ | BLQ |
| Large intestine (content) | BLQ | BLQ | 404 | 483 | 28.9 | 4.90 | 0.664 | BLQ | BLQ | 139 | 35.2 |
| Liver | 11.9 | 62.2 | 52.2 | 29.0 | 6.23 | 1.85 | 0.175 | BLQ | 30.6 | 24.9 | BLQ |
| Lungs | BLQ | BLQ | BLQ | BLQ | BLQ | BLQ | BLQ | BLQ | 0.255 | BLQ | BLQ |
| Small intestine | 99.8 | 104 | 26.2 | 1.65 | 0.425 | 0.095 | BLQ | BLQ | 58.2 | 16.5 | 4.98 |

[10]   PMDA Database.   http://www.pmda.go.jp/drugs/2014/P201400113/index.html (accessed Mar 2016).

*Continued*

| Tissue | Radioactivity Concentration (µg eq./g) | | | | | | | | | | |
| | Pigmented Long-Evans Rat[a] | | | | | | | | Albino Sprague-Dawley Rat[b] | | |
| | 0.5 h | 2 h | 4 h | 8 h | 24 h | 48 h | 96 h | 168 h | 1 h | 8 h | 24 h |
| Small intestine (content) | 278 | 524 | 336 | 19.8 | 3.45 | 1.49 | 0.408 | BLQ | 268 | 7.83 | 9.75 |
| Stomach | 365 | 0.134 | BLQ | 0.343 | BLQ | BLQ | BLQ | BLQ | 8.75 | 0.905 | 0.226 |
| Stomach (content) | 338 | 108 | 34.3 | 0.168 | 0.657 | 0.172 | BLQ | BLQ | 217 | 0.105 | 22.8 |
| Urinary bladder | BLQ | BLQ | BLQ | BLQ | BLQ | BLQ | BLQ | BLQ | 1.44 | 0.375 | BLQ |
| Urinary bladder (content) | BLQ | 0.134 | BLQ | BLQ | BLQ | BLQ | BLQ | BLQ | 1.27 | 0.219 | 0.099 |

BLQ: Below lower limit of quantification (0.075 µg eq./g tissue).   [a] n = 10, the sample time included 0.5, 1, 2, 4, 8, 12, 24, 48, 96 and 168 h.   [b] n = 3.

# Metabolism

Table 16   Asunaprevir Metabolism Formation Rates of Hydroxy Metabolites by Individual Human cDNA-expressed CYP Enzymes[10]

| Isoform | Model | Product | Asunaprevir Metabolism Formation Rate | |
| | | | $K_m$ (µM) | $V_{max}$ (pmol/min/mg protein) |
| HLM | Substrate inhibition | Hydroxy metabolite | 83 | 1005 |
| CYP3A4 | Substrate inhibition | Hydroxy metabolite | 54 | 33 |
| CYP3A5 | Substrate inhibition | Hydroxy metabolite | 294 | 100 |

Asunaprevir (1, 2, 5, 10, 20, 40, 60, 80, 100 and 120 µM) was incubated with HLM and recombinant singly expressed human CYP isozymes (Supersomes™) and NADPH (1 mM) for 30 min.   Samples were analyzed using LC-MS/MS.   HLM: Human liver microsomes.   NADPH: β-Nicotinamide adenine dinucleotide phosphate. CYP: Cytochrome P450.

Table 17   *In Vitro* Metabolites of [$^{14}$C]Asunaprevir in Liver Microsomes, S9 fraction or Hepatocytes of Humans and Animal Species[10]

| Metabolite | Metabolism of [$^{14}$C]Asunaprevir (% of Total) | | | | | | | | | | |
| | Mouse | | Rat | | | Dog | | Monkey | | Human | |
| | H | LM | H | S | LM | H | LM | H | LM | H | LM |
| Parent | 76.7 | 78.8 | 63.3 | 78.7 | 79.7 | 81.4 | 85.1 | 65.5 | 44.0 | 69.1 | 75.9 |
| M1 | 0.4 | ND | 2.6 | 0.8 | ND | MS | ND | 1.5 | ND | 0.9 | ND |
| M2 | 1.5 | 1.5 | MS | 2.0 | 1.4 | 1.7 | 1.6 | 2.0 | 3.2 | 0.7 | 2.0 |
| M3 | MS | MS | 1.4 | 1.5 | 0.9 | 0.3 | MS | 1.5 | 2.9 | 0.3 | 2.1 |
| M4 | MS | MS | 1.5 | 0.9 | 0.8 | MS | ND | 0.8 | 5.1 | MS | 1.9 |
| M5 | ND | MS | MS | MS | MS | ND | ND | 1.0 | MS | ND | MS |
| M6 | 3.1 | 4.6 | 2.4 | 1.4 | 1.3 | 4.8 | 3.1 | 1.9 | 5.7 | 10.0 | 2.3 |
| M7 | 2.3 | 3.1 | 2.8 | 3.6 | 2.6 | 1.0 | 1.6 | 4.2 | 8.3 | 1.4 | 4.7 |
| M8 | ND | 1.8 | 0.3 | ND | 0.2 | ND | MS | 0.4 | 1.1 | ND | MS |
| M9 | 2.6 | 2.1 | 5.4 | 2.6 | 1.0 | 1.3 | 1.2 | 3.0 | 3.4 | 3.5 | 1.0 |
| M10 | ND | ND | MS | ND | ND | MS | ND | ND | ND | ND | ND |
| M11 | MS | 1.8 | 0.2 | 1.2 | 0.8 | 0.9 | 0.2 | 1.1 | 1.5 | 0.6 | 1.4 |
| M12 | 0.5 | 0.1 | 2.4 | 1.4 | 0.4 | 0.8 | MS | 1.7 | 3.5 | 1.7 | 0.8 |
| M15 | 1.2 | 1.1 | 1.4 | 0.7 | MS | 1.1 | MS | 1.2 | 1.4 | 0.9 | 0.9 |

Liver microsomes (1 mg protein/mL): 10 µM [$^{14}$C]asunaprevir, 1 h incubation with NADPH (1 mM), with or without glutathione (5 mM) at 37 °C.   Liver S9 fraction (1 mg protein/mL) from Aroclor 1254-pretreated rats: 10 µM asunaprevir, 1 h incubation at 37 °C.   Hepatocytes (2 million cells/mL): 10 µM asunaprevir, 4 h incubation at 37 °C.   ND: Not detected.   MS: Presence of metabolite detected by LC-MS/MS.   H: Hepatocytes.   LM: Liver microsomes.   S: Hepatic S9 fraction from Aroclor 1254-induced rats, supplemented with NADPH.   NADPH: β-Nicotinamide adenine dinucleotide phosphate.   M6: BMS798430 (an *O*-demethylated metabolite).   M9: BMS558364.

[10]   PMDA Database.   http://www.pmda.go.jp/drugs/2014/P201400113/index.html (accessed Mar 2016).

Table 18   Metabolic Stability of [$^{14}$C]Asunaprevir in Hepatic Microsomal and Hepatocytes Fractions[10]

| Species | Dose (µM) | Gender | Oxidation (pmol/min/mg/protein) | Hepatic Clearance (mL/min/kg) | Species | Dose (µM) | Metabolism Rate (pmol/min/10$^6$ cell) | Hepatic Clearance (mL/min/kg) |
|---|---|---|---|---|---|---|---|---|
| Rat | 0.5 | Male | 4.9 | 13.3 | Rat | 0.5 | ND | ND |
|  |  | Female | ND | ND |  | 3 | ND | ND |
| Dog | 0.5 | Male | 4.7 | 13.3 |  | 10 | ND | ND |
|  |  | Female | ND | ND | Dog | 0.5 | ND | ND |
| Monkey | 0.5 | Male | 50 | 31.7 |  | 3 | ND | ND |
|  |  | Female | 90 | 36.7 |  | 10 | ND | ND |
|  | 3 | Male | 117 | 21.3 | Monkey | 0.5 | 7.8 | 22 |
|  |  | Female | 369 | 33.6 |  | 3 | 14.9 | 10 |
|  | 10 | Male | 152 | 11.6 |  | 10 | 14.2 | 3.6 |
|  |  | Female | 530 | 24.8 |  |  |  |  |
| Human | 0.5 | Male | 7.7 | 10.0 | Human | 0.5 | ND | ND |
|  |  | Female | 29 | 16.1 |  | 3 | ND | ND |
|  | 3 | Male | 54 | 10.8 |  | 10 | ND | ND |
|  |  | Female | 57 | 11.1 |  |  |  |  |
|  | 10 | Male | 117 | 8.6 |  |  |  |  |
|  |  | Female | 96 | 7.6 |  |  |  |  |

Asunaprevir (0.5-10 µM) was incubated with liver microsomes in the presence of NADPH and also with primary hepatocytes.   Metabolism rates were determined based on the disappearance of parent drug, as measured by LC-MS/MS.   Formation of small amounts of M6 (BMS798430) was observed in liver microsomes and the approximate amount formed, relative to the asunaprevir remaining, was <2% in rats and dogs, 3% in humans and 7% in monkeys.   No M6 was detected in hepatocyte incubations.   ND: Not determined due to insufficient metabolism of asunaprevir.

Table 19   Metabolites in Plasma and Excreta in Humans and Animal Species after Oral Dose of Asunaprevir[10]

| Matrix | Species | Dose (mg/kg) | Time (h) | Parent | M1 | M3 | M4 | M5 | M7 | M8 | M9 | M12 | M15 | M20 | M25 | M26 |
|---|---|---|---|---|---|---|---|---|---|---|---|---|---|---|---|---|
| Plasma | Mouse | 100 | 1 | 70.8 | - | 1.6 | MS | 0.6 | 2.5 | 0.4 | 1.5 | 1.3 | 1.3 | 2.6 | 1.5 | - |
|  |  |  | 4 | 53.3 | - | 1.9 | MS | 0.8 | 5.1 | 0.5 | 2.9 | 1.0 | 1.5 | 4.8 | 1.3 | - |
|  |  |  | 8 | 40.3 | - | 1.2 | MS | MS | MS | 0.8 | 9.0 | 0.8 | 1.4 | 2.2 | 1.6 | - |
|  | Rat | 80 | 1 | 74.9 | - | 1.0 | 0.7 | ND | 0.7 | 0.2 | 0.9 | MS | MS | 0.3 | 0.3 | - |
|  |  |  | 4 | 90.8 | - | 0.8 | 0.2 | ND | 0.7 | 0.2 | ND | MS | MS | 0.5 | 0.4 | - |
|  |  |  | 8 | 79.0 | - | 2.3 | 0.3 | ND | 1.2 | ND | ND | MS | 0.3 | 0.7 | MS | - |
|  | Dog | 50 | 1 | 74.2 | - | 0.5 | ND | MS | 0.6 | ND | 0.3 | MS | MS | 1.0 | ND | - |
|  |  |  | 4 | 72.4 | - | 0.6 | ND | 1.0 | 0.8 | ND | 0.4 | MS | 0.7 | 1.7 | ND | - |
|  |  |  | 8 | 74.3 | - | 5.4 | ND | MS | MS | ND | 0.5 | 0.4 | 2.0 | 2.2 | ND | - |
|  | Rabbit[a] | 100 | 1 | 157 | - | 1.52 | 0.02 | 2.36 | 2.47 | - | 3.50 | 0.14 | - | 0.02 | 0.11 | - |
|  |  |  | 4 | 142 | - | 1.02 | 0.11 | 4.64 | 2.99 | - | 13.3 | 0.08 | - | 0.05 | 0.05 | - |
|  |  |  | 12 | 61.5 | - | 0.83 | 0.12 | 1.11 | 0.09 | - | 3.15 | 0.05 | - | 0.03 | 0.03 | - |
|  |  |  | 0-24 | 90.0 | - | 0.52 | 0.28 | 3.24 | 0.45 | - | 3.44 | 0.07 | - | 0.05 | 0.05 | - |
|  | Monkey (BDC) | 100 | 2 | 16.0 | - | 2.8 | 1.8 | MS | 2.6 | 3.7 | 10.2 | 3.2 | 9.6 | 2.3 | 4.3 | - |

[10] PMDA Database.   http://www.pmda.go.jp/drugs/2014/P201400113/index.html (accessed Mar 2016).

*Continued*

| Matrix | Species | Dose (mg/kg) | Time (h) | Parent | M1 | M3 | M4 | M5 | M7 | M8 | M9 | M12 | M15 | M20 | M25 | M26 |
|---|---|---|---|---|---|---|---|---|---|---|---|---|---|---|---|---|
| | | | | % of Radioactivity (ng/mL) | | | | | | | | | | | | |

| Matrix | Species | Dose (mg/kg) | Time (h) | Parent | M1 | M3 | M4 | M5 | M7 | M8 | M9 | M12 | M15 | M20 | M25 | M26 |
|---|---|---|---|---|---|---|---|---|---|---|---|---|---|---|---|---|
| Plasma | Human | 200 | 2 | 73.2 | - | 5.5 | 3.0 | ND | 3.3 | 1.6 | 3.0 | 1.4 | 1.1 | 3.6 | 0.3 | - |
| | | | 4 | 52.7 | - | 1.4 | 9.2 | ND | 3.1 | 5.7 | 2.8 | 0.5 | 9.0 | 0.5 | 8.7 | - |
| | | | 0-24 | 54.9 | - | 2.9 | 2.9 | ND | 3.1 | 1.6 | 4.6 | 1.5 | 2.0 | 1.2 | 4.3 | - |
| Urine | Mouse | 100 | 0-168 | 0.5 | ND | 0.03 | ND | ND | 0.1 | ND | 0.2 | 0.1 | ND | ND | ND | ND |
| Feces | Mouse | 100 | 0-168 | 35.1 | ND | 1.1 | 0.8 | 1.1 | 5.6 | 0.8 | 8.3 | 4.3 | 1.3 | 1.8 | 2.0 | 0.4 |
| | Rat | 80 | 0-168 | 36.2 | ND | 1.8 | 0.3 | 1.1 | 3.7 | 2.2 | 7.0 | 2.8 | 2.3 | 2.3 | 2.1 | 0.8 |
| | Rat (BDC) | 80 | 0-48 | 29.6 | ND | 0.4 | 0.2 | 0.4 | 0.3 | 1.7 | 1.5 | 0.6 | 0.8 | MS | MS | ND |
| | Rabbit | 100 | 0-168 | 66.3 | ND | 1.3 | 0.2 | 0.4 | 3.1 | MS | 0.5 | 0.7 | ND | ND | 0.2 | ND |
| | Dog | 50 | 0-168 | 42.1 | 0.8 | 2.3 | ND | 1.6 | 1.2 | 0.8 | 2.3 | 1.2 | 0.7 | 1.2 | ND | ND |
| | Monkey (BDC) | 100 | 0-72 | 26.8 | ND | 0.9 | 1.2 | 1.0 | 1.1 | 1.6 | 4.6 | 2.6 | 1.1 | 1.2 | 1.8 | 0.4 |
| | Human | 200 | 0-240 | 5.6-7.5 | ND | 2.5-4.9 | 4.5-4.9 | ND | 0.4-0.7 | 14.6-15.5 | 1.8-2.1 | 4.8-8.3 | 1.8-3.8 | 0.3-3.6 | 5.0-5.6 | 0.8-1.8 |
| Bile | Rat (BDC) | 80 | 0-48 | 18.3 | ND | 0.1 | 0.1 | 0.3 | 0.8 | MS | 0.5 | 0.5 | 0.2 | 0.2 | MS | ND |
| | Monkey (BDC) | 100 | 0-72 | 3.1 | ND | 0.5 | 2.0 | 0.2 | 1.0 | 0.8 | 2.3 | 1.7 | 1.0 | 0.4 | 2.8 | 0.1 |
| | Human | 200 | 3-8 | 2.2 | ND | 0.6 | 0.5 | ND | 0.2 | 0.4 | 0.7 | 0.2 | 0.2 | 0.3 | 0.4 | 0.2 |

% of Radioactivity for plasma and % of dose for excreta.   Values were from analysis of pooled samples.   Due to low radioactivity concentrations, metabolites were not profiled in urine of rats, dogs, BDC monkeys or humans.   ND: Not detected.   BDC: Bile duct-cannulated.   MS: Detected only by LC-MS.   M9: BMS558364.
[a] Concentration of asunaprevir and metabolites in plasma (ng/mL).

Table 20    Inhibition of Asunaprevir Metabolism in Human Liver Microsomes by Chemical Inhibitors of CYP450[10]

| Inhibitor | Con. (µM) | CYP Inhibited | %Inhibition |
|---|---|---|---|
| Furafylline | 15 | CYP1A2 | 13 |
| α-Naphthoflavone | 1 | CYP1A2 | 4.0 |
| Sulfaphenazole | 10 | CYP2C9 | 25, 83 |
| Benzylnirvanol | 1 | CYP2C19 | 4.9 |
| Quinidine | 1 | CYP2D6 | 0.0, 4.0 |
| | 10 | CYP2D6 | 39, 31 |
| Ketoconazole | 1 | CYP3A4 | 90, 120 |
| | 10 | CYP3A4 | 123, 81 |
| Troleandomycin | 50 | CYP3A4 | 119, 94 |

Asunaprevir (0.5 µM) was incubated with human liver microsomes (0.9 mg protein/mL) for 80 min to determine the disappearance of asunaprevir in human liver microsome with or without chemical inhibitors selective for major CYP isoforms.

[10]  PMDA Database.   http://www.pmda.go.jp/drugs/2014/P201400113/index.html (accessed Mar 2016).

Table 21　Effects of CYPs on the Formation Rate of Metabolites of Asunaprevir[10]

| Isozyme | Asunaprevir Con. (μM) | Metabolite Formation Rate (pmol/min/pmol protein) | | Inhibitor | Con. (μM) | Enzyme Inhibited | Asunaprevir Con. (μM) | Metabolite Formation Relative to Control[a] (%) | |
|---|---|---|---|---|---|---|---|---|---|
| | | Hydroxy Metabolite | Ether Cleavage Metabolite | | | | | Hydroxy Metabolite | Ether Cleavage Metabolite |
| CYP1A1 | 2 | ND | ND | Furafylline[b] | 10 | CYP1A2 | 2 | 117 ± 8.2 | ND[c] |
| | 20 | 0.092 ± 0.002 | ND | | | | 20 | 92.4 ± 7.5 | 95.8 ± 10.2 |
| CYP1A2 | 2 | ND | ND | Tranylcypromine | 2 | CYP2A6 | 2 | 76.9 ± 6.4 | ND |
| | 20 | 0.064 ± 0.002 | ND | | | | 20 | 75.2 ± 3.5 | 85.4 ± 5.6 |
| CYP1B1 | 2 | ND | ND | Orphenadrine[b] | 50 | CYP2B6 | 2 | 67.3 ± 3.8 | ND |
| | 20 | 0.021 ± 0.004 | ND | | | | 20 | 64.4 ± 2.8 | 78.2 ± 9.1 |
| CYP2A6 | 2 | ND | ND | Montelukast | 3 | CYP2C8 | 2 | 101 ± 5.5 | ND |
| | 20 | 0.030 ± 0.006 | ND | | | | 20 | 90.8 ± 5.4 | 88.4 ± 7.5 |
| CYP2B6 | 2 | ND | ND | Sulfaphenazole | 10 | CYP2C9 | 2 | 33.8 ± 1.8 | ND |
| | 20 | 0.023 ± 0.001 | 0.022 ± 0.002 | | | | 20 | 43.9 ± 6.6 | 74.5 ± 6.6 |
| CYP2C8 | 2 | ND | ND | Benzylnirvanol | 1 | CYP2C19 | 2 | 34.5 ± 0.8 | ND |
| | 20 | ND | ND | | | | 20 | 49.6 ± 5.2 | 75.9 ± 4.8 |
| CYP2C9 | 2 | ND | ND | Quinidine | 1 | CYP2D6 | 2 | 41.7 ± 2.1 | ND |
| | 20 | ND | 0.021 ± 0.003 | | | | 20 | 69.5 ± 0.8 | 67.3 ± 8.2 |
| CYP2C19 | 2 | ND | ND | Diethyldithiocarbamate[b] | 50 | CYP2E1 | 2 | 61.1 ± 5.5 | ND |
| | 20 | 0.020 ± 0.003 | 0.013 ± 0.001 | | | | 20 | 56.8 ± 4.5 | 95.8 ± 7.5 |
| CYP2D6 | 2 | ND | ND | Ketoconazole | 1 | CYP3A4 | 2 | 4.5 ± 0.9 | ND |
| | 20 | 0.044 ± 0.003 | ND | | | | 20 | 5.2 ± 0.5 | 10.6 ± 3.2 |
| CYP3A4 | 2 | 1.49 ± 0.11 | 0.23 ± 0.04 | Troleandomycin[b] | 20 | CYP3A4 | 2 | 4.3 ± 0.7 | ND |
| | 20 | 15.8 ± 1.1 | 2.03 ± 0.26 | | | | 20 | 3.1 ± 0.3 | 8.4 ± 2.7 |
| CYP3A5 | 2 | 0.69 ± 0.09 | 0.13 ± 0.03 | 1-ABT[b] | 1000 | All CYPs | 2 | 3.3 ± 0.5 | ND |
| | 20 | 6.92 ± 0.85 | 1.24 ± 0.10 | | | | 20 | 0.8 ± 0.4 | 7.6 ± 3.5 |

Data were mean ± SD.　Samples were analyzed using LC-MS/MS.　ND: Not determined due to low concentrations of the metabolites.　HLM: Human liver microsomes.　ABT: 1-Aminobenzotraizole.　[a] Incubations in HLM without inhibitors were conducted as the controls.　[b] Time-dependent inhibition study design.　[c] Rate was not determined because of low concentration.

[10]　PMDA Database.　http://www.pmda.go.jp/drugs/2014/P201400113/index.html (accessed Mar 2016).

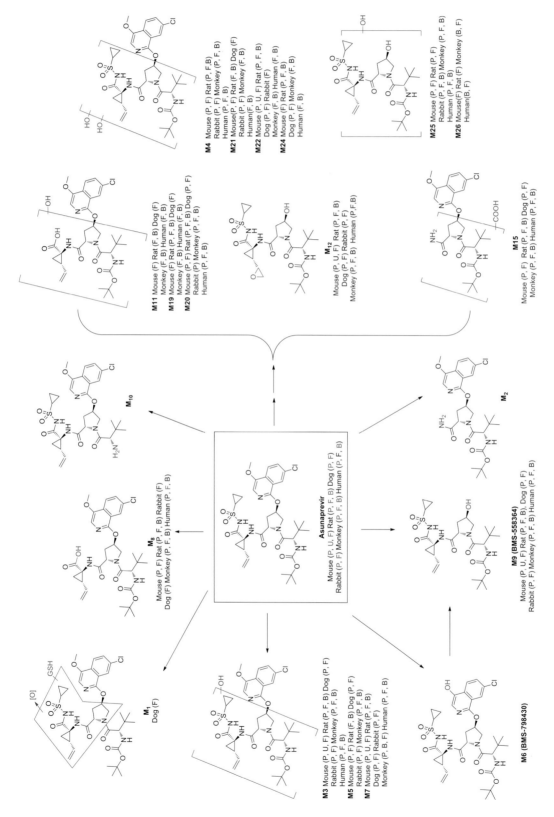

Figure B  Proposed Pathways for *In Vivo* Biotransformation of Asunaprevir in Mice, Rats, Dogs, Rabbits, Monkeys and Humans[10]

The red labels represent the major components in the matrices.    P = Plasma, U = Urine, B = Bile and F = Feces.

[10]  PMDA Database.    http://www.pmda.go.jp/drugs/2014/P201400113/index.html (accessed Mar 2016).

# Excretion

Table 22    Excretion Profiles in Humans and Animal Species after Single Dose of [$^{14}$C]Asunaprevir[10]

| Species | State | Dose (mg/kg) | Route | Time (h) | Bile (% of dose) | Urine (% of dose) | Feces (% of dose) | Total (% of dose) |
|---|---|---|---|---|---|---|---|---|
| Mouse (male) | Intact | 100 | p.o. | 0-168 | - | 1.42 ± 0.82 | 87.9 ± 6.67 | 94.3 ± 5.47[a] |
| Rat (male) | Intact | 80 | p.o. | 0-168 | - | 0.29 ± 0.16 | 86.9 ± 11.5 | 91.2 ± 7.77[a] |
| | BDC | 80 | p.o. | 0-48 | 25.5 ± 1.67 | 1.01 ± 0.81 | 43.0 ± 10.0 | 69.5 |
| | BDC | 5 | i.v. | 0-8 | 38.3 | 2.1 | 0.8 | 41.2 |
| Rabbit (female) | Intact | 100 | p.o. | 0-168 | - | 0.92 ± 0.21 | 84.5 ± 4.68 | 85.8 ± 4.84[a] |
| Dog (male) | Intact | 50 | p.o. | 0-168 | - | 0.42 ± 0.18 | 77.1 ± 13.8 | 97.1 ± 1.22[a] |
| | BDC | 3 | i.v. | 0-72 | 51.4 | 1.0 | 51.3 | 103.7 |
| Monkey (male) | BDC | 6 | p.o. | 0-72 | 32.9 | 1.7 | 18.3 | 52.9[b] |
| | | 100 | p.o. | 0-72 | 26.3 ± 14.7 | 0.40 ± 0.20 | 55.6 ± 12.3 | 82.3 |
| | | 2 | i.v. | 0-72 | 15.9 | 0.7 | 65.1 | 81.7 |
| Human[c] | Intact | 200 | p.o. | 0-240 | 8.14 ± 4.14 | 0.19 ± 0.04 | 73.1 ± 1.66 | 81.4 ± 5.56 |

Values were mean ± SD.    BDC: Bile duct cannulated.    [a] Total includes recovery from matrices, carcass (mouse and rat), cage rinse, wash, wipe and debris collections.    [b] Incomplete dose recovery in orally-dosed monkey may have resulted from diarrhea during the first day.    [c] Samples from clinical study, and human bile was collected between 3-8 h after dosing.

# Drug-Drug Interaction

Table 23    *In Vitro* Evaluation of Asunaprevir as an Inducer of Recombinant CYP450 Isoforms[10]

| Compound | Conc. (µM) | Percent of Positive Control Effect | | | | | |
|---|---|---|---|---|---|---|---|
| | | CYP1A2 | | CYP2B6 | | CYP3A4/5 | |
| | | Activity | mRNA Level | Activity | mRNA Level | Activity | mRNA Level |
| Omeprazole[a] | 50 | 58.9 ± 24.0[b] | 70.2 ± 31.7[b] | - | - | - | - |
| Phenobarbital[a] | 750 | - | - | 21.6 ± 14.9[b] | 9.85 ± 2.70[b] | - | - |
| Rifampin[a] | 10 | - | - | - | - | 20.9 ± 6.5[b] | 17.4 ± 9.0[b] |
| Asunaprevir | 0 | 0 ± 0 | 0 ± 0 | 0 ± 0 | 0 ± 0 | 0 ± 0 | 0 ± 0 |
| | 0.065 | 0.253 ± 0.712 | -0.203[c] | 8.25 ± 13.8 | 2.65[c] | 6.36 ± 11.3 | 4.07[c] |
| | 0.20 | -0.208 ± 0.360 | -0.474 ± 0.552 | 1.60 ± 0.75 | -1.11 ± 1.09 | 0.727 ± 1.41 | 2.97 ± 1.81 |
| | 0.65 | -0.144 ± 0.572 | -0.669 ± 0.614 | 4.07 ± 1.73 | 1.55 ± 4.78 | 7.83 ± 2.08 | 13.6 ± 2.4 |
| | 1.3 | 0.392 ± 0.221 | -0.636 ± 0.636 | 5.05 ± 2.03 | 2.00 ± 5.00 | 13.6 ± 3.3 | 26.8 ± 0.4 |
| | 2.7 | 0.542 ± 0.371 | -0.278[c] | 6.98 ± 3.35 | 5.28[c] | 16.3 ± 5.2 | 33.8[c] |
| | 6.5 | 0.939 ± 0.414 | -0.839 ± 0.745 | 8.21 ± 3.41 | 3.81 ± 7.33 | 13.1 ± 7.1 | 41.4 ± 7.0 |
| | 13.3 | 0.821 ± 0.153 | -0.849 ± 0.658 | 8.25 ± 5.07 | 1.76 ± 7.02 | 2.75 ± 2.27 | 30.1 ± 7.9 |
| | 26.7 | 0.404 ± 0.206 | -0.899 ± 0.553 | 2.60 ± 1.95 | -3.51 ± 3.88 | -3.50 ± 2.29 | 11.4 ± 3.9 |

Cultured human hepatocytes from 3 individual donors were treated once daily for 3 consecutive days with asunaprevir (0.065, 0.20, 0.65, 1.3, 2.7, 6.5, 13.3 and 26.7 µM).    [a] Positive control.    [b] The value was 7 folds increase.    [c] n = 2.

[10]  PMDA Database.    http://www.pmda.go.jp/drugs/2014/P201400113/index.html (accessed Mar 2016).

Table 24    *In Vitro* Evaluation of Asunaprevir as an Inhibitor on the Activity of Recombinant CYP450 Isoforms[10]

| Substrate | Isoform | IC$_{50}$ (µM) | |
|---|---|---|---|
| | | **No Pre-incubation** | **30 min Pre-incubation** |
| Tacrine 1'-hydroxylation | CYP1A2 | >40 | >40 |
| Bupropion hydroxylation | CYP2B6 | >40 | 31.8 |
| Amodiaquine *N*-deethylation | CYP2C8 | 30.9 | 32.5 |
| Diclofenac 4'-hydroxylation | CYP2C9 | >40 | >40 |
| *S*-mephenytoin 4'-hydroxylation | CYP2C19 | >40 | >40 |
| Dextromethorphan *O*-demethylation | CYP2D6 | >40 | 5.7 |
| Midazolam 1'-hydroxylation | CYP3A4 | 27.3 | 5.4 |
| Testosterone 6$\beta$-hydroxylation | CYP3A4 | >45 | 2.4 |

Table 25    *In Vitro* Evaluation of Asunaprevir as a Substrate and an Inhibitor of Uptake Transporter[10]

| Transporter | OAT1 | OAT3 | OCT1 | OCT2 | OATP1B1 | OATP2B1 | OATP1B3 |
|---|---|---|---|---|---|---|---|
| Inhibitor (IC$_{50}$, µM) | 11.8 | 69.6 | 77.6 | >80 | 0.3 | 1.2 | 3.0 |
| Substrate (uptake, % of control) | 13.5-100 | 51.0-132 | 42.6-100 | 80.2-127 | Yes | Yes | No |

Table 26    *In Vitro* Evaluation of Asunaprevir as an Inhibitor of BCRP in MDCK Cell Model[10]

| Compound | Con. (µM) | [$^3$H]Genistein Permeability Coefficient (nm/s) | | B→A/A→B | %Inhibiton | IC$_{50}$ (µM) |
|---|---|---|---|---|---|---|
| | | **A→B** | **B→A** | | | |
| Asunaprevir | 0 | 193 ± 2 | 477 ± 34 | 2.5 | NA | >50 |
| | 0.1 | 178 ± 5 | 434 ± 24 | 2.4 | 9.9 | |
| | 1 | 183 ± 9 | 473 ± 23 | 2.6 | -2.1 | |
| | 5 | 169 ± 7 | 453 ± 6 | 2.7 | -0.2 | |
| | 20 | 184 ± 10 | 384 ± 34 | 2.1 | 30 | |
| | 50 | 186 ± 13 | 369 ± 31 | 2.0 | 36 | |
| FTC[a] | 10 | 207 ± 8 | 218 ± 28 | 1.1 | 96 | NA |
| Cyclosporin A[a] | 10 | 145 ± 9 | 221 ± 13 | 1.5 | 73 | NA |

FTC: Fumitremorgin C.   BCRP: Breast cancer resistance protein.   MDCK: Madin-Darby canine kidney.   [a] Positive control.

[10]   PMDA Database.   http://www.pmda.go.jp/drugs/2014/P201400113/index.html (accessed Mar 2016).

Table 27    *In Vitro* Evaluation of Asunaprevir as an Inhibitor on P-gp in MDCK Cell Model[10]

| Compound | Con. (μM) | [³H]Digoxin Permeability Coefficient (nm/s) | | B→A/A→B | %Inhibiton | IC₅₀ (μM) |
| | | A→B | B→A | | | |
|---|---|---|---|---|---|---|
| Asunaprevir | 0 | 7 ± 0.7 | 196 ± 5 | 27.2 | NA | 50.6 ± 17 |
| | 1 | 6 ± 0.6 | 181 ± 2.7 | 30.1 | 7.6 | |
| | 10 | 11 ± 0.8 | 169 ± 7.8 | 15.8 | 16.3 | |
| | 25 | 30 ± 0.5 | 172 ± 14 | 5.7 | 25.2 | |
| | 50 | 54 ± 0.7 | 162 ± 9.8 | 3.0 | 43.3 | |
| | 75 | 144 ± 7.7 | 146 ± 4.7 | 1.0 | 98.6 | |
| Quinidine[a] | 10 | 30 ± 0.8 | 51 ± 1.8 | 1.7 | 88.4 | NA |
| Ketoconazole[a] | 10 | 22 ± 1.6 | 80 ± 3.8 | 3.6 | 69.3 | NA |

P-gp: P-glycoprotein.    MDCK: Madin-Darby canine kidney.    [a] Positive control.

Table 28    *In Vitro* Evaluation of Asunaprevir as a P-gp Substrate in Caco-2 Cell Monolayer Model[10]

| Compound | Conc. (μM) | $Papp_{(A→B)}$ (nm/s) | $Papp_{(B→A)}$ (nm/s) | Efflux Ratio | Permeability Class |
|---|---|---|---|---|---|
| Asunaprevir | 5 | 11 ± 2 | 341 ± 20 | 31 | Moderate |
| Asunaprevir | 25 | 54 ± 3 | 174 ± 22 | 3.2 | Moderate |
| Asunaprevir | 100 | NA | NA | - | - |
| Asunaprevir + GF120918 | 5 (Asu) + 4 (GF) | 65 ± 4 | 126 ± 2 | 1.9 | High |
| Asunaprevir + MK-571 | 5 (Asu) + 50 (MK) | 141 ± 25 | 100 ± 17 | 1.4 | High |
| Asunaprevir + FTC | 5 (Asu) + 10 (FTC) | 14 ± 3 | 277 ± 40 | 20 | High |

Values were mean ± SD (n = 3).    GF120918 was a P-gp and BCRP inhibitor.    MK-571 was a MRP-2 inhibitor.    FTC was a BCRP inhibitor.    Digoxin (5 μM) was tested as a positive control: The A→B and B→A ratio was 19.    FTC: Fumitremorgin C.

# 6    Non-Clinical Toxicology

## Summary

Single-Dose Toxicity

❖ Single-dose toxicity studies were performed by the oral route in rodent and non-rodent species:
  • Mouse MNLD: 600 mg/kg.
  • Rat MNLD: 2000 mg/kg.
  • Dog MNLD: 300 mg/kg.

Repeated-Dose Toxicity

❖ Pivotal repeated-dose toxicity were evaluated by the oral route in rats (up to 6 months) and dogs (up to 9 months) for asunaprevir alone, and in monkeys (up to 3 months) for asunaprevir/daclatasvir combination:
  • By the chronic studies conducted in rats and dogs, drug-related toxicities across species included reversible hematologic and hepatic changes.    Mean AUC of either species at the NOAEL for toxicity was more than 82 times of that in human.
  • Doses of the combined administration toxicity were set to cover the range of 18 times of the human AUC, at which no pronounced toxicological changes were found.

[10]    PMDA Database.    http://www.pmda.go.jp/drugs/2014/P201400113/index.html (accessed Mar 2016).

Safety Pharmacology

❖ Safety pharmacology was evaluated for cardiotoxicity, CNS toxicity and respiratory effects:
  • Cardiovascular effects: *In vitro* assays evaluated the relative inhibition of ligand binding and enzyme activity of the receptor and ion channel. For hERG/cardiac ion currents and APD, effects were absent to mild. Meanwhile, *in vivo* telemetry assay did not elicited any adverse cardiovascular effects either.
  • Respiratory and central nervous effects: Mainly illustrated as part of the single- and repeated-dose (single-agent and combination) GLP toxicity studies, which exhibited no specific adverse effect.

Genotoxicity

❖ Asunaprevir was neither mutagenic in the *in vitro* Ames assay, nor clastogenic in the *in vitro* CHO cell chromosome aberration assay and the *in vivo* bone marrow micronucleus assay.

Reproductive and Developmental Toxicity

❖ Fertility and early embryonic development in rats:
  • No anomaly emerged on parent fertility or early embryonic endpoints, with 101-105 folds exposure margin to clinical recommended dose.
❖ Embryo-fetal developmental in mice and rabbits:
  • There was no pronounced drug-related maternal toxicity or fetal malformation/variation in either species.
❖ Pre- and postnatal development in rats:
  • Maternal toxicity arose, targeting adrenal, abdomen and GI tract, and survival rate of $F_1$ fetus decreased, with NOAEL exposure 7.26 and 76.4 folds of that in clinical dose, respectively.

Carcinogenicity

❖ The carcinogenic potential was evaluated in Tg-rasH2 transgenic mice and SD rats:
  • No neoplastic but limited non-neoplastic pathology emerged, moreover, the latter was considered spontaneous or adaptive rather than drug-related.

Special Toxicology

❖ Phototoxicity: Probably phototoxic.

## Single-Dose Toxicity

Table 29    Single-Dose Toxicity Studies of Asunaprevir[10]

| Species | Dosage (mg/kg) | MNLD (mg/kg) | Finding |
|---|---|---|---|
| CD-1 mouse | 200, 600, 2000, p.o. | 600 | 2000 mg/kg: Death or moribund euthanasia within 24 h of dosing with clinical signs; Microscopic lesions in gastric and intestinal mucosa, enterocyte extrusion, necrosis of lymphocytes within the mantle zone of the ileal Peyer's patches.<br>200 and 600 mg/kg: Decreased (5%-6%) mean body weight (male, on day 8 and 15). |
| SD rat | 200, 600, 2000, p.o. | 2000 | Clinically well tolerated at ≤600 mg/kg.<br>2000 mg/kg: Body soiling, low incidences of decreased activity, partially closed eyelids, and low body posture in male on day 1 and low incidences of scant feces in male and female; Decreased (6.7%-8.5%) mean body weight in male on day 3-15 and body weight loss (4.3%) in 1 female on day 3. |
| Beagle dog | 30, 100, 300, p.o. | 300 | Clinically well tolerated at ≤100 mg/kg.<br>300 mg/kg: Emesis noted 10-60 min post-dose. |

Vehicle: 60% PEG-400 and 40% TPGS.

[10]  PMDA Database.   http://www.pmda.go.jp/drugs/2014/P201400113/index.html (accessed Mar 2016).

# Repeated-Dose Toxicity

Table 30 Repeated-Dose Toxicity Studies of Asunaprevir by Oral Administration[10]

| Species | Duration | Dose (mg/kg/day) | NOAEL Dose (mg/kg/day) | NOAEL AUC$_{0-24}$ (µg·h/mL) | NOAEL Safety Margin[a] (× MRHD) | Finding |
|---|---|---|---|---|---|---|
| SD rat | 2 weeks | 0, 30, 100, 300, p.o. | 300 | 294 | 79.7 | 30, 100 mg/kg/day: No noteworthy finding. 300 mg/kg: Slightly ↑ urine pH (+ 0.7 pH units), minor ↑ serum bilirubin in females (1.9 × control), ↓ kidney (15%) and heart weights (12%) in males. Tissue toxicokinetics: At necropsy (approximately 24 h after last dose), asunaprevir was detected in liver (35.7-229 µg/g), heart (0.069-1.99 µg/g), and spleen (0.064-1.90 µg/g) at each dose level. |
| | 1 month | 0, 30, 100, 600 p.o. | 100 | Male: 83.2 Female: 98.2 | Male: 22.5 Female: 26.6 | 30, 100 mg/kg/day: Well tolerated. 600 mg/kg/day: Hemoglobin, ↓ MCV, MCH and fibrinogen; ↑ Thyroid, adrenal and liver weight; Hypertrophy of mucosal cells in small intestine. |
| | | Asunaprevir: 0, 30, 60 Daclatasvir: 0, 10, 60, p.o. | 60 | Male: 27.9 Female: 54.9 | Male: 7.6 Female: 14.9 | 60 mg/kg/day: Mild effects including slightly ↑ urine volume, minor ↓ hemoglobin and MCV. |
| | 6 months | 0, 40, 80, 200, p.o. | 200 | Male: 321 Female: 684 | Male: 87 Female: 185 | 200 mg/kg/day: Well tolerated. ↓ Total cholesterol (0.79-0.92 times, reversible); Dose-dependent ↑ liver weight (+ 8% to +23%) in all males, but no associated hepatic pathological finding. |
| Beagle dog | 1 month | 0, 20, 60, 300 | 60 | Male: 102 Female: 98.5 | Male: 27.6 Female: 26.7 | 60 mg/kg/day: Well tolerated. 300 mg/kg/day: ↑ Adrenal and spleen weight; ↑ ALT, GGT and total bilirubin; Necrosis of hepatocyte. Liver toxicity was found at 300 mg/kg/day. |
| | 9 months | 0, 15, 50, 100 | 100 | Male: 223 Female: 380 | Male: 60.4 Female: 103 | Well tolerated at 100 mg/kg/day. Minor ↓ MCV (0.93-0.94 times) and ↓ MCH (0.91 to 0.92 times) in females at HD; ↑ ALP (1.32 to 2.17 times, reversible) in males and females at MD and HD. No associated histopathological finding. |
| Monkey | 1 week | 0, 30, 150, 300 | 300 | Male: 982 Female: 411 | Male: 266 Female: 111 | ≥150 mg/kg: Decreased total cholesterol (0.64-0.82 times) in 1 male at 150 mg/kg and in 1 female and 2 males at 300 mg/kg, increased total bilirubin (4.0-1.93 times) and decreased albumin (0.84-0.91 times) in male at 300 mg/kg. 300 mg/kg/day: Well tolerated with minimal bone marrow hypercellularity (due to an increase in the myeloid component, likely reflecting stimulation of leukocyte cell lines) in the sternum and rib. |
| | 1 month | Asunaprevir: 0, 72, 129.5 Daclatasvir: 0, 15, 50, p.o. | Asunaprevir: 129.5 Daclatasvir: 50 | Male: 73.9 Female: 60.2 | Male: 20 Female: 16.3 | Mild effects including vomiting, mixed cell or eosinophilic infiltration in large intestine with slight necrosis and distension of intestinal crypt at HD. |
| | 3 months | Asunaprevir: 0, 45, 80 Daclatasvir: 0, 15, 50, p.o. | Asunaprevir: 80 Daclatasvir: 50 | Male: 31.7 Female: 13.9 | Male: 8.6 Female: 3.8 | Well tolerated, mild to moderate ↓ vacuoles in adrenal cortex trabecular meshwork cells at HD. |

[a] Animal AUC/Human AUC, the clinical recommended dose AUC was 3.69 µg·h/mL in human.

[10] PMDA Database. http://www.pmda.go.jp/drugs/2014/P201400113/index.html (accessed Mar 2016).

## Safety Pharmacology

Table 31    Safety Pharmacological Studies of Asunaprevir[10]

| Study | System | Dose | Finding |
|---|---|---|---|
| Cardiovascular effect | HEK-293 cell expressing hERG channel | 10, 30 µM | Mild-moderate inhibition of hERG currents (8.2%-20.6% vs pretest); $IC_{50}$ >30 µM. |
| | HEK-293 cell expressing $Na^+$ channel | 10, 30 µM | Mild-moderate inhibition of sodium currents (26.6%-65.9% vs pretest at 1 Hz stimulation frequency and 29.8%-71.6% vs pretest at 4 Hz). |
| | HEK-293 cell expressing L-type $Ca^{2+}$ channel | 30 µM | Mild-moderate inhibition of L-type calcium (Cav 1.2) (18.3% vs pretest). |
| | Rabbit (cardiac Purkinje fiber) | 3, 10, 30 µM | No drug-related finding. |
| | Beagle dog (telemetered) | 0, 100 mg/kg | Unformed and/or liquid stool in 2 males and 2 females on 1 day post-dose, bloody stool on day 6 and unformed/mucoid stool on days 6-9 in 1 male. Maximum asunaprevir plasma concentration (4 h post-dose): 43.68 µg/mL (male); 70.36 µg/mL (female). |

Note: Respiratory and central nervous toxicological endpoints were incorporated into single and repeated toxicity studies, in view of which no specific effects were found.

## Genotoxicity

Table 32    Genotoxicity Studies of Asunaprevir[10]

| Assay | Species/ System | Metabolism Activity | Dose | Finding |
|---|---|---|---|---|
| *In vitro* reverse mutation assay in bacterial cell | *S. typhimurium* TA98, TA100, TA1535, TA1537; *E. coli* WP2 *uvrA* | ±S9 | 1.5-5000 µg/plate | Negative. |
| *In vitro* chromosome aberrations assay in mammalian cell | CHO cell | ±S9 | 2.5-40 µg/mL (+S9) 2.5-60 µg/mL (-S9) | Negative. |
| *In vivo* bone marrow micronucleus assay | SD rat | + | 250, 500, 1000, 2000 mg/kg/day for 3 days, p.o. | Negative. |

## Reproductive and Developmental Toxicity

Table 33    Reproductive and Developmental Toxicology Studies of Asunaprevir by Oral Administration[10]

| Study | Species | Dose (mg/kg/day) | Endpoint | NOAEL Dose (mg/kg/day) | NOAEL $AUC_{0-24}$ (ng·h/mL) | NOAEL Safety Margin[a] (× MRHD) | Finding |
|---|---|---|---|---|---|---|---|
| Fertility and early embryonic development | SD rat | 0, 50, 200, 600 | Male fertility | 600 | 386 | 105 | ↓ BW and BWG in both sexes at HD, ↑ liver weight at MD and HD in females. |
| | | | Female fertility | 600 | 373 | 101 | No effect on parent fertility or early embryonic development. |
| Embryo-fetal development | ICR mouse | 0, 10, 50, 250, 500 | Maternal | 250 | 737 | 200 | Well tolerated at ≤250 mg/kg/day; 1 case of moribund euthanasia at HD, whose relation with drug remained unclear. |
| | | | Fetal | 500 | 1740 | 472 | No fetal malformation/variation. |
| | NZW rabbit | 0, 50, 100, 200 | Maternal/fetal | 200 | 4.40 | 1.19 | No anomaly on either maternal or embryo-fetal endpoint. |
| Pre- and postnatal development | SD rat | 0, 40, 125, 400 | $F_0$ | 40 | 26.8 | 7.26 | ↑ Adrenal weight, abdominal and gastrointestinal distension in dams at MD and HD. |
| | | | $F_1$ | 125 | 282 | 76.4 | ↓ Survival rate of $F_1$ offspring at HD. |

[a] Animal AUC/Human AUC, the clinical recommended dose AUC was 3.69 µg·h/mL in humans.

[10]  PMDA Database.   http://www.pmda.go.jp/drugs/2014/P201400113/index.html (accessed Mar 2016).

# Carcinogenicity

Table 34   Carcinogenicity Studies of Asunaprevir by Oral Administration[10]

| Species | Duration (Week) | Dose (mg/kg/day) | NOAEL | | | Finding |
| | | | Dose (mg/kg/day) | AUC$_{0-24}$ (μg·h/mL) | Safety Margin[a] (× MRHD) | |
|---|---|---|---|---|---|---|
| Tg-rasH2 mouse[b] | 26 | 0, 25, 100, 200 | 200 | 1292 | 350 | Non-neoplastic:<br>Centrilobular liver cell hypertrophy (males only, minimal to minor) and hepatocellular vacuolation (very slight to mild), ↑ chronic mesenteric thrombus in white adipose tissue (males only, minimal to moderate).   But all believed to be advanced spontaneous lesions; Liver cell hypertrophy considered adaptive response in the long-term administration (induction of microsomal enzyme).<br>Neoplastic:<br>Incidental tumor but at the same level as the control. |
| SD rat[c] | 104 | Male: 0, 50, 75, 125<br>Female: 0, 40, 60, 80 | Male: 125<br>Female: 80 | Male: 193<br>Female: 202 | Male: 52.3<br>Female: 54.7 | Non-neoplastic: Increased frequency of bile duct hyperplasia at 125 mg/kg/day in males and 80 mg/kg/day in females (minimal to moderate).<br>Neoplastic: No tumor and proliferative finding in the bile duct. |

Vehicle: 60% PEG-400 and 40% TPGS.   [a] Animal AUC/Human AUC, the clinical recommended dose AUC was 3.69 μg·h/mL in humans.

# Special Toxicology

Table 35   Phototoxicity Studies of Asunaprevir[10]

| Study | Species | Dose | Finding |
|---|---|---|---|
| Neutral red uptake phototoxicity assay | Balb/c 3T3 mouse fibroblast | 0.11-65 mg/L | Phototoxic potential in Balb/c 3T3 cell. |
| Photo-irritation patch test | Long-Evans rat | 0, 60, 325, 600 mg/kg, p.o. | Not phototoxic. |

[10]   PMDA Database. http://www.pmda.go.jp/drugs/2014/P201400113/index.html (accessed Mar 2016).

# CHAPTER

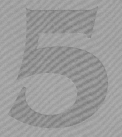

## Ataluren

# Ataluren

## (Translarna®)

Research code: PTC-124

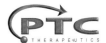

## 1  General Information

❖ Ataluren is an inhibitor of cystic fibrosis transmembrane conductance regulator (CFTR), which was first approved in Jul 2014 by EMA.

❖ Ataluren was developed and marketed by PTC Therapeutics.

❖ Ataluren is an inhibitor of nonsense mutation in DNA, which promotes read-through of premature stop codons, resulting in the formation of a full-length functional protein in patients with nonsense mutation genetic disorders.

❖ Ataluren is indicated for the treatment of Duchenne muscular dystrophy (DMD) resulted from a nonsense mutation in the dystrophin gene, in ambulatory patients aged 5 years and older.    Efficacy has not been demonstrated in non-ambulatory patients.

❖ Available as oral suspension, containing 125 mg, 250 mg, or 1000 mg of granules, and the recommended dose is 10 mg/kg body weight in the morning and afternoon, 20 mg/kg body weight in the evening.

❖ Sales of Translarna® were 1.4 and 33.7 million US$ in 2014 and 2015, respectively, referring to the financial reports of PTC Therapeutics.

### Key Approvals around the World*

|  | EU (EMA) |
| --- | --- |
| First approval date | 07/31/2014 |
| Application or approval No. | EMEA/H/C/002720 |
| Brand name | Translarna® |
| Indication | Duchenne muscular dystrophy (DMD) |
| Authorisation holder | PTC Therapeutics |

* Till Mar 2016, it had not been approved by FDA (US), PMDA (Japan) and CFDA (China).

## Active Ingredient

Molecular formula:  $C_{15}H_9FN_2O_3$
Molecular weight:    284.24
CAS No.:                   775304-57-9 (Ataluren)
Chemical name:       3-[5-(2-Fluorophenyl)-1,2,4-oxadiazol-3-yl]-benzoic acid

Parameters of Lipinski's "Rule of 5"

| MW | $H_D$ | $H_A$ | FRB[a] | PSA[a] | cLogP[a] |
| --- | --- | --- | --- | --- | --- |
| 284.24 | 1 | 5 | 3 | 76.2Å² | 2.67 ± 0.41 |

[a] Calculated by ACD/Labs software V11.02.

## Drug Product*

Dosage route:        Oral
Strength:               125 mg/250 mg/1000 mg (Ataluren)
Dosage form:        Granules for oral suspension
Inactive ingredient:  Polydextrose (E1200), macrogol, poloxamer, mannitol (E421), crospovidone, hydroxyethyl cellulose, artificial vanilla flavour (maltodextrin, artificial flavours and propylene glycol), colloidal anhydrous (E551) silica and magnesium stearate.
Recommended dose:  The recommended dose is 10 mg/kg body weight in the morning, 10 mg/kg body weight at midday and 20 mg/kg body weight in the evening (for a total daily dose of 40 mg/kg body weight).

* Sourced from EMA drug label information

## 2   Key Patents Information

### Summary

❖  Translama® (Ataluren) was approved by EMA on Jul 31, 2014.

❖  Ataluren was originally discovered by PTC Therapeutics, and its compound patent application was filed as PCT application by PTC Therapeutics in 2004.

❖  The compound patent will expire in 2024 foremost, which has been granted in the United States, Japan, China and Europe successively.

Table 1   Ataluren's Compound Patent Protection in Drug-Mainstream Country

| Country | Publication/Patent NO. | Application Date | Granted Date | Estimated Expiry Date |
|---------|------------------------|------------------|--------------|-----------------------|
| WO | WO2004091502A2 | 04/09/2004 | / | / |
| US | US6992096B2 | 04/09/2004 | 01/31/2006 | 05/17/2024[a] |
| | US7419991B2 | 04/09/2004 | 09/02/2008 | 05/17/2024[b] |
| EP | EP1618098B1 | 04/09/2004 | 11/19/2014 | 04/09/2024 |
| JP | JP4851933B2 | 04/09/2004 | 01/11/2012 | 04/09/2024 |
| CN | CN1802360B | 04/09/2004 | 05/07/2014 | 04/09/2024 |

[a] The term of this patent is extended by 38 days.   [b] The term of this patent is extended by 138 days (TD).

Table 2   Originator's International Patent Application List (Patent Family)

| Publication NO. | Title | Applicant/Assignee/Owner | Publication Date |
|-----------------|-------|--------------------------|------------------|
| Technical Subjects | Active Ingredient (Free Base)'s Formula or Structure and Preparation | | |
| WO2004091502A2 | 1,2,4-Oxadiazole benzoic acid compounds and their use for nonsense suppression and the treatment of disease | PTC Therapeutics | 10/28/2004 |
| Technical Subjects | Salt, Crystal, Polymorphic, Solvate (Hydrate), Isomer, Derivative Etc. and Preparation | | |
| WO2008030570A1 | Processes for the preparation of 1,2,4-oxadiazole benzoic acids | PTC Therapeutics | 03/13/2008 |
| WO2008039431A2 | Crystalline forms of 3-[5-(2-fluorophenyl)-[1,2,4]oxadiazol-3-yl]-benzoic acid | PTC Therapeutics | 04/03/2008 |
| WO2015134711A1 | Pharmaceutical compositions and salts of a 1,2,4-oxadiazole benzoic acid | PTC Therapeutics | 09/11/2015 |
| Technical Subjects | Indication or Methods for Medical Needs | | |
| WO2006044682A1 | Compounds for nonsense suppression, and methods for their use | PTC Therapeutics | 04/27/2006 |
| WO2006110483A1 | Compositions of an orally active 1,2,4-oxadiazole for nonsense mutation suppression therapy | PTC Therapeutics | 10/19/2006 |
| WO2007117438A2 | Methods for the production of functional protein from DNA having a nonsense mutation and the treatment of disorders associated therewith | PTC Therapeutics | 10/18/2007 |
| WO2008045566A1 | Methods for dosing an orally active 1,2,4-oxadiazole for nonsense mutation suppression therapy | PTC Therapeutics | 04/17/2008 |
| WO2008130370A1 | Hydroxylated 1,2,4-oxadiazole benzoic acid compounds, compositions thereof and the use for nonsense suppression | PTC Therapeutics | 10/30/2008 |
| WO2011072281A1 | Methods for treating methylmalonic acidemia | PTC Therapeutics | 06/16/2011 |

The data was updated until Jan 2016.

# 3  Chemistry

## Route 1:  Original Discovery Route

*Synthetic Route*:  The sequence to construct ataluren, which was described by the authors at PTC Therapeutics, commenced with commercially available methyl 3-cyanobenzoate **1**.  This ester was exposed to hydroxylamine in aqueous *tert*-butanol and warmed gently until the reaction was deemed complete.  Then this mixture was treated with 2-fluorobenzoyl chloride and subsequently triethylamine.  To minimize exotherm and undesired side products, additions of these liquid reagents should be careful controlled through slow dropwise manner.  Upon complete consumption of starting materials and formation of amidooxime **4**, the aqueous reaction mixture was then heated to 83 °C to facilitate 1,2,4-oxadiazole formation, resulting in the tricyclic ester **5** in 93% yield over three steps.  Finally, saponification of ester **5** with sodium hydroxide, followed by acidic quench gave ataluren in 74% yield over the two-step sequence.  The overall yield was 69%.[1-7]

## Route 2

*Synthetic Route*:  Under the optimized conditions, reaction of commercial 2-fluorobenzoic acid **1** with 3-methyl benzamidine **2** and sequential hydroxylamine-induced cyclization in hot acetic acid resulted in the formation of the desired 1,2,4-oxadiazole **4** as a white solid in 70% across a two-step one-pot procedure.  Subsequent oxidation of the methyl group with aqueous potassium permanganate in pyridine furnished ataluren in 40% yield.  The overall yield was 28%.[8]

[1]  Almstead, N. G.; Hwang, P. S.; Pines, S., et al. WO2008030570A1, **2008**.
[2]  Almstead, N. G.; Hwang, P. S.; Pines, S., et al. US20080139818A1, **2008**.
[3]  Hirawat, S.; Miller, L. WO2008045566A1, **2008**.
[4]  Hirawat, S.; Miller, L. US20080114039A1, **2008**.
[5]  Karp, G. M.; Hwang, S.; Chen, G., et al. WO2004091502A2, **2004**.
[6]  Karp, G. M.; Hwang, S.; Chen, G., et al. US6992096B2, **2006**.
[7]  Lentini, L.; Melfi, R.; Di Leonardo, A., et al. *Mol. Pharm.* **2014**, *11*, 653-664.
[8]  Gupta, P. K.; Hussain, M. K.; Asad, M., et al. *New J. Chem.* **2014**, *38*, 3062-3070.

# Route 3

*Synthetic Route*:   Aryl bromides were successfully transformed into their corresponding *N,N'*-diacylhydrazines *via* a Pd-catalyzed carbonylative coupling with acylhydrazines, which approach could also been applied in a similar protocol for the synthesis of the corresponding 1,2,4-oxadiazoles.   The preparation of ataluren was the representative instance.   Starting from 3-cyanobenzoic acid **1**, protection of the free acid and subsequent preparation of the amidoxime led to **3** with 63% and 94% yield, respectively.   Coupling of (*Z*)-*N'*-hydroxybenzimidamide **3** with 1-bromo-2-fluorobenzene **4** under the well-developed conditions afforded the ataluren precursor **5** in a 74% isolated yield.   Finally, deprotection of the *tert*-butyl ester using TFA furnished ataluren in a near quantitative yield.   The overall yield was 43%.[9]

## 4   Pharmacology

## Summary

Mechanism of Action

❖ As an inhibitor of nonsense mutation in DNA, ataluren can promote read-through of premature stop codons, resulting in the formation of a full-length functional protein in patients with nonsense mutation genetic disorders (The read-through potential: UGA > UAG > UAA).

❖ Ataluren did not lead to read-through of normal stop codons in cultured cells, tissues from rats and dogs, or in PBMCs from patients.

❖ The minimal effect dose was 0.01-0.1 µg/mL (the maximal activity dose = 3 µM) on premature stop codons in transfected HEK293 LUC-190 (UGA) cells.

❖ Ataluren did not significantly block ligand binding to any of the targets (inhibition of >50% was considered significant) in a panel of 62 diverse receptors or enzymes (neurotransmitter receptors, enzymes, steroids, ion channels, secondary messengers, prostaglandins, growth factors, hormones, brain and gut peptides) at 10 µM (2.84 µg/mL) or 30 µM (8.52 µg/mL).[10]

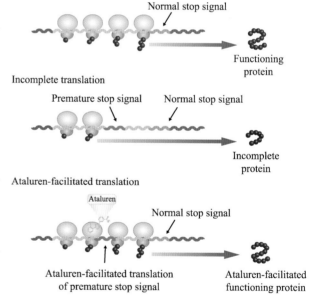

[9]   Andersen, T. L.; Caneschi, W.; Ayoub, A., et al. *Adv. Synth. Catal.* **2014**, *356*, 3074-3082.

[10]   European Medicines Agency (EMA) Database.   http://www.ema.europa.eu/docs/en_GB/document_library/EPAR_Public_assessment_report/human/002720/WC500171816.pdf (accessed Mar 2016).

*In Vitro* Efficacy

❖ Ataluren promotes read-through of premature stop codons with no effect on normal stop codons or cellular mRNA levels in cell-based assays.
  - HEK293 LUC-190 (UGA):
    - Read-through of premature UGA codon: Minimal effect dose at 0.01-0.1 μM, and maximal activity at 3 μM.
    - No effect on LUC-190 mRNA levels at 30 μM.
  - HEK293 LUC-190 CD40 cells: No effect on the read-through of normal stop codons at 100 μM.
❖ Promoted dystrophin production in primary myotubes:
  - From the *mdx* mouse: The maximal effect at 10 μg/mL.
  - From the nmDMD patient: The maximal effect at 10 μg/mL.
❖ Promoted enzyme activities in primary embryonic fibroblasts (MEFs):
  - From the Idua-W392X mouse: The maximal induction of enzyme activity at 10 μg/mL.
  - From CPT1A deficiency patient: Increased 30% enzyme activity.
❖ The fibroblasts isolated from INCL patient: Yielded small increase in PPT1 enzymatic activity at 0.15-15 μg/mL.
❖ In photoreceptor cells from nonsense mutation usher syndrome patients: 8-fold increase in the expression and full-length function of harmonin.

*In Vivo* Efficacy

❖ Ataluren adjusted dystrophin, CFTR and IDUA expression.
❖ In *mdx* mouse model:
  - Reduced functional dystrophin.
  - Significant reductions in serum CK.
❖ In the CF mouse model:
  - Significantly increased hCFTR expression at 60 mg/kg.
  - Partially restored hCFTR expression at both 0.3 and 0.9 mg/kg.
  - Yielded average cAMP-stimulated short-circuit currents: 0.91 μA/cm$^2$ at 0.3 mg/mL and 1.35 μA/cm$^2$ at 0.9 mg/mL.
❖ In nmHurler syndrome mouse model:
  - In Idua-W392X mouse: Increased Idua enzyme activity with a bell-shaped dose response, and the maximal induction at 0.1% (in brain, spleen, heart and lungs) or 0.3% (in liver).
  - In Idua-W402X mouse: Enabled read-through of the premature stopped codon present in the IDUA mRNA at 10 μg/mL.

## *In Vitro* Efficacy

Table 3    The Read-through of Premature and Normal Stop Codons by Ataluren[10-12]

| Model System | Source | Stop Codon | Dose (μg/mL) | Effect(s) | |
|---|---|---|---|---|---|
| | | | | ED$^a$ (μM) | Finding |
| HEK293 LUC-190 (UGA) cell$^b$ | Human | Premature | NA | 0.01-0.1 (mED$^c$ = 3 μM) | Dose-dependent read-through: UGA > UAG > UAA. |
| | | Normal | NA | No altered | No alteration of LUC-190 mRNA levels at 30 μM. |
| Wild type HEK293 LUC-190 CD40 cell$^d$ | Human | Normal | 1, 10, 100 | No altered | No read-through of normal stop codons at 100 μM. |

$^a$ ED: Minimum effect dose.   $^b$ HEK293 cells transfected with the luciferase gene engineer to have premature stop codons at codon 190.   $^c$ mED: Maximal effect dose.
$^d$ HEK293 LUC-190 cells with the normal UAA luciferase-CD40 stop codon changed to a UGA stop codon.

[10]  EMA Database.   http://www.ema.europa.eu/docs/en_GB/document_library/EPAR_-_Public_assessment_report/human/002720/WC500171816.pdf (accessed Mar 2016)
[11]  Welch, E.; Barton, E. C.; Zhuo, J., et al. *Nature* **2007**, *477*, 87-91.
[12]  Peltz, S. W.; Morsy, M.; Welch, E. M., et al. *Annu. Rev. Med.* **2013**, *64*, 407-425.

Table 4    Production of the Expression of Functional Protein with Nonsense Suppression by Ataluren in Cells[10, 12, 13]

| Experimental System | Resource | Targets | Dose (µg/mL) | Effect | |
|---|---|---|---|---|---|
| | | | | mED[a] (µg/mL) | Finding |
| Primary myotube | mdx mouse[b] | DMD gene[c] | 0.1-30 | 10 | Significantly induced dystrophin expression with a bell-shaped dose response. |
| | nmDMD patient | DMD gene | 0.1-40 | 10 | Significantly induced dystrophin expression with a bell-shaped dose response. |
| | Miyoshi patient | DYSF gene[d] | NA | 10 | Resulted in the expression of functional dysferlin expression. |
| Embryonic fibroblast | Idua-W392X mouse[e] | Idua gene | NA | 10 | Significantly increased iduronidase activity. |
| | CPT1A deficiency patient | CPT1A gene[f] | 1.5 | NA | Increased 30% enzyme activity compared to wild-type levels in untreated cells. |
| Photoreceptor cell | Usher syndrome patient | USH1C gene[g] | 2.5-10 | NA | 8-fold increase in harmonin; Increased the functional activity of actin filament bundling compared to untreated controls. |
| Fibroblasts | INCL patient[h] | CLN1 gene[i] | 0.15-15 | NA | Yielded small increase in PPT1 enzymatic activity. |

[a] mED: Maximal effect dose.   [b] mdx mouse model: A UAA codon replaced a glutamine codon in exon 23 of the dystrophin gene.   [c] DMD: Duchenne muscular dystrophy.   [d] DYSF: Dysferlin.   [e] Idua-W392X mouse model: The mouse model of nonsense mutation Hurler syndrome.   [f] CPT1A: Carnitine palmitoyltransferase 1A.   [g] USH1: One of usher syndrome type I gene.   [h] INCL: Infantile neuronal ceroid lipofuscinosis.   [i] CLN1: The gene encod palmitoyl-proteinthioesterase-1 (PPT1).

## *In Vivo* Efficacy

Table 5    *In Vivo* Efficacy of Ataluren in Nonsense Mutation Mouse Model[10-13]

| System | | | Dose (mg/kg) | Route & Duration (Day) | Effect | |
|---|---|---|---|---|---|---|
| Model | Animal | Test | | | mED[a] | Fingding |
| nmDMD mouse model | mdx mouse | Dystrophin expression | NA | p.o., single dose; i.p., single dose; p.o./i.p.[b], single dose; | NA[c] | The production of dystrophin protein: 20% of the normal levels. Resulted in protection from eccentric contraction injury and in reduced serum CK, indicating reduced muscle fragility. |
| nmCF mouse model[d] | Cftr-/-FABP-hCFTR-G542X mouse[e] | Full-length CFTR expression[f] | 15, 30, 60 | s.c. QD × 14-21 | NA | Increased full-length CFTR expression at 60 mg/kg s.c. in the submucosal glands of intestinal tissues. |
| | | | 0.3, 0.9 mg/mL | p.o. QD × 14-21 | NA | Partially restored hCFTR expression |
| | | Chloride channel function[g] | 0.3, 0.9 mg/mL | p.o. QD × 14-21 | NA | Restored CFTR dependent chloride channel function, yielding average cAMP-stimulated short-circuit currents: 0.91 µA/cm² at 0.3 mg/mL and 1.35 µA/cm² at 0.9 mg/mL. |
| nmHurler syndrome mouse model | Idua-W392X mouse | Idua enzyme activity | NA | NA | 0.1% 0.3% | Increased idua enzyme activity with a bell-shaped dose response. The maximal induction: 0.1% (in brain, spleen, heart, and lungs) or 0.3% (in liver), with less activity at 1.0% (w/w). |
| | Idua-W402X mouse[h] | GAG levels in tissues[i] | NA | NA | 10 µg/mL | Reduced GAG levels, indicating enabled read-through of the premature stop codon present in the IDUA mRNA. |

NA: Not available.   [a] mED: Maximal effect dose.   [b] 1.8 mg/mL *via* a liquid diet and 33 mg/kg i.p. TID.   [c] The optimal efficacy of combination (1.8 mg/mL *via* a liquid diet and 33 mg/kg i.p. TID).   [d] nmCF: Nonsense mutant Cystic Fibrosis.   [e] Cftr-/- mice expressing a human CFTR-G542X transgene.   [f] Cftr-/-hCFTR-G542X transgenic mice treated with ataluren by once daily s.c. injection, the expression of hCFTR in submucosal glands of intestinal tissues was detected by immunofluorescence assay.   [g] The data collected from short-circuit current measurements from intestinal tissues harvested from untreated Cftr+/+ mice, Cftr+/+ mice treated with ataluren.   [h] Idua-W402X mouse: Mouse harbor a nonsense mutation in exon 9 of the IDUA gene that corresponds to the human W402X mutation.   [i] GAG: Glycosaminoglycans.

[10]   EMA Database.   http://www.ema.europa.eu/docs/en_GB/document_library/EPAR_-_Public_assessment_report/human/002720/WC500171816.pdf (accessed Mar 2016)
[11]   Welch, E.; Barton, E. C.; Zhuo, J., et al. *Nature* **2007**, *477*, 87-91.
[12]   Peltz, S. W.; Morsy, M.; Welch, E. M., et al. *Annu. Rev. Med.* **2013**, *64*, 407-425.
[13]   Du, M.; Liu, X.; Welch, E. C., et al. *Proc. Natl. Acad. Sci. U. S. A.* **2008**, *105*, 2064-2069.

# 5 ADME & Drug-Drug Interaction

## Summary

Absorption of Ataluren

❖ Exhibited a non-linear pharmacokinetics in mice, rats, dogs and rabbits following oral dosing.   The increases of $C_{max}$ and AUC were less than dose-proportional.

❖ Had low oral bioavailability in dogs (7%), which corresponded to the observed low urinary excretion in dogs (12% of the dose).   In mice and rats, the excretion *via* urine and bile indicated high bioavailability (40% urinary excretion in mice and 90% urinary and bile excretion in rats).

❖ Following oral administrations of ataluren to mice, rats, dogs and rabbits, the drug was rapidly absorbed and eliminated in all species, with peak concentrations after single dose occurring at 0.25 to 4 h post-dose.   The $T_{max}$ tended to increase with increasing dose and with multiple doses.

❖ The half-life was similar across the tested non-clinical species and ranged within 1.1 to 7.6 h after oral administrations.

❖ Had high clearance in dogs (123 ml/h/kg), in contrast to liver blood flow, after intravenous administration.

❖ Exhibited a confined distribution in dogs, with apparent volume of distribution at 0.21 L/kg, after intravenous administration.

Distribution of Ataluren

❖ Exhibited high plasma protein binding in mice (98.4%), rats (98.7%) and dogs (97.5%).

❖ Rats after single oral administration:

• Relatively higher concentration levels were observed in the gastrointestinal tract, the secretion organs (liver and kidneys), adrenal gland, brown fat and lungs.

• Low radioactivity concentration levels were observed in the brain.   The blood-to-plasma ratio of ataluren radioactivity was less than one, indicating that ataluren did not accumulate in erythrocytes.

• At 24 h post-dose, radioactivity was still observed in brown fat, skin, harderian and preputial glands.

Metabolism of Ataluren

❖ The major biotransformation pathway of ataluren included acyl glucuronidation, reductive oxadiazole ring cleavage, oxidative deamination and hydrolysis.

❖ In all species, unchanged ataluren was the major component in plasma (ranging from 70% to 91%).

❖ Ataluren was not metabolized by CYP isozymes, but was directly glucuronidated *via* UGT1A9 in human liver microsomes.

Excretion of Ataluren

❖ Was predominantly excreted in feces in mice, rats and dogs.

Drug-Drug Interaction

❖ *In vitro*, inhibitors of UGT1A9 or drugs metabolized by UGT1A9 may have a clinically relevant effect on the metabolism of ataluren.

❖ *In vitro* studies indicated that ataluren was not a substrate of P-gp.

## Absorption

**Oral Administration:**[10]

❖ Following oral administrations of ataluren to mice, rats, dogs and rabbits, the drug was rapidly absorbed and eliminated in all species, reaching peak concentrations after single doses occurring at 0.25 to 4 h post-dose.   The $T_{max}$ tended to increase with increasing dose and with multiple doses.

❖ The half-life was similar across the non-clinical species tested and ranged within 1.1 to 7.6 h.

❖ There was no accumulation of drug in plasma upon repeated daily dosing.   In rats, two peak plasma concentrations were observed, indicating entero-hepatic recirculation.

❖ Plasma exposure of ataluren in all species, based on $C_{max}$ and AUC, was less than dose proportional.   After multiple dosing, plasma exposure (in particular the AUC values) decreased after Day 1.

**Intravenous Administration:**

❖ Following intravenous administrations of ataluren to dogs, the systemic clearance averaged on 123 mL/h/kg and the volume of distribution at steady state ($V_{ss}$) was 0.21 L/kg.

---

[10]   EMA Database.   http://www.ema.europa.eu/docs/en_GB/document_library/EPAR_-_Public_assessment_report/human/002720/WC500171816.pdf (accessed Mar 2016).

❖ In a bioavailability study conducted in dogs with intravenous and oral doses, low bioavailability (7%) was observed, which corresponded to the observed low urinary excretion in this species (12% of the dose).  In mice and rats, the excretion *via* urine and bile indicated high bioavailability (40% urinary excretion in mice and 90% urinary and bile excretion in rats).

Table 6   *In Vivo* Pharmacokinetic Parameters of Ataluren in Humans after Single Oral Dose of Ataluren[14]

| Species | Route | Dose (mg/kg) | $T_{max}$ (h) | $C_{max}$ (µg/mL) | $AUC_{0-72}$ (µg·h/mL) | $T_{1/2}$ (h) |
|---------|-------|--------------|---------------|-------------------|------------------------|----------------|
| Healthy human | p.o. | 3 | $1.0 \pm 1.0$ | $6 \pm 0.5$ | $27 \pm 6$ | $3.1 \pm 0.2$ |
| | p.o. | 10 | $0.7 \pm 0.3$ | $27 \pm 6$ | $110 \pm 16$ | $3.6 \pm 0.2$ |
| | p.o. | 30 | $0.9 \pm 0.2$ | $90 \pm 22$ | $482 \pm 95$ | $4.7 \pm 0.1$ |
| | p.o. | 100 | $2.2 \pm 1.0$ | $210 \pm 75$ | $2200 \pm 1422$ | $5.4 \pm 1.1$ |
| | p.o. | 150 | $2.0 \pm 1.3$ | $260 \pm 33$ | $3001 \pm 1214$ | $5.1 \pm 0.7$ |
| | p.o. | 200 | $2.7 \pm 0.8$ | $314 \pm 29$ | $2937 \pm 436$ | $6.3 \pm 2.0$ |

Mean ± SD, n = 6.

Figure A   *In Vivo* Plasma Concentration-Time Profiles in Humans after Single Oral Dose of Ataluren (n = 6)[14]

# Distribution[10]

❖ Ataluren showed high plasma protein binding (98.4% in mice, 98.7% in rats and 97.5% in dogs).
❖ After oral administration of radio-labelled ataluren to rats, high concentrations were found in the gastrointestinal tract, the secretion organs (liver and kidneys), adrenal gland, brown fat and lungs.
❖ Low radioactivity concentrations were observed in the brain.  The blood-to-plasma ratio of ataluren radioactivity was less than one, indicating that ataluren did not accumulate in erythrocytes.
❖ At 24 h post-dose, radioactivity was still observed in brown fat, skin, harderian and preputial glands.

# Metabolism[10]

❖ The major biotransformation pathway of ataluren included acyl glucuronidation, reductive oxadiazole ring cleavage, oxidative deamination and hydrolysis.  In all species, unchanged ataluren was the major component in plasma (ranging from 70% to 91%).
❖ Ataluren was not metabolized by CYP isozymes, but was directly glucuronidated *via* UGT1A9 in human liver microsomes.

# Excretion[10]

❖ Following single oral dose of radio-labelled ataluren, the majority of the administered radioactivity was excreted in feces: 54% by mice, 84% by rats and 80% by dogs.  Most of the dose was excreted within 48 h.  The total recovery was >93% in three species.

[10]   EMA Database.   http://www.ema.europa.eu/docs/en_GB/document_library/EPAR_-_Public_assessment_report/human/002720/WC500171816.pdf (accessed Mar 2016).
[14]   Hirawat, S.; Wilch, E. M.; Elfring, G. L., et al. *J. Clin. Pharmacol.* **2007**, *47*, 430-444.

## Drug-Drug Interaction[10]

❖ No non-clinical studies were performed by the applicant to evaluate potential drug-drug interaction, but based on the *in vitro* data, inhibitors of UGT1A9 or drugs metabolized by UGT1A9 may have a clinically relevant effect on the metabolism of ataluren.

❖ *In vitro* studies indicated that ataluren was not a substrate of P-glycoprotein.

# 6   Non-Clinical Toxicology

## Summary

### Single-Dose Toxicity[10]

❖ Single-dose toxicity studies by the oral route in rats and dogs:
  • The rat $LD_{50}$ was >2000 mg/kg with the highest dose tested.
  • In dogs, ataluren was well tolerated up to the highest dose of 1600 mg/kg.
  • No macroscopic abnormality was noted at necropsy.

### Repeated-Dose Toxicity

❖ Sub- and chronic toxicity by the oral route in mice (up to 29 days), rats (up to 26 weeks) and dogs (up to 52 weeks):
  • The most important toxicity identified in mice was nephrotoxicity, and no NOEL or safety margin was established. Despite of its non-universality for other species tested, CHMP was of the view that risk for humans could not be ruled out considering the unknown mechanism.
  • One of main concerns in rats was malignant hibernoma, which could relate to the effects on fat tissue metabolism and plasma lipid parameters.   Similarly, CHMP concluded similar effects in humans could not be excluded, particularly in the young population considering higher quantity of the brown adipose tissue.
  • In addition, several other mild adverse effects included decreased body weight gain, food intake and increased liver weight without a histological correlate were observed.
  • The toxicokinetic data indicated a short $T_{1/2}$ and no significant drug accumulation in plasma upon repeated daily dosing. Ataluren exposure increased with ascending dosage, but less than dose-proportionally at higher doses.   There were no sex-related differences in ataluren exposure in dogs, but exposure was slightly higher in females than in males of rats and mice.

### Safety Pharmacology[10]

❖ A full core battery of standard safety pharmacology studies to assess effects on the CNS, RS and CVS:
  • No relevant effect on the CNS or RS was observed in rats up to 2000 mg/kg/day.
  • *In vitro* and *in vivo* cardiovascular studies exhibited no relevant inhibition on hERG channel in mammalian cells up to 100 μM or biologically important changes in dogs up to 1500 mg/kg.

### Genotoxicity

❖ An adequate battery of genotoxicity tests were conducted and the data did not reveal any special hazard for humans.

### Reproductive and Developmental Toxicity[10]

❖ Fertility and early embryonic development in rats:
  • NOAEL was determined as 300 mg/kg/day (HD), while early embryonic NOAEL was 100 mg/kg/day.
❖ Embryo-fetal development in rats and rabbits:
  • For rats: Maternal NOAEL was 30 mg/kg/day; Embryo-fetal NOAEL was 100 mg/kg/day (4 × RHD exposure), based on increased early resorptions, post-implantation loss and decreased viable fetuses and signs of developmental delay (increased skeletal variations).
  • For rabbits: Maternal and embryo-fetal toxicities were observed at 100 mg/kg/day (HD), consisted of decreased mean fetal weight and increased skeletal variations; NOAEL showed no margin when compared to human exposure.
❖ Pre- and postnatal development in rats:
  • Significant maternal and neonatal toxicities were observed at 150 mg/kg/day (5 × RHD exposure), and maternal systemic exposure at NOAEL was <3 mg/kg/day and at LOEL was <4 mg/kg/day.

### Carcinogenicity[10]

❖ Carcinogenicity bioassays in transgenic mice (26 weeks) and in rats (24 months):

---

[10]   EMA Database.   http://www.ema.europa.eu/docs/en_GB/document_library/EPAR_-_Public_assessment_report/human/002720/WC500171816.pdf (accessed Mar 2016).

- For Tg-rasH2 mouse: Ataluren did not increase the incidence of tumors up to the HDs in males (600 mg/kg/day) or in females (300 mg/kg/day).   The non-neoplastic findings included endometrial hyperplasia and nephropathy in females.
- For rats: Urinary bladder tumors (benign urothelial cell papilloma [2 rats] and malignant urothelial cell carcinoma [1 rat]) were observed in 3/60 female rats dosed at 300 mg/kg/day.   In addition, one case of malignant hibernoma was observed in 1/60 male rats at the dose of 300 mg/kg/day.   The non-neoplastic toxicity consisted of a decrease of body weight.

Special Toxicity
❖ Not available.

## Repeated-Dose Toxicity

Table 7    Repeated-Dose Toxicity Studies of Ataluren by the Oral Route[10]

| Species/Strain | Duration | Dose (mg/kg/day) | NOAEL (mg/kg/day) | Finding |
|---|---|---|---|---|
| Mouse | 29 days[a] | 0, 600, 1200, 1800 | N/A | 1800 mg/kg/day: ↓ Hb (Female), Hct (Female), MCV (Female), ↑ segm neutrophils (Female); ↓ glucose (Male), ↑ AP (Male), Creatine (Male). <br> 1200-1800 mg/kg/day: ↓ BW, ↓ BWG, small ↓ d-r MCH, small ↑ total bilirubin. <br> 600-1800 mg/kg/day: d-r ↑ deaths, temporary ↑ food intake (Male), ↑ BUN, ↓ Cl, both attributed to renal nephrosis or dehydration, ↑ liver weight , ↓ abs and ↑ rel weight of brain, kidneys, heart, ovaries and testes (possibly due to BW). <br> Histopathology: Nephrosis, thymus atrophy. |
| Rat | 26 weeks[a] (starting from 5 weeks old) | 0, 150, 300, 1200 | <150 | 1200 mg/kg/day: ↓ BW, ↓ BWG, ↓ food intake (first week), Urea nitrogen (Male), Ca (Female), mean mandibular salivary gland weights (possibly due to ↓ food intake), ↓ mean prostate weight. <br> 300-1200 mg/kg/day: ↓ RBC, Hb (Female), Hct, ↑ MCHC, WBC (Female), LC, ↓ PTT, ↓ glucose, ↑ albumin (Male), ↓ Triglyceride (Male), ↓ AST (Female), ↑ K, ↑ urine volume. <br> 150-1200 mg/kg/day: ↑ Total protein, ↑ Cholesterd, AP, ↑ liver and kidney weight (without histopath correlate). <br> Malignant hibernoma in 6 animals. <br> (HD: 2 males + 1 female at 20 weeks and 2 males at 26 weeks and LD: 1 male at 26 weeks). <br> 150-300 mg/kg/day: ↓ BW, ↓ BWG. |
|  | 26 weeks[a] (starting from 4 weeks old) | 0, 30, 60, 120, 1200 | 120 | 1200 mg/kg/day: ↓ BW, food intake, ↓ RBC, Hb, Hct, ↑ Ret + anisocytosis/ hyperchromia, ↑ AP, ↓ Triglyceride (Male), ↑ erosion/ulcer (2 Male + 2 Female) in glandular stomach. <br> 120-1200 mg/kg/day: ↓ Neutrophils, ↑ adrenal weight without microsc correlate. <br> 60-1200 mg/kg/day: ↓ Glucose, ↑ renal weight without microsc correlate, ↑ liver weight without microsc correlate. |
| Dog | 52 weeks (starting from 68-83 days old) | 0, 250, 500, 1000 | <250 | 1000 mg/kg/day: ↑ AP, ↑ basal serum ACTH. <br> 500-1000 mg/kg/day: ↓ Serum cortisol response to ACTH stimulation, ↑ aldosterone. <br> 250-1000 mg/kg/day: ↓ RBC, Hb, Ht, PLT, ↑ Chol, ↓ Trigl, ↓ adrenal weight, ↑ liver/gallbladder weight, ↓ spleen weight, ↑ thyroid/ parathyroid weight, ↑ hepatocellular glycogen. <br> Histopathological findings adrenals: <br> Multifocal lymphohistiocytic infiltrates in adrenal cortex and focal degeneration of individual or small groups of adjacent parenchymal cells. <br> Terminal recovery: <br> 1000 mg/kg/day: ↓ Red blood cell parameters and ↑ PLT not fully recovered, ↑ AP not fully recovered, ↓ adrenal weight, ↑ liver/gallbladder weight, ↓ spleen weight, ↑ thyroid/ parathyroid weight; Histopathological findings in adrenals not fully recovered. <br> 250-500 mg/kg/day: Histopathological findings in adrenals not fully recovered. |

[a] Conducted along with toxicokinetic study.

[10]   EMA Database.   http://www.ema.europa.eu/docs/en_GB/document_library/EPAR_-_Public_assessment_report/human/002720/WC500171816.pdf (accessed Mar 2016).

# Genotoxicity

Table 8    Genotoxicity Studies of Ataluren[10]

| Assay | Species | Metabolism Activity | Treatment | Finding |
|---|---|---|---|---|
| *In vitro* chromosome aberration assay in mammalian cells | CHO | ±S9 | 12.5-412 μg/mL (-S9)<br>98.8-300 μg/mL (+S9) | Negative. |
| *In vitro* microbial reverse mutation assay | *Salmonella* and E. *coli* Strains | ±S9 | 33.3-5000 μg/plate | Negative. |
| *In vivo* mouse bone marrow erythrocyte micronucleus assay | PCEs/rat | + | 323-1800 mg/kg | Negative. |

[10]  EMA Database.   http://www.ema.europa.eu/docs/en_GB/document_library/EPAR_-_Public_assessment_report/human/002720/WC500171816.pdf (accessed Mar 2016).

# CHAPTER

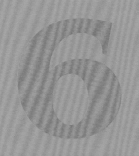

6

## Belinostat

# Belinostat

## (Beleodaq®)

Research code: PX-105684; PXD-101

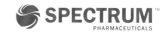

## 1　General Information

❖ Belinostat is a small molecule histone deacetylase (HDAC) inhibitor, which was first approved in Jul 2014 by US FDA.

❖ Belinostat was discovered by TopoTarget, developed and marketed by Spectrum pharmaceuticals.

❖ Belinostat is an intravenously administered HDAC inhibitor that can alter acetylation levels of histone and non-histone proteins, resulting in cell cycle arrest and/or apoptosis of cancer cells.

❖ Belinostat is indicated for the treatment of patients with relapsed or refractory peripheral T-cell lymphoma (PTCL).

❖ Available as lyophilized powder, containing 500 mg of belinostat and the recommended starting dose is 1000 mg/m² reconstitution with 250 mL of sterile 0.9% sodium chloride injection prior to infusion.

❖ The 2014 and 2015 worldwide sales of Beleodaq® were 4.9 and 10.1 million US$, respectively, referring to the financial reports of Spectrum.

## Key Approvals around the World*

|  | US (FDA) |
|---|---|
| First approval date | 07/03/2014 |
| Application or approval No. | NDA 206256 |
| Brand name | Beleodaq® |
| Indication | Peripheral T-cell lymphoma (PTCL) |
| Authorisation holder | Spectrum Pharmaceuticals |

* Till Mar 2016, it had not been approved by EMA (EU), PMDA (Japan) and CFDA (China).

## Active Ingredient

Molecular formula:　$C_{15}H_{14}N_2O_4S$
Molecular weight:　318.35
CAS No.:　　　　　866323-14-0 (Belinostat)
Chemical name:　　(2E)-N-hydroxy-3-[3-(phenylsulfamoyl)phenyl]prop-2-enamide

Parameters of Lipinski's "Rule of 5"

| MW | $H_D$ | $H_A$ | FRB[a] | PSA[a] | cLogP[a] |
|---|---|---|---|---|---|
| 318.35 | 3 | 6 | 5 | 104Å² | 1.46 ± 0.52 |

[a] Calculated by ACD/Labs software V11.02.

## Drug Product*

Dosage route:　　　　Intravenous infusion
Strength:　　　　　　500 mg (Belinostat)
Dosage form:　　　　Lyophilized powder
Inactive ingredient:　L-Arginine
Recommended dose: The recommended starting dose is 1000 mg/m² administered over 30 min by intravenous infusion once daily on days 1-5 of a 21-day cycle.

* Sourced from US FDA drug label information

## 2 Key Patents Information

### Summary

❖ Beleodaq® (Belinostat) has got five-year NCE market exclusivity protection and seven-year orphan drug exclusivity after it was approved by US FDA on Jul 03, 2014.

❖ Belinostat was originally discovered by TopoTarget and then developed by Spectrum, and its compound patent application was filed as PCT application by Prolifix in 2001.

❖ The compound patent will expire in 2021 foremost, which has been granted in the United States, Japan and Europe successively, but has not been filed in China yet.

Table 1　Belinostat's Compound Patent Protection in Drug-Mainstream Country

| Country | Publication/Patent NO. | Application Date | Granted Date | Estimated Expiry Date |
|---|---|---|---|---|
| WO | WO0230879A2 | 09/27/2001 | / | / |
| US | US6888027B2 | 09/27/2001 | 05/03/2005 | 09/27/2021 |
| EP | EP1328510B1 | 09/27/2001 | 11/20/2013 | 09/27/2021 |
| JP | JP4975941B2 | 09/27/2001 | 07/11/2012 | 09/27/2021 |
| CN | NA | / | / | / |

Table 2　Originator's International Patent Application List (Patent Family)

| Publication NO. | Title | Applicant/Assignee/Owner | Publication Date |
|---|---|---|---|
| **Technical Subjects** | **Active Ingredient (Free Base)'s Formula or Structure and Preparation** | | |
| WO0230879A2 | Carbamic acid compounds comprising a sulfonamide linkage as HDAC inhibitors | Prolifix | 04/18/2002 |
| **Technical Subjects** | **Formulation and Preparation** | | |
| WO2005105055A1 | Formulation comprising histone deacetylase inhibitors | TopoTarget | 11/10/2005 |
| WO2006120456A1 | Pharmaceutical formulations of HDAC inhibitors | TopoTarget | 11/16/2006 |
| **Technical Subjects** | **Indication or Methods for Medical Needs** | | |
| WO2005000282A2 | Using inhibitors of histone deacetylases for the suppression therapy of inherited disease predisposing conditions | TopoTarget | 01/06/2005 |
| WO2007112832A1 | Use of valproic acid for the topical treatment of mild to moderate acne vulgaris | TopoTarget | 10/11/2007 |
| WO2009109861A1 | Methods of treatment employing prolonged continuous infusion of belinostat | TopoTarget | 09/11/2009 |
| **Technical Subjects** | **Combination Including at Least Two Active Ingredients** | | |
| WO2006082428A2 | Combination therapies using HDAC inhibitors | TopoTarget | 08/10/2006 |
| WO2007054719A2 | Histone deacetylase (HDAC) inhibitors for the treatment of cancer | TopoTarget | 05/18/2007 |
| WO2007009539A2 | The use of inhibitors of histone deacetylases in combination with compounds acting as nsaid for the therapy of human diseases | TopoTarget | 01/25/2007 |
| WO2010081662A2 | Methods for identifying patients who will respond well to cancer treatment | TopoTarget | 07/22/2010 |
| WO2011112623A1 | Thioxanthone-based autophagy inhibitor therapies to treat cancer | Spectrum | 09/15/2011 |
| WO2014049549A1 | Combination therapy using belinostat and trabectedin | TopoTarget | 04/03/2014 |
| **Technical Subjects** | **Others** | | |
| WO2006082448A1 | Assays for agents with selective cytotoxicty to HDAC resistant cell lines | TopoTarget | 08/10/2006 |

The data was updated until Jan 2016.

# 3 Chemistry

## Route 1: Original Discovery Route

*Synthetic Route*: The reaction of benzaldehyde **1** with oleum gave 3-formylbenzenesulfonic acid sodium salt **2** after basic working up in 51% yield, which upon a Hornor-Wadsworth-Emmons reaction with trimethyl phosphonoacetate **3** gave rise to methyl acrylate **4** in 55% yield. The chloridization of **4** with thionyl chloride furnished the corresponding sulfonyl chloride **5** in 97% yield. The condensation of **5** with aniline took place prior to its subjection to hydrolysis under basic condition to form the corresponding acrylic acid **8**. After acid **8** was activated by oxalyl chloride, oximation was carried out in the presence of hydroxylamine hydrochloride under weak basic condition (*sat.* NaHCO₃) to finally achieve the target belinostat in 36% yield over two steps from acrylic acid **8**. The overall yield was 2%.[1, 2]

## Route 2

*Synthetic Route*: This alternative approach employed commercially available 3-nitrobenzaldehyde **1** and trimethyl phosphonoacetate **2** to prepare methyl acrylate **3** *via* a Hornor-Wadsworth-Emmons reaction, and followed by reduction of **3** using SnCl₂ in hot alcohol to produce the aniline **4** in excellent yield over two steps. Thereafter, diazotization of **4** with NaNO₂ in concentrated hydrochloride, followed by the immediate displacement of diazonium salt by SO₂ in the presence of CuCl provided the key intermediate methyl (2*E*)-3-(3-chlorosulfonylphenyl)prop-2-enoate, which underwent the amination with aniline **5** to generate sulfonamide **6** with the yield of 41% from ester **4**. Finally, the target belinostat was obtained from **6** *via* oximation in 84% yield and the overall yield of 33%.[3]

[1] Watkins, C. J.; Romero-Martin, M.-R.; Moore, K. G., et al. WO2002030879A2, **2002**.
[2] Watkins, C. J.; Romero-Martin, M.-R.; Moore, K. G., et al. US6888027B2, **2005**.
[3] Yang, L.; Xue, X.; Zhang, Y. *Synth. Commun.* **2010**, *40*, 2520-2524.

## Route 3

*Synthetic Route*: Firstly, commercially available 3-bromobenzenesulfonyl chloride **1** was reacted with aniline in the presence of DMAP to deliver sulfonamide **3**. Next, the aryl bromide **3** was subjected to a palladium acetate-catalyzed Heck reaction utilized ethyl acrylate **4** to give the cinnamate ester **5** in 69% yield over two steps, which upon immediately saponification and acidic workup furnished the corresponding acid **6** in 84% yield. Activation of this acid as the corresponding acid chloride took place prior to its subjection to hydroxylamine to form the hydroxamic acid which was then further recrystallized from an 8:1 ethanol:water mixture in the presence of catalytic sodium bicarbonate to finally furnish belinostat in 77% yield over two steps from acid **6**. The overall yield was 45%.[4]

## 4 Pharmacology

## Summary

Mechanism of Action

❖ Belinostat is a potent histone deacetylase (HDAC) inhibitor, which is able to increase the acetylation levels of histones, resulting in cell cycle arrest and/or apoptosis of cancer cells.

❖ HDACs are a family of enzymes that remove acetyl groups from the lysine residues in the *N*-terminal tails of core histone proteins in the nucleosome. The deacetylation of histones by HDACs results in a remodeling of the chromatin structures and affects the access of transcription factors to the chromatin for gene transcription, which is an ongoing process that is required for normal cell growth and differentiation.

❖ Inhibition of belinostat on HDACs 1-11:
  - Class I (HDAC 1, 2, 3): $EC_{50}$ = 30-125 nM.
  - Class II (HDAC 4, 5, 7, 9): $EC_{50}$ = 67-128 nM.
  - Class III (HDAC 6, 10): $EC_{50}$ = 31.3-82 nM.
  - Class IV (HDAC 11): $EC_{50}$ = 44.2 nM.

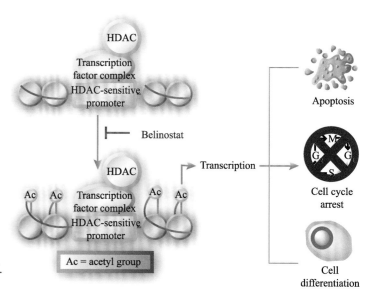

*In Vitro* Efficacy

❖ Belinostat inhibited cancer cell growth:
  - HeLa cells: $EC_{50}$ = 1.92 μM.
  - Bladder carcinoma cell lines: $IC_{50}$ = 1.0-10.0 μM.
❖ Growth-inhibitory activity of belinostat in multidrug resistant cell lines:
  - $IC_{50}$ = 0.345-3.78 μM.
  - Fold change (for $IC_{50}$ of parent cells): 0.92-2.4.

[4] Reisch, H. A.; Leeming, P.; Raje, P. S. WO2009040517A2, **2009**.

❖ Effect of belinostat on relative cell viability of normal and cancer cell lines:
  • Cancer cell viability:
    ♦ 12%-49% at 625 nM.
    ♦ 2%-40% at 2500 nM.
  • Normal cell viability:
    ♦ 28%-77% at 625 nM.
    ♦ 6%-36% at 2500 nM.
❖ *In vitro* pharmacodynamics on histones and cell cycles:
  • Reversibly increased acetylation of histones H3, H4 and acetylated alpha-tubulin.
  • Increased PARP cleavage.
  • Induced p21 expression.
❖ Effect of belinostat on cell cycle:
  • Tumor cells:
    ♦ Increased the proportion of cells in $SubG_1$, $G_2/M$ phase.
    ♦ Decreased the proportion of cells in $G_0/G_1$ and S-phase.
  • Normal cells:
    ♦ Resulted in less $SubG_1$ staining.
    ♦ Decreased in S-phase and $G_2/M$ populations.

*In Vivo* Efficacy

❖ In mouse ascites model:
  • H4 acetylation from 1 to 6 h was above the baseline.
❖ In human ovarian carcinoma xenograft mouse model:
  • No anti-tumor effect on QD dosing groups.
  • Tumor growth delayed in TID dosing groups.
❖ In transgenic mice model:
  • Reduced the weights of Ras-expressing bladders.
  • Decreased hematuria.

## Mechanism of Action

Table 3　*In Vitro* Effect on HDAC Activity by Belinostat and Other HDAC Inhibitors[5, 6]

| Inhibitor | rhHDAC $EC_{50}$ (nM) | | | | | | | | | | |
|---|---|---|---|---|---|---|---|---|---|---|---|
| | 1 | 2 | 3 | 4 | 5 | 6 | 7 | 8 | 9 | 10 | 11 |
| Belinostat | 41 ± 6 | 125 ± 21 | 30 ± 0 | 115 ± 16 | 76.3 | 82 ± 19 | 67 ± 22 | 216 ± 43 | 128 ± 46 | 31.3 | 44.2 |
| TSA | 2 ± 0 | 3 ± 0 | 4 ± 1 | 6 ± 2 | NA | 3 ± 1 | 5 ± 2 | 456 ± 59 | 6 ± 5 | NA | NA |
| NVP-LAQ824 | 5 ± 1 | 5 ± 1 | 12 ± 1 | 23 ± 18 | NA | 7 ± 3 | 18 ± 4 | 162 ± 44 | 6 ± 5 | NA | NA |
| Panobinostat | 3 ± 0 | 3 ± 0 | 4 ± 1 | 12 ± 5 | 7.8 | 61 ± 1 | 14 ± 7 | 248 ± 11 | 3 ± 2 | 2.3 | 2.7 |
| ITF2357 | 28 ± 8 | 56 ± 13 | 21 ± 3 | 52 ± 5 | NA | 27 ± 16 | 163 ± 8 | ND | ND | NA | NA |
| Vorinostat | 68 ± 14 | 164 ± 45 | 48 ± 17 | 101 ± 31 | 163 | 90 ± 26 | 104 ± 35 | 1524 ± 463 | 107 ± 21 | 88.4 | 109 |
| MS-275 | 181 ± 62 | 1155 ± 134 | 2311 ± 803 | >10000 | NA | >10000 | >10000 | >10000 | 505 ± 37 | NA | NA |
| MGCD0103 | 34 ± 17 | 34 ± 8 | 998 ± 431 | >10000 | 1889 | >10000 | >10000 | >10000 | ND | 54.9 | 104 |
| Apicidin | >10000 | 120 ± 28 | 43 ± 7 | >10000 | NA | >10000 | >10000 | 575 ± 111 | >10000 | NA | NA |
| VPA | 1584000 ± 302624 | 3068000 ± 0 | 3071000 ± 0 | ND | NA | >10000 | >10000 | 7442000 ± 2740000 | >10000 | NA | NA |

Belinostat inhibited HDACs 1, 2, 3, 4, 6, 7, 8 and 9 using recombinant human proteins at concentrations <250 nM.　Each compound was assayed in triplicate per plate. $EC_{50}$ values were determined from the average of a minimum of two plates.　Results were means ± S.E.M.

[5]  U.S. Food and Drug Administration (FDA) Database.　http://www.accessdata.fda.gov/drugsatfda_docs/nda/2014/206256Orig1s000PharmR.pdf (accessed Mar 2016).
[6]  Khan, N.; Jeffers, M.; Kumar, S., et al. *Biochem. J.* **2008**, *409*, 581-589.

## *In Vitro* Efficacy

Table 4    Inhibition of Cell Proliferation and Anchorage Independent Growth by Belinostat and the Major Human Metabolites[5]

| Metabolite | WST-1, IC$_{50}$ (nM) | Clonogenic Assay, IC$_{50}$ (nM) | | |
|---|---|---|---|---|
| | HeLa | HeLa | MCF-7 | HCT-116 |
| Belinostat | 700 | 400 | 1300 | 510 |
| Belinostat glucuronide (M18) | >100000 | 26000 | >300000 | 41000 |
| 3-ASBA (M24) | >100000 | >300000 | >300000 | >300000 |
| Belinostat amide (M21) | >100000 | 97000 | 148000 | 224000 |
| Belinostat acid (M26) | >90000 | >300000 | >300000 | >300000 |
| Methyl belinostat | ND | 105000 | 54000 | 199000 |

Three cell lines, HeLa, HCT-116 and MCF-7 were tested.    Cells were incubated with different concentrations of belinostat or metabolites for 48 h.    The number of viable cells was then assessed using the cell proliferation reagent WST-1.    The same three cell lines that were tested in the WST-1 assay were also tested in a clonogenic assay.

Table 5    Inhibition of Cell Proliferation by Belinostat[7]

| Cell Line | Cell Type | Inhibitor | EC$_{50}$ (µM) |
|---|---|---|---|
| HeLa | Cervical carcinoma | Belinostat | 1.92 ± 0.29 |
| 5637 | Bladder carcinoma | Belinostat | 1.0[a] |
| T24 | Bladder carcinoma | Belinostat | 10.0[a] |
| J82 | Bladder carcinoma | Belinostat | 3.5[a] |
| RT4 | Bladder carcinoma | Belinostat | 6.0[a] |

Each compound was assayed in triplicate per plate.    EC$_{50}$ values were determined from the averages of 3-min of two plates.    Results were means ± S.E.M.
[a] IC$_{50}$ value.

Table 6    Growth-Inhibitory Activity of Belinostat and Docetaxel on Multidrug Resistant Cell Lines[8]

| Cell Line | Cancer Type | Belinostat | | Docetaxel | |
|---|---|---|---|---|---|
| | | IC$_{50}$ (µM) | Fold Resistance | IC$_{50}$ (µM) | Fold Resistance |
| KB-3-1 | Cervical | 0.446 | 1 | 0.003 | 1 |
| KB-V1 | Drug-resistant variant | 1.07 | 2.4 | 0.513 | 171 |
| MES-SA | Uterine | 4.12 | 1 | 0.051 | 1 |
| MES-SA/Dx5 | Drug-resistant variant | 3.78 | 0.92 | 7.82 | 153 |
| NOMO-1 | Leukemia | 0.548 | 1 | 0.002 | 1 |
| NOMO-1/ADM | Drug-resistant variant | 0.655 | 1.2 | 0.472 | 236 |
| P388 | Leukemia | 0.183 | 1 | 0.003 | 1 |
| P388/ADR | Drug-resistant variant | 0.345 | 1.9 | 3.34 | 1113 |
| K562 | Leukemia | 1.12 | 1 | 0.064 | 1 |
| K562/ADM | Drug-resistant variant | 2.03 | 1.8 | 0.894 | 14 |

IC$_{50}$ values were extrapolated from growth curves obtained using the Cell Titer-Glo assay following 72 h of treatment with nine different concentrations of drug.    Fold resistance was calculated by dividing the IC$_{50}$ of the drug-resistant variant cell line by that of the corresponding parental cell line.

[5]  FDA Database.   http://www.accessdata.fda.gov/drugsatfda_docs/nda/2014/206256Orig1s000PharmR.pdf (accessed Mar 2016).
[7]  Buckley, M. T.; Yoon, J.; Yee, H., et al. *J. Transl. Med.* **2007**, *5*, 1-12.
[8]  Qian, X.; LaRochelle, W. J.; Ara, G., et al. *Mol. Cancer Ther.* **2006**, *5*, 2086-2095.

Table 7    Activity of Belinostat on Cell Viability of Normal and Cancer Cell Lines[5]

| Cell Line | Cell Type | Number of Viable Cells Relative to No-Drug Control (%) | |
| | | 625 nM | 2500 nM |
|---|---|---|---|
| SW-620 | Colon carcinoma | 48 | 5 |
| HCT-116 | Colon carcinoma | 18 | 8 |
| HT29 | Colon carcinoma | 44 | 2 |
| SK-MEL-2 | Melanoma | 12 | 6 |
| HeLa | Cervical carcinoma | 44 | 40 |
| BT-549 | Breast carcinoma | 49 | 8 |
| NHLF | Primary lung fibroblasts | 28 | 6 |
| HRE | Primary renal epithelial | 56 | 36 |
| APPE-19 | Retinal epithelial | 49 | 31 |
| CCD1070sk | Skin fibroblasts | 77 | 30 |

Cells were treated with 0.625 or 2.5 μM belinostat for 3 days, after which time the number of viable and dead cells in the total populations was determined by trypan-blue dye exclusion.

Table 8    *In Vitro* Pharmacodynamics of Belinostat on Histones and Some Proteins in Cells[5]

| Cell Type /Origin | Cell Line | Conc. & Dose | Incubation Time (h) | Test | Finding |
|---|---|---|---|---|---|
| Ovarian | A2780 | 1000 nM | 0, 0.5, 1, 2, 4, 6, 8, 12, 24, 36 | H3 acetylation | Increased. |
| | | | | H4 acetylation | Increased. |
| | A2780 | 1000 nM | 0, 0.5, 1 h and post-removed (0.5, 1, 2, 3, 4, 5, 6)[a] | H4 acetylation | Decreased in cell previously treated after incubation in drug free medium. |
| | OVCAR-3 | 0, 100, 1000 nM | 24 | Acetylation of α-tubulin | Dose-dependently increased. |
| Ovarian xeno-graft mice model[b] | PBMC | i.p., single dose: 40 mg/kg | 0, 1, 2, 3, 4 | H4 acetylation | Increased at 1 and 2 h, then returned to baseline levels by 3 h. |
| | PBMC | i.p., single dose: 0, 10, 20, 40 or 60 mg/kg | 2 | H4 acetylation | Dose-dependently increased. |
| | A2780 | i.p., 0, 10, 20, 40 or 60 mg/kg | 2 | H4 acetylation | Dose-dependently increased. |
| Human colon cancer[c] | HCT-116 | 0, 0.08, 0.16, 0.3, 0.6, 1.25, 2.5, 5 or 10 μM | 24 | PARP cleavage | A temporal and dose-dependent increase in PARP cleavage starting at 0.16 μM. |
| | | | | p21 expression | Induced expression of p21 starting at 0.08 μM. |
| | | | | H3 acetylation | Dose-dependently increased. |
| | | | | H4 acetylation | Dose-dependently increased. |
| | HCT-116 | 1 μM | 24 | PARP cleavage | Time-dependently increased in PARP cleavage starting at 24 h. |
| | | | | p21 expression | Time-dependent increased from 24 h. |

[a] Removed +: A2780 cells treated for 1 h with belinostat and then incubated in drug-free medium for various times.    [b] *In vivo* acetylation of histone H4 from peripheral blood mononuclear cells in mice with A2780 human tumor xenografts.    Histone H3, H4 and alpha-tubulin were determined by Western blot.    [c] HCT-116 was plated in 25-cm² flasks at sub-confluent density and allowed to establish for 48 h.    The cleavage of PARP, expression of p21 and acetylation of histones H3 and H4 were examined by immunoblot analysis.    PBMC: Peripheral blood mononuclear cells.

[5]  FDA Database.   http://www.accessdata.fda.gov/drugsatfda_docs/nda/2014/206256Orig1s000PharmR.pdf (accessed Mar 2016).

Table 9    Belinostat on Cell Cycle of Normal and Cancer Cell Lines[5, 9]

| Cell Type | Cell Line | Belinostat Conc. (nM) | Cell Cycle Distribution (%) | | | | | | | |
|---|---|---|---|---|---|---|---|---|---|---|
| | | | 24 h | | | | 48 h | | | |
| | | | SubG$_1$ | G$_0$/G$_1$ | S | G$_2$/M | SubG$_1$ | G$_0$/G$_1$ | S | G$_2$/M |
| Pancreatic carcinoma | MiaPaca-2 | 0 | 8 | 51 | 28 | 13 | 10 | 45 | 30 | 15 |
| | | 8000 | 73 | 4 | 0 | 23 | 38 | 10 | 0 | 52 |
| | BxPC-3 | 0 | 19 | 49 | 16 | 16 | 13 | 36 | 25 | 26 |
| | | 8000 | 57 | 11 | 0 | 32 | 31 | 20 | 0 | 49 |
| | Panc-1 | 0 | 19 | 36 | 28 | 17 | 10 | 38 | 29 | 23 |
| | | 8000 | 52 | 21 | 2 | 25 | 59 | 16 | 3 | 22 |
| Lung carcinoma | A549 | 0 | 2 | 36 | 46 | 16 | 14 | 37 | 31 | 18 |
| | | 8000 | ND | ND | ND | ND | 54 | 12 | 3 | 31 |
| | NCI-H460 | 0 | 3 | 39 | 42 | 16 | 11 | 43 | 31 | 15 |
| | | 8000 | 17 | 26 | 0 | 57 | 50 | 15 | 2 | 33 |
| | HCC827 | 0 | 24 | 22 | 32 | 22 | 11 | 40 | 31 | 18 |
| | | 8000 | 93 | 2 | 0 | 5 | 84 | 2 | 0 | 14 |
| Prostate carcinoma | PC-3 | 0 | 16 | 41 | 24 | 19 | 3 | 54 | 24 | 19 |
| | | 8000 | 13 | 31 | 1 | 55 | 22 | 30 | 1 | 47 |
| | DU145 | 0 | 3 | 42 | 24 | 19 | 3 | 54 | 24 | 19 |
| | | 8000 | 60 | 31 | 1 | 55 | 22 | 30 | 1 | 47 |
| | LNCaP | 0 | 31 | 54 | 12 | 3 | 22 | 51 | 19 | 8 |
| | | 8000 | ND | ND | ND | ND | 54 | 23 | 4 | 19 |
| Normal prostate | PREC | 0 | 5 | 70 | 13 | 12 | 7 | 65 | 16 | 12 |
| | | 8000 | 9 | 66 | 1 | 24 | 20 | 60 | 0 | 20 |

SubG$_1$: <2N DNA content.   G$_0$/G$_1$: 2N DNA content.   S-phase: 2N and 4N DNA content.   G$_2$/M: 4N DNA content.   Cells in SubG$_1$ were considered dead or dying. PREC and 9 tumor cells were seeded in 90 mm tissue culture dishes to sub-confluent density and allowed to attach overnight then exposed to 0.5, 2 or 8 µM belinostat. Cells were processed after 24 or 48 h of exposure using propidium iodide for staining and flow cytometry with Cell Quest DNA and Mod Fit LT cell cycle analysis software.   ND: Not done.

## *In Vivo* Efficacy

Table 10    *In Vivo* Effect of Belinostat in Mice Models[5, 7]

| Animal Model | | | | Administration | | Finding |
|---|---|---|---|---|---|---|
| Model | Animal | Cell | Test | Dose (mg/kg) | Route & Duration (Day) | |
| Mouse ascites model | B6D2F1 mouse | P388[a] | H4 histone acetylation | 80 | i.p. single dose on day 7 | H4 acetylation in ascites cells collected from 1 to 6 h was above the baseline. H4 acetylation began to decline after 4 h. Belinostat concentration in ascites fluid declined from approximately 800 µM to 0.5 µM. |
| Human ovarian carcinoma xenograft | NMRI mouse (female) | A2780[b] | Tumor volume | 0, 30, 60 | i.v., QD × 7 | No effect on anti-tumor growth in QD dosing groups. |
| | | | | 10, 20 | i.v., TID × 7 | Tumor delayed in the 10, 20 mg/kg TID groups. |
| Ha-*ras* transgenic model | Transgenic superficial bladder cancer mouse | NA | Bladder weights | 100 mg/kg | i.p., QD × 5, 2 days off, 3 cycles | Decreased the weights of Ras-expressing bladders 50% and 36% in of the male and female mice. Decreased hematuria. Well-tolerated. |

Mice received a single i.p. dose of 80 mg/kg belinostat on Day 7 and 3 mice/time points were sacrificed at 5, 15, 30 min and 1, 2, 4, 5, 6, 7 and 8 h.   Ascites fluid was collected from the abdominal cavity of these mice and centrifuged.   Belinostat concentration was measured in the ascites supernatants and H4 histone acetylation was evaluated in the cell pellet using immunoblotting.   [a] B6D2F1 mice were injected i.p. with 10$^6$ P388 mouse leukemia cells in 200 µL.   [b] NMRI mice were injected s.c. with 10$^7$ A2780 human ovarian cancer cells.

[5]  FDA Database.   http://www.accessdata.fda.gov/drugsatfda_docs/nda/2014/206256Orig1s000PharmR.pdf (accessed Mar 2016).
[7]  Buckley, M. T.; Yoon, J.; Yee, H., et al. *J. Transl. Med.* **2007**. *5*, 1397-1402.
[9]  Qian, X.; Ara, G.; Mills, E., et al. *Int. J. Cancer* **2008**, *122*, 1400-1410.

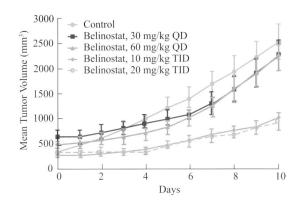

Figure A    Anti-tumor Activities of Belinostat in Human Ovarian Carcinoma Xenograft Models[5]

**Study:** Anti-tumor in A2780 human ovarian carcinoma xenograft mouse models.

**Animal:** Female NMRI mouse.

**Model:** Injected s.c. with $1 \times 10^7$ A2780 ovarian cancer cells into mice.

**Administration:** Treated 7 days, i.v., belinostat: 0, 30 or 60 mg/kg, QD for 7 or 10 days, 10 or 20 mg/kg, TID for 7 days; Vehicle control: NA.

**Starting**: Tumors were established.

**Test:** Measured by tumor volumes every day.

**Results**: Belinostat treated once daily for 7 days at 60 mg/kg did not exhibit an anti-tumor effect.    Because the half-life of belinostat in mice was <50 min, therefore the final tumor volumes were reduced after using 10 and 20 mg/kg, TID.

# 5    ADME & Drug-Drug Interaction

## Summary

### Absorption of Belinostat

❖ Exhibited a linear pharmacokinetics in humans following intravenous dosing.    The increases in $C_{max}$ and AUC appeared to be dose-proportional in the dose range of 150 to 1200 mg/m$^2$ belinostat.

❖ Showed a half-life ranging between 0.45-0.90 h in humans and 0.47-1.58 h in monkeys, after intravenous administrations.

❖ Had high system clearance in humans (58.9-132 L/h/m$^2$) and moderate to high in monkeys (258-677 mL/min/m$^2$), in contrast to liver blood flow, after intravenous administrations.

❖ Exhibited an extensive tissue distribution in humans and confined to extensive in monkeys, with apparent volumes of distribution at 43.4-114 L/m$^2$ and 0.20-1.26 L/kg, respectively, after intravenous administrations.

### Distribution of Belinostat

❖ Exhibited high plasma protein binding in humans (92.9%-95.8%).

❖ The mean $AUC_{inf}^{CSF}/AUC_{inf}^{freeplasma}$ was 9.6%, suggesting limited CSF penetration of belinostat.

### Metabolism of Belinostat

❖ UGT1A1 was the major metabolizing enzyme.    Besides, UGT1A3, UGT1A8, UGT2B4 and UGT2B7 were involved.

❖ M21 (belinostat amide) and M26 (belinostat acid) were formed by CYP2A6, 3A4 and 2C9.

❖ Overall, belinostat-GA represented the most abundant component in human plasma, and four others were identified as belinostat acid, belinostat amide, methyl belinostat and belinostat glucoside.

### Excretion of Belinostat

❖ Was predominantly excreted in feces in dogs.

### Drug-Drug Interaction

❖ Belinostat had no inhibition for CYP2C8 and weak for CYP2C9 ($IC_{50} = 61.8$ μM).

❖ Belinostat had induction for CYP1A2 of 1.2-2.3 folds at 1.5-15 μM.

❖ Belinostat was a substrate of P-gp, but had no inhibition for P-gp.

[5] FDA Database.    http://www.accessdata.fda.gov/drugsatfda_docs/nda/2014/206256Orig1s000PharmR.pdf (accessed Mar 2016).

## Absorption

Table 11  *In Vivo* Pharmacokinetic Parameters of Belinostat in Monkeys after Single Intravenous Dose of Belinostat[10]

| Dose (mg/kg) | AUC$_{inf}$ (ng·h/mL) | T$_{1/2}$ (h) | Cl (mL/min/m$^2$) | V$_{ss}$ (L/kg) | AUC$_{inf}^{CSF}$/AUC$_{inf}^{freeplasma}$ (%) |
|---|---|---|---|---|---|
| 10 | 13000 | 0.47 | 258 | 0.20 | - |
| 25 | 19200 | 1.23 | 435 | 0.31 | 9.8 |
| 35 | 43000 | 1.58 | 274 | 0.38 | 4.7 |
| 50 | 34700 | 0.89 | 481 | 1.11 | 6.3 |
| 60 | 27100 | 0.89 | 677 | 1.26 | 17.9 |

CSF: Cerebrospinal fluid.

Table 12  *In Vivo* Pharmacokinetic Parameters of Belinostat in Humans after Single Intravenous (30-min infusion) Dose of Belinostat on Day 1[11, 12]

| Dose (mg/m$^2$) | T$_{max}$ (h) | C$_{max}$ (ng/mL) | AUC$_{inf}$ (ng·h/mL) | AUC$_{0-t}$ (ng·h/mL) | T$_{1/2}$ (h) | Cl (L/h/m$^2$) | V$_z$ (L/m$^2$) |
|---|---|---|---|---|---|---|---|
| 150 | 0.02 ± 0.02 | 6010 ± 6235 | 1220 ± 1184 | 1212 ± 1177 | 0.45 ± 0.39 | 132 ± 135 | 90.0 ± 82.2 |
| 300 | 0.00 ± 0.00 | 14777 ± 4704 | 3422 ± 1276 | 3414 ± 1275 | 0.54 ± 0.09 | 99.4 ± 43.2 | 80.7 ± 47.0 |
| 600 | 0.00 ± 0.00 | 28611 ± 6425 | 11008 ± 3435 | 11002 ± 3434 | 0.52 ± 0.16 | 58.9 ± 18.4 | 43.4 ± 17.1 |
| 900 | 0.00 ± 0.00 | 46278 ± 17893 | 15181 ± 3748 | 15164 ± 3753 | 0.90 ± 0.32 | 62.3 ± 17.7 | 76.9 ± 16.5 |
| 1000 | 0.00 ± 0.00 | 32124 ± 9128 | 9990 ± 3420 | 9993 ± 3335 | 0.69 ± 0.22 | 110 ± 34.4 | 114 ± 60.9 |
| 1200 | 0.02 ± 0.04 | 53793 ± 11474 | 19240 ± 8895 | 19210 ± 8894 | 0.79 ± 0.25 | 73.4 ± 30.0 | 89.2 ± 58.2 |

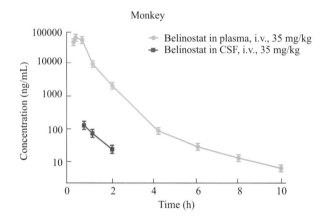

Figure B  *In Vivo* Plasma and CSF Concentration-Time Profiles in Monkeys after Single Intravenous (30-min infusion) Dose of Belinostat[10]

## Distribution

Table 13  *In Vitro* Plasma Protein Binding of Belinostat[13]

| Species | Conc. (ng/mL) | %Bound |
|---|---|---|
| Human | 500-2500 | 92.9-95.8 |

**Key Findings:**[10]

❖ The mean AUC$_{inf}^{CSF}$/AUC$_{inf}^{plasma}$ was 0.67% in monkeys receiving dose of 25 mg/kg and above.   Lumbar CSF belinostat concentration was extremely low in the animal that received 10 mg/kg belinostat.

❖ The mean AUC$_{inf}^{CSF}$/AUC$_{inf}^{freeplasma}$ was 9.6%, suggesting limited CSF penetration of belinostat.

[10]  Warren, K. E.; McCully, C.; Dvinge, H., et al. *Cancer Chemother. Pharmacol.* **2008**, *62*, 433-437.
[11]  FDA Database.   http://www.accessdata.fda.gov/drugsatfda_docs/nda/2014/206256Orig1s000ClinPharmR.pdf (accessed Mar 2016).
[12]  Steele, N. L.; Plumb, J. A.; Vidal, L., et al. *Clin. Cancer Ras.* **2008**, *14*, 804-810.
[13]  FDA Database.   http://www.accessdata.fda.gov/drugsatfda_docs/label/2014/206256lbl.pdf (accessed Mar 2016).

# Metabolism

Table 14    Enzyme Kinetic Parameters for the Glucuronidation of Belinostat in UGT1A1[14]

| UGT | $K_m$ (μM) | $V_{max}$ (pmoL/min/mg protein) | $Cl_{int}$ (μL/min/mg protein) |
|---|---|---|---|
| 1A1 | 99.6 | 353 | 3.5 |

**Key Findings:**[14]

❖ UGT1A1 glucuronidated belinostat significantly, whereas no metabolism was observed after incubation with UGT1A4, UGT1A6, UGT1A7, UGT1A9, UGT1A10, UGT2B15 and UGT2B17.

❖ Minor metabolism (less than 3%) was detected with UGT1A3, UGT1A8, UGT2B4 and UGT2B7.

❖ 73.6% and 89.4% of belinostat were converted to belinostat-GA after 2 h and 4 h of incubation with UGT1A1, respectively.

❖ M21 (belinostat amide) and M26 (belinostat acid) were formed by CYP2A6, 3A4 and 2C9.

Table 15    Metabolites in Plasma, Urine, Bile and Feces of Humans and Animal Species[5, 11, 14]

| Matrix | Species | Route | Dose (mg/m²) | Fold of Belinostat AUC or % of Dose | | | | | | | | | |
|---|---|---|---|---|---|---|---|---|---|---|---|---|---|
| | | | | M0 | M5 | M6 | M11 | M12 | M17 | M18 | M21 | M24 | M26 |
| Plasma | Rat | NA | NA | √ | - | √ | √ | √ | √ | √ | √ | √ | √ |
| | Human[a] | i.v. | 600 | 1 | - | - | - | - | - | 16.2 | 1.0 | 2.7 | 0.5 |
| Urine | Rat | NA | NA | √ | √ | - | √ | √ | √ | √ | √ | √ | √ |
| | Human[b] | i.v. | 1000 | 0.926 | - | - | - | - | - | 30.5 | 0.0929 | 4.61 | 0.925 |
| Bile | Rat | NA | NA | √ | √ | √ | √ | √ | √ | √ | - | √ | - |
| Feces | Rat | NA | NA | √ | - | √ | √ | √ | √ | √ | √ | √ | √ |

√ : Detected.    [a] Fold of belinostat AUC.    [b] % of dose.

**Key Findings:**[14]

❖ Five metabolites of belinostat were identified in human plasma.

❖ Glucuronidation was the most significant pathway of belinostat metabolism.

❖ Two alternate biotransformation pathways involved methylation to methyl belinostat and reduction of the hydroxamic group to its corresponding belinostat amide.

❖ Belinostat acid and belinostat glucoside were the another two minor metabolites detected.

[5]  FDA Database.  http://www.accessdata.fda.gov/drugsatfda_docs/nda/2014/206256Orig1s000PharmR.pdf (accessed Mar 2016).

[11]  FDA Database.  http://www.accessdata.fda.gov/drugsatfda_docs/nda/2014/206256Orig1s000ClinPharmR.pdf (accessed Mar 2016).

[14]  Wang, L. Z.; Ramirez, J.; Yeo, W., et al. *PLoS One* **2013**, *8*, e54522.

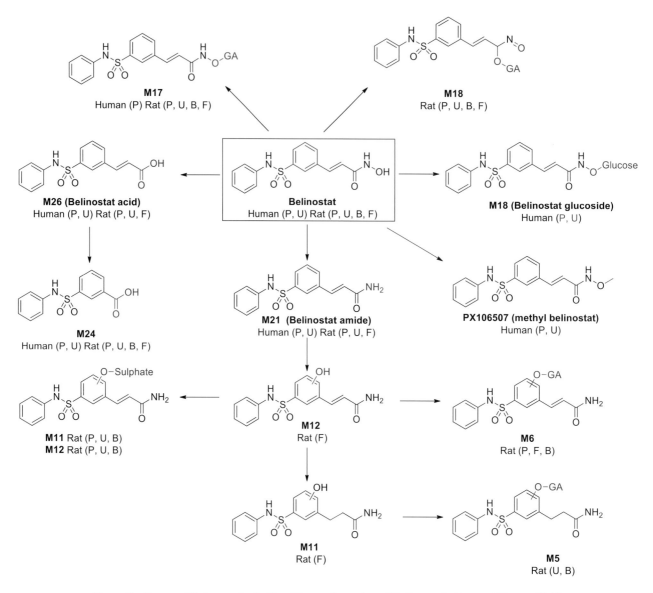

Figure C    Proposed Pathways for *In Vivo* Biotransformation of Belinostat in Rats and Humans[11, 14]

M18 was identified as a different structure in humans and rats above according to US FDA files.    The red labels represent the main components in the matrices.
P = Plasma, U = Urine, F = Feces, B = Bile and GA = Glucuronic acid.

[11]   FDA Database.   http://www.accessdata.fda.gov/drugsatfda_docs/nda/2014/206256Orig1s000ClinPharmR.pdf (accessed Mar 2016).
[14]   Wang, L. Z.; Ramirez, J.; Yeo, W., et al. *PLoS One* **2013**, *8*, e54522.

# Excretion

Table 16    Excretion Profiles of [$^{14}$C]Belinostat in Dogs after Single Dose of Belinostat[11]

| Route | Gender | Dose (mg) | Time (h) | Bile (% of dose) | Urine (% of dose) | Feces (% of dose) | Total Recovery (% of dose) |
|-------|--------|-----------|----------|------------------|-------------------|-------------------|----------------------------|
| i.v. | Male | 25 | 0-168 | - | 28.3 | 64.8 | 95.9 |
|      | Female | 25 | 0-168 | - | 31.7 | 62.6 | 96.0 |
| p.o. | Male | 50 | 0-168 | - | 21.7 | 71.9 | 96.1 |
|      | Female | 50 | 0-168 | - | 17.5 | 76.4 | 95.2 |

Total recovery included the radioactivity in cage wash, residual water and swabs.

# Drug-Drug Interaction

Table 17    *In Vitro* Evaluation of Belinostat and Metabolites as Inhibitors and Inducers of CYP Enzymes[11]

| Compound | As Inhibitors, IC$_{50}$ (μM) | | Conc. (μM) | As Inducers, Fold Induction |
|----------|--------|--------|------------|------------------------------|
|          | CYP2C8 | CYP2C9 |            | CYP1A2 |
| Belinostat | 100 | 61.8 | 1.5/15 | 1.2/2.3 |
| M18 | - | - | - | ND |
| M24 | 49.1 | - | - | ND |
| M21 | 30.8 | 44.4 | - | ND |
| M26 | 22.1 | - | - | ND |
| PX106507 | 13.8 | 11.5 | - | ND |

Table 18    *In Vitro* Evaluation of Belinostat as a Substrate and an Inhibitor of P-gp[11]

| Belinostat as a Substrate | | Belinostat as an Inhibitor |
|-----------------|--------------|----------------------------|
| Conc. (μM) | Efflux Ratio | |
| 2 | 3.11 ± 0.04 | |
| 10 | 2.76 ± 0.46 | No |
| 50 | 2.60 ± 0.50 | |

# 6    Non-Clinical Toxicology

## Summary

Single-Dose Toxicology
❖ Not reviewed.

Repeated-Dose Toxicity
❖ Repeated-dose toxicity studies by cyclic intravenous administration in rats (24 weeks) and dogs (4 weeks):
- Consistent targets of toxicity in rats and dogs: Heart (increased heart rate, cardiomyopathy and increased weight), hematopoietic/lymphocytic system (reduced RBCs and WBCs, atrophy of lymphoid tissues), GI tract (vomiting, liquid feces), male reproductive system (reduced weight of testes and epididymides, immature testes) and injection site reactions.
- No sex differences emerged, but accumulation was identified at HD.

Safety Pharmacology
❖ Both *in vitro* and *in vivo* safety pharmacology studies to assess the effects on nervous, cardiovascular and respiratory system:

[11] FDA Database.   http://www.accessdata.fda.gov/drugsatfda_docs/nda/2014/206256Orig1s000ClinPharmR.pdf (accessed Mar 2016).

- Cardiovascular toxicities included cardiomyopathy (rats) and increased heart weight and heart rate (dogs).
- There were no other findings of toxicity to the cardiovascular, respiratory or central nervous system.

### Genotoxicity

❖ Belinostat demonstrated genotoxicity in all the three assays employed, *in vitro* Ames and mouse lymphoma assay and *in vivo* mouse micronucleus assay.

### Reproductive and Developmental Toxicity

❖ Embryo-fetal development toxicology studies were not conducted since belinostat was genotoxic and cytotoxic towards rapidly dividing cells both *in vitro* and *in vivo* (peripheral blood lymphocytes and gut mucosal epithelium) and therefore, it was expected to cause teratogenicity and/or embryo-fetal lethality.

❖ Belinostat elicited toxicity towards male reproductive organs in dogs, including both delayed testicular maturation and exfoliated spermatid cells in the epididymis.

### Carcinogenicity

❖ Not conducted or needed for clinical indication.

### Special Toxicology

❖ No special toxicology studies had been performed.

## Repeated-Dose Toxicity

Table 19    Repeated-Dose Toxicity Studies of Belinostat by Oral (Gavage) Administration[5]

| Species | Duration (Week) | Dose (mg/kg/day) | Vehicle | Finding |
|---|---|---|---|---|
| Wistar rat | 28 | 10, 25, 100, BID | *L*-Arginine in water | 100 mg/kg/day: 40% mortality in male and 20% in female rats. Tail lesions observed in all early decedents. Bone marrow suppression at HD. Mean body weight and mean food consumption descended in all groups. Dose-proportional and significant ↓ ALT in males at all doses and in females at MD and HD, but no microscopic correlates. Widely observed urine with protein and blood at LD and MD and lower to absent at HD. Microscopically visible minimal thymus atrophies in 48% of male rats. |
| Beagle dog | 4 | 10, 25, 50, BID | 10% w/v ethanol, 15% v/v PEG200 in 0.1 M TRIS buffer (pH 8.5) | Atrophy of the lymphoid tissues, decreased cellularity in the bone marrow and reduced circulating lymphocyte and, possibly, neutrophil counts. Phlebitis and periphlebitis at the dose sites in most animals including controls. MTD approximately 50 mg/kg/day.    NOEL: 10 mg/kg/day. |

## Safety Pharmacology

Table 20    Safety Pharmacology Studies of Belinostat[5]

| Study | System | Dose | Finding |
|---|---|---|---|
| Cardiovascular effect | HEK293 cell expressing hERG channel | 8.4, 105.5, 270 μM | Inhibited hERG potassium current at the two highest concentrations used, but an $IC_{50}$ not reached. Shortened cardiac APD, suggesting mixed ion channel effects would inhibit depolarizing currents. |
| | Anaesthetized Beagle dog | 7, 15, 35 mg/kg/day, i.v. | Increased HR at HD. |
| | Isolated canine cardiac purkinje fibers | 0.01, 0.05, 0.1 mg/mL | Shortened cardiac APD. |
| Respiratory effect | Anaesthetized Beagle dog | 7, 15, 35 mg/kg/day, i.v. | Transient slight increase of respiration rate following 15 and 35 mg/kg administration, but not significantly different from vehicle controls. |
| Neurological effect | Male Wistar rat | 10, 25, 100 mg/kg, i.v. | No significant behavioral or physiological changes. |

Vehicle: 0.3% DMSO in HEPES buffer for *in vitro* studies, *L*-Arginine aqueous solution for *in vivo* studies.

---

[5]  FDA Database.   http://www.accessdata.fda.gov/drugsatfda_docs/nda/2014/206256Orig1s000PharmR.pdf (accessed Mar 2016).

# Genotoxicity

Table 21    Genotoxicity Studies of Belinostat[5]

| Assay | Species/System | Metabolism Activity | Dose | Finding |
| --- | --- | --- | --- | --- |
| *In vitro* reverse mutation assay in bacterial cells (Ames) | *S. typhimurium* TA98, TA100, TA1535, TA1537, TA102 | ±S9 | 78.125-5000 µg/plate<br>39.0625-1250 µg/plate | Positive. |
| *In vitro* assays in mammalian cells (MLA) | L5178Y t/k[+/-] | ±S9 | -S9: 0.05-0.725 µg/mL for 24 h;<br>+S9: 10-180 µg/mL for 3 h | Positive. |
| *In vivo* clastogenicity assay in rodents (Micronucleus assay) | Wistar rat | + | 130-520 mg/kg/day, i.v. for 2 days | Positive at a non-toxic dosage. Myelosuppression at HD. |

Vehicle: DMSO for *in vitro* studies, *L*-Arginine in water on a ratio of 2:1 belinostat by weight for *in vivo* studies.

[5]  FDA Database.   http://www.accessdata.fda.gov/drugsatfda_docs/nda/2014/206256Orig1s000PharmR.pdf (accessed Mar 2016).

# CHAPTER

7

## Ceritinib

# Ceritinib
## (Zykadia®)

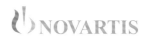

## 1  General Information

- ❖ Ceritinib is a kinase inhibitor, which was first approved in Apr 2014 by US FDA.

- ❖ Ceritinib was discovered by IRM, developed and marketed by Novartis.

- ❖ Ceritinib inhibited autophosphorylation of anaplastic lymphoma kinase (ALK) and ALK-mediated phosphorylation of the downstream signaling protein STAT3, resulting in anti-proliferation of ALK-dependent cancer cells.

- ❖ Ceritinib is indicated for the treatment of patients with ALK-positive metastatic non-small cell lung cancer (NSCLC) who have progressed on or are intolerant to crizotinib.

- ❖ Available as capsule, with each containing 150 mg ceritinib and the recommended dose is 750 mg once daily until disease progression or unacceptable toxicity.

- ❖ The 2014 and 2015 sales of Zykadia® were 31 and 79 million US$, respectively, referring to the financial reports of Novartis.

### Key Approvals around the World*

|  | US (FDA) | EU (EMA) | Japan (PMDA) |
|---|---|---|---|
| First approval date | 04/29/2014 | 05/06/2015 | 03/28/2016 |
| Application or approval No. | NDA 205755 | EMEA/H/C/003819 | 22800AMX00384000 |
| Brand name | Zykadia® | Zykadia® | Zykadia® |
| Indication | NSCLC | NSCLC | NSCLC |
| Authorisation holder | Novartis | Novartis | Novartis |

* Till Mar 2016, it had not been approved by CFDA (China).

## Active Ingredient

Molecular formula:  $C_{28}H_{36}N_5O_3ClS$
Molecular weight:  558.14
CAS No.:  1032900-25-6 (Ceritinib)
Chemical name:  5-Chloro-N4-{2-[(1-methylethyl) sulfonyl]phenyl}-N2-[5-methyl-2-(1-methylethoxy)-4-(4-piperidinyl)phenyl]-2,4-pyrimidine diamine

*Parameters of Lipinski's "Rule of 5"*

| MW | H_D | H_A | FRB^a | PSA^a | cLogP^a |
|---|---|---|---|---|---|
| 558.14 | 3 | 8 | 7 | 114Å² | 4.70 ± 0.95 |

ª Calculated by ACD/Labs software V11.02.

## Drug Product*

Dosage route:  Oral
Strength:  150 mg (Ceritinib)
Dosage form:  Capsule
Inactive ingredient:  Colloidal anhydrous silica, L-hydroxypropylcellulose, magnesium stearate, microcrystalline cellulose, sodium starch glycolate, gelatin, indiogotine and titanium dioxide.
Recommended dose: The recommended starting dose is 750 mg once daily without food (i.e., do not administer within 2 h of a meal).
Discontinue ceritinib for patients unable to tolerate 300 mg daily.
If a dose of ceritinib is missed, make up that dose unless the next dose is due within 12 h.

* Sourced from US FDA drug label information

# 2 Key Patents Information

## Summary

❖ Zykadia® (Ceritinib) has got five-year NCE market exclusivity protection and seven-year orphan drug exclusivity after it was initially approved by US FDA on Apr 29, 2014.

❖ Ceritinib was originally developed by IRM and then licensed to Novartis, and its compound patent application was filed as PCT application by IRM in 2007.

❖ The compound patent will expire in 2027 foremost, which has been granted in the United States, Japan and Europe successively.

Table 1    Ceritinib's Compound Patent Protection in Drug-Mainstream Country

| Country | Publication/Patent NO. | Application Date | Granted Date | Estimated Expiry Date |
|---|---|---|---|---|
| WO | WO2008073687A2 | 11/20/2007 | / | / |
| US | US8039479B2 | 11/20/2007 | 10/18/2011 | 06/29/2030[a] |
| EP | EP2091918B1 | 11/20/2007 | 08/27/2014 | 11/20/2027 |
| JP | JP5208123B2 | 11/20/2007 | 06/12/2013 | 11/20/2027 |
| CN | CN103641816A | 11/20/2007 | Examination | / |

[a] The term of this patent is extended by 952 days.

Table 2    Originator's International Patent Application List (Patent Family)

| Publication NO. | Title | Applicant/Assignee/Owner | Publication Date |
|---|---|---|---|
| **Technical Subjects** | **Active Ingredient (Free Base)'s Formula or Structure and Preparation** | | |
| WO2008073687A2 | Compounds and compositions as protein kinase inhibitors | IRM | 06/19/2008 |
| **Technical Subjects** | **Salt, Crystal, Polymorphic, Solvate (Hydrate), Isomer, Derivative Etc. and Preparation** | | |
| WO2012082972A1 | Crystalline forms of 5-chloro-N2-(2-isopropoxy-5-methyl-4-piperidin-4-yl-phenyl)-N4-[2-(propane-2-sulfonyl)-phenyl]-pyrimidine-2,4-diamine | Novartis | 06/21/2012 |
| **Technical Subjects** | **Indication or Methods for Medical Needs** | | |
| WO2012106540A1 | Methods of using ALK inhibitors | IRM | 08/09/2012 |
| **Technical Subjects** | **Combination Including at Least Two Active Ingredients** | | |
| WO2014074580A1 | Combination therapy | Novartis | 05/15/2014 |
| WO2014203152A1 | Pharmaceutical combinations | Novartis | 12/24/2014 |
| WO2015031666A1 | Combination of an ALK inhibitor and a CDK inhibitor for the treatment of cell proliferative diseases | IRM | 03/05/2015 |
| WO2015097622A1 | Pharmaceutical combinations | Novartis | 07/02/2015 |
| WO2015097621A2 | Pharmaceutical combinations | Novartis | 07/02/2015 |
| **Technical Subjects** | **Formulation and Preparation** | | |
| WO2015181739A1 | Ceritinib formulation | Novartis | 12/03/2015 |

The data was updated until Jan 2016.

# 3   Chemistry

## Route 1:   Original Discovery Route

SPhos: 2-Dicyclohexylphosphine-2',6'-dimethoxybiphenyl

*Synthetic Route*:   The critical step in the original synthesis of ceritinib involved a late-stage Buchwald-Hartwig coupling of two advanced intermediates, anilino piperidine **6** and arylsulfonyl chloro-pyrimidine **7**.   Concurrently, construction of anilino piperidine **6** commenced with 2-chloro-4-fluoro-1-methylbenzene **1**.   Nitration with $KNO_3/H_2SO_4$ and subsequent reaction with *i*-PrOH/$Cs_2CO_3$ at an elevated temperature provided the 5-isopropoxy-4-nitrobenzene intermediate **3** in 67% yield over two steps.   Palladium-catalyzed Suzuki coupling of **3** with 4-pyridine boronic acid **4** under microwave-enabled coupling conditions provided **5** in 73% yield, which was then subjected to platinum oxide-catalyzed hydrogenation conditions in the presence of acetic acid and trifluoroacetic acid, affording the corresponding piperidinyl aniline intermediate which underwent immediate Boc-protection of the crude aniline to provide the Buchwald-Hartwig coupling precursor **6** in 60% yield over two steps.   Next, the critical union of **6** and **7** *via* Buchwald-Hartwig coupling furnished the framework of ceritinib and this was followed by removal of the Boc group with TFA, and subsequent precipitation with 1M HCl to yield ceritinib as the HCl salt in 35% yield from **6**.

Besides, 2,5-dichloropyrimidine derivative **7** was prepared by condensation of 2-(isopropylsulfonyl)aniline **8** and 2,4,5-trichloro-pyrimidine **9** in 60% yield.   The overall yield concerning the whole process was about 6%.[1-3]

[1]   Marsilje, T. H.; Pei, W.; Chen, B., et al. *J. Med. Chem.* **2013**, *56*, 5675-5690.
[2]   Michellys, P. Y.; Pei, W.; Marsilje, T. H., et al. WO2008073687A2, **2008**.
[3]   Michellys, P. Y.; Pei, W.; Marsilje, T. H., et al. US20080176881A1, **2008**.

## Route 2

*Synthetic Route:* This synthetic route as reported was initiated with hydrogenation on the key intermediate 4-(5-isopropoxy-2-methyl-4-nitrophenyl)pyridine **1**, which was identical to the sequence referred to route 1, leading to piperidine derivative **2** in 92% yield. Sandmeyer reaction of amine **2** was carried out in standard conditions (NaNO₂/CuBr/HBr) to give bromobenzene derivative **3** in 83% yield. Buckward-Hartwig coupling of **3** with 5-chloro-4-nitropyrimidin-2-amine **4** yielded the desired *N*-phenylpyrimidin-2-amine **5** in 78% yield, within which nitro group was hydrogenated and allowed for the resultant amine to couple with 1-bromo-2-(isopropylsulfonyl)benzene **7** achieving the target ceritinib in 75% yield over two steps and the overall yield of 44%.[4]

## 4    Pharmacology

## Summary

### Mechanism of Action

❖ As an ALK kinase inhibitor, ceritinib was approximately 50-fold more specific for ALK (IC$_{50}$ = 0.15 nM) than insulin receptor (InsR, IC$_{50}$ = 7 nM) and insulin-like growth factor 1 receptor (IGF-1R, IC$_{50}$ = 8 nM), and other members of the insulin receptor superfamily.

❖ Ceritinib inhibited autophosphorylation of ALK, ALK-mediated phosphorylation of the down-stream signaling protein STAT3, and the proliferation of ALK-dependent cancer cells.

❖ Ceritinib showed no significant off-target activities in off-target assays in a 42-target receptor panel, a 84-broad spectrum screen receptor panel, and a 10-GPCR panel, except MC₄ (IC$_{50}$ = 0.6 μM), rabbit vesicular monoamine transporter (VMAT2, 97% inhibition at 10 μM, IC$_{50}$ = 0.331 μM), rat K⁺ channel (99% inhibition at 10 μM, IC$_{50}$ = 0.68 μM) and dopamine 2 receptor (IC$_{50}$ = 1.2 μM).

### *In Vitro* Efficacy

❖ Phosphorylation of ceritinib in Karpas299 cells:
  • ALK protein: IC$_{50}$ = 46 nM.
  • STAT3 protein: IC$_{50}$ = 150 nM.

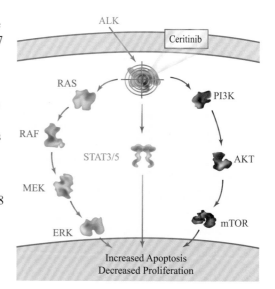

[4]  Xuenong, X. CN103992262A, **2014**.

❖ Anti-proliferative activity in tumor cells:
- Ba/F3 cells containing ALK fusion protein: $IC_{50}$ = 26-56 nM.
- Ba/F3 cells containing EMLA-ALK mutation: $IC_{50}$ = 37.6-940 nM.
- Ba/F3 cells containing other fusion proteins: $IC_{50}$ = 180-400 nM.
- Human NSCLC cell lines: $IC_{50}$ = 3.8-14.6 nM.
- Other human cell lines containing wild type and fusion ALK: $IC_{50}$ = 24-45 nM.
- Cells from crizotinib-resistant patients with ALK mutation: $IC_{50}$ = 25-230 nM.
- Cells from crizotinib-resistant patients without ALK mutation: $IC_{50}$ = 2.6 nM.
- JFCR013-2 cells (from ceritinib-resistant patient): $IC_{50}$ = 192 nM.

*In Vivo* Efficacy

❖ H2228 cells xenograft models:
- In SCID mouse:
  - Tumor growth inhibition: 41% T/C at 3.125 mg/kg.
  - Complete tumor regression at 25 mg/kg after 14 days treatment.
- In nude rat:
  - Tumor growth inhibition 2% T/C at 10 mg/kg.
  - Complete tumor regression at 25 mg/kg.
❖ Crizotinib-resistant H2228 cells carrying the ALK-mutation xenograft model in SCID mouse:
- Non-ALK-mutation:
  - Tumor growth inhibition: T/C% = -15.97% at 50 mg/kg and complete tumor regression at 100 mg/kg.
- I1171T ALK-mutation:
  - Tumor growth inhibition T/C% = 44% at 25 mg/kg and complete tumor regression at 50 mg/kg.
- C1156Y ALK-mutation:
  - Tumor growth inhibition T/C% = 11.7% at 50 mg/kg and complete tumor regression at 100 mg/kg.
❖ Karpas299 cells xenograft models:
- In SCID mouse:
  - Tumor growth inhibition T/C% = 18% at 12.5 mg/kg.
  - Significant tumor regression at 25 mg/kg after 14 days treatment.
- In nude rat:
  - Tumor growth inhibition T/C% = 30% at 12.5 mg/kg.
  - Significant tumor regression at 25 mg/kg after 14 days treatment.

# Mechanism of Action

Table 3　*In Vitro* Inhibition of Ceritinib and Crizotinib on Human Protein Kinases[5, 6]

| Kinase | Type | $IC_{50}$ (nM) | | Kinase | Type | $IC_{50}$ (nM) | |
| --- | --- | --- | --- | --- | --- | --- | --- |
| | | Ceritinib | Crizotinib | | | Ceritinib | Crizotinib |
| EML4-ALK | Y[a] | 31 | 160 | EML4-ALK L1196M | Y | 69 | 1460 |
| EML4-ALK C1156Y | Y | 160 | 440 | EML4-ALK G1202R | Y | 940 | 1370 |
| EPK CE ALK (1066-1459) | Y | 0.15 | 3 | EPK ROCK2 | S/T | 450 | 2500 |
| EPK CE IGF-1R (980-1369) | Y | 8 | 400 | EPK EPHB4 (566-987) | Y | 2600 | 150 |
| EPK CE INSR (871-1343) | Y | 7 | 290 | EPK LCK | Y | 600 | 80 |
| EPK AURORA_A | S/T[b] | 110 | 60 | EPK MET (956-1390) | Y | 3200 | 8 |
| EPK cABLT315 | Y | 130 | 6 | EPK JAK2 | Y | 600 | 60 |
| EPK CE AXL (515-885) | Y | 180 | 13 | EPK CE FGFR3 (411-K650E-806) | Y | 430 | 1700 |
| EPK CE RET (658-1072) | Y | 400 | 2200 | | | | |

The applicant evaluated the selectivity of ceritinib and crizotinib by testing its *in vitro* activity against 36 recombinant human protein kinases using the caliper mobility shift assay, table 3 showed the potency kinases for ceritinib ($IC_{50}$ <500 nM) and crizotinib ($IC_{50}$ <200 nM). [a] Y: Tyrosine-specific protein kinases. [b] S/T: Serine/Threonine-specific protein kinases.

[5] U.S. Food and Drug Administration (FDA) Database. http://www.accessdata.fda.gov/drugsatfda_docs/nda/2014/205755Orig1s000PharmR.pdf (accessed Mar 2016).
[6] European Medicines Agency (EMA) Database. http://www.ema.europa.eu/docs/en_GB/document_library/EPAR_-_Public_assessment_report/human/003819/WC500187506.pdf (accessed Mar 2016).

Table 4    *In Vitro* Off-Target Activity of Ceritinib[5, 6]

| Target Receptor[a] | | | Broad Spectrum Receptor[b] | | | | |
|---|---|---|---|---|---|---|---|
| Receptor | IC$_{50}$ (nM) | Functional IC$_{50}$ (nM) or %Inhibition | Target | Species | Conc. (µM) | %Inhibition | Binding IC$_{50}$ (nM) |
| H$_2$ receptor | 170 | NA | Transporter monoamine | Rabbit | 10 | 97 | 331 |
| Opk receptor | 570 | NA | K$^+$ channel [K$_A$] | Rat | 10 | 99 | 682 |
| MC$_3$ receptor | 670 | NA | Somatostatin sst1 | Human | 10 | 88 | 2420 |
| MC$_4$ receptor | 600 | 35% at 10 µM | Somatostatin sst2 | Human | 10 | 93 | 2250 |
| Ad$_3$ receptor | 730 | 8300 | Somatostatin sst3 | Human | 10 | 76 | 5120 |
| NK$_1$ receptor | 990 | 79% at 30 µM | Somatostatin sst4 | Human | 10 | 90 | 1880 |
| D$_2$ receptor | 1200 | NA | 5-HT$_{5A}$ | Human | 10 | 71 | 5000 |

The off-target activity of ceritinib was evaluated using an *in vitro* safety pharmacology profiling panel including 139 G protein-coupled receptors (GPCRs), ion channels, nuclear receptors, transporters, and enzymes that had been previously linked to potential side effects.    The agonist and antagonist activities of ceritinib were evaluated for 10 GPCRs using a safety pharmacology screen.    A fluorometric imaging plate reader (FLIPR) assay was conducted with a four-fold, eight-point serial dilution of ceritinib up to 10 µM to assess agonist and antagonist activity.    Ceritinib showed weak agonist activity on the dopamine D$_2$ receptor (EC$_{50}$ = 6 µM, IC$_{50}$ = 4 µM), but did not exhibit significant activity against the other GPCRs tested.    [a] Ceritinib interacted with 42 target receptors, table 4 showed the target receptors with IC$_{50}$ <1500 nM.    [b] A safety pharmacology broad spectrum screen with 84 receptors at ceritinib was tested at 10 µM in duplicate, table 4 showed the broad spectrum receptors with >70% inhibition at 10 µM.

## *In Vitro* Efficacy

Table 5    *In Vitro* Anti-Proliferation and Phosphorylation of Ceritinib[5-8]

| Study | Cell Line | Type/Origin | Fusion/Protein/ Mutant Point | IC$_{50}$ (nM) | |
|---|---|---|---|---|---|
| | | | | Ceritinib | Crizotinib |
| ALK enzymatic assay | NA | NA | NA | 0.15 | 3 |
| Endogenous phosphorylation | Karpas299 | Human ALCL | ALK protein | 46 | NA |
| | | | STAT3 protein | 150 | NA |
| Anti-proliferative activity | Ba/F3 | Murine pro-B lymphoma cell with ALK fusion kinase | NPM-ALK | 26, 35[a] | NA |
| | | | TEL-ALK-Q1 | 56 | NA |
| | | | EML4-ALK | 27, 31[a] | 160 |
| | | Murine pro-B lymphoma cell with ALK-mutation | EML4-ALK I1171T | 37.6 | 440 |
| | | | EML4-ALK L1196M | 69 | 1460 |
| | | | EML4-ALK G1202R | 940 | 1370 |
| | | | EML4-ALK C1156 | 160 | 440 |
| | | | EML4-ALK S1206A | 160 | 270 |
| | | | EML4-ALK G1269S | 250 | 2140 |
| | | Murine pro-B lymphoma cell with tyrosine kinase | TEL-ROS1 | 180 | NA |
| | | | TEL-IGF-1R | 220 | NA |
| | | | TEL-InsR | 400 | NA |
| | Karpas299 | Human ALCL | NPM-ALK | 45 (n = 8) | NA |
| | NB-1 | Human neuroblastoma cell | ALK | 24 (n = 3) | NA |
| | NCI-H2228 | Human NSCLC | Wild type | 3.8 | 107 |
| | | | EML4-ALK | 11 (n = 5) | NA |

[5]  FDA Database.  http://www.accessdata.fda.gov/drugsatfda_docs/nda/2014/205755Orig1s000PharmR.pdf (accessed Mar 2016).
[6]  EMA Database.  http://www.ema.europa.eu/docs/en_GB/document_library/EPAR_-_Public_assessment_report/human/003819/WC500187506.pdf (accessed Mar 2016).
[7]  Katayame, R.; Sakashita, T.; Yanagitani, N., et al. *EBioMedicine* **2016**, *3*, 54-66.
[8]  Friboulet, L.; Li, N.; Katayama, R., et al. *Cancer Discov.* **2014**, *4*, 662-673.

*Continued*

| Study | Cell Line | Type/Origin | Fusion/Protein/Mutant Point | IC$_{50}$ (nM) | |
| | | | | Ceritinib | Crizotinib |
|---|---|---|---|---|---|
| Anti-proliferative activity | H3122 | Human NSCLC | Wild type | 6.3, 14.6[a] | 245, 69.7[a] |
| | H3122 CR1 | Crizotinib resistant NSCLC | L1196M | 230 | 2884 |
| | MGH021-4 | Crizotinib resistant patient | ALK-rearranged/G1269A | 80 | 500 |
| | MGH045 | Crizotinib resistant patient | ALK-rearranged/L1196M | 25 | 891 |
| | MGH051 | Crizotinib resistant patient | No ALK resistance mutations | 2.6 | 62 |
| | JFCR013-02 | Ceritinib resistant patient | Wild Type | 192 | 704 |

The cell viability following 48 h of treatment with control compounds or ceritinib serially diluted with DMSO was determined using the Bright-Glo™ luciferase bioluminescent assay and cell proliferation was measured using the Brite Lite™ luciferase assay.   ALCL: Anaplastic large-cell lymphoma.   NSCLC: Non-small cell lung cancer.   NA: Not available.   [a] Two independent experiments.

## *In Vivo* Efficacy

Table 6   *In Vivo* Efficacy of Ceritinib in Different Xenograft Models[5, 6]

| Xenograft System | | | | Dose (mg/kg/day, p.o.) | Duration (Day) | Effect | |
| Cell Line | Type | Animal | ALK-Mutation | | | T/C (%) | Finding |
|---|---|---|---|---|---|---|---|
| H2228 | Human NSCLC | SCID mouse (female) | Wild type | 3.125 | QD × 14 | 41 | Complete tumor regression at 25 mg/kg/day after 14 days administration. |
| | | | | 6.25 | QD × 14 | 36 | |
| | | | | 12.5 | QD × 14 | -64 | |
| | | | | 25 | QD × 14 | -100 | |
| | | RNU nude rat (female) | Wild type | 5 | QD × 14 | 67 | Complete tumor regression at 25 mg/kg/day after 14 days administration. |
| | | | | 10 | QD × 14 | 2 | |
| | | | | 25 | QD × 14 | -100 | |
| Crizotinib resistant H2228 | Human NSCLC | SCID mouse (female) | Wild type | 25 | QD × 22 | 67.2 | Complete tumor regression at 100 mg/kg/day after 22 days administration. |
| | | | | 50 | QD × 147 | -16.0 | |
| | | | | 100 | QD × 147 | -100 | |
| | | | I1171T ALK-mutation | 12.5 | QD × 14 | 78 | Complete tumor regression at 50 mg/kg/day after 14 days administration. |
| | | | | 25 | QD × 14 | 44 | |
| | | | | 50 | QD × 14 | -100 | |
| | | | C1156Y ALK-mutation | 25 | QD × 12 | 61.8 | Complete tumor regression at 100 mg/kg/day after 12 days administration. |
| | | | | 50 | QD × 12 | 11.7 | |
| | | | | 100 | QD × 12 | -100 | |
| Karpas299 | Human ALCL | SCID mouse (female) | Wild type | 6.25 | QD × 14 | 62 | Significant tumor regression at 25 mg/kg after 14 days administration. |
| | | | | 12.5 | QD × 14 | 18 | |
| | | | | 25 | QD × 14 | -93 | |
| | | RNU nude rat (female) | Wild type | 6.25 | QD × 14 | 74 | Significant tumor regression at 25 mg/kg/day after 14 days administration. |
| | | | | 12.5 | QD × 14 | 30 | |
| | | | | 25 | QD × 14 | -33 | |
| | | | | 50 | QD × 14 | -66 | |

NSCLC: Non-small cell lung cancer.   ALCL: Anaplastic large-cell lymphoma.   SCID: Severe combined immunodeficient.

[5]  FDA Database.   http://www.accessdata.fda.gov/drugsatfda_docs/nda/2014/205755Orig1s000PharmR.pdf (accessed Mar 2016).
[6]  EMA Database.   http://www.ema.europa.eu/docs/en_GB/document_library/EPAR_-_Public_assessment_report/human/003819/WC500187506.pdf (accessed Mar 2016).

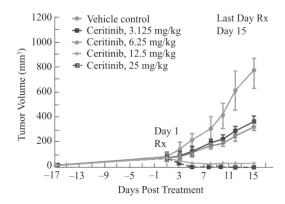

**Study:** Anti-tumor activities in H2228 NSCLC xenograft models.

**Animal:** SCID beige mouse (female, n = 4/group).

**Model:** 2-3 pieces of 1-2 $mm^3$ stock H2228 tumor were subcutaneously implanted into the right flank of SCID beige mice in the matrigel mixture.

**Administration:** Ceritinib: 3.125, 6.25, 12.5 and 25 mg/kg/day, p.o. for 14 days; Vehicle control: 0.5% methylcellulose (MC)/0.5% Tween 80.

**Starting:** Tumors were established (~85 $mm^3$).

**Test:** Measured tumor volumes, 3 times per week.

**Result:** Treatment with 25 mg/kg ceritinib resulted in complete tumor regression after 14 days.

Figure A    Anti-tumor Activities of Ceritinib in Human NSCLC H2228 cell Xenograft Model in SCID Mice[5]

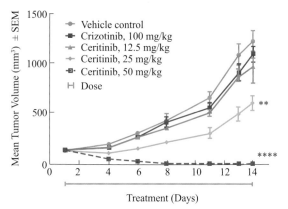

**Study:** Anti-tumor activities in crizotinib-resistant ALK I1171T mutant H2228 cells xenograft models.

**Animal:** SCID beige mouse (female, n = 6/group).

**Model:** Mice were subcutaneously implanted 2-3 pieces of frozen tumor with matrigel.

**Administration:** Ceritinib: 12.5, 25 and 50 mg/kg/day, p.o. for 14 days; Crizotinib: 100 mg/kg/day, p.o. for 14 days.   Vehicle control: 0.5% MC/0.5% Tween 80.

**Starting:** Mice bearing established tumors (mean ~130 $mm^3$).

**Test:** Measured tumor volumes, 3 times per week.

**Result:** Treatment with 50 mg/kg ceritinib resulted in complete tumor regression after 14 days of treatment.   (** $P \leq 0.05$; **** $P \leq 0.0001$).

Figure B    Anti-tumor Activities of Ceritinib in Crizotinib-Resistant with ALK I1171T Mutations Human H2228 NSCLC Xenografts in SCID Mouse Models[5]

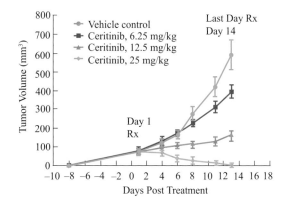

**Study:** Anti-tumor activities in Karpas299 ALCL xenograft models.

**Animal:** SCID beige mouse (female, n = 4/group).

**Model:** 2-3 pieces of 1-2 $mm^3$ stock Karpas299 tumor were subcutaneously implanted into the right flank of SCID beige mice in the matrigel mixture.

**Administration:** Ceritinib: 6.25, 12.5 and 25 mg/kg/day, p.o. for 14 days; Vehicle control: 0.5% MC/0.5% Tween 80.

**Starting:** Mice bearing established tumors (mean ~74 $mm^3$).

**Test:** Measured tumor volumes, 3 times per week.

**Result:** Treatment with 25 mg/kg ceritinib resulted in a significant tumor regression after 14 days of treatment.

Figure C    Anti-tumor Activities of Ceritinib in Human Karpas299 ALCL Xenografts in SCID Mouse Models[5]

[5] FDA Database.   http://www.accessdata.fda.gov/drugsatfda_docs/nda/2014/205755Orig1s000PharmR.pdf (accessed Mar 2016).

# 5   ADME & Drug-Drug Interaction

## Summary

### Absorption of Ceritinib

❖ Exhibited a non-linear pharmacokinetics in humans after oral administrations.   The increase in AUC appeared to be greater than dose-proportional in the dose range of 50 to 750 mg ceritinib.

❖ Had moderate bioavailability in rats (48.3%), but high in mice (54.6%) and monkeys (58%).

❖ Was absorbed slowly ($T_{max}$ = 3.98-15 h) in humans, mice (7 h), rats (12 h) and monkeys (13-18.3 h).

❖ Showed a half-life ranging between 19.4-40.6 h in humans, much longer than those in rats (13.2 h) and monkeys (12.1-16 h), after oral administrations.

❖ Had moderate system clearance in mice (26.6 mL/min/kg), rats (1.49 L/h/kg), but low to moderate in monkeys (0.366-0.78 L/h/kg), in contrast to liver blood flow, after intravenous administrations.   The Cl/F in humans was 44.5-147 L/h after oral administration.

❖ Exhibited an extensive distribution in mice, rats and monkeys, with apparent volumes of distribution at 9.7, 19.9 and 6.53-13.5 L/kg, respectively, after intravenous administrations.   The $V_z$/F in humans was 1880-6230 L after oral administration.

❖ Was classified as a low passive permeability compound.

### Distribution of Ceritinib

❖ Exhibited high plasma protein binding in rats (97.9%-98.4%), dogs (98.3%-98.8%), monkeys (94.4%-95.2%) and humans (96.7%-98.8%).   Note that ceritinib was mainly bound to HSA.

❖ The binding to RBC was 56.9%-58.6% in humans, indicating the drug was distributed more to blood cells than to plasma.

❖ In Long-Evans rats after oral and intravenous administrations:
  • The drug was widely distributed into most tissues including central nervous system with a lower degree compared to other tissues.
  • Relatively higher concentration levels were observed in intestinal wall, uveal tract, pituitary gland, bile, adrenal cortex, harderian gland, liver, spleen, lymph node, lungs, kidneys, thyroid, bone marrow, adrenal medulla, pancreas, thymus and salivary gland.   The concentration in tissues was generally higher than blood concentration.
  • The radioactivity concentration in the uveal tract was 176 times of that in blood, suggesting a high affinity for melanin-rich tissues.
  • Ceritinib-derived radioactivity was retained in several other tissues (including testes epididymis and skin) and the elimination was not yet completed at 168 h post-dose.

### Metabolism of Ceritinib

❖ Could be slightly metabolized in rat, monkey and human hepatocytes.

❖ CYP3A was the major metabolizing enzyme, with CYP2C19, 1A2, 2C8, 2D6 and 2C9 involved in the metabolism of ceritinib.

❖ The metabolism of ceritinib included mono-oxygenation, *O*-dealkylation, *S*-dealkylation and *N*-formylation of ceritinib. Secondary biotransformation pathways involving the primary biotransformation products included glucuronidation, dehydrogenation and the addition of a thiol group to *O*-dealkylation ceritinib.

❖ Overall, the parent drug was the most abundant component in plasma in humans.   Eleven metabolites were found in the human plasma, each at levels ≤2.3% of the total drug-related AUC.

❖ Five of these eleven metabolites were not detected in rat or monkey plasma.   The remaining three unique human metabolites detected at low levels in plasma included M46.6 (1.7%), M48.8 (1.7%) and M52.0 (2%).

### Excretion of Ceritinib

❖ Was predominantly excreted in feces in rats, monkeys and humans, with the parent drug as the significant component in rat, monkey and human feces.

❖ About 24.3% and 65.4% of ceritinib were recovered via biliary excretion in bile duct-cannulated (BDC) rats after oral and intravenous administration, respectively.

### Drug-Drug Interaction

❖ Ceritinib was a strong inhibitor of CYP3A4/5 ($IC_{50}$ = 0.2 μM), moderate of CYP2A6 ($IC_{50}$ = 5 μM), CYP2B6 ($IC_{50}$ = 2 μM), CYP2C8 ($IC_{50}$ = 2 μM, amodiaquine as substrate) and CYP2C9 ($IC_{50}$ = 2 μM), but weak of CYP2C19 ($IC_{50}$ = 70 μM), CYP2D6 ($IC_{50}$ = 20 μM), CYP2E1 ($IC_{50}$ = 30 μM) and CYP2C8 ($IC_{50}$ = 25 μM, paclitaxel as substrate).

❖ Ceritinib had no induction for CYP1A2, CYP2B6 or CYP2C9 mRNA/activities, but had concentration-dependent induction for CYP3A4 mRNA.

❖ Ceritinib was a substrate of P-gp and BCRP, but had no inhibition for them.

❖ Ceritinib was not a substrate of OCT1, OAT2, OATP1B1 or OATP2B1, had weak inhibition for OATP1B1, OATP1B3, OAT1 and OCT2, with $IC_{50}$ >5 μM, but had no inhibition for OCT1 or OAT3.

# Absorption

Table 7    *In Vivo* Pharmacokinetic Parameters of Ceritinib in Mice, Rats and Monkeys after Single Intravenous and Oral Dose of Certinib[5]

| Species | Route | Dose (mg/kg) | $T_{max}$ (h) | $C_{max}$ (ng/mL) | $AUC_{inf}$ (ng·h/mL) | $AUC_{last}$ (ng·h/mL) | $T_{1/2}$ (h) | Cl (L/h/kg) | $V_{ss}$ (L/kg) | F (%) |
|---|---|---|---|---|---|---|---|---|---|---|
| Balb/c mouse (male) | i.v. | 5 | - | 1753 ± 509 nM | 5634 ± 441 nM·h | 5366 ± 379 nM·h[a] | 6.2 ± 0.5 | 26.6 ± 2.2 mL/min/kg | 9.7 ± 0.6 | - |
| | p.o. | 20 | 7.0 ± 0.0 | 695 ± 31 nM | 12296 ± 981 nM·h | 10334 ± 963 nM·h[a] | - | - | - | 54.6 |
| Han Wistar rat (male) | i.v. | 10 | 0.083 ± 0 | 975 ± 139 | 6950 ± 1470 | 6890 ± 1510 | 9.7 ± 1.2 | 1.49 ± 0.342 | 19.9 ± 0.49 | - |
| | p.o. | 25 | 12.0 | 363 | 8390 | 8330 | 13.2 | NA | NA | 48.3 |
| Cynomolgus monkey (male) | i.v. | 5 | 0.083 | 1410 | 6530 | 6450 | 29 | 0.78 | 13.5 | - |
| | i.v. | 10 | 0.083[b] | 3190 | 27800 | 27400 | 14.5 | 0.366 | 6.53 | - |
| | p.o. | 30 | 18.3 ± 9.8 | 881 ± 12 | 35800 ± 3460 | 35500 ± 3520 | 12.1 ± 2.0 | - | - | 43.0 |
| | p.o. | 60 | 13 ± 9.2 | 947 ± 140 | 45300 ± 8860 | 45100 ± 8840 | 16 ± 0.61 | - | - | 58 |

[a] $AUC_{0-24}$.   [b] First sampling time point.

Table 8    *In Vivo* Pharmacokinetic Parameters of Ceritinib in Patients after Single Oral Dose of Ceritinib on Cycle 1 Day 1 during PK-Run-in Period of Dose Escalation Phase[9]

| Dose (mg) | $T_{1/2}$ (h) | $T_{max}$ (h) | $C_{max}$ (ng/mL) | $AUC_{0-24}$ (ng·h/mL) | $AUC_{last}$ (ng·h/mL) | $V_z/F$ (L) | Cl/F (L/h) |
|---|---|---|---|---|---|---|---|
| 50 | 19.5 n = 1 | 5.95 n = 1 | 13.1 n = 1 | 226 n = 1 | 366 n = 1 | 3540 n = 1 | 126 n = 1 |
| 100 | 19.4 n = 1 | 15.0 (6.00-24.0) n = 2 | 29.3 (10.1) n = 2 | 467 (10.7) n = 2 | 938 (24.3) n = 2 | 3250 n = 1 | 116 n = 1 |
| 200 | 33.2 n = 1 | 5.08 (4.17-6.00) n = 2 | 40.2 (88.5) n = 2 | 703 (55.6) n = 2 | 1460 (62.9) n = 2 | 3720 n = 1 | 77.5 n = 1 |
| 300 | 30.1 (10.0) n = 3 | 4.00 (4.00-5.95) n = 3 | 198 (41.5) n = 3 | 3440 (44.7) n = 3 | 7470 (46.5) n = 3 | 1880 (50.7) n = 2 | 44.5 (36.8) n = 2 |
| 400 | 30.7 (39.1) n = 10 | 4.99 (2.97-6.73) n = 12 | 120 (80.9) n = 12 | 1920 (78) n = 12 | 4070 (81.8) n = 12 | 3470 (74.4) n = 5 | 95.9 (58.6) n = 5 |
| 500 | 31.1 (11.1) n = 7 | 3.98 (3.00-23.5) n = 8 | 153 (86.5) n = 8 | 2350 (87.9) n = 8 | 5140 (142) n = 8 | 6230 (219) n = 3 | 147 (170) n = 3 |
| 600 | 37.6 (24.6) n = 6 | 6.00 (3.00-24.1) n = 9 | 212 (59.7) n = 9 | 3590 (53.4) n = 9 | 8180 (57.4) n = 9 | 1990 (4.30) n = 2 | 46.3 (9.60) n = 2 |
| 700 | 38.9 (98.4) n = 3 | 6.00 (4.00-25.0) n = 4 | 206 (146) n = 4 | 3450 (138) n = 4 | 9210 (112) n = 4 | 2340 (56.5) n = 2 | 66.6 (35.8) n = 2 |
| 750 | 40.6 (34.7) n = 9 | 6.02 (3.95-23.8) n = 10 | 186 (127) n = 10 | 3390 (121) n = 10 | 7870 (127) n = 10 | 4230 (164) n = 3 | 88.5 (163) n = 3 |

n: Number of patients with non-missing values.   Values were median (range) for $T_{max}$, geometric mean (CV% of geometric mean) for all others.

# Key Findings:[5]

❖ Ceritinib was classified as a low passive permeability compound.

[5] FDA Database. http://www.accessdata.fda.gov/drugsatfda_docs/nda/2014/205755Orig1s000PharmR.pdf (accessed Mar 2016).
[9] FDA Database. http://www.accessdata.fda.gov/drugsatfda_docs/nda/2014/205755Orig1s000ClinPharmR.pdf (accessed Mar 2016).

# Distribution

Table 9   *In Vitro* Plasma Protein Binding and Blood Partitioning of [$^{14}$C]Ceritinib[5]

| Study | Binding of [$^{14}$C]Ceritinib to Plasma Protein of Different Species (%) | | | Binding of Ceritinib to Isolated Human Serum Protein (%) | | Binding of [$^{14}$C]Ceritinib to RBC of Different Species (%) | | | |
|---|---|---|---|---|---|---|---|---|---|
| Conc. (ng/mL) | 50 | 500 | 10000 | Conc. (ng/mL) | HSA | Conc. (ng/mL) | 50 | 500 | 10000 |
| Rat | 97.9 ± 0.2 | 98.4 ± 0 | 98.4 ± 0.1 | 100 | 97.6 ± 0.6 | Rat | 68.8 ± 0.4 | 64.9 ± 3.7 | 65.3 ± 1.3 |
| Dog | 98.8 ± 0.05 | 98.3 ± 0.21 | 98.4 ± 0.08 | | | Dog | 66.6 ± 1.6 | 67.0 ± 0.4 | 71.6 ± 1.1 |
| Monkey | 94.4 ± 0.05 | 94.5 ± 0.4 | 95.2 ± 0.2 | 10000 | 98.6 ± 0.8 | Monkey | 78.7 ± 1.1 | 77.8 ± 1.5 | 76.4 ± 0.4 |
| Human | 98.8 ± 0.05 | 97.2 ± 0.14 | 96.7 ± 1.8 | | | Human | 58.2 ± 3.5 | 58.6 ± 5.5 | 56.9 ± 4.8 |

Table 10   *In Vivo* Tissue Distribution of Ceritinib in Long-Evans Rats after Single Oral Dose of [$^{14}$C]Ceritinib[5]

| Tissue | Long-Evans Rats, p.o., 25 mg/kg | | | | | | | Long-Evans Rats, i.v., 10 mg/kg | |
|---|---|---|---|---|---|---|---|---|---|
| | Radioactivity (ng eq./g) | | | | | | Tissue/Blood AUC$_{0-168}$ Ratio | Radioactivity (ng eq./g) | Tissue/Blood Radioactivity Ratio |
| | 1 h | 4 h | 8 h | 24 h | 72 h | 168 h | | | |
| Blood | 63.4 | 600 | 220 | 48.0 | NM | NM | 1.00 | 1420 | 1.00 |
| Brain | 29.8 | 42.0 | 20.0 | 13.0 | NM | NM | 0.148 | 137 | 0.096 |
| Bile | NM | 74000 | 29000 | 11000 | NM | NM | 155 | 48800 | 34.4 |
| Lungs | 607 | 18000 | 5900 | 2100 | 28.9 | 21.2 | 37.2 | 23300 | 16.4 |
| Liver | 2720 | 33000 | 8100 | 1800 | 78.7 | 130 | 52.6 | 29500 | 20.8 |
| Kidney cortex | 693 | 17000 | 6400 | 1300 | 20.3 | 28.3 | 32.8 | 23700 | 16.7 |
| Stomach glandular | 13400 | 5200 | 1900 | 310 | NM | NM | 26.3 | 6590 | 4.64 |
| Adrenal cortex | 1870 | 37000 | 11000 | 4100 | 41.4 | NM | 72.4 | 48700 | 34.3 |
| Harderian gland | 31.5 | 1700 | 1800 | 2600 | 1060 | 2990 | 62.8 | 5040 | 3.55 |
| Bone marrow | 198 | 7600 | 3000 | 2700 | 23.3 | NM | 28.0 | 9220 | 6.50 |
| Small intestine wall | 164000 | 490000 | 11000 | 730 | NM | NM | 413 | 6980 | 4.92 |
| Thyroid gland | 843 | 18000 | 7300 | 1200 | NM | NM | 30.3 | 35100 | 24.7 |
| Pituitary gland | 229 | 14000 | 6600 | 15000 | 1810 | 2590 | 211 | 15000 | 10.6 |
| Spleen | 1040 | 27000 | 6400 | 2500 | 42.3 | 41.6 | 47.6 | NA | NA |
| Lymph node | 200 | 19000 | 2900 | 4100 | 183.0 | NM | 45.1 | 8720 | 6.14 |
| Adrenal medulla | 890 | 21000 | 2100 | 1300 | 48.1 | NM | 26.5 | 14600 | 10.3 |
| Pancreas | 388 | 13000 | 4000 | 1300 | 6.6 | NM | 24.6 | 14200 | 9.98 |
| Thymus | 120 | 4300 | 1400 | 2400 | 86.7 | NM | 21.3 | 3860 | 2.72 |
| Salivary gland | 208 | 9700 | 3500 | 1700 | NM | NM | 20.2 | 8740 | 6.16 |
| Uveal tract | 108 | 6500 | 1100 | 8500 | 2880 | 8160 | 176 | 8600 | 6.06 |

NM: Not measured.

[5]   FDA Database.   http://www.accessdata.fda.gov/drugsatfda_docs/nda/2014/205755Orig1s000PharmR.pdf (accessed Mar 2016).

## Metabolism

Table 11    *In Vitro* Intrinsic Clearance of [$^{14}$C]Ceritinib in Monkey, Rat and Human Hepatocytes[5]

| Species | Conc. (μM) | Time Points Used (h) | $T_{1/2}$ (h) | $Cl_{int}$ (μL/h/$10^6$ cells) | $Cl_H$ (mL/h/kg) | Extraction Ratio |
|---|---|---|---|---|---|---|
| Rat | 2.5 | 0-18 | NC | NC | NC | NC |
| | 12.5 | 0-24 | NC | NC | NC | |
| Monkey | 2.5 | 0-4 | 7.02 | 98.7 | 313 | 0.12 |
| | 12.5 | 0-8 | 18.0 | 38.5 | 132 | |
| Human | 2.5 | 0.25-18 | 100 | 6.90 | 17.3 | 0.014 |
| | 12.5 | 0-18 | 67.0 | 10.4 | 25.8 | |

NC: Not calculated.

Table 12    *In Vitro* Metabolic Phenotype of [$^{14}$C]Ceritinib in Human Liver Microsomes[5]

| Inhibitor (main inhibited P450) | Concentration Range Used (μM) | Median Reported $K_i$ or $IC_{50}$ Value (μM) | $IC_{50}$ (μM) | %Maxima Inhibition[a] |
|---|---|---|---|---|
| Ketoconazole (3A) | 0-1 | 0.100 | ~0.03 | 90.5 |
| Azamulin (3A) | 0-5 | 0.15 | ~0.01 | 100 |
| Ticlopidine (2B6/2C19) | 0-10 | 1.70 | >10 | 10.9 |
| S-mephenytoin (2C19) | 0-250 | 95.5 | >250 | 18 |
| Montelukast (2C8) | 0-2 | 0.014 (0.18-0.71) | >2 | 16.5 |
| Furafylline (1A2) | 0-10 | 2.00 | >10 | 19.1 |
| Quinidine (2D6) | 0-1 | 0.0605 | >1 | 17.9 |
| Sulfaphenazole (2C9) | 0-5 | 0.510 | >5 | 11.9 |
| Fluvastatin (2C9) | 0-5 | 0.525 | >5 | 21.6 |

[a] Percent maximal inhibition of total [$^{14}$C]ceritinib metabolism at the concentrations of inhibitor was examined.

Table 13    Apparent Covalent Binding of [$^{14}$C]Ceritinib in Human and Rat Hepatocytes[5]

| Species | Analyte | Drug Equivalents Bound (pmol/$10^6$ cells) or (pmol/mg tissue) | | | |
|---|---|---|---|---|---|
| | | 0.083 h | 0.5 h | 1 h | 4 h |
| Rat[a] | Ceritinib | 108 ± 2.3 | 325 ± 17.1 | 426 ± 63 | 609 ± 32 |
| | L746530 | 168 ± 1.3 | 461 ± 22.3 | 710 ± 43 | 1068 ± 18 |
| Human[a] | Ceritinib | 106 ± 7.02 | 281 ± 0.68 | 504 ± 17 | 702 ± 57 |
| | L746530 | 174 ± 8.8 | 523 ± 0.5 | 684 ± 70 | 1057 ± 76 |
| Rat[b] | Ceritinib | 11.6 ± 0.25 | 34.7 ± 1.83 | 45.6 ± 6.7 | 65.2 ± 3.5 |
| | L746530 | 18.0 ± 0.14 | 49.3 ± 2.38 | 75.9 ± 4.6 | 114 ± 2 |
| Human[b] | Ceritinib | 11.3 ± 0.75 | 30.1 ± 0.07 | 54.0 ± 1.8 | 75.1 ± 6.1 |
| | L746530 | 18.6 ± 0.94 | 56.0 ± 0.05 | 73.2 ± 7.5 | 113 ± 8 |

L746530 was a positive control.    [a] Based on viable cells.    [b] Based on 107 × $10^6$ hepatocytes per gram of tissue.

## Key Findings:[5]

❖ The metabolism of ceritinib included mono-oxygenation, *O*-dealkylation, *S*-dealkylation, *N*-formylation of ceritinib, secondary *di*-oxygenation, glucuronidation, sulfation and dehydrogenation.

[5]  FDA Database.  http://www.accessdata.fda.gov/drugsatfda_docs/nda/2014/205755Orig1s000PharmR.pdf (accessed Mar 2016).

Table 14    Apparent Covalent Binding of [$^{14}$C]Ceritinib in Rat and Human Liver Microsomes[5]

| Analyte | Species | Drug Equivalents Bound (pmol/mg protein[a]) | | | |
|---|---|---|---|---|---|
| | | GSH | NADPH | NADPH + UDPGA | NADPH + UDPGA + GSH |
| Ceritinib | Rat | 10.0 ± 1.2 | 21.2 ± 1.3 | 21.4 ± 0.9 | 15.0 ± 1.9 |
| | Human | 10.4 ± 1.3 | 20.5 ± 0.5 | 12.3 ± 10.7 | 11.3 ± 0.9 |
| L746530 | Rat | 64.4 ± 1.7 | 716 ± 36 | 580 ± 35 | 590 ± 50 |
| | Human | 52.8 ± 2.6 | 254.3 ± 5.2 | 245 ± 24 | 354 ± 34 |

L746530 was a positive control.    Values were mean ± SD (n = 3).    [a] Based on nominal microsomal protein included in incubation.

Table 15    *In Vitro* Metabolism of [$^{14}$C]Ceritinib in Monkey and Human Hepatocytes[5]

| Species | Conc. (μM) | Time (h) | % of Radioactivity | | | | | | | | | |
|---|---|---|---|---|---|---|---|---|---|---|---|---|
| | | | Parent | M21.6 | M23.6 | M25.7 | M27.5/M27.6[a] | M29.5 | M32.9 | M33.4 | M35.8 | M37.3 |
| Monkey | 2.5 | 0.25 | 92.5 | 0.23 | 0.31 | ND | 3.33 | ND | 0.68 | 1.20 | ND | ND |
| | | 0.5 | 89.9 | 0.28 | 0.59 | ND | 4.68 | ND | 0.77 | 1.77 | ND | ND |
| | | 1 | 83.8 | 0.81 | 0.95 | ND | 8.67 | ND | 0.58 | 3.58 | ND | ND |
| | | 2 | 76.9 | 1.96 | 1.26 | ND | 10.6 | 1.00 | 5.15 | ND | ND | ND |
| | | 4 | 69.1 | 2.37 | 2.13 | 2.20 | 13.4 | 1.46 | 7.15 | ND | ND | ND |
| | | 8 | 61.5 | 2.97 | 3.01 | 4.27 | 14.8 | 2.69 | 8.12 | ND | ND | ND |
| | | 18 | 50.6 | 4.06 | 2.40 | 5.11 | 20.4 | 2.68 | 8.21 | ND | 2.51 | 2.91 |
| | | 24 | 32.0 | 7.11 | 4.42 | 11.5 | 25.0 | 5.23 | 8.77 | ND | 2.15 | 2.5 |
| | 12.5 | 0.25 | NA | NA | NA | NA | NA | NA | NA | NA | NA | NA |
| | | 0.5 | 92.7 | 0.23 | 0.24 | ND | 1.95 | 0.20 | 0.37 | 1.92 | ND | ND |
| | | 1 | 89.3 | 0.34 | 0.56 | ND | 3.11 | 0.41 | 0.53 | 3.09 | ND | ND |
| | | 2 | 80.7 | 1.68 | 0.97 | 1.09 | 6.05 | 1.17 | 5.60 | ND | ND | ND |
| | | 4 | 80.6 | 1.12 | 1.21 | 1.56 | 5.32 | 1.81 | 6.12 | ND | ND | ND |
| | | 8 | 74.2 | 2.16 | 1.34 | 4.06 | 5.96 | 3.48 | 5.90 | ND | ND | 0.93 |
| | | 18 | 71.2 | 2.10 | 1.43 | 5.61 | 6.81 | 3.34 | 5.07 | ND | 0.89 | 1.69 |
| | | 24 | 61.9 | 4.05 | 1.81 | 8.11 | 9.31 | 5.82 | 5.41 | ND | 0.87 | 1.40 |
| Human | 2.5 | 0.25 | 90.4 | - | - | - | 0.78 | - | 0.75 | 1.76 | - | ND |
| | | 0.5 | 90.9 | - | - | - | 0.77 | - | 0.98 | 1.19 | - | ND |
| | | 1 | 91.8 | - | - | - | 1.28 | - | 1.35 | 1.14 | - | ND |
| | | 2 | 91.6 | - | - | - | 2.22 | - | 1.18 | 1.02 | - | ND |
| | | 4 | 89.9 | - | - | - | 3.11 | - | 1.46 | 1.26 | - | ND |
| | | 8 | 87.6 | - | - | - | 4.52 | - | 1.47 | 1.55 | - | 1.11 |
| | | 18 | 83.2 | - | - | - | 8.17 | - | 1.61 | 1.52 | - | 1.59 |
| | | 24 | 81.4 | - | - | - | 8.94 | - | 2.62 | 1.38 | - | 2.28 |
| | 12.5 | 0.25 | NA | - | - | - | ND | - | NA | NA | - | NA |
| | | 0.5 | 96.4 | - | - | - | ND | - | ND | 3.60 | - | ND |
| | | 1 | 95.5 | - | - | - | ND | - | ND | 4.47 | - | ND |

[5]    FDA Database.    http://www.accessdata.fda.gov/drugsatfda_docs/nda/2014/205755Orig1s000PharmR.pdf (accessed Mar 2016).

*Continued*

| Species | Conc. (µM) | Time (h) | % of Radioactivity | | | | | | | | | |
|---|---|---|---|---|---|---|---|---|---|---|---|---|
| | | | Parent | M21.6 | M23.6 | M25.7 | M27.5/M27.6[a] | M29.5 | M32.9 | M33.4 | M35.8 | M37.3 |
| Human | 12.5 | 2 | 95.5 | - | - | - | ND | - | ND | 4.55 | - | ND |
| | | 4 | 95.7 | - | - | - | ND | - | ND | 4.26 | - | ND |
| | | 8 | 95.2 | - | - | - | ND | - | ND | 4.81 | - | ND |
| | | 18 | 85.1 | - | - | - | 7.05 | - | ND | 7.89 | - | ND |
| | | 24 | 90.8 | - | - | - | 2.96 | - | 3.93 | 0.67 | - | 1.65 |

-: Not observed.  NA: Not available.  [a] M27.5/M27.6: Co-elute under the LC/MS conditions used.

Table 16  Metabolites in Plasma, Bile and Feces in Rats, Monkeys and Humans after Single Oral and Intravenous Dose of Ceritinib[5, 6]

| Matrix | Species | Route | Dose (mg/kg) | % of Dose | | | | | | | | | | |
|---|---|---|---|---|---|---|---|---|---|---|---|---|---|---|
| | | | | M0 | M21.6 | M23.6 | M27.6 | M32.9 | M33.4 | M35.8 | M46.1 | M46.6 | M48.8 | M52.0 |
| Plasma[a] | Rat | i.v./p.o. | 10/25 | 100 | - | - | - | - | - | - | - | - | - | - |
| | Monkey | i.v. | 10 | 89.9 | 1.4 | - | 1.8 | 0.6 | 1.2 | - | 3 | - | - | - |
| | | p.o. | 30 | 84.4 | 3.6 | - | 2.5 | 0.4 | 1.6 | - | 3.1 | - | - | - |
| | Human | p.o. | 750 mg | 81.6 | - | 1.2 | 1.4 | 1.9 | 1.6 | 1.8 | 2.3 | 1.7 | 1.7 | 2 |
| Bile | Rat | i.v. | 10 | 34.9 | ND | ND | - | 1.09 | 3.26 | 0.83 | - | - | - | - |
| | | p.o. | 25 | 9.19 | 1.71 | 0.84 | - | 0.72 | 1.46 | 0.52 | - | - | - | - |
| Feces | Rat | i.v. | 10 | 12.0 | 3.75 | 4.56 | - | ND | ND | ND | - | - | - | - |
| | | p.o. | 25 | 51.8 | 4.54 | 5.88 | - | ND | 2.82 | ND | - | - | - | - |
| | Monkey | i.v. | 10 | 55.1 | 1.8 | 2.8 | - | 3.7 | 10.9 | 17.9 | 0.3 | - | - | - |
| | | p.o. | 30 | 60.2 | 2.7 | 2.2 | - | 2.7 | 5.9 | >8.7 | 0.4 | - | - | - |
| | Human | p.o. | 750 mg | 68 | - | 3.9 | - | 1.8 | 1.4 | 6.5 | 1.6 | 1.1 | 1.4 | 2.2 |

M0: Ceritinib.  [a] %AUC in plasma.

[5] FDA Database. http://www.accessdata.fda.gov/drugsatfda_docs/nda/2014/205755Orig1s000PharmR.pdf (accessed Mar 2016).
[6] EMA Database. http://www.ema.europa.eu/docs/en_GB/document_library/EPAR_-_Public_assessment_report/human/003819/WC500187506.pdf (accessed Mar 2016).

Figure D   Proposed Pathways for *In Vivo* Biotransformation of [$^{14}$C]Ceritinib in Rats, Monkeys and Humans[6]
The red labels represent the major components in matrices.   P = Plasma, B = Bile and F = Feces.

[6]   EMA Database.   http://www.ema.europa.eu/docs/en_GB/document_library/EPAR_-_Public_assessment_report/human/003819/WC500187506.pdf (accessed Mar 2016).

# Excretion

Table 17   Excretion Profiles of [$^{14}$C]Ceritinib in Rats, Monkeys and Humans after Single Oral and Intravenous Dose of [$^{14}$C]Ceritinib[5, 6]

| Species | State | Dose (mg/kg) | Route | Time (h) | Bile (% of dose) | Urine (% of dose) | Feces (% of dose) |
|---------|-------|--------------|-------|----------|------------------|-------------------|-------------------|
| Rat | Intact | 10 | i.v. | 0-168 | - | $0.241 \pm 0.174$ | $107 \pm 7.8$ |
| | | 25 | p.o. | 0-168 | - | 0.180 | 101 |
| Rat | BDC | 10 | i.v. | 0-72/168 | 65.4 | 0.62 | 29.8 |
| | | 25 | p.o. | 0-72/168 | $24.3 \pm 8.52$ | $1.05 \pm 1.03$ | $65.0 \pm 17.0$ |
| Monkey | Intact | 10 | i.v. | 0-168 | - | 0.59 | 105 |
| | | 30 | p.o. | 0-168 | - | $0.71 \pm 0.45$ | $92.3 \pm 6.94$ |
| Human | Intact | 9.14 | p.o. | 0-168 | - | 1.2 | 91.0 |

# Drug-Drug Interaction

Table 18   *In Vitro* Evaluation of Ceritinib as an Inhibitor and an Inducer of CYP Enzymes[5, 9]

| Ceritinib as an Inhibitor | | | | | Ceritinib as an Inducer | | | | | |
|---------------------------|-----------|----------------|--------------|------------------------|--------|-----------|---------------|------|--------|------------------------|
| CYPs | Substrate | IC$_{50}$ (µM) | K$_i$ (µM) | R$_1$ Value (1+I/K$_i$) | CYPs | Parameter | Conc. (µM) | | | Positive Control[a] |
| | | | | | | | 0.25 | 1 | 2.5 | |
| CYP1A2 | Phenacetin | >100 (2.5) | - | 1.0 | CYP1A2 | mRNA | 1.01 | 1.14 | 1.07 | 32.1 |
| CYP2A6 | Coumarin | 5 (1.5) | 0.03 (0.009) | 61.0 | | Activity | 1.15[d] | 1.22 | 1.01 | 31.7 |
| CYP2B6 | Bupropion | 2 (0.3) | 5.3 (0.780) | 1.3 | CYP2B6 | mRNA | 1.02 | 1.17 | 0.96 | 10.2 |
| CYP2C8 | Paclitaxel | 25 (0.6) | - | 1.1 | | Activity | 1.05 | 1.20 | 0.92 | 4.65 |
| CYP2C8 | Amodiaquine | 2 (0.6) | 16.7 (4.86) | 1.1 | CYP2C9 | mRNA | 1.12 | 1.15 | 1.18 | 2.34 |
| CYP2C9 | Diclofenac | 2 (0.6) | 0.24 (0.0701) | 8.5 | | Activity | 1.27 | 1.77 | 1.10 | 3.50 |
| CYP2C19 | *S*-mephenytoin | 70 (1.8) | - | 1.0 | CYP3A4 | mRNA | 1.27 | 2.73 | 6.03[b] | 31.1 |
| CYP2D6 | Bufuralol | 20 (2.9) | - | 1.2 | | Activity | 0.98 | 1.43 | 1.33[c] | 8.81 |
| CYP2E1 | Chlorzoxazone | 30 (4.4) | - | 1.1 | | | | | | |
| CYP3A4/5 | Midazolam | 0.2 (0.06) | 0.16 (0.0469) | 12.3 | | | | | | |
| CYP3A4/5 | Testosterone | 0.2 (0.06) | – | 19.0 | | | | | | |

Calculation of R$_1$ values based on maximal steady-state concentration of 1010 ng/mL or 1.8 µM.   [I]/K$_i$ assumed to be IC$_{50}$/2 for competitive inhibition for those CYP enzymes without an experimental K$_i$ value.   [a] Omeprazole 50 µM for CYP1A2, phenobarbital 1000 µM for CYP2B6 and CYP2C9, rifampin 10 µM for CYP3A4.   [b] Mean of 3.24-, 8.74- and 6.12-fold change relative to vehicle control in the three human hepatocyte lots.   [c] Mean of 0.936-, 0.983- and 2.06-fold change relative to vehicle control in the three human hepatocyte lots.   [d] Mean of 1.75-, 1.24- and 2.31-fold change relative vehicle control in the three human hepatocyte lots.

[5]  FDA Database.  http://www.accessdata.fda.gov/drugsatfda_docs/nda/2014/205755Orig1s000PharmR.pdf (accessed Mar 2016).
[6]  EMA Database.  http://www.ema.europa.eu/docs/en_GB/document_library/EPAR_-_Public_assessment_report/human/003819/WC500187506.pdf (accessed Mar 2016).
[9]  FDA Database.  http://www.accessdata.fda.gov/drugsatfda_docs/nda/2014/205755Orig1s000ClinPharmR.pdf (accessed Mar 2016).

Table 19   *In Vitro* Evaluation of Ceritinib as an Inhibitor and a Substate of Uptake Transporters[9]

| Ceritinib as an Inhibitor | | | | | Ceritinib as a Substrate | | | | |
|---|---|---|---|---|---|---|---|---|---|
| Transporter | Substrate | IC$_{50}$ (μM) | C$_{max}$[a] /IC$_{50}$ | Unbound C$_{max}$/IC$_{50}$ | Transporter | Conc. (μM) | Cellular Uptake (pmol/mg protein$^{-1}$·min$^{-1}$) | | Fold in Uptake Caused by Transporter |
| | | | | | | | Control Cell | Expressing Cell | |
| OATP1B1 | Estradiol 17β-dglucu-ronide-D- | >5 | <0.36 | - | OCT1 | 5.0 | 396 ± 30 | 386 ± 26 | - |
| OATP1B3 | Estradiol 17β-dglucu-ronide-D- | >5 | <0.36 | - | OAT2 | 5.6 | 360 ± 35 | 517 ± 9 | 1.44 |
| OAT1 | Cidofovir | >5 | - | <0.01 | OATP1B1 | 5.6 | 360 ± 35 | 463 ± 27 | 1.29 |
| OAT3 | Estrone-3-sulfate | ND | - | - | OATP2B1 | 6.3 | 466 ± 5.7 | 470 ± 51 | 1.01 |
| OCT1 | MPP+ | ND | - | - | | | | | |
| OCT2 | Metformin | >5 | - | <0.01 | | | | | |

ND: Not determined.   [a] Plasma maximal steady-state concentration (C$_{max}$) of 1010 ng/mL or 1.8 μM.

Table 20   *In Vitro* Evaluation of Ceritinib as an Inhibitor and a Substrate of Efflux Transporters[9]

| Ceritinib as an Inhibitor | | | | | Ceritinib as a Substrate | | |
|---|---|---|---|---|---|---|---|
| Transporter | Substrate | Conc. (μM) | Parameter | | Transporter | Ceritinib | |
| | | Ceritinib | Ceritinib | Positive Control | | Conc. (μM) | Efflux Ratio |
| P-gp | Rho 123 | 0-1.5 | 12.6-18.2 | 250 or 258 | P-gp | 3.0/14 | 182/19.5 |
| BCRP | BCRP-mediated | 0-1.5 | 15.2-18.2 | 130 or 120 | BCRP | 3 | 121 |

# 6   Non-Clinical Toxicology

## Summary

### Single-Dose Toxicity

❖ Acute toxicity in monkeys: No lethality up to 250 mg/kg.

### Repeated-Dose Toxicity

❖ A series of oral repeated-dose toxicology studies were conducted with ceritinib in rats (up to 13 weeks) and monkeys (up to 13 weeks).
  • By the 13-week studies, the NOAEL was 10 mg/kg/day in monkeys, but not established in rats.
  • Target organ of species-concordance: Pancreas (atrophy and inflammation in both species), biliopancreatic and bile ducts (inflammation and dilatation in rats), GI tract and liver (elevation of liver enzymes in both species).

### Safety Pharmacology

❖ Both *in vitro* and *in vivo* safety pharmacology studies were conducted to assess the effects on cardiovascular, behavioral, general physiological and respiratory function.
  • Ceritinib was unlikely to interfere with vital functions of the respiratory and central nervous systems.
  • It demonstrated sort of potential for causing QT prolongation (modest): Ceritinib inhibited the hERG current at all tested concentrations, with an estimated IC$_{50}$ of 0.4 μM.   The effects were confirmed by the monkey study at a single dose of 100 mg/kg.[6]

### Genotoxicity

❖ The micronucleus test in TK6 cells was considered positive, but no mutagenicity or clastogenicity was confirmed in other *in vitro* and *in vivo* genotoxicity studies with ceritinib.   Therefore, genotoxic risk was not expected in humans.

### Reproductive and Developmental Toxicity

❖ No fertility, early embryonic development, pre- and postnatal or juvenile toxicology studies had been conducted, in line with ICH S9 for the advanced cancer indication.

[6]   EMA Database.   http://www.ema.europa.eu/docs/en_GB/document_library/EPAR_-_Public_assessment_report/human/003819/WC500187506.pdf (accessed Mar 2016).
[9]   FDA Database.   http://www.accessdata.fda.gov/drugsatfda_docs/nda/2014/205755Orig1s000ClinPharmR.pdf (accessed Mar 2016).

❖ Embryo-fetal development in rats and rabbits:
  • No fetotoxicity and teratotoxicity after dosing with ceritinib organogenesis. However, maternal plasma exposure was less than that at the clinical RHD of 50 mg.[6]

Carcinogenicity
❖ No carcinogenicity studies were performed and required for the cancer indication according to ICH S9.

Special Toxicology
❖ Ceritinib showed a low potential for phototoxicity in the 3T3 NRU *in vitro* assay and was confirmed to be non-phototoxic in the UV mouse LLNA.

## Single-Dose Toxicity

Table 21    Single-Dose Toxicity Studies of Ceritinib[5, 9]

| Species | Dose (mg/kg) | MNLD (mg/kg) | Finding |
|---|---|---|---|
| Cynomolgus monkey | 20, 60, 120, 250, p.o. | 250 | ≥120 mg/kg: Diarrhea, ↑ AST (3-5 ×), ↑ ALT (2 ×). 250 mg/kg: Diarrhea, emesis. |

Formulation: 0.5% MC.

## Repeated-Dose Toxicity

Table 22    Repeated-Dose Toxicity Studies of Ceritinib[5, 6]

| Species | Duration (Week) | Dose (mg/kg/day) | Finding |
|---|---|---|---|
| Wistar rat | 2[a] | Male: 0, 10, 25, 100 | 25 mg/kg: ↓ BWG, ↓ reticulocyte counts, ↓ MCV and MCH, ↓ haematocrit and hemoglobin. ↓ Triglycerides, ↓ glucose and albumin, ↑ globulin. Bile duct vacuolation/hypertrophy; Adrenal gland: ↑ cortical vacuolation and/or cortical single cell necrosis; Stomach: (glandular) erosion. 100 mg/kg: Piloerection, ↓ BW, ↑ RBC# and hemoglobin, ↑ PLT#, ↑ total WBC, neutrophil and monocyte counts. ↑ AST, ↑ creatine kinase in one animal, ↓ urea, total bilirubin, and cholesterol, ↓ triglycerides, glucose and albumin, ↑ globulin. ↓ Mean thymic and splenic weights, bile duct vacuolation/hypertrophy; Focal/multifocal or single cell necrosis of hepatocytes, peri-/cholangiolitis. Hypocellularity in bone marrow (sternum), absence of haemopoiesis in spleen. Mesenteric lymph nodes: Focal/multifocal necrosis (cortex/paracortex), abscess formation (paracortex) and increase in aggregates of macrophages, subacute focal inflammation in the mesentery, reduction/absence of germinal center development. Thymus: Cortical atrophy and/or lymphocytosis. Adrenal gland: Increase in cortical vacuolation and/or cortical single cell necrosis. Small intestine: Minimal neutrophilic cell infiltration; Stomach: (glandular) erosion. NOAEL: 10 mg/kg. |
| | 4 | Male & female: 0, 7.5, 25, 75→50[b] | ≥25 mg/kg: ↓ BWG, ↑ neutrophil, ↑ PLT, ↑ serum insulin concentration (male). 50 mg/kg: ↓ BWG, ↓ food consumption; Inflammation (↑ monocyte, ↑ plasma fibrinogen), ↑ lymphocyte counts (male). ↑ Insulin (female), ↑ serum liver enzyme activities (male), ↑ serum phosphorus concentration. 75 mg/kg: Not tolerated and was reduced to 50 mg/kg due to adverse clinical signs. ↓ Reticulocyte counts, ↓ urea, ↓ phosphorus (male) and ↓ magnesium, ↓ glucose (female), ↓ calcium (male), ↑ serum AST and ALT activities (male). NOAEL: 7.5 mg/kg. |
| | 13 | Male & female: 0, 3, 10, 30 | Target: Biliopancreatic duct (chronic inflammation, degeneration/necrosis, erosion, hyperplasia, dilatation, and vacuolation at all doses), the duodenum (degeneration, necrosis, hyperplasia, dilatation, inflammation, and vacuolation), liver (bile duct vacuolation), mesenteric lymph nodes (increased macrophage aggregates) and lungs (macrophage aggregates). 30 mg/kg: Hematology (↑ fibrinogen concentration and ↑ PLT#. ↑ Total protein concentration (male), ↓ albumin concentration (female), ↑ globulin concentration and ↓ albumin-to-globulin ratio. ↑ Cholesterol concentration and ↓ triglyceride concentration. ↑ Thyroid stimulating hormone concentration). ↓ Body weight gain, ↓ food consumption and ↓ body weight. Duodenum (chronic-active inflammation, hyperplasia and luminal dilatation), mesenteric lymph node and lung (↑ number of macrophages). Exposure increased with the minor accumulation of dose following repeat dosing. NOAEL: ND. |

[5]  FDA Database.  http://www.accessdata.fda.gov/drugsatfda_docs/nda/2014/205755Orig1s000PharmR.pdf (accessed Mar 2016).
[6]  EMA Database.  http://www.ema.europa.eu/docs/en_GB/document_library/EPAR_-_Public_assessment_report/human/003819/WC500187506.pdf (accessed Mar 2016).
[9]  FDA Database.  http://www.accessdata.fda.gov/drugsatfda_docs/nda/2014/205755Orig1s000ClinPharmR.pdf (accessed Mar 2016).

*Continued*

| Species | Duration (Week) | Dose (mg/kg/day) | Finding |
|---|---|---|---|
| Cynomolgus monkey | 2[a] | Male & female: 0, 10, 40, 100 | ≥40 mg/kg: Circling, depression, cold to touch, dehydration, hunched posture, decreased loco-motor activity (DLA), soft feces/diarrhoea and emesis. Thymus (lymphoid depletion), pancreas (decreased zymogen).<br>100 mg/kg: ↓ BW, ↓ neutrophils, ↓ reticulocytes, ↓ cellularity in bone marrow smears. ↑ ALT (2-3 fold), ↑ total bilirubin, ↑ urea and ↑ creatinine. Bone marrow (↓ cellularity), pancreas (↓ zymogen).<br>NOAEL: 10 mg/kg. |
| | 4 | Male & female: 0, 3, 10, 30 | ≥10 mg/kg: ↓ Thyroid gland weights (male), small thyroid gland (male), small follicles and colloid depletion in thyroid gland (male). Sinus histiocytosis in mesenteric LN (female).<br>30 mg/kg: ↑ Serum ALT activity, erosion and vacuolation of the lining epithelium of duodenal ampulla, associated with epithelial hyperplasia and foamy macrophage infiltration of the sub-mucosa. Neutrophilic inflammation in duodenal ampulla and adjacent duodenal mucosa, ↓ zymogen in the acinar pancreas, sinus histiocytosis in mesenteric lymph nodes, thymic lymphoid depletion.<br>Recovery: Complete recovery, except for reduced thyroid gland weight (male), small follicles and colloid depletion in the thyroid glands (male).<br>NOAEL: 10 mg/kg. |
| | 13 | Male & female: 0, 3, 10, 30 | Target organ: Cystic bile duct, hepatic bile duct, common bile duct (inflammation and vacuolation) and duodenum (congestion and hemorrhage) of HD males, as well as vacuolation and inflammation of the duodenum of HD monkeys of both genders.<br>≥3 mg/kg: Sporadic vomitus.<br>30 mg/kg: Liquid feces, ↑ ALT activity, ↑ glucose, ↑ insulin (male), ↑ mixed cell inflammation in the cystic bile duct (male), hepatic bile duct (male), and the common bile duct (male). Mixed cell inflammation (mononuclear cells and neutrophils) in major duodenal papilla. Fine cytoplasmic vacuoles in duct epithelium of the cystic bile duct (male), hepatic bile duct (male), common bile duct (male), and lining cells of the major duodenal papilla (male). Minimal mixed cell peribiliary inflammation in the liver.<br>Recovery: Complete recovery.<br>In general, exposure increased with dose, and drug accumulation was more pronounced with increasing dose on Day 73.<br>NOAEL: 10 mg/kg. |

Vehicle: 0.5% (w/v) MC in RODI Water. [a] Non-GLP study. [b] The HD was reduced from 75 to 50 mg/kg/day on Day 13 due to significant weight loss, and not dosed on Day 9-12.

# Safety Pharmacology

Table 23　Safety Pharmacology Study Summary of Ceritinib[5]

| Study | System | Dose | Finding |
|---|---|---|---|
| Neurological effect[a] | Male Wistar rat (n = 10) | 0, 100 mg/kg, p.o. | No significant neurologic changes during FOB. |
| Respiratory effect[a] | Male Wistar rat (n = 10) | 0, 100 mg/kg, p.o. | No effect on respiratory rate, tidal volume, minute volume. |
| Cardiovascular effect[a] | HEK293 cell expressing hERG[b] | 0, 0.3, 0.4, 1, 2.4 μM | $IC_{50}$ = 0.4 μM (233 ng/mL). |
| | Male Cynomolgus monkey (Telemetry) | 0, 10, 30, 100 mg/kg, p.o. | 100 mg/kg: QT/QTc prolongation of 14-44 minutes at 10-19 h post-dose in 1 of 4 monkeys.<br>No drug-related effect on blood pressure, heart rate, body temperature, PR or QRS intervals, or arrhythmias. |

[a] Vehicle: HEPES-buffered physiological saline (HB-PS) + 0.3% DMSO. [b] Positive control: Terfenadine.

[5] FDA Database. http://www.accessdata.fda.gov/drugsatfda_docs/nda/2014/205755Orig1s000PharmR.pdf (accessed Mar 2016).

# Genotoxicity

Table 24    Genotoxicity Studies of Ceritinib[5, 6]

| Assay | Species/System | Metabolism Activity | Dose | Finding |
|---|---|---|---|---|
| *In vitro* reverse mutation assay (Ames) | *S. typhimurium*: TA97, TA98, TA100, TA1535, TA102 | ±S9 | 0-1000 µg/plate | Negative. |
| *In vitro* miniscreen Ames test | *S. typhimurium*: TA98, TA100 | ±S9 | 30-1000 µg/well | Negative[a]. |
| *In vitro* chromosome aberration assay | HPBL | 3 or 17 h: ±S9 20 h: -S9 | 0-16 µg/mL | Negative. |
| | | | 0-22 µg/mL | Incomplete[b]. |
| *In vitro* miconucleus assay | HPBL | 3 or 20 h: -S9 3 h: +S9 | 0-18.6 µg/mL | Negative. |
| | TK6 cell | 3 or 20 h: -S9 3 h: +S9 | 0-33 µg/mL | Positive for 20 h treatment[c]. |
| *In vivo* micronucleus assay | Rat bone marrow | - | 0-2000 mg/kg, p.o. × 2 | Negative. |

[a] Positive and negative control results were not provided for comparative purposes.    [b] 2nd assay cancelled (-S9: 20 h; +S9: 3 + 17 h) by the applicant.    [c] Increased number of cells containing micronuclei after 20 h treatment -S9, but not after 3 h treatment ± S9.

# Reproductive and Developmental Toxicity

Table 25    Reproductive and Developmental Toxicology Studies of Ceritinib by Oral (Gavage) Administration[5]

| Study | Species | Dose (mg/kg/day) | Endpoint | Finding |
|---|---|---|---|---|
| Embryonic-fetal development | Wistar rat | 0, 1, 10, 50 | Maternal | Depressed gestational body weight at MD and HD. |
| | | | Fetal developmental | No embryo lethality or fetotoxicity. |
| | NZW rabbit | 0, 2, 10, 25 | Maternal | Mildly depressed gestational body weight and food consumption at HD. |
| | | | Fetal developmental | No significant embryo lethality or fetotoxicity. Significant incomplete ossification of sternebrae at all doses. Incidence of visceral anomalies in a small number of fetuses. |

Vehicle: 0.5% (w/v) MC in RODI water.

# Special Toxicology

Table 26    Special Toxicology Studies of Ceritinib[5]

| Assay | System | Dose | Finding |
|---|---|---|---|
| *In vitro* phototoxicity test | Balb/c 3T3 fibroblast cell | 0.125-16 µg/mL | Phototoxic at ≥4.4 µg/mL. |
| *In vivo* phototoxic potential in local LN assay | Female Balb/c mouse | 10-100 mg/kg/day, p.o. | No phototoxic potential. |

[5]   FDA Database.   http://www.accessdata.fda.gov/drugsatfda_docs/nda/2014/205755Orig1s000PharmR.pdf (accessed Mar 2016).
[6]   EMA Database.   http://www.ema.europa.eu/docs/en_GB/document_library/EPAR_-_Public_assessment_report/human/003819/WC500187506.pdf (accessed Mar 2016).

# CHAPTER

8

## Chidamide

# Chidamide

## (Epidaza®)

微芯生物
CHIPSCREEN

## 1 General Information

❖ Chidamide is a histone deacetylase (HDAC) inhibitor, which was first approved in Dec 2014 by CFDA.

❖ Chidamide was originally discovered, developed and marketed by Chipscreen.

❖ Chidamide increases the acetylation levels of histones and produces epigenetic regulation by inhibiting HDAC subtypes, resulting in the arrest of lymphatic and blood tumor cells at $G_1$ phase of the cell cycle and promoting apoptosis.

❖ Chidamide is indicated for the treatment of patients with relapsed or refractory peripheral T-cell lymphoma.

❖ Available as tablets, with each containing 5 mg of chidamide and the recommended dose is 30 mg orally twice weekly until disease progression or unacceptable toxicity.

❖ The sale of Epidaza® was not available up to Mar 2016.

### Key Approvals around the World*

|  | China (CFDA) |
| --- | --- |
| First approval date | 12/23/2014 |
| Application or approval No. | 国药准字 H20140129 |
| Brand name | Epidaza® |
| Indication | Relapsed or refractory peripheral T-cell lymphoma |
| Authorisation holder | Chipscreen |

* Till Mar 2016, it has not been approved by PMDA (Japan), EMA (EU) and FDA (US).

### Active Ingredient

*Molecular formula*: $C_{22}H_{19}FN_4O_2$
*Molecular weight*: 390.41
*CAS No.*: 743438-44-0 (Chidamide)
*Chemical name*: (*E*)-*N*-(2-amino-4-fluorophenyl)-4-((3-(pyridin-3-yl)acrylamido)methyl)benzamide

*Parameters of Lipinski's "Rule of 5"*

| MW | $H_D$ | $H_A$ | FRB[a] | PSA[a] | cLogP[a] |
| --- | --- | --- | --- | --- | --- |
| 390.41 | 4 | 6 | 7 | 97.1Å$^2$ | 3.78 ± 0.65 |

[a] Calculated by ACD/Labs software V11.02.

### Drug Product*

*Dosage route*: Oral
*Strength*: 5 mg (Chidamide)
*Dosage form*: Tablet
*Recommended dose*: The recommended starting dose is 30 mg twice weekly for adult after taking breakfast 30 min, and two dosing intervals of not less than 3 days.

* Sourced from CFDA drug label information

## 2　Key Patents Information

### Summary

❖ Epidaza® (Chidamide) was approved by CFDA on Dec 23, 2014.

❖ Chidamide was originally discovered by Shenzhen Chipscreen, and its compound patent application was filed as PCT application by Shenzhen Chipscreen in 2004.

❖ The compound patent will expire in 2023 foremost, which has been granted in China, the United States and Japan successively.

Table 1　Chidamide's Compound Patent Protection in Drug-Mainstream Country

| Country | Publication/Patent NO. | Application Date | Granted Date | Estimated Expiry Date |
|---|---|---|---|---|
| WO | WO2004071400A3 | 02/09/2004 | / | / |
| US | US7550490B2 | 02/02/2004 | 06/23/2009 | 02/02/2024 |
| EP | EP1592665A4 | 02/09/2004 | Refused | / |
| | EP2860174A2 | 02/09/2004 | Examination | / |
| JP | JP4637821B2 | 02/09/2004 | 02/23/2011 | 02/09/2024 |
| CN | CN1284772C | 07/04/2003 | 11/15/2006 | 07/04/2023 |

Table 2　Originator's International Patent Application List (Patent Family)

| Publication NO. | Title | Applicant/Assignee/Owner | Publication Date |
|---|---|---|---|
| **Technical Subjects** | **Active Ingredient (Free Base)'s Formula or Structure and Preparation** | | |
| WO2004071400A2 | Histone deacetylase inhibitors of novel benzamide derivatives with potent differentiation and anti-proliferation activity | Shenzhen Chipscreen | 08/26/2004 |
| **Technical Subjects** | **Salt, Crystal, Polymorphic, Solvate (Hydrate), Isomer, Derivative Etc. and Preparation** | | |
| WO2014082354A1 | Crystal form of chidamide, preparation method and use thereof | Shenzhen Chipscreen | 06/05/2014 |

The data was updated until Jan 2016.

## 3　Chemistry

### Route1:　Original Discovery Route

*Synthetic Route:*　The scalable synthetic approach to chidamide followed closely to the discovery route: The sequence began with the Knoevenagel condensation of commercial available nicotinaldehyde **1** and malonic acid **2** in a refluxing mixture of pyridine and piperidine to afford 3-(3-pyridinyl)-2-propenoic acid **3** in 82% yield.　Next, activation of acid **3** with CDI and subsequent condensation with 4-aminomethyl benzoic acid **4** under the base condition of 1 M NaOH afforded amide **5** in 62% yield after quenching with concentrated HCl.　Finally, activation of **5** with CDI prior to the exposure to 2-amino-4-fluorobenzamide **6** yielded chidamide in an overall yield of 29% after deprotection with TFA.[1-3]

[1]　Yin, Z. H.; Wu, Z. W.; Lan, Y. K., et al. *Chin. J. New Drugs* **2004**, *13*, 536-538.
[2]　Lu, X.; Li, Z.; Xie, A., et al. US7244751B2, **2007**.
[3]　Lu, X.; Li, Z.; Xie, A., et al. CN1513839A, **2004**.

# 4 Pharmacology

## Summary

### Mechanism of Action

❖ Chidamide is an HDAC inhibitor, which inhibited HDAC subtypes 1 ($IC_{50}$ = 95 nM), 2 ($IC_{50}$ = 160 nM), 3 ($IC_{50}$ = 67 nM) and 10 ($IC_{50}$ = 78 nM), resulting in abnormal regulation of tumor epigenetic function.

❖ Histone deacetylases (HDACs) are a family of enzymes that can remove the lysine residues in the $N$-terminal tails of core histone proteins in the nucleosome.    The deacetylation of histones by HDACs results in a remodeling of the chromatin structures and affects the access of transcription factors to the chromatin for gene transcription, which is an ongoing process that is required for normal cells growth and differentiation.

❖ Chidamide increases the acetylation levels of histone H3 and inhibits the PI3K/Akt and MAPK/Ras signaling pathways, resulting in the arrest of tumor cells at the $G_1$ phase of the cell cycle and promoting apoptosis.

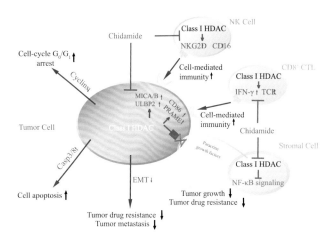

### In Vitro Efficacy

❖ Anti-proliferation in cells:
  • Chidamide against transformed and normal human cultured cells:
    ◆ Transformed cell lines: $GI_{50}$ = 0.4-8.2 μM.
    ◆ Normal cells: $GI_{50}$ >100 μM.
  • Pancreatic cancer cell lines: $IC_{50}$ <50 μM.
  • A375 cell line: $IC_{50}$ = 250 μM.
  • CAL-51 cells: $IC_{50}$ = 19.6 μM.

❖ Effect of chidamide on apoptosis related proteins in HL60 and K562 cell lines:
  • Dose-dependently down-regulated H3.
  • Decreased Cyclin E1/2.
  • PARP and pro-caspase 3, 8 and 9 were cleaved by chidamide.    Pro-survival Bcl-2 family proteins Mcl-1, Bcl-2 and Bcl-xL were decreased in a dose-dependent manner.

❖ Efficacy of chidamide on cell apoptosis in tumor cell lines:
  • Leukaemia cell lines: >30%-35% apoptosis at 4 μM.
  • Pancreatic cancer cell lines: ~5%->5% apoptosis at 25 μM.
  • Human colon cancer cell lines: >20%-25% apoptosis at 4 μM.
  • Malignant melanoma cell A375: 79.5%-83.1% at 62.5-250 μM.
  • TNBC CAL-51: 20.5%-50.1% apoptosis at 10-20 μM.

❖ Efficacy of chidamide on cell cycle in tumor cell lines:
  • Human colon cancer, leukaemia, malignant melanoma cell lines: Dose-dependently increased the proportion of cells in $G_0/G_1$ phase.
  • Pancreatic cancer cell lines: No increase of the proportion of $G_0/G_1$ phase cells.

*In Vivo* Efficacy

- ❖ In Patu8988 pancreatic xenograft tumor mouse model:
  - Tumor growth inhibition: 46.7% at 12.5 mg/kg and 60.4% at 25 mg/kg.
  - Significantly decreased tumor weight at 12.5 mg/kg.
  - Well-tolerance: No gross body weight loss.
- ❖ In HL60 myelogenous leukaemia xenograft tumor mouse model:
  - Tumor growth inhibition: 41.8% at 50 mg/kg.
  - Significantly decreased tumor weight at 50 mg/kg.
  - Well-tolerance: No gross body weight loss.
- ❖ In other xenograft tumor mouse model:
  - Significantly inhibited tumor volumes and weight at 12.5 mg/kg.
  - Well-tolerance: No gross body weight loss.

# Mechanism of Action

Table 3    The Inhibition of Recombinant Human HDACs by Chidamide[4]

| Compound | IC$_{50}$ (nM) | | | | | | | | | | |
| | Class I | | | | Class IIa | | | | Class IIb | | Class IV |
| | 1 | 2 | 3 | 8 | 4 | 5 | 7 | 9 | 6 | 10 | 11 |
|---|---|---|---|---|---|---|---|---|---|---|---|
| Chidamide | 95 | 160 | 67 | 733 | >30000 | >30000 | >30000 | >30000 | >30000 | 78 | 432 |
| Entinostat | 262 | 306 | 499 | 2700 | >30000 | >30000 | >30000 | >30000 | >30000 | 254 | 649 |
| Vorinostat | 38 | 144 | 6 | 38 | >30000 | >30000 | >30000 | >30000 | 10 | 21 | 28 |

The results were expressed as mean from three independent experiments.    Chidamide significantly induced histone H3 acetylation in both HeLa human cervical adenocarcinoma cells and human PBMC and the extent of induction was similar to that observed with entinostat and vorinostat.    When HeLa cells were incubated with chidamide at 1 μM concentration, H3 acetylation increased as early as 30-60 min after treatment and reached maximal levels at 24-72 h after treatment.

# *In Vitro* Efficacy

Table 4    *In Vitro* Anti-proliferation of Chidamide against Transformed and Normal Human Cultured Cells[4]

| Cell Type | Cell Line | Source | GI$_{50}$ (μM) | |
| | | | Chidamide | Entinostat |
|---|---|---|---|---|
| Transformed cell line | A549 | Lungs | 8.2 ± 2.9 | 10.8 ± 3.4 |
| | LNCaP | Prostrate | 4.0 ± 1.2 | 2.5 ± 0.8 |
| | MCF-7 | Breast | 5.0 ± 1.3 | 6.3 ± 1.7 |
| | MB-231 | Breast | 7.9 ± 2.1 | 5.0 ± 2.0 |
| | HCT-8 | Colon | 7.2 ± 1.7 | 1.2 ± 0.3 |
| | HepG2 | Liver | 4.0 ± 1.5 | 3.2 ± 1.1 |
| | PANC-1 | Pcancreas | 6.3 ± 2.1 | 5.0 ± 1.7 |
| | U2OS | Osteosarcoma | 2.0 ± 0.6 | 1.0 ± 0.3 |
| | Raji | B-cell lymphoma | 4.0 ± 0.9 | 6.3 ± 1.4 |
| | HL60 | Myelogenous leukemia | 0.4 ± 0.1 | 0.32 ± 0.1 |
| | 28SC | Myelomonocytic leukemia | 5.8 ± 1.2 | 4.0 ± 0.8 |
| | Jurkat | T-cell lymphoma | 6.3 ± 0.9 | 6.3 ± 1.1 |
| Normal cell | CCC-HEK | Human fetal kidney cell | >100 | 30 ± 6.9 |
| | CCC-HEL | Human liver cell | >100 | 40 ± 5.7 |

The results were expressed as mean ± SE from at least three independent experiments.

[4]  Ning, Z. Q.; Li, Z. B.; Newman, M. J., et al. *Cancer Chemother. Pharmacol.* **2012**, *69*, 901-909.

Table 5　*In Vitro* Pharmacodynamics of Chidamide in Chronic Myelogenous Leukaemia Cells[5]

| Assay | Cell Line | Conc. (μM) | Test Content | Finding |
|---|---|---|---|---|
| Histone acetylation | HL60, K562 | 0, 1, 2, 3, 4 | Ace-H3K9 acetylation | Significantly increased the acetylation of histone H3 at Lys$^9$ and Lys$^{18}$, and histone H4 at Lys$^8$. No effect on the level of total histone H3 and H5. |
| | | | Ace-H3K18 acetylation | |
| | | | Ace-H4K8 acetylation | |
| Cell-cycle arrest | HL60, K562 | 0 (DMSO), 0.1, 0.2, 0.4, 0.8 | Cyclin E1 | Down-regulated the protein expression of cyclin E1 and E2 after chidamide treatment. |
| | | | Cyclin E2 | |
| Caspase-dependent apoptosis | HL60, K562 | 0, 1, 2, 3, 4 | PARP cleavage | PARP and pro-caspase 3, 8 and 9 were cleaved following chidamide treatment in HL60 and K562 cells.　In addition, Bid, a protein involved in intrinsic and extrinsic apoptotic signalling, was cleaved. |
| | | | Pro-caspase 3 cleavage | |
| | | | Pro-caspase 8 cleavage | |
| | | | Pro-caspase 9 cleavage | |
| | | | Bid cleavage | |

Table 6　*In Vitro* Efficacy of Chidamide on Apoptosis and Cell Cycle in Cancer Cells[5-9]

| Source | Cell Line | IC$_{50}$ (μM) | Apoptosis | | Cell Cycle Distribution (%) | | | |
|---|---|---|---|---|---|---|---|---|
| | | | Conc. (μM) | %Apoptosis | Conc. (μM) | G$_0$/G$_1$ | G$_2$/M | S |
| Human colon cancer | LoVo | NA | 0 | >5 | 0 | >39 | >10 | >50 |
| | | | 4 | >20 | 4 | >45 | >5 | >45 |
| | | | 8 | >30 | 8 | >60 | >2 | >30 |
| | | | 16 | >50 | 16 | >75 | >3 | >15 |
| | HT-29 | NA | 0 | >15 | 0 | >30 | >10 | >55 |
| | | | 4 | >25 | 4 | >35 | >2 | >57 |
| | | | 8 | >40 | 8 | >55 | >5 | >35 |
| | | | 16 | >50 | 16 | >65 | >3 | >25 |
| Leukaemia | HL60 | NA | 0 | >1 | 0 | 27.2 | 3.6 | 69.1 |
| | | | 1 | >5 | 0.1 | 47.4 | 6 | 46.6 |
| | | | 2 | >15 | 0.2 | 66.6 | 8.3 | 25.1 |
| | | | 3 | >25 | 0.4 | 76.1 | 7.7 | 16.1 |
| | | | 4 | >30 | 0.8 | 82.7 | 6.8 | 10.5 |
| | K562 | NA | 0 | >0.1 | 0 | 43.3 | 8.4 | 48.3 |
| | | | 1 | >10 | 0.1 | 47.8 | 7.8 | 44.4 |
| | | | 2 | >12 | 0.2 | 51.4 | 11.2 | 37.4 |
| | | | 3 | >20 | 0.4 | 67.6 | 11.7 | 20.7 |
| | | | 4 | >35 | 0.8 | 75.2 | 11.4 | 13.4 |

[5]　Gong, K.; Xie, J.; Yi, H., et al. *Biochem. J.* **2012**, *443*, 735-746.
[6]　Liu, L.; Chen, B.; Qin, S., et al. *Biochem. Biophys. Res. Commun.* **2010**, *392*, 190-195.
[7]　Qiao, Z.; Ren, S.; Li, W., et al. *Biochem. Biophys. Res. Commun.* **2013**, *434*, 95-101.
[8]　Shi, X. X.; Ma, F.; Li, H. H., et al. *Chin. Clin. Oncol.* **2013**, *18*, 1057-1062.
[9]　Chen, J.; Zhou, W. Q.; Chen, H., et al. *Chin. J. Dermatol.* **2009**, *42*, 255-261.

*Continued*

| Source | Cell Line | IC$_{50}$ (μM) | Apoptosis | | Cell Cycle Distribution (%) | | | |
|---|---|---|---|---|---|---|---|---|
| | | | Conc. (μM) | %Apoptosis | Conc. (μM) | G$_0$/G$_1$ | G$_2$/M | S |
| Pancreatic cancer | BxPC-3 | <25 | 25 | ~5 | 0 | >80 | >10 | >2 |
| | | | | | 12.5 | >70 | >15 | >5 |
| | | | | | 25 | >65 | >20 | >1 |
| | | | | | 50 | >60 | >20 | >1 |
| | PANC-1 | <50 | 25 | >5 | 0 | >70 | >10 | >10 |
| | | | | | 12.5 | >70 | >15 | >15 |
| | | | | | 25 | >75 | >20 | >5 |
| | | | | | 50 | >75 | >20 | >1 |
| Malignant melanoma | A375 | 250 | 0 | 10.4 ± 0.96 | 0 | 38.7 ± 3.36 | 15.7 ± 0.23 | 45.5 ± 3.50 |
| | | | 62.5 | 80.3 ± 3.06 | 62.5 | 76.3 ± 6.06 | 12.2 ± 2.68 | 11.4 ± 3.38 |
| | | | 125 | 79.5 ± 5.70 | 125 | 82.8 ± 0.74 | 10.4 ± 0.62 | 6.81 ± 1.34 |
| | | | 250 | 83.1 ± 6.90 | 250 | 88.9 ± 5.29 | 8.57 ± 4.42 | 2.52 ± 0.87 |
| TNBC | CAL-51 | 19.6 | 0 | 0.65 ± 0.07 | NA | NA | NA | NA |
| | | | 10 | 20.5 ± 1.41 | NA | NA | NA | NA |
| | | | 15 | 32.4 ± 2.12 | NA | NA | NA | NA |
| | | | 20 | 50.1 ± 2.05 | NA | NA | NA | NA |

TNBC: Three negative breast cancer.

Table 7    The Combination of Chidamide and Platinum Drugs in NSCLC Cells[10]

| Compound | Cell Line | Sensitivity, IC$_{50}$ (μM) | | Combination Index Value | | | |
|---|---|---|---|---|---|---|---|
| | | Treated Alone | Combined with 0.3 μM Chidamide | ED$_{25}$ | ED$_{50}$ | ED$_{75}$ | Mean |
| Chidamide | A549 | 8.69 | NA | NA | NA | NA | NA |
| | NCI-H157 | 27.7 | NA | NA | NA | NA | NA |
| Carboplatin | A549 | 152 | 67.8 | 0.550 | 0.874 | NA | 0.712 |
| | NCI-H157 | 90.0 | 56.3 | 0.640 | 0.637 | 0.639 | 0.639 |
| Cisplatin | A549 | 39.4 | 25.1 | 0.627 | 0.671 | 0.787 | 0.695 |
| | NCI-H157 | 22.0 | 10.3 | 0.388 | 0.477 | 0.600 | 0.488 |
| Oxaliplatin | A549 | >50 | >50 | 0.880 | NA | NA | 0.880 |
| | NCI-H157 | >50 | 35.8 | 0.290 | NA | NA | 0.290 |

Combination index values <1.0 were consistent with synergism, thus the lower the value was, the greater the synergism achieved.

[10]  Zhou, Y.; Pan, D. S.; Shan, S., et al. *Biomedicine & pharmacotherapy* **2014**, *68*, 483-491.

## *In Vivo* **Efficacy**

Table 8    *In Vivo* Anti-tumor Effect of Chidamide in Human Tumor Xenografts Models[4, 5, 11]

| Xenograft System | | | Dose (mg/kg) | Route & Schedule (Day) | Effect | |
|---|---|---|---|---|---|---|
| Cell Line | Type | Animal | | | ED (mg/kg/day) | Finding |
| PaTu8988 | Human pancreatic carcinoma | Balb/c nude mouse | 12.5, 50 | i.p., QD × (day 7-21) | 12.5 | Tumor growth inhibition: 46.7% and 60.4%. Tumor weight: 0.20 g at 12.5 mg/kg (vehicle: 0.37 g, $P$ <0.01). No gross body weight loss. |
| HL60 | Human chronic myelogenous leukaemia | Balb/c nude mouse | 12.5, 25, 50 | p.o., QD × 20 | NA | Tumor growth inhibition: 19.5%, 23.8% and 41.8%. Tumor weight: 5.4 g at 50 mg/kg (vehicle: 9.4 g, $P$ <0.01). No gross body weight loss. |
| HCT-8[a] | Human colorectal carcinoma | Balb/c nude mouse (male) | 12.5, 25, 50 | p.o., QD × 20-28 | 12.5 | Inhibited tumor size and weight in dose-dependent manner. Well-tolerated: No gross body weight loss. |
| A549[a] | Human lung carcinoma | Balb/c nude mouse (male) | 12.5, 25, 50 | p.o., QD × 20-28 | 12.5 | |
| BEL-7402[a] | Human liver carcinoma | Balb/c nude mouse (male) | 12.5, 25, 50 | p.o., QD × 20-28 | 12.5 | |
| MCF-7[a] | Human breast carcinoma | Balb/c nude mouse (female) | 12.5, 25, 50 | p.o., QD × 20-28 | 12.5 | |

[a] Tumor cells as a tumor fragment (about 1 mm³) were transplanted subcutaneously into the flank of a mouse with a trocar needle.    Treatment was started 3 days after inoculation, orally once daily for 20-28 days, depending on the tumor type.

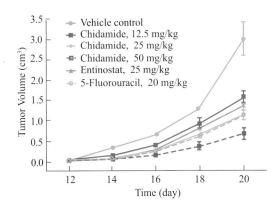

**Study:** Anti-tumor in human HCT-8 tumor xenograft mouse models.

**Animal:** Athymic nude mouse.

**Model:** HCT-8 cells as tumor fragments (1 mm³) were transplanted s.c. into the flank of a mouse with a trocar needle.

**Administration:** Treated daily for 20 days, p.o., chidamide: 12.5, 25 and 50 mg/kg/day; Vehicle control: NA.

**Starting:** 3 days after inoculation.

**Test:** Tumor volume, every 3 days.

**Result:** Treatment with 12.5-50 mg/kg chidamide resulted in dose-dependent reduction of tumor size and tumor weight.

Figure A    Anti-tumor Activity of Chidamide in Human Tumor Xenografts Models[4]

[4]  Ning, Z. Q.; Li, Z. B.; Newman, M. J., et al. *Cancer Chemother. Pharmacol.* **2012**, *69*, 901-909.
[5]  Gong, K.; Xie, J.; Yi, H., et al. *Biochem. J.* **2012**, *443*, 735-746.
[11]  Zhao, B.; He, T. *Oncology reports* **2015**, *33*, 304-310.

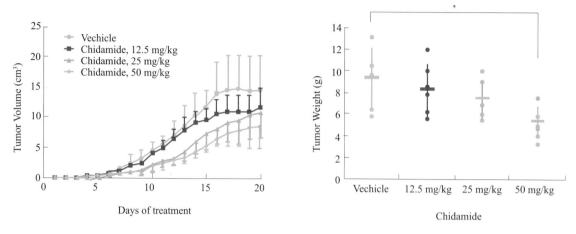

Figure B  Anti-tumor Activity of Chidamide in HL60 Tumor Xenografts Models[5]

**Study:** Anti-tumor in HL60 human chronic myelogenous leukaemia tumor xenograft mouse models.

**Animal:** Balb/c nude mouse (male).

**Model:** $2 \times 10^7$ HL60 cells were transplanted s.c. into the flank of a mouse.

**Administration:** Orally treated daily for 20 days, chidamide: 12.5, 25 and 50 mg/kg/day; Vehicle: NA.

**Starting:** Tumors were established ($200 \text{ mm}^3$).

**Test:** Tumor volume and body mass, every day.

**Result:** 41.8% tumor growth inhibition and tumor mass decreases at 50 mg/kg/day.   No gross body mass loss.

## 4   ADME & Drug-Drug Interaction

### Summary

Absorption of Chidamide

❖ Exhibited dose-related increases in AUC and $C_{max}$ in the dose range of 25 to 50 mg after oral administration in humans.

❖ Was absorbed slowly ($T_{max} = 3.5\text{-}10$ h) in patients.

❖ Plasma drug concentrations generally returned to close to baseline level within 48 h, but remained quantifiable at 72 h after single dose.

❖ Showed a long half-life ranging between 16.8-18.3 h in patients, longer than that in rats (11.9 h), after oral administrations.

❖ The apparent volumes of distribution were 118 L/kg in rats and 790-1517 L in humans, after oral administrations.

❖ The values of clearance were 6.8 L/h in rats and 35-59 L/h in patients after oral administrations.

Distribution of Chidamide

❖ The drug was extensively distributed into most tissues at 2 h post-dose, and relatively higher concentration levels were observed in gastrointestinal tract, liver, pancreas and kidneys.

❖ Small amounts of the drug was detected in gastrointestinal tract at 96 h post-dose.

Metabolism of Chidamide

❖ The metabolites of [$^3$H]chidamide were found in plasma, feces, urine and bile of rats after intragastric administration, and 50% of parent drug was excreted from rats.

Excretion of Chidamide

❖ Was predominantly excreted in feces in rats, accounting for the majority of the administered dose (63.3%) following oral administration to rats at 336 h post-dose and urinary excretion accounted for 18.8% of the administered dose, indicating the drug was eliminated completely with no accumulation.

❖ Bile excretion accounted for 4.28% of the administered dose at 48 h post-dose in rats.

❖ The parent drug and metabolites were detected in plasma, feces, urine and bile of rats, and the parent drug accounted for approximately 50% of the total radioactivity.

[5]  Gong, K.; Xie, J.; Yi, H., et al. *Biochem. J.* **2012**, *443*, 735-746.

## Absorption

Table 10   *In Vivo* Pharmacokinetic Parameters of Chidamide in Rats after Single Oral Dose of Chidamide[12]

| Species | Route | Dose (mg/kg) | $T_{max}$ (h) | $C_{max}$ (ng/mL) | $AUC_{inf}$ (ng·h/mL) | $AUC_{0-t}$ (ng·h/mL) | $T_{1/2}$ (h) | Cl/F (L/h) | $V_d$/F (L/kg) |
|---|---|---|---|---|---|---|---|---|---|
| SD rat (male) | p.o. | 30 | NA | 4986 ± 2826 | 5013 ± 2095 | 4600 ± 2121 | 11.9 ± 5.4 | 6.8 ± 2.5 | 118 ± 65.5 |

Mean ± SD (n = 6).

Table 11   *In Vivo* Pharmacokinetic Parameters of Chidamide in Humans after Single Oral Dose of Chidamide[13]

| Species | Route | Dose (mg) | $T_{max}$ (h) | $C_{max}$ (ng/mL) | $AUC_{0-t}$ (ng·h/mL) | $AUC_{inf}$ (ng·h/mL) | $T_{1/2}$ (h) | Cl/F (L/h) | $V_d$/F (L) |
|---|---|---|---|---|---|---|---|---|---|
| Patient (male & female) | p.o. | 25 | 10.0 ± 10.5 | 39.7 ± 12.4 | 809 ± 390 | 867 ± 398 | 16.8 ± 4.9 | 35 ± 18 | 790 ± 321 |
| | | 32.5 | 3.5 ± 4.5 | 122 ± 126 | 828 ± 509 | 875 ± 512 | 17.5 ± 4.2 | 59 ± 46 | 1517 ± 1241 |
| | | 50 | 4.0 ± 4.3 | 163 ± 156 | 1120 ± 438 | 1180 ± 461 | 18.3 ± 4.2 | 50 ± 24 | 1285 ± 580 |

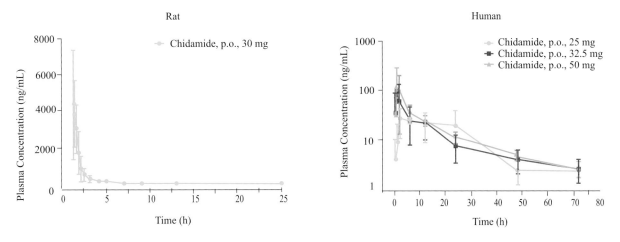

Figure C   *In Vivo* Plasma Concentration-Time Profiles of Chidamide in Rats and Humans after Single Oral Dose Of Chidamide[12, 13]

## Distribution

### Key Findings:[14]

❖ In rats after single oral administration of [³H]chidamide:
- The drug was extensively distributed into most tissues at 2 h post-dose, and relatively higher concentration levels were observed in gastrointestinal tract, liver, pancreas and kidneys.
- Small amounts of the drug was detected in gastrointestinal tract at 96 h post-dose.

## Metabolism

Table 12   Radioactivity of Chidamide in Plasma and Feces of Rats after Single Oral Dose of [³H]Chidamide[13]

| Matrix | Time (h) | Percentage of Total Radioactivity (%) |
|---|---|---|
| Plasma | 2 | 40.2 |
| Bile | 0-5 | 53.4 |
| Feces | 0-24 | 50.4 |
| Urine | 0-24 | 49.9 |

[12]   Wang, X. Q.; Chen, M. C.; Wen, C. C., et al. *Biomed. Chromatogr.* **2013**, *27*, 1801-1806.
[13]   Dong, M.; Ning, Z. Q.; Xing, P. Y., et al. *Cancer Chemother. Pharmacol.* **2012**, *69*, 1413-1422.
[14]   Wang, X.; Meng, X. M.; Meng, Z. Y., et al. *Pharm. J. Chin. PLA* **2006**, *22*, 113-115.

**Key Findings:**[15]

❖ The metabolites of [³H]chidamide were found in plasma, feces, urine and bile of rats after intragastric administration, and 50% of parent drug was excreted from rats.

## Excretion

Table 13    Excretion Profiles of [³H]Chidamide in Rats after Single Oral Dose of Chidamide[15]

| Species | Dose (mg/kg) | Time (h) | Bile (% of dose) | Urine (% of dose) | Feces (% of dose) | Recovery of Feces and Urine (% of dose) |
|---|---|---|---|---|---|---|
| Wistar rat (male) | 1.2 | 5 | 1.92 ± 1.15 | - | - | - |
| | | 24 | 2.77 ± 1.87 | 4.06 ± 2.28 | 51.1 ± 16.6 | 55.2 ± 17.0 |
| | | 48 | 4.28 ± 2.72 | 13.4 ± 3.70 | 59.7 ± 12.1 | 73.1 ± 13.3 |
| | | 72 | - | 13.6 ± 3.57 | 60.2 ± 12.2 | 73.8 ± 13.3 |
| | | 96 | - | 14.3 ± 3.63 | 60.5 ± 12.2 | 74.8 ± 13.8 |
| | | 120 | - | 14.6 ± 3.54 | 60.8 ± 12.2 | 75.3 ± 13.8 |
| | | 144 | - | 15.4 ± 3.87 | 61.0 ± 12.2 | 76.4 ± 14.4 |
| | | 192 | - | 16.4 ± 3.76 | 62.0 ± 12.5 | 78.3 ± 14.3 |
| | | 216 | - | 18.8 ± 3.21 | 62.3 ± 12.6 | 81.1 ± 13.2 |
| | | 336 | - | 18.8 ± 3.21 | 63.3 ± 12.4 | 82.2 ± 13.2 |

Vehicle: 0.2% CMCNa and 0.1% Tween 80 solution, n = 5.    Recovery included urine and feces.

## 5    Non-Clinical Toxicology

The data of non-clinical toxicology was not available.

[15]  Wang, X.; Zhou, M. X.; Meng, Z. Y., et al. *Bull. Acad. Mil. Med. Sci.* **2006**, *30*, 440-442.

# CHAPTER

## 9

---

## Daclatasvir Dihydrochloride

# Daclatasvir Dihydrochloride

## (Daklinza®)

Research code: BMS-790052

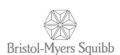
Bristol-Myers Squibb

## 1 General Information

❖ Daclatasvir dihydrochloride is an inhibitor of NS5A, which was first approved in Jul 2014 by PMDA of Japan.

❖ Daclatasvir dihydrochloride was discovered, developed and marketed by Bristol-Myers Squibb.

❖ Daclatasvir dihydrochloride is a hepatitis C virus (HCV) NS5A inhibitor, which binds to the N-terminus of NS5A and inhibits both viral RNA replication and virion assembly.

❖ Daclatasvir dihydrochloride is indicated for the treatment of patients with chronic HCV infection.

❖ Available as tablet, with each containing 60 mg of daclatasvir and the recommended dose is 60 mg orally once daily until disease progression or unacceptable toxicity.

❖ Sales of Daklinza® were 201 and 1315 million US$ in 2014 and 2015, respectively, referring to the financial reports of Bristol-Myers Squibb.

## Key Approvals around the World*

|  | Japan (PMDA) | EU (EMA) | US (FDA) |
|---|---|---|---|
| First approval date | 07/04/2014 | 08/22/2014 | 07/24/2015 |
| Application or approval No. | 22600AMX 00764000 | EMEA/H/C/ 003768 | NDA 206843 |
| Brand name | Daklinza® | Daklinza® | Daklinza® |
| Indication | HCV infection | HCV infection | HCV infection |
| Authorisation holder | BMS | BMS | BMS |

BMS: Bristol-Myers Squibb.

* Till Mar 2016, it had not been approved by CFDA (China).

## Active Ingredient

*Molecular formula*: $C_{40}H_{50}N_8O_6 \cdot 2HCl$
*Molecular weight*: 811.80
*CAS No.*: 1009119-64-5 (Daclatasvir)
1009119-65-6 (Daclatasvir dihydro-chloride)
*Chemical name*: Dimethyl N, N'-([1,1'-biphenyl]-4,4'-diylbis{1H-imidazole-5,2-diyl-[(2S)-pyrrolidine-2,1-diyl][(1S)-3-methyl-1-oxobutane-1,2-diyl]}) dicarbamate dihydrochloride

*Parameters of Lipinski's "Rule of 5"*

| MW[a] | $H_D$ | $H_A$ | FRB[b] | PSA[b] | cLogP[b] |
|---|---|---|---|---|---|
| 738.88 | 4 | 14 | 13 | 175Å² | 2.51 ± 1.35 |

[a] Molecular weight of daclatasvir. [b] Calculated by ACD/Labs software V11.02.

## Drug Product*

*Dosage route*: Oral
*Strength*: 60 mg (Daclatasvir)
*Dosage form*: Tablet
*Inactive ingredient*: Anhydrous lactose, microcrystalline cellulose, croscarmellose sodium, silicon dioxide, magnesium stearate, hypromellose, titanium oxide, macrogol 400, FD&C blue #2/indigo carmine aluminum lake and yellow ferric oxide.
*Recommended dose*: The recommended dose is 60 mg once daily with or without food in combination with asunaprevir.
The recommended treatment duration is 24 weeks.

* Sourced from Japan PMDA drug label information

# 2 Key Patents Information

## Summary

❖ Daklinza® (Daclatasvir dihydrochloride) was initially approved by PMDA of Japan on Jul 04, 2014.

❖ Daclatasvir was developed by Bristol-Myers Squibb, and its compound patent application was filed as PCT application by Bristol-Myers Squibb in 2007.

❖ The compound patent will expire in 2027 foremost, which has been granted in the United States, Japan, Europe and China successively.

Table 1    Daclatasvir's Compound Patent Protection in Drug-Mainstream Country

| Country | Publication/Patent NO. | Application Date | Granted Date | Estimated Expiry Date |
|---------|------------------------|------------------|--------------|-----------------------|
| WO | WO2008021927A2 | 08/09/2007 | / | / |
| US | US8329159B2 | 08/08/2007 | 12/11/2012 | 04/13/2028[a] |
| | US8642025B2 | 08/08/2007 | 02/04/2014 | 08/11/2027[b] |
| EP | EP2049522B1 | 08/09/2007 | 05/14/2014 | 08/09/2027 |
| JP | JP5235882B2 | 08/09/2007 | 07/10/2013 | 11/06/2028[c] |
| | JP5769749B2 | 08/09/2007 | 08/26/2015 | 08/09/2027 |
| CN | CN101558059B | 08/09/2007 | 12/03/2014 | 08/09/2027 |

[a] The term of this patent is extended by 249 days.    [b] The term of this patent is extended by 3 days (TD).    [c] The term of this patent is extended by 455 days.

Table 2    Originator's International Patent Application List (Patent Family)

| Publication NO. | Title | Applicant/Assignee/Owner | Publication Date |
|-----------------|-------|--------------------------|------------------|
| **Technical Subjects** | **Active Ingredient (Free Base)'s Formula or Structure and Preparation** | | |
| WO2008021927A2 | Hepatitis C virus inhibitors | Bristol-Myers Squibb | 02/21/2008 |
| **Technical Subjects** | **Salt, Crystal, Polymorphic, Solvate (Hydrate), Isomer, Derivative Etc. and Preparation** | | |
| WO2009020825A1 | Process for synthesizing compounds useful for treating hepatitis C | Bristol-Myers Squibb | 02/12/2009 |
| WO2009020828A1 | Crystalline form of methyl ((1S)-1-(((2S)-2-(5-(4'-(2-((2S)-1-((2S)-2-((methoxycarbonyl)amino)-3-methylbutanoyl)-2-pyrro-lidinyl)-1H-imidazol-5-yl)-4-biphenylyl)-1H-imidazol-2-yl)-1-pyrrolidinyl)carbonyl)-2-methylpropyl)carbamate dihydrochloride salt | Bristol-Myers Squibb | 02/12/2009 |
| WO2009102325A1 | Imidazolyl biphenyl imidazoles as hepatitis C virus inhibitors | Bristol-Myers Squibb | 08/20/2009 |
| **Technical Subjects** | **Combination Including at Least Two Active Ingredients** | | |
| WO2011046811A1 | Combinations of a specific HCV NS5A inhibitor and an HCV NS3 protease inhibitor | Bristol-Myers Squibb | 04/21/2011 |
| WO2012018829A1 | Combinations of hepatitis C virus inhibitors | Bristol-Myers Squibb | 02/09/2012 |
| WO2013106520A1 | Hepatitis C virus inhibitors | Bristol-Myers Squibb | 07/18/2013 |

The data was updated until Jan 2016.

# 3 Chemistry

## Route 1: Original Discovery Route

*Synthetic Route*: Bromination of commercial 4,4'-diacetylbiphenyl **1** gave 4,4'-bis(bromoacetyl)biphenyl **2** in 82% yield. Alkylation of *N*-Boc-L-proline **3** with **2** gave symmetric diester **4** which was treated with ammonium acetate to effect cyclization of the bis-ketoester to provide bis-imidazole **5** in 63% yield over two steps. Acidic removal of the Boc protecting groups followed by recrystallization provided bis-pyrrolidine hydrochloride **6** in 74% yield. Acylation of **6** with *N*-(methoxycarbonyl)-L-valine **7** using EDCI and HOBt furnished declatasvir. The dihydrochloride salt was then prepared and purified with Cuno Zet Carbon® followed by crystallization to give declatasvir dihydrochloride in 74% yield across two steps with the overall yield of 28%.[1-9]

[1]  Pack, S. K.; Geng, P.; Smith, M. J., et al. WO2009020825A1, **2009**.
[2]  Pack, S. K.; Geng, P.; Smith, M. J., et al. US7728027B2, **2010**.
[3]  Kim, S.; Gao, Q.; Yang, F. WO2009020828A1, **2009**.
[4]  Kim, S.; Gao, Q.; Yang, F. US8629171B2, **2014**.
[5]  Bachand, C.; Belema, M.; Deon, D. H., et al. WO2008021927A2, **2008**.
[6]  Belema, M.; Nguyen, V. N. US8329159B2, **2012**.
[7]  Bachand, C.; Belema, M.; Deon, D. H., et al. US8303944B2, **2012**.
[8]  Bachand, C.; Belema, M.; Deon, D. H., et al. US20090068140A1, **2009**.
[9]  Kim, S.; Gao, Q.; Yang, F. US20100158862A1, **2010**.

## Route 2

*Synthetic Route*: Huenig's base-promoted condensation of 2-bromo-1-(4-bromophenyl)ethanone **1** with Boc-L-proline **2** in MeCN and then ammonium acetate-mediated thermal cyclization afforded **3**. Acidic liberation of free amine accompanied by successively amine trapping with 4M HCl to provide pyrrolidine hydrochloride **4**. Peptide coupling general procedure then delivered amide **6**, which converted to the crucial boronate **8** for the key Suzuki coupling with another amide molecule **6** ultimately to give rise to daclatasvir.[10]

## 4  Pharmacology

### Summary

Mechanism of Action

❖ Daclatasvir, a small molecule inhibitor of HCV NS5A, binds to the new *N*-terminus of NS5A and inhibits both viral RNA replication and virion assembly.

❖ In biochemical assay daclatasvir *S*-stereoisomer inhibited NS5A ($EC_{50}$ = 33 nM), but *R*-stereoisomer did not ($EC_{50}$ >10 μM).

❖ Daclatasvir had no significant inhibition or induction in a panel of 36 targets assay at 10 μM, including standard receptors, enzymes and ion channels or a panel of receptors for rat aldosterone, human angiotensin, atrial natriuretic factor and vasopressin, except the sodium ion channel (65% inhibition).[11]

*In Vitro* Efficacy

❖ Anti-HCV replicon in Huh-7 cell line:
  • HCV genotype 1a/1b/2a/4a/5a/6a: $EC_{50}$ = 1.2-54 pM.
  • HCV genotype 3a: $EC_{50}$ = 140-190 pM.
❖ The antiviral activity in presence of 40% human serum:
  • 1a/1b: 1.7-fold increase of $EC_{50}$.

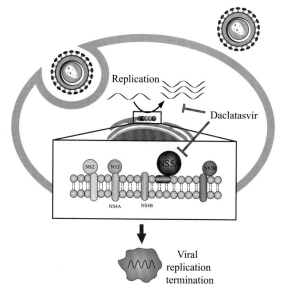

[10]  Thibeault, C.; Edwards, P. J.; Kuhn, C., et al. WO2012048421A1, **2012**.
[11]  Japan Pharmaceuticals and Medical Devices Agency (PMDA) Database.  http://www.pmda.go.jp/drugs/2014/P201400112/index.html (accessed Mar 2016).

❖ Resistant development of daclatasvir in HCV genotype 3-6 (NS5A substitutions):
- HCV-3a: L31F + Y93H.
- HCV-4a: L30H, R30G/H/S, L30H + Y93H.
- HCV-5a: L31F/V, L31F + K56R.
- HCV-6a: P32S + T58A/S, L31M + P32L/S.

❖ Antiviral activities against HCV containing NS5A substitutions (fold change for $EC_{50}$):
- HCV Genotype 1a:
  - Q30, Y93: 1227->330000 folds; M28, L31: 340-4596 folds.
  - Double substitutions: >10707 folds (except T21I-L31M/M28T-Q30H/H58P-Y93H: 318-1205 folds).
- HCV Genotype 1b:
  - P32del: 389105 folds.
  - Double and triple: 2521-18949 folds.

## Mechanism of Action

Table 3  Binding Efficacy of NS5A Inhibitors[11]

| Type | Inhibitor | $EC_{50}$ (nM) |
|---|---|---|
| Biotinylated NS5A inhibitor | BMS-634671 | 33 |
| | BMS-666690 | >10000 |
| Radioactive and photoaffinity labeled NS5A inhibitor | BMS-642194 | 7 |
| Biotin and photocrosslinking labeled NS5A inhibitor | BMS-642350 | 29 |

BMS-634671: Daclatasvir S-stereoisomer.   BMS-666690: Daclatasvir R-stereoisomer.

## *In Vitro* Efficacy

Table 4  Anti-HCV Activities of Daclatasvir and Its Metabolites in Replicon Cell Lines[11, 12]

| HCV Replicon Genotype | Strain | Method | $EC_{50}$ (nM) | | |
|---|---|---|---|---|---|
| | | | Daclatasvir | Metabolite 2 | Metabolite 4 |
| 1a | H77c | Luciferase | 0.020 ± 0.009 | ND | ND |
| | | FRET | 0.050 ± 0.013 | 19 ± 5 | 14 ± 2 |
| | | Taqman | 0.003 ± 0.0006 | 17 ± 5 | 14 ± 2 |
| 1b | Con1 | Luciferase | 0.004 ± 0.002 | 0.4 ± 0.20 | ND |
| | | FRET | 0.009 ± 0.004 | 0.82 ± 0.23 | 0.07 ± 0.03 |
| | | Taqman | 0.0012 ± 0.0007 | 0.63 ± 0.10 | ND |
| 2a | JFH-1 | Luciferase | 0.034 ± 0.019 | ND | ND |
| 3a | - | FRET | 0.146 ± 0.034 | 3.8 ± 1 | 50 ± 30 |
| | 1-100 in Con1 replicon | Luciferase | 0.19 ± 0.07 | ND | ND |
| | 3 additional clinical isolates in JFH-1 replicon 1, 2, 4 | Luciferase | 0.14-1.25 | ND | ND |
| 4a | - | FRET | 0.012 ± 0.004 | 0.66 ± 0.13 | 1.6 ± 1.4 |
| | Full genotype in Con1 replicon | Luciferase | 0.007 ± 0.003 | ND | ND |
| | 2 additional clinical isolates 21, 23 | Luciferase | 0.007-0.013 | ND | ND |
| 5a | - | FRET | 0.033 ± 0.010 | 0.0019 ± 0.0004 | 0.416 ± 0.065 |
| | 1-100 in JFH-1 replicon | Luciferase | 0.019 ± 0.007 | ND | ND |
| | 2 additional clinical isolates 7, 9 | Luciferase | 0.003-0.004 | ND | ND |
| 6a | 1-429 in JFH-1 replicon | Luciferase | 0.054 ± 0.008 | ND | ND |

Metabolite 2: Pyrrolidine-hydroxylated rearraged daclatasvir.   Metabolite 4: Descarboxymethyl daclatasvir.   FRET: Fluorescent resonance energy transfer.   Therapeutic index: Daclatasvir dihydrochloride = 1900000 nM, Metabolite 2 = 21000 nM, Metabolite 4 >330000 nM.   Therapeutic index = Genotype 1b (Con1) in replicon cells $CC_{50}/EC_{50}$ (FRET), $CC_{50}$: 50% Cytotoxic concentration, $EC_{50}$: 50% Effective concentration.   ND: Not determined.

[11]  PMDA Database.   http://www.pmda.go.jp/drugs/2014/P201400112/index.html (accessed Mar 2016).
[12]  U.S. Food and Drug Administration (FDA) Database.   http://www.accessdata.fda.gov/drugsatfda_docs/nda/2015/206843Orig1s000MicroR.pdf (accessed Mar 2016).

Table 5    *In Vitro* Activity of Daclatasvir-resistant in HCV Genotype 3-6 NS5A[13-15]

| Replicon | Selection Conc. (nM) | EC$_{50}$ (nM) | NS5A Amino Acid Substitution |
|---|---|---|---|
| HCV3a-1 | 0 | 0.47 ± 0.08 | None |
| | 10 | >1000 | L31F, Y93H |
| | 100 | >1000 | L31F, Y93H |
| HCV4a-20 | 0 | 0.01 ± 0.004 | None |
| | 0.2 | 0.64 ± 0.35 | L30H |
| | 1.0 | 1.32 ± 0.78 | L30H |
| HCV4a-21 | 0 | 0.01 ± 0.002 | None |
| | 0.1 | 2.55 ± 0.07 | R30G/H/S |
| | 1.0 | 1.00 ± 0.06 | R30G/H/S |
| | 10 | 21.1 ± 0.25 | R30G |
| HCV4a-23 | 0 | 0.02 ± 0.001 | None |
| | 0.1 | 4.4 ± 1.5 | L30H, Y93H |
| | 1.0 | 14.2 ± 0.4 | L30H, Y93H |
| | 10 | 16.0 ± 3.0 | L30H |
| HCV5a-7 | DMSO | 0.0054 ± 0.0002 | None |
| | 1 | 14 ± 0.22 | L31F/V |
| | 10 | 37 ± 0.51 | L31F, K56R |
| | 100 | No cells survived | NA |
| HCV5a-9 | DMSO | 0.0042 ± 0.0006 | None |
| | 1 | 4.5 ± 0.35 | L31F/V |
| | 10 | No cells survived | NA |
| | 100 | No cells survived | NA |
| HCV6a-16 | DMSO | 0.041 ± 0.004 | None |
| | 1 | 6.4 ± 1.3 | P32S, T58A/S |
| | 10 | 59.2 ± 8.2 | L31M, P32L/S |
| | 100 | 323 ± 6.5 | P32L |

Table 6    *In Vitro* Antiviral Effects of Daclatasvir with 40% Human Serum[11]

| HCV Genotype | %Serum | EC$_{50}$ (nM) | Effect (fold increase of the EC$_{50}$ value) |
|---|---|---|---|
| 1a | 10 | 41 ± 13 | 1 |
| 1a | 40 | 68 ± 16 | 1.7 |
| 1b | 10 | 7 ± 2 | 1 |
| 1b | 40 | 12 ± 3 | 1.7 |

[11]  PMDA Database.   http://www.pmda.go.jp/drugs/2014/P201400112/index.html (accessed Mar 2016).
[13]  Wang, C.; Valera, L.; Jia, L., et al. *Antimicrob. Agents Chemother.* **2013**, *57*, 611-613.
[14]  Wang, C.; Jia, L.; Huang, H., et al. *Antimicrob. Agents Chemother.* **2012**, *56*, 1588-1590.
[15]  Wang, C.; Jia, L.; O'Boyle, D. R., et al. *Antimicrob. Agents Chemother.* **2014**, *58*, 5155-5163.

Table 7    Antiviral Selectivity of Daclatasvir in Cell Lines[11, 12]

| Replicon/Virus | Cell Line | Effect | | Replicon/Virus | Cell Line | Effect | |
| | | EC$_{50}$ (nM) | Selectivity Index | | | EC$_{50}$ (nM) | Selectivity Index |
| --- | --- | --- | --- | --- | --- | --- | --- |
| HCV replicon (1b) | HuH-7 | 0.009 | NA | Influenza | MDBK | >100000 | >11000000 |
| HCV genotype 2a (JFH-1) virus | HuH-7 | 0.020 | NA | CPIV | Vero | 26000 | 2900000 |
| BVDV replicon | HuH-7 | 9000 | 1000000 | Human rhinovirus | MRC5 | >29000 | >3200000 |
| BVDV | MDBK | 12000 | 1300000 | Coxsackie virus | MRC5 | >29000 | >3200000 |
| HIV | MT2 | >20 | >2200000 | Poliovirus | MRC5 | >29000 | >3200000 |
| HSV-1/HSV-2 | Vero | >11000 | >1200000 | Human coronavirus | MRC5 | >29000 | >3200000 |

BVDV: Bovine viral diarrhea virus.   HIV: Human immunodeficiency virus.   HSV-1, 2: Herpes simplex virus type 1, 2.   CPIV: Canine parainfluenza virus.   HuH-7: Human hepatoma cell line.   MDBK: Madin-Darby bovine kidney cells.   MT2: Human T cell line.   MRC5: Lung fibroblast cell line.   Vero: Monkey kidney epithelial cells.   Selectivity index = Other replicon or virus EC$_{50}$/HCV replicon (genotype 1b) EC$_{50}$.

Table 8    *In Vitro* Resistance Profile of Daclatasvir in Transient Replicon Replication Assays[11, 12]

| Type | Amino Acid Substitution | Replication Rate (%) | Anti-HCV | |
| | | | EC$_{50}$ (nM) | Fold Increase of the EC$_{50}$ Value |
| --- | --- | --- | --- | --- |
| | Wild type | 100 | 0.00594 | 1 |
| | M28A | 27 | 27.3 | 4596 |
| | M28T | 31 | 4.05 | 682 |
| | Q30D | 171 | >1999 | 336532 |
| | Q30E | 130 | 150 | 25252 |
| | Q30G | 54 | 51.0 | 8586 |
| | Q30H | 75 | 8.78 | 1478 |
| | Q30K | 19 | 146 | 24579 |
| | Q30R | 41 | 7.29 | 1227 |
| | L31M | 55 | 2.02 | 340 |
| | L31V | 117 | 20.1 | 3384 |
| | H58D | 92 | 2.97 | 500 |
| | Y93C | 11 | 11.1 | 1869 |
| | Y93H | 18 | 32.3 | 5438 |
| Genotype 1a | Y93N | 13 | 282 | 47475 |
| | T21I-L31M | 82 | 3.23 | 544 |
| | M28T-Q30H | 31 | 622 | 104714 |
| | M28T-Q30K | 15 | >1999 | >336532 |
| | M28T-Q30R | 76 | 356 | 59933 |
| | M28V-Q30R | 147 | 1.89 | 318 |
| | Q30E-Y93H | 6 | 404 | 68013 |
| | Q30H-H58D | 28 | >1999 | >336532 |
| | Q30H-Y93H | 20 | 553 | 93098 |
| | Q30R-L31M | 54 | 1172 | 197306 |
| | Q30R-H58D | 60 | 2520 | 424242 |
| | Q30R-E62D | 30 | 151 | 25421 |
| | Q30R-Y93H | 6 | 341 | 57407 |
| | L31M-H58D | 41 | 398 | 67003 |

[11]  PMDA Database.   http://www.pmda.go.jp/drugs/2014/P201400112/index.html (accessed Mar 2016).
[12]  FDA Database.   http://www.accessdata.fda.gov/drugsatfda_docs/nda/2015/206843Orig1s000MicroR.pdf (accessed Mar 2016).

*Continued*

| Type | Amino Acid Substitution | Replication Rate (%) | Anti-HCV | |
|---|---|---|---|---|
| | | | EC$_{50}$ (nM) | Fold Increase of the EC$_{50}$ Value |
| Genotype 1a | L31V-V37A | 10 | 63.6 | 10707 |
| | L31V-H58P | 100 | 72.9 | 12273 |
| | L31V-Y93H | 20 | >1000 | 168350 |
| | H58P-Y93H | 22 | 7.16 | 1205 |
| Genotype 1b | Wild type | 100 | 0.00257 | 1 |
| | P32del | 29.1 | >1000 | 389105 |
| | L31I-Y93H | 43 | 6.48 | 2521 |
| | L31M-Y93H | 70 | 18.2 | 7082 |
| | L31V-Y93H | 49.9 | 37.9 | 14747 |
| | L31V-Q54H-Y93H | 189 | 48.7 | 18949 |

Replicon cells were culturing for 4-5 weeks with daclatasvir dihydrochloride.    Genotype 1a: H77c with P1496L and S2204I mutations that enhance the replication of cells in culture.    Genotype 1b: Con1 with S2204I mutations that enhance replication in cultured cells.

Table 9    *In Vitro* Anti-HCV Activity of Compounds against Mutation Genotype 1a HCV Replicon[11, 12]

| Genotype 1a Mutation | EC$_{50}$ (nM) | | | |
|---|---|---|---|---|
| | Daclatasvir | Asunaprevir | HCV-796 | pegIFNα |
| Wild type | 0.009-0.050 | 0.74-9.9 | 43.2 | 2.30 |
| Q30E/K/D | 217-239/82/>2000 | 2.1-4.4/3.4/2.4 | 27.8/ND/ND | 3.10/ND/ND |
| Y93N/H | 354-465/52 | 1.4-4.1/2.3 | 17.4/ND | 2.30/ND |
| M28A-Q30R | >2000 | 2.4 | ND | ND |
| M28T-Q30H | 768->1000 | 3-4.6 | 25.2 | 3.92 |
| Q30R-L31M | 442 | 1.4 | ND | ND |
| Q30H-Y93H | 471-561 | 1.6-2.7 | 15.5 | 4.05 |
| Q30R-H58D | >2000 | 2.9 | ND | ND |

HCV-796: NS5B polymerase site II inhibitors.    pegIFNα: Polyethylene glycol interferon alpha.    ND: Not determined.

# 5    ADME & Drug-Drug Interaction

## Summary

Absorption of Daclatasvir

❖ Exhibited a non-linear pharmacokinetics in hepatitis C infected humans following oral dosing.    The increase in AUC appeared to be greater than dose-proportional in the dose range of 1-100 mg daclatasvir.

❖ Had high oral bioavailability in humans (67%), mice (123%), rats (50.4%), dogs (48%-144%), but moderate in monkeys (38%).

❖ Was absorbed rapidly to moderately in mice, rats, dogs, monkeys and humans ($T_{max}$ = 0.5-2.9 h).

❖ Showed a half-life of 9.51 h in humans, longer than that in animals (1.1-4.7 h), after intravenous administrations.

❖ Had low clearance in humans (4.24 L/h), mice (9.3 mL/min/kg), rats (9.1-14.8 mL/min/kg), but moderate in dogs (5.5-20.3 mL/min/kg) and monkeys (12.4 mL/min/kg), in contrast to liver blood flow, after intravenous administrations.

❖ Exhibited an extensive distribution in humans, rats, dogs and monkeys, but confined in mice, with apparent volumes of distribution at 47.1 L, 1.2-3.6, 1.4-5.4, 2.2 and 0.61 L/kg, respectively, after intravenous administrations.

❖ Showed a moderate permeability, with a Papp$_{(A \to B)}$ of (<1.5) × 10$^{-6}$ cm/s in Caco-2 cell monolayer model and 44.2-48.6 × 10$^{-6}$ cm/s in PAMPA monolayer model.

[11]  PMDA Database.    http://www.pmda.go.jp/drugs/2014/P201400112/index.html (accessed Mar 2016).
[12]  FDA Database.    http://www.accessdata.fda.gov/drugsatfda_docs/nda/2015/206843Orig1s000MicroR.pdf (accessed Mar 2016).

Distribution of Daclatasvir

❖ Exhibited high serum protein binding in humans (95.6%), mice (98.2%), rats (98.3%), dogs (96.5%), rabbits (99.5%) and monkeys (95.1%).

❖ Pigmented Long-Evans rats after single oral administration:
  • [$^{14}$C]Daclatasvir was rapidly absorbed and widely distributed into tissues.
  • In Long-Evans rats, [$^{14}$C]daclatasvir was highest in the adrenal gland, bile, liver, cecum, small intestine and stomach. Similar effects were observed in non-pigmented rats.
  • However, in pigmented skin, the elimination of radioactivity was slower than that in non-pigmented tissue.
  • Elimination was complete at 840 h post-dose in most tissues.

Metabolism of Daclatasvir

❖ Low metabolism was observed in liver microsomes and hepatocytes of humans and animal species.

❖ The formation of metabolites mainly involved oxidation.

❖ CYP3A4 was the primary enzyme involved in the metabolism of daclatasvir.

❖ Overall, the parent drug represented the most abundant component, with M2 (BMS-805215) as the only metabolite in human plasma.   M2 was the major plasma metabolite in monkeys but was minor in mice, rats, rabbits and dogs.

❖ *In vivo* metabolite profiles were qualitatively similar in animals and humans, and there was on unique human metabolite.

Excretion of Daclatasvir

❖ Was predominantly excreted in feces in humans and tested animals, with the parent drug as the most significant component in feces of mice, rats, dogs, monkeys and humans.

❖ Biliary clearance was an important elimination pathway in bile-duct cannulated rats, dogs and monkeys.

Drug-Drug Interaction

❖ *In vitro* results indicated that daclatasvir was a weak, reversible and time-dependent inhibitor of CYP3A4.   In human hepatocytes, daclatasvir was an inducer of CYP3A4, but not an inducer of CYP1A2 or CYP2B6.

❖ Daclatasvir was a substrate and an inhibitor of P-gp.

❖ Daclatasvir was not a substrate of OATP2B1, OATP1B1, OATP1B3 or BCRP, but had inhibition for OATP1B1, OATP1B3 and BCRP, and weak inhibition for OATP2B1.

❖ Daclatasvir had inhibition for OCT1, OCT2, OAT1 and OAT3.

# Absorption

Table 10   *In Vivo* Pharmacokinetic Parameters of Daclatasvir in Mice, Rats, Dogs and Monkeys after Single Intravenous and Oral Dose of Daclatasvir[11]

| Species | Vehicle | Route | Dose (mg/kg) | $T_{max}$ (h) | $C_{max}$ (μg/mL) | $AUC_{inf}^a$ (μg·h/mL) | $T_{1/2}$ (h) | Cl or Cl/F (mL/min/kg) | $V_{ss}$ (L/kg) | F (%) |
|---|---|---|---|---|---|---|---|---|---|---|
| P-gp knockout mouse (male) | PEG400/propylene glycol/ ethanol/water (30:25:10:35) | i.v. | 3 | NA | NA | 12.4 | 1.6 | 4.0 | 0.61 | - |
| | | p.o. | 3 | 2.0 | 1.8 | 11.2 | NA | NA | NA | 91[b] |
| Wild type mouse (male) | | i.v. | 3 | NA | NA | 5.4 | 1.1 | 9.3 | NC | - |
| | | p.o. | 3 | 0.5 | 2.3 | 6.6 | NA | NA | NA | 123[b] |
| SD rat (male) | PEG400 | i.v. | 2 | NA | NA | 3.7 ± 0.15 | 3.3 + 0.58 | 9 1 ± 0.36 | 1.2 ± 0.10 | - |
| | | i.v. | 5 | NA | NA | 5.66 ± 0.63 | 4.7 ± 1.0 | 14.8 ± 1.6 | 3.6 ± 1.1 | - |
| | | p.o. | 5 | 2.7 ± 1.2 | 0.59 ± 0.10 | 3.6 ± 0.97 | NA | NA | NA | 50.4[c] |
| | | IPT | 2 | 0.5 ± 0.0 | 1.6 ± 0.25 | 2.8 ± 0.49 | 1.2 ± 0.05 | NA | NA | - |
| Beagle dog (male) | PEG400/water (85:15) | i.v. | 1 | NA | NA | 1.31 ± 0.75 | 3.9 ± 1.4 | 20.3 ± 21.3 | 5.4 ± 4.6 | - |
| | PEG400/povidone K-30/vita-min E TPGS/Tween 80 (95:2:2:1) | p.o. | 3 | 2.9 ± 1.6 | 0.85 ± 0.51 | 5.66 ± 3.64 | NA | NA | NA | 144 |
| | PEG400/ethanol/10 mM phosphate buffer pH 6.8 (60:10:30) | i.v. | 1 | NA | NA | 3.3 ± 1.4 | 3.5 ± 0.68 | 5.5 ± 2.1 | 1.4 ± 0.29 | - |
| | PEG400/ethanol/water (60:10:30) | p.o. | 3 | 1.8 ± 2.0 | 1.8 ± 0.30 | 13 ± 3.8 | NA | NA | NA | 130 ± 25 |
| | Powder in capsule | p.o. | 3 | 2.3 ± 1.6 | 1.5 ± 0.58 | 9.1 ± 4.3 | NA | NA | NA | 89 ± 14 |
| | Powder in capsule | p.o. | 3 | 2.3 ± 1.5 | 1.3 ± 1.0 | 5.4 ± 4.4 | NA | NA | NA | 48 ± 24 |

[11]  PMDA Database.   http://www.pmda.go.jp/drugs/2014/P201400112/index.html (accessed Mar 2016).

*Continued*

| Species | Vehicle | Route | Dose (mg/kg) | $T_{max}$ (h) | $C_{max}$ (µg/mL) | $AUC_{inf}{}^a$ (µg·h/mL) | $T_{1/2}$ (h) | Cl or Cl/F (mL/min/kg) | $V_{ss}$ (L/kg) | F (%) |
|---|---|---|---|---|---|---|---|---|---|---|
| Cynomolgus monkey (male) | PEG400/water (85:15) | i.v. | 1.13 | NA | NA | 1.63 ± 0.47 | 3.7 ± 0.31 | 12.4 ± 4.2 | 2.2 ± 0.88 | - |
| | PEG400/povidone K-30/ TPGS/Tween 80 (95:2:2:1) | p.o. | 2.83 | 2.0 ± 0.0 | 0.20 ± 0.03 | 1.45 ± 0.32 | NA | NA | NA | 38 ± 17 |

NC: Not calculated as the terminal profile was not well characterized.    IPT: Intraportal vein.    [a] $AUC_{0-8}$ for mice.    [b] Bioavailability was calculated using the $AUC_{0-8}$ after oral and i.v. administration of daclatasvir.    [c] Bioavailability was calculated using the dose-normalized $AUC_{inf}$ after oral and 2 mg/kg i.v. administration of daclatasvir.

Table 11    *In Vivo* Pharmacokinetic Parameters of Daclatasvir in Humans after Single Intravenous and Oral Dose of Daclatasvir[11]

| Species | Route | Dose | $AUC_{inf}{}^a$ (ng·h/mL) | $AUC_{0-t}{}^a$ (ng·h/mL) | $C_{max}{}^a$ (ng/mL) | $T_{1/2}{}^b$ (h) | $T_{max}{}^c$ (h) | $Cl^a$ (L/h) or $Cl/F^a$ (mL/min) | $V_{ss}{}^b$ (L) | F (%) |
|---|---|---|---|---|---|---|---|---|---|---|
| Healthy human | i.v. | 100 µg[d] | 23.6 (24%) | 23.0 (24%) | 6.57 (26%) | 9.51 (1.93) | 0.133 (0.133-0.167) | 4.24 (21%) | 47.1 (9.78) | - |
| | p.o. | 60 mg | 9486 (33%) | 9396 (33%) | 928 (41%) | 11.9 (2.12) | 1.38 (1.13-2.02) | NA | NA | 67.0 (20%) |
| Healthy human | p.o. | 1 mg (n = 6) | 162 (24%) | 160 (24%) | 16.4 (31%) | 9.83 (2.06) | 1.5 (1.0-2.0) | 103 (23%) | NA | NA |
| | p.o. | 10 mg (n = 6) | 2075 (38%) | 2053 (38%) | 200 (40%) | 11.0 (2.36) | 1.0 (1.0-6.0) | 80.3 (50%) | NA | NA |
| | p.o. | 25 mg (n = 6) | 4000 (20%) | 3962 (21%) | 406 (25%) | 11.3 (2.21) | 1.0 (1.0-2.0) | 104 (24%) | NA | NA |
| | p.o. | 50 mg (n = 6) | 13471 (13%) | 13255 (14%) | 1226 (19%) | 13.5 (6.99) | 1.0 (1.0-1.5) | 61.9 (13%) | NA | NA |
| | p.o. | 100 mg (n = 6) | 22614 (25%) | 22240 (25%) | 1921 (17%) | 12.3 (2.58) | 1.0 (1.0-2.0) | 73.7 (27%) | NA | NA |
| | p.o. | 200 mg (n = 6) | 31793 (45%) | 31473 (44%) | 2816 (30%) | 10.9 (1.11) | 1.0 (1.0-2.0) | 105 (48%) | NA | NA |
| Chronic HCV GT-1 infected human | p.o. | 1 mg (n = 6) | 129 (49%) | 127 (49%) | 15.7 (56%) | 9.7 (2.65) | 1.0 (0.5-3.0) | 129 (48%) | NA | NA |
| | p.o. | 10 mg (n = 5)[e] | 1431 (45%) | 1414 (45%) | 178 (52%) | 12.1 (1.97) | 1.0 (1.0-1.5) | 116 (43%) | NA | NA |
| | p.o. | 100 mg (n = 5) | 29256 (53%) | 28239 (48%) | 2416 (27%) | 14.0 (6.43) | 1.5 (1.0-3.0) | 57.0 (49%) | NA | NA |

The i.v. dose of 100 µg and p.o. dose of 60 mg in healthy humans were Cl, the others were Cl/F.    [a] Geo. Mean (CV%).    [b] Mean (SD).    [c] Median (min-max).
[d] [$^{13}$C, $^{15}$N]daclatasvir.    [e] n = 4 for $AUC_{0-t}$, $AUC_{inf}$, Cl/F and $T_{1/2}$.

Table 12    *In Vitro* Permeability of Daclatasvir in PAMPA Model and Caco-2 Cell Monolayer Model[11]

| PMAPA Model[a] | | | Caco-2 Model[b] | | |
|---|---|---|---|---|---|
| pH | $P_{app(A \to B)}$ ($1 \times 10^{-6}$ cm/s) | Permeability Class | pH | $P_{app(A \to B)}$ ($1 \times 10^{-6}$ cm/s) | Permeability Class |
| 5.5 | 44.2 | Moderate | 5.5 | <1.5 | Moderate |
| 7.4 | 48.6 | Moderate | 6.5 | <1.5 | Moderate |
| | | | 7.4 | <1.5 | Moderate |

Mean ± SD.    [a] The concentration of daclatasvir was 100 µM.    [b] The concentration of daclatasvir was 0.3 µM.

[11]    PMDA Database.    http://www.pmda.go.jp/drugs/2014/P201400112/index.html (accessed Mar 2016).

# Distribution

Table 13  *In Vitro* Plasma Protein Binding and Blood Partitioning of Daclatasvir in Various Species[11]

| Study | Serum Protein Binding[a] | Human Plasma Protein Binding | | Blood Partitioning[a] ($C_b$:$C_p$, n = 3) | | | |
|---|---|---|---|---|---|---|---|
| Species | %Bound | Conc. (μM) | %Bound | Species | 0 h | 0.5 h | 2 h |
| Mouse | 98.2 ± 0.8 | 0.1 | 97.9 | Mouse | 0.83 ± 0.01 | 0.81 ± 0.10 | 0.66 ± 0.02 |
| Rat | 98.3 ± 0.1 | | | Rat | 0.71 ± 0.05 | 0.76 ± 0.10 | 0.68 ± 0.06 |
| Dog | 96.5 ± 0.7 | 1 | 98.0 | Dog | 0.45 ± 0.04 | 0.56 ± 0.05 | 1.08 ± 0.57 |
| Rabbit | 99.5 ± 0.1 | | | Monkey | 0.52 ± 0.08 | 0.65 ± 0.20 | 0.63 ± 0.11 |
| Monkey | 95.1 ± 0.1 | 10 | 97.7 | Human | 0.68 ± 0.06 | 0.77 ± 0.01 | 0.82 ± 0.11 |
| Human | 95.6 ± 0.3 | | | | | | |

[a] The concentration of daclatasvir was 10 μM.

Table 14  *In Vivo* Tissue Distribution of Daclatasvir in SD and Long-Evans Rats after
Single Oral Dose of 10.5 mg/kg [[14]C]Daclatasvir[11]

| Species | Long-Evans Rat (Male) | | | | | | | SD Rat (Male) | | |
|---|---|---|---|---|---|---|---|---|---|---|
| | Radioactivity (μg eq./g) | | | | | | | Radioactivity (μg eq./g) | | |
| Tissue | 0.5 h | 1 h | 2 h | 8 h | 24 h | 168 h | 840 h | 1 h | 8 h | 24 h |
| Blood | 1.06 | 0.89 | 0.51 | BLQ | BLQ | BLQ | NS | 0.43 | BLQ | BLQ |
| Adrenal gland | 6.85 | 9.13 | 6.26 | 0.598 | 0.13 | 0.10 | 0.15 | 3.54 | 0.35 | 0.14 |
| Bile | 29.8 | 59.5 | 67.5 | 3.61 | 0.27 | NS | NS | 25.3 | 1.13 | 0.69 |
| Brain (entire) | BLQ | BLQ | BLQ | BLQ | BLQ | NS | NS | BLQ | BLQ | BLQ |
| Cecum | 2.13 | 5.12 | 4.97 | 21.4 | 0.16 | NS | NS | 1.47 | 22.3 | 0.28 |
| Cecum content | BLQ | 1.57 | 154 | 775[a] | 11.6 | NS | NS | BLQ | 337 | 4.75 |
| Kidneys | 3.38 | 3.03 | 1.93 | 0.43 | 0.11 | 0.16 | BLQ | 1.66 | 0.44 | 0.20 |
| Liver | 8.77 | 8.52 | 4.81 | 1.42 | 0.21 | 0.11 | BLQ | 3.70 | 0.96 | 0.18 |
| Lungs | 1.54 | 1.62 | 0.76 | BLQ | BLQ | BLQ | NS | 0.64 | 0.09 | BLQ |
| Skin (pigmented) | 0.74 | 0.85 | 0.83 | 0.18 | 0.13 | 0.11 | 0.210 | NA | NA | NA |
| Skin (non-pigmented) | 0.49 | 0.97 | 0.70 | 0.18 | BLQ | NS | NS | 0.33 | 0.20 | 0.07 |
| Small intestine | 19.1 | 17.3 | 8.50 | 1.16 | 0.11 | NS | NS | 12.3 | 0.88 | 0.395 |
| Small intestinal content | 177 | 71.3 | 32.7 | 12.0 | 0.81 | NS | NS | 97.1 | 18.9 | 4.47 |
| Stomach | 7.33 | 16.1 | 5.30 | 0.44 | BLQ | NS | NS | 1.18 | 0.56 | 0.18 |
| Stomach content | 486 | 82.4 | 24.9 | 0.76 | BLQ | NS | NS | 456 | BLQ | 1.78 |

Vehicle: PEG400/povidone K-30/vitamin E TPGS/0.1 M $H_3PO_4$ buffer pH 3 (15:5:5:75, w/w/w/w).  BLQ: Below limit of quantification (0.069 μg eq./g).  NS: Not sampled.  [a] Value was higher than upper limit of quantification (595 μg eq./g).

Table 15  *In Vivo* Tissue Distribution of Daclatasvir in Mice, Rats, Dogs and Monkeys
after Intravenous and Oral Dose of Daclatasvir[11]

| Species | Tissue/Plasma $AUC_{0-t}$ Ratio | | | | | | | | |
|---|---|---|---|---|---|---|---|---|---|
| | Route | Vehicle | Dose (mg/kg) | Liver | Brain | Heart | Spleen | Atrium | Ventricle | Bile |
| Wild type mouse (male) | i.v. | PEG400/propylene glycol/ethanol/water (30:25:10:35, w/w/w/w) | 3 | 2.35 | 0.0876 | NA | NA | NA | NA | NA |
| | p.o. | | 3 | 1.9 | 0.037 | NA | NA | NA | NA | NA |
| P-gp knockout (MDR 1a/1b) mouse (male) | i.v. | | 3 | 1.61 | 0.310 | NA | NA | NA | NA | NA |
| | p.o. | | 3 | 1.88 | 0.198 | NA | NA | NA | NA | NA |

[11]  PMDA Database.  http://www.pmda.go.jp/drugs/2014/P201400112/index.html (accessed Mar 2016).

*Continued*

| Species | Route | Vehicle | Tissue/Plasma AUC$_{0-t}$ Ratio | | | | | | | |
|---|---|---|---|---|---|---|---|---|---|---|
| | | | Dose (mg/kg) | Liver | Brain | Heart | Spleen | Atrium | Ventricle | Bile |
| SD rat (male) | i.v. | PEG400 (100) | 2 | 5.9 | 0.03 | 1.6 | 2.2 | NA | NA | NA |
| | p.o. | PEG400/povidone K-30/vitamin E TPGS/Tween 80 (95:2:2:1) | 5 | 6.8 | NC | 1.3 | 1.4 | NA | NA | NA |
| Beagle dog (male) | p.o. | PEG400/ethanol/water (60:10:30) | 3 | 10.6 | NA | NA | 0.5 | 1.3 | 1.5 | NA |
| Cynomolgus monkey (male) | p.o. | PEG 400/povidone K-30/TPGS/Tween 80 (95:2:2:1, w/w/w/w) | 2.8 | 17 | NA | NA | NA | NA | NA | 681 |

BLQ: Below limit of quantification (0.069 μg eq./g). NC: Not calculated (concentrations were below limit of quantification, 23 ng/mL). PEG: Polyethylene glycol. TPGS: *d-α*-tocopheryl polyethylene glycol 1000 succinate.

# Metabolism

Table 16 *In Vitro* Metabolism Rate of Daclatasvir in Liver Microsomes and Hepatocytes[11]

| Species | Metabolism Rate in Liver Microsomes (pmol/min/mg protein) | Metabolism Rate in Hepatocytes (pmol/min/10$^6$ cells) |
|---|---|---|
| Mouse | 6.5 | 31.7 |
| Rat | 3.6 | 5.6 |
| Dog | 6.1 | 52.6 |
| Monkey | 6.8 | 43.8 |
| Human | 4.0 | 7.0 |

Daclatasvir (0.5 μM) was incubated with liver microsomes in the presence of NADPH (1 mM) at 37 °C for 120 min. Daclatasvir (3 μM) was also incubated with hepatocytes at 37 °C for 2 h.

Table 17 *In Vitro* Metabolism of Daclatasvir in Liver Microsomes and Hepatocytes[11]

| Metabolite | Percent of Sample Radioactivity | | | | | | | | | | | | | | | | | |
|---|---|---|---|---|---|---|---|---|---|---|---|---|---|---|---|---|---|---|
| | Mouse | | | Rat | | | Rabbit | Dog | | | Monkey | | | Human | | |
| | H | LM | S9 | H | LM | S9 | LM | H | LM | S9 | H | LM | S9 | H | LM | S9 |
| Daclatasvir | 83.2 | 84.4 | 82.7 | 78.4 | 82.1 | 73.6 | 73.8 | 82.3 | 81.0 | 86.6 | 57.5 | 72.8 | 73.3 | 88.9 | 77.6 | 79.8 |
| M1 | ND | ND | ND | MS | ND | ND | MS | MS | ND | ND | MS | ND | ND | MS | 4.2 | 2.4 |
| M2 | 1.6 | 2.4 | 1.4 | 10.6 | 8.3 | 6.3 | 12.2 | 2.1 | 1.9 | 2.0 | 23.2 | 17.8 | 14.9 | 6.3 | 11.1 | 9.2 |
| M4 | 6.4 | 4.0 | 3.8 | 2.2 | MS | 1.0 | 1.0 | 10.2 | 4.0 | 2.8 | 7.4 | 1.5 | 1.0 | MS | 0.3 | 0.4 |
| M6 | ND | MS | MS | ND | MS | 0.9 | ND | ND | MS | MS | ND | ND | ND | ND | 0.2 | ND |
| M9 | MS | MS | MS | MS | MS | ND | MS | MS | MS | MS | 2.9 | MS | MS | ND | ND | ND |
| M11 | 0.7 | MS | ND | MS | ND | ND | MS | MS | ND | ND | ND | ND | ND | MS | MS | MS |
| M12 | ND | ND | ND | ND | ND | ND | ND | ND | ND | ND | 2.7 | ND | ND | ND | ND | ND |
| M13 | ND | ND | ND | ND | ND | ND | ND | ND | ND | ND | MS | ND | ND | ND | ND | ND |
| M20 | MS | MS | 0.4 | MS | MS | 1.4 | MS | MS | ND | ND | MS | 0.3 | MS | MS | 0.3 | MS |
| M27 | MS | MS | MS | MS | ND | ND | MS | ND | ND | ND | MS | ND | ND | MS | ND | ND |
| M28 | MS | MS | 0.3 | MS | MS | 3.2 | 2.4 | 0.4 | MS | MS | MS | 0.3 | 0.2 | 0.3 | MS | MS |

Liver microsomes (1 mg protein/mL): 10 μM [$^{14}$C]daclatasvir, 1 h incubation with NADPH (1 mM), with or without glutathione (5 mM) at 37 °C. Hepatocytes: 10 μM daclatasvir, 4 h incubation at 37 °C. ND: Not detected. MS: Presence of metabolite detected by LC-MS/MS. H: Hepatocytes. LM: Liver microsomes. S9: Hepatic S9 fraction from mouse, Aroclor 1254-pretreated rats, dogs, monkeys, and humans. M1: BMS821647 (hydroxy daclatasvir). M2: BMS805215 (pyrrolidine-hydroxylated, rearranged daclatasvir). M4: BMS795853 (descarboxymethyl daclatasvir). M11: BMS798820 (hydroxy daclatasvir). M20: BMS952328 (desimidazo-daclatasvir-2-oxo-napthyl ethanoic acid).

[11] PMDA Database. http://www.pmda.go.jp/drugs/2014/P201400112/index.html (accessed Mar 2016).

Table 18    *In Vitro* Metabolic Phenotype of Daclatasvir[11]

| | Recombinant Enzyme | | | | HLM, Chemical Inhibitor | | | | | | | |
|---|---|---|---|---|---|---|---|---|---|---|---|---|
| Isozyme | Relative Percentage of BMS821647 Formation | | Relative Percentage of BMS805216 Formation | | Isozyme | BMS821647 Formation Rate (Percent of Control) | | BMS805215 Formation Rate (Percent of Control) | | CYP Inhibited | % Inhibition | |
| | 2 µM[c] | 10 µM[c] | 2 µM[c] | 10 µM[c] | | 2 µM[c] | 20 µM[c] | 2 µM[c] | 20 µM[c] | Isozyme | Isozyme | 0.5 µM |
| CYP1A2 | 0 | 0 | <0.1 | <0.1 | CYP1A2 | 92.4 ± 9.6 | 97.5 ± 2.6 | 94.0 ± 6.4 | 101 ± 3.7 | CYP2C9[a] | 38 |
| CYP2A6 | 0 | 0 | <0.1 | <0.1 | CYP2A6 | 104 ± 14 | 96.5 ± 2.0 | 98.7 ± 11 | 97.2 ± 0.8 | CYP1A2[b] | 0 |
| CYP2B6 | 0 | 0 | <0.1 | <0.1 | CYP2B6 | 121 ± 9.0 | 105 ± 5.6 | 96.8 ± 10 | 87.0 ± 4.5 | CYP2C19[b] | 0 |
| CYP2C8 | 93.1 ± 1.8 | 61.7 ± 6.2 | 0.422 ± 0.008 | 0.829 ± 0.105 | CYP2C8 | 14.5 ± 0.6 | 14.7 ± 1.4 | 92.2 ± 5.3 | 91.8 ± 7.2 | CYP2D6[b] | 0 |
| CYP2C9 | 0 | 0 | <0.1 | <0.1 | CYP2C9 | 104 ± 11 | 91.0 ± 6.3 | 106 ± 9.8 | 94.1 ± 6.0 | CYP3A4[d] | 82 |
| CYP2C19 | 0 | 0 | 0.104 ± 0.012 | 0.214 ± 0.010 | CYP2C19 | 110 ± 12 | 94.5 ± 3.0 | 103 ± 8.5 | 98.0 ± 3.8 | CYP3A4[e] | 100 |
| CYP2D6 | 0 | 0 | <0.1 | <0.1 | CYP2D6 | 102 ± 12 | 90.2 ± 6.0 | 105 ± 12 | 92.0 ± 3.8 | | |
| CYP2E1 | 0 | 0 | <0.1 | <0.1 | CYP2E1 | 47.9 ± 3.7 | 55.8 ± 0.9 | 63.8 ± 1.0 | 73.8 ± 2.9 | | |
| CYP2J2 | 0 | 0 | <0.1 | <0.1 | CYP3A4[d] | 85.3 ± 12 | 77.3 ± 5.0 | 6.92 ± 0.66 | 11.9 ± 0.33 | | |
| CYP3A4 | 6.23 ± 0.54 | 3.49 ± 0.07 | 100 ± 2.16 | 100 ± 4.48 | CYP3A4[e] | 93.3 ± 9.5 | 88.8 ± 5.4 | 4.44 ± 0.19 | 12.9 ± 1.2 | | |
| CYP3A5 | 3.01 ± 0.40 | 1.50 ± 0.27 | 7.60 ± 6.19 | 10.9 ± 1.8 | All CYPs | 3.34 ± 0.26 | 5.14 ± 0.25 | 2.93 ± 0.46 | 5.12 ± 0.24 | | |
| FMO3 | 0 | 0 | <0.1 | <0.1 | | | | | | | |
| FMO5 | 0 | 0 | <0.1 | <0.1 | | | | | | | |
| HLM | 100 ± 11 | 100 ± 2.4 | 18.2 ± 1.6 | 28.8 ± 2.3 | | | | | | | |

[a] Percent inhibition of BMS805215 formation.    [b] Percent inhibition of daclatasvir.    [c] Concentration of daclatasvir.    [d] Inhibitor was ketoconazole.    [e] Inhibitor was troleandomycin.

Table 19    *In Vitro* Covalent Binding of Daclatasvir[11]

| | [³H]Daclatasvir Covalent Binding Rate (pmol/mg/h) | | | | [¹⁴C]Daclatasvir Covalent Binding Rate (pmol/mg/h) | | |
|---|---|---|---|---|---|---|---|
| Species | Without NADPH | With NADPH | With NADPH and GSH | Species | Without NADPH | With NADPH | With NADPH and GSH |
| Human | 15.8 ± 5.0 | 55.2 ± 8.1 | 40.9 ± 7.2 | Human | 25.6 ± 3.0 | 59.0 ± 1.8 | 40.9 ± 9.1 |
| Rat | 13.0 ± 0.1 | 57.6 ± 10.7 | 22.4 ± 3.0 | Rat | 34.7 ± 8.1 | 71.7 ± 19.1 | 24.9 ± 2.0 |
| Monkey | 19.6 ± 2.3 | 67.8 ± 21.0 | 25.2 ± 5.8 | Dog | 29.2 ± 4.2 | 40.5 ± 3.1 | 21.6 ± 8.6 |

[³H]daclatasvir and [¹⁴C]daclatasvir were 10 µM.

Table 20    Metabolites in Plasma, Urine and Feces in Humans and Non-clinical Species after Single Oral Dose of Daclatasvir[11]

| Matrix | Species | Dose (mg/kg) | Time (h) | % of Dose | | | | | | | | | |
|---|---|---|---|---|---|---|---|---|---|---|---|---|---|
| | | | | M0 | M2 | M4 | M9 | M28 | M11 | M12 | M15 | M20 | M27 |
| Plasma | Mouse | 50 | 1 | 89.8 | 1.6 | 3.2 | 1.5 | 1.5 | 2.8 | ND | MS | ND | MS |
| | | | 4 | 74.6 | 4.0 | 2.1 | 3.0 | 3.0 | 6.7 | ND | 1.5 | ND | 2.4 |
| | Rat | 30 | 1 | 84.6 | 2.9 | 2.0 | ND | 4.5 | ND | ND | 0.3 | 1.5 | ND |
| | | | 4 | 88.2 | 2.6 | 1.9 | ND | 3.5 | ND | ND | 0.7 | 1.5 | ND |
| | Monkey | 30 | 1 | 78.2 | 21.8 | ND | ND | ND | ND | MS | ND | ND | ND |
| | | | 8 | 85.6 | 14.4 | ND | ND | ND | ND | MS | ND | ND | ND |
| | Rabbit | 40 | 1 | 92.0 | 1.2 | 0.8 | 0.8 | 0.4 | NA | 0.1 | MS | 0.7 | MS |
| | | | 12 | 92.8 | 1.9 | 0.7 | 0.1 | 0.1 | NA | 0.7 | MS | 0.2 | 0.4 |
| | Human | 25 | 1 | 96.8 | 1.4 | ND | ND | ND | ND | ND | ND | ND | ND |
| | | | 12 | 100 | MS | ND | ND | ND | ND | ND | ND | ND | ND |

[11] PMDA Database.    http://www.pmda.go.jp/drugs/2014/P201400112/index.html (accessed Mar 2016).

*Continued*

| Matrix | Species | Dose (mg/kg) | Time (h) | % of Dose | | | | | | | | | | | |
|---|---|---|---|---|---|---|---|---|---|---|---|---|---|---|---|
| | | | | M0 | M2 | M4 | M6 | M9 | M12 | M13 | M15 | M16 | M20 | M21 | M24 |
| Urine | Mouse | 50 | 0-168 | 0.4 | 0.1 | 0.4 | ND | 0.2 | ND | ND | ND | ND | 0.1 | ND | ND |
| | Rat | 30 | 0-168 | 0.8 | 0.2 | ND | ND | ND | ND | ND | ND | ND | 0.4 | ND | ND |
| | Monkey | 30 | 0-168 | 0.5 | 0.7 | ND | ND | ND | ND | ND | ND | ND | 0.4 | ND | ND |
| | Human | 25 | 0-72 | 6.4 | 0.2 | 0.1 | ND | ND | ND | ND | ND | ND | ND | ND | ND |
| Feces | Mouse | 50 | 0-168 | 34.0 | 1.1 | 5.9 | 3.1 | ND | ND | ND | 1.0 | ND | 7.3 | ND | ND |
| | Rat | 30 | 0-168 | 24.5 | 2.0 | 3.7 | 4.9 | ND | ND | ND | ND | ND | 9.4 | 4.1 | 2.8 |
| | Monkey | 30 | 0-168 | 32.3 | 16.8 | 0.9 | 1.0 | ND | 1.9 | 2.2 | 0.6 | 1.0 | 1.0 | ND | ND |
| | Rabbit | 40 | 0-168 | 51.9 | 3.6 | 2.5 | 1.3 | 1.3 | 0.6 | 2.9 | 0.7 | 1.5 | 1.0 | 2.1 | 2.0 |
| | Human | 25 | 0-144 | 52.5 | 15.2 | 4.0 | 1.0 | ND | ND | 1.9 | 0.9 | 1.0 | 3.4 | 2.4 | ND |

Vehicle: 0.1 M Phosphoric acid buffer, pH 3.0/PEG400/povidone K-30/vitamin E TPGS (75:15:5:5, %w/w) for non-clinical species, and 33.3% (w/w) simple syrup, NF, and 66.6% 0.1 M citrate buffer (pH 3) for humans.   MS: Presence of metabolite detected by LC-MS/MS.   ND: Not detected by radioactivity detection.   M0: Daclatasvir.   M2: BMS805215 (pyrrolidine-hydroxylated rearranged daclatasvir).   M4: BMS795853 (descarboxymethyl daclatasvir).   M20: BMS952328 (desimidazodaclatasvir-2-oxo-napthyl ethanoic acid).

Table 21    Metabolites in Plasma, Urine and Feces in Bile Duct-Cannulated Animals after Single Oral Dose of Daclatasvir[11]

| Matrix | Species | Dose (mg/kg) | Time (h) | % of Dose | | | | | | | | | |
|---|---|---|---|---|---|---|---|---|---|---|---|---|---|
| | | | | M0 | M2 | M4 | M9 | M28 | M11 | M12 | M15 | M20 | M27 |
| Plasma | Dog | 50 | 1.5 | 87.5 | MS | MS | MS | MS | ND | ND | 2.9 | ND | ND |
| | | | 4 | 92.4 | MS | 2.3 | 1.2 | 1.2 | ND | ND | MS | ND | ND |
| | | | 8 | 93.9 | MS | 2.0 | 0.6 | 0.6 | ND | ND | MS | ND | ND |

| Matrix | Species | Dose (mg/kg) | Time (h) | % of Dose | | | | | | | | | | | | | |
|---|---|---|---|---|---|---|---|---|---|---|---|---|---|---|---|---|---|
| | | | | M0 | M2 | M4 | M6 | M9 | M28 | M11 | M12 | M16 | M17 | M20 | M21 | M23 | M24 |
| Urine | Rat | 30 | 0-48 | 0.03 | 0.1 | 0.1 | ND | ND | ND | ND | ND | ND | ND | 0.2 | ND | ND | ND |
| | Dog | 50 | 0-72 | 7.4 | 0.2 | 0.3 | ND | 0.2 | ND | ND | ND | ND | ND | ND | ND | ND | ND |
| | Monkey | 100 | 0-72 | 0.1 | 2.1 | 0.3 | ND | 0.04 | ND | ND | 0.4 | ND | ND | ND | ND | ND | ND |
| Bile | Rat | 30 | 0-48 | 11.5 | 10.1 | 2.2 | ND | 2.5 | 2.5 | 2.5 | 0.4 | 0.7 | 0.1 | 1.6 | ND | ND | ND |
| | Dog | 50 | 0-72 | 12.5 | 2.9 | 2.6 | ND | 0.6 | ND | ND | 0.1 | ND | ND | ND | ND | ND | ND |
| | Monkey | 100 | 0-72 | 1.4 | 7.2 | 0.2 | ND | 0.4 | 0.4 | 0.1 | 1.6 | 0.1 | 0.1 | 0.1 | ND | ND | ND |
| Feces | Rat | 30 | 0-48 | 5.3 | 0.3 | 1.1 | 2.6 | ND | ND | ND | ND | 1.1 | 0.7 | 3.1 | 2.5 | ND | 2.8 |
| | Dog | 50 | 0-72 | 16.6 | 2.0 | 3.1 | 0.2 | 1.1 | ND | ND | ND | 0.5 | ND | 1.6 | ND | ND | ND |
| | Monkey | 100 | 0-72 | 12.3 | 3.3 | 1.5 | 0.8 | ND | ND | ND | 1.1 | 0.9 | 1.4 | 4.7 | ND | 2.7 | 1.5 |

Vehicle: 0.1 M Phosphoric acid buffer, pH 3.0/PEG400/povidone K-30/vitamin E TPGS (75:15:5:5, %w/w) for non-clinical species.   MS: Presence of metabolite detected by LC-MS/MS.   ND: Not detected by radioactivity detection.   M0: Daclatasvir.   M2: BMS805215 (pyrrolidine-hydroxylated rearranged daclatasvir).   M4: BMS795853 (descarboxymethyl daclatasvir).   M11: BMS798820 (hydroxy daclatasvir).   M20: BMS952328 (desimidazo-daclatasvir-2-oxo-napthyl ethanoic acid).

[11]  PMDA Database.   http://www.pmda.go.jp/drugs/2014/P201400112/index.html (accessed Mar 2016).

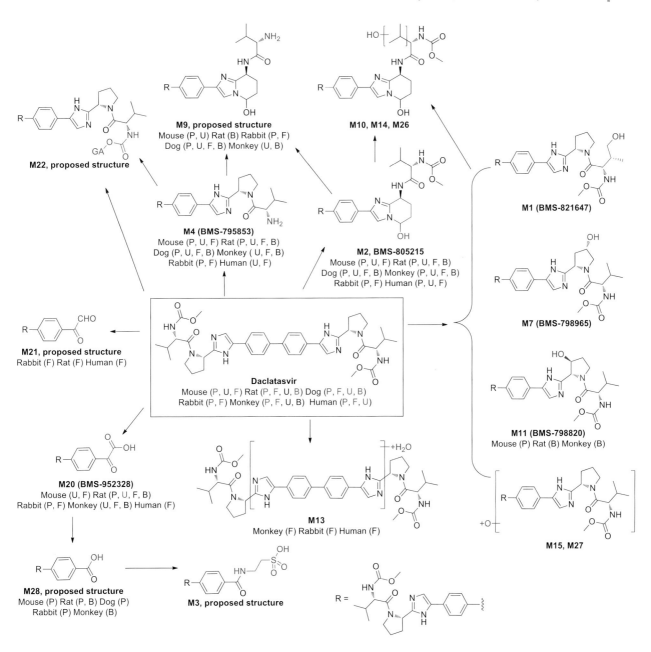

Figure A   Proposed Pathways for *In Vivo* Biotransformation of Daclatasvir in Mice, Rats, Dogs, Monkeys, Rabbits and Humans[11]
The red labels represent the major components in matrices.   P = Plasma, U = Urine, B = Bile, F = Feces and GA = Glucuronic acid.

## Excretion

Table 22   Excretion Profiles of [$^{14}$C]Daclatasvir in Mice, Rats, Rabbits, Monkeys and
Humans after Single Oral Dose of [$^{14}$C]Daclatasvir[11]

| Species | Dose (mg/kg) | Route | Time (h) | Urine (% of dose) | Feces (% of dose) | Total (% of dose) |
|---|---|---|---|---|---|---|
| RasH2 mouse (male) | 50 | p.o. | 0-168 | 1.40 ± 0.20 | 87.4 ± 1.96 | 92.4 ± 0.33[a] |
| SD rat (male) | 30 | p.o. | 0-168 | 1.55 ± 1.23 | 91.1 ± 6.65 | 96.3 ± 1.94[a] |
| NZW rabbit (female) | 40 | p.o. | 0-168 | 0.73 ± 0.20 | 91.6 ± 1.32 | 92.4 ± 1.14[a] |
| Cynomolgus monkey (male) | 30 | p.o. | 0-168 | 1.35 ± 0.70 | 69.4 ± 16.0 | 90.5 ± 1.85[b] |
| Human (male) | 25 mg | p.o. | 0-240 | 6.60 ± 2.38 | 87.6 ± 2.79 | 94.2 ± 1.66 |

Vehicle: 0.1 M Phosphoric acid buffer, pH 3.0/PEG400/povidone K-30/vitamin E TPGS (75:15:5:5, %w/w) for non-clinical species, and 33.3% (w/w) simple syrup, NF, and 66.6% 0.1 M citrate buffer (pH 3) for humans.   [a] Included cage wash, cage wipe and cage debris.   [b] Included cage wash, cage wipe and cage debris (total 19.7% of dose).

[11]  PMDA Database.   http://www.pmda.go.jp/drugs/2014/P201400112/index.html (accessed Mar 2016).

Table 23    Excretion Profiles in Bile of [$^{14}$C]Daclatasvir in Bile Duct-cannulated Animals after Single Dose of [$^{14}$C]Daclatasvir[11]

| Species | Dose (mg/kg) | Route | Time (h) | Analyte | Bile (% of dose) | Urine (% of dose) | Feces (% of dose) | Total (% of dose) |
|---|---|---|---|---|---|---|---|---|
| SD rat (male) | 5[a] | i.v. bolus | 0-24 | Daclatasvir | 29.5 | 0.49 | 27.2 | 57.2 |
| | 30[d] | p.o. | 0-48 | Total radioactivity | 38.5[e] | 1.22 | 42.3 | 83.7[f] |
| Beagle dog (male) | 1[b] | i.v. infusion, 10 min | 0-72 | Daclatasvir | 11.4 | 0.26 | 8.05 | 19.7 |
| | 50[d] | p.o. | 0-72 | Total radioactivity | 24.5 ± 4.33[e] | 8.75 ± 4.61 | 29.7 ± 8.54 | 63.0 ± 8.26 |
| Cynomolgus monkey (male) | 1[c] | i.v. infusion, 10 min | 0-72 | Daclatasvir | 6.9 | 0.11 | 1.9 | 8.9 |
| | 100[d] | p.o. | 0-72 | Total radioactivity | 14.7 ± 3.28[e] | 4.53 ± 3.54 | 52.5 ± 3.98 | 71.8 ± 3.98 |

[a] Vehicle: Propylene glycol/ethanol/cremophor EL/water (40:10:10:40) for rats.    [b] Vehicle: PEG400/water (85:15) for dogs.    [c] Vehicle: PEG400/ethanol/phosphate buffer (60:10:30) for monkeys.    [d] Vehicle: 0.1 M $H_3PO_4$ buffer (pH 3)/PEG400/povidone K-30/vitamin E TPGS (75:15:5:5).    [e] The percents of dose recovered in bile as parent compound were 11.5%, 12.5% and 1.4% in rat, dog and monkey, respectively.    [f] Included cage wash, cage wipes and cage rinse.

## Drug-Drug Interaction

Table 24    *In Vitro* Evaluation of Daclatasvir as an Inhibitor and an Inducer of CYP Enzymes[11]

| Enzyme Isoform | As an Inhibitor | | | Enzyme | Conc. (µM) | As an Inducer | |
|---|---|---|---|---|---|---|---|
| | IC$_{50}$ (µM)[a] | Reversible IC$_{50}$ (µM)[b] | Metabolism-Dependant IC$_{50}$ (µM)[b] | | | % of Positive Control[c] | |
| | | | | | | Activity | mRNA Level |
| CYP1A2 | >40 | >40 | >40 | CYP1A2 | 0.22 | 1.28 | 0.60 |
| CYP2C9 | 16.1 | >40 | >40 | | 2.2 | 2.18 | 0.50 |
| CYP2C19 | >40 | >40 | >40 | | 13 | 2.56 | 0.35 |
| CYP2D6 | >40 | >40 | >40 | CYP2B6 | 0.22 | -1.22 | 1.13 |
| CYP3A4 | 14.8[d] | 31.8[f] | 13.5[f] | | 2.2 | 4.07 | 2.33 |
| | 7.9[e] | 11.0[g] | 8.9[g] | | 13 | 9.93 | 3.63 |
| CYP2C8 | NA | >40 | >40 | CYP3A4 | 0.22 | -0.223 | 0.54 |
| UGT | 12.7[h] | NA | NA | | 2.2 | 0.72 | 7.56 |
| | | | | | 13 | 1.83 | 21.7 |

[a] Inhibition of recombinant CYP450: The concentration of daclatasvir was 0.002-40 µM.    [b] Inhibition of microsomal CYP450: The concentration of daclatasvir was 0.002-40 µM.    [c] Induction of CYPP450 in human hepatocytes: The concentration of daclatasvir was 0.22-13 µM.    [d] Substrate was 7-benzyloxy-4-trifluromethylcoumarin.    [e] Substrate was resorufin benzyl ester.    [f] Reaction was midazolam 1'-hydroxylation.    [g] Reaction was testosterone 6β-hydroxylation.    [h] Inhibition of human liver microsomes.

Table 25    *In Vitro* Evaluation of Daclatasvir as a Substrate of Transporters[11]

| SLC | Uptake | Substrate | ABC | pH | Efflux Ratio | Substrate |
|---|---|---|---|---|---|---|
| OATP2B1[a] | 1.03 ± 0.10/0.95 ± 0.04 pmol/mg/2 min | No | BCRP[d] | - | 12.4/10.8 | No |
| OATP1B1[a] | 1.02 ± 0.02/0.88 ± 0.01 pmol/mg/2 min | No | P-gp | 5.5 | >44 | Yes |
| OATP1B3[a] | 0.93 ± 0.02/0.79 ± 0.06 pmol/mg/2 min | No | | 6.5 | >25 | |
| MRP2[b] | 69.8 ± 14.0/74.4 ± 8.1 pmol/50 µg/10 min | No | | 7.4 | >24 | |
| MRP2[b, c] | 78.7 ± 0.0/75.2 ± 20.8 pmol/50 µg/10 min | No | | | | |

BSP: Bromosulfophthalein.    AMP: Adenosine mono-phosphate.    ATP: Adenosine tri-phosphate.    [a] Without BSP/With BSP.    [b] +AMP/+ATP.    [c] + MK-571 (a known inhibitor of MRP2).    [d] Wild type MDCK/BCRP-transfected MDCK.

[11]  PMDA Database.    http://www.pmda.go.jp/drugs/2014/P201400112/index.html (accessed Mar 2016).

Table 26   *In Vitro* Evaluation of Daclatasvir as an Inhibitor of Transporters[11]

| Parameter | Inhibition, IC$_{50}$ (µM) | | | | | | | | | | | | |
|---|---|---|---|---|---|---|---|---|---|---|---|---|---|
| | OAT1 | OAT3 | OCT1 | OCT2 | OATP1B1 | OATP1B3 | OATP2B1 | BSEP | NTCP | MRP2 | BCRP | P-gp$^a$ | P-gp$^b$ |
| Daclatasvir | >8$^c$ | >8$^d$ | 1.4 | 7.3 | 2.3 | 5.7 ± 1.3 | 41.8 ± 4.0 | 6.39 | ND | 32 ± 7.7 | 10.9 ± 8.6 | 4.4 | >7$^e$ |

BSEP: Bile salt export pump.   NTCP: Sodium taurocholate cotransporting polypeptide.   ND: Not determined.   $^a$ Caco-2 cells.   $^b$ Human P-gp-transfected MDCK cells.   $^c$ Maximum inhibition of 27.9% at the highest tested concentration (8 µM) was observed.   $^d$ Maximum inhibition of 25.8% at the highest tested concentration (8 µM) was observed.   $^e$ 18.7% inhibition at 7 µM was observed.

# 6   Non-Clinical Toxicology

## Summary

### Single-Dose Toxicity

❖ Single-dose toxicity studies by oral administrations in mice, rats, dogs and monkeys:
  • Mouse MNLD: 1000 mg/kg.
  • Rat MNLD: 1000 mg/kg.
  • Dog MNLD: 150 mg/kg.
  • Monkey MNLD: 150 mg/kg.

### Repeated-Dose Toxicity

❖ Pivotal repeated-dose toxicity studies by oral administration for up to 1 month in mice, up to 6 months in rats, up to 1 month in dogs, and up to 9 months in monkeys:
  • The main target organs cross species included the adrenal gland and liver.   Other daclatasvir-related effects were noted in bone marrow (dogs and monkeys) and prostate and/or testes (dogs) occurred with either minimal severity or were associated with overtly toxic doses.

### Safety Pharmacology

❖ Safety pharmacology was evaluated for cardiotoxicity, CNS toxicity, and respiratory effects as part of the single- and repeated-dose (single-agent and combination) GLP toxicity studies:
  • *In vitro* assays evaluated effects on receptor and ion channel ligand binding and relative inhibition of enzyme activity. No significant safety pharmacology signal were detected.
  • Minor *in vivo* cardiovascular effects were noted in rabbits with an exposure margin of 91 compared to the C$_{max}$ at RHD.[13]

### Genotoxicity

❖ Daclatasvir was neither mutagenic in the *in vitro* Ames assay nor clastogenic in the *in vitro* assays in CHO cells, or the *in vivo* bone marrow micronucleus assay.

### Reproductive and Developmental Toxicity [13]

❖ Fertility and early embryonic development in rats:
  • There were no effect on female reproductive parameters.
  • In male rats, there were no effects on mating performance but reduced prostate/seminal vesicle weights and minimally increased dysmorphic sperm, which were observed at 200 mg/kg/day.
❖ Embryo-fetal development in rats and rabbits:
  • Daclatasvir is markedly embryotoxic in rats and is considered teratogenic in both rats and rabbits.
  • The findings in the rat and rabbit embryo-fetal development toxicity studies, including malformations in both species at the lowest dose levels 50 mg/kg/day for rats and 40/20 mg/kg/day for rabbits tested raised concerns for use in pregnancy and in women of child-bearing potential.
❖ Pre- and postnatal development in rats:
  • Maternal toxicity was evident at the highest dose (100 mg/kg/day) and included mortality of 1 dam during parturition, reduced body weight gains, reductions in food consumption and gross findings in adrenal glands.   This dose associated with reductions in offspring birth weight and viability.
❖ Juvenile toxicity:
  • There were no novel toxicity, and the profile of daclatasvir-related changes in juvenile rats was similar to that observed previously in adult rats.

---

[11]   PMDA Database.   http://www.pmda.go.jp/drugs/2014/P201400112/index.html (accessed Mar 2016).
[13]   FDA Database.   http://www.accessdata.fda.gov/drugsatfda_docs/nda/2015/206843Orig1s000PharmR.pdf (accessed Mar 2016).

Carcinogenicity

❖ The carcinogenic potential of daclatasvir was evaluated in a 26-week study in Tg-rasH2 transgenic mice and a 2-year study in SD rats:

   • Daclatasvir was not carcinogenic in mice at doses ≤300 mg/kg/day (≤8.7-fold clinical exposure based on AUC) or in rats at doses ≤50 mg/kg/day (≤4.7-fold clinical exposure based on AUC).

Special Toxicology

❖ Phototoxicity: Probably phototoxic.

## Single-Dose Toxicity

Table 27   Single-Dose Toxicity Studies of Daclatasvir[11, 13]

| Species | Dose/Route (mg/kg) | MNLD (mg/kg) | Finding |
|---|---|---|---|
| CD1 mouse | 100, 300, 1000, p.o. | 1000 | All mice survived to the end of the study and there was no drug related finding or change in clinical signs, body weight, food consumption, physical examinations, and gross pathology at any dose. The NOEL was 1000 mg/kg. |
| SD rat | 100, 300, 1000, p.o. | 1000 | All animals survived to the end of the study, and there were no drug-related gross- or microscopic-pathology findings. Transient decreases in food consumption occurred during days 1-3 in all groups. Transient body weight losses occurred at 300 and 1000mg/kg. At 1000 mg/kg a low incidence of transient hair coat soiling was observed. Due to the transient weight loss at 300 and 100 mg/kg, the NOAEL was 100 mg/kg. |
| Beagle dog | 15, 50, 150, p.o. | 150 | There was no drug-related body weight change, and no clinical-pathology, or physical examination findings. Although there was vomiting in the dogs at 50 and 150 mg/kg, there was no other effect. The NOAEL was considered to be 150 mg/kg. |
| Cynomolgus monkey | 15, 50, 150, p.o. | 150 | All animals survived the study. There were no drug-related clinical observation, effect on body weight or feeding behavior, or change in serum chemistry parameters. The NOEL was considered to be 150 mg/kg. |

## Repeated-Dose Toxicity

Table 28   Repeated-Dose Toxicity Studies of Daclatasvir by Oral Administration[11, 13]

| Species | Duration | Dose (mg/kg/day) | NOAEL | | | Finding |
|---|---|---|---|---|---|---|
| | | | Dose (mg/kg/day) | $AUC_{0-24}$ (µg·h/mL) | Safety Margin[a] (× MRHD) | |
| CByB6F1 Hybrid mouse | 1 month | 0, 100, 300, 600, 1000 | 300 | Male: 365 Female: 332 | NA | Body weight loss and deaths were noted. The deaths included 1 TK male at 600 mg/kg and 2 mice at 1000 mg/kg (1 male, and 1 female). Organ weights increased in the spleen and liver with increasing doses. Liver vacuolation (attributed to decreased glycogen) with increasing doses. Liver enzyme changes which increased with dose. Minimal to mild increased extramedullary hematopoiesis in the spleen was noted at all doses in females and at 1000 mg/kg/day in males, and was considered to represent the correlate for the increased spleen weights. |

[11]  PMDA Database.  http://www.pmda.go.jp/drugs/2014/P201400112/index.html (accessed Mar 2016).
[13]  FDA Database.  http://www.accessdata.fda.gov/drugsatfda_docs/nda/2015/206843Orig1s000PharmR.pdf (accessed Mar 2016).

*Continued*

| Species | Duration | Dose (mg/kg/day) | NOAEL | | | Finding |
|---------|----------|------------------|-------|-------|------|---------|
| | | | Dose (mg/kg/day) | AUC$_{0-24}$ (μg·h/mL) | Safety Margin[a] (× MRHD) | |
| SD rat | 1 month | 0, 10, 30, 100, p.o. | 10 | Male: 5.39 Female: 4.75 | 0.3 | Effects at 30 and 100 mg/kg: Cortical hypertrophy/hyperplasia of the adrenal gland (with associated gross findings). The adrenal findings were associated with increased urine corticosterone levels. At 100 mg/kg, there was stomach erosion and discoloration. |
| | | Daclatasvir: 0, 10, 60; Asunaprevir: 0, 30, 60 | 60 | Male: 34.5 Female: 35.6 | NA | Increase in adrenal gland vacuolation (4 of 10 males and 4 of 10 females) at the 60 mg/60 mg combination dose. All of the affected females were grade 1. The males were more affected with 1 male at grade 1, 2 males at grade 2, and 1 male at grade 3. Lung alveolar space histiocytosis (4 of 10 males and 4 of females; All grade 1/mild) at the 60 mg/60 mg combination dose. |
| | 6 months | 0, 12.5, 25, 50 | 25 | Male: 15.6 Female: 17.2 | 1.1 | At doses of 50 mg/kg, the most significant finding was cortical hypertrophy/hyperplasia of the adrenal gland. |
| Beagle dog | 1 month | 0, 3, 15, 100/50 | 3 | Male: 1.23 Female: 2.36 | 0.1 | Dose reduction to 50 mg/kg. Four animals in the high dose group had to be euthanized early due to poor condition (with liver and bone-marrow findings). Of the surviving animals: Bone marrow effects, liver enzyme changes, minimal/slight seminiferous tubule degeneration in the testes. |
| Monkey | 1 month | 0, 10, 30, 100, 300 | 10 | Male: 2.31 Female: 1.65 | 0.1 | Drug-related finding at 30 to 300 mg/kg/day were limited to minimal perivascular inflammation in the liver which was morphologically similar to that observed in dogs. There was no evidence of bone marrow toxicity. |
| | 4 months | 0, 15, 50, 300 | 15 | Male: 2.55 Female: 2.07 | 0.2 | In males and females at 50 and 300 mg/kg/day, macroscopic changes correlated with histopathology in liver and adrenal gland. Microscopic changes were also noted in bone marrow. |
| | 9 months | 0, 15, 30, 150 | 15 | Male: 2.91 Female: 3.61 | 0.2 | Target organs were liver and adrenal gland. At 30 and 150 mg/kg/day, histopathology was noted in the liver and adrenal gland. All changes were at least partially reversible after a 2-month recovery period. Mortality: One high-dose (150 mg/kg/day) male was euthanized on day 28 due to a poor and deteriorating condition attributed to inflammatory changes in lymphoid tissue, liver and skin. |
| | 3 months | Daclatasvir: 0, 15, 50; Asunaprevir: 0, 45, 80 | Daclatasvir: 50; Asunaprevir: 80 | Male: 29.4 Female: 27.9 | NA | There were no toxicologically significant drug-related effect or toxicologic interactions. All drug-related findings were minor and were consistent with the findings from previous single-agent studies. |

[a] animal AUC/human AUC, the clinical recommended dose was 60 mg in human mg steady-state AUC (15.1 μg·h/mL).

## Safety Pharmacology

Table 29    Safety Pharmacological Studies of Daclatasvir[11, 13]

| Study | System | Dosage | Finding |
|---|---|---|---|
| Cardiovascular effect | hERG channel/HEK293 cell | 10, 30 μM | The $IC_{50}$ value for the inhibitory effect on hERG current was 29.2 μM.   The inhibition was 26.2% and 50.6% at 10 and 30 μM daclatasvir, respectively. |
| | Sodium channels/HEK293 cell | 10 μM | Daclatasvir was also a mild inhibitor of sodium channels (inhibition: 50.5% and 59.4% at 10 μM). |
| | L-type calcium channels/ HEK293 cell | 10, 30 μM | Daclatasvir was not an inhibitor of L-type calcium channels (inhibition: 31.9% at 10 μM, and 42.6% at 30 μM). |
| | Rabbit | 0, 1, 3, 10, 30 mg/kg, i.v. | There was no effect on ECG parameters at 1, 3 or 10 mg/kg (plasma concentrations ≤72.9 μg/mL), but at 30 mg/kg (156.9 μg/mL), daclatasvir moderately increased QRS duration (29 ± 1%) and mildly increased PR (19 ± 3%), AH (16 ± 4%) and HV (10 ± 1%) intervals.   These effects indicated a slowed cardiac conduction within His-Purkinje system and ventricles, as well as in the atrioventricular (AV) node at 30 mg/kg of daclatasvir. |
| | Beagle dog | 0, 15, 100 mg/kg, p.o. 0, 3, 15, 100 mg/kg/day for 1 month, p.o. | Daclatasvir exposures in dogs was ~9.6 × (AUC) recommended daily human exposure. |
| | Cynomolgus monkey | 0, 15, 50, 300 mg/kg/day for 4 months, p.o. 0, 15, 30, 150 mg/kg/day for 9 months, p.o. | Daclatasvir exposures in monkeys was ~2.7 × (AUC) recommended daily human exposure. |
| Central nervous and respiratory effect | ICR mouse | 0, 100, 300, 1000 mg/kg, p.o. | No CNS or respiratory effect. |
| | SD rat | 0, 100, 300, 1000 mg/kg, p.o. | No CNS or respiratory effect. |
| | Beagle dog | 0, 3, 15, 100 mg/kg/day for1 month, p.o. | No CNS or respiratory effect. |
| | Cynomolgus monkey | 0, 15, 50, 300 mg/kg/day for 4 months, p.o. 0, 15, 30, 150 mg/kg/day for 9 months, p.o. | No CNS or respiratory effect. |

AH: Interval between atrial wave to His wave.    HV: Interval between the His wave to ventricular wave.    PR: Atrioventricular conduction time.

## Genotoxicity

Table 30    Genotoxicity Studies of Daclatasvir[11, 13]

| Assay | Species/ System | Metabolism Activity Administration | Dose | Finding |
|---|---|---|---|---|
| *In vitro* ames reverse mutation assay in bacterial cells | *S. typhimurium* TA98, TA100, TA1535, TA1537; *E. coli* WP2 *uvrA* | ±S9 | Up to 5000 μg/plate | Negative. |
| *In vitro* chromosome aberrations assay in CHO cells | CHO cell | ±S9 | Up to 40 μg/mL (+S9) Up to 30 μg/mL (-S9) | Negative. |
| *In vivo* bone marrow micronucleus assay | SD rat | + | Single dose, p.o., 0, 500, 1000, 2000 mg/kg | Negative. |

[11]   PMDA Database.    http://www.pmda.go.jp/drugs/2014/P201400112/index.html (accessed Mar 2016).
[13]   FDA Database.    http://www.accessdata.fda.gov/drugsatfda_docs/nda/2015/206843Orig1s000PharmR.pdf (accessed Mar 2016).

# Reproductive and Developmental Toxicity

Table 31    Reproductive and Developmental Toxicology Studies of Daclatasvir by Oral (Gavage) Administration[11, 13]

| Study | Species | Dose (mg/kg/day) | NOAEL | | | | Finding |
|-------|---------|------------------|-------|---|---|---|---------|
| | | | Endpoint | Dose (mg/kg/day) | $AUC_{0-24}$ (μg·h/mL) | Safety Margin[a] (× MRHD) | |
| Fertility and early embryonic development | SD rat | 0, 15, 50, 200 | Male fertility | 50 | 51.8 | 3.4 | Daclatasvir caused clinical findings in dams at 50 and 200 mg/kg/day with no effects on the offspring.    In Males, reproductive effects were noted at 200 mg/kg.    This dose also produced overt toxicity. |
| | | | Female fertility | 200 | 267 | 17.7 | |
| Embryo-fetal development | SD rat | 0, 50, 200, 1000 | Maternal/Fetal | 50 | 70.1 | 4.6 | Daclatasvir did not produce development effects at a dose that did not produce maternal toxicity (50 mg/kg).    Findings among dams at doses ≥200 mg/kg/day (AUC ≥364 μg·h/mL) included mortality, adverse clinical signs, body-weight losses, and reduced food consumption.    In the offspring at 200 and 1000 mg/kg, fetal malformations were observed.    Additionally, the dose of 1000 mg/kg/day was associated with profound embryolethality and fetal body-weight decrements. |
| | Rabbit | 40, 200, 750 for 3-6 doses; Dose reduction to 20, 99, 370 | Maternal/Fetal | 40/20 | 245 | 16 | Maternal toxicity included mortality, adverse clinical signs, decrements in body weight and food consumption.<br><br>Developmental toxicity consisted of increased embryo-fetal lethality, reduced fetal body weights, and increased incidences of fetal malformations of the ribs and variations, notably affecting the developing head and skull. |
| Pre- and postnatal development | SD rat | 0, 25, 50, 100 | $F_0/F_1$ | 50 | 39.5 | 2.6 | Daclatasvir produced changes in the offspring at the maternally toxic dose of 100 mg/kg/day. |
| Juvenile | Rat | 0, 25, 50, 100 | N/A | 50 | 46.5 | 3.1 | Well-tolerated at all doses.<br>No novel toxicity, and similar profile of drug-related changes to that in adult rats.<br>Adrenal hypertrophy/enlargement at 100 mg/kg. |

[a] Animal AUC/human AUC, the clinical recommended dose was 60 mg in human mg steady-state AUC (15.1 μg·h/mL).

[11]  PMDA Database.    http://www.pmda.go.jp/drugs/2014/P201400112/index.html (accessed Mar 2016).
[13]  FDA Database.    http://www.accessdata.fda.gov/drugsatfda_docs/nda/2015/206843Orig1s000PharmR.pdf (accessed Mar 2016).

# Carcinogenicity

Table 32    Carcinogenicity Studies of Daclatasvir by Oral Administration[11, 13]

| Species | Duration | Dose (mg/kg/day) | Vehicle | NOAEL | | | Finding |
|---|---|---|---|---|---|---|---|
| | | | | Dose (mg/kg/day) | AUC$_{0-24}$ ($\mu$g·h/mL) | Safety Margin[a] ($\times$ MRHD) | |
| CByB6F1-Tg (HRAS) 2Jic hemizygous mouse | 26 weeks | 0, 30, 100, 300 | 15% PEG-400, 5% PVP K-30, 5% TPGS, 75% 0.1 M H$_3$PO$_4$, pH~3 in Milli-Q gradient A10 water | 300 | 131 | 8.7 | There was no daclatasvir related mortality, and clinical signs were limited to non-dose dependent instances of rough coat primarily in males. Tumor incidences in the water- and vehicle-control groups were similar and there were no daclatasvir-related neoplastic microscopic findings at any dose. |
| SD rat | 2 years | 0, 5, 15, 50 | 15% PEG-400, 5% PVP K-30, 5% TPGS, 75% 0.1 M H$_3$PO$_4$, pH~3 in ultra-pure water | 50 | 70.3 | 4.7 | There were no daclatasvir-related effects on the incidence, distribution, or nature of neoplastic change. Daclatasvir was not carcinogenic in the 2-year studies in rats. |

[a] Animal AUC/human AUC, the clinical recommended dose was 60 mg in human mg steady-state AUC (15.1 $\mu$g·h/mL).

# Special Toxicology

Table 33    Special Toxicology Studies of Daclatasvir[13]

| Study | Species | Finding |
|---|---|---|
| Neutral red uptake phototoxicity assay | Murine (Balb/c 3T3) fibroblast | Daclatasvir elicited reductions in cell viability in the presence of UVA exposure indicative of a phototoxic potential. |
| Phototoxicity study with the eyes and skin | Long-Evans pigmented rat | Non-phototoxic at doses of ≤100 mg/kg. |

[11]  PMDA Database.   http://www.pmda.go.jp/drugs/2014/P201400112/index.html (accessed Mar 2016).
[13]  FDA Database.   http://www.accessdata.fda.gov/drugsatfda_docs/nda/2015/206843Orig1s000PharmR.pdf (accessed Mar 2016).

# CHAPTER

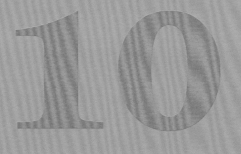

## Delamanid

# Delamanid

## (Deltyba®)

Research code: OPC-67683

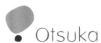

## 1　General Information

❖ Delamanid is an orphan antibiotic specific for mycobacteria, which was first approved in Apr 2014 by EMA.

❖ Delamanid was discovered, developed and marketed by Otsuka.

❖ Delamanid is a nitro-dihydro-imidazo-oxazole derivative, which inhibits the synthesis of the mycobacterial cell wall components, methoxy-mycolic and keto-mycolic acid, thereby exhibiting antibacterial activities for mycobacteria.

❖ Delamanid is indicated for the treatment of multidrug-resistant tuberculosis (MDR-TB) in adult patients.

❖ Available as tablet, with each containing 50 mg of delamanid and the recommended dose is 100 mg orally twice daily until disease progression or unacceptable toxicity.

❖ The sale of Deltyba® was not available up to Mar 2016.

### Key Approvals round the World*

|  | EU (EMA) | Japan (PMDA) |
|---|---|---|
| First approval date | 04/28/2014 | 07/04/2014 |
| Application or approval No. | EMEA/H/C/002552 | 22600AMX00741 |
| Brand name | Deltyba® | Deltyba® |
| Indication | MDR-TB | MDR-TB |
| Authorisation holder | Otsuka | Otsuka |

MDR-TB: multidrug-resistant tuberculosis.
*Till Mar 2016, it had not been approved by FDA (US) and CFDA (China).

## Active Ingredient

*Molecular formula*:　$C_{25}H_{25}F_3N_4O_6$
*Molecular weight*:　534.48
*CAS No.*:　681492-22-8 (Delamanid)
*Chemical name*:　(2*R*)-2-methyl-6-nitro-2-[(4-{4-[4-(trifluoromethoxy)phenoxy]piperidin-1-yl}phenoxy)methyl]-2,3-dihydroimidazo[2,1-*b*]oxazole

*Parameters of Lipinski's "Rule of 5"*

| MW | H_D | H_A | FRB[a] | PSA[a] | cLogP[a] |
|---|---|---|---|---|---|
| 534.48 | 0 | 10 | 8 | 104Å$^2$ | 5.53 ± 0.66 |

[a] Calculated by ACD/Labs software V11.02.

## Drug Product*

*Dosage route*:　Oral
*Strength*:　50 mg (Delamanid)
*Dosage form*:　Tablet
*Inactive ingredient*: Hypromellose phthalate, povidone, all-rac-α-tocopherol, microcrystalline cellulose, sodium starch glycolate (type A), carmellose calcium, colloidal hydrated silica, magnesium stearate, lactose monohydrate, hypromellose, macrogol 8000, titanium dioxide, talc and iron oxide yellow (E172).
*Recommended dose*: The recommended dose for adults is 100 mg twice daily for 24 weeks.

* Sourced from EMA drug label information

## 2   Key Patents Information

## Summary

❖ Deltyba® (Delamanid) was initially approved by EMA on April 28, 2014.

❖ Delamanid was originally discovered by Otsuka, and its compound patent application was filed as PCT application by Otsuka in 2003.

❖ The compound patent will expire in 2023 foremost, which has been granted in the United States, China, Japan and Europe successively.

Table 1   Delamanid's Compound Patent Protection in Drug-Mainstream Country

| Country | Publication/Patent NO. | Application Date | Granted Date | Estimated Expiry Date |
|---|---|---|---|---|
| WO | WO2004033463A1 | 10/10/2003 | / | / |
| US | US7262212B2 | 10/10/2003 | 08/28/2007 | 02/22/2024[a] |
| EP | EP1555267B1 | 10/10/2003 | 01/16/2013 | 10/10/2023 |
| JP | JP4186065B2 | 10/14/2003 | 11/26/2008 | 10/14/2028[b] |
| CN | CN100366624C | 10/10/2003 | 02/06/2008 | 10/10/2023 |

[a] The term of this patent is extended by 135 days.   [b] The term of this patent is extended by 5 years.

Table 2   Originator's International Patent Application List (Patent Family)

| Publication NO. | Title | Applicant/Assignee/Owner | Publication Date |
|---|---|---|---|
| Technical Subjects | Active Ingredient (Free Base)'s Formula or Structure and Preparation | | |
| WO2004033463A1 | 2,3-Dihydro-6-nitroimidazo[2,1-b]oxazoles | Otsuka | 04/22/2004 |
| Technical Subjects | Salt, Crystal, Polymorphic, Solvate (Hydrate), Isomer, Derivative Etc. and Preparation | | |
| WO2004035547A1 | 1-Substituted-4-nitroimidazole compound and process for producing the same | Otsuka | 04/29/2004 |
| WO2005092832A1 | Method of producing aminophenol compounds | Otsuka | 10/06/2005 |
| WO2008140090A1 | Epoxy compound and method for manufacturing the same | Otsuka | 11/20/2008 |
| WO2011093529A1 | Synthetic intermediate of oxazole compound and method for producing the same | Otsuka | 08/04/2011 |
| Technical Subjects | Formulation and Preparation | | |
| WO2007013477A1 | Pharmaceutical composition comprising 2,3-dihydro-6-nitro-imidazo[2,1-b]oxazole derivatives | Otsuka | 02/01/2007 |
| Technical Subjects | Combination Including at Least Two Active Ingredients | | |
| WO2007043542A1 | Antituberculous composition comprising oxazole compounds | Otsuka | 04/19/2007 |

The data was updated until Jan 2016.

# 3 Chemistry

## Route 1: Original Discovery Route

DBU: 1,8-Diazabicyclo[5.4.0]undec-7-ene
ADDP: 1,1'-(Azodicarbonyl)dipiperidine
*rac*-BINAP: Racemic-2,2'-bis(diphenylphosphino)-1,1'-binaphthyl
PPTS: Pyridinium *p*-toluenesulfonate

*Synthesis Route*: Preparation of **6** proceeded through a Payne-like rearrangement in which commercial epoxide **2** was attacked by commercial imidazole **1** in the presence of triethylamine, giving rise to tertiary alcohol **3** in 87% yield. Next, saponification of the *p*-nitrobenzoyl ester **3** followed by mesylation of the resulting primary alcohol and subsequent exposure to DBU facilitated the formation of the desired epoxide synthon **6** in 73% yield for the four-step sequence. Finally, a cascade reaction involving epoxide **6** and phenol **7** furnished delamanid directly: The initial alkylation of the epoxide **6** by phenol **7** proceeded under basic conditions which facilitated the intramolecular nucleophilic substitution reaction by the resulting alcohol on the pendant imidazole chloride. The reaction proceeded in 48% yield to provide delamanid as a free base.[1-3]

Hereof, the key synthon **7** could be constructed *via* firstly the Mitsunobu reaction of alcohol **8** with phenol **9** in the presence of ADDP and (*n*-Bu)$_3$P in benzene, secondly amine liberation for the further Buchwald-Hartwig cross coupling with bromobenzene **12** to provide **13** in 64% yield, in which THP group was removed using PPTS in ethanol to achieve **7** in 94% yield.[1-3]

[1] Sasaki, H.; Haraguchi, Y.; Itotani, M., et al. *J. Med. Chem.* **2006**, *49*, 7854-7860.
[2] Tsubouchi, H.; Sasaki, H.; Kuroda, H., et al. WO2004033463A1, **2004**.
[3] Tsubouchi, H.; Sasaki, H.; Kuroda, H., et al. US20060094767A1, **2006**.

## Route2

i. **1**, L-DIPT, Ti($i$-PrO)$_4$, Toluene
4Å MS, -16 to -18 °C
ii. 80% CHP, -18 to -10 °C
iii. DMSO, 11 to 13 °C, then r.t.
iv. **2**, 25% NaOH, Toluene, 40 °C
76% over 2 steps

Pd$_2$(dba)$_3$, $t$-Butyl XPhos
Toluene, $t$-BuONa, 70 °C

**3**
92.2% *ee*

MsCl, EtOAc, TEA, 0 °C

**5**

K$_2$CO$_3$, MeOH
0 °C to r.t.
76% over 3 steps

**6**

i. **7**, **8**, NaOAc, $t$-BuOAc, 100 °C
ii. 25% NaOH, MeOH, 0 °C to r.t.
73%

**7**
94.3% *ee*

**Delamanid**
99.4% *ee*

L-DIPT: D-(-)-Diisopropyl tartrate
CHP: Cumene hydroperoxide
$t$-Butyl XPhos: 2-*Di-tert*-butylphosphino-2',4',6'-triisopropyl-1,1'-biphenyl

*Synthesis Route*:    Sharpless asymmetric epoxidation of $\beta$-methylallyl alcohol **1** with cumene hydroperoxide (CMNOOH) in the presence of ($i$-PrO)$_4$Ti and (+)-DET in toluene gave ($S$)-methylglycidyl alcohol, which upon condensation with 4-bromophenol **2** in basic conditions yielded 1,2-diol **3** in 76% yield over two steps with 92.2% *ee*.    Buchwald-Hartwig coupling of aryl bromide **3** with 4-[4-(trifluoromethoxy)phenoxy]piperidine **4** afforded tertiary amine **5**.    Activation of the primary hydroxyl group in diol **5** with MsCl facilitated by TEA was prior to cyclization by means of K$_2$CO$_3$ in MeOH, generating oxirane **7** in 76% yield over three steps with 94.3% *ee*.    Finally, coupling of epoxide **7** with 2-chloro-4-nitroimidazole **8** in the presence of NaOAc in $t$-BuOAc at 100 °C and further basic workup furnished the target delamanid in 73% yield with 99.4% *ee*.    The overall yield was 42%.[4, 5]

## 4  Pharmacology

### Summary

Mechanism of Action

❖ Delamanid is a nitro-dihydro-imidazo-oxazole derivative that inhibits the biosynthesis of methoxy-mycolic acid (IC$_{50}$ = 0.036 µg/mL) and keto-mycolic acid (IC$_{50}$ = 0.021 µg/mL), which are mycobacterial cell wall components.

❖ The antibacterial activity of delamanid is specific for mycobacteria (*M. tuberculosis*, MIC = 0.006-0.024 µg/mL), and there is no cross-resistance with any of the currently used anti-tuberculosis (anti-TB) drugs.

❖ The anti-TB activity of delamanid is possibly mediated *via* F420 coenzyme system and the biological reduction of the nitro aromatic.    In delamanid resistant BCG Tokyo strain, the mutation in coenzyme F420-related genes fgd, Rv3547, fbiA, fbiB, and fbiC are found to be resistant mechanism against delamanid.[6]

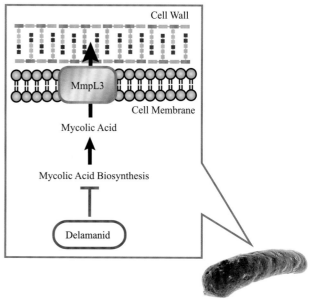

*M. tuberculosis*

[4]  Yamamoto, A.; Shinhama, K.; Fujita, N., et al. WO2011093529 A1, **2011**.
[5]  Yamamoto, A.; Shinhama, K.; Fujita, N., et al. US20120302757A1, **2012**.
[6]  Japan Pharmaceuticals and Medical Devices Agency (PMDA) Database.    http://www.pmda.go.jp/drugs/2014/P201400075/index.html (accessed Mar 2016).

❖ Delamanid had no significant binding inhibition on a panel of receptors (53 types), ion channels (3 types) and transporters (3 types) at 3 μM.[6]

*In Vitro* Efficacy

❖ Antibacterial activity in different strains from clinical:
- In agar dilution method:
  - TB and BCG strains: $MIC_{90}$ = 0.012-0.024 μg/mL.
  - Susceptible-TB strains and MDR-TB strains: $MIC_{90}$ = 0.024 μg/mL.
- Proportion method:
  - *M. tuberculosis*: MIC = ≤0.0005-0.004 μg/mL.
  - TB strains: $MIC_{90}$ = 0.004-0.0125 μg/mL.
  - Resistant TB strains: $MIC_{90}$ = 0.008-0.0125 μg/mL.
  - H37Rv strains: $MIC_{90}$ = 0.002-≤0.00625 μg/mL.
❖ Antibacterial activity of intracellular mycobacteria in cultured cell lines:
- In THP-1 cell lines: $IC_{90}$ = 0.199-0.215 μg/mL.
- In A549 cell lines: Strong activity against intracellular parasite.
❖ Antibacterial activity against multidrug resistant *M. tuberculosis*:
- Susceptible strains: $MIC_{90}$ = 0.01054-0.01535 μg/mL.
- Resistant strains: $MIC_{90}$ = 0.01050-0.02450 μg/mL.

*In Vivo* Efficacy

❖ Efficacy of delamanid in animal models with Kurono strains *M. tuberculosis*:
- In ICR mouse models:
  - Effective dose: 0.52 mg/kg/day.
  - Significantly reduced the number of pulmonary bacteria at 0.313 mg/kg/day.
  - Delamanid showed an initial bactericidal effect corresponding with isoniazid.
- Balb/c nude mouse and Balb/c mouse models:
  - Balb/c nude mice: Significantly reduced TB at 0.625 mg/kg/day in lungs and spleen, 0.313 mg/kg/day in liver.
  - Balb/c mice: Significantly reduced TB at 0.313 mg/kg/day in lungs, spleen and liver.

## Mechanism of Action

Table 3    Inhibition of Synthesis of Mycolic Acid and Fatty Acid by Delamanid[6, 7]

| Subclass Mycolic Acid and Fatty Acid | IC (μg/mL) | |
| --- | --- | --- |
| | $IC_{50}$ | 95% Confidence Interval |
| Fatty acid | >0.25 | NA |
| α-Mycolic acid[a] | >0.25 | NA |
| Methoxy-mycolic acid[a] | 0.036 | 0.020-0.068 |
| Keto-mycolic acid[a] | 0.021 | 0.009-0.059 |

[a] Mycobacterium bovis Bacillus Calmette-Guérin strain.

[6] PMDA Database.   http://www.pmda.go.jp/drugs/2014/P201400075/index.html (accessed Mar 2016).
[7] Matsumoto, M.; Hashizume, H.; Tomishige, T., et al. *PLoS Med.* **2006**, *3*, 2131-2144.

## *In Vitro* Efficacy

Table 4  *In Vitro* Anti-TB Activity of Delamanid against Tuberculosis Strains and Clinical Isolates[6]

| Method | Origin | Strain | Effect | |
|---|---|---|---|---|
| | | | MIC$_{90}$ (µg/mL) | MIC (µg/mL) |
| Agar dilution | NA | 11 tubercle bacillus and 4 clinical BCG | 0.012 | 0.006-0.024 |
| | | 67 tubercle bacillus[a] | 0.024 | 0.006-0.024 |
| | | 35711 *Mycobacterium africanum* ATCC and 17 Atypical mycobacterium | 0.024-1.56 | |
| | | 35711 *Mycobacterium africanum* ATCC isolated clones | ≤0.002/1->8 | |
| | Patients from Japan and overseas[a] | 34 clinical susceptible tubercle bacillus | 0.024 | 0.006-0.024 |
| | | 33 MDR tubercle bacillus | 0.024 | 0.006-0.024 |
| Proportion | Patients from South Africa | 23 clinical tubercle bacillus[a] | 0.0125 | ≤0.00625-0.0125 |
| | | H37Rv | ≤0.00625 | |
| | | 7 susceptible tubercle bacillus[a] | NA | ≤0.00625-0.0125 |
| | | 10 MDR tubercle bacillus[a] | 0.0125 | ≤0.00625-0.0125 |
| | | 6 XDR tubercle bacillus[a] | NA | ≤0.00625-0.0125 |
| | Patients from Japan | 25 tubercle bacillus[a] | 0.004 | 0.002-0.008 |
| | | H37Rv (ATCC 25618)[b] | 0.004 | |
| | | 37 MDR tubercle bacillus[a] | 0.008 | 0.002-0.008 |
| | | 8 XDR tubercle bacillus[a] | NA | 0.002-0.004 |
| | Patient | 128 tubercle bacillus[a] | 0.008 | 0.001->8 |
| | | H37Rv (ATCC 25618)[b] | 0.002, 0.004 | |
| | | 99 MDR tubercle bacillus[a] | 0.008 | 0.002->8 |
| | | 29 XDR tubercle bacillus[a] | 0.008 | 0.001-0.008 |
| | Tubercle bacillus complex | *M. africanum* | ≤0.0005 | |
| | | *M. bovis* | 0.004 | |
| | | *M. caprae* | 0.002 | |
| | | *M. pinnipedii* | 0.002 | |
| | | *M. microti* | 0.002 | |
| | | H37Rv (ATCC 25618)[b] | 0.002 | |

[a] The test of strains were separated from clinical.   [b] Tubercle bacillus H37Rv (ATCC 25618).   MDR: Multi-drug resistance.   XDR: Extensively-drug resistant. MIC: Minimum inhibitory concentration.

Table 5  *In Vitro* Antibacterial Activity of Delamanid against Intracellular Mycobacteria in Cell Lines[6]

| Cell Line | Type | Strain | Delamanid | |
|---|---|---|---|---|
| | | | IC$_{90}$ (µg/mL) | 95% CI |
| THP-1 | *Tubercle bacillus* | H37Rv | 0.215 | 0.178-0.261 |
| | *M. bovis* | BCG | 0.199 | 0.133-0.298 |
| A549 | *Tubercle bacillus* | H37Rv | Delamanid had strong activity against intracellular parasite in A549 cells, and the activity was beneficial in the treatment of tuberculosis. | |
| | *M. bovis* | BCG | | |

THP-1: Human acute mononuclear leukemia cell line.   A549: Human lung epithelial cells.   BCG: Bacillus Calmette-Guérin.   IC$_{90}$: 90% inhibitory concentration. CI: Confidence interval.

[6]  PMDA Database.   http://www.pmda.go.jp/drugs/2014/P201400075/index.html (accessed Mar 2016).

Table 6    *In Vitro* Antibacterial Activity of Delamanid, Metabolites and Control Compounds[6, 8]

| Compound | Type | MIC (µg/mL) | |
|---|---|---|---|
| | | TB Strain | Aerobic and Anaerobic Bacteria Strain[a] |
| Delamanid | Parent | 0.006-0.012 | >100 |
| (R)-DM-6701 | Metabolite | 6.25-50 | 12.5->100 |
| (R)-DM-6702 | Metabolite | 12.5 | 6.25->100 |
| (R)-DM-6703 | Metabolite | ≥50 | 50->100 |
| RFP | Control | 0.05-100 | ≤0.006-25 |
| SM | Control | NA | 1.56->100 |
| PA-824 | Control | NA | 6.25->100 |

[a] The test were against 24 aerobic bacteria strains and 10 anaerobes bacteria strains using the agar dilution method.    TB: Tubercle bacillus.    RFP: Rifampicin.    SM: Streptomycin.    MIC: Minimum inhibitory concentration.

Table 7    *In Vitro* Antibacterial Activity of Delamanid against Multidrug Resistant *M. Tuberculosis*[7]

| M. Tuberculosis | MIC (µg/mL) | |
|---|---|---|
| | MIC$_{90}$ | 95% Confidence Interval |
| RFP-susceptible | 0.01248 | 0.01097-0.01535 |
| RFP-resistant | 0.01221 | 0.01050-0.01583 |
| INH-susceptible | 0.01194 | 0.01054-0.01452 |
| INH-resistant | 0.01279 | 0.01094-0.01679 |
| EB-susceptible | 0.01213 | 0.01081-0.01440 |
| EB-resistant | 0.01341 | 0.01073-0.02450 |
| SM-susceptible | 0.01203 | 0.01077-0.01416 |
| SM-resistant | 0.0134 | 0.01068-0.02298 |

RFP: Rifampicin.    INH: Isoniazid.    EB: Ethambutol.    SM: Sreptomycin.

Table 8    *In Vitro* Resistant Development of Delamanid in Different Mycobacteria Strains[6-8]

| Method | Type | Strain | Conc. (µg/mL) | Natural Resistant Bacteria Frequency | MIC (µg/mL) |
|---|---|---|---|---|---|
| Agar dilution | Tubercle bacillus | H37Rv | 0.192 | $6.44 \times 10^{-6}$-$4.19 \times 10^{-5}$ | 0.006-0.012 |
| | | Kurono | 0.05-0.7825 | $1.35 \times 10^{-4}$-$1.57 \times 10^{-4}$ | 0.006-0.012 |
| | | Erdman | NA | NA | NA |
| | *M.bovis* | Pasteur | NA | NA | 0.006-0.012 |
| | | BCG Tokyo | 0.05-0.7825 | $2.51 \times 10^{-5}$-$3.95 \times 10^{-5}$ | 0.006-0.012 |
| | | BCG Tokyo (dormancy) | NA | NA | NA |
| Proportion | *M. tuberculosis* | NA | NA | NA | 0.003-0.012 |

BCG: Bacillus Calmette-Guérin.    MIC: Minimum inhibitory concentration.

[6]  PMDA Database.    http://www.pmda.go.jp/drugs/2014/P201400075/index.html (accessed Mar 2016).
[7]  Matsumoto, M.; Hashizume, H.; Tomishige, T., et al. *PLoS Med.* **2006**, *3*, 2131-2144.
[8]  European Medicines Agency (EMA) Database.    http://www.ema.europa.eu/docs/en_GB/document_library/EPAR_-_Public_assessment_report/human/002552/WC500166234.pdf (accessed Mar 2016).

## *In Vivo* Efficacy

Table 9    *In Vivo* Efficacy of Delamanid in Animal Models with Kurono Strains *M. Tuberculosis*[6-8]

| Animal Model | | | Dose (mg/kg/day, p.o.) | Duration (Day) | Effect | | |
|---|---|---|---|---|---|---|---|
| Study | Location | Animal | | | Viable Bacteria Count/EBA[a] | ED (mg/kg) | Finding |
| The effect in chronic tuberculosis model | Lung | ICR mouse (male) | Saline | QD × 28 | $7.187 \pm 0.182$ | 0.52 | Delamanid significantly reduced the number of pulmonary bacteria at 0.313 mg/kg/day ($P$ <0.01) at the end of treatment. EB: ED >160 mg/kg/day. INH: ED = 2.96 mg/kg/day. PZA: ED = 165.28 mg/kg/day. RFP: ED = 3.5 mg/kg/day. SM: ED = 48.38 mg/kg/day. |
| | | | 0.156 | QD × 28 | $6.506 \pm 0.132^{NS}$ | | |
| | | | 0.313 | QD × 28 | $5.959 \pm 0.195^{**}$ | | |
| | | | 0.625 | QD × 28 | $5.457 \pm 0.122^{**}$ | | |
| | | | 1.25 | QD × 28 | $4.867 \pm 0.179^{**}$ | | |
| | | | 2.5 | QD × 28 | $4.753 \pm 0.133^{**}$ | | |
| | | | 5 | QD × 28 | $4.272 \pm 0.207^{**}$ | | |
| | | | 10 | QD × 28 | $3.943 \pm 0.208^{**}$ | | |
| | | | 20 | QD × 28 | $3.495 \pm 0.233^{**}$ | | |
| | | | 40 | QD × 28 | $2.791 \pm 0.300^{**}$ | | |
| The EBA in chronic tuberculosis model | BALF | ICR mouse (male) | 0.156 | QD × 7 | $0.150 \pm 0.209^{b}$ | NA | Delamanid showed an initial bactericidal effect corresponding with INH. EBA: INH (2.5-10 mg/kg/day: 0.352-0.514). |
| | | | 0.313 | QD × 7 | $0.123 \pm 0.234^{b}$ | | |
| | | | 0.625 | QD × 7 | $0.355 \pm 0.215^{b}$ | | |
| | | | 1.25 | QD × 7 | $0.424 \pm 0.375^{b}$ | | |
| | | | 2.5 | QD × 7 | $0.529 \pm 0.255^{b}$ | | |
| | | | 10 | QD × 7 | $0.648 \pm 0.228^{b}$ | | |
| The effect in immunodeficient mouse model | Lung | Balb/c nude mouse | Solvent | QD × 10 | $5.543 \pm 0.116$ | NA | Significantly reduced the number of viable bacteria in lungs and spleen at 0.625 mg/kg/day, in liver at 0.313 mg/kg/day in a dose-dependent manner. The same tests were studied in SCID mice, (NOD)-SCID mice, and MDR mice models. Delamanid showed the similar therapeutic effect in them. |
| | | | 0.313 | QD × 10 | $5.399 \pm 0.107^{NS}$ | | |
| | | | 0.625 | QD × 10 | $4.233 \pm 0.545^{**}$ | | |
| | | | 1.25 | QD × 10 | $2.793 \pm 0.438^{**}$ | | |
| | | | 2.5 | QD × 10 | $2.308 \pm 0.194^{**}$ | | |
| | | | 5 | QD × 10 | $1.980 \pm 0.382^{**}$ | | |
| | | | 10 | QD × 10 | $1.992 \pm 0.279^{**}$ | | |
| | | Balb/c mouse | Solvent | QD × 10 | $5.559 \pm 0.034$ | NA | |
| | | | 0.313 | QD × 10 | $4.591 \pm 0.181^{**}$ | | |
| | | | 0.625 | QD × 10 | $3.394 \pm 0.208^{**}$ | | |
| | | | 1.25 | QD × 10 | $2.407 \pm 0.210^{**}$ | | |
| | | | 2.5 | QD × 10 | $2.369 \pm 0.236^{**}$ | | |
| | | | 5 | QD × 10 | $1.989 \pm 0.053^{**}$ | | |
| | | | 10 | QD × 10 | $1.998 \pm 0.130^{**}$ | | |

$^{**}P$ <0.01.    [a] Viable bacteria count: Log.    [b] EBA ± SD.    EBA: Early bactericidal activity defined as the daily average of the decrease value in log CFU from pre-treatment (Day 1) to therapy third day (Day 3).    NS: No significant difference.    BALF: Broncho alveolar lavage fluid.    RFP: Rifampicin.    INH: Isoniazid.    EB: Ethambutol.    SM: Sreptomycin.    PZA: Pyrazinamide.    SCID: Severe-combined immunodeficient mice.    NOD: Non-obese diabetic.    Viable bacteria count = log CFU/organ.    CFU: Colony forming unit.

[6] PMDA Database.   http://www.pmda.go.jp/drugs/2014/P201400075/index.html (accessed Mar 2016).
[7] Matsumoto, M.; Hashizume, H.; Tomishige, T., et al. *PLoS Med.* **2006**, *3*, 2131-2144.
[8] EMA Database.   http://www.ema.europa.eu/docs/en_GB/document_library/EPAR_-_Public_assessment_report/human/002552/WC500166234.pdf (accessed Mar 2016).

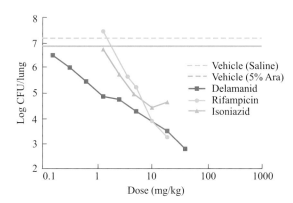

**Study:** Effects of delamanid in an experimental mouse model of TB.

**Animal:** ICR mouse.

**Model:** ICR mice were inoculated intravenously with $8.6 \times 10^4$ CFU of *M. tuberculosis* Kurono.

**Administration:** p.o., QD for 28 days.    Delamanid: 0.156-40 mg/kg; Rifampicin: 1.25-20 mg/kg; Isoniazid: 1.25-20 mg/kg.

**Test:** Bacterial burden in lungs at the end of treatment.

**Result:** Delamanid significantly reduced the number of pulmonary bacteria at 0.313 mg/kg/day ($P < 0.01$) at the end of treatment.

Figure A    Effects of Delamanid in an Experimental Mouse Model of Kurono Strains[7]

## 5  ADME & Drug-Drug Interaction

### Summary

Absorption of Delamanid

❖ Exhibited a non-linear pharmacokinetics in humans following oral dosing.    The increases of $C_{max}$ and $AUC_{inf}$ appeared to be less than dose-proportional in the dose range of 100 to 400 mg delamanid.

❖ Had moderate oral bioavailability in mice (42.2%).

❖ Was absorbed moderately to slowly in humans ($T_{max}$ = 2-5 h) and mice ($T_{max}$ = 2-4 h), and much more slowly in rats ($T_{max}$ = 4-8 h) and dogs ($T_{max}$ = 9.5-17.5 h).

❖ Showed a half-life ranging between 16.6-41.1 h in humans after oral administration, longer than that in mice (4.5-6.8 h), rats (6.4-8.2 h) and dogs (14.3-20.6 h).

❖ Had low clearance in mice (222 mL/h/kg), rats (139-162 mL/h/kg) and dogs (215 mL/h/kg), in contrast to liver blood flow, after intravenous administrations.

❖ Exhibited an extensive distribution in mice, rats and dogs, with apparent volumes of distribution at 2026, 1841-2055 and 5388 mL/kg, respectively, after intravenous administrations.

Distribution of Delamanid

❖ Exhibited high protein binding in mice, rats, rabbits, dogs and humans (≥99.3%).    Note that delamanid was highly bound to $\alpha_1$-AGP (68.7%-87.9%), $\gamma$-GLB (77.6%-97.1%), VLDL (97.3%) and LDL (97.6%).

❖ Had a blood partitioning ratio of 0.04-0.76 in rats and 0.26-0.32 in dogs, indicating rare penetration into red blood cells.

❖ SD rats and Long-Evans rats after single oral administration:

• Delamanid was widely distributed into most tissues including the central nervous system (CNS) in SD rats.

• Relatively high concentration tissues were observed in liver, small intestine, stomach, pituitary, brown fat, pancreas and kidneys in SD rats.

• The radioactivity retention in the eyes of pigmented rats was longer than that observed in non-pigmented ones, which suggested an association with melanin.

Metabolism of Delamanid

❖ The metabolism of delamanid was stable in human liver microsomes.

❖ Transformation delamanid was metabolized primarily by plasma albumin, and to a lesser extent by CYP3A4, CYP1A1, CYP2D6 and CYP2E1.

❖ Overall, the parent drug represented the most abundant component in human plasma, with no significant metabolite observed.

[7] Matsumoto, M.; Hashizume, H.; Tomishige, T., et al. *PLoS Med.* **2006**, *3*, 2131-2144.

Excretion of Delamanid

❖ Was predominantly excreted in feces in rats and dogs, with the parent drug as the significant component in rat and dog feces.

❖ Biliary excretion accounted for 34.1%-36.9% in BDC rats.

Drug-Drug Interaction

❖ Delamanid had rare inhibitory potency against CYPs ($IC_{50}$ >100 μM). (R)-DM-6702 inhibited CYP1A2, CYP2A6, CYP2B6, CYP2C8/9, CYP2C19, CYP2D6 and CYP3A4 activities with $IC_{50}$ values ranging from 18.3 to 87.5 μM.

❖ Delamanid did not induce CYP1A2, CYP2C9 or CYP3A4/5 enzyme activities and mRNA levels at 0.1 and 10 μM.

❖ Delamanid was not a substrate of P-gp.

❖ Delamanid inhibited P-gp, BCRP, OAT1, OAT3, OATP1B1, OATP1B3, OCT1, OCT2 and BSEP ($IC_{50}$ >5 μM).

# Absorption

Table 10　*In Vivo* Pharmacokinetic Parameters of Delamanid in Rats, Mice and Dogs after Single Intravenous and Oral Dose of Delamanid[6]

| Species | Feeding Conditions | Route | Dose (mg/kg) | Vehicle | $T_{max}$ (h) | $C_{max}$ (ng/mL) | $AUC_{inf}$ (ng·h/mL) | $T_{1/2}$ (h) | Cl or Cl/F (mL/h/kg) | $V_{ss}$ (mL/kg) | F (%) |
|---|---|---|---|---|---|---|---|---|---|---|---|
| ICR mouse (male) | Non-fasting | i.v. | 3 | DMSO | - | $C_{5min}$ = 1199 | 13490 | 6.3 | 222 | 2026 | - |
| | | p.o. | 0.3 | 5% (w/v) GA Water/Suspension | 2.0 | 54.4 | 515 | 4.5 | 582 | 3803 | NA |
| | | p.o. | 1 | | 2.0 | 155 | 1818 | 5.2 | 550 | 4146 | NA |
| | | p.o. | 3 | | 4.0 | 431 | 5697 | 5.9 | 527 | 4477 | 42.2 |
| | | p.o. | 10 | | 4.0 | 820 | 10945 | 6.8 | 914 | 8992 | NA |
| | | p.o. | 30 | | 4.0 | 1199 | 22100 | 5.8 | 1358 | 11386 | NA |
| SD rat (male) | Non-fasting | p.o. | 3 | 5% (w/v) GA Water/Suspension | 6.0 | 494 | 7529 | 6.4 | 398 | 3673 | 34.9 |
| | | p.o. | 10 | | 6.0 | 983 | 13934 | 8.2 | 718 | 8444 | NA |
| | | p.o. | 30 | | 4.0 | 1469 | 19950 | 7.5 | 1504 | 16233 | NA |
| | | p.o. | 100 | | 8.0 | 1619 | 27189 | 6.9 | 3678 | 36559 | NA |
| SD rat (male) | Non-fasting | i.v | 3 | DMSO/Solution | - | 13923 | 21566 | 9.2 | 139 | 1841 | NA |
| SD rat (female) | Non-fasting | i.v | 3 | DMSO/Solution | - | 2190 | 18531 | 8.8 | 161.9 | 2056 | NA |
| Beagle dog (male) | Non-fasting | p.o. | 3 | Gelatin capsule | 9.5 | 325 | 8488 | 17.0 | 386 | 9621 | 60.0 |
| | | p.o. | 10 | | 16.0 | 297 | 10590 | 20.6 | 1275 | 34491 | NA |
| | | p.o. | 30 | | 14.0 | 506 | 14381 | 17.3 | 2168 | 55435 | NA |
| | | p.o. | 100 | | 17.5 | 493 | 17900 | 14.3 | 5792 | 120000 | NA |
| | Non-fasting | i.v | 3 | DMSO | - | 1321 | 14140 | 17.6 | 215 | 5388 | NA |

GA: Gum arabic.　DMSO: Dimethyl sulfoxide.

Table 11　*In Vivo* Pharmacokinetic Parameters of Delamanid in Humans after Single Oral Dose of Delamanid[6]

| Species | Feeding Condition | Dose (mg) | $C_{max}$ (ng/mL) | $AUC_{inf}$ (ng·h/mL) | $T_{1/2}$ (h) | $T_{max}$ (h) |
|---|---|---|---|---|---|---|
| Healthy Chinese (male) | Fasting | 100 | 80.7 | 1130 | 16.6 | 3.00 |
| | Fasting | 200 | 108 | 1630 | 22.4 | 2.00 |
| | Fasting | 400 | 126 | 2010 | 24.3 | 3.00 |
| Healthy British (female) | Standard | 100 | 78.4 | 1344 | 41.1 | 3.50 |
| | Standard | 400 | 121 | 2841 | 38.5 | 4.03 |
| Healthy British (male) | Standard | 100 | 103 | 1357 | 24.6 | 3.00 |
| | Standard | 400 | 172 | 2814 | 30.1 | 4.00 |
| | High-fat | 400 | 263 | 4610 | 25.3 | 5.00 |

[6]　PMDA Database.　http://www.pmda.go.jp/drugs/2014/P201400075/index.html (accessed Mar 2016).

# Distribution

Table 12  *In Vitro* Plasma Protein Binding of [$^{14}$C]Delamanid and Metabolites in Several Species[6]

| Species | Conc. (ng/mL) | Total Plasma Protein Binding (%) | | | | Human Serum Protein Binding (%) | | |
|---|---|---|---|---|---|---|---|---|
| | | [$^{14}$C]Delamanid | (*R*)-DM-6701 | (*R*)-DM-6702 | (*R*)-DM-6703 | Protein | Conc. (ng/mL) | [$^{14}$C]Delamanid |
| Rat | 500-5000 | 99.58-99.59 | NC-99.66 | NC-99.40 | NC-98.90 | $\alpha_1$-AGP | 50-5000 | 68.7-87.9 |
| Rabbit | 500-5000 | 99.46-99.50 | NC-99.25 | NC-98.38 | 97.42-98.30 | $\gamma$-GLB | 50-5000 | 77.6-97.1 |
| Dog | 500-5000 | 99.34-99.45 | NC-99.79 | NC-99.62 | NC-99.30 | VLDL | 500 | 97.3 |
| Human | 500-5000 | 99.54-99.57 | NC-99.60 | NC-99.70 | NC-99.21 | LDL | 500 | 97.6 |

Table 13  *In Vivo* Blood Partitioning of [$^{14}$C ]Delamanid in SD Rats and Beagle Dogs after Single Oral Dose of [$^{14}$C]Delamanid[6]

| Species | Route | Dose (mg/kg) | Tissues/Time (h) | Radioactivity (ng eq./mL) | | | | |
|---|---|---|---|---|---|---|---|---|
| | | | | 2 h | 8 h | 24 h | 72 h | 168 h |
| SD rat (male) | p.o. | 3 | Plasma | 431 | 553 | 245 | 43.3 | 7.1 |
| | | | Blood | 283 | 403 | 196 | 52.5 | 18.5 |
| | | | Blood partitioning rate% | 4 | 13 | 22 | 49 | 76 |
| SD rat (female) | p.o. | 3 | Plasma | 464 | 416 | 273 | 96.9 | 34.2 |
| | | | Blood | 320 | 294 | 185 | 83.8 | 47.4 |
| | | | Blood partitioning rate% | 10 | 12 | 9 | 32 | 60 |
| Beagle dog (male) | p.o. | 10 | Plasma | 331 | 1026 | 1029 | 756 | 457 |
| | | | Blood | 253 | 806 | 818 | 648 | 435 |
| | | | Blood partitioning rate% | NA | 26.2 | 27.5 | 32.0 | NA |

Vehicle: 0.5% (w/v) aqueous solution of gum arabic/[$^{14}$C]delamanid suspension.  Each value represented three cases of average value.  Feeding conditions: Non-fasting.  NA: Not available.

Table 14  *In Vivo* Tissue Distribution of [$^{14}$C ]Delamanid in SD Rats and Long-Evans Rats after Single Oral Dose of 3 mg/kg [$^{14}$C ]Delamanid[6]

| Species | SD Rat/Male | | | | | Long-Evans Rat/Male | | | | | |
|---|---|---|---|---|---|---|---|---|---|---|---|
| Tissue | Radioactivity (ng eq./mL or ng eq./g) | | | | Tissue/Plasma AUC$_{0-168}$ Ratio | Radioactivity (ng eq./mL or ng eq./g) | | | | | Tissue/Plasma AUC$_{0-168}$ Ratio |
| | 2 h | 8 h | 24 h | 168 h | | 2 h | 8 h | 24 h | 72 h | 168 h | |
| Plasma | 431 | 553 | 245 | 7.1 | 1.00 | 611 | 847 | 370 | 55.1 | 11.8 | 1.00 |
| Blood | 283 | 403 | 196 | 18.5 | 0.86 | 374 | 518 | 258 | 59.9 | 27.5 | 0.69 |
| Brain | 483 | 1226 | 588 | 185 | 3.07 | ND | ND | ND | ND | ND | 0.00 |
| Kidneys | 1146 | 2034 | 1258 | 301 | 6.28 | 1724 | 2076 | 1460 | 549 | 407 | 4.50 |
| Liver | 2751 | 5194 | 2747 | 354 | 13.0 | 4278 | 6059 | 3652 | 1046 | 516 | 7.71 |
| Spleen | 469 | 1073 | 653 | 91.4 | 2.78 | ND | ND | ND | ND | ND | - |
| Lungs | 817 | 1563 | 833 | 88.2 | 3.38 | ND | ND | ND | ND | ND | - |
| Heart | 815 | 1365 | 518 | 119 | 2.92 | ND | ND | ND | ND | ND | - |
| Stomach | 2165 | 1082 | 372 | 82.3 | 2.42 | ND | ND | ND | ND | ND | - |
| Small intestine | 2545 | 1451 | 428 | 45.2 | 2.55 | ND | ND | ND | ND | ND | - |
| Brown fat | 1609 | 2395 | 702 | 119 | 3.94 | ND | ND | ND | ND | ND | - |
| Pituitary | 1595 | 1892 | 1505 | 194 | 6.31 | ND | ND | ND | ND | ND | - |

[6]  PMDA Database.   http://www.pmda.go.jp/drugs/2014/P201400075/index.html (accessed Mar 2016).

*Continued*

| Species | SD Rata/Male | | | | | Long-Evans Rata/Male | | | | | |
|---|---|---|---|---|---|---|---|---|---|---|---|
| **Tissue** | Radioactivity (ng eq./mL or ng eq./g) | | | | Tissue/Plasma AUC$_{0-168}$ Ratio | Radioactivity (ng eq./mL or ng eq./g) | | | | | Tissue/Plasma AUC$_{0-168}$ Ratio |
| | **2 h** | **8 h** | **24 h** | **168 h** | | **2 h** | **8 h** | **24 h** | **72 h** | **168 h** | |
| Eyeballs | 144 | 264 | 132 | 29.9 | 0.71 | 402 | 866 | 915 | 486 | 408 | 3.15 |
| Muscle | 425 | 860 | 341 | 82.4 | 1.86 | 566 | 813 | 507 | 165 | 106 | 1.34 |
| Pancreas | 1231 | 2088 | 1113 | 92.2 | 4.36 | ND | ND | ND | ND | ND | 0.00 |

Vehicle: 0.5% (w/v) Aqueous solution of gum arabic/[$^{14}$C]delamanid suspension.   ND: Not detected.   Feeding conditions: Non-fasting.

Table 15   *In Vivo* Distribution of Delamanid in Lung in Mice after Single Intravenous and Oral Dose of Delamanid[6]

| Route | Dose (mg/kg) | $K_p$ (lung/plasma, mL/g tissue) | | | | | | | |
|---|---|---|---|---|---|---|---|---|---|
| | | **0.08 h** | **1 h** | **4 h** | **8 h** | **12 h** | **24 h** | **32 h** | **48 h** |
| p.o. | 0.3 | NA | 4.9 | 4.2 | 5.2 | NC | NC | NC | NC |
| | 1 | NA | 2.2 | 3.7 | 2.4 | 2.9 | NC | NC | NC |
| | 3 | NA | 2.1 | 3.3 | 3.2 | 2.6 | 3.3 | NC | NC |
| | 10 | NA | 3.5 | 2.8 | 3.6 | 3.3 | 3.6 | 3.4 | NC |
| | 30 | NA | 4.6 | 4.5 | 3.8 | 4.5 | 20.4 | 3.8 | NC |
| i.v. | 3 | 28.1 | 24.5 | 10 | 9.5 | 5.4 | 8.2 | 4.4 | 20.2 |

NA: Not available.   NC: Not caculated.

## Metabolism

Table 16   *In Vitro* Metabolic Stability of Delamanid in Human Plasma, Albumin and Liver Microsomes[6]

| Matrix | $K_m$ (µM) | $V_{max}$ (pmol/min/mg) | Cl (µL/min/mg) | %Remaining |
|---|---|---|---|---|
| Plasma | 67.8 | 7.55 | 0.111 | 34.2 |
| Albumin | 51.5 | 11.7 | 0.227 | 55.7 |
| Liver microsomes | ND | ND | 0.941 | 92.2 |
| Liver microsomes (with NADH or NADPH) | ND | ND | 4.28 | 66.9 |

ND: Not determined.

Table 17   Metabolism Stability of Delamanid in Liver Microsomes and S9[6]

| Species | Matrix | S9, 2 mg/mL | | Liver Microsomes, 1 mg/mL | |
|---|---|---|---|---|---|
| | | [$^{14}$C]Delamanid Remaining% | DM-6702 Formation% | [$^{14}$C]Delamanid Remaining% | DM-6702 Formation% |
| Mouse | Control | 93.9 | NC | 92.7 | 2.1 |
| | Standard matrices | 95.0 | NC | 91.8 | 1.3 |
| Rat | Control | 96.5 | NC | 92.0 | NC |
| | Standard matrices | 93.2 | NC | 89.6 | 1.0 |
| Rabbit | Control | 97.9 | NC | 91.1 | NC |
| | Standard matrices | 93.7 | NC | 91.5 | NC |
| Dog | Control | 94.1 | NC | 93.9 | NC |
| | Standard matrices | 93.7 | NC | 91.1 | 1.7 |
| Monkey | Control | 94.5 | NC | 88.7 | NC |
| | Standard matrices | 94.4 | NC | 88.7 | 1.3 |

[6]  PMDA Database.   http://www.pmda.go.jp/drugs/2014/P201400075/index.html (accessed Mar 2016).

*Continued*

| Species | Matrix | S9, 2 mg/mL | | Liver Microsomes, 1 mg/mL | |
|---|---|---|---|---|---|
| | | [$^{14}$C]Delamanid Remaining% | DM-6702 Formation% | [$^{14}$C]Delamanid Remaining% | DM-6702 Formation% |
| Human | Control | 92.5 | NC | 93.3 | NC |
| | Standard matrices | 90.7 | NC | 90.1 | NC |

Table 18　*In Vitro* Metabolic Phenotype of Delamanid[6]

| Methods | Recombinant Enzyme | Specific Chemical Inhibitor |
|---|---|---|
| Delamanid | 1 μM, 20 min | 10 μM, 60 min |
| Parameters | %Remaining | %Inhibition |
| CYP1A1 | 53.0 | - |
| CYP1A2 | 89.4 | -47.4 |
| CYP2A6 | 79.4 | NA |
| CYP2B6 | 81.7 | -41.9 |
| CYP2C8 | 79.1 | NA |
| CYP2C9 | 82.7 | -14.8 |
| CYP2C19 | 83.7 | -21.5 |
| CYP2D6 | 85.3 | 48.7 |
| CYP2E1 | 90.6 | NA |
| CYP3A4 | 64.1 | 52.5 |
| CYP3A5 | 94.1 | NA |

NA: Not available.

Table 19　*In Vivo* Metabolites of [$^{14}$C]Delamanid in Plasma and Lungs after Single Oral Dose of [$^{14}$C]Delamanid[6]

| Species | Route | Dose (mg/kg) | Vehicle | Matrix | Time (h) | The Ratio of Total Radioactivity (%) | | | | | | RC (ng eq./mL or g) |
|---|---|---|---|---|---|---|---|---|---|---|---|---|
| | | | | | | Total Radioactivity | Parent | DM-6701 | DM-6702 | DM-6703 | UK-1 | |
| ICR mouse (male) | p.o. | 3 | 5% (w/v) GA/DS | Plasma | 2 | - | 82.3 | - | - | - | - | 413 |
| | | | | | 4 | - | 63.9 | - | - | - | - | 559 |
| | | | | | 8 | - | 76.2 | - | - | - | - | 745 |
| | | | | | 24 | - | 31.0 | - | - | - | - | 196 |
| SD rat (male) | p.o. | 3 | 5% (w/v) GA/DS | Plasma | 2 | 85.9 | 85.9 | - | - | - | - | 431 |
| | | | | | 8 | 73.7 | 73.7 | - | - | - | - | 553 |
| | | | | | 24 | 31.1 | 31.1 | - | - | - | - | 245 |
| | | | | Lungs | 2 | 81.5 | 81.5 | - | - | - | - | 817 |
| | | | | | 8 | 108 | 66.0 | - | 41.6 | - | - | 1563 |
| | | | | | 24 | 67.0 | - | - | 67.0 | - | - | 833 |
| SD rat (female) | p.o. | 3 | 5% (w/v) GA/DS | Plasma | 2 | 86.9 | 86.9 | - | - | - | - | 464 |
| | | | | | 8 | 77.1 | 77.1 | - | - | - | - | 416 |
| | | | | | 24 | 39.1 | 39.1 | - | - | - | - | 273 |
| | | | | Lungs | 2 | 96.9 | 96.9 | - | - | - | - | 846 |
| | | | | | 8 | 98.2 | 72.3 | - | 25.9 | - | - | 2185 |
| | | | | | 24 | 105 | 51.6 | - | 53.2 | - | - | 2113 |

[6] PMDA Database. http://www.pmda.go.jp/drugs/2014/P201400075/index.html (accessed Mar 2016).

*Continued*

| Species | Route | Dose (mg/kg) | Vehicle | Matrix | Time (h) | The Ratio of Total Radioactivity (%) | | | | | | RC (ng eq./mL or g) |
| | | | | | | Total Radioactivity | Parent | DM-6701 | DM-6702 | DM-6703 | UK-1 | |
|---|---|---|---|---|---|---|---|---|---|---|---|---|
| Beagle dog (male) | p.o. | 10 | 5% (w/v) GA/DS | Plasma | 4 | 64.6 | 64.6 | - | - | - | - | 545 |
| | | | | | 12 | 49.3 | 49.3 | - | - | - | - | 1002 |
| | | | | | 24 | 32.7 | 28.6 | - | - | - | 4.1 | 1029 |
| | | | | | 48 | NA | NA | - | - | - | - | 847 |
| | | | | | 72 | NA | NA | - | - | - | - | 756 |
| | | | | | 96 | NA | NA | - | - | - | - | 627 |
| | | | | | 120 | NA | NA | - | - | - | - | 562 |
| | | | | | 144 | NA | NA | - | - | - | - | 506 |
| | | | | | 168 | NA | NA | - | - | - | - | 457 |

Feeding conditions: Non-fasting.    NA: Not available.    GA: Aqueous solution of gum arabic.    DS: Delamanid suspension.    RC: Radioactivity concentration.

Table 20    Metabolites in Urine, Bile and Feces in Non-Clinical Species after Single Oral Dose of Delamanid[6]

| Species | Dose (mg/kg) | Matrix | Time (h) | % of Dose | | | | | | | | | | |
| | | | | Parent | DM-6701 | DM-6702 | RM-1 | RM-4 | RM-10 | RM-11 | RM-12 | RM-15 | RM-17 | UK-2 |
|---|---|---|---|---|---|---|---|---|---|---|---|---|---|---|
| SD rat (male) | 3 | Urine | 0-24 | - | - | 0.29 | 0.41 | 0.92 | - | - | - | - | - | - |
| | | Bile | 0-72 | - | - | 0.35 | 1.47 | - | - | - | - | 1.32 | 3.45 | - |
| | | Feces | 0-24 | 28.2 | 1.06 | 4.95 | 1.82 | - | 0.98 | 1.11 | 0.26 | - | - | - |
| SD rats (female) | 3 | Urine | 0-24 | - | - | 0.25 | 0.31 | 1.30 | - | - | - | - | - | - |
| | | Bile | 0-72 | - | - | 0.54 | 1.66 | - | - | - | - | 2.21 | 2.61 | - |
| | | Feces | 0-24 | 32.1 | 0.85 | 3.11 | 1.97 | - | 0.58 | 0.44 | - | - | - | - |
| Beagle dog (male) | 10 | Urine | 0-24 | - | - | - | - | - | - | - | - | - | - | 0.13 |
| | | Feces | 0-24 | 60.4 | 0.44 | 2.30 | - | - | - | - | - | - | - | - |

Feeding conditions: Non-fasting.    Vehicle: 5% (w/v) GA/DS.    GA: Aqueous solution of gum arabic.    DS: Delamanid suspension.

[6]  PMDA Database.    http://www.pmda.go.jp/drugs/2014/P201400075/index.html (accessed Mar 2016).

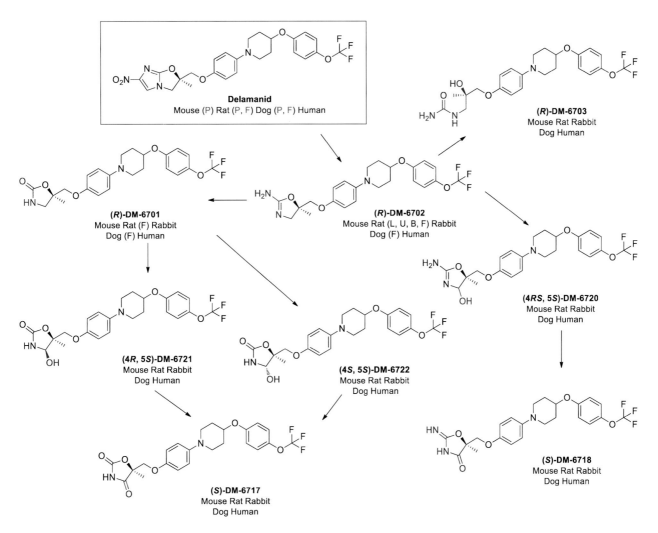

Figure B    Proposed Pathways for *In Vitro* and *In Vivo* Biotransformation of Delamanid in Rats, Mice, Dogs, Rabbits and Humans[6]
The red labels represent the major components in matrices.    P = Plasma, L = Lung, U = Urine, B = Bile and F = Feces.

## Excretion

Table 21    Excretion Profiles of [$^{14}$C]Delamanid in Rats and Dogs after Single Oral Dose of [$^{14}$C]Delamanid[6]

| Species | State | Route | Dose (mg/kg) | Time (h) | Bile (% of dose) | Urine (% of dose) | Feces (% of dose) | Recovery (% of dose) |
|---|---|---|---|---|---|---|---|---|
| SD rat (male) | Intact | p.o. | 3 | 0-168 | - | 6.29 | 91.6 | 97.9 |
| SD rat (female) | Intact | p.o. | 3 | 0-168 | - | 6.45 | 92.2 | 98.7 |
| Beagle dog (male) | Intact | p.o. | 10 | 0-168 | - | 3.0 | 89.8 | 93.6 |
| SD rat (male) | BDC | p.o. | 3 | 0-72 | 34.1 | 6.49 | NA | 40.6 |
| SD rat (female) | BDC | p.o. | 3 | 0-72 | 36.9 | 7.63 | NA | 44.5 |
| SD rat (male) | BDC | i.d. | 1 mL/body bile[a] | 0-72 | 8.54 | 1.94 | NA | 10.5 |

Feeding conditions: Non-fasting.    Vehicle: 5% (w/v) gum arabic solution/suspension.    [a] Following a single oral dose of 3 mg/kg [$^{14}$C]delamanid to rats, bile collected up to 24 h after administration was administered intraduodenally to a different set of rats.

[6]   PMDA Database.    http://www.pmda.go.jp/drugs/2014/P201400075/index.html (accessed Mar 2016).

## Drug-Drug Interaction

Table 22    *In Vitro* Evaluation of Delamanid and Metabolites as Inhibitors and Inducers of Enzymes[6]

| | Delamanid and its Metabolites as Inhibitors | | | | | | | Delamanid as an Inducer | | | | |
| | Remaining Activity (%) | IC$_{50}$ (µM) | | | | | | | Enzyme Activity | | Enzyme Activity | |
| Enzyme | Delamanid | (R)-DM-6701 | (R)-DM-6702 | (R)-DM-6703 | (S)-DM-6718 | (4RS,5S)-DM-6720 | Enzyme | Conc. (µM) | Fold Induction | Positive Control (%) | Fold Induction | Positive Control (%) |
|---|---|---|---|---|---|---|---|---|---|---|---|---|
| CYP1A2 | 98.6 | >100 | 41.0 | >100 | >100 | >100 | CYP1A2 | 0.1 | 1.01 | NC | 0.908 | NC |
| CYP2A6 | 100.8 | >100 | 87.5 | >100 | >100 | 42.3 | | 10 | 1.05 | NC | 1.22 | NC |
| CYP2B6 | 122.3 | 25.2 | 24.3 | 32.8 | >100 | 32.7 | CYP2C9 | 0.1 | 1.04 | NC | 0.911 | NC |
| CYP2C8/9 | 108.5 | 42.9 | 30.7 | 90.6 | >100 | >100 | | 10 | 1.05 | NC | 1.04 | NC |
| CYP2C19 | 107.6 | 89.4 | 18.3 | 54.0 | >100 | >100 | CYP3A4/5 | 0.1 | 1.17 | NC | 1.09 | NC |
| CYP2D6 | 97.8 | >100 | 28.9 | >100 | >100 | >100 | | 10 | 0.672 | NC | 1.49 | 5.84 |
| CYP2E1 | 112.5 | >100 | >100 | >100 | >100 | >100 | | 0.1 | NA | NA | 1.12 | 1.4 |
| CYP3A4[a] | 115.6 | >100 | 35.8 | >100 | >100 | 10.9 | CYP2B6 | 1 | NA | NA | 1.24 | 2.9 |
| CYP3A4[b] | 100.3 | >100 | 53.6 | >100 | >100 | >100 | | 10 | NA | NA | 1.48 | 5.5 |

[a] Testosterone 6β-hydroxylation.    [b] Nifedipine oxidation.    NC: Not calculated.    NA: Not available.

Table 23    *In Vitro* Evaluation of Delamanid as an Inhibitor and a Substrate of Transporters[6]

| | Transporter Inhibition, IC$_{50}$ (µM) | | | | | | | | |
| | ABC | | | SLC | | | | | |
| Inhibitor | P-gp | BCRP | BSEP | OAT1 | OAT3 | OCT1 | OCT2 | OATP1B1 | OATP1B3 |
|---|---|---|---|---|---|---|---|---|---|
| Delamanid | >5 | >5 | >5 | >5 | >5 | >5 | >5 | >5 | >5 |
| (R)-DM-6701 | >3 | >3 | >3 | >3 | >3 | >3 | >3 | >3 | >3 |
| (R)-DM-6702 | 4.65 | 5.71 | >10 | >10 | >10 | >10 | >10 | >10 | >10 |
| (S)-DM-6718 | >3 | >3 | >5 | >3 | >3 | >3 | >3 | >3 | >3 |
| (4RS,5S)-DM-6720 | 7.80 | 6.02 | >10 | >10 | >10 | >10 | >10 | >10 | >10 |
| Delamanid as a substrate | No | NA | NA | NA | NA | NA | NA | NA | NA |

NA: Not available.

Tabel 24    *In Vitro* Evaluation of Delamanid as a Substrate of P-gp and BCRP Transpoters[6]

| Transporter | Compound | Conc. (µM) | Efflux Ratio | | ER | Transporter | Compound | Conc. (µM) | Metablism (µL/mg protein) | | Uptake Ratio |
| | | | Control Cell | LLC-PK1 Cell | | | | | Control Cell | LLC-PK1 Cell | |
|---|---|---|---|---|---|---|---|---|---|---|---|
| P-gp | [14C]Delamnid | 5 | 1.0 | 1.1 | 1.1 | OATP1B1 | [14C]Delamnid | 1 | 25.1 | 34.8 | 1.4 |
| | (R)-DM-6702 | 3 | 2.9 | 9.6 | 3.3 | | (R)-DM-6702 | 1 | 474 | 614 | 1.3 |
| | (R)-DM-6702+ Quinidine | 3, 30 | 1.7 | 1.6 | 0.9 | OATP1B3 | [14C]Delamnid | 1 | 25.1 | 24.9 | 1.0 |
| | | | | | | | (R)-DM-6702 | 1 | 474 | 204 | 0.4 |
| BCRP | [14C]Delamanid | 5 | 1.1 | 1.2 | 1.1 | OCT1 | [14C]Delamnid | 1 | 70.9 | 66.1 | 0.9 |
| | (R)-DM-6702 | 3 | 1.6 | 1.1 | 0.7 | | (R)-DM-6702 | 1 | 474 | 547 | 1.2 |

[6]  PMDA Database.   http://www.pmda.go.jp/drugs/2014/P201400075/index.html (accessed Mar 2016).

# 6  Non-Clinical Toxicology

## Summary

### Single-Dose Toxicity

❖ Single-dose toxicity studies by oral administration in rats and dogs:
- Rat ALD: >1000 mg/kg.
- Dog ALD: >900 mg/kg.

### Repeated-Dose Toxicity

❖ Pivotal repeated-dose toxicity studies by the oral route for up to 26 weeks in rats, and up to 39 weeks in dogs:
- The systemic exposures at the NOAEL from the 26-week rat study were 4.3- to 16.7-fold higher than the proposed clinical AUC.
- Meanwhile, the exposure margin in the 39-week dog study ranged from 0.5 to 0.9, primarily based upon the QT prolongation observed.
- Pronounced cross-species inhibitory effects on blood coagulation were demonstrated.  Moreover, there were also species-specific lesions at exposures in excess of those proposed clinically, e.g., alternations in RBC parameters in rats as well as liver disorder and foamy macrophages in the lymphoid follicles of various organs in dogs.

### Safety Pharmacology

❖ Safety pharmacology to evaluate the effects of delamanid and its metabolites for the cardiotoxicity, CNS toxicity and respiratory effects:
- Cardiovascular system: Some degree of hERG channel inhibition (35.4% at 1.6 µg/mL).  No effect on action potential duration at up to 1.6 µg/mL.  No effect on dog QT interval where plasma levels of delamanid were ≤3.2-fold higher than those observed in man.
- Central nervous system: No treatment related effect at ~18.5-fold higher plasma levels than that proposed clinically (following 100 mg BID).
- Respiratory system: No treatment-related effect on respiratory rate at 3.2-fold higher exposures than the maximum proposed $C_{max}$ in humans.

### Genotoxicity

❖ Delamanid and its metabolites were demonstrated non-mutagenic, and the data therefore suggested that administration of delamanid would not pose a genotoxic risk to humans.

### Reproductive and Developmental Toxicity

❖ Fertility and early embryonic development in rats:
- No effect on male or female fertility at up to 300 mg/kg/day.

❖ Embryo-fetal developmental in rats and rabbits:
- Delamanid was not teratogenic at the doses evaluated in both species.  However, a slight increase in resorption incidences was noted at 10 mg/kg/day in rabbits.

❖ Pre  and postnatal development in rats:
- NOAEL was 300 mg/kg/day for both the $F_0$ dams and fetal organogenesis, with exposure margin as 13 × MRIID.

❖ Repeated-dose toxicity in juvenile rats:
- No additional toxicological effect when compared with adult animals.

### Carcinogenicity

❖ Delamanid did not appear to be carcinogenic in the regular 104-week repeated oral study with mice and rats.

### Special Toxicology

❖ Phototoxicity: Negative at concentrations well in excess of those proposed clinically (0.41 µg/mL).

## Single-Dose Toxicity

Table 25    Single-Dose Toxicity Studies of Delamanid by the Oral Route[6]

| Species | Dose (mg/kg) | ALD (mg/kg) | Finding |
|---|---|---|---|
| SD rat | 1000 | >1000 | No death.    In the general state observation of up to Day 7, loose stools or white stools over the 8-9 h and the next day after the administration in male fasting group was observed. |
| Beagle dog | 900 | >900 | No death.    In the general state observation of up to Day 15, white stools were observed after 2-3 h of the second dose in both animals until Day 3.    Mild decrease in the female in food consumption to Day 2 (56%). Drug-related change in body weight was not observed. |

Vehicle: 5% (w/v) Arabic gum for rats; Gelatin capsule for dogs.

## Repeated-Dose Toxicity

Table 26    Repeated-Dose Toxicity Studies of Delamanid by Oral Administrations[6]

| Species | Duration (Week) | Dose (mg/kg/day) | NOAEL | | | Finding[b] |
| | | | Dose (mg/kg/day) | $AUC_{0-24}$ (µg·h/mL) | Safety Margin[a] (× MRHD) | |
|---|---|---|---|---|---|---|
| SD rat | 4 | 0, 3, 30, 300 | 300 | Male: 67.2 Female: 102.8 | Male: 8.48 Female: 12.98 | ↑ Neutrophil count in HD females. In electron microscopy, rare anomalies (1 case) was observed in liver, kidneys and adrenal gland at HD. |
| | 26 | 0, 3, 30, 300 | Male: 30 Female: 300 | Male: 34.2 Female: 132.7 | Male: 4.3 Female: 16.7 | ↓ Hematocrit and red blood cell count and ↑ reticulocyte ratio; Prolonged PT and APTT mostly in HD males. |
| Beagle dog | 13 | 0, 3, 10, 30, 100 | 3 | Male: 6.97 Female: 3.53 | Male: 0.88 Female: 0.45 | ↓ Body weight associated with ↓ food consumption. ↑ QT and QTc interval and ↑ ALT at HD. |
| | 39 | 0, 1, 3, 30 | Male: 1 Female: 3 | Male: 3.88 Female: 7.28 | Male: 0.5 Female: 0.9 | ↓ ST amplitude and ↑ QT and QTc interval in HD females. Mild to moderate histopathological findings in the liver; Foamy macrophages in the lymphoid follicles of various organs. |

[a] Compared to the AUC at clinical recommended dose, 7.92 µg·h/mL.    [b] The metabolite of delamanid, DM-6717 observed at the effective doses were substantially higher than those in man.

[6]  PMDA Database.    http://www.pmda.go.jp/drugs/2014/P201400075/index.html (accessed Mar 2016).

## Safety Pharmacology

Table 27    Safety Pharmacological Studies of Delamanid and Metabolites[6]

| Study | System | Compound | Dose (mg/kg) | Finding |
|---|---|---|---|---|
| Cardiovascular effect | HEK293 cell expressing hERG channel | Delamanid | 0.03, 0.1, 0.3, 1, 3 μM | Inhibition of hERG: 19.6%-23.2% vs pretest at 0.03-1 μM, and 35.4% inhibition at 1.6 μg/mL (3 μM). |
| | | DM-6701 | 0.01, 0.1, 1, 3 μM | hERG current: Reduced to 33.2% at 3 μM, $IC_{50}$ = 1.6 μM. |
| | | DM-6702 | 0.001, 0.01, 0.1, 1 μM | Significant inhibition at 0.1-1 μM, $IC_{50}$ = 0.0822 μM. |
| | | DM-6717 | 1 μM | No effect. |
| Central nervous effect | SD rat | Delamanid | 10, 100, 1000 | No effect. |
| Respiratory effect | Beagle dog | Delamanid | 50, 150, 450 | No effect. Mean maximum plasma concentration: 1.292 μg/mL. |

## Genotoxicity

Table 28    Genotoxicity Studies of Delamanid and Metabolites[6]

| Assay | Species/System | Test Article | Metabolism | Dose | Finding |
|---|---|---|---|---|---|
| In vitro bacterial reverse mutation assay (Ames) | S. typhimurium TA98, TA100, TA1535, TA1537, YG1041, YG1042 | Delamanid | ±S9 | 5.00-5000 μg/plate, for 48 h | Negative. |
| | S. typhimurium TA98, TA100, TA1535, TA1537 | (R)-DM-6702 | ±S9 | 0.500-150 μg/plate, for 48 h | Negative. |
| | | (S)-DM-6718 | ±S9 | 5.00-5000 μg/plate, for 48 h | Negative. |
| | | (R)-DM-6701 | ±S9 | 0.05-5000 μg/plate, for 48 h | Negative. |
| | | (R)-DM-6703 | ±S9 | 5.00-5000 μg/plate, for 48 h | Negative. |
| In vitro mammalian cell gene mutation assay | L5178Y t/k$^{+/-}$ | Delamanid | ±S9 | 1.0-300 mg/L for 3 h 0.3-300 mg/L for 24 h | Negative. |
| In vivo bone marrow micronuclei assay | SD rat | Delamanid | + | 0, 100, 300, 1000 mg/kg, p.o. | Negative. |
| | | (R)-DM-6702 | + | 0, 7.5, 15, 30 mg/kg, p.o. | Negative. |
| | | (S)-DM-6718 | + | 0, 2, 4, 8 mg/kg, p.o. | Negative. |
| | | (R)-DM-6701 | + | 0, 2.5, 5, 10 mg/kg, p.o. | Negative. |
| | | (R)-DM-6703 | + | 0, 0.25, 0.5, 1.0 mg/kg, p.o. | Negative. |
| In vivo UDS assay | SD rat | Delamanid | + | 0, 1000, 2000 mg/kg, p.o. | Negative. |

[6]  PMDA Database.    http://www.pmda.go.jp/drugs/2014/P201400075/index.html (accessed Mar 2016).

## Reproductive and Developmental Toxicity

Table 29    Reproductive and Developmental Toxicology Studies of Delamanid by Oral (Gavage) Administration[6]

| Studies | Species | Dose (mg/kg/day) | NOAEL | | | | Finding |
|---------|---------|------------------|-------|---|---|---|---------|
| | | | Endpoint | Dose (mg/kg/day) | $AUC_{0-24}$ (µg·h/mL) | Safety Margin[a] (× MRHD) | |
| Fertility and early embryonic development | SD rat | 0, 3, 30, 300 | Male fertility | 300 | 67.2 | 8.5 | The general toxicity of male and female was observed at 300 mg/kg/day. |
| | | | Female fertility | 300 | 102.8 | 13 | |
| Embryo-fetal development | SD rat | 0, 3, 30, 300 | Mater/Fetal development | 300 | 102.8 | 13 | No effects. |
| | NZW rabbit | 0, 1, 5 10 | Mater/Fetal development | 5 | 8.3) | 1 | ↓ Body weight gain and food consumption at 10 mg/kg/day, as well as mild ↑ early resorptions that were considered secondary effects of maternal toxicity was observed. |
| Pre- and postnatal development | SD rat | 0, 3, 30, 300 | $F_0/F_1$ | 300 | 102.8 | 13 | No effects. |
| Juvenile toxicity | 4-day SD rat | 0, 3, 30, 300 for 10 weeks | Male | 3 | 18.8 | 2.37 | ↓ Body weight associated with ↓ food consumption. |
| | | | | | | | ↑ Neutrophil count in HD females. |
| | | | Female | 30 | 49.1 | 6.20 | ↑ QT and QTc interval and ↑ ALT in HD males. |

[a] Compared to the AUC at clinical recommended dose, 7.92 µg·h/mL.

## Carcinogenicity

Table 30    104-Week Carcinogenicity Studies of Delamanid by Oral Administration[6]

| Species | Dose (mg/kg/day) | Finding |
|---------|------------------|---------|
| ICR mouse | 0, 3, 30, 300 | Pre- and neoplasm lesions at all doses, including negative control. |
| SD rat | 0, 3, 30, 300 | Pre- and neoplasm lesions at all doses, including negative control. |

Vehicle: 5% (w/v) Arabic gum.    [a] Animal AUC/human AUC, the clinical recommended dose AUC was 3.69 µg·h/mL in human.

## Special Toxicology

Table 31    Special Toxicology Studies of Delamanid[6]

| Study | Species | Conc. (µg/mL) | Finding |
|-------|---------|---------------|---------|
| Phototoxicity assay-in vitro neutral red uptake assay | Murine (Balb/c 3T3) fibroblast | 2.13-31.6 | No phototoxic potential. |

[6]  PMDA Database.   http://www.pmda.go.jp/drugs/2014/P201400075/index.html (accessed Mar 2016).

# CHAPTER

11

---

## Eliglustat Tartrate

# Eliglustat Tartrate

## (Cerdelga®)

Research code: Genz-112638

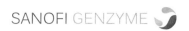

## 1  General Information

❖ Eliglustat tartrate is a glucosylceramide synthase inhibitor, which was first accelerated approved in the worldwide in Aug 2014 by US FDA.

❖ Eliglustat tartrate was discovered and marketed by Genzyme Corp. (now a subsidiary of Sanofi).

❖ Eliglustat tartrate is a selective inhibitor of glucosylceramide synthase, as a substrate reduction therapy (SRT) for Gaucher disease type 1 (GD1).

❖ Eliglustat tartrate is indicated for the treatment of adult patients with GD1 who are CYP2D6 extensive metabolizers (EMs), intermediate metabolizers (IMs), or poor metabolizers (PMs).

❖ Available as capsule, with each containing 84 mg of eliglustat and the recommended starting dose is 84 mg taken orally twice daily in CYP2D6 EMs and IMs, the recommended dose in CY2D6 PMs is 84 mg once daily.

❖ The 2014 and 2015 worldwide sales of Cerdelga® were 5.3 and 73.3 million US$, respectively, referring to the financial reports of Sanofi.

### Key Approvals around the World*

|  | US (FDA) | EU (EMA) | Japan (PMDA) |
|---|---|---|---|
| **First approval date** | 08/19/2014 | 01/19/2015 | 03/26/2015 |
| **Application or approval No.** | NDA 205494 | EMEA/H/C/003 724 | 22700AMX0065 4000 |
| **Brand name** | Cerdelga® | Cerdelga® | Cerdelga® |
| **Indication** | Gaucher disease type 1 | Gaucher disease type 1 | Gaucher disease type 1 |
| **Authorization holder** | Genzyme | Genzyme | Genzyme |

*Till Mar 2016, it had not been approved by CFDA (China).

## Active Ingredient

*Molecular formula*: $C_{23}H_{36}N_2O_4 \cdot 1/2C_4H_6O_6$
*Molecular weight*: 479.59
*CAS No.*: 491833-29-5 (Eliglustat)
928659-70-5 (Eliglustat tartrate)
*Chemical name*: $N$-((1$R$,2$R$)-1-(2,3-dihydrobenzo[$b$][1,4]dioxin-6-yl)-1-hydroxy-3-(pyrrolidin-1-yl)propan-2-yl)octanamide (2$R$,3$R$)-2,3-dihydroxysuccinate

*Parameters of Lipinski's "Rule of 5"*

| MW[a] | H$_D$ | H$_A$ | FRB[b] | PSA[b] | cLogP[b] |
|---|---|---|---|---|---|
| 404.54 | 2 | 6 | 12 | 71.0Å$^2$ | 2.97 ± 0.61 |

[a] Molecular weight of eliglustat.  [b] Calculated by ACD/Labs software V11.02.

## Drug Product*

*Dosage route*:  Oral
*Strength*:  84 mg (Eliglustat)
*Dosage form*:  Capsule
*Inactive ingredient*:  Microcrystalline cellulose, lactose monohydrate, hypromellose and glyceryl behenate, gelatin, candurin silver fine, yellow iron oxide and FD&C blue 2.
*Recommended dose*:  The recommended starting dose is 84 mg taken orally twice daily in CYP2D6 EMs or IMs, the recommended dose in CY2D6 PMs is 84 mg once daily. Dosage reduced to 84 mg once daily for: CYP2D6 EMs and IMs taking strong or moderate CYP2D6 inhibitors, CYP2D6 EMs taking strong or moderate CYP3A inhibitors.

*Sourced from US FDA drug label information

## 2  Key Patents Information

### Summary

❖ Cerdelga® (Eliglustat tartrate) has got five-year NCE market exclusivity protection and seven-year orphan drug exclusivity protection, after it was initially approved by US FDA on Aug 19, 2014.

❖ Eliglustat was originally discovered by Genzyme, and its compound patent application was filed as PCT application by Genzyme in 2002.

❖ The compound patent will expire in 2022 foremost, which has been granted in the United States, Europe and Japan successively, but has not been filed in China yet.

Table 1  Eliglustat's Compound Patent Protection in Drug-Mainstream Country

| Country | Publication/Patent NO. | Application Date | Granted Date | Estimated Expiry Date |
|---------|------------------------|------------------|--------------|------------------------|
| WO | WO03008399A1 | 07/16/2002 | / | / |
| US | US7196205B2 | 07/16/2002 | 03/27/2007 | 04/29/2022[a] |
| EP | EP1409467B1 | 07/16/2002 | 04/18/2012 | 07/16/2022 |
| EP | EP2067775B1 | 07/16/2002 | 04/25/2012 | 07/16/2022 |
| JP | JP5038582B2 | 07/16/2002 | 10/03/2012 | 03/28/2025[b] |
| CN | NA | / | / | / |

[a] The term of this patent is extended by 0 days (the patent is subject to a terminal disclaimer of US6916802B2).   [b] The term of this patent is extended by 986 days.

Table 2  Originator's International Patent Application List (Patent Family)

| Publication NO. | Title | Applicant/Assignee/Owner | Publication Date |
|-----------------|-------|--------------------------|------------------|
| **Technical Subjects** | **Active Ingredient (Free Base)'s Formula or Structure and Preparation** | | |
| WO03008399A1 | Synthesis of UDP-glucose: *N*-acylsphingosine glucosyltransferase inhibitors | Genzyme | 01/30/2003 |
| **Technical Subjects** | **Salt, Crystal, Polymorphic, Solvate (Hydrate), Isomer, Derivative Etc. and Preparation** | | |
| WO2011066352A1 | An amorphous and a crystalline form of Genz 112638 hemi-tartrat as inhibitor of glucosylceramide synthase | Genzyme | 06/03/2011 |
| **Technical Subjects** | **Indication or Methods for Medical Needs** | | |
| WO2007134086A2 | Methods of treating fatty liver disease | Genzyme | 11/22/2007 |

The data was updated until Jan 2016.

## 3 Chemistry

### Route 1: Original Discovery Route

MIBK: Methylisobutyl ketone

*Synthesis Route:* Condensation of commercially available *S*-(+)-2-phenyl glycinol **1** with phenyl bromoacetate **2** in acetonitrile in the presence of DIPEA provided morpholin-2-one hydrochloride **3** in 53% yield upon treatment with HCl. Neutralization with aqueous $NaHCO_3$ followed by coupling with aldehyde **4** in refluxing EtOAc/toluene yielded oxazine adduct **5**, which was isolated as a precipitate from MTBE in 58% yield. Opening of oxazine **5** with pyrrolidine in refluxing THF followed by addition of aqueous HCl in refluxing MeOH gave amide **6** in 81% yield over two steps, which was then reduced to amine **7** using $LiAlH_4$ in refluxing THF in 89% yield. Subsequent hydrogenation cleaved the phenylethanol group to give the free amine, which was converted to dioxalate salt **8** in 77% yield over two steps by treatment with oxalic acid in MIBK. Subjection of aminoethanol **8** to aqueous sodium hydroxide followed by coupling with HOSu activated-ester **10** gave eliglustat as the corresponding freebase in 38% yield from **8** with 99.8% *ee*. Salt formation with L-tartaric acid (0.5 equiv.) then provided eliglustat tartrate in overall yield of 6% from **1**.[1-4]

[1] Hirth, B. H.; SiegeL, C. WO03008399A1, **2003**.
[2] Hirth, B. H.; SiegeL, C. US6855830B2, **2005**.
[3] Liu, H.; Willis, C.; Bhardwaj, R., et al. WO2011066352A1, **2011**.
[4] Liu, H.; Willis, C.; Bhardwaj, R., et al. US20130137743A1, **2013**.

## Route 2

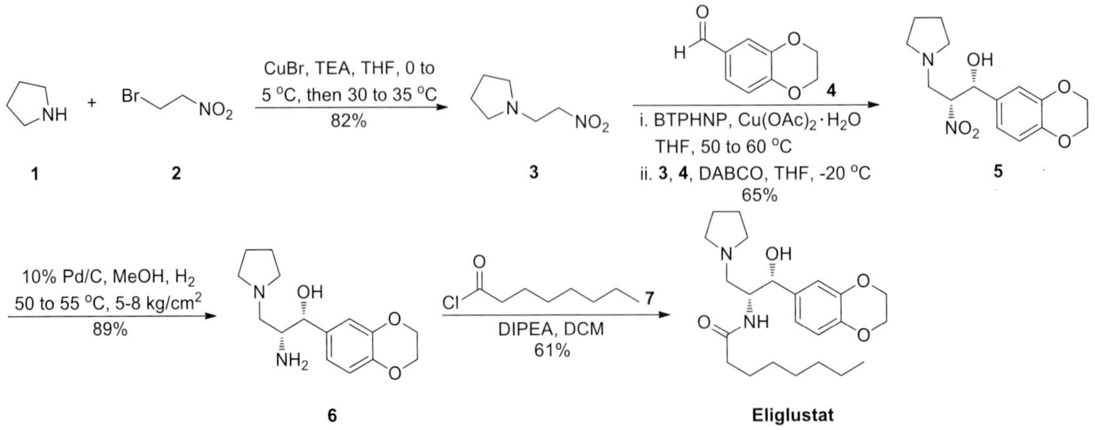

BTPHNP: (11R,13S)-11-(1H-benzo[d][1,2,3]triazol-1-yl)-13-phenyl-7a,8,9,10,11,13-hexahydronaphtho[1,2-e]pyrido[2,1-b][1,3]oxazine
DABCO: 1,4-Diazabicyclo(2.2.2)octane

*Synthesis Route*:   This optimized synthesis referred to a key asymmetric Henry reaction of 1-(2-nitroethyl)pyrolidine **3**, which was prepared by union between 1-bromo-2-nitroethane **2** and pyrrolidine **1**, with aldehyde **4** catalyzed by chiral copper( II ) species with BTPHNP as ligand and DABCO as base to afford α-hydroxyl nitro derivative **5** in 65% yield.   Hydrogenative reduction of nitro group within **5** offered free amine **6** in 89% yield.   Eventually, condensation of amine **6** with acyl chloride **7** furnished eliglustat in 61% yield with the overall yield of 29%.[5]

## 4   Pharmacology

## Summary

Mechanism of Action

❖ Eliglustat selectively inhibits glucosylceramide synthase, and reduces the rate of synthesis of glucosylceramide to match its impaired rate of catabolism in patients with GD1, thereby preventing glucosylceramide accumulation and alleviating clinical manifestations.

❖ Eliglustat inhibited glucosylceramide synthase in A375 cell-derived microsomes ($IC_{50}$ = 19.6 nM) and cell surface expression of GM3 in B16 cells ($IC_{50}$ = 56.7 nM).

❖ Eliglustat had significant inhibition of ligands binding at 9 targets in screening assays in a panel of 80 different receptors, transporters, and ion channels at 10 μM.   The targets with significant inhibition of eliglustat included the dopamine receptors D3 and D4.4, the serotonin receptors 5-HT$_{1A}$, 5-HT$_{2A}$, 5-HT$_{2B}$ and 5-HT$_6$, the μ-opioid receptor, the nonspecific sigma receptor, and the $Ca^{2+}$ ion channel (L, verapamil site).

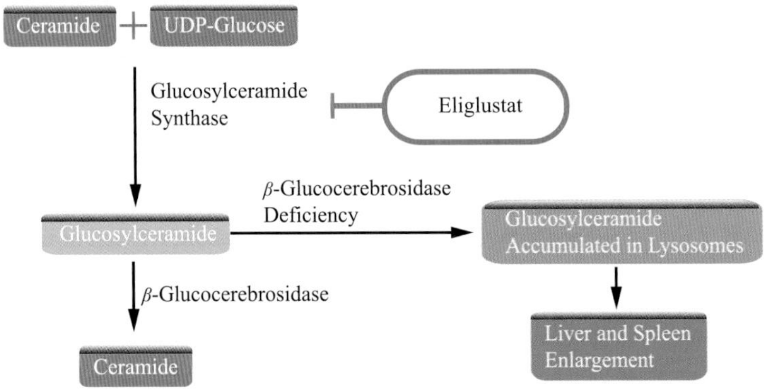

*In Vitro* Efficacy

❖ The inhibition of glucosylceramide synthase in cell lines:
  • Cell homogenates of dog kidney cells: $IC_{50}$ = 115 nM (GM1 level).
  • K562 cells: $IC_{50}$ = 14 or 28 nM (GM1 level).
  • DH82 cells: $IC_{50}$ = 78 or 79 nM (GM1 level).
  • B16 cells: $IC_{50}$ = 56.7 nM (GM3 level).

❖ GL-1 synthase inhibition of the metabolites in human:
  • GL-1 synthesis: $IC_{50}$ = 1.09->30 μM.
  • GM3 synthesis: $IC_{50}$ = 1.54->10 μM.

[5]  Xu, X. CN104557851A, **2015**.

*In Vivo* Efficacy

❖ In normal SD rat models:
- Significantly decreased glucosylceramide levels in liver, kidneys and spleen at 37.5 mg/kg BID (75 mg/kg/day).

❖ In normal beagle dog models:
- Significantly decreased glucosylceramide levels in liver homogenates at 2.5 mg/kg BID (5 mg/kg/day).

❖ In Fabry disease mouse models:
- Significantly reduced GL-3 in the kidneys at 75 mg/kg QD.

❖ In D490V/null Gaucher mouse models:
- Reduced GL-1 levels in liver, lungs and spleen.
- Significantly reduced CD68 staining in liver at 150 mg/kg/day in food.

## Mechanism of Action and *In Vitro* Efficacy

Table 3    Enzyme Inhibition of Eliglustat[6-8]

| Cell Line | Cell Type/Origin | Test | IC$_{50}$ (nM) |
|---|---|---|---|
| Microsomes | Human melanoma cell A375 derived | GL-1 synthase s | $19.6 \pm 0.68$ |
| B16 | Mice melanoma cell | GM3 | $56.7 \pm 22.7$ |
| K562 | Human erythroleukemic cell | GM1 | 28/14[a] |
| DH82 | Canine macrophage cell | GM1 | 78/79[a] |
| Cell homogenates | Dog kidney cell derived | GM1 | 115 |

Inhibition of NBD-C6-glucosylceramide formation was determined in A375 cell-derived microsomes (lysed cell assay) and inhibition of cell surface expression of GM3 was determined using intact B16 cells (intact cell assay).    The inhibition of glycosphingolipid biosynthesis by eliglustat was determined by quantitating GM1 (monosialo-tetrahexosylganglioside) on human K562 cells and on canine DH82 cells.    The cells were harvested and assayed for GM1 expression using the cholera toxin B subunit labeled with fluorescein in isothiocyanate (FITC).    The level of fluorescence was quantitated using fluorescence activated cell sorting (FACS).    GM1: Galactosyl-*N*-acetylgalactosaminyl-(*N*-acetylneuraminyl)-galactosylglucosylceramide, a complex glycosphingolipid synthesized from glucosylceramide in four sequential enzymatic steps.    GM3: (*N*-acetylneuraminyl)-galactosylglucosylceramide.    [a] From 2 separate experiments.

Table 4    Inhibition of Glucosylceramide Synthase (GCS) Enzyme by Metabolites of Eliglustat[6-8]

| Metabolite Structure | IC$_{50}$ (μM) | |
|---|---|---|
| | GL-1 Synthesis | GM3 |
| *N*-oxide | 9.45 | 1.54 |
| Amino | 6.87 | 2.47 |
| 7-keto | 1.09 | 2.24 |
| 5-carboxy | >30 | 4.97 |
| 6-carboxy | >30 | 1.87 |
| 7-hydroxyl | 1.35 | >10 |
| 6-keto | 1.78 | >10 |
| 6-hydroxyl | 2.92 | 3.81 |
| 5-hydroxyl | 2.14 | 3.25 |
| 4-carboxy | >30 | >10 |

The objective of this study was to define a concentration response relationship and IC$_{50}$ determination for GL-1 synthase enzyme inhibition by ten eliglustat metabolites in microsomes from A375 human melanoma cells (lysed cell assay using HPLC) and in intact B16 cells (intact cell assay using immunofluorescence for surface expression of GM3).

[6]   Pharmaceuticals and Medical Devices Agency (PMDA) Database.    http://www.pmda.go.jp/drugs/2015/P20150604001/index.html (accessed Mar 2016).
[7]   U.S. Food and Drug Administration (FDA) Database.    http://www.accessdata.fda.gov/drugsatfda_docs/nda/2014/205494Orig1s000PharmR.pdf (accessed Mar 2016).
[8]   European Medical Agency (EMA) Database.    http://www.ema.europa.eu/docs/en_GB/document_library/EPAR_-_Public_assessment_report/human/003724/WC500182389.pdf (accessed Mar 2016).

Table 5    The Off-Target Ligands Binding Inhibition of Eliglustat[6-8]

| Target | Dose (μM) | %Inhibition |
|---|---|---|
| Dopamine receptor D3 | 10 | >50 |
| Dopamine receptor D4.4 | 10 | >50 |
| 5-HT$_{1A}$ | 10 | >50 |
| 5-HT$_{2A}$ | 10 | >50 |
| 5-HT$_{2B}$ | 10 | >50 |
| 5-HT$_6$ | 10 | >50 |
| Mu opioid receptor | 10 | >50 |
| Nonspecific sigma receptor | 10 | >50 |
| Ca$^{2+}$ ion channel | 10 | >50 |

In a receptor screening, eliglustat showed significant inhibition of ligands binding at 9 targets in a panel of 80 receptors, transporters and ion channels at 10 μM.

## *In Vivo* Efficacy

Table 6    The Effect of Eliglustat on Animal Models[6-8]

| Model | Animal | Administration Dose (mg/kg, p.o.) | Administration Duration (Day) | ED (mg/kg/day) | Finding |
|---|---|---|---|---|---|
| Normal animal | SD rat | 37.5, 125, 250 | BID × 3 | 75 | Significant depletion of glucosylceramide levels (-50% in the liver and kidneys and -20% in the spleen) at 37.5 mg/kg. |
| | | 10, 25, 50 | QD × 4 | NA | Reduced plasma GL-1 30% after four days of treatment at 50 mg/kg/day (6 h post dose). |
| | Beagle dog | 2.5, 5, 12.5 | BID × 3 | 5 | Induced decreases of glucosylceramide levels in liver homogenates (52%, 55% and 40% of vehicle levels, respectively), *P* <0.01 for all doses. |
| Fabry disease model | Fabry mouse[a] | 75, 125, 175 | QD × 56 | 75 | Significantly decreased the concentration of GL-3 in the kidneys, *P* <0.0001. |
| | | α-galactosidase 1 (i.v.) + 0, 75, 125, 175[b] | QD × 56 | NA | Dose-dependent inhibition of re-accumulation of GL-3 levels (without statistically significant). |
| Gaucher model | D409V/null Gaucher mouse | 75, 100, 125, 150[c] | QD × 3; QD × 5-10 weeks | NA | GL-1 was reduced by 50%-60% in the lungs, 55%-65% in the liver and 45%-50% in the spleen. The number of Gaucher cells in the liver were reduced by 60% at 5 weeks and 72% at 10 weeks. |
| | D409V/null Gaucher mouse | 150 | QD × 7 weeks | 150 | Significant reduction in CD68 staining in the liver at 150 mg/kg (p.o.) and at 450 mg/kg in food. |
| | | 150, 300, 450/mg/kg/day mixed in food | QD × 7 weeks | 150 | Reduced GL-1 accumulation in the lungs at 300 and 450 mg/kg mixed in food. Gaucher cells only in the spleens of untreated control group. |
| | D409V/null Gaucher mouse | 0 (vehicle), 150 | QD × 8 weeks | NA | Reduced GL-1 levels at 150 mg/kg (14%, 50% and 36% in the liver, lungs and spleen). |
| | | 450/mg/kg/day in food | QD × 8 weeks | 450 | Reduced GL-1 levels in the 450 mg/kg/day (71%, 73% and 73% in liver, lungs and spleen). |

CD68: A monoclonal antibody to highlight Gaucher cells.    [a] The murine model of Fabry disease (complete α-galactosidase knock-out) in 2 cohorts: monotherapy and maintenance therapy, GL-3 levels were determined for testing the efficacy.    [b] In the maintenance therapy, Fabry mice were treated with a single i.v. dose of α-galactosidase (1 mg/kg) prior to dosing with eliglustat for 56 consecutive days by oral gavage at 0, 75, 125 or 175 mg/kg.    [c] D409V/null mice were a heterozygous model of Type 1 Gaucher.    Animals were dosed once per day for 3 days at 75 mg/kg, followed by 3 days at 100 mg/kg, and 3 days at 125 mg/kg, followed by 5 weeks or 10 weeks at the full dose of 150 mg/kg.    Following the completion of dosing tissue samples were collected for histological and glycolipid analysis.

[6]    PMDA Database.    http://www.pmda.go.jp/drugs/2015/P20150604001/index.html (accessed Mar 2016).
[7]    FDA Database.    http://www.accessdata.fda.gov/drugsatfda_docs/nda/2014/205494Orig1s000PharmR.pdf (accessed Mar 2016).
[8]    EMA Database.    http://www.ema.europa.eu/docs/en_GB/document_library/EPAR_-_Public_assessment_report/human/003724/WC500182389.pdf (accessed Mar 2016).

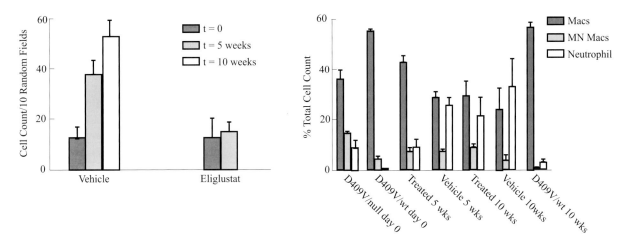

Figure A　Evaluation of the Efficacy of Eliglustat in Treating D409V/null Gaucher Mouse[7]

**Study:** Effects of eliglustat on D409V/null mouse Models.

**Animal:** D409V/null mouse, D409V/wt (male and female).

**Model:** D409V/null mice were heterozygous models of Type 1 Gaucher.　Glucosylceramide in these mice began to accumulate starting at three months of age and Gaucher cells began to appear by four months of age.　In this model, administration was starting at 7 month of age.

**Administration:** Eliglustat, p.o. for 3 days at 75 mg/kg, followed by 3 days at 100 mg/kg, and p.o. for 3 days at 125 mg/kg, followed by 5 weeks or 10 weeks at the full dose of 150 mg/kg.　Vehicle control: D409V/null Gaucher mouse.

**Test:** Gaucher cell number in liver, cell differentials in BALFs (broncho-alveolar gavage fluid).

**Results:**　The number of Gaucher cells in the liver was significantly reduced.　Gaucher cell number was reduced by 60% at 5-week time point and 72% at 10-week time point following treatment with eliglustat.　Neutrophils and multi-nucleated macrophages in BALF were increased several folds in D409V/null mice.　There was no effect of treatment on macrophage and multinucleated (MN) macrophage counts.

# 5　ADME & Drug-Drug Interaction

## Summary

### Absorption of Eliglustat

❖ Exhibited a non-linear pharmacokinetics in CYP2D6 extensive metabolizers (EMs).　Eliglustat pharmacokinetics was highly dependent on CYP2D6 phenotype, and the increases in $C_{max}$ and AUC appeared to be more than dose-proportional in the dose range of 50 to 350 mg eliglustat in CYP2D6 EMs.

❖ Had low bioavailability in all non-clinical species (4.68%-18.4%), especially in monkeys (0.8%), suggesting the involvement of transporters and/or extensive first-pass metabolism.

❖ Was absorbed very rapidly ($T_{max}$ = 0.08-0.7 h) in all non-clinical species, but moderately in humans ($T_{max}$ = 1.5-3.5 h).

❖ Showed a half-life ranging between 6.56-6.87 h in humans, longer than those in mice (0.546-0.557 h), rats (0.240-0.266 h), dogs (0.83-1.03 h) and monkeys (1.43 h), after intravenous administrations.

❖ Had high system clearance in EMs (88.2 L/h), intermediate metabolizers (IMs, 64.6 L/h), male mice (96 mL/min/kg), female mice (268 mL/min/kg), male dogs (31.1 mL/min/kg), female dogs (38.6 mL/min/kg) and monkeys (77.8 mL/min/kg), but moderate in male rats (32.7 mL/min/kg) and female rats (21.4 mL/min/kg), in contrast to liver blood flow, after intravenous administrations.

❖ Exhibited an extensive tissue distribution in dogs, mice and monkeys, but moderate in rats, with apparent volumes of distribution at 2.4, 2.07-9.44, 5.13 and 0.3-0.56 L/kg, respectively, after intravenous administrations.　Eliglustat was widely distributed into tissues in CYP2D6 EMs and IMs with the apparent volumes of distribution at 835 and 641 L, respectively, after intravenous administrations.

❖ Showed a high permeability, with a $Papp_{(A \to B)}$ of (22-23) $\times$ $10^{-6}$ cm/s in Caco-2 cell monolayer model.

[7]　FDA Database.　http://www.accessdata.fda.gov/drugsatfda_docs/nda/2014/205494Orig1s000PharmR.pdf (accessed Mar 2016).

## Distribution of Eliglustat

❖ Exhibited moderate plasma protein binding in humans (76.4%-82.9%), rats (79.7%-99.0%), dogs (91.5%-98.2%), monkeys (80.7%-92.2%) and mice (95.3%-98.9%).

❖ Had a $K_{RBC/Plasma}$ of 1.7-1.9 in humans, suggesting the drug mainly distributed in plasma and not in red blood cells.

❖ Cyclosporin-A pretreated and untreated CF-1 and untreated P-gp deficient mice after single oral administration:
  • In all groups, the highest tissue radioactivity concentrations were observed in gall bladder, kidneys, urinary bladder stomach, small intestine and liver but limited exposure in the brain.
  • In P-gp deficient mice, brain tissues showed an approximately 10-fold increase in radioactivity compared to normal mice, indicating that eliglustat was a substrate for the mouse P-gp transporter.

❖ Pigmented male rats after single oral administration:
  • The drug was rapidly and well distributed into most tissues except for the central nervous system since the blood-brain barrier was crossed by no radioactivity in the brain.
  • Relatively higher concentration levels were observed in liver, lungs, adrenal grand, kidneys and spleen compared to other organs, at 0.5 h post-dose.
  • The concentration in the pigmented skin remained measurable through 168 h post-dose suggested that eliglustat-related radioactivity was selectively associated with melanin-containing tissues.
  • Radioactivity concentrations eliminated completely from most tissues at 168 h post-dose.

## Metabolism of Eliglustat

❖ Could be extensively metabolized in liver microsomes and hepatocytes of different species.

❖ Was extensively metabolized with high clearance, mainly by CYP2D6 and to a lesser extent by CYP3A4.

❖ The primary metabolic pathways of eliglustat involved sequential oxidation of the octanoyl moiety followed by oxidation of the 2,3-dihydro-1,4-benzodioxane moiety, or a combination of the two pathways, resulting in multiple oxidative metabolites.

❖ Overall, the parent drug represented the most abundant component in rat and dog plasma, with octanoyl hydroxyl eliglustat (Genz-256416, M5) and benzodioxane oxidated eliglustat (M10) as the major metabolites in rat plasma and Genz-258162 (M17) in dog plasma.

❖ No active metabolites had been identified.

## Excretion of Eliglustat

❖ Was excreted in feces (51.4%) and urine (41.8%) in humans, mainly as metabolites.

❖ Was predominantly excreted in feces in the non-clinical species.

❖ About 53.4% of eliglustat was recovered *via* biliary excretion in bile duct-cannulated (BDC) rats.

## Drug-Drug Interaction

❖ Eliglustat was a competitive inhibitor of CYP2D6 ($K_i$ = 5.82 μM) and CYP3A4 ($K_i$ = 27.0 μM) (using midazolam as the probe substrate).

❖ Eliglustat was not an inducer of CYP enzyme *in vitro*.

❖ Eliglustat was a substrate of P-gp, and had inhibition for P-gp (IC$_{50}$ = 22 μM).

❖ Eliglustat was not a substrate of other transporters (BCRP, OAT1B1, OAT1B3, MRPs or OAT1), and had no inhibition for BCRP, OAT1B1, OAT1B3, MRP or OAT1.

# Absorption

Table 7  *In Vivo* Pharmacokinetic Parameters of Eliglustat in Several Species after Single Oral and Intravenous Dose of Eliglustat[6]

| Species | Route | Dose (mg/kg) | $T_{max}$ (h) | $C_{max}$ (ng/mL) | $AUC_{0-t}$ (ng·h/mL) | $AUC_{inf}$ (ng·h/mL) | $T_{1/2}$ (h) | Cl (mL/min/kg) | $V_{ss}$ (L/kg) | F (%) |
|---|---|---|---|---|---|---|---|---|---|---|
| C57BL/6 mouse (male) | i.v. | 1[a] | NA | NA | 141 | 146 | 0.546 | 96.0 | 2.07 | - |
| | p.o. | 3[b] | 0.0833 | 115 | 18.8 | 20.5 | 0.214 | NA | NA | 4.68 |
| C57BL/6 mouse (female) | i.v. | 1[a] | NA | NA | 49.6 | 52.5 | 0.557 | 268 | 9.44 | - |
| | p.o.[c] | 3[b] | NA | NA | NA | NA | NA | NA | NA | NA |
| Gaucher mouse (male) | p.o. | 150[b] | 0.667 ± 0.289 | 1450 ± 429 | 4220 ± 1560 | 4230 ± 1590 | 0.975 ± 0.180 | NA | NA | NA |
| Gaucher mouse (female) | p.o. | 150[b] | 0.250 ± 0.00 | 1420 ± 211 | 2570 ± 1770 | 2600 ± 1770 | 1.16 ± 0.209 | NA | NA | NA |
| SD rat (male) | i.v. | 1[d] | NA | NA | 431 ± 64.2 | 436 ± 61.4 | 0.266 ± 0.06 | 32.7 ± 4.5 | 0.556 ± 0.104 | - |
| | p.o. | 3[d] | 0.292 ± 0.144 | 109 ± 52 | 84.3 ± 50.1 | 114 ± 34 | 0.407 ± 0.048 | NA | NA | 8.70 ± 2.60 |
| | p.o. | 5[e] | 0.5 | 28.2 | 22.2[f] | NA | NA | NA | NA | NA |
| | p.o. | 10[d] | 0.438 ± 0.125 | 643 ± 127 | 599 ± 104 | 616 ± 102 | 0.461 ± 0.201 | NA | NA | 14.1 ± 2.3 |
| | p.o. | 15[e] | 0.5 | 257 | 275[f] | NA | NA | NA | NA | NA |
| | p.o. | 50[e] | 0.5 | 650 | 1089[f] | NA | NA | NA | NA | NA |
| SD rat (female) | i.v. | 1[d] | NA | NA | 666 ± 111 | 670 ± 108 | 0.240 ± 0.058 | 21.4 ± 3.7 | 0.301 ± 0.013 | - |
| | p.o. | 3[d] | 0.250 ± 0.00 | 381 ± 150 | 231 ± 69 | 237 ± 67 | 0.369 ± 0.089 | NA | NA | 11.8 ± 3.3 |
| | p.o. | 5[e] | 0.5 | 37.7 | 23.8[f] | NA | NA | NA | NA | NA |
| | p.o. | 10[d] | 0.500 ± 0.00 | 1130 ± 311 | 1210 ± 357 | 1230 ± 362 | 0.497 ± 0.104 | NA | NA | 18.4 ± 5.4 |
| | p.o. | 15[e] | 0.5 | 151 | 286[f] | NA | NA | NA | NA | NA |
| | p.o. | 50[e] | 0.25 | 1058 | 1686[f] | NA | NA | NA | NA | NA |
| New Zealand White rabbit (female) | p.o. | 30[d] | 0.708 ± 0.878 | 88.5 ± 144 | 102 ± 79 | 128 ± 128 | 3.90 ± 2.08 | NA | NA | NA |
| Beagle dog (male) | i.v. | 1[a] | NA | NA | 443 ± 63 | 459 ± 64 | 1.03 ± 0.26 | 31.1 ± 4.4 | 2.38 ± 0.85 | - |
| | p.o. | 2[e] | 0.63 | 433 | 891[g] | NA | NA | NA | NA | NC |
| | p.o. | 3[b] | 0.583 ± 0.382 | 66.2 ± 40.7 | 148 ± 82 | 171 ± 80 | 1.39 ± 0.63 | NA | NA | 12.3 ± 4.7 |
| Beagle dog (male) | p.o. | 5[e] | 0.38 | 1262 | 1687[g] | NA | NA | NA | NA | NA |
| | p.o. | 10[e] | 0.42 | 2078 | 3504[g] | NA | NA | NA | NA | NA |
| Beagle dog (female) | i.v. | 1[a] | NA | NA | 351 ± 57 | 371 ± 63 | 0.830 ± 0.287 | 38.6 ± 6.9 | 2.37 ± 1.04 | - |
| | p.o. | 2[e] | 0.44 | 161 | 132[g] | NA | NA | NA | NA | NC |
| | p.o. | 3[b] | 0.306 ± 0.173 | 69.9 ± 33.8 | 75.9 ± 33.0 | 90.6 ± 34.7 | 0.741 ± 0.179 | NA | NA | 7.92 ± 1.93 |
| | p.o. | 5[e] | 0.63 | 522 | 832[g] | NA | NA | NA | NA | NA |
| | p.o. | 10[e] | 0.50 | 1497 | 2510[g] | NA | NA | NA | NA | NA |
| Cynomolgus monkey (male) | i.v. | 1.18[b] | NA | NA | 220 ± 49 | 222 ± 49 | 1.43 ± 0.16 | 77.8 ± 17.9 | 5.13 ± 0.76 | - |
| | p.o. | 3.57[b] | 0.250 ± 0.000 | 4.66 ± 2.65 | 2.98 ± 1.75 | 4.74 ± 0.49 | 0.737 ± 0.028 | NA | NA | 0.803 ± 0.071 |
| | p.o. | 5[e] | 0.38 | 1262 | 1687[g] | NA | NA | NA | NA | NA |

[a] Vehicle: Normal saline.  [b] Vehicle: Water.  [c] Pharmacokinetic parameters were not available as only one plasma sample had a result greater than the LLOQ.  [d] Vehicle: Sterile water.  [e] Vehicle: Purified water.  [f] $AUC_{0-4}$.  [g] $AUC_{0-6}$.

[6] PMDA Database.  http://www.pmda.go.jp/drugs/2015/P20150604001/index.html (accessed Mar 2016).

Table 8    *In Vivo* Pharmacokinetic Parameters of Eliglustat in Healthy Humans after Single Oral and Intravenous Dose of Eliglustat Tartrate[9]

| Species | Route | Dose (mg) | $T_{max}$ (h) | $C_{max}$ (ng/mL) | $AUC_{inf}$ (ng·h/mL) | $T_{1/2}$ (h) | Cl (L/h) | $V_z$ (L) | F (%) |
|---|---|---|---|---|---|---|---|---|---|
| Healthy human (EMs) | i.v. | 50 | 1.0 (0.05-1.50) | 108 (24.1) | 482 (8.2) | 6.56 (6.86) | 88.2 (8.81) | 835 (12.7) | - |
| | p.o. | 50 | 1.5 (0.5-3) | 2.48 (33.7) | 19.1 (41.1) | 3.69 (33.3) | NA | NA | NA |
| | p.o. | 100 | 1.5 (0.5-3.1) | 10.3 (110) | 77.2 (123) | 5.23 (25.4) | NA | NA | NA |
| | p.o. | 200 | 1.75 (1-4) | 33.0 (91.1) | 294 (110) | 5.36 (25.0) | NA | NA | NA |
| | p.o. | 350 | 2.5 (1-3.1) | 107 (55.3) | 678 (62.7) | 5.65 (7.09) | NA | NA | NA |
| Healthy human (IMs) | i.v. | 50 | 1.08 | 93.2 | 653 | 6.87 | 64.6 | 641 | - |
| | p.o. | 100 | 3.5 (3.0-4.0) | 25.4 (42.3) | 253 (39.4) | 6.99 (8.91) | NA | NA | NA |
| Healthy human (URM) | p.o. | 100 | 1.26 (1.02-1.50) | 1.82 (35.5) | 9.61 (0.29) | 3.07 (32.1) | NA | NA | NA |

Median (min-max) for $T_{max}$, Mean (CV%) for other parameters.    EM: Extensive Metabolizer.    IM: Intermediate Metabolizer.    URM: Ultra Rapid Metabolizer.

Table 9    *In Vitro* Permeability of Eliglustat in Caco-2 Cell Monolayer Model and *In Situ* Permeability of Eliglustat in Rat Perfusion Model[6, 7]

| **In Vitro Permeability in Caco-2 Cell Monolayer Model** | | | | **In Situ Permeability in Rat Perfusion Model** | | | |
|---|---|---|---|---|---|---|---|
| Compound | Conc. (μM) | $Papp_{(A→B)}$ ($1 \times 10^{-6}$ cm/s) | Permeability Class | Compound | Conc. (μg/mL) | Permeability ($1 \times 10^{-6}$ cm/s) | T/R Ratio[c] |
| Eliglustat | 12.5 | 23 ± 2.3 | High | Eliglustat tartrate | 6 | 3.0 ± 5.1 | 0.19 ± 0.219 |
| | 125 | 22 ± 1.8 | High | | 60 | 16.8 ± 4.7 | 1.50 ± 0.319 |
| | 1250 | 22 ± 2.0 | High | | 600 | 26.3 ± 5.6 | 1.64 ± 0.196 |
| Labetalol[a] | 10 | 12 ± 1.7 | High | Metoprolol | 68 + 6 μg/mL eliglustat tartrate | 12.0 ± 5.7 | - |
| Terbutaline[b] | 10 | 0.066 ± 0.015 | Low | | 68 + 60 μg/mL eliglustat tartrate | 12.3 ± 4.7 | - |
| | | | | | 68 + 600 μg/mL eliglustat tartrate | 16.4 ± 3.1 | - |

[a] Co-incubated with 10 μM terbutaline and 12.5 μM eliglustat.    [b] Co-incubated with 10 μM labetalol and 12.5 μM eliglustat.    [c] Test-to-reference (T/R) ratio of the effective permeability of eliglustat to that of metoprolol.

## Distribution

Table 10    *In Vitro* Plasma Protein Binding and Blood Partitioning of Eliglustat in Several Species[6, 7]

| | **Plasma Protein Binding** | | | | | **Blood Partitioning** | | |
|---|---|---|---|---|---|---|---|---|
| | **%Bound** | | | | | **$K_{RBC/Plasma}$** | | |
| Species | 0.01 μM | 0.1 μM | 1 μM | 10 μM | Species | 0.1 μM | 1 μM | 10 μM |
| Human | 82.9 ± 1.6 | 79.5 ± 1.1 | 76.4 ± 2.5 | - | Human (male) | 1.7 ± 0.3 | 1.8 ± 0.2 | - |
| Rat | - | 99.0 ± 0.3 | 97.2 ± 0.4 | 79.7 ± 1.5 | Human (female) | 1.8 ± 0.1 | 1.9 ± 0.2 | - |
| Dog | - | 98.2 ± 0.1 | 97.4 ± 0.4 | 91.5 ± 1.2 | Rat | 0.7 ± 0.1 | 0.8 ± 0.3 | 1.8 ± 0.2 |
| Monkey | - | 92.2 ± 0.1 | 92.0 ± 0.6 | 80.7 ± 2.0 | Dog | 0.9 ± 0.2 | 0.8 ± 0.3 | 1.4 ± 0.4 |
| Mouse | - | 98.9 ± 0.2 | 98.7 ± 0.2 | 95.3 ± 0.2 | Mouse | - | - | - |

[6]  PMDA Database.    http://www.pmda.go.jp/drugs/2015/P20150604001/index.html (accessed Mar 2016).
[7]  FDA Database.    http://www.accessdata.fda.gov/drugsatfda_docs/nda/2014/205494Orig1s000PharmR.pdf (accessed Mar 2016).
[9]  FDA Database.    http://www.accessdata.fda.gov/drugsatfda_docs/nda/2014/205494Orig1s000ClinPharmR.pdf (accessed Mar 2016).

Table 11    *In Vivo* Tissue Distribution of [$^{14}$C]Eliglustat in Mice after Single Oral Dose of 125 mg/kg [$^{14}$C]Eliglustat[6]

| Species | Normal Mouse | | | Normal Pre-Treated with Cyclosporine A | | | P-gp Deficient Mouse | | |
|---|---|---|---|---|---|---|---|---|---|
| | 125 mg/kg, p.o. | | | 125 mg/kg, p.o. | | | 125 mg/kg, p.o. | | |
| Tissue | Radioactivity (µg eq./g) | | | Radioactivity (µg eq./g) | | | Radioactivity (µg eq./g) | | |
| | 0.5 h | 1 h | 2 h | 0.5 h | 1 h | 2 h | 0.5 h | 1 h | 2 h |
| Blood | 15.7 | 24.1 | 12.5 | 20.4 | 31.0 | 17.0 | 21.5 | 25.1 | 26.5 |
| Brain cerebrum | 1.40 | 0.99 | 0.9 | 1.0 | 1.4 | 1.1 | 17.1 | 14.6 | 20.0 |
| Bile (gall bladder) | 757 | 1546 | 2839 | 273 | 230[a] | 666 | 632 | 744 | 1726 |
| Urinary bladder | 497 | 1956 | 3458 | 630 | 2236 | 1514 | 793 | 3552 | 429 |
| Liver | 279 | 752 | 150 | 159 | 178 | 119 | 382 | 291 | 295 |
| Kidneys | 125 | 166 | 120 | 105 | 237 | 113 | 157 | 141 | 131 |
| Small intestine | 27.7 | 118 | 230 | 125 | 113 | 83.5 | 176 | 281 | 324 |
| Stomach | 80.9 | 126 | 61.1 | 84.0 | 90.2 | 58.8 | 156 | 96.2 | 72.2 |
| Spleen | 35.7 | 23.7 | 17.0 | 31.0 | 38.2 | 28.5 | 41.9 | 33.9 | 32.4 |

Data was mean of two different animals.    Vehicle: Sterile water.    [a] Data from only one animal.

Table 12    *In Vivo* Tissue Distribution of [$^{14}$C]Eliglustat in Rats after Single Oral Dose of [$^{14}$C]Eliglustat[6]

| Tissue | Long-Evans Rat (male) | | | | Tissue | SD Rat (male) | | | |
|---|---|---|---|---|---|---|---|---|---|
| | [$^{14}$C]Eliglustat Tartrate, 50 mg/kg | | | | | [$^{14}$C]Eliglustat Tartrate, 100 mg/kg | | | |
| | Radioactivity (µg eq./g)[a] | | | Tissue/Blood AUC$_{0-168}$ Ratio | | Radioactivity (µg eq./g)[b] | | | |
| | 0.5 | 24 h | 168 h | | | 24 h | 48 h | 96 h | 168 h |
| Adrenal gland | 27.2 | 0.582 | ND | 99.6 | Brain | NC | NC | NC | NC |
| Blood | 3.40 | ND | ND | 7.58 | Eyes | NC | NC | NC | NC |
| Brain | BLQ | ND | ND | 0 | Heart | NC | NC | NC | NC |
| Eyes | 2.46 | 1.19 | 0.573 | 163 | Kidneys | 3.27 ± 0.67 | 2.32 ± 0.69 | NC | NC |
| Kidneys | 23.8 | 1.46 | BLQ | 1346 | Liver | 11.2 ± 1.7 | 7.15 ± 1.33 | 3.38 ± 0.43 | 1.92 ± 0.31 |
| Liver | 128 | 5.56 | 0.713 | 8166 | Lungs | 1.35 ± 1.17 | NC | NC | 0.553 ± 0.497 |
| Lungs | 29.7 | ND | ND | 59.7 | Stomach | 14.0 ± 3.1 | 9.78 ± 1.43 | NC | NC |
| Skin (nonpigmented) | 2.71 | BLQ | BLQ | 6.98 | Small intestine | 11.0 ± 5.4 | NC | NC | NC |
| Skin (pigmented) | 3.16 | 1.47 | 1.06 | 2256 | Large intestine | 80.1 ± 23.0 | 18.7 ± 18.1 | NC | NC |
| Spleen | 21.9 | BLQ | ND | 48.8 | Testes | 2.25 ± 0.46 | 0.863 ± 0.752 | 0.788 ± 0.688 | 0.820 ± 0.136 |

Sample time for Long-Evans rats: 0.5, 2, 6, 12, 24, 48, 96 and 168 h post-dose.    [a] Vehicle: Reverse Osmosis water.    [b] Vehicle: Sterile isotonic saline solution.

[6]   PMDA Database.   http://www.pmda.go.jp/drugs/2015/P20150604001/index.html (accessed Mar 2016).

## Metabolism

Table 13    *In Vitro* Metabolic Stability of Eliglustat in Hepatocytes and Liver Microsomes[6]

| Parameter | Conc. (μM) | Hepatocyte | | | | | Liver Microsomes | | | | |
|---|---|---|---|---|---|---|---|---|---|---|---|
| | | Mouse | Rat | Dog | Monkey | Human | Mouse | Rat | Dog | Monkey | Human |
| Cl$_{int}$ (μL/min/mg protein) | 0.05 | 608 ± 55 | 531 ± 44 | 119 ± 6 | 451 ± 43 | 49.9 ± 4.6 | 1870 ± 12 | 2200 ± 53 | 1180 ± 43 | 5020 ± 189 | 99.5 ± 0.5 |
| | 0.2 | 674 ± 15 | 299 ± 45 | 130 ± 10 | 432 ± 42 | 49.0 ± 6.5 | 1550 ± 34 | 913 ± 80 | 1240 ± 3 | 4030 ± 138 | 136 ± 4 |
| | 1.0 | 436 ± 38 | 121 ± 18 | 89.7 ± 10.5 | 159 ± 11 | 30.0 ± 2.3 | 617 ± 20 | 257 ± 3 | 829 ± 49 | 1052 ± 54 | 122 ± 0.8 |
| Extrapolated hepatic metabolic blood Cl (mL/min/kg) | 0.05 | 33.0 ± 1.9 | 27.0 ± 1.1 | 11.3 ± 0.4 | 41.7 ± 0.1 | 10.1 ± 0.5 | 36.7 ± 0.1 | 33.6 ± 0.3 | 20.0 ± 0.2 | 38.6 ± 0.2 | 9.57 ± 0.03 |
| | 0.2 | 35.2 ± 0.5 | 19.3 ± 1.9 | 11.9 ± 0.6 | 41.3 ± 0.1 | 10.0 ± 0.7 | 32.8 ± 0.5 | 23.1 ± 1.2 | 20.2 ± 0.0 | 38.1 ± 0.2 | 11.0 ± 0.2 |
| | 1.0 | 26.4 ± 1.6 | 9.87 ± 1.24 | 9.30 ± 0.78 | 35.9 ± 0.3 | 7.59 ± 0.36 | 16.6 ± 0.4 | 8.65 ± 0.10 | 17.8 ± 0.4 | 27.4 ± 0.5 | 10.6 ± 0.0 |
| Percent of hepatic blood flow (%) | 0.05 | 37 | 49 | 36 | 96 | 49 | 41 | 61 | 65 | 89 | 46 |
| | 0.2 | 39 | 35 | 38 | 95 | 48 | 36 | 42 | 65 | 87 | 53 |
| | 1.0 | 29 | 18 | 30 | 82 | 37 | 18 | 16 | 58 | 63 | 51 |

Table 14    *In Vitro* Metabolic Phenotype of Eliglustat[6]

| Recombinant Human CYP450 Enzyme | % of Radioactivity | | | | | | | | | | | |
|---|---|---|---|---|---|---|---|---|---|---|---|---|
| | Eliglustat | M2 | M3 | M4 | M5 | M6 | M9 | M10 | M11 | M17 | M59 | M69 |
| CYP2C19 | 81.6 | - | - | - | 4.5 | - | 1.1 | 1.6 | 9.6 | - | - | 1.7 |
| CYP2D6 | - | 22.1 | 2.2 | 7.5 | 47.3 | 11.0 | - | - | - | 7.7 | 2.3 | - |
| CYP3A4 | 77.8 | - | - | - | 3.4 | 16.4 | - | - | 2.4 | - | - | - |

[a] The concentration of [$^{14}$C]eliglustat tartrate was 5 μM, incubated for 1 h.

Table 15    *In Vitro* Metabolites of Eliglustat in Hepatocytes and Liver Microsomes[6]

| Analyte | % of Radioactivity | | | | % of Radioactivity | | | |
|---|---|---|---|---|---|---|---|---|
| | Hepatocytes | | | | Liver Microsomes | | | |
| | Rat | Dog | Monkey | Human | Rat | Dog | Monkey | Human |
| Eliglustat | - | - | - | - | 33.1 | 8.13 | - | 44.0 |
| M2 | - | - | 3.78 | 2.45 | 5.28 | 1.58 | 25.9 | - |
| M3 | - | - | - | - | 1.34 | - | 7.43 | - |
| M4 | 1.36 | 1.78 | - | - | 5.33 | √ | √ | - |
| M4 & M45 | √ | √ | - | - | √ | 8.21 | 16.9 | - |
| M5 (Genz-256416) | 9.30 | 44.2 | 26.0 | 34.9 | 20.9 | 59.9 | 26.3 | 31.3 |
| M6 (Genz-311752) | 2.99 | 1.65 | 6.67 | 16.1 | - | 3.70 | 1.53 | 13.8 |
| M9 | - | 2.27 | - | - | 10.7 | 5.04 | - | 3.18 |
| M10 | - | - | - | - | 23.3 | 6.98 | 3.37 | 4.93 |
| M15 | - | 1.14 | 3.70 | 5.84 | - | - | 1.37 | - |
| M16 | 3.19 | 7.41 | - | - | - | 1.56 | - | - |
| M17 (Genz-258162) | - | 22.5 | 13.6 | 12.9 | - | 2.91 | 3.31 | - |
| M24 (Genz-399240) & M54 | √ | √ | 8.28 | 2.76 | - | - | - | - |
| M32 | 6.61 | 2.07 | 12.2 | 5.87 | - | - | - | - |
| M39 & M55 | 6.84 | 2.33 | 7.31 | 1.26 | - | - | - | - |
| M51 & M52 | 21.1 | - | - | - | - | - | - | - |
| M53 & M54 | 13.5 | √ | √ | √ | - | - | - | - |
| Total | 65 | 85 | 82 | 82 | 100 | 98 | 86 | 97 |

√: Metabolites detected but no quantifiable percentage of radioactivity.

[6]  PMDA Database.   http://www.pmda.go.jp/drugs/2015/P20150604001/index.html (accessed Mar 2016).

Table 16    Metabolites in Plasma, Urine in Humans and Non-clinical Test Species after Single Oral and Intravenous of [$^{14}$C]Eliglustat[6]

| Matrix | Species | Administration | Dose (mg/kg) | Time (h) | % of Radioactivity |  |  |  |  |  |  |  |  |  |  |
|--------|---------|----------------|--------------|----------|------------|------|------|------|--------|------|------|------|------|------|------|
|  |  |  |  |  | Eliglustat | M4 | M5 | M6 | M7 | M10 | M17 | M72 | M73 | M74 | M75 |
| Plasma | Rat (male) | p.o. | 50 | 1 | 24.8 | 3.16 | 7.08 | 3.04 | 3.24[a] | 3.76 | 3.89 | NA | NA | NA | NA |
|  | Rat (female) | p.o. | 50 | 1 | 41.5 | 1.82 | 3.92 | - | 1.47[a] | 6.86 | 1.19 | NA | NA | NA | NA |
|  | Dog (male) | p.o. | 10 | 1 | 22.2 | 1.59 | 14.4 | 3.19 | 1.41 | 1.50 | 16.3 | NA | NA | NA | NA |
|  | Dog (female) | p.o. | 10 | 1 | 16.2 | 1.89 | 9.23 | 3.38 | - | 1.15 | 19.7 | NA | NA | NA | NA |
| Urine | Rat | i.v. | 1 | 0-24 | √ | NA | NA | NA | NA | NA | NA | - | - | - | - |
|  | Monkey | i.v. | 1 | 0-8 | √ | NA | NA | NA | NA | NA | NA | √ | √ | √ | √ |

M5: Genz-256416.   M6: Genz-311752.   M7: Genz-258179.   M17: Genz-258162.   √: Metabolite detected but no quantifiable percentage of radioactivity.   –: Not applicable.   [a] Refer to M7 & M62.

[6]  PMDA Database.   http://www.pmda.go.jp/drugs/2015/P20150604001/index.html (accessed Mar 2016).

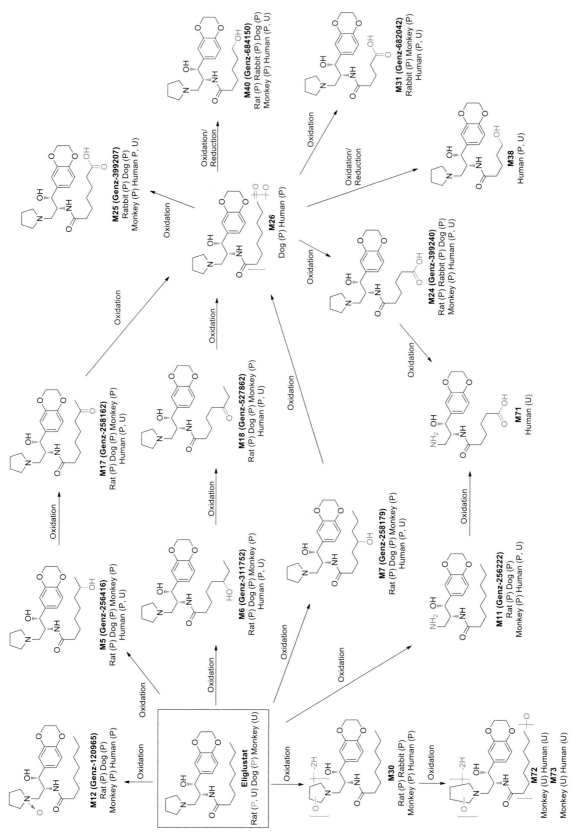

Figure B    Proposed Pathways for *In Vivo* Biotransformation of Eliglustat in Rats, Rabbits, Dogs, Monkeys and Humans (in the Octanoyl and Pyrrolidine Moieties)[6]
The red labels represent the major components in the matrices.  P = plasma and U = urine.

[6]    PMDA Database.    http://www.pmda.go.jp/drugs/2015/P20150604001/index.html (accessed Mar 2016).

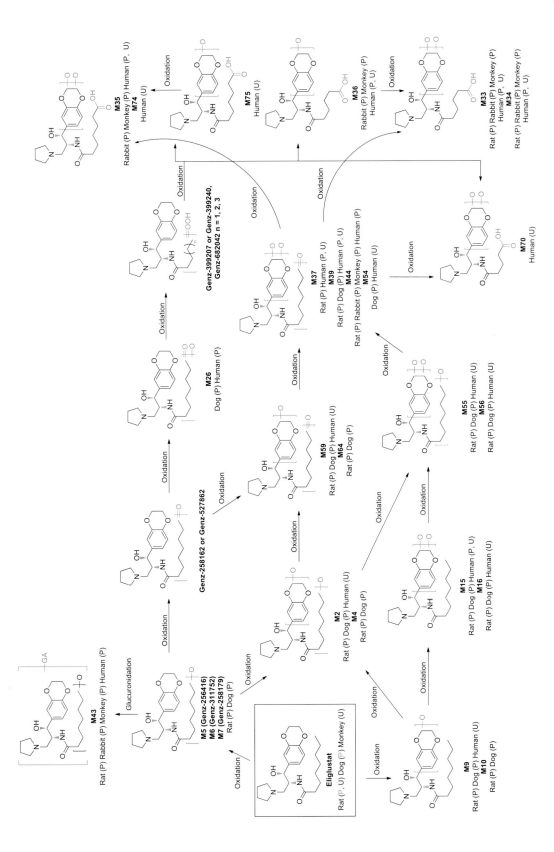

Figure C    Proposed Pathways for *In Vivo* Biotransformation of Eliglustat in Rats, Rabbits, Dogs, Monkeys and Humans (in the Octanoyl and 2,3-Dihydro-1,4-benzodioxane Moieties)[6]

P = plasma, U = urine and GA = glucuronic acid.

[6] PMDA Database.    http://www.pmda.go.jp/drugs/2015/P20150604001/index.html (accessed Mar 2016).

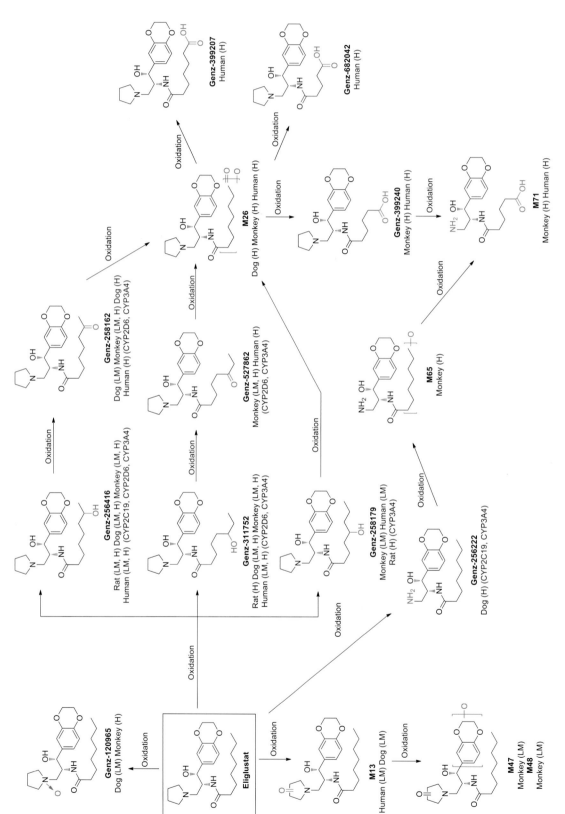

Figure D    Proposed Pathways for *In Vitro* Biotransformation of Eliglustat in Rat, Dog, Monkey and HumanLiver Microsomes and Recombinant
CYP2D6, CYP2C19 and CYP3A4 (in the Octanoyl and Pyrrolidine Moieties)[6]
LM = liver microsomes and H = hepatocytes.

[6]    PMDA Database.    http://www.pmda.go.jp/drugs/2015/P20150604001/index.html (accessed Mar 2016).

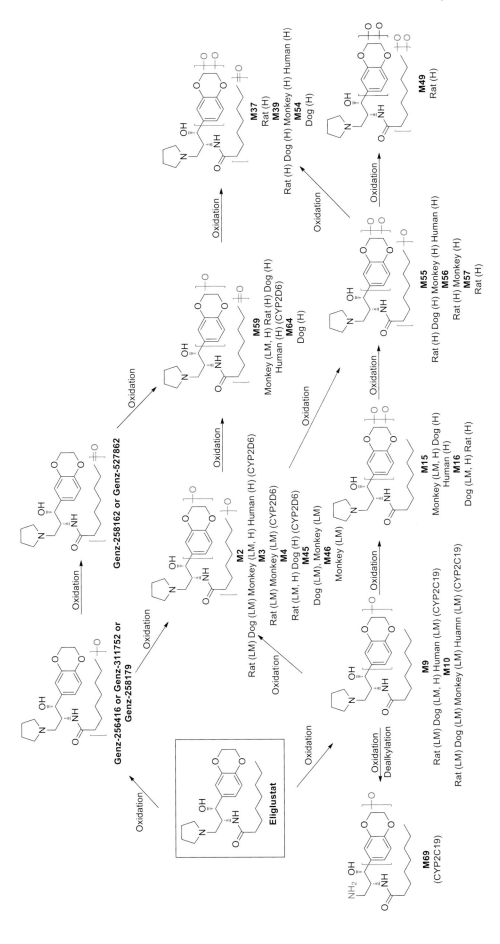

Figure E    Proposed Pathways for *In Vitro* Biotransformation of Eliglustat in Rat, Dog, Monkey and Human Liver microsomes and Recombinant CYP2D6, CYP2C19 and CYP3A4 (in the Octanoyl and 2,3-Dihydro-1,4-benzodioxane Moieties)[6]
LM = livermicrosomes and H = hepatocytes.

[6]  PMDA Database.    http://www.pmda.go.jp/drugs/2015/P20150604001/index.html (accessed Mar 2016).

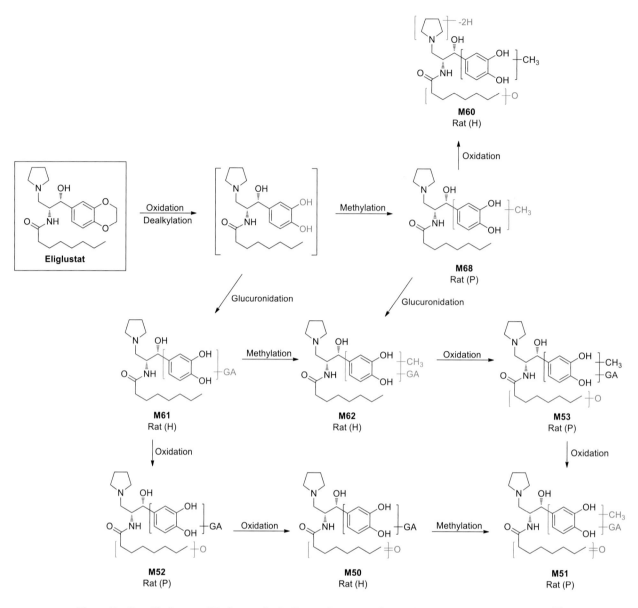

Figure F    Specific Proposed Pathways for *In Vivo* and *In Vitro* Biotransformation of Eliglustat in Rats[6]

P = plasma, H = hepatocytes and GA = glucuronic acid.    M50, M51, M52, M53, M60, M61, M62 and M68 were found *in vivo* biotransformation.

[6]   PMDA Database.    http://www.pmda.go.jp/drugs/2015/P20150604001/index.html (accessed Mar 2016).

# Excretion

Table 17    Excretion Profiles of [$^{14}$C]Eliglustat in Various Species after Single Oral and Intravenous Dose of [$^{14}$C]Eliglustat[6, 9]

| Species | State | Route | Dose (mg/kg) | Time (h) | Urine (% of dose) | Feces (% of dose) | Bile (% of dose) | Cage Wash (% of dose) | Recovery (% of dose) |
|---|---|---|---|---|---|---|---|---|---|
| Rat (male) | Intact | i.v. | 10 | 0-168 | 11.4 ± 3.6 | 82.1 ± 1.1 | - | 1.15 ± 0.60 | 94.5 ± 3.5 |
| | | p.o. | 100 | 0-168 | 16.6 ± 1.1 | 77.0 ± 1.4 | - | 2.30 ± 0.85 | 95.3 ± 1.7 |
| Rat (female) | Intact | i.v. | 10 | 0-168 | 14.2 ± 1.6 | 81.3 ± 1.6 | - | 0.96 ± 0.40 | 96.5 ± 0.9 |
| | | p.o. | 100 | 0-168 | 12.5 ± 0.6 | 83.2 ± 1.2 | - | 1.36 ± 0.45 | 97.1 ± 1.5 |
| Rat (male) | BDC | i.v. & p.o. | 8.44 for i.v. and 84.4 for p.o. | 0-24 | - | - | 53.4 ± 19.9 | - | 53.4 ± 19.9 |
| Dog (male) | Intact | i.v. | 2.5 | 0-168 | 25.6 ± 3.0 | 63.9 ± 4.9 | - | 1.94 ± 0.36 | 91.4 ± 1.8 |
| | | p.o. | 25 | 0-168 | 30.0 ± 8.6 | 49.7 ± 3.0 | - | 3.55 ± 1.73 | 91.7 ± 7.9[a] |
| Dog (female) | Intact | i.v. | 2.5 | 0-168 | 25.0 ± 4.8 | 66.5 ± 6.2 | - | 2.57 ± 1.62 | 94.1 ± 0.4 |
| | | p.o. | 25 | 0-168 | 25.6 ± 4.8 | 56.5 ± 6.1 | - | 3.36 ± 1.25 | 90.3 ± 1.2[a] |
| Human | Intact | p.o. | 100 | 0-168 | 41.8 ± 5.1 | 51.4 ± 4.0 | - | - | 93.2 ± 2.1 |

[a] Including vomit.

# Drug-Drug Interaction

Table 18    *In Vitro* Evaluation of Eliglustat as an Inhibitor of CYP450 Enzymes[9]

| Enzyme | CYP2D6 | CYP3A4[a] | CYP3A4[b] | CYP2C8 | CYP2C9 | CYP2C19 |
|---|---|---|---|---|---|---|
| $K_i$ (µM) | 5.82 | 27.0 | >50 | >50 | >50 | >50 |

[a] Using midazolam as the probe substrate.    [b] Using testosterone as the probe substrate.

Table 19    *In Vitro* Evaluation of Eliglustat Tartrate as a Substrate and an Inhibitor of P-gp in MDCKII-MDR1 Cell[9]

| Treatment | Eliglustat as a Substrate | | | Eliglustat as an Inhibitor | | | |
|---|---|---|---|---|---|---|---|
| | Conc. (µM) | Efflux Ratio | Net Efflux Ratio | Substrate (µM) | Inhibitor (µM) | Efflux Ratio | IC$_{50}$ (µM) |
| Eliglustat tartrate | 1 | 5.7 | ND | [$^3$H]Digoxin (10) | - | 18 | 22 ± 12 |
| | 10 | 4.6 | ND | | | | |
| | 100 | 1.5 | ND | | | | |
| Eliglustat tartrate + PSC833 | 1 + 10 | 1.4 | 1.0 | | Eliglustat tartrate (50) | 7.7 | |
| Eliglustat tartrate + verapamil | 1 + 60 | 1.2 | 1.1 | | | | |

ND: Not determined.

## Key Findings:[9]

❖ Eliglustat was not an inducer of CYP enzyme *in vitro*.
❖ Eliglustat was not a substrate of other transporters (BCRP, OAT1B1, OAT1B3, MRPs or OAT1) and had no inhibition for BCRP, OAT1B1, OAT1B3, MRP or OAT1.

[6]  PMDA Database.    http://www.pmda.go.jp/drugs/2015/P20150604001/index.html (accessed Mar 2016).
[9]  FDA Database.    http://www.accessdata.fda.gov/drugsatfda_docs/nda/2014/205494Orig1s000ClinPharmR.pdf (accessed Mar 2016).

# 6   Non-Clinical Toxicology

## Summary

### Single-Dose Toxicity

❖ Single-dose toxicity studies by the oral or intravenous route in the rodent and non-rodent species:
  • Rat MNLD: 200 mg/kg (p.o.), 20 mg/kg (i.v.).
  • Dog MNLD: 100 mg/kg (p.o.).

### Repeated-Dose Toxicity

❖ Repeated-dose toxicity studies in mice (up to 13 weeks), rats (up to 26 weeks) and dogs (up to 52 weeks):
  • In view of the longest studies employed in each species, the NOAEL was not established in mice, was 50 mg/kg/day in rats and 10 mg/kg/day in dogs.
  • The major target organs in rats and dogs were the lymph node, eyes and thymus.

### Safety Pharmacology

❖ Safety pharmacology studies to investigate the effects on cardiovascular, central nervous and respiratory system.
  • No test article-related behavior, autonomic and motor change were observed in SD rats at doses up to 400 mg/kg.
  • Eliglustat inhibited the hERG tail current with an $IC_{50}$ of 0.35 μg/mL, indicative of QT prolongation, yet there were no statistically significant changes of cardiovascular or respiratory parameters in Beagle dogs at doses up to 80 mg/kg.
  • No statistically significant changes were observed on renal and GI functions in rats at doses up to 20 mg/kg.

### Genotoxicity

❖ Eliglustat was negative in the Ames test, chromosome aberration assay using human peripheral blood lymphocytes and oral *in vivo* mouse micronucleus test.
❖ In addition, Genz-399240, a human metabolite of eliglustat, was negative in the Ames test and chromosome aberration assay using human peripheral blood lymphocytes.

### Reproductive and Developmental Toxicity

❖ Fertility and early embryonic development in rats:
  • Mating/fertility NOAELs were 30 mg/kg/day, at which preimplantation losses increased.
❖ Embryo-fetal development in rats and rabbits:
  • Eliglustat was embryo-toxic and teratogenic when administered to pregnant rats at 120 mg/kg/day during organogenesis.
  • Major fetal malformations included dilated cerebral ventricles and fetal skeletal malformations, fetal skeletal variations.
❖ Pre- and postnatal development in rats:
  • Maternal toxicity was evident at 100 mg/kg/day, including mortality of two dams during parturition, reduced body weight gains associated with reductions in food consumption, and mean post implantation loss.   Consistently, reductions in offspring birth weight occurred at the same dose.

### Carcinogenicity

❖ The carcinogenic potential was evaluated in CD-1 mice and SD rats:
  • Eliglustat tartrate did not produce any treatment-related neoplasm in rats or mice.

## Single-Dose Toxicity

Table 20　Single-Dose Toxicity Studies of Eliglustat by Intravenous or Oral Administration[6-8]

| Species | Dose (mg/kg) | MNLD (mg/kg) | Finding |
|---|---|---|---|
| SD rat | 200, 400, 800, 900, 1000, p.o. | 200 | Mortality at ≥ 400 mg/kg.<br>All doses animals showed signs of salivation, wet fur, areas of fur staining, thin fur, labored and/or abnormal sneezing and breathing, decreased fecal output and/or abdominal distention. |
| | 0, 3, 10, 20, i.v. | 20 | No mortality.<br>No significant treatment-related effect on clinical signs, body weights, food consumption, clinical pathology parameters, organ weights and gross necropsy. |
| Beagle dog | 25, 35, 50, 100, p.o. | 100 | No mortality.<br>Emesis at doses of 25, 35, 50 and 100 mg/kg.<br>Body weight effect at single dose of 25 mg/kg. |

Vehicle: 0.9% NaCl for injection.

## Repeated-Dose Toxicity

Table 21　Repeated-Dose Toxicity Studies of Eliglustat by Oral (Gavage) Administration[6-8]

| Species | Duration (Week) | Dose (mg/kg/day) | NOAEL (mg/kg/day) | Finding |
|---|---|---|---|---|
| CD-1 mouse | 13 | 0, 50, 150, 350 | ND | Adverse effect only observed in males and females treated at HD.<br>No target organ identified in any animal either sacrificed prematurely or at scheduled necropsy. |
| SD rat | 4 | 0, 10, 30, 100 | 10[a], 30[b] | Well tolerated with oral doses up to 100 mg/kg/day (50 mg/kg, BID).<br>BWG ↓ in MD and HD females (↓ 18% and 22%).<br>Moderate increases of ALT (↑ 63% and 50%, M/F) and K (↑ 10% and 10%, M/F) in HD males and females.<br>No histopathology finding correlated with observations in the HD animals. |
| | 26 | 5, 15, 50 | 50 | Three animals died (one male and one female at 50 mg/kg/day and one male at 15 mg/kg/day) and deaths of males were attributed to gavage accident.<br>No significant treatment-related effect on body consumption, hematology, serum chemistry, urinalysis, gross pathology, organ weights or histopathology.<br>The MTD to be higher than 50 mg/kg/day. |
| Beagle dog | 4 | 0, 5, 10, 25 | 5 | No treatment-related finding on clinical signs, body weights and clinical pathology parameters.<br>No ECG finding at the dose levels tested.<br>Histologically, atrophy of lymphoid organs/tissues in 10 and 25 mg/kg/day treatment and was reversed after 2-week recovery. |
| | 13 | 0, 2, 5, 10 | 5 | Histopathological changes were observed in the thymus at all doses including the control.<br>The target organ appeared to be the thymus. |
| | 52 | 0, 2, 5, 10 | 10 | At 10 mg/kg, there was a decrease in the thymus weight and size.<br>The target organ of toxicity appeared to be the lungs, heart and seminiferous epithelial degeneration and segmental hypoplasia in the treated groups. |

ND: Not detected.　[a] The NOAEL data by FDA.　[b] The NOAEL data by PMDA.

[6]　PMDA Database.　http://www.pmda.go.jp/drugs/2015/P20150604001/index.html (accessed Mar 2016).
[7]　FDA Database.　http://www.accessdata.fda.gov/drugsatfda_docs/nda/2014/205494Orig1s000PharmR.pdf (accessed Mar 2016).
[8]　EMA Database.　http://www.ema.europa.eu/docs/en_GB/document_library/EPAR_-_Public_assessment_report/human/003724/WC500182389.pdf (accessed Mar 2016).

## Safety Pharmacology

Table 22   Safety Pharmacology Studies of Eliglustat[6-8]

| Study | System | Dose | Finding |
|---|---|---|---|
| Neurological effect | SD rat (Irwin's method) | 0, 20, 100, 400 mg/kg, p.o. | No significant gross behavioral or physiological change observed during a 240 min post-dose period compared to control. |
| Cardiovascular effect | CHO cell (L-type calcium current inhibition) | 10, 30, 100 μM | hERG $IC_{50}$ = 24.8 μM; Eliglustat inhibited Cav 1.2 current by 30.2% at 10 μM (n = 3), 48.9% at 30 μM (n = 3) and 88.0% at 100 μM (n = 4). |
| | HEK293 cell (*In vitro* perfusion) | 0.01, 0.1, 0.3, 1, 10, 100 μg/mL | Inhibition of hERG, $IC_{25}$ = 0.11 μg/mL, $IC_{50}$ = 0.35 μg/mL, $IC_{75}$ = 1.02 μg/mL. |
| | HEK293 cell (*In vitro* perfusion) | 0.3, 1, 3, 10, 100 μg/mL | Inhibition of Nav1.5 with $IC_{25}$, $IC_{50}$ and $IC_{75}$ as 1.8, 5.2 and 15.0 μg/mL. |
| | Beagle dog | 0, 1, 2.5, 5 mg/kg, i.v. for over 2 min | Dose-related decreases in heart rate and increases in RR interval were observed following all three doses.<br><br>Dose-related increases in atrio-ventricular (A-V) and intra-ventricular (I-V) conduction time measured at all three doses.<br><br>In the ECG, 1 mg/kg caused only a slight increase in the RR interval, 2.5 and 5 mg/kg caused significant increases in multiple ECG parameters, including prolongation of corrected QT interval. |
| | Beagle dog | 0, 1, 3, 10, 25, 50, 80 mg/kg, p.o. | Doses up to 80 mg/kg had no effect on blood pressure over 360 min following dosing.<br><br>80 mg/kg: ↑ Heart rate, ↓ RR interval at 30-90 min post-dose.   PR interval prolongation was observed at 30-120 min following 50 mg/kg (HED = 1667 mg) and at 60-120 min following 80 mg/kg dosing.   QRS duration was prolonged at 60-90 min following 10 mg/kg (HED = 333 mg), at 60-180 min following 25 mg/kg and at 30-360 min following 50 and 80 mg/kg dosing.<br><br>No effect on QT, QTcF and QTcQ intervals.<br><br>NOAEL = 3 mg/kg (HED = 1.67 mg/kg). |
| | Beagle dog Purkinje fibers | 0[a], 0.03, 0.1, 0.3, 1, 10, 100 μg/mL | Dose-related decreases in the action potential duration at doses of 0.3, 1, and 10 μg/mL.   A total block of action potential at 100 μg/mL.<br><br>Dose-related decrease in the up stroke amplitude of the action potential at concentrations of 1, 10 and 100 μg/mL. |
| Pulmonary effect | Male rat | 20, 100, 400 mg/kg, p.o. | At dose of 20 or 100 mg/kg had no significant effect on the respiratory rate or tidal volume of conscious rats at 30 and 100 min post-dose.<br><br>At 400 mg/kg significantly decreased respiration rate at 30 min post-dose. |
| Renal effect | SD rat | 20, 100, 400 mg/kg, p.o. | At 100 mg/kg increased urinary pH at 3-6 h post-dose.<br><br>At 400 mg/kg decrease in potassium and chloride excretion (6-24 h post-dose) and an increase in urinary pH (0-3 and 3-6 h post-dose) were observed. |
| Gastrointestinal effect | SD rat | 20, 100, 400 mg/kg, p.o. | 20 mg/kg has no effect on the endpoints.<br><br>100 and 400 mg/kg resulted in a profound inhibitory effect on GI transit and gastric emptying time. |

[a] Vehicle: 0.1% DMSO.

[6]  PMDA Database.   http://www.pmda.go.jp/drugs/2015/P20150604001/index.html (accessed Mar 2016).
[7]  FDA Database.   http://www.accessdata.fda.gov/drugsatfda_docs/nda/2014/205494Orig1s000PharmR.pdf (accessed Mar 2016).
[8]  EMA Database.   http://www.ema.europa.eu/docs/en_GB/document_library/EPAR_-_Public_assessment_report/human/003724/WC500182389.pdf (accessed Mar 2016).

# Genotoxicity

Table 23    Genotoxicity Studies of Eliglustat and Metabolites[6]

| Assay | Compound | Species/System | Metabolism Activity | Dose | Finding |
|---|---|---|---|---|---|
| *In vitro* reverse mutation assay in bacterial cells (Ames) | Eliglustat | *S. typhimurium* TA1535, TA1537, TA98, TA100; *E. coli* WP2P, WP2P*uvr*A | ±S9 | 50-5000 µg/plate | Negative. |
| | Genz-399240-AA (M24 & M54) | *S. typhimurium* (TA1535, TA1537, TA98, TA100, TA102) | ±S9 | 312.5-5000 µg/plate | Negative. |
| *In vitro* mammalian cell cytogenetic test | Eliglustat | HPBL | ±S9 | 1.56-80 µg/mL | Negative. |
| | Genz-399240-AA (M24 & M54) | HPBL | ±S9 | 3.91-500 µg/mL | Negative. |
| *In vivo* micronucleus assay in rodent | Eliglustat | Swiss mouse | + | 68.75, 137.5, 275 mg/kg/day, for 2 days | Negative. |

# Reproductive and Developmental Toxicity

Table 24    Reproductive and Developmental Toxicology Studies of Eliglustat[6-8]

| Studies | Species | Dose (mg/kg/day) | NOAEL (mg/kg/day) | Finding |
|---|---|---|---|---|
| Fertility and early embryonic development | SD rat | 10, 30, 100 | $F_0 = 30$ (male and female) | 100 mg/kg/day produced very slight maternal toxicity and slightly low fetal weights. Pre-implantation losses were increased at 30 and 100 mg/kg/day compared to control. |
| Embryo-fetal development | SD rat | 10, 30, 120[a] | $F_0 = 30$, $F_1 = 30$ | Maternal toxicities (decreased body weight and food consumption) were observed at 120 mg/kg/day. At 120 mg/kg/day, an increase in the number of late resorptions, dead fetuses and post implantation loss, respectively.    The fetal body weight was also reduced at 120 mg/kg/day. At 120 mg/kg/day, fetal visceral variations included dilated cerebral ventricles and fetal skeletal malformations included abnormal number of ribs or lumbar vertebra and fetal skeletal variations included poor bone ossification. At 30 and 10 mg/kg/day, no litter parameter at cesarean section. |
| | NZW rabbit | 10, 30, 100[b] | $F_0 = 30$, $F_1 = 100$ | At 100 mg/kg/day, three females were dead on GD 11, 17 and 18. Significant adverse effects on embryo fetal development up to 100 mg/kg/day. |
| Pre- and postnatal develpment | SD rat | 10, 30, 100 | $F_0 = 30$, $F_1 = 100$ | $F_0$ generation: Two females at 100 mg/kg and two females at 30 mg/kg/day and one female at 10 mg/kg/day were sacrificed prematurely. Body weight (7%) and food consumption (4%-14%) were reduced at 100 mg/kg/day. The mean duration of gestation was longer at 100 mg/kg/day (22.0 days vs. 21.5 days in control) compared to control. At 100 mg/kg/day, animals had a lower number of delivered pups per litter and decreasing of the mean post-implantation loss. $F_1$ generation: Body weights were reduced by approximately 10% in both sexes at 100 mg/kg/day. The mean numbers of corpora lutea and implantations were lower at 100 mg/kg/day (15.9 vs. 17.3 in control and 14.3 vs. 16.1 in control) and the mean pre-implantation loss was higher (9.9 vs. 6.9 in control). Statistically significantly lower absolute testes and epididymides weights were observed in $F_1$ males at 100 mg/kg/day. |

Vehicle: Purified water.    NA: Not applicable.    [a] Animals were treated at 10, 30 and 120 mg/kg/day from GD 6 to GD 17.    [b] Animals were treated at 10, 30 and 100 mg/kg/day from GD 6 to GD 18.

[6] PMDA Database.    http://www.pmda.go.jp/drugs/2015/P20150604001/index.html (accessed Mar 2016).
[7] FDA Database.    http://www.accessdata.fda.gov/drugsatfda_docs/nda/2014/205494Orig1s000PharmR.pdf (accessed Mar 2016).
[8] EMA Database.    http://www.ema.europa.eu/docs/en_GB/document_library/EPAR_-_Public_assessment_report/human/003724/WC500182389.pdf (accessed Mar 2016).

## Carcinogenicity

Table 25    Carcinogenic Toxicity Studies of Eliglustat[6-8]

| Test | Species | Dose (mg/kg/day) | | | |
|---|---|---|---|---|---|
| **105-week Carcinogenic Study in CD-1 Mice** | | | | | |
| | | 0[a] | 10 | 25 | 75 |
| Survival (%) | Male | 50, 43 | 45 | 37 | 38 |
| | Female | 30, 40 | 48 | 35 | 33 |
| Amyloidosis (number) | Male | 1, 5 | NA | NA | NA |
| | Female | 3, 6 | 4 | 4 | 6 |
| Malignant lymphoma (number) | Male | 5, 3 | 4 | 1 | 4 |
| | Female | 14, 4 | 10 | 10 | 12 |
| Histiocytic sarcoma (number) | Male | NA, 1 | 1 | 1 | NA |
| | Female | 2, 4 | 1 | 5 | 4 |
| Carcinoma/adenoma (number) | Male | 4, 6 | 3 | 10 | 8 |
| | Female | 2, 5 | 3 | 3 | 4 |
| Sarcoma (number) | Male | NA, 1 | NA | 1 | 3 |
| | Female | 5, 0 | 3 | 0 | 4 |

| Dose (ppm) | Species | Dose (mg/kg/day) | | | |
|---|---|---|---|---|---|
| **103/105-week Carcinogenic Studies in Rats[b]** | | | | | |
| | | 0[a] | 10 (M)/5 (F) | 25 (M)/15 (F) | 75 (M)/50 (F) |
| Pituitary neoplasia (number) | Male | 10, 11 | 10 | 9 | 5 |
| | Female | 18, 19 | 21 | 22 | 10 |
| Mammary neoplasia (number) | Male | NA | NA | 1 | 1 |
| | Female | 5, 5 | 12 | 10 | 9 |

Basis of high dose selection: The Carcinogenicity Assessment (CAC) recommended to select on 10, 25 and 75 mg/kg/day for male rats based on mortality observed in the 28-day study and concurred with the dose-levels of 5, 15 and 50 mg/kg/day for the females based on AUC comparisons (the exposure at the high-dose being about 30-fold higher than human AUC of 128 ng·h/mL at 100 mg BID).    M: Male.    F: Female.    NA: Not applicable.    [a] Two groups of dose on 0 mg/kg/day.    [b] Duration of dosing, 105 weeks for males and 103 weeks for females.

[6]  PMDA Database.    http://www.pmda.go.jp/drugs/2015/P20150604001/index.html (accessed Mar 2016).
[7]  FDA Database.    http://www.accessdata.fda.gov/drugsatfda_docs/nda/2014/205494Orig1s000PharmR.pdf (accessed Mar 2016).
[8]  EMA Database.    http://www.ema.europa.eu/docs/en_GB/document_library/EPAR_-_Public_assessment_report/human/003724/WC500182389.pdf (accessed Mar 2016).

# CHAPTER

## 12

## Empagliflozin

# Empagliflozin

## (Jardiance®)

Research code: BI-10773

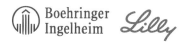

## 1  General Information

❖ Empagliflozin is a SGLT2 (sodium-glucose cotransporter 2) inhibitor, which was initially approved in May 2014 by EMA.

❖ Empagliflozin was discovered by Boehringer Ingelheim, co-developed and co-marketed through a research collaboration with Eli Lilly.

❖ Empagliflozin inhibits the reuptake of glucose by selective inhibition of SGLT2 in kidneys, and increases urine glucose excretion (UGE), thereby reducing blood glucose.

❖ Empagliflozin is indicated for the treatment of patients with type 2 diabetes mellitus to improve glycaemic control in adults.

❖ Available as oral tablet, with each containing 10 mg or 25 mg of empagliflozin and the recommended starting dose is 10 mg once daily before or after breakfast.

❖ The 2014 worldwide sale of Jardiance® was 10.1 million US$, referring to the 2014 financial report of Lilly, yet the 2015 sale was not available up to Mar 2016.

### Key Approvals around the World*

|  | EU (EMA) | US (FDA) | Japan (PMDA) |
|---|---|---|---|
| First approval date | 05/22/2014 | 08/01/2014 | 12/26/2014 |
| Application or approval No. | EMEA/H/C /002677 | NDA 204629 | 22600AMX01387000; 22600AMX01386000 |
| Brand name | Jardiance® | Jardiance® | Jardiance® |
| Indication | Type 2 diabetes | Type 2 diabetes | Type 2 diabetes |
| Authorisation holder | Boehringer Ingelheim & Lilly | | |

* Till Mar 2016, it had not been approved by CFDA (China).

## Active Ingredient

*Molecular formula*:  $C_{23}H_{27}ClO_7$
*Molecular weight*:  450.91
*CAS No.*:  864070-44-0 (Empagliflozin)
*Chemical name*:  (1$S$)-1,5-anhydro-1-$C$-{4-chloro-3-[(4-{[(3$S$)-oxolan-3-yl]oxy}phenyl)methyl]phenyl}-D-glucitol

*Parameters of Lipinski's "Rule of 5"*

| MW | $H_D$ | $H_A$ | FRB[a] | PSA[a] | cLogP[a] |
|---|---|---|---|---|---|
| 450.91 | 4 | 7 | 10 | 109Å$^2$ | 1.16 ± 0.53 |

[a] Calculated by ACD/Labs software V11.02.

## Drug Product*

*Dosage route*:  Oral
*Strength*:  10 mg/25 mg
*Dosage form*:  Film-coated tablet
*Inactive ingredient*:  Lactose monohydrate, microcrystalline cellulose, hydroxypropylcellulose, croscarmellose sodium, colloidal anhydrous silica, magnesium stearate, hypromellose, titanium dioxide (E171), talc, macrogol (400) and iron oxide yellow (E172).
*Recommended dose*: The recommended dose for adults is 10 mg once daily, taken in the morning with or without food.

Dose may be increased to 25 mg once daily.

Assess renal function before initiating Jardiance®. Do not initiate Jardiance® if eGFR is below 60 mL/min/1.73 m².

Discontinue Jardiance® if eGFR falls persistently below 45 mL/min/1.73 m².

* Sourced from EMA drug label information

# 2 Key Patents Information

## Summary

❖ Jardiance® (Empagliflozin) has got five-year NCE market exclusivity protection after it was initially approved by US FDA on Aug 01, 2014.

❖ Empagliflozin was originally discovered by Boehringer Ingelheim and co-developed through a research collaboration with Eli Lilly, and its compound patent application was filed as PCT application by Boehringer Ingelheim in 2005.

❖ The compound patent will expire in 2025 foremost, which has been granted in Japan, the United States, Europe and China, successively.

Table 1    Empagliflozin's Compound Patent Protection in Drug-Mainstream Country

| Country | Publication/Patent NO. | Application Date | Granted Date | Estimated Expiry Date |
|---------|------------------------|------------------|--------------|-----------------------|
| WO | WO2005092877A1 | 03/11/2005 | / | / |
| US | US7579449B2 | 03/11/2005 | 08/25/2009 | 11/05/2025[a] |
| EP | EP1730131B1 | 03/11/2005 | 05/09/2012 | 03/11/2025 |
| JP | JP4181605B2 | 03/11/2005 | 11/19/2008 | 03/11/2030[b] |
| | JP5147314B2 | 03/11/2005 | 02/20/2013 | 03/11/2025 |
| CN | CN103450129B | 03/11/2005 | 08/12/2015 | 03/11/2025 |

[a] The term of this patent is extended by 235 days.    [b] The term of this patent is extended by 5 years.

Table 2    Originator's International Patent Application List (Patent Family)

| Publication NO. | Title | Applicant/Assignee/Owner | Publication Date |
|-----------------|-------|--------------------------|------------------|
| **Technical Subjects** | **Active Ingredient (Free Base)'s Formula or Structure and Preparation** | | |
| WO2005092877A1 | Glucopyranosyl-substituted benzol derivatives, drugs containing said compounds, the use thereof and method for the production thereof | Boehringer Ingelheim | 10/06/2005 |
| **Technical Subjects** | **Salt, Crystal, Polymorphic, Solvate (Hydrate), Isomer, Derivative Etc. and Preparation** | | |
| WO2006117359A1 | Crystalline form of 1-chloro-4-($\beta$-D-glucopyranos-1-yl)-2-[4-(($S$)-tetrahydrofuran-3-yloxy)-benzyl]-benzene, a method for its preparation and the use thereof for preparing medicaments | Boehringer Ingelheim | 11/09/2006 |
| WO2006120208A1 | Processes for preparing of glucopyranosyl-substituted benzylbenzene derivatives and intermediates therein | Boehringer Ingelheim | 11/16/2006 |
| WO2011039108A2 | Processes for preparing of glucopyranosyl-substituted benzylbenzene derivatives | Boehringer Ingelheim | 04/07/2011 |
| WO2011039107A1 | Method for the preparation of a crystalline form of 1-chloro-4-(beta-D-glucopyranos-1-yl)-2-(4-(($S$)-tetrahydrofuran-3-yloxy)benzyl)benzene | Boehringer Ingelheim | 04/07/2011 |
| **Technical Subjects** | **Indication or Methods for Medical Needs** | | |
| WO2010092123A1 | SGLT-2 inhibitor for treating type 1 diabetes mellitus, type 2 diabete mellitus, impaired glucose tolerance or hyperglycemia | Boehringer Ingelheim | 08/19/2010 |
| WO2010092126A1 | Pharmaceutical composition comprising glucopyranosyl diphenylmethane derivatives, pharmaceutical dosage form thereof, process for their preparation and uses thereof for improved glycemic control in a patient | Boehringer Ingelheim | 08/19/2010 |
| WO2012163990A1 | SGLT-2 inhibitors for treating metabolic disorders in patients treated with neuroleptic agents | Boehringer Ingelheim | 12/06/2012 |
| WO2013007557A1 | Pharmaceutical composition, methods for treating and uses thereof | Boehringer Ingelheim | 01/17/2013 |
| WO2014161836A1 | Treatment of metabolic disorders in equine animals | Boehringer Ingelheim | 10/09/2014 |
| WO2014161918A1 | Therapeutic uses of empagliflozin | Boehringer Ingelheim | 10/09/2014 |
| WO2014161919A1 | Therapeutic uses of empagliflozin | Boehringer Ingelheim | 10/09/2014 |
| WO2014170383A1 | Pharmaceutical composition, methods for treating and uses thereof | Boehringer Ingelheim | 10/23/2014 |

*Continued*

| Publication NO. | Title | Applicant/Assignee/Owner | Publication Date |
|---|---|---|---|
| **Technical Subjects** | **Combination Including at Least Two Active Ingredients** | | |
| WO2008055940A2 | Combination therapy with SGLT-2 inhibitors and their pharmaceutical compositions | Boehringer Ingelheim | 05/15/2008 |
| WO2009022007A1 | Pharmaceutical composition comprising a glucopyranosyl-substituted benzene derivative | Boehringer Ingelheim | 02/19/2009 |
| WO2010092124A1 | Pharmaceutical composition comprising linagliptin and optionally a SGLT2 inhibitor, and uses thereof | Boehringer Ingelheim | 08/19/2010 |
| WO2011039337A1 | Pharmaceutical composition, pharmaceutical dosage form, process for their preparation, methods for treating and uses thereof | Boehringer Ingelheim | 04/07/2011 |
| WO2011120923A1 | Pharmaceutical composition comprising an SGLT2 inhibitor and a PPAR- gamma agonist and uses thereof | Boehringer Ingelheim | 10/06/2011 |
| WO2012059416A1 | Pharmaceutical combinations for the treatment of metabolic disorders | Boehringer Ingelheim | 05/10/2012 |
| WO2012062698A1 | Pharmaceutical composition, methods for treating and uses thereof | Boehringer Ingelheim | 05/18/2012 |
| WO2012107476A1 | Pharmaceutical composition, methods for treating and uses thereof | Boehringer Ingelheim | 08/16/2012 |
| WO2012120040A1 | Pharmaceutical compositions comprising metformin and a DPP-4 inhibitor or a SGLT-2 inhibitor | Boehringer Ingelheim | 09/13/2012 |
| WO2013131967A1 | Pharmaceutical compositions comprising metformin and a DPP-4 inhibitor or a SGLT-2 inhibitor | Boehringer Ingelheim | 09/12/2013 |
| WO2013139777A1 | Pharmaceutical composition comprising empagliflozin and antiobesity drug | Boehringer Ingelheim | 09/26/2013 |
| WO2013167554A1 | Pharmaceutical combinations for the treatment of metabolic disorders | Boehringer Ingelheim | 11/14/2013 |

The data was updated until Jan 2016.

## 3   Chemistry

### Route 1:   Original Discovery Route

Et$_3$SiH, BF$_3$·Et$_2$O, DCM
MeCN, 10 to 20 °C to r.t.
then 45 to 50 °C
61%

i. **1**, (COCl)$_2$, DMF, DCM
ii. **2**, AlCl$_3$, DCM, -5 to 5 °C
64%

**1**   **2**   **3**   **4**

BBr$_3$, DCM, 0 °C to r.t.
98%

TBDMSCl, TEA, DMAP
DCM, 0 °C to r.t.
87%

TMSO ... OTMS **7**

i. **6**, 1.7M *t*-BuLi in Pentane
Et$_2$O, -80 °C
ii. **7**, Et$_2$O, -80 to -78 °C
iii. MsOH, MeOH, -78 °C to r.t.

**5**   **6**

i. Et$_3$SiH, BF$_3$·Et$_2$O, DCM
MeCN, -10 to -5 °C
ii. (Ac)$_2$O, Pyridine, DCM
iii. 4M KOH, MeOH
46% over 4 steps

**8**   **9**

TsO ... **10**
Cs$_2$CO$_3$, DMF, 75 °C
49%

**Empagliflozin**

- - - - - - - - - - - - - - - - - - - - - - - - - - - - - - - - - - - - - - - - -

TMSCl, NMP, THF, -5 to
5 °C to r.t., then 35 °C
90%

**11**   **7**

*Synthetic Route*:   Friedel-Crafts reaction of *in situ* generated acyl chloride from commercial 5-bromo-2-chlorobenzoic acid **1** with anisole **2** in the presence of AlCl$_3$ optionally at 5 °C afforded benzophenone derivative **3** in 64% yield, which upon reduction using triethylsilane in the presence of boron trifluoride etherate provided diphenylmethane **4** with the yield of 61%. Nearly quantitative borontribromide-induced demethylation of ether **4** yielded the corresponding phenol **5**, in which phenol group was transformed to silyl ether in 85% yield.   Lithiation of either bromobenzene derivative **6** prior to the exposure to 2,3,4,6-*tetrakis-O*-(trimethylsilyl)-D-glucopyranone **7** (obtained by treating D-glucono-1,5-lactone **11** with TMSCl under basic conditions) in ether at -78 °C, furnished the corresponding lactol, ready for global deprotection with methylsulfonic acid yielded methyl pyranoketal **8**.   Enantiospecific reduction of **8** by a second use of triethylsilane in the presence of boron trifluoride etherate cleaved methoxy group in ketal **8** as an approximate 6:1 mixture of *β/α* and their *tetra*-hydroxyl groups were acylated with Ac$_2$O in order to easy isolation of the pure *β*-anomer from recrystallization by ethanol.   Deacetylation of this *β*-anomer under basic conditions gave rise to *β*-D-glucopyranosyl derivative **9** with 46% yield across a four-step sequence, which upon S$_N$2 displacement with tosylate **10** achieved the desired empagliflozin in 49% yield and 7% overall yield.[1-8]

[1]  Eckhardt, M.; Himmelsbach, F.; Schmid, S., et al. WO2006117359A1, **2006**.
[2]  Himmelsbach, F.; Schmid, S.; Schuehle, M., et al. US7713938B2, **2010**.
[3]  Himmelsbach, F.; Eckhardt, M.; Eickelmann, P., et al. WO2005092877A1, **2005**.
[4]  Eckhardt, M.; Eickelmann, P.; Himmelsbach, F., et al. US7579449B2, **2009**.
[5]  Eckhardt, M.; Eickelmann, P.; Himmelsbach, F., et al. WO2007093610A1, **2007**.
[6]  Eckhardt, M.; Himmelsbach, F.; Eickelmann, P., et al. US7745414B2, **2010**.
[7]  Eckhardt, M.; Himmelsbach, F.; Eickelmann, P., et al. WO2007128749A1, **2007**.
[8]  Eckhardt, M.; Himmelsbach, F.; Eickelmann, P., et al. US7776830B2, **2010**.

# Route 2

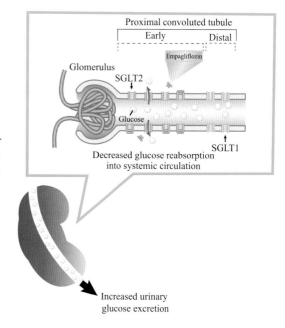

TMDS: 1,1,3,3-Tetramethyldisiloxane

*Synthetic Route*: Commercial 5-iodo-2-chlorobenzoic acid **1** was first converted to the corresponding acid chloride, prior to subjection to fluorobenzene **2** under Friedel-Crafts conditions to generate the desired fluorobenzophenone **3** in 94% yield, which could be isolated by recrystallization from aqueous isopropanol. The fluorobenzophenone **3** was then reacted with commercially available (*S*)-3-hydroxytetrahydrofuran **4** and potassium *tert*-butoxide in THF to afford ethereal benzophenone **5** in 92% yield. Next, removal of the ketone functionality within **5** was achieved through the use of 1,1,3,3-tetramethyl disiloxane (TMDS) in the presence of aluminum chloride in toluene to deliver diaryl iodide **6** with the yield of 83%. This iodide was subsequently converted to the corresponding Grignard and subjected to gluconolactone **7** to give rise to an intermediate lactol which was then sequentially treated with aqueous citric acid, methanolic HCl, and then triethylsilyl hydride and aluminum trichloride to ultimately furnish empagliflozin in 73% yield across the three-step protocol. The overall yield concerning this route was 52%.[9-11]

# 4   Pharmacology

## Summary

### Mechanism of Action

❖ Empagliflozin is an inhibitor of SGLT2, which is the major transporter involved in the reabsorption of glucose in the kidneys.

❖ Empagliflozin selectively inhibited SGLT2 ($IC_{50} = 1.3$ nM), resulting in decrease renal reabsorption of glucose, and thereby increasing urinary glucose excretion (UGE) and reducing plasma glucose (PG) in patients with type 2 diabetes.

[9]  Weber, D.; Renner, S.; Fiedler, T., et al. WO2011039107A1, **2011**.
[10]  Weber, D.; Renner, S.; Fiedler, T., et al. US8802842B2, **2014**.
[11]  Wang, X. J.; Zhang, L.; Byrne, D., et al. *Org. Lett.* **2014**, *16*, 4090-4093.

❖ Empagliflozin showed no activities up to 10 µM in a panel of 98 human, rat, mouse, and rabbit enzymes and receptors, in 106 assays consist of 49 receptors and 21 ion channels binding assays, 29 enzymes and uptake assays, 7 *in vitro* metabolism assays and one receptor function assay, as well as in 50 kinases assays.[12]

*In Vivo* Efficacy

❖ Increased urinary glucose excretion (UGE) and urine volume:
  • In *db/db* mouse: ED = 3 mg/kg.
  • In ZDF diabetic rat: ED = 3 mg/kg.
  • In DIO rat: ED = 10 mg/kg.
  • In beagle dog: $ED_{50}$ = 0.9 mg/kg.
  • In BTBR *ob/ob* mouse: Induced UGE at 300 ppm for 12 weeks.
❖ Decreased blood glucose concentration and blood glucose AUC:
  • In *db/db* mouse:
    ◆ Normal test: Dose-dependently reduced blood glucose during 0-7 h, $ED_{50}$ = 0.6 mg/kg.
    ◆ OGTT: Dose-dependently reduced glucose $AUC_{0-2}$ at ≥0.3 mg/kg.
  • In ZDF rat:
    ◆ Normal test: Significantly reduced blood glucose, $ED_{50}$ = 0.6-1 mg/kg.
    ◆ OGTT: Reduced blood glucose $AUC_{0-3}$ at ≥1 mg/kg in chronic treatments.
  • In BTBR *ob/ob* mouse: Significantly lowered blood glucose at 300 ppm.
  • In DIO rat: Significantly lowered blood glucose at 60 mg/kg.
❖ Protection of insulin secretion: Increased insulin levels in ZDF rat.
❖ Decreased HbA1c level in ZDF rat from 7.93 to 6.84 at 3 mg/kg ($P$ <0.006).
❖ Attenuated body weight gain in DIO rat by 8.2% compared to control at 60 mg/kg ($P$ <0.001).

## Mechanism of Action

Table 3  *In Vitro* Inhibition of Empagliflozin on SGLT1 and SGLT2[12-14]

| Species | Cell line | Type | $IC_{50}$ (nM) | |
| | | | SGLT2 | SGLT1 |
|---|---|---|---|---|
| Human | HEK293 | Human embryonic kidney | 1.3 | 6278 |
| Mouse | HEK293 | Human embryonic kidney | 1.7 | 28000 |
| Rat | CHO | Chinese hamster ovary cell | 1.7 | NA |
| Mouse | CHO | Chinese hamster ovary cell | 1.7 | NA |

HEK293 and CHO cells were stably transfected with cDNA for human, rat or mouse SGLT1 or hSGTL2, respectively, and used to measure the uptake of the glucose analogue [$^{14}$C]alpha-methyl-glucopyranoside ([$^{14}$C]AMG).

[12] U.S. Food and Drug Administration (FDA) Database.  http://www.accessdata.fda.gov/drugsatfda_docs/nda/2014/204629Orig1s000PharmR.pdf (accessed Mar 2016).
[13] Japan Pharmaceuticals and Medical Devices Agency (PMDA) Database.  http://www.pmda.go.jp/drugs/2014/P201400167/index.html (accessed Mar 2016).
[14] European Medicines Agency (EMA) Database.  http://www.ema.europa.eu/docs/en_GB/document_library/EPAR_-_Public_assessment_report/human/002708/WC500139858.pdf (accessed Mar 2016).

Table 4    Binding Affinity of [³H]Empagliflozin for hSGLT2[15]

| Glucose | Kinetic Parameter | | | |
| --- | --- | --- | --- | --- |
| | $K_d$ (nM) | $T_{1/2}$ (min) | $K_{on}$ (mol$^{-1}$·min$^{-1}$) | $K_{off}$ (min$^{-1}$) |
| No | 57.0 ± 37.3 | 59 ± 5 | 314747.7 ± 265243 | 0.01181 ± 0.00098 |
| 20 mM | 194 ± 98.7 | 62 ± 5 | 68302.7 ± 29471.0 | 0.01132 ± 0.00101 |

Data shown were the mean ± SD of three independent experiments.    Every experiment was performed in triplicate and with three different concentrations of [³H]empagliflozin.    $K_d$: Equilibrium dissociation constant.    $K_{on}$: Association rate constant.    $K_{off}$: Dissociation rate constant.    SD: Standard deviation.    SGLT: Sodium glucose cotransporter.    $T_{1/2}$: Terminal elimination half-life.

Table 5    *In Vitro* Inhibition and Selectivity of Empagliflozin on SGLT2 and Other Targets[13, 15]

| Glucoside | Compound | IC$_{50}$ (nM) | | | | |
| --- | --- | --- | --- | --- | --- | --- |
| | | SGLT2 (AMG) | SGLT1 (AMG) | SGLT4 (AMG) | SGLT5 (mannose) | SGLT6 (myo-inositol) |
| *C*-glucoside | Empagliflozin | 3.1 | 8300 | 11000 | 1100 | 2000 |
| | Dapagliflozin | 1.2 | 1400 | 9100 | 820 | 1300 |
| | Canagliflozin | 2.7 | 710 | 7900 | 1700 | 240 |
| | Ipragliflozin | 5.3 | 3000 | 16000 | 740 | 7800 |
| | Tofogliflozin | 6.4 | 12000 | 14000 | 3000 | ND |
| *O*-glucoside | Sergliflozin | 7.5 | 2100 | 6000 | 1100 | 14000 |
| | Remogliflozin | 12 | 6500 | 1500 | 190 | 6200 |
| | T-1095A | 4.4 | 260 | 2300 | 1100 | 3300 |
| | Phlorizin | 21 | 290 | 6100 | 1500 | 10000 |

[¹⁴C]AMG was used as a substrate for hSGLT1, 2 and 4.    [¹⁴C]Mannose was used as a substrate for hSGLT5 and [¹⁴C]myo-inositol for hSGLT6.    Data were derived from at least three independent experiments unless indicated otherwise.    Empagliflozin was also screened *in vitro* for binding activity against a panel of unrelated receptors, ion channels, proteases, growth factors and transporters.    Empagliflozin at 10 μM was found to have minimal (less than 30%) activity in this screening panel.    AMG: Alpha-methyl glucopyranoside.    ND: Not determined.

## *In Vivo* Efficacy

Table 6    *In Vivo* Efficacy of Empagliflozin in the Treatment of Diabetes Mellitus[12-14, 16-18]

| Study | Animal | Dose (mg/kg, p.o.) | Duration (Day) | Glucose Loading (OGTT) | Effect | |
| --- | --- | --- | --- | --- | --- | --- |
| | | | | | ED (mg/kg) | Finding |
| Urinary glucose excretion (UGE) | *db/db* mouse (male) | 3 | Single dose | No | 3 | Increased UGE and urine volume. |
| | ZDF diabetic rat (male) | 3 | Single dose | No | 3 | Increased UGE and urine volume. |
| | DIO rat (female) | 10, 30, 60 | QD × 28 | No | 10 | Dose-dependently increased UGE on Day 21 ($P$ <0.001) and improved glucose tolerance. |
| | Beagle dog | 10 | Single dose | No | ED$_{50}$ = 0.9 | Increased UGE (the maximum voided volume = 600 μM/kg/h) and urine volume. |
| | BTBR *ob/ob* mouse | 300 ppm | 12 weeks | No | 300 ppm | Induced strong and persisting UGE. |

[12]  FDA Database.    http://www.accessdata.fda.gov/drugsatfda_docs/nda/2014/204629Orig1s000PharmR.pdf (accessed Mar 2016).
[13]  PMDA Database.    http://www.pmda.go.jp/drugs/2014/P201400167/index.html (accessed Mar 2016).
[14]  EMA Database.    http://www.ema.europa.eu/docs/en_GB/document_library/EPAR_-_Public_assessment_report/human/002708/WC500139858.pdf (accessed Mar 2016).
[15]  Grempler, R.; Thomas, L.; Eckhardt, M., et al. *Diabetes Obes. Metab.* **2012**, *14*, 83-90.
[16]  Vickers, S. P.; Cheetham, S. C.; Headland, K. R., et al. *Diabetes Metab. Syndr. Obes.* **2014**, *7*, 265-275.
[17]  Gembardt, F.; Bartaun, C.; Jarzebska, N., et al. *Am. J. Physiol. Renal. Physiol.* **2014**, *307*, F317-F325.
[18]  Hansen, H. H.; Jelsing, J.; Hansen, C. F., et al. *J. Pharmacol. Exp. Ther.* **2014**, *350*, 657-664.

*Continued*

| Study | Animal | Dose (mg/kg, p.o.) | Duration (Day) | Glucose Loading (OGTT) | Effect ED (mg/kg) | Finding |
|---|---|---|---|---|---|---|
| Blood glucose | *db/db* mouse (male) | 0.03, 0.1, 0.3, 1, 3, 10, 30 | Single dose | No | $ED_{50} = 0.6$ | Dose-dependently reduced blood glucose at 0-7 h. |
| | | | | Yes | 3 | Dose-dependently reduced glucose $AUC_{0-2}$ at ≥0.3 mg/kg after an OGTT and significantly reduced by 40%-65% at 3 mg/kg at 2 h post administration. |
| | ZDF rat (male) | 0.03, 0.1, 0.3, 1, 3, 10, 30 | Single dose | No | $ED_{50} = 0.6$ | Significantly reduced blood glucose concentration at ≥0.3mg/kg during 0-24 h. |
| | | | | Yes | 1 | Reduced blood glucose $AUC_{0-3}$ at ≥0.3 mg/kg in an OGTT study and significantly reduced by 81% at 30 mg/kg at 3 h after administration. |
| | | 5, 10 | QD × (4 or 8 weeks) | No | NA | Significantly decreased blood glucose. |
| | | | | Yes[a] | NA | Significantly decreased blood glucose $AUC_{0-4}$, as well as peak blood glucose level during the OGTT ($P < 0.001$). |
| | ZDF rat (male) | 0.3, 1, 3 | QD × (5 weeks) | No[b] | 1 | Dose-dependently lowered the blood glucose by 4%-39% on Day 37. |
| | | 0.3, 1, 3 | QD × 23 | Yes | 1 | Dose-dependently reduced blood glucose $AUC_{0-3}$ by 6%-36% in OGTT. |
| | BTBR *ob/ob* mouse | 300 ppm | 12 weeks | No | 300 ppm | Significantly lowered blood glucose. |
| | DIO rat (female) | 10, 30, 60 | QD × 28 | No | 60 | Significantly lowered blood glucose at 60 mg/kg. |
| Plasm Insulin level | ZDF rat (male) | 5, 10 | QD × (4 or 8 weeks) | No | NA | Significantly increased plasma insulin level. |
| | | | | Yes | NA | Significantly increased plasma insulin $AUC_{0-4}$ indicating the improvement of insulin release. |
| | DIO rat (female) | 10, 30, 60 | QD × 28 | No | NA | Reduced plasma insulin level. |
| HbA1c level | ZDF rat (male) | 5, 10 | QD × (4 or 8 weeks) | No | NA | Significantly decreased circulating HbA1c level. |
| | | 0.3, 1, 3 | QD × 37 | No | 3 | HbA1c had decreased from 7.93 to 6.84, representing 14% reduction at 3 mg/kg ($P < 0.006$). |
| Body weight gain | DIO rat (female) | 10, 30, 60 | QD × 28 | No | 60 | Reduced weight gain by 8.2% compared to control at 60 mg/kg ($P < 0.001$). |
| | ZDF rat (female) | 300 ppm | 12 weeks | No | 300 ppm | Showed no impact on body weight gain. |

Vehicle: 0.5% hydroxyethylcellulose.    [a] Subjected to OGTTs on Day 28 and Day 56.    [b] Animals were fasted.

[12]  FDA Database.   http://www.accessdata.fda.gov/drugsatfda_docs/nda/2014/204629Orig1s000PharmR.pdf (accessed Mar 2016).
[13]  PMDA Database.   http://www.pmda.go.jp/drugs/2014/P201400167/index.html (accessed Mar 2016).
[14]  EMA Database.   http://www.ema.europa.eu/docs/en_GB/document_library/EPAR_-_Public_assessment_report/human/002708/WC500139858.pdf (accessed Mar 2016).
[16]  Vickers, S. P.; Cheetham, S. C.; Headland, K. R., et al. *Diabetes Metab. Syndr. Obes.* **2014**, *7*, 265-275.
[17]  Gembardt, F.; Bartaun, C.; Jarzebska, N., et al. *Am. J. Physiol. Renal. Physiol.* **2014**, *307*, F317-F325.
[18]  Hansen, H. H.; Jelsing, J.; Hansen, C. F., et al. *J. Pharmacol. Exp. Ther.* **2014** *350*, 657-664.

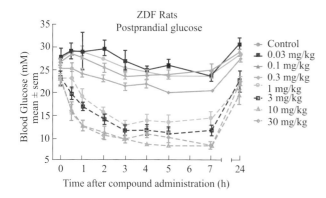

Figure A　Blood Glucose Reduction in ZDF Rats Following Single Dose of Empagliflozin[13]

**Study:** Blood glucose reduction in ZDF rats with empagliflozin.

**Animal:** ZDF diabetic rat (male).

**Administration:** Empagliflozin: Single dose, 0.03-30 mg/kg, p.o.; Vehicle control: NA.

**Test:** Blood glucose reduction in 0-24 h after treated empagliflozin.

**Result:** Significantly reduced blood glucose concentration in 0-7 h.

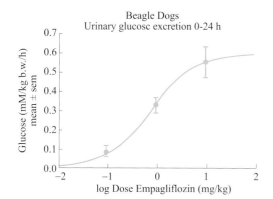

Figure B　Urinary Glucose Excretion in Beagle Dogs Following Single Dose of Empagliflozin[13]

**Study:** Urinary glucose excretion (UGE) in beagle dogs with empagliflozin.

**Animal:** Beagle dog.

**Administration:** Empagliflozin: Single dose, 0.1, 1 and 10 mg/kg, p.o.; Vehicle control: NA.

**Test:** UGE in 0-24 h after treated empagliflozin.

**Result:** Empagliflozin increased UGE, and the maximum voided volume = 600 μM/kg/h.

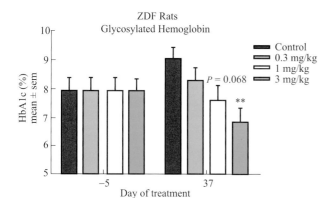

Figure C　Glycosylated Hemoglobin in ZDF Rats Following Multiple Doses of Empagliflozin[13]

**Study:** Glycosylated hemoglobin in ZDF rats with empagliflozin.

**Animal:** ZDF rat.

**Administration:** Empagliflozin: 0.3-3 mg/kg, p.o., QD for 37 days; Vehicle control: NA.

**Test:** The blood HbA1c values on Day 5 before treatment and Day 37 after treatment.

**Result:** HbA1c had decreased from a baseline value of 7.93 to 6.84, representing 2.2% reduction at 3 mg/kg empagliflozin.

[13] PMDA Database.　http://www.pmda.go.jp/drugs/2014/P201400167/index.html (accessed Mar 2016).

# 5 ADME & Drug-Drug Interaction

## Summary

### Absorption of Empagliflozin

❖ Exhibited a linear pharmacokinetics in humans following oral dosing. The increase of AUC appeared to be dose-proportional in the dose range of 10-100 mg empagliflozin.

❖ Had high oral bioavailability in mice (89.8%-96.7%) and dogs (92.1%-102%), but moderate in rats (31.0%).

❖ Was absorbed rapidly ($T_{max} = 0.33$-$0.67$ h) in mice, rats and dogs, but moderately in humans ($T_{max} = 1$-$2$ h).

❖ Showed a half-life ranging between 8.57-13.1 h in humans, much longer than those in mice (4.31-5.59 h), rats (6.32 h) and dogs (3.6-5.16 h), after oral administrations.

❖ Had moderate clearance in rats (14.8 mL/min/kg) and mice (33.0-40.1 mL/min/kg), but low in dogs (1.65-1.76 mL/min/kg), in contrast to liver blood flow, after intravenous administrations. The Cl/F in humans was 167-177 mL/min after oral administration.

❖ Exhibited an extensive distribution in mice, rats and dogs, with apparent volumes of distribution at 0.868-1.17, 0.818 and 0.868-1.08 L/kg, respectively, after intravenous administrations. The apparent volume of distribution in humans was 168-172 L after oral administration.

### Distribution of Empagliflozin

❖ Exhibited moderate plasma protein binding in humans (82%-84.5%), rats (89.9%-91.2%), dogs (88.2%-89.3%) and mice (87.5%-88.5%). Note that the drug was mainly bound to HSA.

❖ Had a $C_b{:}C_p$ ratio of 0.3 in humans, suggesting rare penetration into red blood cells.

❖ Rats after single oral administration:
  • The drug was rapidly and well distributed into some tissues, except for the central nervous system (CNS).
  • Relatively higher concentration levels were observed in tissues involved with absorption and elimination processes such as the gastrointestinal tract, liver and kidneys, compared to other organs.
  • All tissues with measurable concentrations of empagliflozin had maximum concentrations at 1 h post-dose.
  • Tissues where empagliflozin concentrations were absent included the brain, spinal cord, bone, bone marrow, eyes, eye lens, testes and uveal tract.
  • The empagliflozin concentrations in all organs declined over 24-168 h indicating a lack of drug accumulation.

### Metabolism of Empagliflozin

❖ Was metabolized moderately in rat and dog liver microsomes and hepatocytes, but lowly in human liver microsomes and hepatocytes.

❖ Overall, the parent drug represented the most abundant component, with glucuronide metabolites (empagliflozin-2-*O*-, 3-*O*- and 6-*O*-glucuronide) as the major metabolites in the human plasma (3%-7%). Oxidative metabolism predominated in nonclinical species with up to 31%, 20% and 17% oxidative metabolism occurring in mice, rats and dogs, respectively.[13]

❖ The recombinant UGT isoforms responsible for the formation of empagliflozin glucuronides were UGT1A3, 1A8, 1A9 and 2B7.

### Excretion of Empagliflozin

❖ Was predominantly excreted in urine in humans, with parent as the most significant component in human urine.

❖ Was predominantly excreted in feces of mice, rats and dogs, with parent as the most significant component in mouse, rat and dog feces.

### Drug-Drug Interaction

❖ Empagliflozin and its three glucuronide metabolites minimally inhibited human liver microsomal CYP1A2, 2B6, 2C8, 2C9, 2C19, 2D6 and 3A4.

❖ Empagliflozin had no induction on human hepatocyte CYP1A2, 2B6 or 3A4 mRNA expression or enzyme activity.

❖ Empagliflozin was a substrate of both P-gp and BCRP, but did not inhibit P-gp or BCRP.

❖ Empagliflozin was a substrate of transporters OAT3, OATP1B1 and OATP1B3, but not OAT1 or OCT2.

❖ Empagliflozin inhibited OATP1B1, OATP1B3 and OAT2B1 with an $IC_{50}$ in the range of 45-295 μM, but not inhibit OAT1 or OCT2.

[13] PMDA Database. http://www.pmda.go.jp/drugs/2014/P201400167/index.html (accessed Mar 2016).

# Absorption

Table 7  *In Vivo* Pharmacokinetic Parameters of Empagliflozin in Different Species after Single
Intravenous and Oral Dose of Empagliflozin[13]

| Species | Route | Gender | Dose (mg/kg) | $T_{max}$ (h) | $C_{max}$ (nM) | $AUC_{inf}$ (nM·h) | $V_{ss}$ (L/kg) | $T_{1/2}$ (h) | Cl or Cl/F (mL/min/kg) | F (%) |
|---|---|---|---|---|---|---|---|---|---|---|
| CD-1 mouse | p.o. | Male | 250 | 0.67 | 97700 | 207000 | NA | 5.59 | 44.6 | 89.8 |
| | | Female | 250 | 0.33 | 91500 | 273000 | NA | 4.31 | 33.8 | 96.7 |
| | i.v. | Male | 5 | NA | NA | 4610 | 1.17 | 1.26 | 40.1 | - |
| | | Female | 5 | NA | NA | 5600 | 0.868 | 0.654 | 33.0 | - |
| Wistar rat | p.o. | Male | 5 | 1 | $326 \pm 54^a$ | $1798 \pm 293^b$ | NA | $6.32 \pm 2.29$ | $47.2 \pm 7.4$ | $31.0 \pm 5.1$ |
| | i.v. | Male | 0.5 | NA | NA | $595 \pm 160^b$ | $0.818 \pm 0.711$ | $3.64 \pm 1.57$ | $14.8 \pm 3.9$ | - |
| Dog | p.o. | Male | 5 | 1 | $16100 \pm 781$ | 101000 | NA | $3.60 \pm 0.16$ | $1.73 \pm 0.22$ | 102 |
| | | Female | 5 | 1 | $15500 \pm 1500$ | 96800 | NA | $5.16 \pm 1.88$ | $1.80 \pm 0.13$ | 92.1 |
| | i.v. | Male | 0.5 | NA | NA | 10200 | $0.836 \pm 0.192$ | $22.0 \pm 3.9$ | $1.76 \pm 0.13$ | - |
| | | Female | 0.5 | NA | NA | 10800 | $1.08 \pm 0.56$ | $31.2 \pm 13.3$ | $1.65 \pm 0.03$ | - |

Intravenous dosed in PEG400: Saline (80:20), oral dosed in 100% PEG400.   [a] The unit was ng/mL.   [b] The unit was ng·h/mL.

Table 8  *In Vivo* Pharmacokinetic Parameters of Empagliflozin in Humans after Single
Oral Dose of Empagliflozin[13, 19]

| Species | Route | Dose (mg) | $T_{max}$ (h) | $C_{max}$ (nM) | $AUC_{inf}$ (nM·h) | $V_{ss}$ (L) | $T_{1/2}$ (h) | Cl/F (mL/min) |
|---|---|---|---|---|---|---|---|---|
| Human/ caucasian | p.o. | 10 | $1.09 \pm 27.3$ | $377 \pm 26.2$ | $2360 \pm 26.7$ | $168 \pm 41.4$ | $11.9 \pm 40.7$ | $167 \pm 26.2$ |
| | | 25 | $1.38 \pm 60.6$ | $867 \pm 26.8$ | $5550 \pm 26.0$ | $172 \pm 38.5$ | $11.5 \pm 35.9$ | $177 \pm 25.1$ |
| Healthy human | p.o. | 2.5 | 1.75 | 53.2 | 396 | NA | 8.57 | NA |
| | | 10 | 1.5 | 226 | 1730 | NA | 13.1 | NA |
| | | 25 | 2.05 | 505 | 3830 | NA | 10.2 | NA |
| | | 100 | 1.0 | 2500 | 16500 | NA | 10.6 | NA |

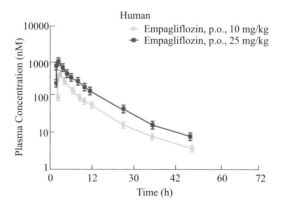

Figure D  *In Vivo* Plasma Concentration-Time Profiles of Empagliflozin in Humans after Single Oral Dose of Empagliflozin[19]

[13]  PMDA Database.   http://www.pmda.go.jp/drugs/2014/P201400167/index.html (accessed Mar 2016).
[19]  FDA Database.   http://www.accessdata.fda.gov/drugsatfda_docs/nda/2014/204629Orig1s000ClinPharmR.pdf (accessed Mar 2016).

Table 9    *In Vitro* Permeability of Empagliflozin in Caco-2 Cell Monolayer Model[13]

| Analyte | Conc. (µM) | Papp$_{(A\to B)}$ (1 × 10$^{-6}$ cm/s) | Permeability Class |
|---|---|---|---|
| Empagliflozin | 1 | 0.85 ± 0.33 | Low |

## Distribution

Table 10    *In Vitro* Plasma Protein Binding and Blood Partitioning of [$^{14}$C]Empagliflozin[13, 19]

| | Protein Binding (%) | | Human Isolated Plasma Protein Binding (%) | | Blood Cell Partitioning | | |
|---|---|---|---|---|---|---|---|
| Species | Conc. (µg/mL) | %Bound | 4% HSA | 0.07% AAG | Species | Conc. (µg/mL) | C$_b$:C$_p$ |
| Mouse | 0.1-40 | 87.5-88.5 | NA | NA | Rat | 1, 10 | 0.296, 0.360 |
| Rat | 0.1-40 | 89.9-91.2 | NA | NA | Dog | 1, 10, 50 | 0.253, 0.243, 0.343 |
| Dog | 0.1-40 | 88.2-89.3 | NA | NA | Human | 0.3, 1 | 0.323, 0.301 |
| Human | 0.01-1.0 | 82.0-84.5 | 80.3-83.6 | 10.6-16.6 | | | |

C$_b$:C$_p$: Blood to plasma concentration ratio.

Table 11    *In Vivo* Tissue Distribution of [$^{14}$C]Empagliflozin in Male Long-Evans Rats after Single Oral Dose of 5 mg/kg [$^{14}$C]Empagliflozin[13]

| Tissue | Long-Evans Rat | | | | |
|---|---|---|---|---|---|
| | Radioactivity (ng eq./g) | | | | |
| | 1 h | 8 h | 24 h | 72 h | 168 h |
| Plasma | 447 | 50.4 | 1.91 | BLQ | BLQ |
| Brain | ND | ND | ND | ND | ND |
| Cecum contents | 35900 | 37300 | 43900 | 103 | ND |
| Large intestine contents | 19900 | 68300 | 4840 | 138 | ND |
| Small intestine contents | 70000 | 7620 | 766 | ND | ND |
| Stomach contents | 17700 | 711 | ND | ND | ND |
| Liver | 4060 | 379 | ND | ND | ND |
| Lungs | 290 | ND | ND | ND | ND |
| Kidneys | 2540 | 880 | 251 | ND | ND |
| Spleen | 158 | BLQ | ND | ND | ND |
| Stomach | 259 | ND | ND | ND | ND |

Vehicle: PEG400.

## Metabolism

Table 12    *In Vitro* Metabolism of Empagliflozin in Liver Microsomes and Hepatocytes of Different Species[13]

| Species | Liver Microsomes | | Hepatocytes | |
|---|---|---|---|---|
| | Cl$_{int}$ (mL/min/kg) | Cl$_h$ (mL/min/kg) | Cl$_{int}$ (mL/min/kg) | Cl$_h$ (mL/min/kg) |
| Wistar rat | 22.0 | 16.7 | 15.8 | 12.9 |
| Dog | 5.66 | 4.78 | 7.70 | 6.17 |
| Human | 3.13 | 2.72 | <2.7 | <2.4 |

[13]  PMDA Database.   http://www.pmda.go.jp/drugs/2014/P201400167/index.html (accessed Mar 2016).
[19]  FDA Database.   http://www.accessdata.fda.gov/drugsatfda_docs/nda/2014/204629Orig1s000ClinPharmR.pdf (accessed Mar 2016).

Table 13    *In Vitro* Metabolic Phenotype of Glucuronide Conjugation for Empagliflozin[13]

| Metabolite | Empagliflozin (10 μM) | Empagliflozin (687 nM) |
|---|---|---|
| CD00006134 (Empagliflozin-6-*O*-glucuronide) | BLOQ | BLOQ |
| CD00006135 (Empagliflozin-2-*O*-glucuronide) | rUGT2B7 | BLOQ |
| CD00006136 (Empagliflozin-3-*O*-glucuronide) | rUGT1A3, rUGT1A8, rUGT1A9, rUGT2B7 | rUGT1A3, rUGT1A8, rUGT1A9 |

Table 14    Metabolites in Plasma and Hepatocytes of Different Species[13]

| Species | Matrix | M555 | M481/1 | M625/1 | M481/2 | M625/2 | M467 | M463 | M625/3 | M379 | M625/4 |
|---|---|---|---|---|---|---|---|---|---|---|---|
| Mouse | Plasma | √ | - | √ | √ | √ | √ | - | √ | √ | - |
| Rat | Hepatocytes | - | - | - | √ | √ | - | - | √ | √ | - |
| | Plasma | √ | - | √ | √ | √ | √ | - | √ | √ | - |
| Dog | Hepatocytes | - | - | - | √ | - | - | - | √ | √ | - |
| | Plasma | √ | √ | √ | √ | √ | √ | √ | √ | √ | - |
| Human | Hepatocytes | - | - | - | √ | - | - | - | √ | √ | - |
| | Plasma | - | - | √ | √ | √ | - | - | √ | √ | √ |

Table 15    Metabolites in Plasma, Urine, Bile and Feces in Humans and Animal Species after Single Oral Dose of Empagliflozin[13]

| Matrix | Species | Dose (mg/kg) | Time (h) | % of Radioactivity or % of Dose | | | | | | | |
|---|---|---|---|---|---|---|---|---|---|---|---|
| | | | | Parent | R-2 M498/1 | R-1 M556/1 | R-3 M482/1 | R-4+R-5 M468+M380 | R-6 M416 | R-7 M464/1 | M626/3 |
| Plasma | Mouse (male) | 250 | 1 | 47.5 | ND | 2.8 | 30.3 | 6.0 | - | 3.5 | 7.7 |
| | | 1000 | 1 | 63.2 | - | 2.3 | 19.2 | 2.2 | - | 6.0 | 6.0 |
| | Rat (male) | 700 | 0.5 | 62.8 | NA | NA | 20.4 | 3.8 | - | 10.9 | |
| | | 5 | 1 | 50.8 | ND | ND | 28.9 | 8.7 | 1.1 | 4.7 | - |
| | Dog | 5 | 1 | 88.7 | - | 0.3 | 2.1 | 1.4 | - | 1.6 | 1.2 |
| | Human | 50 mg | 2 | 77.4 | - | - | 1.2 | 0.4 | - | 0.5 | 3.7 |
| Urine | Mouse (male) | 250 | NA | 2.2 | 0.9 | 1.3 | 17.5 | 7.4 | - | 4.7 | ND |
| | | 1000 | NA | 0.3 | - | ND | 8.0 | 5.4 | - | 1.5 | |
| | Rat (male) | 700 | NA | 1.2 | - | - | 1.3 | 0.6 | - | 0.4 | |
| | | 15 | NA | 6.9 | 0.1 | 0.5 | 9.8 | 5.0 | 0.9 | 3.6 | - |
| | Dog | 5 | NA | 9.6 | | 1.7 | 11.3 | 2.2 | - | 1.2 | |
| | Human | 50 mg | NA | 23.7 | - | - | 2.8 | 2.1 | - | 0.9 | 13.2 |
| Bile | Rat (male) | 15 | NA | ND | 0.3 | 0.7 | 28.4 | 0.6 | ND | 1.3 | - |
| Feces | Mouse (male) | 250 | NA | 9.5 | ND | ND | 23.6 | 5.3 | ND | 8.1 | ND |
| | | 1000 | NA | 63.6 | - | - | 13.8 | 2.7 | - | 1.0 | ND |
| | Rat (male) | 700 | NA | 68.9 | - | - | 7.7 | 2.3 | - | ND | ND |
| | | 15 | NA | 18.0 | 0.5 | ND | 21.4 | 8.0 | 1.0 | 11.7 | - |
| | Dog | 5 | NA | 19.5 | 1.5 | ND | 21.0 | 7.1 | - | 0.6 | ND |
| | Human | 50 mg | NA | 34.2 | - | - | 1.9 | 0.6 | - | 1.1 | ND |

% of radioactivity for plasma, % of dose for urine, bile and feces.

[13] PMDA Database.    http://www.pmda.go.jp/drugs/2014/P201400167/index.html (accessed Mar 2016).

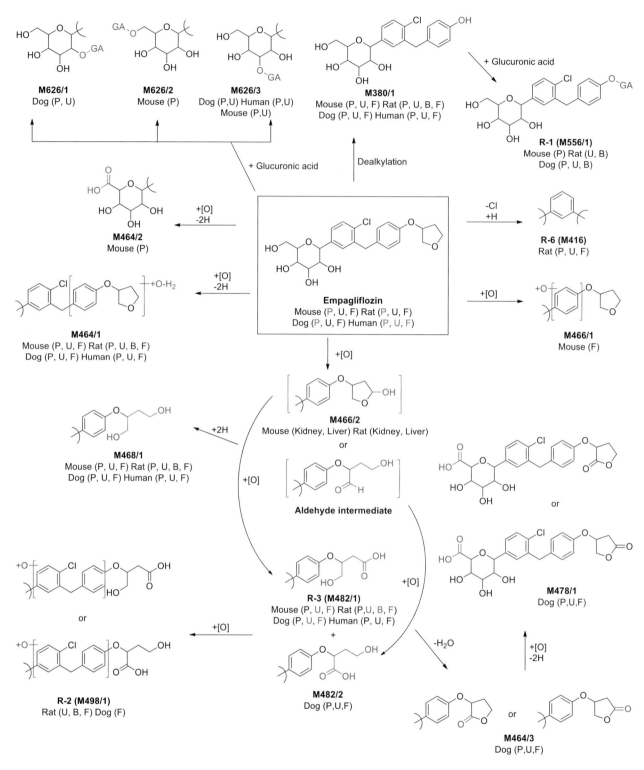

Figure E    Proposed Pathways for *In Vivo* Biotransformation of Empagliflozin in Mice, Rats, Dogs and Humans[13, 19]

The red labels represent the major components in matrices (at the lower dose).    P = Plasma, U = Urine, B = Bile, F = Feces and GA = Glucuronic acid.

[13]  PMDA Database.    http://www.pmda.go.jp/drugs/2014/P201400167/index.html (accessed Mar 2016).

[19]  FDA Database.    http://www.accessdata.fda.gov/drugsatfda_docs/nda/2014/204629Orig1s000ClinPharmR.pdf (accessed Mar 2016).

# Excretion

Table 16    Excretion Profiles of [$^{14}$C]Empagliflozin in Rats, Dogs and Healthy Foreigner Humans after Single Oral and Intravenous Dose of [$^{14}$C]Empagliflozin[13]

| Species | Dose (mg/kg) | Route | Time (h) | Cage Wash (% of dose) | Urine (% of dose) | Feces (% of dose) | Recovery (% of dose) |
|---|---|---|---|---|---|---|---|
| Mouse (male) | 1000 | p.o. | 0-96 | 3.0 | 15.4 | 81.7 | 100 |
| Mouse (female) | 1000 | p.o. | 0-96 | 3.9 | 19.9 | 79.4 | 103 |
| Rat (male) | 0.5 | i.v. | 0-168 | NA | 27.5 | 64.4 | 92.2[a] |
| | 5 | p.o. | 0-168 | NA | 27.4 | 62.9 | 92.9[a] |
| Rat (male) | 700 | p.o. | 0-168 | 0.2 | 3.5 | 79.7 | 83.4 |
| Rat (female) | 700 | p.o. | 0-168 | 1.0 | 7.2 | 69.4 | 77.6 |
| Dog (male) | 0.5 | i.v. | 0-168 | NA | 17.4 | 70.9 | 92.4[a] |
| | 5 | p.o. | 0-168 | NA | 29.6 | 61.4 | 93.7[a] |
| Human | 50 mg | p.o. | NA | NA | 54.4 | 41.2 | 95.6 |

[a] Recovery included cage wash.

# Drug-Drug Interaction

Table 17    *In Vitro* Evaluation of Empagliflozin and Metabolites as Inhibitors and Inducers of Enzymes[13]

| Enzyme | IC$_{50}$ (µM) | | | | Enzyme | Conc.(µM) | Activity/mRNA | |
|---|---|---|---|---|---|---|---|---|
| | Empagliflozin | M626/2 | M626/1 | M626/3 | | | % of Positive | Fold Induction |
| CYP1A2 | >100 | - | - | - | | 0.1 | 0.05/0.02 | 1.1/1.04 |
| CYP2B6 | >50 | - | - | - | CYP1A2 | 3 | 0.05/0.17 | 1.1/1.93 |
| CYP2C8 | >100 | >100 | >20 | >20 | | 30 | 0.71/0.05 | 1.2/1.24 |
| CYP2C9 | ~150 | - | - | - | | 0.1 | -0.06/0.03 | 1.0/0.97 |
| CYP2C19 | >150 | - | - | - | CYP2B6 | 3 | -0.02/1.4 | 1.0/1.73 |
| CYP2D6 | >150 | - | - | - | | 30 | 0.68/2.8 | 1.2/2.46 |
| CYP3A4[a] | >150 | >100 | >100 | >95 | | 0.1 | 0.79/0.46 | 1.3/1.21 |
| CYP3A4[b] | >150 | >100 | >100 | >95 | CYP3A4 | 3 | -0.05/1.0 | 1.0/1.58 |
| UGT1A1 | >150 | - | - | - | | 30 | 2.2/5.0 | 2.0/4.27 |

[a] Testosterone as substrate.    [b] Midazolam as substrate.

[13]  PMDA Database.   http://www.pmda.go.jp/drugs/2014/P201400167/index.html (accessed Mar 2016).

Table 18   *In Vitro* Evaluation of Empagliflozin as a Substrate and an Inhibitor of P-gp and BCRP[13]

| As Substrates of P-gp and BCRP | | | | As an Inhibitor of P-gp | | |
| Caco-2 Cell Monolayer Model | | | | MDCK-MDR1 Cell Monolayer Model | | |
| Compound | Papp(A→B) (1 × 10⁻⁶ cm/s) | Papp(B→A) (1 × 10⁻⁶ cm/s) | Efflux Ratio | Compound | Permeability B→A (%Control) | |
| | | | | | Paclitaxel | Digoxin |
|---|---|---|---|---|---|---|
| Mannitol | 0.39 ± 0.02 | 0.34 ± 0.07 | NA | Control | 100 | 100 |
| Digoxin | 0.97 ± 0.07 | 16.1 ± 0.88 | NA | LY335979 (5 μM) | 18.2 | 16.0 |
| Estrone-3-sulfate | NA | 31.0 ± 4.71 | NA | Empagliflozin (1 μM) | 110 | 127 |
| Empagliflozin (1 μM, P-gp) | 0.85 ± 0.33 | 19.4 ± 0.41 | NA | Empagliflozin (3 μM) | 118 | 122 |
| Empagliflozin (1 μM) + LY335979 | 0.86 ± 0.18 | 15.0 ± 1.04 | 22.6 | Empagliflozin (10 μM) | 105 | 124 |
| Empagliflozin (1 μM, BCRP) | NA | 18.9 ± 1.19 | NA | Empagliflozin (30 μM) | 121 | 126 |
| Empagliflozin (1 μM) + Prazosin (80 μM) | NA | 9.36 ± 1.18 | 50.4 | Empagliflozin (80 μM) | 116 | 142 |
| Empagliflozin (1 μM) + Prazosin (80 μM) +LY335979 (5 μM) | - | 3.20 ± 0.37 | 83.5 | Empagliflozin (100 μM) | 124 | 141 |

Table 19   *In Vitro* Evaluation of Empagliflozin as a Substrate and an Inhibitor of Various Transporters[13, 19]

| Transporter | Substrate | Inhibitor | IC₅₀ (μM) |
|---|---|---|---|
| P-gp | Yes | No | >200 |
| BCRP | Yes | No | 114 |
| MRP2 | No | No | 1399 |
| OATP1B1 | Yes | Yes | 71.8 |
| OATP1B3 | Yes | Yes | 58.6 |
| OATP2B1 | ND | Yes | 45.2 |
| OAT1 | No | No | >1000 |
| OAT3 | Yes | No | 295 |
| OCT2 | No | No | >1000 |

# 6   Non-Clinical Toxicology

## Summary

Single-Dose Toxicity

❖ Few acute toxicity of the p.o./i.p. route was identified in rodents.
  • Mouse $LD_{50}$ by p.o. ≥2000 mg/kg, $LD_{50}$ by i.p. was not definite.
  • Rat $LD_{50}$ of both routes ≥2000 mg/kg.

Repeated-Dose Toxicity

❖ Sub- and chronic toxicological information of the oral route was comprehensively accounted through the 13-week (mice), 26-week (rats) and 52-week (monkeys) studies, the longest one employed in each species.
  • For mice, NOAELs were 62 × and 98 × MRHD for males and females, respectively.
  • For rats, NOAEL was not established due to adrenal and hepatic vacuolation in all treatment groups, and the major target organs included the kidneys, adrenal gland and liver.
  • For dogs, NOAELs were 55 × and 50 × MRHD for males and females, respectively; Dose-related increase in severity of vacuolation of adrenal gland was observed; Nephritis and cortical tubular degeneration with fibrosis were noted (≥ 30 mg/kg).

Safety Pharmacology

❖ No cardiovascular, neurological, pulmonary, renal and gastrointestinal effects.

[13]  PMDA Database.   http://www.pmda.go.jp/drugs/2014/P201400167/index.html (accessed Mar 2016).
[19]  FDA Database.   http://www.accessdata.fda.gov/drugsatfda_docs/nda/2014/204629Orig1s000ClinPharmR.pdf (accessed Mar 2016).

Genotoxicity
- ❖ Empagliflozin possessed least potential for genotoxicity, confirmed by a sufficient battery of genotoxicological studies.

Reproductive and Developmental Toxicity
- ❖ Fertility and early embryonic development in rats:
  - • Putting paternal and maternal systemic toxicities aside, there was no effect on fertility or reproductive performance in both sexes, as the NOAEL was approximately 155 × MRHD at 700 mg/kg.
- ❖ Fetal-embryonic development in rats and rabbits:
  - • The maternal toxicities in cross-species concordance, reduced body weight gain, etc., occurred at high exposure multiples in both rat (48 × MRHD) and rabbit (139 × MRHD). Empagliflozin was also not teratogenic at 48 × and 128 × MRHD in the rat and rabbit, respectively.
  - • The limited findings and the high safety margins suggested empagliflozin unlikely to be teratogenic in humans at the MRHD.
- ❖ Pre- and postnatal development in rats:
  - • Likely due to lactational exposure, reduced body weight/body weight gain were observed in $F_1$ pups during weaning, which in turn led to deficits in memory and learning at PND 22. This might be a sign of risk that nursing or exposure to empagliflozin should be discontinued in nursing mothers.
- ❖ Empagliflozin was able to transfer through placental barrier and presented in fetal tissues.
- ❖ Milk excretion of empagliflozin was also found in lactating rats, and the milk-to-plasma ratio of emplagliflozin ranged from 0.6 to 5 and was greater than 1.0 from 2 to 24 h post-dose.

Carcinogenicity
- ❖ Empagliflozin posed minimal carcinogenic risk to humans based on the high exposure multiples at the NOAELs in the rat (17-21 × MRHD) and the mouse (4-7 × MRHD).

## Single-Dose Toxicity

Table 20    Single-Dose Toxicity Studies of Empagliflozin[12]

| Species | Dose (mg/kg) | NOAEL (mg/kg) | Finding |
|---|---|---|---|
| CD-1 mouse | 2000, p.o. | 2000 | Loose feces in females on Day 2 post-dose; $LD_{50} \geq 2000$ mg/kg. |
| | 300, 2000, i.p. | 300 | 2000 mg/kg: Death of 2/3 females on Day 4 post-dose and one female on Day 5 post-dose.    Fluid filled intestines (red) were found in 2/3 females at necropsy. ↓ activity, ↓ body tone, abnormal gait, abnormal stance, piloerection, prostration, eyes shut and yellow wet fur (urogenital). |
| Wistar rat | 2000, p.o. | 2000 | $LD_{50} \geq 2000$ mg/kg.<br>2000 mg/kg: Abnormal gait, yellow stained fur, soft stool/loose stool and poor grooming. |
| | 300, 2000, i.p. | 2000 | $LD_{50} \geq 2000$ mg/kg.<br>300 mg/kg: Abnormal gait, abnormal stance, soft stool/loose stool and ↓ activity.<br>2000 mg/kg: Piloerection, soft stool/loose stool and poor grooming. |

## Repeated-Dose Toxicity

Table 21    Repeated-Dose Toxicity Studies of Empagliflozin by Oral (Gavage) Administrations[12, 13]

| Species | Duration (Week) | Dose (mg/kg/day) | NOAEL Dose (mg/kg/day) | NOAEL Safety Margin[a] (× MRHD) | Finding |
|---|---|---|---|---|---|
| CD-1 mouse | 13 | 0, 500, 750, 1000 | ≤500 | 27/77 | Mortality at 1000 mg/kg.<br>MTD: 750 mg/kg/day. |
| Wistar rat | 13 | 0, 30, 100, 700 | 100 | 11 | Mortality at 700 mg/kg.<br>Increased BUN at 100 mg/kg without pathology correlate.<br>Dose-related mineralization in the kidneys. |
| | 26 | 0, 30, 100, 700 | 100 | 10/19 | Mortality 1 male and 1 female at 700 mg/kg.<br>All empagliflozin treatment groups: Adrenal gland vacuolation, hepatic vacuolation, kidney corticomedullary tubular dilatation and mineralization.<br>Kidney vacuolation at ≥100 mg/kg. |

[12]  FDA Database.    http://www.accessdata.fda.gov/drugsatfda_docs/nda/2014/204629Orig1s000PharmR.pdf (accessed Mar 2016).
[13]  PMDA Database.    http://www.pmda.go.jp/drugs/2014/P201400167/index.html (accessed Mar 2016).

*Continued*

| Species | Duration (Week) | Dose (mg/kg/day) | NOAEL | | Finding |
|---|---|---|---|---|---|
| | | | Dose (mg/kg/day) | Safety Margin[a] (× MRHD) | |
| Beagle dog | 13 | 0, 10, 30, 100 | 10 | 15/24 | Nephritis and cortical tubular nephropathy at 30 mg/kg that irreversible at 100 mg/kg. Hepatic vacuolation at 30 mg/kg. |
| | 26 | 0, 10, 30, 100 | 10 | 15/12 | Reduced BW/BWG at 30 and 100 mg/kg. Hepatic vacuolation, degeneration and Kupffer cell hypertrophy at 100 mg/kg. |
| | 52 | 0, 10, 30, 100 | 10 | 19/17 | Mortality at 30 mg/kg. Nephritis and cortical tubular at nephropathy 30 and 100 mg/kg. Dose-dependently reduced BW. Adrenal gland vacuolation at 30 and 100 mg/kg. |

Safety margins to expected human exposure were estimated using $AUC_{0-24}$ = 4740 nM·h plasma exposure in T2DM subjects at the proposed MRHD of 25 mg empagliflozin.   [a] Male/female.

## Safety Pharmacology

Table 22    Overall Safety Pharmacological Evaluation of Empagliflozin[12]

| Study | Test System | Dose | Safety Margin[a] (× MRHD) | Finding |
|---|---|---|---|---|
| Neurological effect | Male SD rat | 0, 500, 1000, 2000 mg/kg, p.o. | 0.5-779 | No effect on CNS or ANS. |
| | Irwin test in male mouse | 0, 3, 10, 30 mg/kg, p.o. | | |
| Cardiovascular effect | hERG inhibition test HEK293 cell | NA | NA | hERG: $IC_{50} \geq 30$ μM. |
| | Isolated guinea pig papillary muscle | Up to 10 μM | NA | No effect on action potentials. |
| | Conscious telemetered dog | 10, 30, 100 mg/kg, p.o. | 4-39 | No effect on HR, BP, ECG (QTc interval) or contractility. |
| | Conscious telemetered male Wistar rat | 3, 10, 30 mg/kg, p.o. | 0.5-12 | No effect on systolic or diastolic blood pressure, heart rate or body temperature. |
| Respiratory effect | Conscious male Wistar rat (plethysmography chamber) | 3, 10, 30 mg/kg, p.o. | 0.5-12 | No effect on respiration rate, tidal volume or body temperature. |
| | | 0, 500, 1000, 2000 mg/kg, p.o. | 194-779 | No effect on respiratory rate, tidal volume or min volume. |
| Renal effect | Wistar rat | 3, 10, 30 mg/kg, p.o. | 0.5-12 | 3-30 mg/kg: No impact on urine volume, potassium, calcium, magnesium, protein, albumin or urinary pH. 10 mg/kg and 30 mg/kg: Dose-dependently and significantly increased serum FFA, a compensatory mechanism for urinary glucose loss. |
| Gastrointestinal effect | Wistar rat | 3, 10, 30 mg/kg, p.o. | 0.5-12 | No effect on intestinal transit. 30 mg/kg: Increased gastric emptying by 33%. |
| | Male Wistar rat | 3, 10, 30 mg/kg, i.d. | 1-12 | A minimal effect on gastric acid secretion and thereby ulcerogenic activity. |

[a] On a body surface area basis.   i.d.: Intraduodenal.

[12]  FDA Database.   http://www.accessdata.fda.gov/drugsatfda_docs/nda/2014/204629Orig1s000PharmR.pdf (accessed Mar 2016).

# Genotoxicity

Table 23  Genotoxicity Studies of Empagliflozin[12]

| Assay | Species/System | Metabolism Activity | Dose | Finding |
|---|---|---|---|---|
| *In vitro* reverse mutation assay in bacterial cells (Ames) | *S. Typhimurium* TA100, TA1535, TA98, TA1537; *E. coli* WP2*uvr*A | ±S9 | 156, 313, 625, 1250, 2500, 5000 µg/plate | Negative. |
| *In vitro* mutagenicity testing | L5178Y t/k $^{+/-}$ cell | ±S9 | 4 h, ±S9: 50-400 µg/mL<br>24 h, -S9: 12.5-175 µg/mL | Negative. |
| *In vivo* micronucleus assay in rodents | SD/Wistar rat/Sex | + | 0, 100, 300, 1000, 2000 mg/kg/day, p.o. for 3 days | Negative. |
| | Wistar rat/Sex | + | 0, 30, 100, 300, 500 mg/kg, p.o. for 2 weeks | Negative. |

Vehicle: DMSO for *in vitro* assays and 0.2% natrosol (HEC) for *in vivo* studies.

# Reproductive and Developmental Toxicity

Table 24  Embryonic and Fetal Developmental Toxicity Studies of Empagliflozin by the Oral Routes[12, 13]

| Study | Species | Dose (mg/kg/day) | NOAEL Endpoint | NOAEL Dose (mg/kg/day) | NOAEL $AUC_{0-24}$ (nM·h) | NOAEL Safety Margin (× MRHD) | Finding |
|---|---|---|---|---|---|---|---|
| Fertility and early embryonic development | Wistar rat | 100, 300, 700 | Male and female fertility | 700 | 734000 | 155 | ↓ BWG (>10%) at MD and HD in both sexes. |
| Embryo-fetal development | Wistar rat | 30, 100, 300, 700 | Maternal | 100 | 102000 | 22 | ↓ Maternal BWG (>10%) associated with ↓ food consumption at MD and HD. |
| | | | Fetal development | 300 | 228000 | 48 | Bent limb bone malformation at HD. |
| | NZW rabbit | 30, 100, 300, 700 | Maternal | 300 | 608000 | 128 | Abortion at HD associated with ↓ BWG. ↓ Viable fetuses (post-implantation loss due to early resorption). |
| | | | Fetal development | 700 | 658860 | 139 | No effect on malformations or developmental variations. |
| Pre- and postnatal development | Wistar rat | 10, 30, 100 | $F_0$ fertility | 100 | 102000 | 16 | No observed maternal toxicity. ↓ BWG of $F_1$ pups at all doses during the lactation period, particularly at HD. |
| | | | $F_1$ development | 30 | 18800 | 4 | Deficits of learning and memory at PND 22 in HD males. |
| | | | $F_1$ reproductivity | 100 | 102000 | 16 | No effect on $F_1$ mating or reproductive performance and no morphological changes in the $F_2$ pups. |

Vehicle: 0.5% HEC.  Safety margins to expected human exposure were estimated using $AUC_{0-24}$ = 4740 nM·h plasma exposure in T2DM subjects at the proposed MRHD of 25 mg empagliflozin.

[12] FDA Database.  http://www.accessdata.fda.gov/drugsatfda_docs/nda/2014/204629Orig1s000PharmR.pdf (accessed Mar 2016).
[13] PMDA Database.  http://www.pmda.go.jp/drugs/2014/P201400167/index.html (accessed Mar 2016).

## Carcinogenicity

Table 25    104-Week Carcinogenic Toxicity Studies of Empagliflozin[12]

| Species | Dose (mg/kg/day) | NOAEL | | | Finding |
|---|---|---|---|---|---|
| | | Dose (mg/kg/day) | AUC$_{0-24}$ (nM·h) | Safety Margin (× MRHD) | |
| Wistar rat | 0, 100, 300, 700 | 100 | Male, 79800 Female, 100000 | Male, 17; Female, 21 | No increase of tumor incidence in females. Dose-dependently increased whole body/cavity hemangioma incidence, which became significant at 700 mg/kg. Numerically increased testicular Leydig cell tumors in the 300 and 700 mg/kg males, consistent with the results of several SGLT2 inhibitors. |
| CD-1 mouse | 0, 100, 300, 1000 | 100 | Male, 20700 Female, 32700 | Male, 4; Female, 7 | No increase of drug-related neoplasms in females. Renal tubular adenoma and carcinoma (combined), accompanied by a high incidence of renal atypical hyperplasia. Renal cystic tubular hyperplasia increased at all doses. Renal neoplasms also occurred in the presence of renal tubular injury (single cell necrosis, karyomegaly, hypertrophy, atrophy, cysts and pelvic dilatation). |

Vehicle: 0.5% HEC.    Safety margins to expected human exposure were estimated using AUC$_{0-24, ss}$ = 4740 nM·h plasma exposure in T2DM subjects at the MRHD of 25 mg.

[12]  FDA Database.   http://www.accessdata.fda.gov/drugsatfda_docs/nda/2014/204629Orig1s000PharmR.pdf (accessed Mar 2016).

# CHAPTER

## 13

## Finafloxacin

# Finafloxacin

## (Xtoro®)

Research code: AL-60371

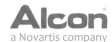

## 1    General Information

❖ Finafloxacin is a quinolone antimicrobial, which was first approved in Dec 2014 by US FDA.

❖ Finafloxacin was originally developed by Bayer, developed and marketed by Alcon Research.

❖ Finafloxacin is a member of the fluoroquinolone class of antibiotics which inhibits bacterial DNA gyrase and topoisomerase IV, resulting in inhibition of bacterial cell division and bacterial cell death.

❖ Finafloxacin is indicated for the treatment of acute otitis externa (AOE) caused by susceptible strains of *Pseudomonas aeruginosa* and *Staphylococcus aureus*.

❖ Available as topical otic suspension, containing 0.3% finafloxacin and the recommended starting dose is 4 drops in the affected ear(s) twice daily for 7 days.

❖ The sale of Xtoro® was not available up to Mar 2016.

### Key Approvals around the World*

|  | US (FDA) |
|---|---|
| First approval date | 12/17/2014 |
| Application or approval No. | NDA 206307 |
| Brand name | Xtoro® |
| Indication | Acute Otitis Externa (AOE) |
| Authorisation holder | Alcon |

* Till Mar 2016, it had not been approved by EMA (Europe), PMDA (Japan) and CFDA (China).

### Active Ingredient

Molecular formula:   $C_{20}H_9FN_4O_4$
Molecular weight:   398.39
CAS No.:   209342-40-5 (Finafloxacin)
Chemical name:   (-)-8-cyano-1-cyclopropyl-6-fluoro-7-[(4aS,7aS)-hexahydropyrrolo[3,4-b]-1,4-oxazin-6(2H)-y]-4-oxo-1,4-dihydroquinoline-3-carboxylic acid

*Parameters of Lipinski's "Rule of 5"*

| MW | $H_D$ | $H_A$ | FRB[a] | PSA[a] | cLogP[a] |
|---|---|---|---|---|---|
| 398.39 | 2 | 8 | 3 | 106Å² | 1.83 ± 1.30 |

[a] Calculated by ACD/Labs software V11.02.

### Drug Product*

Dosage route:   Topical otic
Strength:   5 mL of 0.3% finafloxacin otic suspension.
Dosage form:   Suspension
Inactive ingredient:   Sodium chloride, hydroxyethyl cellulose, tyloxapol, magnesium chloride and purified water.
Recommended dose:   The recommended dose is 4 drops instilled in the affected ear(s) twice daily for 7 days.
    For patients requiring use of an otowick: The initial dose can be doubled (to 8 drops), followed by 4 drops instilled into the affected ear twice daily for 7 days.

* Sourced from US FDA drug label information

# 2 Key Patents Information

## Summary

❖ Xtoro® (Finafloxacin) has got five-year NCE market exclusivity protection after it was approved by US FDA on Dec 17, 2014.

❖ Finafloxacin was originally developed by Bayer and then registered by Alcon Research, and its compound patent application was filed as PCT application by Bayer in 1997.

❖ The compound patent will expire in 2017 foremost, which has been granted in the United States, Europe, Japan and China successively.

Table 1    Finafloxacin's Compound Patent Protection in Drug-Mainstream Country

| Country | Publication/Patent NO. | Application Date | Granted Date | Estimated Expiry Date |
|---------|------------------------|------------------|--------------|------------------------|
| WO | WO9826779A1 | 12/04/1997 | / | / |
| US | US6133260A | 12/04/1997 | 10/17/2000 | 12/04/2017 |
| EP | EP946176B1 | 12/04/1997 | 03/27/2002 | 12/04/2017 |
| JP | JP3463939B2 | 12/04/1997 | 11/05/2003 | 12/04/2017 |
| | JP5112395B2 | 12/04/1997 | 01/09/2013 | 12/04/2017 |
| CN | CN100335054C | 12/04/1997 | 09/05/2007 | 12/04/2017 |

Table 2    Originator's International Patent Application List (Patent Family)

| Publication NO. | Title | Applicant/Assignee/Owner | Publication Date |
|-----------------|-------|--------------------------|------------------|
| **Technical Subjects** | **Active Ingredient (Free Base)'s Formula or Structure and Preparation** | | |
| WO9826779A1 | The use of 7-(2-oxa-5,8-diazabicyclo[4.3.0]non-8-yl)-quinolone carboxylic acid and naphthyridon carboxylic acid derivatives for the treatment of helicobacter pylori infections and associated gastroduodenal diseases | Bayer | 06/25/1998 |
| **Technical Subjects** | **Formulation and Preparation** | | |
| WO2014088838A1 | Finafloxacin suspension compositions | Alcon Research | 06/12/2014 |
| **Technical Subjects** | **Indication or Methods for Medical Needs** | | |
| WO2011003091A1 | Compositions comprising finafloxacin and methods for treating ophthalmic, otic, or nasal infections | Alcon Research | 01/06/2011 |

The data was updated until Jan 2016.

# 3   Chemistry

## Route 1:   Original Discovery Route

**Finafloxacin**

**Finafloxacin Hydrochloride**
**99.6% ee**

TBAHS:   Tetrabutylammonium hydrogensulphate

*Synthetic Route*:   Synthesis of the 8-cyanofluoroquinolone core of finafloxacin has been reported on kilogram scale starting from 5-fluoro-1,3-xylene **1**.   Catalytic chlorination through the use of FeCl₃ in DCE was followed by a photochemical chlorination at elevated temperatures to generate the polychlorinated intermediate **3** in 45% yield over two steps.   The trichlorobenzyl derivative **3** was then hydrolyzed with concentrated sulfuric acid to arrive at 3-formylbenzoic acid **4**.   Conversion of the formyl group within **4** to the corresponding nitrile **6** was achieved in a two-step sequence, *via* firstly condensation of the aldehyde **4** with hydroxylamine hydrochloride in the presence of aqueous NaOH and subsequent treatment with refluxing thionyl chloride.  Acid chloride **6** was converted to quinolone **11** through the following four-step sequence which was conducted without isolation of intermediates as: **6** was first coupled with ethyl 3-dimethylamino-acrylate **7** followed by condensation with cyclopropylamine **9** in the presence of acetic acid and this was followed by treatment with potassium carbonate in warm NMP and upon acidification, ethyl ester **11** was furnished in a remarkable 90% yield over the four steps.  Acidic hydrolysis of ester **11** generated acid **12** which underwent coupling with pyrrolo-oxazine **13** in the presence of triethylamine and warm acetonitrile to provide finafloxacin in 90% yield from **11**.  Finafloxacin hydrochloride was then synthesized as the final API in 95% yield with >99% *ee*.[1, 2]

The synthesis of pyrrolo-oxazine fragment **13** was commenced with (*Z*)-butene-1,4-diol **14**.  Mesylation of this diol followed by reaction with tosylamide under phase transfer conditions afforded dihydropyrrole **15**.  Epoxidation of the olefin using *m*-CPBA followed by subjection to ethanolamine affected an epoxide ring opening to give rise to the trans aminoalcohol **18** which was then tosylated and cyclized upon treatment with methanolic sodium hydroxide to give the bis-toluenesulfonamide **20** which at this point was resolved to >99% *ee* by chiral chromatography to arrive at the desired (*S,S*)-enantiomer **21**. Removal of the tosyl protecting groups within **21** through the use of hydrobromic acid in glacial acetic acid preceded the treatment with KOH to finally furnish pyrrolo-oxazine **13**.

[1]  Michael, M.; Uwe, P.; Thomas, J., et al. WO9826779A1, **1998**.
[2]  Michael, M.; Uwe, P.; Thomas, J., et al. US6133260A, **2000**.

## Route 2

*Synthetic Route*:   The synthesis of quinoline ester unit **14** began with commercially available dichlorofluorobenzene **1**.   The dichloro-fluoro-benzoic acid **3** was prepared from **1** by a two-step reaction sequence (Friedel-Craft's acetylation, followed by the oxidation) in moderate yield.   The nitro-group of **4** was introduced smoothly in 90% yield.   The aniline **6** was prepared by reduction of the corresponding nitro-unit in 80% yield.   A mild Sandmayer reaction condition was used to install cyano-moiety in ester **7** in 43% yield.   The ester **7** upon hydrolysis followed by thionyl chloride treatment led to the acyl chloride **9** which upon the reaction with *N,N*-dimethyl ethyl acrylate **10** in the presence of triethyl amine at an elevated temperature (80 °C) led to the acrylate intermediate **11** in 70% yield over two steps.   The addition of the cyclopropyl amine **12** furnished the *β*-ketoacrylate ester **13** at room temperature and it was easily cyclized to the quinolone structure **14** in the presence of $K_2CO_3$ with an overall yield of 89% for two steps.   **14** was then coupled with chiral pyrrolidine *N*-Boc **15** to give the 7-substituted quinolone ester **16** in 76% yield.   Hydrolysis of the ester followed by Boc-deprotection was completed in two steps with good yield to afford the desired final product finafloxacin hydrochloride.[3, 4]

An improved ten-step route to Boc-protected pyrrolo-oxazine fragment **15** has been published by Hong et al., albeit with limited synthetic detail, featuring separation of diastereomers by extraction and crystallization instead of chiral chromatography. As before, this route commenced with conversion of (*Z*)-butene-1,4-diol **18** to epoxide **21** in three steps.   Epoxide opening with (*R*)-1-phenyl-ethanamine **22** generated a mixture of diastereomers; it was found that the minor diastereomer was more soluble than **23** in ethyl acetate.   Amidation of **23** with chloroacetyl chloride **24**, followed by ring closure with *t*-BuOK afforded amide **26** in moderate yield.   The lactam was then reduced using $LiAlH_4$ to oxazine **27** in 60% yield.   A series of three protecting group manipulation steps (hydrogenation, Boc protection, detosylation) then led to Boc-protected pyrrolo-oxazine **15**.   The overall yield involving this route was 4%.[3, 4]

# 4   Pharmacology

## Summary

### Mechanism of Action

❖ Finafloxacin is a broad spectrum fluoroquinolone antibiotic which involves the inhibition of bacterial type II topoisomerase enzymes, DNA gyrase and topoisomerase IV, which are required for bacterial DNA replication, transcription, repairation and recombination.

❖ Finafloxacin was highly selective for bacterial type II topoisomerases, and exhibited superior activity against *E. coli* DNA gyrase ($CL_{50}$ = 25 ng/mL) and topoisomerase IV ($CL_{50}$ = 8 ng/mL).

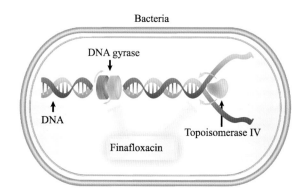

Termination of bacterial DNA replication, transcription, repair and recombination

### *In Vitro* Efficacy

❖ Antibacterial spectrum:
  - MICs at pH 5.8 were shown to be 2-3 folds lower than that at pH 7.3.
  - MICs at pH 5.8:
    ◆ *Staphylococcus*: $MIC_{50}$ = 0.016-4 µg/mL.
    ◆ *Streptococcus*: $MIC_{50}$ = 0.125-0.25 µg/mL.
    ◆ *Enterobacteriaceae*: $MIC_{50}$ = 0.125-8 µg/mL.
    ◆ *Pseudomonas*: $MIC_{50}$ = 0.125-16 µg/mL.
  - MICs at pH 7.3:
    ◆ *Staphylococcus*: $MIC_{50}$ = 0.125-16 µg/mL.
    ◆ *Streptococcus*: $MIC_{50}$ = 0.5 µg/mL.
    ◆ *Enterobacteriaceae*: $MIC_{50}$ = 1-128 µg/mL.
    ◆ *Pseudomonas*: $MIC_{50}$ = 0.5-512 µg/mL.
❖ The bactericidal activity:
  - $G^+$ and $G^-$ bacteria: MBC = 0.03-2 µg/mL (pH 5.8); 1-2 µg/mL (pH 7.2).
  - MBC/MIC = 1-2.
  - The MBC/MIC relationship was not altered at lower pH.

[3]   Hong, J.; Zhang, Z.; Lei, H., et al. *Tetrahedron Lett.* **2009**, *50*, 2525-2528.
[4]   Vasilou, S.; Vicente, M.; Castaner, R. *Drug Future* **2009**, *34*, 451-457.

❖ The activity against drug-resistant mutants:[5]
- *E.coli*:
  - *E.coli* WT: MIC = 0.008-0.06 µg/mL.
  - *E.coli* single mutant: MIC = 0.015-32 µg/mL.
  - *E.coli* double mutations: MIC = 1-16 µg/mL.
- *S. aureus:*
  - *S. aureus* WT: MIC ≤0.03-0.06 µg/mL.
  - *S. aureus* mutations: MIC = 0.06-32 µg/mL.
- *S. pneumoniae:*
  - *S. pneumoniae* WT: MIC = 0.06-0.125 µg/mL.
  - *S. pneumoniae* mutations: MIC = 4-8 µg/mL.
- *S. pyogenes* mutations: MIC = 8-32 µg/mL.
- *P. aeruginosa* mutations: MIC ≤0.125-16 µg/mL.

*In Vivo* Efficacy

❖ Acute otitis externa models:
- *P. aeruginosa* CFU reduction at 0.3% finafloxacin: 4-6 folds (at 24 h) or 0.5-1.5 folds (at 48 h).

❖ Sepsis models:
- *S. aureus*: ED = 10 mg/kg (immunocompetent mouse) or 50 mg/kg (neutropenic mouse).
- *E. coli*: ED = 0.5 mg/kg (immunocompetent mouse) or 1 mg/kg (neutropenic mouse).

❖ Respiratory tract infection: Finafloxacin showed a bacteriostatic effect in mouse or rat model infected by *Streptococcus pneumoniae*, *H. influenza* and *P. aeruginosa.*

❖ Gastrointestinal and intra-abdominal infection:
- Peritonitis model: 100% survival at 25 mg/kg.
- Enteritis model: 83%-100% survival at 0.1-10 mg/kg.
- Cecal ligation model: 100% survival at 10 mg/kg.
- LPS-induced shock model: 83% survival at 10 mg/kg.

❖ Skin and soft tissue infection: Finafloxacin showed similar efficacy as comparator fluoroquinolones in reducing the bacterial load in *S. aureus* and *P. aeruginosa* infection.

❖ Urinary tract infection:
- *E. coli*: >3 $\log_{10}$ reduction in CFU in kidneys at 10 mg/kg.
- *Proteus mirabilis*: >4 $\log_{10}$ reduction in CFU in kidneys at 100 mg/kg.

# Mechanism of Action

Table 3    The Activity of Finafloxacin and Comparator Fluoroquinolones Against Bacterial Type II Topoisomerases[6]

| Test | Drug | DNA Gyrase | | DNA Topoisomerase IV | |
|---|---|---|---|---|---|
| | | CDL (ng/mL) | $CL_{50}$ (ng/mL) | CDL (ng/mL) | $CL_{50}$ (ng/mL) |
| Quantitative plasmid DNA cleavage assay | Finafloxacin | 1 | 25 | 1 | 8 |
| | Clinafloxacin | 1 | 10 | 1 | 52 |
| | Ciprofloxacin | 1 | 120 | 10 | 200 |
| | Moxifloxacin | 1 | 70 | 1 | 200 |
| | Enoxacin | 10 | 50 | 50 | 500 |

CDL: Defined as the lowest concentration of drug yielding detectible cleavage product.    $CL_{50}$: Defined as the concentration that induces 50% maximum cleavage. Inhibition of *E. coli* DNA gyrase or DNA topoisomerase IV activity was measured by quantification of released, linear DNA.

[5]  U.S. Food and Drug Administration (FDA) Database.    http://www.accessdata.fda.gov/drugsatfda_docs/nda/2014/206307Orig1s000MicroR.pdf (accessed Mar 2016).

[6]  MerLion Pharmaceuticals Database.    http://merlionpharma.com/sites/default/files/file/PPS/F1-2046_Muller.pdf (accessed Mar 2016).

## *In Vitro* Efficacy

Table 4    Antibacterial Spectrum of Finafloxacin[5]

| Organism | Species | MIC (µg/mL) | | | | | |
|---|---|---|---|---|---|---|---|
| | | pH 5.8 | | | pH 7.3 | | |
| | | MIC50 | MIC90 | Ranging | MIC50 | MIC90 | Ranging |
| G+ bacteria | *Staphylococcus* | | | | | | |
| | S. aureus | ≤0.03 | 0.06 | ≤0.03-0.06 | 0.125 | 0.125 | 0.06-0.125 |
| | Ciprofloxacin-resistant *S. aureus* | 4 | 8 | 0.125-16 | 16 | 16 | 0.5-32 |
| | Ciprofloxacin-susceptible *S. aureus* | 0.06 | 0.125 | 0.03-0.125 | 0.125 | 0.25 | 0.06-0.5 |
| | *S. aureus* community associate *MRSA* | 0.06 | 1 | 0.03-1 | 0.125 | 2 | 0.125-4 |
| | Ciprofloxacin-resistant *S. epidermidis* | 2 | 6 | 0.5-16 | 8 | 512 | 2-512 |
| | Ciprofloxacin-susceptible *S. epidermidis* | 0.016 | NA | 0.008-0.125 | 0.125 | NA | 0.016-0.25 |
| | Other *coagulase negative staphylococci* | 0.016 | 4 | 0.008-4 | 0.25 | 16 | 0.016-16 |
| | *Streptococcus* | | | | | | |
| | S. pneumoniae | 0.25 | 0.5 | 0.125-0.5 | 0.5 | 2 | 0.25-2 |
| | Beta-hemolytic streptococci | 0.125 | 1 | 0.125-1 | 0.5 | 1 | 0.25-1 |
| | Non-pneumococcal streptococci | NA | NA | NA | 0.5 | 0.5 | 0.25-0.5 |
| | Other | | | | | | |
| | E. faecalis | 8 | 16 | 0.25-16 | 4 | 32 | 0.5-32 |
| | C. amycolatum[a] | 32 | 256 | 0.008-256 | 128 | 512 | 0.03-512 |
| | P. acnes[a] | 0.125 | 4 | 0.06-4 | 0.25 | 4 | 0.125-4 |
| G- bacteria | *Enterobacteriaceae* | | | | | | |
| | Enterobacter cloacae | 0.125 | 0.5 | 0.016-0.5 | 1 | 2 | 0.25-2 |
| | E. coli | 0.25 | 8 | 0.06-8 | 1 | 16 | 0.25-16 |
| | Fluoroquinolone-resistant *E. coli* | 8 | 32 | 2-64 | 128 | 256 | 16->256 |
| | Klebsiella pneumoniae | 0.25 | 1 | 0.008-1 | 1 | 4 | 0.125-4 |
| | P. mirabilis | 0.25 | 8 | 0.25-8 | 1 | 16 | 0.5-16 |
| | Providencia spp. | 1 | 8 | ≤0.03-8 | 8 | 16 | 0.06-16 |
| | Salmonella spp. | 0.5 | 4 | 0.06-4 | 2 | 16 | 0.5-16 |
| | Serratia marcescens | 0.25 | 2 | 0.06-4 | 1 | 8 | 0.125-8 |
| | *Pseudomonas* | | | | | | |
| | P. aeruginosa | NA | NA | NA | 4 | 32 | 1-64 |
| | Ciprofloxacin-resistant *P. aeruginosa* | 16 | 512 | 2-512 | 512 | >512 | 8->512 |
| | Ciprofloxacin-susceptible *P. aeruginosa* | 1 | 4 | 0.25-4 | 4 | 16 | 2-16 |
| | P. otitidis | 0.125 | 0.25 | 0.03-0.25 | 0.5 | 2 | 0.5-2 |
| | Other | | | | | | |
| | M. catarrhalis | NA | NA | NA | 0.008 | 1 | 0.008-1 |
| | H. influenzae | 0.008 | 0.125 | ≤0.004-0.125 | 0.008 | 0.125 | ≤0.004-0.125 |
| | Stenotrophomonas maltophilia | 0.25 | 4 | 0.125-4 | 2 | 8 | 0.5-8 |
| | Acinetobacter spp. | NA | NA | NA | 0.06 | 0.25 | 0.004-8 |

MIC: Minimum inhibitory concentrations.    G+: Gram-positive.    G-: Gram-negative.    MRSA: Methicillin-resistant *S. aureus*.    Antibiotic susceptibilities of finafloxacin were determined by broth microdilution following Clinical Laboratory Standards Institute (CLSI) method.    The antibacterial activity of finafloxacin was enhanced at lower pH (5.8) than normal pH (7.3).    [a] Anaerobes.

[5]  FDA Database.   http://www.accessdata.fda.gov/drugsatfda_docs/nda/2014/206307Orig1s000MicroR.pdf (accessed Mar 2016).

Table 5    Antimicrobial Activities of Finafloxacin and Comparator Drugs Tested against MSSA Strain Pairs Consisting of SCVs and Their Clonally Identical Strains with NP[7]

| Antimicrobial Agent | pH | MIC Range | | MIC$_{50}$ (mg/L) | | MIC$_{90}$ (mg/L) | |
|---|---|---|---|---|---|---|---|
| | | NP | SCV | NP | SCV | NP | SCV |
| Finafloxacin | 7.2 | 0.023-0.38 | 0.064-0.38 | 0.125 | 0.125 | 0.25 | 0.25 |
| | 5.8 | 0.006-0.25 | 0.032-0.19 | 0.064 | 0.064 | 0.125 | 0.094 |
| Clinafloxacin | 7.2 | 0.047-3 | 0.064-3 | 0.25 | 0.38 | 0.5 | 1 |
| | 5.8 | 0.064-6 | 0.19-8 | 0.5 | 0.75 | 1.5 | 2 |
| Levofloxacin | 7.2 | 0.047-0.5 | 0.064-0.75 | 0.19 | 0.19 | 0.38 | 0.38 |
| | 5.8 | 0.064-2 | 0.125-2 | 0.38 | 0.38 | 0.75 | 0.5 |
| Moxifloxacin | 7.2 | 0.012-0.125 | 0.016-0.125 | 0.032 | 0.032 | 0.064 | 0.125 |
| | 5.8 | 0.023-0.38 | 0.047-0.38 | 0.125 | 0.19 | 0.25 | 0.25 |

MSSA: Methicillin-susceptible *S. aureus*.    SCV: Small colony variant.    NP: Normal phenotype.

Table 6    Bactericidal Activity of Finafloxacin[5]

| Strain | pH 5.8 | | | pH 7.2 | | |
|---|---|---|---|---|---|---|
| | MIC (µg/mL) | MBC (µg/mL) | MBC/MIC | MIC (µg/mL) | MBC (µg/mL) | MBC/MIC |
| *Staphylococcus. aureus* ATCC 29213 | 0.06 | 0.125 | 2 | 0.25 | 2 | 1 |
| *Staphylococcus. aureus* NRS 384 | 0.06 | 0.125 | 2 | 0.25 | 2 | 2 |
| *Staphylococcus saprophyticus* ATCC 15305 | 0.06 | 0.06 | 1 | 0.25 | 2 | 2 |
| *Staphylococcus epidermidis* ATCC 12228 | 0.06 | 0.06 | 1 | 0.125 | 2 | 2 |
| *Enterococcus faecalis* ATCC 29212 | 0.25 | 0.5 | 2 | 1 | 2 | 2 |
| *Streptococcus pneumoniae* ATCC 49619 | ND | ND | ND | 0.5 | 2 | 2 |
| *Escherichia coli* ATCC 700928 | 0.016 | 0.03 | 2 | 0.125 | 1 | 1 |
| *Pseudomonas aeruginosa* ATCC 27853 | 1 | 2 | 2 | 8 | 2 | 2 |
| *Enterobacter cloacae* ATCC 13047 | 0.06 | 0.06 | 1 | 0.25 | 1 | 1 |
| *Proteus mirabilis* ATCC 14153 | 0.25 | 0.5 | 2 | 1 | 1 | 2 |
| *Acinetobacter baumannii* ATCC 19606 | 0.06 | 0.125 | 2 | 0.5 | 1 | 2 |
| *Escherichia coli* 2C35_06 (FQ-R) | 0.5 | 0.5 | 1 | 2 | 1 | 1 |

MIC: Minimum inhibitory concentrations.    MBC: Minimal bactericidal concentrations.    FQ-R: Fluoroquinolone resistant.    The MBC was defined as the lowest concentration of drug which killed ≥99.9% equivalent to 3 log$_{10}$ reductions in CFU of the initial inoculum of $5 \times 10^5$ CFU/mL within 24 h.

[5]    FDA Database.    http://www.accessdata.fda.gov/drugsatfda_docs/nda/2014/206307Orig1s000MicroR.pdf (accessed Mar 2016).
[7]    Idelevich, E. A.; Kriegeskorte, A.; Stubbings, W., et al. *J. Antimicrob. Chemother.* **2011**, *66*, 2809-2813.

Table 7    Activity of Finafloxacin and Comparator Fluoroquinolones against Drug-Resistant Mutants[5, 8, 9]

| Strain | Mutant | MIC (µg/mL) in Different pH | | | |
|---|---|---|---|---|---|
| | | Finafloxacin | Ciprofloxacin | Levofoxacin | Moxifloxacin |
| | - | 0.015[a], 0.008[c], 0.06[d] | 0.125[a], 0.06[c], 0.016[d] | 0.25[a], 0.06[c], 0.03[d] | 0.25[a], 0.125[c], 0.06[d] |
| *E. coli* WT | gyrA (S83L) | 0.25[c], 0.5[d] | 2[c], 0.5[d] | 2[c], 0.5[d] | 2[c], 0.5[d] |
| | gyrA (S83L), parC (S80I) | 4[c], 16[d] | 32[c], 4[d] | 16[c], 4[d] | 32[c], 8[d] |
| | gyrA (S83L, D87N), parC (S80R) | 4[c], 16[d] | 32[c], 4[d] | 16[c], 4[d] | 32[c], 8[d] |
| | gyrA (S83L, D87N), parC (S80I) | 8[c], 16[d] | >32[c], 8[d] | 32[c], 8[d] | 32[c], 16[d] |
| | gyrA (S83L, D87Y), parC (S80I) | 4[c], 16[d] | >32[c], 8[d] | 16[c], 8[d] | 32[c], 8[d] |
| | qepA | 0.015[a], 0.06[d] | 2[a], 0.125[d] | 0.5[a], 0.06[d] | 1[a], 0.06[d] |
| | qnrA1 | 0.125[a], 1[d] | 1[a], 0.06[d] | 2[a], 0.125[d] | 2[a], 0.5[d] |
| | qnrB1 | 0.5[a], 2[d] | 2[a], 0.25[d] | 2[a], 0.25[d] | 4[a], 0.5[d] |
| *E. coli* MI | gyrA (S83L) | 0.25[a], 1[d] | 2[a], 0.25[d] | 4[a], 0.5[d] | 4[a], 0.25[d] |
| | qepA | 0.25[a], 1[d] | 64[a], 4[d] | 8[a], 1[d] | 8[a], 1[d] |
| | qnrA1 | 2[a], 4[d] | 16[a], 1[d] | 8[a], 1[d] | 16[a], 2[d] |
| | qnrB1 | 2[a], 8[d] | 8[a], 1[d] | 8[a], 1[d] | 16[a], 2[d] |
| *E. coli* MII | gyrA (S83L) + marR (Δ175bp) | 1[a], 4[d] | 16[a], 1[d] | 16[a], 2[d] | 16[a], 2[d] |
| | qepA | 1[a], 4[d] | ≥256[a], 64[d] | 64[a], 4[d] | 32[a], 8[d] |
| | qnrA1 | 8[a], 32[d] | 128[a], 4[d] | 64[a], 4[d] | 64[a], 8[d] |
| | qnrB1 | 8[a], 32[d] | 32[a], 4[d] | 32[a], 4[d] | 64[a], 4[d] |
| FREC WT-3-M21 | gyrA (S83L, D87G), parC (E84K) | 16[a], 128[d] | >256[a], 128[d] | 256[a], 32[d] | >256[a], 32[d] |
| FREC MII-4T2 | gyrA (S83L), parC (S80I), marR (+) | 2[a], 16[d] | >256[a], 4[d] | 64[a], 8[d] | 128[a], 8[d] |
| FREC MIII | gyrA (S83L, D87G), parC (S80I), marR (+) | 32[a], 256[d] | >256[a], >256[d] | >256[a], 128[d] | >256[a], 128[d] |
| *S. aureus* WT | - | ≤0.03[b], 0.06[d] | 0.25 | 0.125 | 0.06 |
| *S. aureus* WT | gyrA (S84L), grlA(S80Y, E84K) | 16[b], 32[d] | 512 | 128 | 32 |
| *S. aureus* WT | gyrA (S84L), grlA(E84K) | 8[b], 16[d] | 128 | 64 | 32 |
| *S. aureus* BB 27 | gyrA (S84L), grlA(S80F) | 2[b], 4[d] | 128 | 32 | 4 |
| *S. aureus* BB 25 | gyrA (S84L), grlA(E84K) | 4[b], 4[d] | 64 | 32 | 2 |
| *S. aureus* 1758 (ermC cassette) | Efflux (norA disruption) | 0.12 | 0.25 | NA | 0.12 |
| *S. aureus* MT 23142 | Efflux (norA overexpression) | 0.06 | 0.25 | 0.125 | 0.03 |
| *S. pneumoniae* WT | - | 0.06[b], 0.125[d] | 0.5 | 0.25 | 0.06 |
| *S. pneumoniae* WT | gyrA (S81F), grlA/parC (S79Y) | 2[b], 4[d] | 64 | 32 | 16 |
| *S. pneumoniae* 3C172 | gyrA (S81F) | 2[b], 4[d] | 0.25 | 32 | 4 |
| *S. pneumoniae* 4A245 | gyrA (S81F), grlA/parC (S79Y) | 4[b], 4[d] | 64 | 32 | 4 |
| *S. pneumoniae* 4A245 | gyrA (S81Y), grlA/parC (S79F) | 4[b], 4[d] | 128 | 64 | 4 |
| *S. pneumoniae* 85B | gyrA (S81F), grlA/parC (S79Y) | 8[b], 8[d] | 64 | 32 | 2 |
| *S. pyogenes* 30A21 | gyrA (S82F), grlA/parC (D78N) | 8[b], 8[d] | 64 | 32 | 8 |
| *S. pyogenes* 30A21 | gyrA (E85K), grlA/parC (S79V) | 16[b], 32[d] | 128 | 64 | 16 |
| *S. pyogenes* 30A118 | gyrA (E85K), grlA/parC (S79V) | 16[b], 16[d] | 64 | 32 | 16 |

[5]  FDA Database.   http://www.accessdata.fda.gov/drugsatfda_docs/nda/2014/206307Orig1s000MicroR.pdf (accessed Mar 2016).
[8]  Emrich, N. C.; Heisig, A.; Stubbings, W., et al. *J. Antimicrob. Chemother.* **2010**, *65*, 2530-2533.
[9]  Dalhoff, A.; Stubbings, W.; Schubert, S. *Antimicrob. Agents Chemother.* **2011**, *55*, 1814-1818.

*Continued*

| Strain | Mutant | MIC (µg/mL) in Different pH | | | |
|---|---|---|---|---|---|
| | | Finafloxacin | Ciprofloxacin | Levofoxacin | Moxifloxacin |
| *S. pyogenes* 30A118 | gyrA (S81F), grlA/parC (N83Y) | 16[b], 16[d] | 128 | 64 | 16 |
| *S. pyogenes* 7A2 | gyrA (E85K), grlA/parC (S79F) | 8[b], 16[d] | 16 | 16 | 8 |
| *P. aeruginosa* PAO 200 | Efflux (ΔmexAB) | ≤0.125 | ≤0.125 | ≤0.125 | ≤0.125 |
| *P. aeruginosa* PAO 200 | Efflux (ΔmexAB), Plasmid (mexCD overexpression) | 8 | 2 | 4 | 64 |
| *P. aeruginosa* PAO 200 | Efflux (ΔmexAB), Plasmid (mexCD hyperexpression) | 16 | 4 | 8 | 64 |
| *P. aeruginosa* K 1121 | Efflux (ΔmexAB) | 0.5 | ≤0.125 | 1 | 2 |
| *P. aeruginosa* K 1121 | Plasmid (mexAB overexpression) | 4 | 1 | 2 | 8 |

MIC: Minimum inhibitory concentrations.   FREC: Fluorquinolone-resistant *E. coli*.   [a] pH 5.8.   [b] pH 6.   [c] pH 6.2.   [d] pH 7.2.

## *In Vivo* Efficacy

Table 8    Effect of Finafloxacin in the Animal Infection Models[5]

| Study | Bacterial Species | Animal | Dose (mg/kg) | Route | Finding |
|---|---|---|---|---|---|
| Acute otitis externa[a] | *P. aeruginosa* | Guinea pig | 0, 0.03%, 0.3%, 100 µL | Drops, single, 16 h p.i. | 0.3%: 4-6 folds reduction in CFU at 24 h and 0.5-1.5 folds reduction at 48 h. |
| Sepsis model[b] | *S. aureus* DSM 11823 | Mouse (female) | 1, 10, 25 | p.o., single, 30 min p.i. | ED = 10 mg/kg. |
| | | Neutropenic mouse[c] (female) | 6.25, 12.5, 25, 50 | i.v., single, 30 min p.i. | ED = 50 mg/kg. Similar in activity as comparator fluoroquinolones. |
| | *E. coli* DSM 10650 | Mouse (female) | 0.1, 0.5, 1, 10 | p.o., single, 30 min p.i. | ED = 0.5 mg/kg. |
| | | Neutropenic mouse[c] (female) | 0.1, 0.5, 1, 10, 25 | i.v., single, 30 min p.i. | ED = 1 mg/kg. Less effective than comparator fluoroquinolones. |
| Respiratory tract infection (pneumonia model)[d] | *Streptococcus pneumoniae* L3TV | Mouse (female) | 10, 25 | p.o. or i.v., BID | MIC = 2 µg/mL. Bacteriostatic effect was showed either orally or intravenously up to 25 mg/kg. |
| | *H. influenzae* | Rat (female) | 1, 2.5, 5 | p.o., 1h & 4 h p.i. | ≥5 log10 reduction in CFU at 2.5 mg/kg. |
| | *P. aeruginosa* DSM 12055 | Rat (female, acute model) | 1, 10, 25 | i.p., BID | Bacteriostatic effect (<0.5 log10 reduction in CFU) in acute model at 1 and 10 mg/kg. |
| | | Rat (female, chronic model) | 10, 25 | i.p., starting on day 7 p.i. | Weak bacteriostatic effect in chronic model at 25 mg/kg. |
| Gastrointestinal and intra-abdominal infection[e] | *Listeria Monocytogenes* | Mouse (female) | 1, 10, 25 | p.o., 2 h, 18 h & 24 h p.i. | Complete survival (100% survival) at doses of 25 mg/kg in peritonitis model. |
| | *Salmonella typhimurium* | Mouse (female) | 0.1, 0.5, 1, 10 | p.o., 2 h, 18 h & 24 h p.i. | Effective (83%-100% survival) at doses between 0.1-10 mg/kg in enteritis model. |
| | Multi microorganism | Mouse (female) | 10 | p.o. or i.v., 4 h, 18 h & 24 h p.s. | Complete survival (100% survival) after 7 days in cecal ligation model. |
| | LPS fro *S. typhimurium* | Mouse (female) | 10 | i.v., 15 min p.c. | 83% survival in LPS-induced shock model. |

[5]  FDA Database.   http://www.accessdata.fda.gov/drugsatfda_docs/nda/2014/206307Orig1s000MicroR.pdf (accessed Mar 2016).

*Continued*

| Study | Bacterial Species | Animal | Dose (mg/kg) | Route | Finding |
|---|---|---|---|---|---|
| Skin and soft tissue infection[f] | *S. aureus* DSM 18823 | Mouse | 10 | p.o., BID, 2 h p.i. | MIC = 0.125 µg/mL, similar effective as comparator fluoroquinolones in reducing the bacterial load. |
| | | | 2, 10, 50 | s.c., 0.5 h & 4 h p.i. | Greater reduction in CFU at 10 mg/kg and 50 mg/kg in thigh infection model. |
| | *S. aureus* A12 | Mouse | 3.1, 12.5, 50 | p.o., 0.5 h, 4 h, 24 h & 32 h p.i. | Similar effective as comparator fluoroquinolones in reducing the bacterial load at 12.5 mg/kg and 50 mg/kg in granuloma pouch model. |
| | *P. aeruginosa* DSM 12055 | Mouse | 10 | p.o., BID, 2 h p.i. | Marginal effect ($\Delta\log_{10}$ -0.5) was observed at Day 4 post-infection. Similar or better effectiveness compared to other fluoroquinolones in reducing bacterial count at Day 7 post-infection. |
| Urinary tract infection[g] | *E. coli* | Mouse | 1, 10 | p.o., 2 h p.i. | >3 $\log_{10}$ reduction in CFU in kidneys at 10 mg/kg in pyelonephritis model, similar effective as comparator fluoroquinolones. |
| | *Proteus mirabilis* | Mouse | 0.1, 1, 10, 100 | p.o., 2 h, 5 h, 24 h & 32 h p.i. | MIC = 0.5 µg/mL. Greater than 4 $\log_{10}$ reduction in CFU in kidneys at 100 mg/kg in cystitis model. |

[a] Guinea pig ears were infected with approximately $10^7$ CFU of *P. aeruginosa*. [b] CFW-1 mice were infected with long-phase cultures of organisms by intraperitoneal injections. [c] CFW-1 mice were rendered neutropenic by two intraperitoneal injections of cyclophosphamide 4 days (150 mg/kg) and 1 day (100 mg/kg) prior to infection. [d] CFW-1 mice or Wistar rats were inoculated intranasally (mouse) or by intratracheal injection (rat). [e] CFW-1 mice were inoculated with *Listeria Monocytogenes* and LPS from *S. typhimurium* by intraperitoneal injection, while infected with *Salmonella typhimurium* orally. [f] CFW-1 mice were infected with *S. aureus* and *P. aeruginosa* by subcutaneous infections that modeled abscess formation (Gelfoam® model), foreign body infection (with implanted catheter) and tissue infection (granuloma pouch and thigh infection). [g] Pyelonephritis was induced by direct injection of *E. coli* into the right kidney of mice, while *Proteus mirabilis* was injected into bladder to build cystitis model. FU: Colony Forming Units. p.o.: Oral. i.v.: Intravenous injection. i.p.: Intraperitoneal. s.c.: Subcutaneous. BID: Twice daily. p.i.: Post-infection. p.s.: Post surgery. p.c.: Post challenge. ED: Effective dose (protecting 100% infected animals).

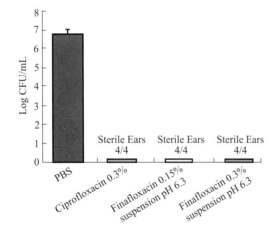

**Study:** Antibacterial activities in acute otitis externa model.

**Animal:** Guinea pig.

**Model:** Guinea pig ears were infected with approximately $10^7$ CFU of the *P. aeruginosa* strains.

**Administration:** Finafloxacin: Drops, 100 µL (0.15% or 0.3%), at 16 h post-infection; Ciprofloxacin: Drops, 100 µL (0.3%), at 16 h post-infection; Vehicle: Saline.

**Test:** Bacterial counts in ears.

**Results:** Concentration of 0.15% or greater at pH 6.3 resulted in complete eradication of *P. aeruginosa* at 24 h post-infection.

Figure A　The Antibacterial Activity of Finafloxacin at pH 6.3 in Experimental AOE Guinea Pig Models[5]

[5] FDA Database. http://www.accessdata.fda.gov/drugsatfda_docs/nda/2014/206307Orig1s000MicroR.pdf (accessed Mar 2016).

# 5 ADME & Drug-Drug Interaction

## Summary

### Absorption of Finafloxacin

❖ Due to insufficient oto topical plasma concentration data, it was not possible to characterize systemic PK parameters or assess the relative bioavailability of finafloxacin by oto topical route.[10]

❖ Had high oral bioavailability in rats (57%) and dogs (73%).

❖ Was absorbed rapidly with the $T_{max}$ occurring at 0.5 to 1 h after oral administrations in rats and humans.

❖ Showed a half-life ranging between 1.28-10.5 h in humans, 2.47 h in rats and 5.7 h in dogs after oral administrations.

### Distribution of Finafloxacin

❖ Exhibited moderate plasma protein binding in humans (82%-84%), rats (44%-55%) and dogs (70%-79%).

❖ Pigmented male Long-Evans rats following repeated oral administrations:
  • The drug was rapidly and well distributed into most tissues except for the central nervous system (CNS) since the blood-brain barrier was crossed by a very small extent.
  • Relatively higher concentration levels were observed in urine > bile > eye uveal tract > kidneys > liver > cartilage > epiphyseal line > small intestine > periosteum > arterial wall > other tissues.[10]
  • The concentration in eye uveal tract was very high at 24 h post-dose.

❖ Guinea Pigs following repeated otic administrations:
  • On Day 1, the concentration levels in tissues in order were tympanic membrane > external ear canal > tympanic bulla wall.
  • On Day 7, the concentration levels in tissues in order were malleus > external ear canal > tympanic membrane > tympanic bulla wall > cochlea.

### Metabolism of Finafloxacin

❖ Finafloxacin was stable in hepatocytes from non-clinical species. No metabolism was detected in human, rat, rabbit or monkey hepatic microsomes.

❖ Overall, the parent drug represented the most abundant component, with AL-91591 ($\beta$-glucuronide ester, conjugated at the carboxylic acid of finafloxacin) as the major metabolite in human plasma. Other two metabolites were detected in human plasma, but not in rat and dog plasma.

❖ CYP1A2, 2D6, 2C19 and 3A4 were the major metabolizing enzymes.

### Excretion of Finafloxacin

❖ Was predominantly excreted in urine in rats after intravenous administration.

### Drug-Drug Interaction

❖ Finafloxacin did not inhibit the human CYP450 isoforms tested (CYP1A2, 2D6, 2C9, 2C19 or 3A4).

## Absorption

Table 9  *In Vivo* Pharmacokinetic Parameters of [$^{14}$C]Finafloxacin in Rats and Dogs after Single Intravenous and Oral Dose of [$^{14}$C]Finafloxacin[10]

| Species | Route | Dose (mg/kg) | $T_{max}$ (h) | $C_{max}$ (μg eq./g) | $AUC_{inf}$ (μg eq. · h/g) | $T_{1/2}$ (h) | F (%) |
|---------|-------|--------------|---------------|----------------------|----------------------------|---------------|-------|
| Long-Evans rat (male) | i.v. | 2 | - | 2.19 | 1.69 | 1.15 | - |
|  | p.o. | 2 | 0.5 | 0.38 ± 0.068 | 0.986 | 2.47 | 57.1 |
| Beagle dog (male) | i.v. | 1 | NA | NA | NA | 7.26 | - |
|  | p.o. | 2 | NA | NA | NA | 5.7 | 73 |

[10] FDA Database. http://www.accessdata.fda.gov/drugsatfda_docs/nda/2014/206307Orig1s000PharmR.pdf (accessed Mar 2016).

Table 10  *In Vivo* Pharmacokinetic Parameters of Finafloxacin in Humans after Single Oral Dose of Finafloxacin[11]

| Species | Route | Dose (mg) | $T_{max}$ (h) | $C_{max}$ (mg/L) | $AUC_{inf}$ (mg·h/L) | $T_{1/2}$ (h) | Cl/F (L/h) | Vz/F (L) |
|---|---|---|---|---|---|---|---|---|
| | p.o. | 25 | 1.00 | 0.24 | 0.42 | 1.28 | 59.0 | 109 |
| | p.o. | 50 | 0.88 | 0.44 ± 0.16 | 1.26 ± 0.48 | 3.8 ± 2.7 | 45.0 ± 17.1 | 220 ± 127 |
| Healthy human | p.o. | 100 | 0.50 | 1.32 ± 0.62 | 2.80 ± 0.72 | 7.2 ± 3.2 | 37.2 ± 7.5 | 389 ± 202 |
| | p.o. | 200 | 0.75 | 1.90 ± 0.73 | 4.08 ± 1.05 | 4.6 ± 1.9 | 51.5 ± 11.7 | 348 ± 194 |
| | p.o. | 400 | .00 | 5.06 ± 2.09 | 14.2 ± 4.44 | 10.0 ± 4.4 | 30.8 ± 10.4 | 487 ± 363 |
| | p.o. | 800 | 0.88 | 11.1 ± 2.96 | 29.2 ± 7.50 | 10.5 ± 2.2 | 29.0 ± 7.7 | 435 ± 130 |

## Distribution

Table 11  *In Vitro* Plasma Protein Binding of Finafloxacin in Several Species[10]

| Species | Conc. (ng/mL) | %Bound |
|---|---|---|
| Rat | 10-1000 | 44.1-55.3 |
| Dog | 10-1000 | 70.4-79 |
| Human | 10-1000 | 82.1-84.3 |

Table 12  *In Vivo* Tissue Distribution of [$^{14}$C]Finafloxacin in Pigmented Male Long-Evans Rats and Guinea Pigs after Repeated Oral and Otic Doses of [$^{14}$C]Finafloxacin[10]

| Pigmented Rat/Male | | | | | | | Guinea Pig Head/Male | | | |
|---|---|---|---|---|---|---|---|---|---|---|
| Oral, [$^{14}$C]Finafloxacin 2 mg/kg for 7 days | | | | | | | Otic, [$^{14}$C]Finafloxacin ~0.2 mg/kg BID for 7 days | | | |
| Tissue | Radioactivity (ng eq./g) | | | | | | Duration | Tissue | Radioactivity (ng eq./g) | |
| | 1 h | 2 h | 4 h | 8 h | 12 h | 24 h | | | 4 h | 24 h |
| Blood | 190 | 183 | 22.7 | BLQ | ND | ND | Day 1 | Tympanic membrane | 730 | 300 |
| Brain | BLQ | BLQ | ND | ND | ND | ND | | External ear canal | 560 | 1280 |
| Eye uveal tract | 2600 | 3870 | 3680 | 4080 | 2430 | 3910 | | Tympanic bulla wall | 235 | 230 |
| Kidneys | 2330 | 2580 | 379 | 110 | 56.1 | ND | | Below LLOQ for other tissues | | |
| Liver | 1280 | 1180 | 136 | 61.2 | 23.8 | ND | Day 7 | Tympanic membrane | 950 | 480 |
| Cartilage | 1150 | 1120 | 1030 | 129 | 75.6 | 71.0 | | External ear canal | 3600 | 1530 |
| Epiphyseal line | 954 | 876 | 308 | 107 | 67.1 | 98.2 | | Tympanic bulla wall | 220 | 140 |
| Small intestine | 458 | 326 | 82.0 | 40.5 | 41.4 | ND | | Malleus | 5400 | BLQ |
| Periosteum | 374 | 369 | 147 | 72.8 | 43.8 | 77.5 | | Cochlea | 57 | BLQ |
| Arterial wall | 292 | 295 | ND | ND | ND | ND | | Below LLOQ for other tissues | | |

BLQ: Below the limit of quantitation.   ND: Not detected.   LLOQ: Lower limit of quantitation was 36.4 ng/g of tissue.

## Metabolism

### Metabolic Stability[10]

❖ Chromatographic profiles of [$^{14}$C]finafloxacin following incubation with rat, rabbit, monkey and human liver microsomes and hepatocytes:
- Incubation of finafloxacin with hepatocytes from humans, rats, rabbits and monkeys observed minor metabolism.
- No clear species differences were apparent.
- No metabolism was detected when finafloxacin was incubated with hepatic microsomes from humans, rats, rabbits or monkeys for up to 60 min.

[10] FDA Database.   http://www.accessdata.fda.gov/drugsatfda_docs/nda/2014/206307Orig1s000PharmR.pdf (accessed Mar 2016).
[11] Patel, H.; Andresen, A.; Vente, A., et al. *Antimicrob. Agents Chemother.* **2011**, *55*, 4386-4393.

Table 13    Metabolites in Humans and Non-clinical Test Species Plasma after Single Oral Dose of Finafloxacin[10]

| Matrix | Species | Route | Dose (mg/kg) | Time (h) | %Amount of Finafloxacin | | | | |
|---|---|---|---|---|---|---|---|---|---|
| | | | | | M0 | M1 | M2 | AL-60317 | AL-91591 |
| | Rat | p.o. | 10 | 1 | √ | - | - | 1215 ng/mL | 150 ng/mL |
| Plasma | Dog | p.o. | 10 | 1 | √ | - | - | 1510 ng/mL | 7.31 ng/mL |
| | Human | p.o. | 200 mg | 1 | 100 | 5.6 | 29 | NA | 66 |

AL-91591: β-glucuronide ester, conjugated at the carboxylic acid of finafloxacin.

Table 14    *In Vitro* Metabolic Phenotype of Finafloxacin[10]

| | Finafloxacin Hydrochloride (1 μM) Incubated in Six Recombinant Human CYP Enzymes for 30 min | | | | | | |
|---|---|---|---|---|---|---|---|
| CYP Enzyme | Control | 1A2 | 2B6 | 2C9 | 2C19 | 2D6 | 3A4 |
| %Metabolism | 0 | 45 | 18 | 4 | 27 | 29 | 23 |

## Excretion

Table 15    Excretion Profiles of [14C]Finafloxacin in Rats after Single Intravenous Dose of [14C]Finafloxacin[10]

| Species | State | Route | Dose (mg/kg) | Time (h) | Bile (% of dose) | Urine (% of dose) | Feces (% of dose) | Cage Rinse[a] (% of dose) | Recovery (% of dose) |
|---|---|---|---|---|---|---|---|---|---|
| Rat (male) | Intact | i.v. | 2 | 0-120 | - | 57.5 | 38.7 | 5.50 | 102 |

[a] Cage rinse was collected from 0-96 h.

## Drug-Drug Interaction

### CYP Enzymes Based DDI[10]

❖ Finafloxacin did not inhibit the human cytochrome P450 isoforms tested (CYP1A2, 2D6, 2C9, 2C19 or 3A4).

# 6    Non-Clinical Toxicology

## Summary

### Topical Otic Dosing Safety (Repeated-Dose)[10]

❖ The safety of the AOE indication supported by two 14-day toxicology studies in NZW rabbits:
  • The first study detected minimal-to-mild local toxicity with finafloxacin hydroxide in phosphate buffer at pH 7.5.   The high-dose (1.0% finafloxacin, ~2.18 mg/animal/day, 3.3 × MRHD) was the NOAEL for systemic toxicity.
  • The second study tested finafloxacin.   The NOAEL was the highest dose tested, 1.2% (~2.78 mg/animal/day, 4 × MRHD).

### Safety of Middle Ear Dosing Safty (Single-Dose and Repeated-Dose)

❖ Middle-ear dosing safety profile was identified by two single-dose middle-ear dosing studies in chinchillas, and two repeated-dose middle-ear dosing studies in guinea pigs.   Toxicity endpoints focused on hearing loss and middle ear necropsy.
  • The first (28-day) study tested finafloxacin hydrochloride.   The NOAEL for hearing loss was the high dose, 1.2% (~1.2 mg/animal/day).   This study did not identify a NOAEL for local toxicity.   The lowest dose (0.6%, ~0.6 mg/animal/day) was associated with minimal hyperplasia of the tympanic membrane, minimal hemorrhage, and increased incidence of pericanular bone fibrosis.
  • The second (30-day) study tested finafloxacin free base in a different formulation (similar to the clinical formulation).   Compared to saline control, the vehicle control was associated with hearing loss (at all frequencies tested) and local toxicity (bulla thickening, periosteal bone proliferation, and thickened tympanic membrane stroma).   Finafloxacin did not exacerbate these toxicities.

### Safety Pharmacology[10]

❖ Safety pharmacology studies were not required to support the AOE indication, but studies were completed to support other routes of exposure, and these studies were submitted to this NDA for completeness.   The results were of concern for the AOE indication.

### Genotoxicity

❖ Finafloxacin was positive for *in vitro* mutagenicity, and for *in vitro* and *in vivo* clastogenicity as well.

---

[10]  FDA Database.   http://www.accessdata.fda.gov/drugsatfda_docs/nda/2014/206307Orig1s000PharmR.pdf (accessed Mar 2016).

Reproductive and Developmental Toxicity[10]

❖ Fertility: No finafloxacin-toxicity was apparent.
  • The rat toxicity studies consistently observed finafloxacin-toxicity in the male reproductive tract.  A 4-week intravenous study identified the NOAEL as 30 mg/kg, based on decreased sperm counts and motility ≥40 mg/kg.  The $C_{max}$ for males at 30 mg/kg was 34900 ng/mL (149000 × MRHD).
  • A stand-alone fertility study in rats was conducted.  The NOAEL for male and female fertility was 100 mg/kg/day.  The male 500 mg/kg group was completely infertile, and exhibited reduced sperm counts, essentially no sperm motility.
❖ In oral-dosing embryo-fetal studies, finafloxacin was clearly teratogenic.
  • In rabbits: No developmental NOAEL was established.  The NOAEL for reproductive toxicity was 3 mg/kg (based on increased preimplantation loss at 9 mg/kg).  NOAEL for maternal general toxicity was 9 mg/kg.
  • In rats: Developmental NOAEL = 30 mg/kg, LOAEL = 100 mg/kg, based on exencephaly.  Reproductive NOAEL = 100 mg/kg, LOAEL = 500 mg/kg, based on increased preimplantation loss.
❖ Pre- and postnatal development studies with finafloxacin had not been conducted.
❖ The concentration of finafloxacin was higher in milk than in dams blood or plasma.

Carcinogenicity[10]

❖ No carcinogenicity testing was performed for finafloxacin, according to the current ICH SIA guidance.
  • Carcinogenicity studies should be performed for any pharmaceutical whose expected clinical use was continuous for at least 6 months.
  • Pharmaceuticals showing poor systemic exposure from topical routes in humans which might not need studies by the oral route to assess the carcinogenic potential to internal organs.

Phototoxicity

❖ Finafloxacin was not phototoxic under the *in vitro* or *in vivo* conditions tested.

## Single-Dose Toxicity

Table 16    Single-Dose Toxicity Studies of Finafloxacin by Transbullar Injection[a][10]

| Species | Dose (%Finafloxacin) | Finding |
|---|---|---|
| Laniger chinchillas | 0.3% (acetate, pH 5.5) | No finafloxacin-related toxicity was observed following a single dose (0.6 mg/kg) administered directly into the middle ear (transbullar). |
| | 0.33% (acetate) 0.33%, 0.66%, 1.1% (phosphate) | Single-dose administration of 500 μL of fluid into the middle ear of chinchillas resulting in hearing loss. Beyond the vehicle-related hearing loss, finafloxacin (1.1%, equivalent to 5.5 mg/animal, and 9.2 mg/kg) was not associated with additional hearing loss. |

[a] Under anesthesia, the skin was prepared (hair plucked, surgical scrub) over both ears; A ~1 cm incision was made into the skin over the upper chamber of the middle ear cavity (bulla), to reach the thin bony covering of the superior chamber of the bulla; A 16 gauge needle was inserted through the bone, into the superior chamber of each bulla, resulting in a ~2 mm diameter hole; After instillation of test article, the tissue and skin were closed with sutures.

## Repeated-Dose Toxicity

Table 17    Repeated-Dose Toxicity Studies of Finafloxacin Hydrochloride by Topical Otic Route (*via* Drop-Tainer)[10]

| Species | Duration (Week) | Dose (%Finafloxacin) | Finding |
|---|---|---|---|
| NZW rabbit | 2 | 0.3% (acetate, pH 5.75) 0.3%, 0.6%, 1.0% (phosphate, pH 7.5) | All finafloxacin doses were well tolerated. 0.3% finafloxacin in acetate buffer (pH 7.5) was not associated with toxicity (no systemic histopathology was performed). The effect associated with finafloxacin in the phosphate buffer (pH 7.5) was minimal-to-mild epithelial nerosis of the ear canal at the 0.3%, 0.6% and 1% finafloxacin groups (phosphate formulations). No NOAEL was identified for the phosphate buffer. |
| | 2 | 0.15%, 0.3%, 0.6%, 1.2% (phosphate) | No apparent treatment-related histopathology in the tympanic membrane or ear canal. No epithelial necrosis of the ear canal. The NOAEL was the high-dose, 1.2% finafloxacin (2.79 mg/animal/day). |

[10] FDA Database.  http://www.accessdata.fda.gov/drugsatfda_docs/nda/2014/206307Orig1s000PharmR.pdf (accessed Mar 2016).

*Continued*

| Species | Duration (Week) | Dose (%Finafloxacin) | Finding |
|---------|-----------------|----------------------|---------|
| Guinea pig | 4 | 0, 0.6%, 1.2% (suspension) | No apparent hearing loss. No NOAEL for local toxicity was observed. The low-dose (0.6 mg/day) was associated with minimal hyperplasia of the tympanic membrane, minimal hemorrhage, and increased incidence of pericanular bone fibrosis. The high dose (1.2 mg/day) was also associated with mild thickening of the tympanic membrane, more severe (mild) tympanic membrane hyperplasia, and more severe (moderate) pericanular bone fibrosis, and increased incidence of pericanular bone proliferation. |
|  | 4 | 0, 0.3%, 0.6%, 1.2% (suspension) | No treatment-related cochlear histology change were reported in the finafloxacin-or vehicle-treated groups. No drug-related hearing loss. No NOEL was identified. Finafloxacin was associated grossly with bulla thickening, which correlated microscopically with increased severity of periosteal bone proliferation. |

Frequency of dosing: Twice daily.

# Genotoxicity

Table 18　Genotoxicity Studies of Finfloxacin Hydrochloride[10]

| Assay | Species/System | Metabolism Activity | Dose | Finding |
|-------|----------------|---------------------|------|---------|
| *In vitro* bacterial reverse mutation assay (Ames) | *S. typhimurium* TA1535, TA1537, TA98, TA100, TA102 *E. coli* WP2PuvrA | ±S9 | 0.01-1 μg/plate | Positive ±S9 in TA102 Negative in any other strains. |
| *In vitro* mammalian cell mutation assay | L5178Y t/k$^{+/-}$ cell | ±S9 | 125-2500 μg/mL | Positive. |
|  | L5178Y t/k$^{+/-}$ cell | ±S9 | 75-200 μg/mL | Positive. |
| *In vitro* mammalian cell chromosome aberration assay | V7 CHL cell | ±S9 | 125-1000 μg/mL | Inconclusive. |
| *In vivo* rodent bone marrow micronucleus assay | NMRI Mouse | + | 500-2000 mg/kg | Positive. |
|  | ICR Mouse | + | 1000-4000 mg/kg | Positive. |

Vehicle: 1 to 10 dilution of DMSO for *in vitro* test, 10% HP$\beta$CD in PBS for *in vivo* test.

# Reproductive and Developmental Toxicity

Table 19　Reproductive and Developmental Toxicology Studies of Finafloxacin Hydrochloride[10]

| Study | Species | Dose (mg/kg) | NOAEL Endpoint | NOAEL Dose (mg/kg) | NOAEL $C_{max}^{a}$ (ng/mL) | NOAEL Exposure Margin[b] |
|-------|---------|--------------|----------|-------------|------------------|----------------------|
| Fertility and early embryonic development | Wistar rat | 0, 20, 100, 500, p.o. | Male fertility | 100 | 34900 | 149145 |
|  |  |  | Female fertility | 100 | 13900 | 59402 |
| Embryo-fetal development | Himalaya rabbit | 0, 1, 3, 9, i.v. | Maternal | 9 | 1870 | 7991 |
|  |  |  | Development | 3 | NA | NA |
|  | Wistar rat | 0, 20, 100, 500, p.o. | Maternal | 100 | 13900 | 59402 |
|  |  |  | Development | 100 | 5089 | 21748 |

Note: Data present here was integrated with rat oral repeated-dose toxicity studies by FDA reviewer, yet which were not fully publicly available. Vehicle: Xanthan (aqueous suspension), pH 7.0 to 7.5 in rats toxicity study, water for injection, pH adjusted to 8.0 to 8.5 in rabbits toxicity study. $^{a}$ Ineterpolated/extrapolated $C_{max}$ levels (based on oral does rat TK data) $^{b}$ Compared to the patient benchmark of 0.234 ng/mL.

[10] FDA Database. http://www.accessdata.fda.gov/drugsatfda_docs/nda/2014/206307Orig1s000PharmR.pdf (accessed Mar 2016).

Table 20   Finafloxacin Concentration in Blood, Plasma and Milk of Lactating Long-Evans Rats after Single
Oral Dose of 2 mg/kg [$^{14}$C]Finfloxacin Hydrochloride at 12 days Postpartum[10]

| Time (h) | Finafloxacin Conc. (ng/g) | | |
|---|---|---|---|
| | **Blood** | **Plasma** | **Milk** |
| 0.5 | 430 ± 86 | 439 ± 86 | 1020 ± 220 |
| 1 | 360 ± 87 | 357 ± 81 | 1220 ± 394 |
| 4 | 64 ± 30 | 66 ± 31 | 378 ± 175 |
| 8 | 6.1 ± 3.3 | 6.8 ± 3.3 | 44 ± 27 |
| 12 | 2.3 ± 1.9 | 3.2 ± 1.7 | 17.3 ± 11.3 |
| 24 | BLQ | BLQ | BLQ |
| 48 | BLQ | BLQ | BLQ |

BLQ: Below the limit of quantitation.

## Special Toxicity

Table 21   Special Toxicology Studies of Finafloxacin[10]

| Study | Finding |
|---|---|
| Testing for sensitizing properties of finafloxacin hydrochloride in female guinea pig | Dermal finafloxacin exposure was not sensitizing under the tested conditions. |
| Local tolerance testing in female New Zealand White rabbits after a single intravenous (0, 5 mg/animal), intraarterial (0, 5 mg/animal) and paravenous (0, 1.25 mg/animal) administrations of finafloxacin versus vehicle (0.01 M trometamol (Tris buffer), 0.75% sodium chloride, pH 8.5) | No treatment-related local effect (no erythema, edema, apparent pain, gross pathology or histopathology change). |
| *In vitro* cytotoxic, phototoxic, and convulsive potentials of gastro-fluoroquinolones analogous compounds | Finaloxacin was not phototoxic in mouse fibrolast Balb/c 3T3 cells after UVA irradiation.<br>2 μM of finafloxacin did not affect the excitatory potential of rat hippocampus *ex vivo*. |
| Photoreactive potential in guinea pig | Single oral doses of 30 or 100 mg/kg finafloxacin followed by UVA irradiation (20 J/cm$^2$) caused transient redness of the back and ears of treated female guinea pigs.<br>These data showed that finafloxacin produced a photoreaction. |
| *In vitro* cytotoxicity of finafloxacin on cartilage cells from dogs and men (1, 3, 10, 30, 100 μg/mL) | Finafloxacin was not chondrotoxic under the tested conditions.<br>Fluoroquinolones, as a class, potentially target juvenile cartilage.<br>This *in vitro* screening study was performed to assess the potential chondrotoxicity of finaloxacin. |
| Comparison of cytotoxicity of finafloxacin in primary hepatocytes of rat | Finafloxacin did not induce AST, ALT or LDH, and released into the media of rat primary hepatocytes exposed *in vitro*.<br>This screening assay was conducted because some fluoroquinolones targeted the liver. |

[10]   FDA Database.   http://www.accessdata.fda.gov/drugsatfda_docs/nda/2014/206307Orig1s000PharmR.pdf (accessed Mar 2016).

# CHAPTER

## 14

## Idelalisib

# Idelalisib

(Zydelig®)

Research code: CAL-101; GS-1101

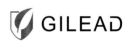 

## 1   General Information

❖ Idelalisib is a small molecule PI3K$\delta$ inhibitor, which was first approved in Jul 2014 by US FDA.

❖ Idelalisib was discovered by IWS Corp., then developed and marketed by Gilead Science.

❖ Idelalisib is an inhibitor of PI3K$\delta$ kinase, which is a downstream signal molecule for multiple receptors involving in B-cell proliferation, mobilization, and in homing to and maintenance of the tumor microenvironment.

❖ Idelalisib is indicated for the treatment of patients with chronic lymphocytic leukemia (CLL) and indolent non-Hodgkin lymphoma (iNHL).

❖ Available as tablet, with each containing 150 mg or 100 mg of idelalisib and the recommended starting dose is 150 mg twice daily.

❖ The 2014 and 2015 worldwide sales of Zydelig® were 23 and 132 million US$, respectively, referring to the financial reports of Gilead.

### Key Approvals around the World*

|  | US (FDA) | EU (EMA) |
| --- | --- | --- |
| First approval date | 07/23/2014 | 09/18/2014 |
| Application or approval No. | NDA 206545; NDA 205858 | EMEA/H/C/003843 |
| Brand name | Zydelig® | Zydelig® |
| Indication | CLL & iNHL | CLL & iNHL |
| Authorisation holder | Gilead Science | Gilead Science |

* Till Mar 2016, it had not been approved by PMDA (Japan) and CFDA (China).

### Active Ingredient

*Molecular formula*: $C_{22}H_{18}FN_7O$
*Molecular weight*: 415.42
*CAS No.*: 870281-82-6 (Idelalisib)
*Chemical name*: 5-Fluoro-3-phenyl-2-[(1$S$)-1-(9$H$-purin-6-ylamino)propyl]quinazolin-4(3$H$)-one

*Parameters of Lipinski's "Rule of 5"*

| MW | $H_D$ | $H_A$ | FRB[a] | PSA[a] | cLogP[a] |
| --- | --- | --- | --- | --- | --- |
| 415.42 | 2 | 8 | 4 | 99.2Å$^2$ | 3.15 ± 0.68 |

[a] Calculated by ACD/Labs software V11.02.

### Drug Product*

*Dosage route*:      Oral
*Strength*:          100 mg/150 mg (Idelalisib)
*Dosage form*:       Film-coated tablet
*Inactive ingredient*:  Microcrystalline cellulose, hydroxypropyl cellulose, croscarmellose sodium, sodium starch glycolate, magnesium stearate, polyethylene glycol, talc, polyvinyl alcohol, titanium dioxide and of FD&C Yellow#6/Sunset Yellow FCF aluminum lake (for the 100 mg tablet) and red iron oxide (for the 150 mg tablet).
*Recommended dose*: The recommended starting dose is 150 mg twice daily.

* Sourced from US FDA drug label information

## 2 Key Patents Information

## Summary

❖ Zydelig® (Idelalisib) has got five-year NCE market exclusivity protection after it was initially approved by US FDA on Jul 23, 2014.

❖ Idelalisib was originally discovered by ICOS Corp., then acquired by Calistoga.    In 2011, Gilead acquired the Calistoga bolsters areas of oncology and inflammation.

❖ Idelalisib's compound patent application was filed as PCT application by ICOS Corp. in 2005.

❖ The compound patent will expire in 2025 foremost, which has been granted in China and the United States successively.

Table 1    Idelalisib's Compound Patent Protection in Drug-Mainstream Country

| Country | Publication/Patent NO. | Application Date | Granted Date | Estimated Expiry Date |
|---------|------------------------|------------------|--------------|-----------------------|
| WO | WO2005113556A1 | 05/12/2005 | / | / |
| US | US7932260B2 | 05/12/2005 | 04/26/2011 | 08/05/2025[a] |
| EP | EP2612862A2 | 05/12/2005 | Examination | / |
| JP | JP2007537291A | 05/12/2005 | Withdraw | / |
| CN | CN101031569B | 05/12/2005 | 06/22/2011 | 05/12/2025 |

[a] The term of this patent is extended by 85 days.

Table 2    Originator's International Patent Application List (Patent Family)

| Publication NO. | Title | Applicant/Assignee/Owner | Publication Date |
|-----------------|-------|--------------------------|------------------|
| **Technical Subjects** | **Active Ingredient (Free Base)'s Formula or Structure and Preparation** | | |
| WO2005113556A1 | Quinazolinones as inhibitors of human phosphatidylinositol 3-kinase delta | ICOS Corp. | 12/01/2005 |
| **Technical Subjects** | **Salt, Crystal, Polymorphic, Solvate (Hydrate), Isomer, Derivative Etc. and Preparation** | | |
| WO0181346A2 | Inhibitors of human phosphatidyl-inositol 3-kinase delta | ICOS Corp. | 11/01/2001 |
| WO2013134288A1 | Polymorphic forms of (S)-2-(1-(9H-purin-6-ylamino)propyl)-5-fluoro-3-phenylquinazolin-4(3H)-one | Gilead | 09/12/2013 |
| WO2015095601A1 | Process methods for phosphatidylinositol 3-kinase inhibitors | Gilead | 06/25/2015 |
| WO2015095605A1 | Polymorphic forms of a hydrochloride salt of (S)-2-(9H-purin-6-ylamino)propyl)-5-fluoro-3-phenylquinazolin-4(3H)-one | Gilead | 06/25/2015 |
| **Technical Subjects** | **Indication or Methods for Medical Needs** | | |
| WO2010057048A1 | Therapies for hematologic malignancies | Calistoga | 05/20/2010 |
| WO2011156759A1 | Methods of treating hematological disorders with quinazolinone compounds in selected patients | Calistoga | 12/15/2011 |
| **Technical Subjects** | **Combination Including at Least Two Active Ingredients** | | |
| WO2012125510A1 | Combination therapies for hematologic malignancies | Gilead | 09/20/2012 |
| WO2015081127A2 | Therapies for treating myeloproliferative disorders | Gilead | 06/04/2015 |
| WO2015109286A1 | Therapies for treating cancers | Gilead | 07/23/2015 |

The data was updated until Jan 2016.

# 3   Chemistry

## Route 1:   Original Discovery Route

*Synthetic Route*:   Commercial 2-fluoro-6-nitrobenzoic acid **1** was treated with oxalyl chloride in the presence of catalytic amount of DMF in DCM to give the corresponding 2-fluoro-6-nitrobenzoyl chloride as a brown syrup, which was subsequently coupled with aniline **2** under Schotten-Baumann conditions to yield 2-fluoro-6-nitro-*N*-phenylbenzamide **3** in 99% yield.   Coupling of **3** with commercial *N*-Boc-2(*S*)-aminobutyric acid **4** in the presence of TEA in DCM generated imide **5** in 66% yield.   Reductive cyclization of nitro imide **5** by means of zinc dust in acetic acid gave the cyclized quinazolinone **6** in 69% yield, which underwent immediate *N*-deprotection with TFA in DCM to furnish the corresponding free amine **7**.   Finally, a substitution reaction involving amine **7** and 6-bromopurine **8** in the presence of DIPEA in *t*-BuOH gave idelalisib as a solid in 50% yield and with 99.6% *ee*.[1-3]

## Route 2

[1]   Fowler, K. W.; Huang, D.; Kesicki, E. A., et al. WO2005113556A1, **2005**.
[2]   Fowler, K. W.; Huang, D.; Kesicki, E. A., et al. US7932260B2, **2011**.
[3]   Li, G.; Liu, X.; Fan, M., et al. CN104130261A, **2014**.

*Synthetic Route*:   Synthesis of idelalisib using ethyl 2(*S*)-hydroxybutyrate ester **1** as starting material was described in the sequence involved nucelophilic substitution of activated hydroxybutyrates with adenine **2**, condensation with 2-amino-6-fluorobenzoic acid **4**, cyclization and finally substitution with aniline **6**.   Treatment of ethyl 2(*S*)-hydroxybutyrate **1** with MsCl in the presence of TEA yielded the corresponding sulfonate ester, which upon nucleophilic substitution reaction with xadenine **2** in the presence of pyridine in hot DMF furnished 2(*S*)-(purin-6-ylamino)butyrates **3** with 82% yield over two steps.

Lewis acid facilitated condensation of esters **3** with 2-amino-6-fluorobenzoic acid **4** gave rise to the corresponding carbox-amide **5** in 92% yield, which went through cyclization in refluxing Ac2O, followed by substitution by aniline **6** in refluxing AcOH to access the titled compound in 73% yield over two steps.[4]

## Route 3

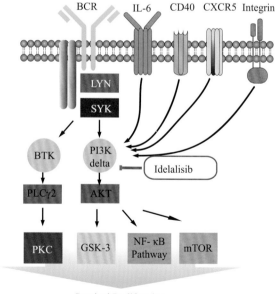

**Idelalisib**

*Synthetic Route*:   A one-pot preparation of (*S*)-*tert*-butyl (1-(5-fluoro-4-oxo-3-phenyl-3,4-dihydroquinazolin-2-yl)propyl) carbamate **4** as a key intermediate of idelalisib relied on firstly condensation between **1** and **2** mediated by P(OPh)3 in hot pyr-idine, secondly treatment of the reaction sphere with aniline **3**.   Boc group was removed using TFA to afford amine **5** in 70% yield over two steps.   Condensation of **5** with 6-chloropurine **6** under standard conditions provided idelalisib in 69% yield.[5, 6]

## 4   Pharmacology

### Summary

Mechanism of Action

❖ Idelalisib is an inhibitor of PI3Kδ, binding to the ATP binding site of the catalytic subunit p110δ.[7]

❖ Idelalisib inhibits PI3Kδ ($IC_{50}$ = 19 nM), which is a downstrean signal molecule for several receptors including B-cell receptor (BCR), CD40 receptors, chemokine receptors CXCR4/5, IL-6 receptor and integrins, which are involved in B-cell prolifera-tion, mobilization, and in homing to and maintenance of the tumor microenvironment.

[4]  Xu, X. CN104262344A, **2015**.
[5]  Dong, Y. CN104876931A, **2015**.
[6]  Bremner, S.; Evarts, J.; Sujino, K., et al. WO2015095601A1, **2015**.
[7]  European Medicines Agency (EMA) Database.   http://www.ema.europa.eu/docs/en_GB/document_library/EPAR-Public_assessment_ report/human/003843/WC500175379.pdf (accessed Mar 2016).

❖ The primary of human metabolite, GS-563117, did not show inhibitory activity at any of PI3K kinases, but exhibited the binding affinities to lymphocyte-oriented kinase (LOK, $IC_{50}$ = 110 nM) and Ste2-like kinase (SLK, $IC_{50}$ = 50 nM), respectively.

❖ Idelalisib had no significant effect on a panel of 61 receptors including GPCRs, ion channels, receptor tyrosine kinases, steroid receptors, and transporters in the radioligand displacement assay at 10 μM.[7]

*In Vitro* Efficacy

❖ PI3Kδ activity in cells:
  • CD63 expression in human basophil cell lines: $EC_{50}$ = 8.9 nM.
  • Anti-proliferation in B-lymphocytes: $EC_{50}$ = 6 nM.

❖ Phosphorylation of PI3K signaling in cells from lymphoma and leukaemia patients:
  • Reduced phosphorylation of $Akt^{S473}$, $Akt^{T308}$ and the downstream target S6 ribosomal protein (S6RP).

❖ Cell cycle and apoptosis:
  • In WSU-FS-CCL and WSU-NHL cell lines: Arrested in $G_1$ phase and $IC_{50}$ = 30 nM.
  • In cells from lymphoma and leukaemia patients: Increased caspase/PARP cleavage/Annexin V positivity.

❖ Inhibition of CLL cells chemotaxis, migration and secretion of chemokines.

❖ Significantly inhibited TNFα-stimulated adhesion of EC/MBSC cells.

*In Vivo* Efficacy

❖ The applicant did not provide.

## Mechanism of Action

Table 3     Inhibition of Idelalisib against PI3Kδ Isoforms[7-9]

| PI3K Isoforms | $K_m$ (μM) | $IC_{50}$ (nM)[a] | Selectivity (fold) |
|---|---|---|---|
| PI3Kδ | 118 | 19 | 1 |
| PI3Kα | 48 | 8600 | 453 |
| PI3Kβ | 279 | 4000 | 211 |
| PI3Kγ | 37 | 2100 | 110 |

Enzymatic activity was measured using a time resolved fluorescence resonance energy transfer (TR-FRET) assay.    [a] At steady-state concentrations of adenosine triphosphate (ATP).

Table 4     Kinase Selectivity of Idelalisib and Its Metabolite in Different Assays[8, 9]

| Compound | Kinase | $IC_{50}$ (nM)[a] | Conc. (μM) | %Inhibition |
|---|---|---|---|---|
| Idelalisib | PIK3CA (PI3Kα)[a] | 8600 | 10 | 17 |
| | PIK3CA (E545K)[a] | NA | 10 | 18 |
| | PIK3CB (PI3Kβ)[a] | 4000 | 10 | 0 |
| | PIK3CD (PI3Kδ)[a] | 19 | 10 | 0.35 |
| | PIK3CG (PI3Kγ)[a] | 2100 | 10 | 2.7 |
| | LOK | NA | 100 | 33 |
| | SLK | NA | 100 | 27 |

[7] EMA Database. http://www.ema.europa.eu/docs/en_GB/document_library/EPAR_-_Public_assessment_report/human/003843/WC500175379.pdf (accessed Mar 2016).
[8] U.S. Food and Drug Administration (FDA) Database. http://www.accessdata.fda.gov/drugsatfda_docs/nda/2014/205858Orig1s000PharmR.pdf (accessed Mar 2016).
[9] Somoza, J. R.; Koditek, D.; Villasenor, A. G., et al. *J. Biol. Chem.* **2015**, *290*, 8439-8446.

*Continued*

| Compound | Kinase | IC$_{50}$ (nM)[a] | Conc. (µM) | %Inhibition |
|---|---|---|---|---|
| GS-563117 | LOK | 110 | 100 | NA |
| | SLK | 50 | 100 | NA |
| | ABL1(H396P)-nonphosphorylated[b] | NA | 10 | 18 (%vehicle control) |
| | LCK[b] | NA | 10 | 27 (%vehicle control) |
| | LIMK2[b] | NA | 10 | 26 (%vehicle control) |
| | MAP3K1[b] | NA | 10 | 4.2 (%vehicle control) |
| | PIK3CD (PI3Kδ)[b] | NA | 10 | 27 (%vehicle control) |
| | QSK[b] | NA | 10 | 20 (%vehicle control) |
| | SIK2[b] | NA | 10 | 34 (%vehicle control) |
| | TNNI3K[b] | NA | 10 | 19 (%vehicle control) |

[a] Six compounds at 10 µM, including IDELA (CAL-101), were screened against panels of 353 kinases. The cutoff for being a positive hit was greater than 35% of the vehicle control, or greater than 65% of the kinase inhibition. Any inhibition below the cutoff for a positive hit was listed as "no hit" in the study report and actual values for % kinase inhibition were not provided. [b] The primary human metabolite of idelalisib, CAL-244 (GS-563117, Lot # 805-DJA-28K) at 10 µM, was screened against a panel of 442 kinases using KINOMEscan[TM] *in vitro* competitive binding assay.

## *In Vitro* Efficacy

Table 5    Inhibition of Efficacy of PI3K Isoforms in Cell Lines[7, 8]

| Study | PI3K Isoform | Cell | Stimulus | Primary Endpoint | EC$_{50}$ (nM)[a] | Selectivity (fold) |
|---|---|---|---|---|---|---|
| Cell-based potency assays[b] | PI3Kδ | Human basophil | Anti-FcεRI | CD63 expression | 8.9 | 1 |
| | PI3Kα | Murine embryonic fibroblsat | PDGF | pAKT | >10000 | >1124 |
| | PI3Kβ | Murine embryonic fibroblsat | LPA | pAKT | 1419 | 159 |
| | PI3Kγ | Human basophil | fMLP | CD63 expression | 2500 | 281 |
| Human whole blood cell assays | PI3Kδ | Human basophil | Anti-FcεRI | NA | 39 | 1 |
| | PI3Kγ | Human basophil | fMLP | NA | 2833 | 70 |
| Human lymphocyte proliferation assay | PI3Kδ | B-lymphocyte | Anti-IgM | Proliferation | 6 | 1 |
| | PI3Kδ/γ | T-lymphocyte | Anti-CD3ε | Proliferation | 973 | 160 |

PDGF: Platelet-derived growth factor.    LPA: Lysophosphatidic acid.    fMLP: Formyl methionyl leucyl phenylalanine.    [a] EC$_{50}$ represented geometric mean values. [b] In the presence of human plasma.

[7]  EMA Database.   http://www.ema.europa.eu/docs/en_GB/document_library/EPAR_-_Public_assessment_report/human/003843/WC500175379.pdf (accessed Mar 2016).
[8]  FDA Database.   http://www.accessdata.fda.gov/drugsatfda_docs/nda/2014/205858Orig1s000PharmR.pdf (accessed Mar 2016).

Table 6 *In Vitro* Pharmacodynamics of Idelalisib in Cells[7, 8, 10]

| Study | Cell | Source | Stimulator | Endpoint | Effect |
|---|---|---|---|---|---|
| Phosphorylation of PI3K signaling | SU-DHL-5/10[a] | DLBCL patient | - | pAkt$^{T308}$/pS6RP | Dose-dependent reduction, EC$_{50}$ = 0.1-1.0 μM. |
| | KARPAS[a] | FL patient | - | pAkt$^{T308}$/pS6RP | Dose-dependent reduction, EC$_{50}$ = 0.1-1.0 μM. |
| | CCRF-SB[a] | B-ALL patient | - | pAkt$^{T308}$/pS6RP | Dose-dependent reduction, EC$_{50}$ = 0.1-1.0 μM. |
| | Primary tumor[b] | CLL patient | CD40 | pAkt$^{S473}$/pAkt$^{T308}$ | p-Akt$^{T308}$: EC$_{50}$ <100 nM. |
| | Primary tumor[b] | MCL patient | BCR | pAkt$^{S473}$/pAkt$^{T308}$ | p-Akt$^{T308}$: EC$_{50}$ <100 nM. |
| | Malignant B-cell[c] | FL patient | - | pAkt$^{S473}$ | 86% inhibition at 0.1 μM. |
| Cell viability | B-ALL | Leukemia patient | - | Proliferation | Percentage of sensitive cell (defined: EC$_{50}$ <1 μM): B-ALL cells: 23% (5/22). |
| | CLL | Leukemia patient | - | Proliferation | Percentage of sensitive cells (defined: EC$_{50}$ <1 μM): CLL cells: 26% (11/42). |
| | AML | Leukemia patient | - | Proliferation | Percentage of sensitive cells (defined: EC$_{50}$ <1 μM): AML cell: 3% (1/31). |
| | MPN | Leukemia patient | - | Proliferation | No sensitive cell (defined: EC$_{50}$ <1 μM). |
| | PBMCs | Healthy volunteer | - | Proliferation | No sensitivity to idelalisib. |
| Cell cycle | WSU-FSCCL | FL patient | - | Cell cycle/proliferation | Arrested in G$_1$ phase, IC$_{50}$ = 30 nM. |
| | WSU-NHL | FL patient | - | Cell cycle/proliferation | Arrested in G$_1$ phase, IC$_{50}$ = 30 nM. |
| Induction of apoptosis | SU-DHL-5 | DLBCL patient | - | Caspase 3/PARP cleavage/ Annexin V positivity | Increased: Caspase, PARP cleavage (2-8 ×), and Annexin V positivity. |
| | WSU-NHL | FL patient | - | Caspase 3/PARP cleavage/ Annexin V positivity | Increased: Caspase, PARP cleavage (2-8 ×), and Annexin V positivity. |
| | CCRF-SB | B-ALL patient | - | Caspase 3/PARP cleavage/ Annexin V positivity | Increased: Caspase, PARP cleavage (2-8 ×), and Annexin V positivity. |
| Migration assay | 9-15C cell | NA | Anti-IgM | Migration | Significantly reduced to 39.1% (± 4.6%). |
| | TSt-4 cell | NA | Anti-IgM | Migration | Significantly reduced from 191.1% (± 50.3%) to 52.3% (± 7.3%). |
| Chemotaxis assay | CLL | NA | Anti-IgM | Migration | Reduced the number of cells migrating toward CXCL12 and CXCL13 at 5 μM. |
| Secretion of chemokine | CLL | NA | BCR with anti-IgM | CCL3 & CCL4 | Significant inhibition of secretion at 1 μM. |
| | | | NLCs | CCL3 & CCL4 | Significant inhibition of secretion at 0.5 μM. |
| Cell adhesion | HUVEC | EC | TNF$\alpha$ | Adhesion | Significantly reduced from 162.8%-95.7%. |
| | HMEC-1 | EC | TNF$\alpha$ | Adhesion | Significantly reduced from 144.3%-99.4%. |
| | 9-15c | BMSC | TNF$\alpha$ | Adhesion | Significantly reduced from 128.9%-94.1%. |
| | CLL-MSC | BMSC | TNF$\alpha$ | Adhesion | Significantly reduced from 143.9%-100.7%. |

Caspase: Cysteinyl aspartate specific proteinase.　PARP: Poly (ADP-ribose) polymerase.　S6RP: S6 ribosomal protein, the downstream target of the PI3Kδ signaling pathway.　DLBCL: Diffuse large B-cell lymphoma.　FL: Follicular lymphoma.　[a] Evaluated by immunoblot and ELISA analyses to measure the levels of p-Akt and pS6RP.　[b] Measured by flow cytometry.　[c] Prepared from biopsy specimens of 7 patients and measured by flow cytometry and anti-IgM/IgG was used for BCR stimulation.

[7] EMA Database. http://www.ema.europa.eu/docs/en_GB/document_library/EPAR_-_Public_assessment_report/human/003843/WC500175379.pdf (accessed Mar 2016).

[8] FDA Database. http://www.accessdata.fda.gov/drugsatfda_docs/nda/2014/205858Orig1s000ClinPharmR.pdf (accessed Mar 2016).

[10] Fiorcari, S.; Brown, W. D.; Maintyre, B. W., et al. *PLoS One* **2013**, *8*, e83830.

# 5 ADME & Drug-Drug Interaction

## Summary

### Absorption of Idelalisib

❖ The increase of $AUC_{inf}$ appeared to be dose-proportional in humans in the dose range of 50 to 200 mg idelalisib after oral administration, but the increase of $C_{max}$ was disproportional.

❖ Had moderate oral bioavailability in rats (39%) and dogs (48%).

❖ Was absorbed rapidly with the $T_{max}$ occurring 1 to 3 h in non-clinical species and humans.

❖ Showed a half-life ranging between 3-3.5 h in healthy humans, longer than that in rats (1.52 h) and dogs (1.99 h), after oral administrations.

❖ Had high clearance in rats (478 mL/min/kg), but low in dogs (0.76 mL/min/kg), in constrast to liver blood flow, after intravenous administrations.

❖ Exhibited an extensive tissue distribution in rats and dogs, with apparent volumes of distribution at 2.49 and 1.23 L/kg, respectively, after intravenous administrations. The apparent volume of distribution was 23 L in humans after oral administration.

❖ Showed a high permeability with $Papp_{(A \to B)}$ of $(4.6-17) \times 10^{-6}$ cm/s in Caco-2 cell monolayer model.

### Distribution of Idelalisib

❖ Exhibited moderate plasma protein binding in humans (83.7%), rats (81.3%), mice (80.2%) and dogs (79.3%).

❖ Had a $C_b:C_p$ ratio of 0.7 in humans, suggesting rare penetration into red blood cells.

❖ SD and Long-Evans rats after single oral administration:
  • The drug was widely distributed into most tissues except for the central nervous system (CNS) since the blood-brain barrier was crossed by a very small extent.
  • Relatively higher concentration levels were observed in small intestine, liver, cecum, stomach, kidneys, adrenals, harderian gland and brown adipose.
  • The lowest concentrations (<500 ng eq./g) of [$^{14}$C]idelalisib in SD rats were observed in the bone, brain, spinal cord and eye lens.
  • At 72 h post-dose, most tissues were BLQ except for kidney medulla, liver, kidney cortex, testis, thyroid, stomach gastric mucosa, lymph node and bone marrow.
  • In LE rats, pigmented skin and pigmented eye uvea showed higher concentrations of idelalisib than those observed for the similar tissues in SD rats, suggesting some associations of drug-derived radioactivity with melanin.

### Metabolism of Idelalisib

❖ Overall, the metabolite (M30A, GS-563117) represented the most abundant component in human plasma, but the parent in rat and dog plasma.

❖ Idelalisib underwent metabolism by aldehyde oxidase (~70%) and CYP3A4 (~30%) to form its major metabolite GS-563117.

❖ The metabolism by aldehyde oxidase accounted for ~43% of the overall metabolism of idelalisib and CYP3A4 accounted for ~19%. Other metabolic pathways included glucuronide conjugation with involvement of UGT1A4.

❖ GS-563117 was inactive against PI3Kδ *in vitro*.[11]

### Excretion of Idelalisib

❖ Was predominantly excreted in feces in humans, with GS-653117 as the significant component in human feces.

❖ A large percentage of radioactivity was eliminated in rat bile (63.5%) and dog bile (71.7%).

### Drug-Drug Interaction

❖ Idelalisib and its metabolite GS-563117 inhibited CYP3A ($IC_{50}$ = 44/>100 and 5.1/16.6 µM), CYP2C8 ($IC_{50}$ = 13 and 39.8 µM) and CYP2C19 ($IC_{50}$ = 76 and 60.4 µM).

❖ Idelalisib was an inducer of CYP2B6, 2C8, 2C9, 3A4, UGT1A1 and UGT1A4 at 10 µM, but had no induction for CYP1A2, 2C19 or aldehyde oxidase. GS-563117 did not induce UGTs or CYP450 enzymes at 10 µM.

❖ Idelalisib and its metabolite GS-563117 were substrates of P-gp and BCRP.

❖ Idelalisib was not a substrate of OATP1B1, OATP1B3, OAT1, OAT3 or OCT2. GS-563117 was not a substrate of OATP1B1 or OATP1B3.

❖ Idelalisib and its metabolite GS-563117 inhibited P-gp ($IC_{50}$ = 8 µM), OATP1B1 ($IC_{50}$ = 10 µM) and OATP1B3 ($IC_{50}$ = 7 µM) *in vitro*.

---

[11] FDA Database. http://www.accessdata.fda.gov/drugsatfda_docs/nda/2014/205858Orig1s000ClinPharmR.pdf (accessed Mar 2016).

# Absorption

Table 7   *In Vivo* Pharmacokinetic Parameters of Idelalisib in Rats and Dogs after Single Intravenous and Oral Dose of Idelalisib[8]

| Species | Route | Dose (mg/kg) | Vehicle | $T_{max}$ (h) | $C_{max}$ (ng/mL) | $AUC_{inf}$ (ng·h/mL) | $T_{1/2}$ (h) | Cl (mL/min/kg) | $V_{ss}$ (L/kg) | F (%) |
|---|---|---|---|---|---|---|---|---|---|---|
| Rat (female) | i.v. | 3 | 10% ethanol/citrix acid buffer solution | 0.08 | 1437 ± 4220 | 1151 ± 407 | 1.89 | 478 ± 19 | 2.49 | - |
| | p.o. | 3 | 0.5% w/v carboxymethylcellu-lose/0.1% v/v Tween 80 | 3.0 | 129 ± 49 | 422 ± 67 | 1.52 | NA | NA | 39 ± 13 |
| Beagle dog (female) | i.v. | 1 | 10% ethanol/citrix acid buffer solution | 0.08 | 977 ± 314 | 1432 ± 509 | 2.31 ± 0.43 | 0.76 ± 0.25 | 1.23 ± 0.3 | - |
| | i.v. followed by p.o. | 1 | Capsule | 0.5 | 510 ± 62 | 1081 ± 284 | 2.31 ± 0.43 | NA | NA | 79 ± 23 |
| | p.o. | 1 | Capsule | 1.0 | 209 ± 68 | 671 ± 277 | 1.99 ± 0.10 | NA | NA | 48 ± 23 |

Mean ± SD, n = 3.

Table 8   *In Vivo* Pharmacokinetic Parameters of Idelalisib in Humans after Single Oral Dose of Idelalisib[11]

| Species | Route | Dose (mg) | $T_{max}$ (h) | $C_{max}$ (ng/mL) | $AUC_{inf}$ (ng·h/mL) | $T_{1/2}$ (h) |
|---|---|---|---|---|---|---|
| Healthy human (male & female) | p.o. | 50 | NA | 598 (29%) | 2301 (36%) | 3.0 (33%) |
| | p.o. | 100 | NA | 1425 (30%) | 4547 (17%) | 3.3 (30%) |
| | p.o. | 200 | NA | 1769 (27%) | 8110 (36%) | 3.5 (43%) |
| Japanese | p.o. | 150 | 1.25 (1.00-2.50)[a] | 2535 (32.4%) | 9828 (26.7%) | 8.42 (5.63-10.64)[a] |
| Caucasian | p.o. | 150 | 2.75 (1.50-3.00)[a] | 1947 (22.6%) | 8325 (37.8%) | 10.0 (5.32-17.4)[a] |

[a] Median (range).   Geometric mean (CV%) for other values.

## Other Findings:[8]

❖ The population estimated apparent central volume of distribution of idelalisib and GS-563117 (M30) were 23 L and 7.5 L, respectively, suggesting idelalisib and GS-563117 were predominantly distributed to plasma.

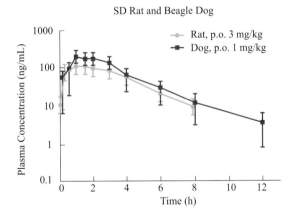

Figure A   *In Vivo* Plasma Concentration-Time Profiles in Plasma of Idelalisib in Female Rats and Dogs (n = 3) after Single Oral Dose of Idelalisib[8]

[8] FDA Database.   http://www.accessdata.fda.gov/drugsatfda_docs/nda/2014/205858Orig1s000PharmR.pdf  (accessed Mar 2016).
[11] FDA Database.   http://www.accessdata.fda.gov/drugsatfda_docs/nda/2014/205858Orig1s000ClinPharmR.pdf  (accessed Mar 2016).

Table 9    *In Vitro* Permeability of Idelalisib in Caco-2 Cell Monolayer Model[12]

| Compound | Conc. (µM) | Papp (1 × 10⁻⁶ cm/s) | Permeability Class |
|---|---|---|---|
| Idelalisib | 1-50 | 4.6-17 | Moderate to high |

## Distribution

Table 10    *In Vitro* Plasma Protein Binding and Blood Partitioning of [$^{14}$C]Idelalisib and Metabolite (GS-563117) in Several Species[8, 11]

| Analyte | Plasma Protein Binding (%) | | | | Blood Partitioning ($C_b$:$C_p$) | |
|---|---|---|---|---|---|---|
| | CD-1 Mouse | SD Rat | Dog | Human | Analyte | Human |
| Idelalisib | 80.2 | 81.3 | 79.3 | 83.7 | Idelalisib | 0.7 |
| GS-563117 | NA | NA | NA | 88.4 | GS-563117 | 0.6 |

$C_b$:$C_p$ = Blood to plasma concentration ratio.    The concentrations of idelalisib were 0.5 and 2 µM in the mice and rats and 0.5-20 µM in the dogs and humans, GS-563117, was assessed in humans at a concentration of 10 µM.

### Key Findings:[8]

❖ SD rats after single oral administration:
- Idelalisib was widely distributed into most tissues except for the central nervous system (CNS) since the blood-brain barrier was crossed by a very small extent.
- The highest concentrations of [$^{14}$C]idelalisib in SD rats at 1 h post-dose were small intestine, liver, cecum, stomach, kidneys, adrenals, harderian gland and brown adipose.
- The lowest concentrations (<500 ng eq./g) of [$^{14}$C]idelalisib in SD rats were observed in the bone, brain, spinal cord and eye lens.
- At 72 h post-dose, most tissues were BLQ except for kidney medulla (2178 ng eq./g), liver (1189 ng eq./g), kidney cortex (766 ng eq./g), testis (451 ng eq./g), thyroid (415 ng eq./g), stomach gastric mucosa (GM) (286 ng eq./g), lymph node (198 ng eq./g) and bone marrow (196 ng eq./g).
- All tissues in SD rats, except large intestine and cecum, had reached maximal concentration at 1 h post-dose (35 of 37 tissues) and decreased at 24-48 h post-dose.
- In SD rats, $T_{max}$ in blood and plasma were observed at 1 h post-dose, then declined in 93% during 4 h and then rose in 29%-39% during 8 h before declining steadily to the 72 h time point.

❖ LE rats after single oral administration:
- In LE rats, pigmented skin and pigmented eye uvea showed higher concentrations of idelalisib than that observed for the similar tissues in SD rats, suggesting some associations of drug-derived radioactivity with melanin.
- Kinetics was similar in LE rats between 8 and 72 h.
- The patterns and tissue concentrations observed in LE rats appeared similar to that observed in the SD rats, except that the pigmented skin of the LE rats showed a tissue concentration of 609 ng eq./g at 72 h post-dose compared to the BLQ for non-pigmented skin in the SD rats at 72 h post-dose; The eye uvea showed a tissue concentration of 594 ng eq./g at 72 h post-dose compared to the BLQ for eye uvea in the SD rats at 72 h post-dose.

[8]    FDA Database.    http://www.accessdata.fda.gov/drugsatfda_docs/nda/2014/205858Orig1s000PharmR.pdf (accessed Mar 2016).
[11]    FDA Database.    http://www.accessdata.fda.gov/drugsatfda_docs/nda/2014/205858Orig1s000ClinPharmR.pdf (accessed Mar 2016).
[12]    Ramanathan, S.; Jin, F.; Sharma, S., et al. *Clin. Pharmacokinet.* **2016**, *55*, 33-45.

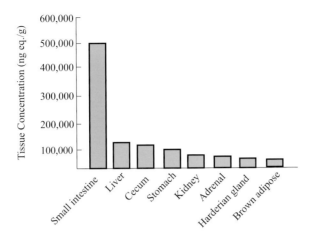

Figure B    Relatively Higher Concentrations of [$^{14}$C]Idelalisib in the Tissues of SD Rats after Single Oral Dose of Idelalisib[8]

## Metabolism

Table 11    Metabolites in Plasma, Urine, Bile and Feces in Humans and Non-clinical Test Species after Single Oral Dose of Idelalisib[8, 11]

| Matrix | Species | Dose (mg/kg) | Time (h) | % of Dose | | | | | | | | | | | | |
|--------|---------|--------------|----------|-----|-----|-----|-----|-----|-----|-----|-----|-----|------|-----|-----|-----|
| | | | | M0 | M1 | M7 | M8 | M10 | M12 | M20 | M21 | M22 | M30A | M31 | M36 | M40 |
| Plasma | Rat | 50 | 0-8 | 91-93 | NA | NA | NA | NA | NA | NA | NA | NA | 1.4 | NA | NA | NA |
| | Dog | 5 | 0-24 | 59 | NA | NA | NA | NA | NA | NA | NA | NA | 34 | NA | NA | NA |
| | Human | 150 mg | 0-168 | NA | NA | NA | NA | NA | NA | NA | NA | NA | 62 | NA | NA | NA |
| Urine | Rat (intact) | 50 | 0-24 | NA | 1.4 | NA | NA | NA | NA | 0.104 | NA | NA | 0.477 | NA | NA | NA |
| | Rat (BDC) | 1.95 | 0-24 | NA | 1.3 | NA | NA | NA | NA | 0.193 | NA | NA | 1.93 | NA | NA | NA |
| | Human | 150 mg | 0-168 | NA | NA | NA | <7a | NA | NA | NA | NA | NA | 49 | NA | NA | NA |
| Bile | Rat (BDC) | 50 | 0-24 | 1.77 | NA | 3.99 | 6.37 | 1.52 | 31.6 | NA | NA | 4.43 | 2.02 | NA | NA | NA |
| | Dog | 5 | 0-24 | 6.23 | NA | NA | NA | NA | NA | NA | NA | 5.35 | NA | NA | NA | NA |
| Feces | Rat (intact) | 50 | 0-48 | 10 | NA | NA | NA | 8.21 | NA | NA | 3.93 | NA | 9.38 | 2.68 | 6.50 | 6.12 |
| | Rat (BDC) | 1.95 | 0-72 | 13.5 | NA | NA | NA | NA | NA | NA | NA | NA | 1.72 | 1.38 | 0.356 | NA |
| | Human | 150 mg | 0-168 | NA | NA | NA | NA | NA | NA | NA | NA | NA | 44 | NA | NA | NA |

M0: Unchanged parent.    M1: Structure not proposed.    M4: Hydroxy-purine.    M7: Desfluoro-idelalisib-glutathione conjugate.    M8: GS-563129/hydroxyl-idelalisib-glucuronide-1/hydroxyl-idelalisib-cysteine glycine conjugate.    M10: Desfluoro-hydroxy-idelalisib-cysteine conjugate.    M12: Desfluoro-oxy-idelalisib-glutathione conjugate.    M20: Unknown structure.    M21: Hydroxyl-idelalisib-3.    M22: Idelalisib-glutathione conjugate/desfluoro-dioxy-idelalisib-glutathione conjugate.    M30: GS-563117.    M31: Idelalisib-C$_5$H$_8$O$_3$-adduct.    M36: Desfluoro-mercapto-methoxy-idelalisib/desfluoro-mercapto-hydroxy-methoxy-idelalisib.    M40: [desfluoro-hydroxy-idelalisib-S-S-desfluorohydroxy-idelalisib]-dimer.    % of radioactivity for humans.    a M8A.

[8]  FDA Database.   http://www.accessdata.fda.gov/drugsatfda_docs/nda/2014/205858Orig1s000PharmR.pdf  (accessed Mar 2016).
[11]  FDA Database.   http://www.accessdata.fda.gov/drugsatfda_docs/nda/2014/205858Orig1s000ClinPharmR.pdf  (accessed Mar 2016).

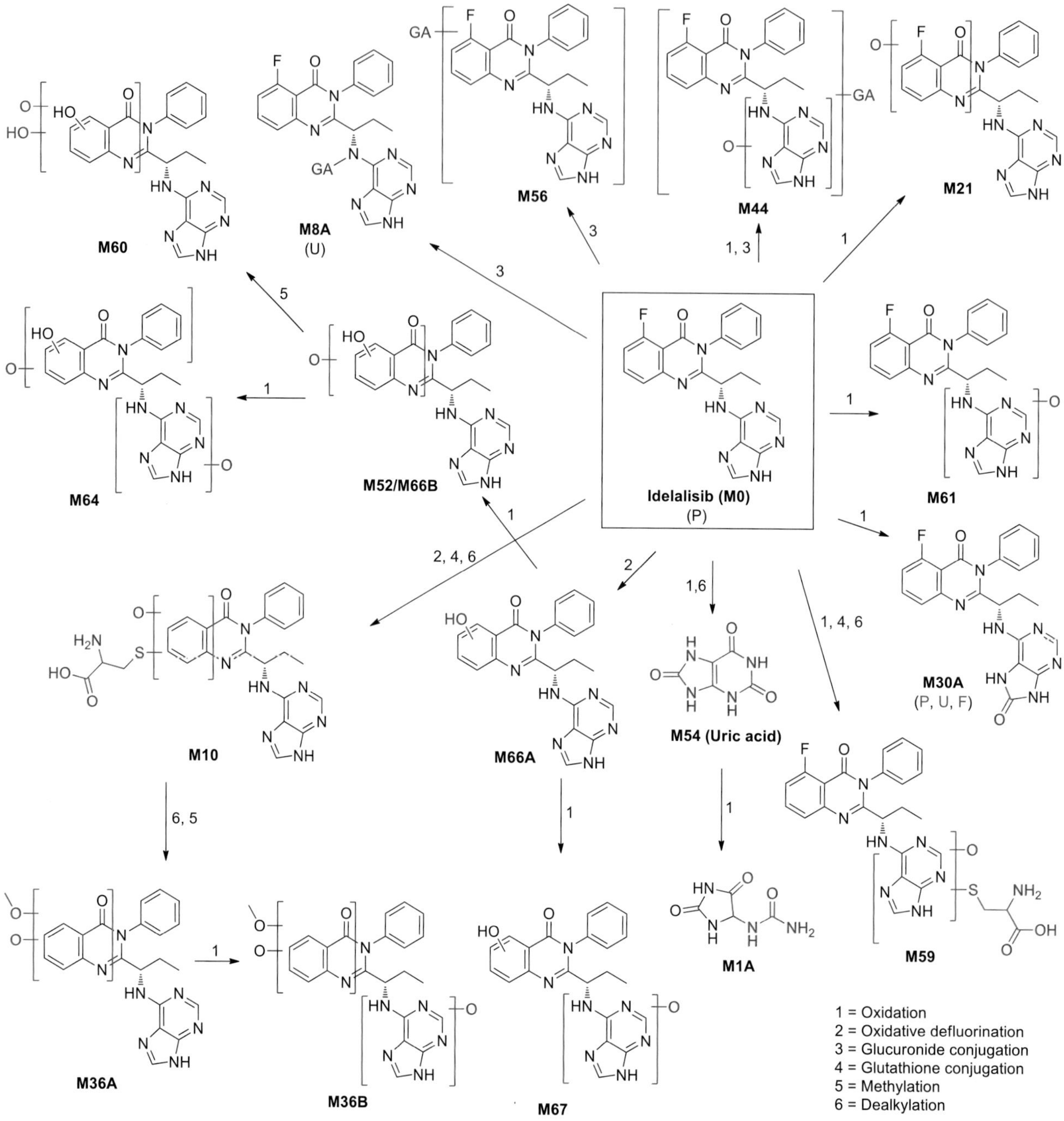

Figure C    Proposed Pathways for *In Vivo* Biotransformation of Idelalisib in Humans after Single Oral Dose of Idelalisib[11]

The red labels represent the major components in matrices.    P = Plasma, U = Urine, F = Feces and GA = Glucuronic acid.

[11]   FDA Database.   http://www.accessdata.fda.gov/drugsatfda_docs/nda/2014/205858Orig1s000ClinPharmR.pdf (accessed Mar 2016).

Figure D   Proposed Pathways for *In Vivo* Biotransformation of Idelalisib in Rats after Single
Oral Dose of Idelalisib[8]

The red labels represent the major components in matrices.   P = Plasma, U = Urine, B = Bile, F = Feces and GA = Glucuronic acid.

[8]  FDA Database.   http://www.accessdata.fda.gov/drugsatfda_docs/nda/2014/205858Orig1s000PharmR.pdf (accessed Mar 2016).

**Key findings:**

Metabolizing enzyme identification:[11]

❖ Idelalisib underwent metabolism by aldehyde oxidase (~70%) and CYP3A4 (~30%) to form its major metabolite GS-563117.   Therefore, the metabolism by aldehyde oxidase accounted for ~43% of the overall metabolism of idelalisib and CYP3A4 accounted for ~19%.

❖ Other metabolic pathways included glucuronide conjugation with involvement of UGT1A4.

## Excretion

Table 12    Excretion Profiles of [$^{14}$C]Idelalisib in Various Species after Single Oral Dose of Idelalisib[8, 11]

| Species | State | Route | Dose (mg/kg) | Time (h) | Bile (% of dose) | Urine (% of dose) | Feces (% of dose) | Recovery (% of dose) |
|---|---|---|---|---|---|---|---|---|
| Rat (male) | Intact | p.o. | 50 | 0-24 | - | 3.04 | 83.9 | 86.9 |
| | BDC | p.o. | 50 | 0-24 | 63.5 | 5.54 | 19.2 | 88.2 |
| Dog (male) | BDC | p.o. | 5 | 0-24 | 71.7 ± 4.9 | 6.04 ± 1 | 20.2 ± 5 | 97.9 |
| Human (male) | Intact | p.o. | 150 mg | NA | - | 14 ± 2.9 | 78 ± 3.9 | 92 |

Vehicle: 0.5% w/v carboxymethylcellulose/0.1% v/v Tween 80 for animals.

## Drug-Drug Interaction

Table 13    *In Vitro* Evaluation of Idelalisib and Metabolite as Inhibitors and Inducers of Enzymes[11]

| | Idelalisib and Metabolite as Inhibitors | | | | Idelalisib and Metabolite as Inducers | | |
|---|---|---|---|---|---|---|---|
| | IC$_{50}$ (µM) | | | | | % of Positive or Fold Induction$^e$ | |
| Enzyme | Control Inhibitor | Idelalisib | Control Inhibitor | GS-563117 | Enzyme | Idelalisib | GS-563117 |
| CYP1A/1A2$^b$ | 37 | >100$^a$ | 0.11 ± 0.02 | >100 | CYP1A2 | 2% | 2% |
| CYP2B6 | 4.3 | >25 | 0.89 ± 0.13 | >100 | CYP2B6 | 46% | 10% |
| CYP2C8 | 2.0 | 13 | 0.91 ± 0.22 | 39.8 ± 4.06 | CYP3A4 | 54% | 5% |
| CYP2C9 | 0.83 | >100$^a$ | 0.45 ± 0.07 | 90.7 ± 9.80 | CYP2C8 | 3.9-fold | 1.4-fold |
| CYP2C19 | 8.1 | 76 | 10.1 ± 2.55 | 60.4 ± 7.69 | CYP2C9 | 3.1-fold | 1.5-fold |
| CYP2D6 | 0.12 | >100$^a$ | 0.05 ± 0.005 | >100 | CYP2C19 | 1.3-fold | 1.0-fold |
| CYP3A$^c$ | 0.89 | 44 | 0.06 ± 0.007 | 5.1 ± 1.0 | UGT1A1 | 2.4-fold | 1.3-fold |
| CYP3A$^d$ | 2.0 | >100$^a$ | 0.23 ± 0.05 | 16.6 ± 2.14 | UGT1A4 | 2.1-fold | 1.2-fold |
| UGT1A1 | - | 42 | - | 22 | Aldehyde oxidase | 1.5-fold | 1.0-fold |

$^a$ The concentration-response curve showed <25% inhibition at 100 µM.    $^b$ CYP1A for idelalisib, CYP1A2 for GS-563117.    $^c$ Midazolam as substrate.    $^d$ Testosterone as substrate.    $^e$ At 10 µM.

[8]  FDA Database.   http://www.accessdata.fda.gov/drugsatfda_docs/nda/2014/205858Orig1s000PharmR.pdf  (accessed Mar 2016).

[11]  FDA Database.   http://www.accessdata.fda.gov/drugsatfda_docs/nda/2014/205858Orig1s000ClinPharmR.pdf  (accessed Mar 2016).

Table 14    *In Vitro* Evaluation of Idelalisib and Metabolite as Substrates, Inhibitors and Inducers of Transporters[11]

| Transport | As Substrates | | As Inhibitors IC$_{50}$ (μM) | | As Inducers | |
|---|---|---|---|---|---|---|
| | Idelalisib | GS-563117 | Idelalisib | GS-563117 | Idelalisib | GS-563117 |
| P-gp | Yes | Yes | 8 | >100 | 1.6-fold | 1.2-fold |
| BCRP | Yes | Yes | >100 | >100 | NA | NA |
| OATP1B1 | No | No | 10 | 26 | NA | NA |
| OATP1B3 | No | No | 7 | 36 | NA | NA |
| OAT1 | No | NA | >10 | >100 | NA | NA |
| OAT3 | No | NA | >10 | >100 | NA | NA |
| OCT2 | No | NA | >10 | 50 | NA | NA |

# 6   Non-Clinical Toxicology

## Summary

### Single-Dose Toxicity

❖ Single-dose toxicity studies in rats and dogs following oral administrations:
  • MTD was not established in rats, while was <25 mg/kg in dogs.

### Repeated-Dose Toxicity

❖ Repeated-dose toxicity study by oral administrations of idelalisib for up to 6 months in rats, and 9 months in dogs:
  • Primary target organ toxicities in rats and/or dogs: Hematopoietic/lymphoid system, liver, male reproductive system, heart (in rats only) and GI tract.

### Safety Pharmacology

❖ Both *in vitro* and *in vivo* safety pharmacology studies to assess the effects of idelalisib on neurological, cardiovascular, and respiratory system:
  • hERG potassium current IC$_{50}$ >50 μM, hardly suggesting QT prolongation.
  • In addition, no clear drug-related effect were observed on neurological, cardiovascular, or respiratory function.
  • However, drug-related cardiomyopathy and increased in the heart weight were observed in the repeated-dose toxicity studies.

### Genotoxicity

❖ Idelalisib did not induce mutation in the bacterial mutagenesis (Ames) assay, and was not clastogenic in the *in vitro* HPBL chromosome aberration assay, however, was genotoxic in males in the *in vivo* rat micronucleus study.

### Reproductive and Developmental Toxicity

❖ Fertility and early embryonic development in rats:
  • For males: No effect was considered on reproductive function or fertility despite decreased testicular and epididymal weights at all doses and sperm concentrations at MD (50 mg/kg/day) and HD (100 mg/kg/day).
  • For females: There was an increase in pre-implantation and post-implantation loss, and early embryolethality, resulting in a 20% decrease in the number of live embryos at HD.
❖ Embryo-fetal development in rats:
  • Idelalisib was maternally toxic based on reduction in net body weight (>10%) at MD (75 mg/kg/day) and HD (150 mg/kg/day), and clinical signs of maternal toxicity, most evident at HD.[8]
  • As a kinase inhibitor, the teratogenic effects of idelalisib were expected and observed in rats at MD and HD.   Adverse embryo-fetal findings at MD and HD included decreased fetal weights, external malformations and skeletal variations. At HD, idelalisib resulted in spontaneous abortion and malformations in live fetuses.[8]
  • Based on teratogenicity findings, an embryo-fetal developmental study on a second species was not needed.[8]

---

[8]  FDA Database.   http://www.accessdata.fda.gov/drugsatfda_docs/nda/2014/205858Orig1s000PharmR.pdf (accessed Mar 2016).
[11]  FDA Database.   http://www.accessdata.fda.gov/drugsatfda_docs/nda/2014/205858Orig1s000ClinPharmR.pdf (accessed Mar 2016).

Carcinogenicity

❖ Carcinogenicity studies with idelalisib had not been conducted and were not necessary for the proposed indications.

Special Toxicology

❖ Impurity qualification study:
  • No additional toxicity related to the impurities.
❖ Phototoxicity:
  • An *in vitro* photo-toxicity study was conducted in the embryonic murine fibroblast Balb/c 3T3 cell line using Neutral Red uptake as a marker of cellular viability in the presence and absence of UVA light exposure.[7]
  • Results for idelalisib were inconclusive, while the primary human metabolite, GS-563117, induced photo-toxicity in the presence of UVA exposure.

## Single-Dose Toxicity

Table 15    Single-Dose Toxicity Studies of Idelalisib after Orally Administrations[7, 8]

| Species | Dose (mg/kg) | MTD (mg/kg) | Finding |
|---------|--------------|-------------|---------|
| SD rat | 300, 900, 1500 | NA | No mortality.    BW loss (≤20%) at MD and HD. Clinical signs: Ruffled haircoat and/or squinted eyes at HD (Day 5). Histopathologic findings (Day 5) in all treated groups: Depletion/necrosis of hematopoietic cells (bone marrow and spleen), lymphocytes (lymphoid organs, thymus, spleen, lymph node, and gut-associated lymphoid tissue), and neutrophilic inflammation (intestine).    Hypertrophic centrilobular hepatocytes in HD males. |
| Beagle dog | 10, 25, 50, 200 | 25 | At dose 200 mg/kg: 2 deaths (female). Clinical signs for the toxicity were observed at 25 and 50 mg/kg including weight loss (>10%), loose black stool containing yellow mucus, emesis and decreased food consumption. Females showed higher $AUC_{last}$ than males at 25 (3.4-fold) and 50 (1.5-fold) mg/kg. |

[7] EMA Database.  http://www.ema.europa.eu/docs/en_GB/document_library/EPAR_-_Public_assessment_report/human/003843/WC500175379.pdf (accessed Mar 2016).
[8] FDA Database.  http://www.accessdata.fda.gov/drugsatfda_docs/nda/2014/205858Orig1s000PharmR.pdf (accessed Mar 2016).

# Repeated-Dose Toxicity

Table 16    Repeated-Dose Toxicity Studies of Idelalisib by Oral (Gavage) Administrations[7, 8]

| Species | Duration (Week) | Dose (mg/kg/day) | Finding |
|---------|-----------------|------------------|---------|
| SD rat | 4 | 0, 50, 100, 150 | No effect on body weights, food consumption, ophthalmologic findings, coagulation parameters or urinalysis results.   No toxicological relevant changes in serum chemistry were observed among animals that survived to the conclusion of the 4-week dosing period.<br>Mortality:<br>Several deaths at 100 (3 deaths) and 150 mg/kg (5 deaths).<br>Clinical signs:<br>>100 mg/kg/day: Excessive salivation leading to wet fur and/or dry, red material on the fur due to porphyrin staining.<br>Histopathology and organ weights:<br>Overall, the microscopic findings among animals that died or were euthanized in moribund condition reflected more severe presentations of similar and milder findings observed among animals from these dose groups that survived to the conclusion of the 4-week dosing period: Increases in serum ALT, AST, ALP and GGT in several of these animals correlated with hepatic necrosis and/or tongue ulceration.   In general, severe bone marrow depletion with marked myeloid hyperplasia and erythroid depletion were also observed in these early deaths.<br>TK:<br>Exposure was greater than dose-proportional, accumulative, and higher in females than males. |
| | 13 | 0, 25, 50, 90 | No idelalisib-related effect on mortality, body weight, food consumption, ophthalmic examination results, haematology, coagulation, or urinalysis parameters in males and females and no clearly idelalisib-related clinical chemistry change.<br>Clinical signs:<br>90 mg/kg: Wet fur and discolored material around the eyes and nose, and an unkempt appearance (2/15F).   Three female rats had inflammatory changes in the skin and mucocutaneous junction, associated with changes in haematological and/or clinical chemistry parameters.   No similar effects were observed in males or after the recovery period.<br>Histopathology and organ weights:<br>Statistically significant increase (14%-15%) in the absolute weights in the heart at 90 mg/kg/day compared to controls.   There was a slight increase in the incidence and severity of cardiomyopathy in the heart in males at 90 mg/kg/day and in females at all dose levels compared to controls.<br>Organs of toxicity: Heart, pancreas, tongue and testes. |
| | 26 | 0, 25, 50, 90 | No idelalisib-related effect on body weights, food consumption, ophthalmic findings, coagulation or urinalysis parameters, or macroscopic observations at necropsy.<br>Mortality:<br>5 mortalities, four of which were likely drug-related but one at the low dose was due to malignant lymphoma, which might be incidental.<br>Histopathology and organ weights:<br>Common microscopic findings in animals found dead were decreased lymphocytes in the spleen, hemorrhage of the thymus, and dilatation of the urinary bladder.   Other microscopic findings in the 90 mg/kg/day males found dead were cardiomyopathy, hypertrophy of the adrenal cortex, inflammation of the pancreas, and alveolar macrophages in the lungs.<br>At all doses, there were increases in WBC (lymphocytes, neutrophils, monocytes, and basophils).<br>Organs of toxicity: hematopoietic system, reproductive organs, kidneys, heart, liver, lungs, and pancreas.   Axonal degeneration in the peripheral nerves and hemorrhage in the brain of one male were also observed at low incidence in males at 90 mg/kg/day.<br>TK:<br>Readily absorbed, accumulated with repeat-dosing, and exposures (AUC and $C_{max}$) were dose dependent with greater than 2-fold higher exposures in females.   The toxicokinetic profile of the metabolite GS-563117 was similar to the parent, despite the fact that the parent compound was not readily converted to its metabolite in rats. |

[7]  EMA Database.   http://www.ema.europa.eu/docs/en_GB/document_library/EPAR_-_Public_assessment_report/human/003843/WC500175379.pdf (accessed Mar 2016).
[8]  FDA Database.   http://www.accessdata.fda.gov/drugsatfda_docs/nda/2014/205858Orig1s000PharmR.pdf (accessed Mar 2016).

*Continued*

| Species | Duration (Week) | Dose (mg/kg/day) | Finding |
|---------|-----------------|-------------------|---------|
| Beagle dog | 4 | 0, 2.5, 5, 20 | No idelalisib-related effect on ophthalmology or electrocardiography observations, coagulation or urinalysis parameters.<br><br>Mortality:<br><br>One death at 20 mg/kg/day on Day 29.<br><br>Clinical signs:<br><br>20 mg/kg: Soft feces and apparent fecal blood.　Decreased food consumption and lowered body weights in females (-8.3%).　Nasal or ocular discharge more frequent.<br><br>Clinical pathology, hematology and histopathology:<br><br>Primary toxicities to the GI, liver and lymphoid tissues.　Evident bone marrow toxicities in hematology findings. |
| | 13 | 0, 2.5, 5, 7.5 | There were no early mortality; No effects on body weights, food consumption, haematology, clinical chemistry, coagulation or urinalysis parameters, or in ophthalmic and electrocardiographic examinations.<br><br>Immunophenotyping was performed, showing inconsistent changes in lymphocyte subsets; These data were considered of limited or no value for characterizing the toxicity of idelalisib.<br><br>Histopathology and organ weights:<br><br>≥2.5 mg/kg: Decreases in lymphocyte numbers in predominantly B cell-dependent areas.　Following recovery, there was generally a hyperplastic response, indicating reversal of the idelalisib-related reduction of lymphoid tissues.<br><br>Dose-dependent decreases in testicular organ weights (5.3%-44.9%), correlating microscopically with reduced spermatogenesis incompletely reversible.<br><br>Non-adverse minimal to mild subacute inflammation in alveolar spaces of the lungs (male). |
| | 39 | 0, 2.5, 5, 7.5 | In animals surviving until the scheduled necropsy, no idelalisib-related effect on food consumption, serum chemistry, coagulation, urinalysis, ophthalmic and electrocardiographic examinations or organ weights.<br><br>Mortality:<br><br>Two unscheduled deaths related to idelalisib, which were attributed to systemic inflammation in multiple organs and decreased lymphocytes in peripheral lymphoid tissues.<br><br>Hematology and histopathology:<br><br>Decreased lymphocytes and inflammation in the immune system, as well as red areas, inflammatory changes, and crypt dilatation in GI tract.<br><br>TK:<br><br>Exposure to idelalisib generally increased with the elevation in dosage level from 2.5-7.5 mg/kg/day. |

Vehicle: 0.5% CMC, 0.1% Tween 80 in rats.

## Safety Pharmacology

Table 17　Safety Pharmacology Studies of Idelalisib[7, 8]

| Study | System | Dose | Vehicle | Finding |
|-------|--------|------|---------|---------|
| Cardiovascular effect | HEK293 cell expressing hERG channel | 0.0977-50 μM | DMSO | Up to 50 μM: No inhibitory effect on hERG channel, $IC_{50}$ >50 μM. |
| | Telemetered beagle dog (male) | Single, p.o. 0, 1, 5, 20 mg/kg/day | Lactose monohydrate | At 5 and 20 mg/kg: ↑ SAP up to 6%, ↑ MAP up to 4% after 60-90 min.<br><br>These changes were small, transient and not considered adverse. |
| Respiratory effect | Telemetered beagle dog (male) | Single, p.o. 0, 1, 5, 20 mg/kg/day | Lactose monohydrate | Unremarkable. |
| Neurological effect | SD Rat (male & female) | Single, i.g. 0, 50, 100, 150 mg/kg | 0.5% (w/v) CMC and 0.1% (v/v) Tween 80 in water | No drug-induced neurobehavioral effect. |

[7] EMA Database.　http://www.ema.europa.eu/docs/en_GB/document_library/EPAR_-_Public_assessment_report/human/003843/WC500175379.pdf (accessed Mar 2016).

[8] FDA Database.　http://www.accessdata.fda.gov/drugsatfda_docs/nda/2014/205858Orig1s000PharmR.pdf (accessed Mar 2016).

# Genotoxicity

Table 18    Genotoxicity Studies of Idelalisib[7, 8]

| Assay | Species/ System | Metabolism | Dose | Finding |
|---|---|---|---|---|
| *In vitro* bacterial reverse mutation assay (Ames) | *S. typhimurium* TA98, TA100, TA1535, TA1537, *E. coli* WP2 *uvr*A | ±S9 | 0-5000 µg/plate | Negative. |
| *In vitro* mammalian cell chromosome aberration assay | HPBL | ±S9 | 32, 64, 128, 256 µg/mL, -S9 64, 128, 256, 500 µg/mL, +S9 | Negative. |
| *In vivo* rodent micronucleus clastogenicity assay | SD rat | + | Single, p.o., 500, 1000, 2000 mg/kg | Positive in HD males, but not females. |

Vehicle *in vitro* was DMSO, and vehicle in vivo was 0.5% CMC and 0.1% Tween 80.

# Reproductive and Developmental Toxicity

Table 19    Reproductive and Developmental Toxicology Studies of Idelalisib by Oral (Gavage) Administration[7, 8]

| Studies | Species | Dose (mg/kg/day) | NOAEL Endpoint | NOAEL Dose (mg/kg/day) | Finding |
|---|---|---|---|---|---|
| Fertility and early embryonic development | SD rat | 0, 25, 50, 100, QD | Male fertility | NA | 2 mortalities at 25 mg/kg/day; 1 mortality at 50 mg/kg/day. Decreased testicular and epididymal weights (at all doses) and sperm concentrations (at MD and HD). No effect on reproductive indices. |
| | | | Female fertility | 100 | One female dosed at 100 mg/kg had a completely resorbed litter. An increase in post-implantation loss and early embryo lethality at 100 mg/kg, resulting in a 20% decrease in the number of live embryos was observed. No test-article related effect on female reproductive function. |
| Embryo-fetal development | SD rat | 0, 25, 75, 150, QD | Maternal | 75 | One test-article related maternal death at 150 mg/kg/day. Clinical signs at 150 mg/kg/day/group: Urogenital blood loss correlated with complete resorptions, increased post-implantation loss, and decreased mean litter size. |
| | | | Fetal development | 25 | At doses ≥75 mg/kg/day, the net reduction in the maternal body weight gain was >10% compared to controls, and the presence of external malformations and skeletal variations in fetuses were observed. $AUC_{0-t}$ for idelalisib increased greater than dose-proportionally and there was accumulation with repeated dosing. |

# Special Toxicology

Table 20    Special Toxicology Studies of Idelalisib[7, 8]

| Study | Species | Dose | Finding |
|---|---|---|---|
| Impurity qualification study | SD rat | 90 mg/kg lower impurity levels 25 and 90 mg/kg higher impurity levels | Targets including organs of the lymphatic system and digestive tract, eyes, heart, organs of the exocrine system (including the kidneys) and testis. No additional toxicity related to the impurities. |
| Phototoxicity | Balb/c 3T3 cell | 0-100 µg/mL | Inconclusive for idelalisib, while positive for the primary human metabolite, GS-563117. |

[7]  EMA Database.   http://www.ema.europa.eu/docs/en_GB/document_library/EPAR_-_Public_assessment_report/human/003843/WC500175379.pdf (accessed Mar 2016).

[8]  FDA Database.   http://www.accessdata.fda.gov/drugsatfda_docs/nda/2014/205858Orig1s000PharmR.pdf (accessed Mar 2016).

# CHAPTER

## 15

# Ipragliflozin L-proline

# Ipragliflozin L-proline

## (Suglat®)

Research code: ASP-1941

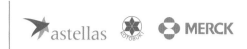

## 1  General Information

❖ Ipragliflozin is a SGLT2 (sodium-glucose cotransporter 2) inhibitor, which was first approved in Jan 2014 by PMDA of Japan.

❖ Ipragliflozin was discovered by Kotobuki and Astellas, co-developed and co-marketed by Kotobuki, Merck & Co. and Astellas.

❖ Ipragliflozin reduces blood glucose levels by inhibiting the reuptake of glucose *via* selectively inhibiting SGLT2.

❖ Ipragliflozin is indicated for the treatment of patients with type 2 diabetes, which is the third approved drug of this class launched after dapagliflozin (Farxiga®/Forxiga®) and canagliflozin (Invokana®/Canaglu®).

❖ Available as oral tablet, with each containing 25 mg or 50 mg of ipragliflozin and the recommended starting dose is 50 mg once daily before or after breakfast.

❖ The 2014 and 2015 worldwide sales of Suglat® were 30.8 and 51.6 million US$, respectively, referring to the financial reports of Astellas.

### Key Approvals around the World[*]

|  | Japan (PMDA) |
| --- | --- |
| First approval date | 01/17/2014 |
| Application or approval No. | 22600AMX00009; 22600AMX00010 |
| Brand name | Suglat® |
| Indication | Type 2 diabetes mellitus |
| Authorisation holder | Astalles/Kotobuki/Merck & Co. |

[*] Till Mar 2016, it had not been approved by FDA (US), EMA (EU) or CFDA (China).

## Active Ingredient

*Molecular formula*: $C_{21}H_{21}FO_5S \cdot C_5H_9NO_2$
*Molecular weight*: 519.58
*CAS No.*: 761423-87-4 (Ipragliflozin)
951382-34-6 (Ipragliflozin L-proline)
*Chemical name*: (1S)-1,5-anhydro-1-C-{3-[(1-benzothiophen-2-yl)methyl]-4-fluorophenyl}-D-glucitol (2S)-pyrrolidine-2-carboxylic acid (1:1)

*Parameters of Lipinski's "Rule of 5"*

| MW[a] | $H_D$ | $H_A$ | FRB[b] | PSA[b] | cLogP[b] |
| --- | --- | --- | --- | --- | --- |
| 404.45 | 4 | 5 | 8 | 118Å² | 1.96 ± 0.59 |

[a] Molecular weight of ipragliflozin.  [b] Calculated by ACD/Labs software V11.02.

## Drug Product

*Dosage route*:      Oral
*Strength*:      25 mg/50 mg (Ipragliflozin)
*Dosage form*:      Film-coated tablet
*Inactive ingredient*:  D-Mannitol, crystalline cellulose, sodium starch glycolate, hydroxypropyl cellulose, magnesium stearate, hypromellose, macrogol, titanium dioxide, talc and yellow ferric oxide/black iron oxide.

*Recommended dose*: The recommended starting dose for adults is 50 mg once daily, taken before or after breakfast. If the effects are insufficient, dosage may be increased up to 100 mg once daily while carefully monitoring the progress of the disease.

[*] Sourced from Japan PMDA drug label information

# 2　Key Patents Information

## Summary

❖ Suglat® (Ipragliflozin L-proline) has got five-year patent term extension after it was approved by PMDA of Japan on Jan 17, 2014.

❖ Ipragliflozin was discovered by Kotobuki and Astellas, co-developed and co-marketed by Kotobuki, Merck & Co. and Astellas, and its compound patent application was filed as PCT application by Astellas and Kotobuki in 2004.

❖ The compound patent will expire in 2024 foremost, which has been granted in the United States, Japan, China and Europe successively.

Table 1　Ipragliflozin's Compound Patent Protection in Drug-Mainstream Country

| Country | Publication/Patent NO. | Application Date | Granted Date | Estimated Expiry Date |
|---|---|---|---|---|
| WO | WO2004080990A1 | 03/12/2004 | / | / |
| US | US7202350B2 | 03/12/2004 | 04/10/2007 | 05/27/2024[a] |
| | US7772407B2 | 03/12/2004 | 08/10/2010 | 05/27/2024[b] |
| | US7977466B2 | 03/12/2004 | 07/12/2011 | 05/27/2024[c] |
| EP | EP1980560B1 | 03/12/2004 | 05/25/2011 | 03/12/2024 |
| JP | JP4222450B2 | 03/12/2004 | 11/28/2008 | 03/12/2029[d] |
| | JP4913104B2 | 03/12/2004 | 01/27/2012 | 03/04/2026[e] |
| CN | CN1802366B | 03/12/2004 | 12/22/2010 | 03/12/2024 |

[a] The term of this patent is extented by 76 days.　[b] The term of this patent is extented by 474 days (TD).　[c] The term of this patent is extented by 327 days (TD).　[d] The term of this patent is extented by 5 years.　[e] The term of this patent is extented by 722 days.

Table 2　Originator's International Patent Application List (Patent Family)

| Publication NO. | Title | Applicant/Assignee/Owner | Publication Date |
|---|---|---|---|
| **Technical Subjects** | **Active Ingredient (Free Base)'s Formula or Structure and Preparation** | | |
| WO2004080990A1 | C-glycoside derivatives and salts thereof | Astellas, Kotobuki | 09/23/2004 |
| **Technical Subjects** | **Salt, Crystal, Polymorphic, Solvate (Hydrate), Isomer, Derivative Etc. and Preparation** | | |
| WO2007114475A1 | Cocrystal of C-glycoside derivative and L-proline | Astellas, Kotobuki | 10/11/2007 |
| WO2008075736A1 | Method for producing C-glycoside derivative and synthetic intermediate thereof | Astellas, Kotobuki | 06/26/2008 |
| WO2015012110A1 | Method for manufacturing C-glycoside derivative | Kotobuki | 01/29/2015 |
| **Technical Subjects** | **Formulation and Preparation** | | |
| WO2011049191A1 | Pharmaceutical composition for oral administration | Astellas, Kotobuki | 04/28/2011 |
| WO2012144592A1 | Solid pharmaceutical composition | Astellas, Kotobuki | 10/26/2012 |
| **Technical Subjects** | **Indication or Methods for Medical Needs** | | |
| WO2009096455A1 | Pharmaceutical composition for treatment of fatty liver diseases | Astellas, Kotobuki | 08/06/2009 |

The data was updated until Jan 2016.

# 3    Chemistry

## Route 1:    Original Discovery Route

*Synthetic Route*:    In this original route, the target ipragliflozin was synthesized from commercial 5-bromo-2-fluorobenzaldehyde **1** through six steps: Condensation of benzaldehyde **1** with the lithiated derivative of 1-benzothiophene **2** gave secondary alcohol **3** in 84% yield, which upon *O*-silylated protection to generate silyl ether **4** in 78% yield.    Successive lithiation of **4** accompany with addition to gluconolactone **5** provided the protected 1-aryl glucitol **6** in 50% yield, and subsequent desilylation yielded the corresponding alcohol **7** in 75% yield, which then underwent deoxygenation by means of triethylsilane and trifluroboron diethyl etherate to provide intermediate **8** in 30% yield.    Thus, ipragliflozin was achieved finally relied on smoothly global debenzylation in 88% yield.    The overall yield hereof was 6%.[1-4]

[1]  Komenoi, K.; Nakamura, A.; Kasai, M., et al. WO2008075736A1, **2008**.
[2]  Komenoi, K.; Nakamura, A.; Kasai, M., et al. US8198464B2, **2012**.
[3]  Imamura, M.; Murakami, T.; Shiraki, R., et al. WO2004080990A1, **2004**.
[4]  Imamura, M.; Murakami, T.; Shiraki, R., et al. US2006122126A1, **2006**.

## Route 2

*Synthetic Route*: In this optimized process, commercial 5-bromo-2-fluorobenzaldehyde **1** was subjected to nucleophilic attack upon subjection to lithiated benzo[*b*]thiophene **2** to afford the diaryl methanol **3** in 85% yield. Quantitative halogenation by means of thionyl chloride was prior to the reduction of the corresponding chloride **4** to give rise to benzothiophene **5** in 81% yield, which was further purified by crystallization from 2-propanol and methanol. Bromide **5** next underwent lithium-halogen exchange then was exposed to 2,3,4,6-*tetrakis-O*-(trimethylsilyl)-*D*-glucono-1,5-lactone **6** in toluene. Without workup, the resulting mixture was subjected to a solution of aqueous HCl in methanol to give a globally desilylated $\alpha$-glucopyranoside **7** that was then subjected to acetylation along with deoxygenation by means of TfOH/TBDMS/MeCN conditions to furnish *tetra-O*-acetyl ipragliflozin **9** in 75% yield over three steps. Polyacetate **9** was then saponified using aqueous sodium hydroxide, and ipragliflozin was crystallized from methanol and water in 97% yield. Subsequent treatment with L-Proline **10** in refluxing ethanol provided ipragliflozin L-proline in 64% yield with the overall yield of 33%.[1, 2, 5, 6]

[1] Komenoi, K.; Nakamura, A.; Kasai, M., et al. WO2008075736A1, **2008**.
[2] Komenoi, K.; Nakamura, A.; Kasai, M., et al. US8198464B2, **2012**.
[5] Imamura, M.; Nakanishi, T.; Shiraki, R., et al. WO2007114475A1, **2007**.
[6] Imamura, M.; Nakanishi, K.; Shiraki, R., et al. US20090143316A1, **2009**.

# 4   Pharmacology

## Summary

Mechanism of Action

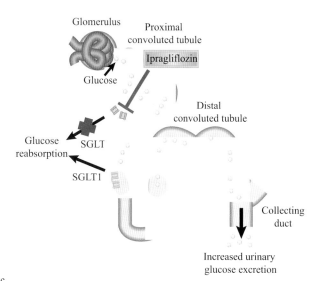

- ❖ Ipragliflozin is an inhibitor of SGLT2, which is the major transporter involved in the reabsorption of glucose in the kidneys.
- ❖ Ipragliflozin selectively inhibited hSGLT2 ($IC_{50}$ = 7.38 nM, selectivity: 254-fold), resulting in decrease of renal glucose reabsorption, and thereby increasing urinary glucose excretion (UGE) and lowering plasma glucose (PG) in patients with type 2 diabetes.
- ❖ Ipragliflozin exhibited no significant affinity and inhibition at 10 μM in a panel of 54 types of transporters, ion channels and enzymes (3 types), except weak affinity for 5-$HT_{2B}$ ($IC_{50}$ = 9.21 μM), serotonin dopamine transporter ($IC_{50}$ = 5.54 μM).[7]

*In Vivo* Efficacy

- ❖ Increased urinary glucose excretion (UGE) and volume of urine:
  - Normal ICR mouse: Increased UGE at 0.3 mg/kg and urine volume at 3 mg/kg, respectively.
  - NA/STZ diabetic mouse: Increased UGE at 0.3 mg/kg and urine volume at 3 mg/kg, respectively.
  - KK-A$^y$ diabetic mouse:
    - ◆ Normal test: Significantly increased UGE at 0.3 mg/kg, but had no effect on the volume of urine.
    - ◆ After 28 days treatment: Significantly increased UGE at 1 mg/kg/day on Day 30.
- ❖ Decreased blood glucose concentration and blood glucose AUC:
  - KK-A$^y$ diabetic mouse:
    - ◆ Normal test: Decreased blood glucose $AUC_{0-8}$ at 0.1 mg/kg.
    - ◆ Glucose loading: Decreased blood glucose $AUC_{0-8}$ at 0.1 mg/kg (single dose) and 1 mg/kg (p.o., QD × 28 days).
  - NA/STZ diabetic mouse: Decreased blood glucose $AUC_{0-12}$ at 0.1 mg/kg.
  - Normal ICR mouse:
    - ◆ Glucose loading: Decreased blood glucose $AUC_{0-6}$ at 0.1 mg/kg.
    - ◆ Fasting: Decreased blood glucose $AUC_{0-6}$ at 10 mg/kg.
  - Wistar diabetic rat: Significantly reduced blood glucose $AUC_{0-8}$, MED = 0.1 mg/kg.
- ❖ Decreased HbA1c level:
  - KK-A$^y$ diabetic mouse: MED = 0.3 mg/kg.
  - *db/db* mouse MED = 0.1 mg/kg.
- ❖ Ipragliflozin improved pancreatic *β* cell protection and insulin secretion:
  - KK-A$^y$ diabetic mouse: Significantly increased pancreatic insulin content at 1 mg/kg/day.
  - *db/db* mouse: Inhibited the decrease in insulin-positive granules in the pancreas at ≥0.1 mg/kg and significantly increased the pancreatic insulin content and plasma insulin levels at 1 mg/kg.

---

[7] Japan Pharmaceuticals and Medical Devices Agency (PMDA) Database.   http://www.pmda.go.jp/drugs/2013/P201300172/index.html (accessed Mar 2016).

# Mechanism of Action

Table 3    *In Vitro* Inhibition and Selectivity of Ipragliflozin and Its Metabolites on Human SGLT2 and SGLT1[7, 8]

| Compound | IC$_{50}$ (nM) | | Selectivity |
| --- | --- | --- | --- |
| | SGLT2 | SGLT1 | |
| Ipragliflozin | 7.38 | 1880 | 254 |
| M1 | 686 | 99500 | 145 |
| M2 | 1870 | >100000 | >53 |
| M3 | 7110 | >100000 | >14 |
| M4 | 3690 | >100000 | >27 |
| M5 | 392 | >100000 | >255 |
| M6 | 399 | 47500 | 119 |
| Dapagliflozin | 1.12 | 1391 | 1242 |
| Phlorizin | 34.6 | 210 | 6 |

Human recombinant SGLT2 and SGLT1 were expressed in CHO cell line and enzyme activities were determined by measuring [$^{14}$C]methyl-$\alpha$-D-glucopyranoside ([$^{14}$C]AMG) transportation efficacy.

# *In Vivo* Efficacy

Table 4    *In Vivo* Effects of Ipragliflozin in Non-Clinical Pharmacology Studies[7-10]

| Study | Model | | Dose$^a$ (mg/kg, p.o.) | Duration (Day) | Effect | |
| --- | --- | --- | --- | --- | --- | --- |
| | Animal | System | | | MED (mg/kg) | Finding |
| Urinary glucose excretion | Normal ICR mouse | Normal | 0.01, 0.3, 0.1, 0.3, 1, 3, 10 | Single dose | 0.3 | Increased urinary glucose excretion at ≥0.3 mg/kg. Increased the volume of urine at ≥3 mg/kg. |
| | NA/STZ mouse | Type II diabetes | 0.01, 0.3, 0.1, 0.3, 1, 3, 10 | Single dose | 0.3 | Increased urinary glucose excretion at ≥0.3 mg/kg. Increased the amount of urine at ≥3 mg/kg. |
| | KK-A$^y$ mouse | Type II diabetes | 0.01, 0.3, 0.1, 0.3, 1, 3, 10 | Single dose | 0.3 | Increased urinary glucose excretion at ≥0.3 mg/kg. No effect on the volume of urine. |
| | | Day 30 | 0.3, 1$^b$ | QD × 28 | 1 | Significantly promoted urinary glucose excretion at 1 mg/kg. |
| Blood glucose | KK-A$^y$ mouse | Type II diabetes | 0.1, 0.3, 1 | Single dose | 0.1 | Dose-dependently decreased blood glucose levels and significantly decreased blood glucose AUC$_{0-8}$ at 0.1 mg/kg. |
| | | Glucose loading | 0.1, 0.3, 1 | Single dose | 0.1 | Dose-dependently decreased blood glucose concentration. Significantly decreased blood glucose AUC at ≥0.1 mg/kg. |
| | | Glucose loading on Day 30 | 0.3, 1$^b$ | QD × 28 | 1 | Significantly promoted blood glucose reduction at 1mg/kg. |
| | NA/STZ rat | Type II diabetes | 0.1, 0.3, 1 | Single dose | 0.1 | Dose-dependently decreased blood glucose concentration. Significantly decreased blood glucose AUC$_{0-8}$ at ≥0.1 mg/kg. |
| | NA/STZ mouse | Glucose loading | 0.1, 0.3, 1 | Single dose | 0.1 | Dose-dependently decreased blood glucose concentration. Significantly decreased blood glucose AUC at ≥0.1 mg/kg. |

[7]  PMDA Database.   http://www.pmda.go.jp/drugs/2013/P201300172/index.html (accessed Mar 2016).
[8]  Kurosaki, E.; Ogasawara, H. *Pharmacol. Ther.* **2013**, *139*, 51-59.
[9]  Tahara, A.; Kurosaki, E.; Yokono, M., et al. *Naunyn-Schmiedeberg's Arch. Pharmacol.* **2012**, *385*, 423-436.
[10]  Tahara, A.; Kurosaki, E.; Yokono, M., et al. *Eur. J. Pharmacol.* **2013**, *715*, 246-255.

*Continued*

| Study | Model | | Dose[a] (mg/kg, p.o.) | Duration (Day) | Effect | |
|---|---|---|---|---|---|---|
| | Animal | System/Condition | | | MED (mg/kg) | Finding |
| Blood glucose | ICR mouse | Glucose loading | 0.03, 0.1, 0.3, 1, 3, 10, 30, 100 | Single dose | 0.1 | Dose-dependently decreased blood glucose level. Significantly decreased blood glucose $AUC_{0-6}$ at ≥0.1 mg/kg. |
| | | Fasting | 0.03, 0.1, 0.3, 1, 3, 10, 30, 100 | Single dose | 10 | Dose-dependently decreased blood glucose level. Significantly decreased blood glucose $AUC_{0-6}$ at ≥10 mg/kg. |
| | | Glucose loading | 0.1, 0.3, 1 | Single dose | 0.1 | Dose-dependently decreased blood glucose concentration. Significantly decreased blood glucose $AUC_{0-12}$ at ≥0.1 mg/kg. |
| | STZ Wistar rat | Type I diabetic | 0.1, 0.3. 1 | Single dose | 0.1 | Significantly decreased blood glucose $AUC_{0-8}$ reduced at ≥0.1 mg/kg. |
| HbA1c level | KK-A[y] mouse | On Day 30 | 0.3, 1[b] | QD × 28 | 0.3 | Significantly reduced HbA1c at 0.3 mg/kg/day. |
| | | Type II diabetes | 0.03-3 | QD × 21 | 0.3 | Significantly reduced HbA1c value at ≥0.3 mg/kg. |
| | db/db mouse | Type II diabetes | 0.1, 0.3, 1 | QD × 28 | 0.1 | Reduced the HbA1c value at ≥0.1 mg/kg. |
| Pancreatic β cell protection and insulin secretion | KK-A[y] mouse | After treatment | 0.03-3 | QD × 21 | 1 | Significant increased pancreatic insulin content after 3 weeks administration at 1 mg/kg/day. |
| | db/db mouse | Type II diabetes | 0.1, 0.3, 1 | QD × 28 | 0.1 | Inhibited the decrease in insulin-positive granules in the pancreas at ≥0.1 mg/kg. Significantly increased the pancreatic insulin content and plasma insulin level at 1mg/kg. |
| Body weight effect | Normal SD rat | High-fat diet | 1-10 | QD × 30 | 10 | Decreased body weight gain and epididymal fat weight at 10 mg/kg. |

NA/STZ mice: Nicotinamide/Streptozotocin-induced diabetic mice.　MED: Minimum effective dose.　[a] Ipragliflozin L-proline.　[b] Ipragliflozin (free state).

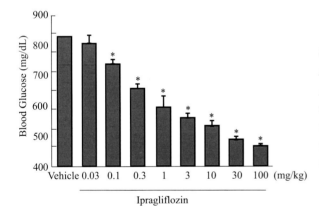

**Study:** Effects of ipragliflozin on blood glucose levels.

**Animal:** Male ICR mouse.

**Administration:** p.o., single dose, ipragliflozin: 0.03, 0.1, 0.3, 1, 3, 10 or 100 mg/kg; Vehicle: 0.5% MC.

**Test:** Blood glucose levels were investigated at 0-6 h after dosing.

**Result:** Ipragliflozin dose-dependently reduced blood glucose, with significance at 0.1-100 mg/kg.　*$P$ <0.05 vs. vehicle group.

Figure A　Effects of Ipragliflozin on Blood Glucose in ICR Mouse[7]

[7] PMDA Database. http://www.pmda.go.jp/drugs/2013/P201300172/index.html (accessed Mar 2016).

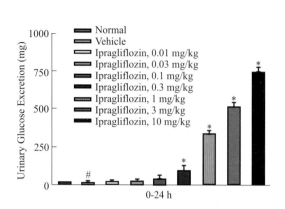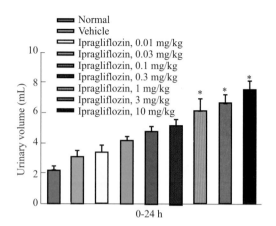

Figure B    Effects of Ipragliflozin on Urinary Glucose Excretion and Urine Volume in NA/STZ Type 2 Diabetic Mouse[10]

**Study:** Effect of ipragliflozin on urinary glucose in diabetic mouse.

**Animal:** Male ICR mouse.

**Modeling:** High-fat diet and streptozotocin-nicotinamide-induced (NA/STZ-induced).

**Administration:** p.o., single dose, ipragliflozin: 0.01, 0.03, 0.1, 0.3, 1, 3 or 10 mg/kg; Vehicle: NA.

**Test:** Spontaneously voided urine was collected for 24 h while the animals were kept in metabolic cages.    After urine volume had been measured, the glucose concentration in the urine was measured using the Glucose CII test reagent (Wako Pure Chemical Industries, Ltd., Osaka, Japan).

**Result:** Ipragliflozin dose-dependently increased urinary glucose excretion and this effect was significant at ≥0.3 mg/kg, and even at 12 h after administration at ≥1 mg/kg.    Also significantly increased urine volume.    $^{\#} P < 0.05$ vs. normal group, $^{*} P < 0.05$ vs. vehicle group.

# 4    ADME & Drug-Drug Interaction

## Summary

### Absorption of Ipragliflozin

❖ Had high oral bioavailability in rats (78.2%-90.7%), monkeys (74.5%-75.3%) and humans (90.2%).

❖ Was absorbed rapidly ($T_{max} = 0.5$-1 h) in rats, moderately in monkeys (1.75-2 h), but rapidly to moderately in humans (0.75-2.60 h).

❖ Showed a half-life of 16.8 h in humans, much longer than those in rats (3.85 h) and monkeys (9.45 h), after intravenous administrations.

❖ Had low clearance in humans (10.9 L/h), rats (0.433 L/h/kg) and monkeys (0.252 L/h/kg), in contrast to liver blood flow, after intravenous administrations.

❖ Exhibited an extensive tissue distribution in rats, monkeys and humans, with apparent volumes of distribution at 1.68, 2.32 L/kg and 127 L, respectively, after intravenous administrations.

### Distribution of Ipragliflozin

❖ Exhibited high plasma protein binding in humans and in all nonclinical species (92%-97%).

❖ Had a blood cell partition ratio range between 16.9%-19.1% in humans, suggesting low penetration into red blood cells.

❖ Albino rats and pigmented rats after oral administration:

  • The drug was rapidly and well distributed into most tissues except for the central nervous system (CNS), with trace or no radioactivity in the brain.

  • Relatively higher concentration levels were observed in kidneys, liver, adrenal gland and stomach.

  • Radioactivity concentrations decreased below the lower limit of quantification in all tissues at 24 h post-dose.

### Metabolism of Ipragliflozin

❖ Ipragliflozin underwent low oxidative metabolism by numerous human cytochrome P450 enzymes.

❖ Overall, the parent drug represented the most abundant component, with the glucuronide conjugate of ipragliflozin (M2) as the major metabolite in human plasma.

[10]    Tahara, A.; Kurosaki, E.; Yokono, M., et al. *Eur. J. Pharmacol.* **2013**, *715*, 246-255.

❖ M2 and M4 were the major human metabolites formed in the kidneys and the liver.
❖ Ipragliflozin was metabolized by multiple UGT enzymes and primary metabolic enzyme was UGT2B7, with UGT2B4, 1A8 and 1A9 involved in metabolism of ipragliflozin.
❖ No unique ipragliflozin human metabolites were identified.

### Excretion of Ipragliflozin

❖ Was predominantly excreted in urine in humans, with M2 as the significant component in human urine.
❖ About 83.6% of ipragliflozin was recovered *via* biliary excretion in bile duct-cannulated (BDC) rats.

### Drug and Drug Interaction

❖ Ipragliflozin minimally inhibited multiple CYP450 enzymes with an $IC_{50}$ of >58 µM *in vitro*.
❖ Ipragliflozin was not an inducer of CYP3A4 or CYP1A2 *in vitro*.
❖ Ipragliflozin was not an inhibitor of UGT2B7, UGT1A1, UGT1A4, UGT1A6 or UGT1A9 with an $IC_{50}$ > 100 µM *in vitro*.
❖ Ipragliflozin was a substrate of P-gp, but had no inhibition for P-gp.
❖ Ipragliflozin was not a substrate of BCRP, MRP2, OATP1B1 or OATP1B3 *in vitro*.
❖ Ipragliflozin was a weak inhibitor of OATP1B1, OAT3 and OCT1, but did not inhibit the activities of transporters of BCRP, MRP2, MATE, OAT1 or OCT2 *in vitro*.

## Absorption

Table 5    *In Vivo* Pharmacokinetic Parameters of Ipragliflozin in Different Species after Single Intravenous and Oral Dose of Ipragliflozin L-proline[7]

| Species | Route | Dose (mg/kg) | $C_{max}$ (ng/mL) | $T_{max}$ (h) | $T_{1/2}$ (h) | $AUC_{inf}$ (ng·h/mL) | Cl (L/h/kg) | $V_{ss}$ (L/kg) | F (%) |
|---|---|---|---|---|---|---|---|---|---|
| SD rat[a] (male) | i.v. | 0.3 | NA | NA | 3.85 | 692 | 0.433 | 1.68 | - |
| | p.o. | 0.3 | 114 | 0.5 | 4.43 | 541 | NA | NA | 78.2 |
| | p.o. | 1 | 331 | 1 | 3.61 | 1654 | NA | NA | 71.7 |
| | p.o. | 3 | 832 | 0.5 | 3.93 | 6277 | NA | NA | 90.7 |
| Cynomolgus monkey[b] (male) | i.v. | 0.3 | NA | NA | 9.45 ± 2.02 | 1271 ± 367 | 0.252 ± 0.072 | 2.32 ± 0.76 | - |
| | p.o. | 0.3 | 133 ± 12 | 2.0 ± 0.0 | 8.65 ± 0.65 | 952 ± 343 | NA | NA | 74.5 ± 8.5 |
| | p.o. | 1 | 444 ± 144 | 1.75 ± 0.50 | 10.1 ± 1.1 | 3231 ± 1204 | NA | NA | 75.3 ± 7.1 |
| | p.o. | 3 | 1358 ± 380 | 1.75 ± 0.50 | 9.56 ± 1.23 | 9564 ± 3184 | NA | NA | 74.8 ± 5.0 |

[a] The parameters were calculated from the curve of average plasma concentration time (n = 3).    [b] The parameters were the mean ± SD.

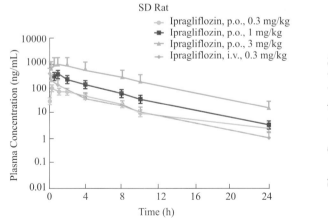
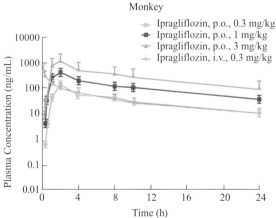

Figure C    *In Vivo* Plasma Concentration-Time Profiles of Ipragliflozin in Rats and Monkeys after Single Oral and Intravenous Dose of Ipragliflozin L-Proline[7]

[7]  PMDA Database.   http://www.pmda.go.jp/drugs/2013/P201300172/index.html (accessed Mar 2016).

Table 6  *In Vivo* Pharmacokinetic Parameters of Ipragliflozin and Metabolite M2 in Humans after Single
Intravenous and Oral Dose of Ipragliflozin[7]

| Species | Analyte | Route | Dose (mg) | $C_{max}$ (ng/mL) | $T_{max}$ (h) | $T_{1/2}$ (h) | $AUC_{inf}$ (ng·h/mL) | Cl or Cl/F (L/h) | $V_{ss}$ (L) | F (%) |
|---------|---------|-------|-----------|-------------------|---------------|---------------|----------------------|------------------|--------------|-------|
| Healthy human (male & female) | Ipragliflozin | i.v. | 25 | 612 ± 90 | 0.972 ± 0.004 | 16.8 ± 5.0 | 2374 ± 429 | 10.9 ± 2.0 | 127 ± 34 | - |
| | | p.o. | 100 | 1406 ± 338 | 1.50 ± 0.88 | 16.3 ± 5.5 | 8457 ± 1320 | 12.1 ± 2.0 | NA | 90.2 ± 5.3 |
| | M2 | i.v. | 25 | 207 ± 32 | 1.38 ± 0.13 | 16.3 ± 4.0 | 1309 ± 210 | 12.4 ± 2.4 | NA | - |
| | | p.o. | 100 | 927 ± 221 | 2.04 ± 0.89 | 16.8 ± 5.4 | 5577 ± 1003 | 11.3 ± 2.5 | NA | - |
| Japanese (male) | Ipragliflozin | p.o. | 1 | 17.9 ± 4.0 | 0.75 ± 0.27 | 4.35 ± 1.05 | 58.9 ± 11.2 | 17.4 ± 3.0 | NA | NA |
| | | p.o. | 3 | 53.7 ± 15.6 | 0.92 ± 0.20 | 10.0 ± 2.3 | 245 ± 35 | 12.5 ± 1.9 | NA | NA |
| | | p.o. | 10 | 174 ± 14 | 0.92 ± 0.20 | 13.3 ± 5.0 | 855 ± 168 | 12.1 ± 2.8 | NA | NA |
| | | p.o. | 30 | 524 ± 103 | 1.58 ± 1.11 | 12.4 ± 5.0 | 2896 ± 363 | 10.5 ± 1.3 | NA | NA |
| | | p.o. | 100 | 1392 ± 423 | 2.33 ± 1.21 | 11.7 ± 2.0 | 9696 ± 2242 | 11.0 ± 3.6 | NA | NA |
| | | p.o. | 300 | 3421 ± 690 | 2.60 ± 1.34 | 10.3 ± 1.6 | 27298 ± 4622 | 11.3 ± 2.0 | NA | NA |

The parameters were the mean ± SD.

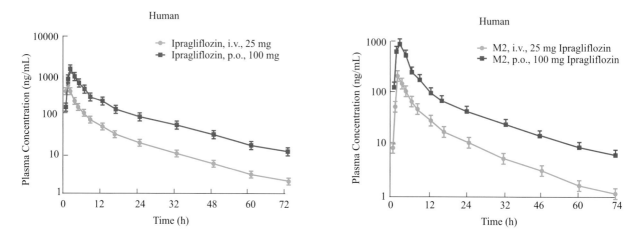

Figure D  *In Vivo* Plasma Concentration-Time Profiles of Ipragliflozin and Metabolite M2 in Humans after
Single Oral and Intravenous Dose of Ipragliflozin[7]

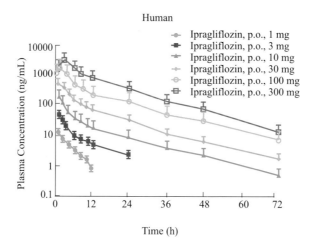

Figure E  *In Vivo* Plasma Concentration-Time Profiles of Ipragliflozin in Humans after Single Oral Dose of Ipragliflozin[7]

[7]  PMDA Database.   http://www.pmda.go.jp/drugs/2013/P201300172/index.html (accessed Mar 2016).

# Distribution

Table 7    *In Vitro* Plasma Protein Binding and Blood Partitioning of Ipragliflozin in Different Species[7]

| Species | Plasma Protein Binding (%) | | | | Blood Cell Partitioning (%) | | |
|---|---|---|---|---|---|---|---|
| | 0.05 μg/mL | 2 μg/mL | 20 μg/mL | 200 μg/mL | 0.02 μg/mL | 2 μg/mL | 200 μg/mL |
| Mouse | 95.4 ± 0.16 | 95.0 ± 0.23 | 94.7 ± 0.12 | 93.2 ± 0.13 | 32.2 ± 6.4 | 35.2 ± 0.7 | 38.7 ± 1.1 |
| Rat | 96.1 ± 0.19 | 96.1 ± 0.17 | 96.0 ± 0.03 | 94.6 ± 0.16 | 43.0 ± 2.2 | 41.7 ± 1.7 | 44.5 ± 1.9 |
| Rabbit | 92.9 ± 3.12 | 93.8 ± 0.09 | 94.0 ± 0.02 | 92.2 ± 0.42 | NA | NA | NA |
| Dog | 95.7 ± 0.26 | 95.7 ± 0.14 | 95.5 ± 0.11 | 93.8 ± 0.30 | NA | NA | NA |
| Monkey | 95.3 ± 0.18 | 94.4 ± 0.26 | 94.7 ± 0.12 | 93.2 ± 0.14 | 25.4 ± 4.4 | 24.3 ± 1.5 | 27.5 ± 4.5 |
| Human | 96.5 ± 0.31 | 95.1 ± 0.14 | 95.8 ± 0.12 | 94.6 ± 0.12 | 19.1 ± 9.4 | 16.9 ± 2.0 | 17.2 ± 3.4 |

Table 8    *In Vivo* Tissue Distribution of [$^{14}$C]Ipragliflozin in SD and Long-Evans Rats after Single Oral Dose of Ipragliflozin[7]

| | Concentration of Radioactivity (ng eq./mL) of [$^{14}$C]Ipragliflozin in Major Tissues | | | | | | | | | |
|---|---|---|---|---|---|---|---|---|---|---|
| Species | Sprague-Dawley Rat (male, n = 3) | | | | Long Evans Rat (male, n = 1) | | | | | |
| Dose | 1 mg/kg, p.o., single dose | | | | 1 mg/kg, p.o., single dose | | | | | |
| Time | 0.25 h | 1 h | 4 h | 24 h | 1 h | 24 h | 168 h | 336 h | 504 h | 672 h |
| Blood | 439 ± 260 | 352 ± 62 | 162 ± 21 | 4 ± 1 | 288 | 6.30 | ND | ND | ND | ND |
| Plasma | 461 ± 275 | 362 ± 66 | 166 ± 12 | 6 ± 1 | 278 | 5.79 | ND | ND | ND | ND |
| Brain | 20 ± 13 | 40 ± 12 | 40 ± 3 | 3 ± 0 | 18.8 | 4.07 | ND | ND | ND | ND |
| Lungs | 530 ± 289 | 694 ± 66 | 321 ± 39 | 9 ± 1 | 514 | 12.1 | ND | ND | ND | ND |
| Heart | 655 ± 396 | 881 ± 212 | 366 ± 47 | 8 ± 0 | 556 | 9.50 | ND | ND | ND | ND |
| Liver | 3981 ± 2751 | 2233 ± 288 | 1116 ± 134 | 28 ± 6 | 2156 | 42.5 | ND | ND | ND | ND |
| Kidneys | 2798 ± 1472 | 3435 ± 856 | 2298 ± 124 | 236 ± 19 | 4016 | 321 | ND | ND | ND | ND |
| Adrenal gland | 1519 ± 1037 | 1399 ± 316 | 693 ± 94 | 14 ± 1 | 1014 | 13.8 | ND | ND | ND | ND |
| Stomach | 2667 ± 2169 | 1187 ± 623 | 817 ± 594 | 5 ± 0 | ND | ND | ND | ND | ND | ND |
| Eyeballs | 59 ± 34 | 95 ± 17 | 63 ± 13 | 3 ± 0 | 73.1 | 8.97 | 1.59 | 1.40 | 1.08 | <LLOD |
| Thyroid | 506 ± 312 | 253 ± 141 | 256 ± 28 | 5 ± 1 | 476 | 12.2 | ND | ND | ND | ND |

ND: Not detected.    LLOD: Lower limit of detection.

# Metabolism

Table 9    *In Vitro* Metabolic Rate of Ipragliflozin L-proline in Liver Microsomes with NADPH of Different Species[7]

| Species | Dose (μM) | Residual Rate of Ipragliflozin | | | | | Cl$_{int}$ (mL/min/mg protein) |
|---|---|---|---|---|---|---|---|
| | | 0 min | 15 min | 30 min | 60 min | 120 min | |
| Mouse | 0.05 | 100 | 98.7 | 92.2 | 90.5 | 87.4 | 0.0046 |
| Rat | 0.05 | 100 | 86.4 | 75.9 | 66.2 | 51.2 | 0.0142 |
| Dog | 0.05 | 100 | 101 | 97.1 | 93.1 | 92.7 | 0.0033 |
| Monkey | 0.05 | 100 | 93.8 | 91.0 | 83.2 | 74.1 | 0.0062 |
| Human | 0.05 | 100 | 89.8 | 84.8 | 84.5 | 69.8 | 0.0067 |

# Other Findings:[7]

❖ Ipragliflozin was metabolized by multiple UGT enzymes and the primary metabolic enzyme was UGT2B7, with UGT2B4, 1A8 and 1A9 involved in metabolism of ipragliflozin.

[7]  PMDA Database.    http://www.pmda.go.jp/drugs/2013/P201300172/index.html (accessed Mar 2016).

Table 10    Metabolites Formation Following Microsomes Incubation with Ipragliflozin in Human Different Tissues[7]

| Microsome | Conc. (μM) | Metabolite Formation Rate (pmol/min/mg protein) | | |
|---|---|---|---|---|
| | | M2 | M3 | M4 |
| Liver | 2 | 5.14 ± 0.34 | NA | 1.15 ± 0.04 |
| | 20 | 49.4 ± 1.2 | 2.28 ± 0.12 | 11.4 ± 0.2 |
| Kidneys | 2 | 6.78 ± 0.23 | NA | 3.16 ± 0.03 |
| | 20 | 67.9 ± 2.6 | 0.595 ± 0.031 | 33.2 ± 1.9 |
| Small intestine | 2 | 0.415 ± 0.027 | NA | NA |
| | 20 | 3.76 ± 0.13 | NA | 1.61 ± 0.16 |

Table 11    Metabolites in Plasma, Urine and Bile in Non-clinical Test Species after Single Oral Dose of Ipragliflozin[7]

| Matrix | Species | Dose (mg/kg) | Time (h) | % of Radioactivity or % of Dose | | | | | | | |
|---|---|---|---|---|---|---|---|---|---|---|---|
| | | | | M0 | M1 | M2 | M3 | M4 | M5 | M6 | M7 |
| Plasma | SD rat | 1 | 4 | 82.2 | ND | 0.4 | 1.0 | ND | ND | ND | 1.9 |
| | Monkey | 1 | 24 | 47.6 | ND | 6.3 | ND | 6.3 | ND | ND | ND |
| | Human | 100 mg | 0-∞ | 7326 | 524 | 5065 | 1404 | 1064 | NA | 678 | NA |
| Urine | SD rat | 1 | 0-24 | 5.5 | ND | 0.1 | 0.0 | ND | ND | ND | 6.2 |
| | Monkey | 1 | 0-72 h | 0.9 | ND | 20.7 | 2.5 | 5.8 | ND | 0.7 | 7.2 |
| | Human | 100 mg | 0-∞ | √ | 4.2 | 39.7 | 3.7 | 10.8 | - | 0.96 | - |
| Bile | SD rat | 1 | 0-24 | 2.0 | ND | 41.2 | 5.1 | 2.7 | 5.8 | ND | 5.7 |
| | Monkey | 1 | 0-72 | 6.9 | ND | 9.1 | 0.2 | 9.3 | 0.1 | 2.4 | 0.6 |

ND: Not detected.    The value was $AUC_{inf}$ (ng·h/mL) for plasma in humans.    % of radioactivity for plasma in rats and monkeys.    % of dose for urine and bile.    M0: Ipragliflozin L-proline.    M1: AS2551864.    M2: AS2364093.    M3: AS2551840.    M4: AS2551844.    M5: AS2556836.    M6: AS2551868.    M7: AS2054727.

[7]    PMDA Database.    http://www.pmda.go.jp/drugs/2013/P201300172/index.html (accessed Mar 2016).

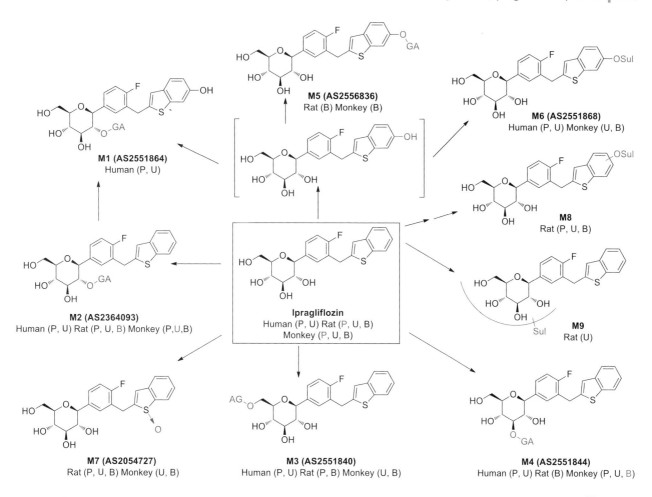

Figure F    Proposed Pathways for *In Vivo* Biotransformation of Ipragliflozin in Rats, Monkeys and Humans[7]
The red labels represent the main components in matrices.    P = Plasma, U = Urine, F = Feces, B = Bile, GA = Glucuronic acid and Sul = SO3H.

## Excretion

Table 12    Excretion Profiles of Ipragliflozin in Rats, Monkeys and Humans after Single Oral Dose of [$^{14}$C]Ipragliflozin L-proline[7]

| Species | State | Dose (mg/kg) | Time (h) | Urine (% of dose) | Feces (% of dose) | Bile (% of dose) | Recovery (% of dose) |
|---|---|---|---|---|---|---|---|
| Rat (male) | Intact | 1 | 0-168 | 13.2 ± 0.7 | 86.9 ± 2.6 | NA | 100 ± 2.4 |
|  | BDC | 1 | 0-72 | 13.7 ± 4.6 | NA | 83.6 ± 7.4 | 97.3 ± 2.8 |
|  | BDC | 0.5 mL bile[a] | 0-72 | 6.5 ± 1.2 | NA | 55.3 ± 8.5 | 61.8 ± 9.4 |
| Monkey | Intact | 1 | 0-168 | 44.7 ± 8.2 | 48.4 ± 11.6 | NA | 93.1 ± 3.5 |
|  | BDC | 1 | 0-72 | 45.6 ± 8.8 | NA | 32.3 ± 14.2 | 77.8 ± 5.5 |
| Human | Intact | 100 mg | 0-144 | 67.9 | 32.7 | NA | 101 |

[a] Following a single oral dose of 1 mg/kg [$^{14}$C]ipragliflozin to rats, bile collected up to 6 h after administration was administered intraduodenally to a different set of rats.

[7]  PMDA Database.    http://www.pmda.go.jp/drugs/2013/P201300172/index.html (accessed Mar 2016).

## Drug and Drug Interaction

Table 13    *In Vitro* Evaluation of Ipragliflozin as an Inhibitor and an Inducer of Enzymes[7]

| Ipragliflozin as a CYP Inhibitor[a] | | | Ipragliflozin as a CYP Inducer | | | Ipragliflozin as a UGTs Inhibitor[d] | |
|---|---|---|---|---|---|---|---|
| **CYPs** | **IC$_{50}$ (µM)** | | **CYPs** | **Conc. (µM)** | **Fold Induction** | **Isoform** | **IC$_{50}$ (µM)** |
| | **Direct Inhibition** | **Time-dependent Inhibition (30-min)** | | | | | |
| CYP1A2 | >250 | >250 | | DMSO | 1 | UGT1A1 | >100 |
| CYP2A6 | >250 | - | | 0.1 | 0.886-1.07 | | |
| CYP2B6 | 58.4 | 67.6 | CYP1A2 | 1 | 0.898-1.19 | UGT1A4 | >100 |
| CYP2C8 | 129 | 151 | | 10 | 1.10-1.54 | | |
| CYP2C9 | 218 | 250 | | 100 | 1.29-1.87 | UGT1A6 | >100 |
| CYP2C19 | 183 | 185 | | DMSO | 1 | | |
| CYP2D6 | 206 | >250 | | 0.1 | 0.947-1.05 | UGT1A9 | >100 |
| CYP2E1 | >250 | - | CYP3A4 | 1 | 0.943-1.09 | | |
| CYP3A4[b] | 116 | 121 | | 10 | 0.959-1.14 | UGT2B7 | >100 |
| CYP3A4[c] | >250 | >250 | | 100 | 1.57-2.39 | | |

[a] Tested concentration of ipragliflozin was 1.03-250 µM.    [b] Substrate was testosterone.    [c] Substrate was midazolam.    [d] Tested concentration of ipragliflozin was 0.1-100 µM.

Table 14    *In Vitro* Evaluation of Ipragliflozin as a Substrate and an Inhibitor of P-gp in MDCKII Cell Monolayer Model[7]

| Ipragliflozin as a Substrate | | | | | | | Ipragliflozin as an Inhibitor |
|---|---|---|---|---|---|---|---|
| **Ipragliflozin** | **Inhibitor** | **Cell** | **Papp (1 × 10$^{-6}$ cm/s)** | | **Papp Ratio** | **Efflux Ratio** | **IC$_{50}$ (µM)** |
| | | | **A→B** | **B→A** | | | **Ipragliflozin[a]** |
| 1 µM | None | P-gp transfected cell | 5.98 ± 0.26 | 28.8 ± 0.75 | 4.8 | 3.2 | >100 |
| | | Control cell | 12.4 ± 0.32 | 18.2 ± 0.34 | 1.5 | | |
| | Verapamil 200 µM | P-gp transfected cell | 9.72 ± 0.29 | 13.2 ± 0.33 | 1.4 | 1.3 | |
| | | Control cell | 17.2 ± 0.31 | 18.3 ± 0.44 | 1.1 | | |
| | Ketoconazole 50 µM | P-gp transfected cell | 11.3 ± 0.13 | 15.2 ± 0.57 | 1.4 | 1.3 | |
| | | Control cell | 17.1 ± 0.47 | 19.4 ± 0.38 | 1.1 | | |
| 10 µM | None | P-gp transfected cell | 6.17 ± 0.13 | 30.6 ± 1.51 | 5.0 | 3.6 | |
| | | Control cell | 12.7 ± 0.18 | 18.3 ± 0.32 | 1.4 | | |
| | Verapamil 200 µM | P-gp transfected cell | 9.65 ± 0.42 | 12.8 ± 0.53 | 1.3 | 1.2 | |
| | | Control cell | 16.2 ± 0.19 | 17.7 ± 0.60 | 1.1 | | |
| | Ketoconazole 50 µM | P-gp transfected cell | 11.3 ± 0.39 | 14.6 ± 0.34 | 1.3 | 1.2 | |
| | | Control cell | 17.0 ± 0.36 | 18.5 ± 0.18 | 1.1 | | |

[a] Tested concentration of ipragliflozin was 0.412-100 µM.

Table 15    *In Vitro* Evaluation of Ipragliflozin as a Substrate and an Inhibitor of Transporters[7]

| Transporter | BCRP | MRP2 | MATE | OATP1B1 | OATP1B3 | OAT1 | OAT3 | OCT1 | OCT2 |
|---|---|---|---|---|---|---|---|---|---|
| **Substrate** | No | No | ND | No | No | ND | ND | ND | ND |
| **Inhibition (IC$_{50}$, µM)** | >100 | >100 | >100 | 23.2 | 96.1 | >100 | 28.5 | 70.9 | >500 |

[7]  PMDA Database.    http://www.pmda.go.jp/drugs/2013/P201300172/index.html (accessed Mar 2016).

# 5  Non-Clinical Toxicology

## Summary

### Single-Dose Toxicity

❖ Single-dose toxicities by the oral route in rodent and non-rodent species:
  • Rat MTD (p.o.): 2000 mg/kg (male); 500 mg/kg (female).
  • Monkey MTD (p.o.): 2000 mg/kg.

### Repeated-Dose Toxicity

❖ Sub- and chronic toxicity by the oral route in rats (up to 26 weeks) and monkeys (up to 52 weeks):
  • Osmotic diuretic-like effects in all species, and ipragliflozin induced food and water consumption.
  • For the 26-week rat study, NOAEL was 0.1 mg/kg/day as 0.02-fold of MRHD for males and 0.03-fold of MRHD for females, determined by the increase of urinary $\beta$2-microglobulin excretion, urinary NAG excretion, and the increase of kidney weight at 1 mg/kg/day.   Most toxicities found were kidneys and bladder lesions derived from osmolality changes, nevertheless, bone marrow, lungs, GI track, liver, and spleen lesions were also observed.[7]
  • For the 52-week monkey study, NOAEL was 10 mg/kg/day as 5-fold of MRHD in males and 1 mg/kg/day as 0.4-fold of MRHD in females, determined by the increase of urinary $\beta$2-microglobulin excretion, urinary NAG excretion, and the primary target organs were liver and GI tract.

### Safety Pharmacology

❖ Core battery of studies to evaluate safety pharmacology:
  • Least potential for QT prolongation, based on 17.4 % inhibition of hERG tail current at 10 μM.
  • In Cynomolgus monkeys dosed up to 1000 mg/kg, no effect was observed on BP, HR, ECG, blood gas and respiratory rate.

### Genotoxicity

❖ Based on *in vitro* studies, while ipragliflozin was negative for mutagenicity in Ames assay, and chromosome structural aberrations occurred in mammalian cells, which were associated with severe cytotoxicity.   Furthermore, the positive results were not repeated in the *in vivo* study, with the weights of evidence, thus ipragliflozin was considered no genotoxic risk.

### Reproductive and Developmental Toxicity

❖ Fertility and early embryonic development in rats:
  • NOAEL was 300 mg/kg/day as 86-174 folds exposure of MRHD.
❖ Embryo-fetal development in rats and rabbits:
  • NOAEL was 100 mg/kg/day for dam and does, whilst 300 mg/kg/day for fetal development in both species.
❖ Pre- and postnatal developmental in rats:
  • NOAEL was 100 mg/kg/day as 25 folds of MRHD.
❖ Ipragliflozin distributed through placenta to fetus in pregnant rats.[7]
❖ Milk excretion of ipragliflozin was also found in lactating rats.[7]

### Carcinogenicity

❖ No significant malignant or benign neoplasia found in 2-year standard carcinogenicity studies of mice.
❖ Tumorigenicity to adrenal medulla emerged in rats, as for humans, it was not considered to be an indicator of carcinogenic risk.

[7]  PMDA Database.   http://www.pmda.go.jp/drugs/2013/P201300172/index.html (accessed Mar 2016).

## Single-Dose Toxicity

Table 16    Single-Dose Toxicology Studies of Ipragliflozin by Oral Administration[7]

| Species | Dose (mg/kg) | MTD (mg/kg) | ALD (mg/kg) | Finding |
|---|---|---|---|---|
| SD rat | Male: 1000, 2000<br>Female: 250, 500, 1000, 2000 | Male, 2000<br>Female, 500 | Male, >2000<br>Female, 1000 | ≥1000 mg/kg: Pancreas and stomach toxicity.<br>≤500 mg/kg: No abnormalities. |
| Cynomolgus monkey | 300, 1000, 2000 | 2000 | >2000 | Vomiting and GI tract reaction. |

Vehicle: 0.5% MC.

## Repeated-Dose Toxicity

Table 17    Repeated-Dose Toxicology Studies of Ipragliflozin by Oral Administration[7]

| Species | Duration (Week) | Dose (mg/kg/day) | NOAEL Dose (mg/kg/day) | NOAEL AUC$_{0-24}$ (ng·h/mL) | NOAEL Safety Margin[a] (× MRHD) | Finding |
|---|---|---|---|---|---|---|
| SD rat | 2 | 1, 10, 100, 1000 | 1 | Male: 1550<br>Female: 2760 | Male: 0.17<br>Female: 0.3 | ↑ Urine amount, ↓ osmolality, ↑ urine glucose, ↑ food and water consumption, ↓ body weight at ≥1 mg/kg/day group. |
| | 13 | 0.1, 1, 10, 100 | 0.1 | Male: 139<br>Female: 310 | Male: 0.02<br>Female: 0.03 | Kidney toxicity at 10 mg/kg/day group (13 weeks), and 1 mg/kg/day group (26 weeks). |
| | 26 | 0.1, 1, 10, 100 | 0.1 | Male: 175<br>Female: 432 | Male: 0.02<br>Female: 0.05 | ↑ Urinary NAG excretion at 1 mg/kg/day group (13 weeks and 26 weeks).<br>Liver and GI track toxicity at 100 mg/kg/day group (13 weeks) and 10 mg/kg/day group (26 weeks). |
| Cynomolgus monkey | 2 | 10, 100, 1000 | 100 | Male: 315000<br>Female: 341000 | Male: 34<br>Female: 37 | ↑ Urine amount, ↑ food and water consumption, hypertrophy of adrenal cortex. |
| | 13 | 10, 100, 300 | 10 | Male: 33500<br>Female: 29300 | Male: 4<br>Female: 3 | ↑ Urine amount, ↓ osmolality, ↑ urine glucose, ↑ food and water consumption, ↑ urinary electrolyte excretion, ↓ creatinine clearance. |
| | 52 | 1, 10, 300 | Male: 10<br>Female: 1 | Male: 46200<br>Female: 3780 | Male: 5<br>Female: 0.4 | ↑ β2-Microglobulin excretion and ↑ urinary NAG excretion in the female at 10 mg/kg/day group. Histological change included kidneys, liver and GI track.<br>↑ Urine amount, ↓ osmolality, ↑ urine glucose, ↑ food and water consumption, ↓ body weight at ≥1 mg/kg/day group. |

Vehicle: 0.5% CMC.    [a] Calculated based on MRHD exposure estimated for 100 mg QD (AUC$_{0-24}$ = 9213 ng·h/mL).

## Safety Pharmacology

Table 18    Summary of Safety Pharmacology Studies of Ipragliflozin[7]

| Study | System | Dose | Finding |
|---|---|---|---|
| Neurological Safety | SD rat | 10, 100, 1000 mg/kg, p.o, | None. |
| Cardiovascular Safety | hERG-transfected HEK293 cell | 0.1, 1, 10 μM | 17.4% inhibition of hERG current at 10 μM. |
| | Papillary muscle<br>Cardiac action potential test (*in vitro*) | 0.1, 1, 10 μM | No inhibition at 10 μM. |
| | Cynomoglus monkey (*in vivo*) | 10, 100, 1000 mg/kg<br>p.o, single dose | No effect on blood pressure, heart rate, ECG, blood gas up to 1000 mg/kg. |
| Respiratory Safety | Cynomoglus monkey (*in vivo*) | 10, 100, 1000 mg/kg | No effect on respiratory rate. |

Vehicle: 0.5% MC for *in vivo* tests, DMSO for *in vitro* tests.

[7]  PMDA Database.    http://www.pmda.go.jp/drugs/2013/P201300172/index.html (accessed Mar 2016).

# Genotoxicity

Table 19    Summary of Genetic Toxicology Studies of Ipragliflozin[7]

| Assay | System | Metabolism | Dose | Finding |
|---|---|---|---|---|
| *In vitro* reverse mutation assay in bacterial cells (Ames) | *S. typhimurium* TA98, TA100, TA1535, TA1537; *E. coli* WP2uvTA | ±S9 | 100-5000 μg/plate | Negative. Cytotoxicity: 750 μg/plate. |
| *In vitro* chromosomal aberration assays in mammalian cells | CHL/IU | ±S9 | 0-270 μg/mL | Positive at 270 μg/mL +S9, 210 μg/mL -S9. |
| *In vivo* micronucleus assay in rodent | SD rat | + | 500-2000 mg/kg | Negative. |
| *In vivo* measurement of unscheduled DNA synthesis | SD rat | + | 500-2000 mg/kg | Negative. |

Vehicle: 0.5% methyl cellulose in water for *in vivo* tests, while DMSO for *in vitro* tests.

# Reproductive and Developmental Toxicity

Table 20    Embryonic and Developmental Toxicology Studies of Ipragliflozin[7]

| Study | Species | Dose (mg/kg/day) | NOAEL | | | | Finding |
|---|---|---|---|---|---|---|---|
| | | | Endpoint | Dose (mg/kg/day) | $AUC_{0-24}$ (ng·h/mL) | Safety Margin[a] (× MRHD) | |
| Fertility and early embryonic development | SD rat | 100, 300, 1000 | Fertility & embryo | 300 | Male: 794000 Female: 1600000 | Male: 86 Female: 174 | Fertility and early embryonic development not evaluated at HD due to high mortality rate premating. |
| Embryo-fetal development | SD rat | 100, 300, 600 | Maternal | 100 | 603000 | 65 | ↓ Maternal BW associated with ↓ food consumption at MD and HD. ↓ Placental weight and fetal birth weight , ↑ incidence of residual neck at HD. |
| | | | Fetal | 300 | 1310000 | 142 | |
| | NZW rabbit | 30, 100, 300 | Maternal | 100 | 303000 | 33 | ↓ Maternal BW associated with ↓ food consumption, ↓ placental weight at HD. |
| | | | Fetal | 300 | 2340000 | 254 | |
| Pre- and postnatal development | SD rat | 30, 100, 300 | $F_0$ | 100 | 226000 | 25 | ↓ Food consumption at all doses. Delayed physical development at HD. |
| | | | $F_1$ | 100 | 226000 | 25 | |

[a] Calculated based on MRHD exposure estimated for 100 mg QD ($AUC_{0-24}$ = 9213 ng·h/mL).

# Carcinogenicity

Table 21    Carcinogenic Toxicity Studies of Ipragliflozin after 104-Week Oral QD Administration[7]

| Species | Dose (mg/kg/day) | NOAEL | | | Finding |
|---|---|---|---|---|---|
| | | Dose (mg/kg/day) | $AUC_{0-24}$ (ng·h/mL) | Safety Margin (× MRHD) | |
| Mouse | 0, 50, 150, 500 | Male: 150 Female: 500 | Male: 448000 Female: 1960000 | Male: 49 Female: 213 | No carcinogenic. |
| SD rat | 12.5, 40, 125, 250 | Male: 12.5 Female: 40 | Male: 28300 Female: 158000 | Male: 3 Female: 17 | Showed pro-tumor against adrenal medulla of rats. |

Vehicle: 0.5% MC.    MRHD was considered 9213 ng·h/mL based on the average AUC at 100 mg QD administration.

[7]  PMDA Database.    http://www.pmda.go.jp/drugs/2013/P201300172/index.html (accessed Mar 2016).

# CHAPTER

## 16

### Luseogliflozin Hydrate

# Luseogliflozin Hydrate

## (Lusefi®)

Research code: TS-071

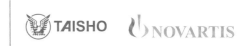

## 1  General Information

- ❖ Luseogliflozin hydrate is a sodium-glucose cotransporter 2 (SGLT2) inhibitor, which was approved by PMDA of Japan.

- ❖ Luseogliflozin hydrate was discovered by Taisho, co-developed and co-marketed by Taisho and Novartis.

- ❖ Luseogliflozin hydrate is a selective SGLT2 inhibitor, which inhibits the reuptake of glucose and increases glucose excretion through urine, thereby reducing blood glucose levels.

- ❖ Luseogliflozin hydrate is indicated for the treatment of type 2 diabetes.

- ❖ Available as tablet, with each containing 2.5 mg or 5 mg of luseogliflozin and the recommended dose is 2.5 mg once daily before or after breakfast.

- ❖ The 2014 and 2015 worldwide sales of Lusefi® were 22.4 and 5.7 million US$, respectively, referring to the financial reports of Taisho.

### Key Approvals around the World*

|  | Japan (PMDA) |
| --- | --- |
| First approval date | 03/24/2014 |
| Application or approval No. | 22600AMX00540000; 22600AMX00541000 |
| Brand name | Lusefi® |
| Indication | Type 2 diabetes mellitus |
| Authorisation holder | Taisho/Novartis |

* Till Mar 2016, it had not been filed to FDA (US), EMA (EU) or CFDA (China).

## Active Ingredient

*Molecular formula*:  $C_{23}H_{30}O_6S \cdot xH_2O$
*Molecular weight*:  434.55 (Luseogliflozin)
*CAS No.*:  898537-18-3 (Luseogliflozin)
*Chemical name*:  (2S,3R,4R,5S,6R)-2-{5-[(4-ethoxyphenyl)methyl]-2-methoxy-4-methylphenyl}-6-(hydroxymethyl)thiane-3,4,5-triol hydrate

*Parameters of Lipinski's "Rule of 5"*

| MW[a] | H_D | H_A | FRB[b] | PSA[b] | cLogP[b] |
| --- | --- | --- | --- | --- | --- |
| 434.55 | 4 | 6 | 11 | 125Å² | 4.73 ± 0.64 |

[a] Molecular weight of luseogliflozin.  [b] Calculated by ACD/Labs software V11.02.

## Drug Product*

*Dosage route*:  Oral
Strength:  2.5 mg/5 mg (Luseogliflozin)
*Dosage form*:  Film-coated tablet
*Inactive ingredient*:  Lactose hydrate, crystalline cellulose, sodium starch glycolate, hydroxypropyl cellulose, magnesium stearate, hypromellose, titanium oxide, macrogol 400, carnauba wax and light anhydrous silicic acid.
*Recommended dose*: The recommended starting dose for adults is 2.5 mg once daily, taken before or after breakfast.  If the effects are insufficient, dosage may be increased up to 5 mg once daily while carefully monitoring the progress of the disease.

* Sourced from Japan PMDA drug label information

## 2  Key Patents Information

### Summary

❖ Lusefi® (Luseogliflozin hydrate) was approved by PMDA of Japan on Mar 24, 2014 initially.
❖ Luseogliflozin was originally discovered by Taisho, co-developed and co-marked by Taisho and Novartis, and its compound patent application was filed as PCT application by Taisho in 2006.
❖ The compound patent will expire in 2026 foremost, which has been granted in Japan, the United States, Europe and China successively.

Table 1    Luseogliflozin's Compound Patent Protection in Drug-Mainstream Country

| Country | Publication/Patent NO. | Application Date | Granted Date | Estimated Expiry Date |
|---|---|---|---|---|
| WO | WO2006073197A1 | 01/10/2006 | / | / |
| US | US7910619B2 | 01/10/2006 | 03/22/2011 | 04/04/2028[a] |
| EP | EP1845095B1 | 01/10/2006 | 09/07/2011 | 01/10/2026 |
| JP | JP5187592B2 | 01/10/2006 | 04/24/2013 | 01/10/2026 |
| | JP4492968B2 | 01/10/2006 | 06/30/2010 | 12/17/2029[b] |
| CN | CN101103013B | 01/10/2006 | 05/23/2012 | 01/10/2026 |

[a] The term of this patent is extended by 815 days.    [b] The term of this patent is extended by 1437 days.

Table 2    Originator's International Patent Application List (Patent Family)

| Publication NO. | Title | Applicant/Assignee/Owner | Publication Date |
|---|---|---|---|
| **Technical Subjects** | **Active Ingredient (Free Base)'s Formula or Structure and Preparation** | | |
| WO2006073197A1 | 1-Thio-D-glucitol derivatives | Taisho | 07/13/2006 |
| **Technical Subjects** | **Combination Including at Least Two Active Ingredients** | | |
| WO2010119990A1 | Pharmaceutical compositions | Taisho | 10/21/2010 |
| WO2014034842A1 | Combination of SGLT2 inhibitor and anti-hypertension drug | Taisho | 03/06/2014 |

The data was updated until Jan 2016.

# 3 Chemistry

## Route 1: Original Discovery Route

3,4-DHP: 3,4-Dihydro-2*H*-pyran
PPTS: Pyridinium *p*-toluenesulfonate

*Synthetic Route*: Commercially available 4-methoxy-2-methyl benzoic acid **1** was brominated in the presence of a catalytic amount of iron powder, generating a 1:1 mixture of 3- and 5-bromo derivatives which were separable by recrystallization from methanol, providing the desired regioisomer **2** in 34% yield. Afterwards, benzoic acid **2** was treated with oxalyl chloride to give the corresponding acyl chloride which underwent a Friedel-Crafts reaction with ethoxybenzene **3** to afford benzophenone **4** in 82% yield for the two-step sequence. Reduction of **4** using triethylsilane and boron trifluoride diethyletherate gave aglycon **5** in 99% yield. The preparation of Grignard reagent from bromide **5** was prior to alkylation with thiolactone **6** to afford hemithioacetal **7** in 75% yield, which underwent stereoselective reduction to provide thioglycoside **8** in 77% yield. Hydrogenation of **8** resulted in global debenzylation to provide the luseogliflozin hydrate in 81% yield.

The preparation of key thiolactone **6** was started from commercially available polyacetate **9**. Subjection of this carbohydrate derivative to methyl hydrazine in acetic acid followed by converting the resultant hemithioacetal to the corresponding THP ether **12** and then globally saponification prior to benzylation furnished tetrabenzyloxy derivative **13** in excellent yield from **10**. Quantitative removal of the THP protecting group and further oxidation gave rise to the key luseogliflozin thioglycoside fragment **6** in 82% yield. The overall yield concerning this route was 7%.[1-3]

## 4 Pharmacology

### Summary

*Mechanism of Action*

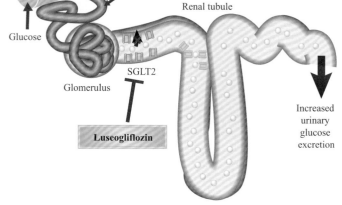

- ❖ Luseogliflozin is an inhibitor of SGLT2, which is the major transporter involved in the reabsorption of glucose in kidneys.
- ❖ Luseogliflozin selectively inhibited hSGLT2 ($K_i$ = 1.10 nM, $IC_{50}$ = 2.26 nM, >1200 folds selectivity for hSGLT1), resulting in decrease of renal glucose re-absorption, and thereby increasing urinary glucose excretion (UGE) and lowering plasma glucose (PG) in patients with type 2 diabetes.
- ❖ The metabolites had pharmacological profiles similar to luseogliflozin on inhibiting SGLT2 with less potent (M2, $IC_{50}$ = 4.01 nM; M17, $IC_{50}$ = 201 nM).
- ❖ Luseogliflozin showed very faint ligand binding inhibition activity in a panel of transporters (3 types), ion channels (5 types) and receptors (6 types) up to 100 μM, except $Na^+$ channel site 2 (66.96% inhibition at 100 μM) and Neurokinin 1 (58.75% inhibition at 100 μM).

*In Vivo Efficacy*

- ❖ Increased urinary glucose excretion (UGE):
  - *db/db* mouse: MED = 1 mg/kg.
  - ZDF diabetic rat: MED = 0.3 mg/kg.
  - DIO rat: MED = 3 mg/kg.
  - Beagle dog: MED = 150 μg/kg/h for infusion, and 0.03 mg/kg after OGTT.
- ❖ Decreased blood glucose concentration and blood glucose AUC:
  - *db/db* mouse: Significantly reduced $AUC_{0-8}$ at ≥0.3 mg/kg (single dose) and blood glucose levels at ≥3 mg/kg (QD × 4 weeks).
  - ZDF rat: Significantly decreased blood glucose concentration and $AUC_{0-2}$ at ≥3 mg/kg in OGTT.
  - STZ SD rat:
    - ✦ Significantly reduced plasma glucose levels and $AUC_{0-8}$ at ≥0.3 mg/kg (single dose).
    - ✦ Significantly reduced plasma glucose levels at ≥0.001% mixed in diet for 4 weeks.
  - Non-diabetic SD rat: Significantly reduced plasma glucose levels at 1 mg/kg (no-fasted) and 3 mg/kg (fasted).
- ❖ Improved Pancreatic *β* cell protection and insulin secretion:
  - STZ diabetic SD rat: MED = 0.01%.
- ❖ Decreased GHb level:
  - *db/db* mouse: Significantly at 3 mg/kg.
  - GK non-fatty diabetic rat: Significantly at 0.002%.
  - STZ diabetic SD rat: Significantly at 0.001%.

[1] Kakinuma, H.; Oi, T.; Hashimoto-Tsuchiya, Y., et al. *J. Med. Chem.* **2010**, *53*, 3247-3261.
[2] Kakinuma, H.; Hashimoto, Y.; Oi, T., et al. WO2006073197A1, **2006**.
[3] Kakinuma, H.; Hashimoto, Y.; Oi, T., et al. US2008132563A1, **2008**.

# Mechanism of Action

Table 3　*In Vitro* Binding Affinity and Inhibition of Luseogliflozin and Its Major Metabolites on SGLT2 and Other Targets[4]

| Target | Source | Cell line | Luseogliflozin | | | M2 | | M17 | | Phlorizin | |
|--------|--------|-----------|------------------|-----------------|-----------------------|-----------------|-----------------------|-----------------|-----------------------|-----------------|-----------------------|
| | | | $K_i$ (nM) | $IC_{50}$ (nM) | Selectivity to SGLT2 | $IC_{50}$ (nM) | Selectivity to SGLT2 | $IC_{50}$ (nM) | Selectivity to SGLT2 | $IC_{50}$ (nM) | Selectivity to SGLT2 |
| SGLT2 | Human | CHO-K1 | 1.10 | 2.26 | 1 | 4.01 | 1 | 201 | 1 | 27.8 | 1 |
| SGLT1 | Human | CHO-K1 | - | 2900 | 1283 | 1410 | 352 | >30000 | >149 | 165 | 5.9 |
| SGLT3 | Human | HEK293 | - | 47.3%[a] | - | - | - | - | - | 65.1%[b] | - |
| SGLT5 | Monkey | Kidney Cos-7 | - | 1310 | 580 | - | - | - | - | 1730 | 62 |
| SMIT1 | Monkey | Kidney Cos-7 | - | 23300 | 10309 | - | - | - | - | 370000 | 13309 |
| SMIT2 | Monkey | Kidney Cos-7 | - | 584 | 258 | - | - | - | - | 47200 | 1698 |

[a] 47.3% at 100000 nM.　[b] % inhibition at 500000 nM.

Table 4　*In Vitro* Selectivity of Luseogliflozin on Human SGLT2 and Other Targets[5]

| Inhibitor | $IC_{50}$ (nM) | SGLT2 Selectivity | | | | | |
|-----------|----------------|-------------------|---------|---------|---------|---------|---------|
| | hSGLT2 | hSGLT1 | hSGLT3 | hSGLT4 | hSGLT5 | hSGLT6 | hSMIT1 |
| Luseogliflozin | 3.1 ± 0.1 | 1600 | 8100 | 9800 | 280 | 220 | 7800 |
| Tofogliflozin | 2.9 ± 0.7 | 2900 | 19000 | 1500 | 540 | 6200 | 28000 |
| Dapagliflozin | 1.3 ± 0.2 | 610 | 190000 | 3000 | 210 | 1300 | 22000 |
| Canagliflozin | 6.7 ± 2.9 | 290 | 52000 | 2800 | 180 | 200 | 5600 |
| Ipragliflozin | 2.8 ± 0.5 | 860 | 7700 | 4500 | 87 | 3500 | 21000 |
| Empagliflozin | 3.6 ± 1.6 | 1100 | 62000 | 2200 | 110 | 1100 | 8300 |
| PF-04971729 | 1.4 ± 0.1 | 1300 | >71000 | 2300 | 3400 | 980 | 26000 |
| Phlorizin | 16.4 ± 5.2 | 11 | 1300 | 490 | 36 | 1000 | 25000 |

The inhibitory activities of luseogliflozin and other SGLT inhibitors against the seven human SGLTs (hSGLT1, hSGLT2, hSGLT3, hSGLT4, hSGLT5, hSGLT6 and hSMIST1) were compared in SGLT-overexpressing cells (CHO, HEK293 or Cos-7) by measuring sodium-dependent sugar (AMG, fructose or MI) uptake.

Table 5　Binding Affinity of Luseogliflozin on hSGLT2[6]

| Glucose | hSGLT2 Selectivity | | | |
|---------|--------------------|--------|--------|--------|
| | $K_d$ (nM) | $K_{on}$ (M$^{-1}$·min$^{-1}$) | $K_{off}$ (min$^{-1}$) | Dissociation Half-time (min) |
| - | 1.3 ± 0.13 | $1.4 \times 10^6 \pm 1.5 \times 10^5$ | $1.8 \times 10^{-3} \pm 5.4 \times 10^{-5}$ | 420 ± 10 |
| 20 mM | 7.0 ± 0.70 | $2.4 \times 10^5 \pm 6.9 \times 10^3$ | $1.7 \times 10^{-3} \pm 1.6 \times 10^{-4}$ | 430 ± 39 |

Each of the values was calculated from the association and dissociation curves.　Data represented the mean ± SEM of three experiments.

[4]　Japan Pharmaceuticals and Medical Devices Agency (PMDA) Database.　http://www.pmda.go.jp/drugs/2014/P201400033/index.html (accessed Mar 2016).

[5]　Suzuki, M.; Honda, K.; Fukazawa, M., et al. *J. Pharmacol. Exp. Ther*. **2012**, *341*, 692-701.

[6]　Uchida, S.; Mitani, A.; Gunji, E., et al. *J. Pharmacol. Sci*. **2015**, *128*, 54-57.

Table 6    Off-Target Activities of Luseogliflozin[4]

| Target | Source | System | Luseogliflozin | | Positive Control | |
|---|---|---|---|---|---|---|
| | | | Conc. (µM) | Inhibition (%) | Compound Conc. (µM) | Inhibition (%) |
| GLUT1/GLUT4 | Mouse | Adipocyte like 3T3-L1 cell | 100 | 43.3 | Cytochalasin B (10 µM) | 96.3 |
| GLUT2 | Mouse | Pancreatic $\beta$ and MIN6 cell line | 100 | 2.44 | Phlorizin (400 µM) | 92.6 |
| Na+ channel site 2 | Rat | Recombinant protein | 10 | 15.0 | Dibucaine | 95.8 |
| | | | 100 | 67.0 | | |
| Neurokinin 1 | Human | Recombinant protein | 100 | 58.8 | L-703, 606 | 98.6 |

The study used human recombinant protein or rat tissue, transporter (3 types), ion channel (five types) and receptor (six types).    Other receptor and transporter inhibited all <35% (100 µM ) or <18% (10 µM ).    Each of the values was calculated from the association and dissociation curves.    Mean ± SEM of three experiments.

## *In Vivo* Efficacy

Table 7    *In Vivo* Efficacy on Blood Glucose Regulation by Luseogliflozin[4, 5, 7, 8]

| Study | System | | Dose (mg/kg) | Route & Duration | Efficacy | |
|---|---|---|---|---|---|---|
| | Animal | Type | | | MED (mg/kg) | Finding |
| Urine glucose excretion (UGE) | *db/db* mouse | Type II diabetes | 0.1, 0.3, 1, 3 | p.o., single dose | 1 | Significantly increased UGE at 1 and 3 mg/kg. |
| | Zucker fatty rat | Type II diabetes | 0.1, 0.3, 1, 3 | p.o., single dose | 0.3 | Significantly increased UGE at ≥0.3 mg/kg in OGTT. |
| | DIO rat | Non-diabetic | 3, 10 | p.o., QD × 32 days | 3 | Significantly increased urine glucose excretion. |
| | Beagle dog | Non-diabetic | 150, 500 µg/kg/h | i.v. infusion × 35 min | 150 | Significantly increased UGE. |
| | | | 0.003, 0.01, 0.03, 0.1, 0.3, 1 | p.o., single dose | 0.03 | Increased UGE at ≥0.03 mg/kg in OGTT. |
| Blood glucose | *db/db* mouse | Type II diabetes | 0.1, 0.3, 1, 3 | p.o., single dose | 0.3 | Significantly reduced plasma glucose $AUC_{0-8}$ at ≥0.3 mg/kg. |
| | *db/db* mouse | Type II diabetes | 0.3, 1, 3, 10 | p.o., QD × 4 weeks | 3 | Significantly reduced plasma glucose levels at 3 and 10 mg/kg. |
| | Zucker fatty rat | Type II diabetes | 0.1, 0.3, 1, 3 | p.o., single dose | 0.3 | Significantly decreased blood glucose concentration and blood glucose $AUC_{0-2}$ at ≥3 mg/kg in OGTT. |
| | STZ induced SD rat | Type I diabetes | 0.1, 0.3, 1, 3 | p.o., single dose | 0.3 | Significantly reduced plasma glucose levels and blood glucose $AUC_{0-8}$ at ≥ 0.3 mg/kg. |
| | STZ induced SD rat | Type I diabetes | 0.001%, 0.003%, 0.01% with diet | p.o., 4 weeks | 0.001% | Significantly reduced plasma glucose levels at 0.001%. |
| | Normal SD rat | Non-diabetic No-fasted | 0.3, 1, 3 | p.o., single dose | 1 (no-fasted) 3 (fasted) | Reduced no-fasted plasma glucose level at 1 mg/kg. Significantly reduced fasted plasma glucose levels at 3 mg/kg. |

[4]  PMDA Database.    http://www.pmda.go.jp/drugs/2014/P201400033/index.html (accessed Mar 2016).
[5]  Suzuki, M.; Honda, K.; Fukazawa, M., et al. *J. Pharmacol. Exp. Ther.* **2012**, *341*, 692-701.
[7]  Yamamoto, K.; Uchida, S.; Kitano, K., et al. *Br. J. Pharmacol.* **2011**, *164*, 181-191.
[8]  Kurosaki, E.; Ogasawara, H. *Pharmacol. Ther.* **2013**, *139*, 51-59.

*Continued*

| Study | System | | Dose (mg/kg) | Route & Duration | Efficacy | |
|---|---|---|---|---|---|---|
| | Animal | Type | | | MED (mg/kg) | Finding |
| GHb level | *db/db* mouse | Type II diabetes | 0.1, 0.3, 1, 3 | p.o., QD × 4 weeks | 3 | Significantly decreased GHb level at ≥3 mg/kg in OGTT. |
| | GK rat | Non-fatty type II diabetes | 0.002%, 0.06%, 0.02% | p.o., QD × 20 weeks | 0.002% | Significantly decreased GHb at ≥0.002%. |
| | STZ-induced SD rat | Type I diabetes | 0.001%, 0.003%, 0.01% | p.o., TID × 4 weeks with diet test | 0.001% | Significantly decreased GHb at ≥0.001%. |
| Body weight growth reduction | DIO rat | Obesity | 3, 10 | p.o., QD × 32 days | 3 | Significantly reduced body weight. |
| Pancreatic β cell protection and insulin secretion | STZ-induced SD rat | Type I diabetes | 0.001%, 0.003%, 0.01% | p.o., TID × 4 weeks with diet test | 0.01% | Attenuated pancreatic β cells reduction, indicating improvement of insulin resistance at 0.01%. |

Vehicle for i.v. infusion was lactate Ringer's solution containing 40% w/v glucose.    Vehicle for oral administration was 0.5 % CMC-Na.    DIO: Diet induced obesity.
GHb: Glycated hemoglobin.

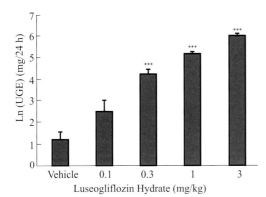

**Study**: Effects of luseogliflozin on urinary glucose excretion in Zucker fatty rats.

**Animal**: Zucker fatty rat.

**Administration**: Luseogliflozin: 0.01, 0.3, 1 or 3 mg/kg, p.o., single dose. Vehicle: 0.5% CMC, 5 mL/kg.

**OGTT**: Thirty minutes after the administration, the rats were orally dosed with an aqueous 40% solution of glucose (2 g/5 mL·kg⁻¹).

**Test**: Urinary samples were collected 0-24 h after administration.

**Results**: Significantly reduced UGE at 0.3 mg/kg.    *** $P < 0.001/4$.

Figure A    Effects of Luseogliflozin on Urinary Glucose Excretion after Oral Glucose Loading in Zucker Fatty Rats[8]

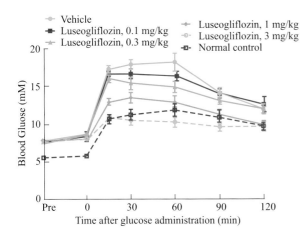

**Study**: Effects of luseogliflozin on oral glucose tolerance test in type II diabetic rats.

**Animal**: Zucker fatty rat.

**Administration**: Luseogliflozin: 0.1, 0.3, 1 or 3 mg/kg, p.o., single dose. Vehicle: 0.5% CMC, 5 mL/kg.

**OGTT**: Thirty minutes after the administration, the rats were orally dosed with an aqueous 40% solution of glucose (2 g/5 mL·kg⁻¹).

**Test**: Blood samples were collected from the tail vein immediately at 0 (before administration), 1, 2, 4, 6, 8, 10, 12, and 24 h after administration.

**Results**: Decreased plasma glucose in a dose-dependent manner.

Figure B    Effects of Luseogliflozin on Plasma Glucose and Insulin Levels after Oral Glucose Loading in Zucker Fatty Rats[8]

[8]    Kurosaki, E.; Ogasawara, H. *Pharmacol. Ther.* **2013**, *139*, 51-59.

# 5 ADME & Drug-Drug Interaction

## Summary

### Absorption of Luseogliflozin

❖ Had moderate oral bioavailability in male rats (30.3%-37.8%), but high in dogs (92.7%-101.6%) and female rats (58.2%).

❖ Was absorbed rapidly ($T_{max}$ = 0.5-1.33 h) in rats and dogs, but rapidly to moderately in humans.

❖ Showed a half-life ranging between 9.23-13.8 h in humans, much longer than those in rats (2.52-4.51 h) and dogs (3.84-4.25 h), after oral administrations.

❖ Had moderate clearance in rats (1.61-2.18 L/h/kg), but low in dogs (0.19 L/h/kg), in contrast to liver blood flow, after intravenous administrations.

❖ Exhibited an extensive tissue distribution in rats, but moderate in dogs, with apparent volumes of distribution at 2.63-2.88 and 0.8 L/kg, respectively, after intravenous administrations.

❖ Showed a high permeability, with a $Papp_{(A\rightarrow B)}$ of $14 \times 10^{-6}$ cm/s at 10 μM in Caco-2 cell monolayer model.

### Distribution of Luseogliflozin

❖ Exhibited high plasma protein binding (96.0%-96.3%) in humans and all nonclinical species.

❖ Had a blood cell association of 4.8%-6.9% in humans, suggesting low penetration into red blood cells.

❖ Rats after oral administration:

- The drug was rapidly and well distributed into most tissues except for the central nervous system (CNS), with trace or no radioactivity in brain.
- Relatively higher concentration levels were observed in small intestine, stomach, kidneys, lungs and liver, compared to other organs.
- Radioactivity concentrations decreased below the low limit of quantification in all tissues at 168 h post-dose.
- The distribution of luseogliflozin in male rats was similar to female rats.

### Metabolism of Luseogliflozin

❖ Could be largely metabolized in rat and monkey hepatocytes, but rare in dog and human hepatocytes.

❖ CYP3A4 was the major metabolizing enzyme, with 4A11, ADL and ALDH involved in the metabolism of luseogliflozin.

❖ Overall, the parent drug represented the most abundant component, with M2 as the major metabolite in human plasma.

### Excretion of Luseogliflozin

❖ Was predominantly excreted in feces in humans.

❖ Was predominantly excreted in feces in rats and dogs, but in urine in monkeys.

❖ About 75.8%-76.6% of luseogliflozin was recovered *via* biliary excretion in bile duct-cannulated (BDC) rats.

### Drug-Drug Interaction

❖ Luseogliflozin weakly inhibited CYP2C19, but did not inhibit other human CYP450 enzymes.

❖ Luseogliflozin was not an inducer of CYP3A4, CYP1A2 or CYP2B6.

❖ Luseogliflozin was a substrate of P-gp, but not of OATP1B1, OATP1B3, OAT1, OAT3 or OCT2.

❖ Luseogliflozin did not inhibit P-gp, BCRP, OATP1B1, OATP1B3, OAT1, OAT3 or OCT2.

# Absorption

Table 8    *In Vivo* Pharmacokinetic Parameters of Luseogliflozin in Different Species after Single Intravenous and Oral Dose of Luseogliflozin Hydrate[4]

| Species | Route[a] | Dose (mg/kg) | $T_{max}$ (h) | $C_{max}$ (ng/mL) | $AUC_{inf}$ (ng·h/mL) | $T_{1/2}$ (h) | Cl (L/h/kg) | $V_{ss}$ (L/kg) | F (%) |
|---|---|---|---|---|---|---|---|---|---|
| Rat (male) | i.v. | 1 | NA | NA | 462 ± 34.0 | 4.92 ± 2.61 | 2.18 ± 0.16 | 2.63 ± 0.565 | NA |
| | p.o. | 0.3 | 0.83 ± 0.29 | 8.02 ± 1.28 | 42.0 ± 7.60 | 3.17 ± 0.38 | NA | NA | 30.3 |
| | p.o. | 1 | 0.50 ± 0.00 | 35.7 ± 17.0 | 163 ± 40.6 | 2.93 ± 2.00 | NA | NA | 35.3 |
| | p.o. | 3 | 0.67 ± 0.29 | 136 ± 32.3 | 524 ± 98.3 | 2.52 ± 0.38 | NA | NA | 37.8 |
| Rat (female) | i.v. | 1 | NA | NA | 625 ± 29.1 | 4.41 ± 0.34 | 1.61 ± 0.075 | 2.88 ± 0.546 | NA |
| | p.o. | 1 | 0.83 ± 0.29 | 64.0 ± 16.3 | 364 ± 26.2 | 4.51 ± 1.47 | NA | NA | 58.2 |
| Dog (male) | i.v. | 1 | NA | NA | 5250 ± 445 | 3.89 ± 0.25 | 0.19 ± 0.016 | 0.80 ± 0.060 | NA |
| | p.o. | 0.3 | 0.67 ± 0.29 | 301 ± 44.8 | 1480 ± 319 | 3.84 ± 0.41 | NA | NA | 94.0 |
| | p.o. | 1 | 0.67 ± 0.29 | 914 ± 73.4 | 4880 ± 654 | 4.07 ± 0.25 | NA | NA | 92.7 ± 7.1 |
| | p.o. | 3 | 1.33 ± 0.58 | 2760 ± 50.3 | 16000 ± 1950 | 4.25 ± 0.45 | NA | NA | 101.6 |

Rats were under non-fasted conditions, and dogs were under fasted conditions.    [a] Vehicle: 0.5% CMC-Na (p.o.); 22.5% HP$\beta$CD (i.v.).

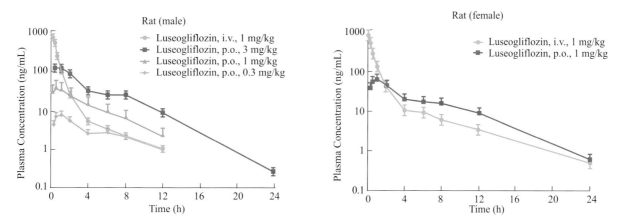

Figure C    *In Vivo* Plasma Concentration-Time Profiles of Luseogliflozin in Rats after Single Oral and Intravenous Dose of Luseogliflozin[4]

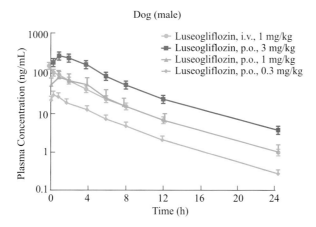

Figure D    *In Vivo* Plasma Concentration-Time Profiles of Luseogliflozin in Dogs after Single Oral and Intravenous Dose of Luseogliflozin[4]

[4]  PMDA Database.    http://www.pmda.go.jp/drugs/2014/P201400033/index.html (accessed Mar 2016).

Table 9    *In Vivo* Pharmacokinetic Parameters of Luseogliflozin in Humans after Single Intravenous or
Oral Dose of Luseogliflozin Hydrate[4]

| Species | Route[a] | Dose (mg) | $T_{max}$ (h) | $C_{max}$ (ng/mL) | $AUC_{inf}$ (ng·h/mL) | $T_{1/2}$ (h) |
|---|---|---|---|---|---|---|
| Healthy human (male) | p.o. | 1 | 0.667 ± 0.289 | 38.2 ± 4.86 | 337 ± 51.9 | 10.4 ± 0.552 |
| | | 3 | 0.750 ± 0.267 | 116 ± 24.6 | 1000 ± 260 | 9.23 ± 0.950 |
| | | 5 | 1.06 ± 0.496 | 187 ± 27.3 | 1830 ± 322 | 9.72 ± 1.17 |
| | | 9 | 1.25 ± 0.598 | 312 ± 45.2 | 3050 ± 326 | 9.87 ± 0.72 |
| | | 15 | 1.56 ± 1.02 | 544 ± 143 | 5140 ± 834 | 13.8 ± 5.76 |
| | | 25 | 2.25 ± 1.46 | 721 ± 123 | 8510 ± 1180 | 12.6 ± 2.13 |

Table 10    *In Vitro* Permeability of [14C]Luseogliflozin in Caco-2 Cell Monolayer Model[9]

| Compound | Conc. (μM) | $Papp_{(A \to B)}$ ($1 \times 10^{-6}$ cm/s) | Permeability Class |
|---|---|---|---|
| Luseogliflozin | 10 | 14 | High |

## Distribution

Table 11    *In Vitro* Plasma Protein Binding and Blood Cell Partitioning of [14C]Luseogliflozin
in Different Species[4]

| Plasma Protein Binding (%) | | | Isolated Human Plasma Protein Binding (%) | | | | Blood Cell Partitioning (%) | | |
|---|---|---|---|---|---|---|---|---|---|
| Species | Conc. (ng/mL) | %Bound | Protein | Conc. (ng/mL) | %Bound | | Species | Conc. (ng/mL) | Blood Cell Association (%) |
| Mouse | 500-50000 | 94.0-94.4 | HSA | 50 | 95.3 ± 0.3 | | Human | 50-5000 | 4.8-6.9 |
| Rat | 50-50000 | 93.8-95.3 | | 500 | 95.4 ± 0.1 | | | | |
| Rabbit | 500-50000 | 95.6-95.9 | | 5000 | 95.5 ± 0.1 | | | | |
| Dog | 50-50000 | 91.7-95.6 | α-AGP | 50 | 53.8 ± 2.9 | | | | |
| Monkey | 50-5000 | 94.7-94.8 | | 500 | 47.8 ± 1.7 | | | | |
| Human | 50-5000 | 96.0-96.3 | | 5000 | 39.5 ± 1.0 | | | | |

Table 12    *In Vivo* Tissue Distribution of [14C]Luseogliflozin in Male
Rats after Single Oral Dose of 1 mg/kg of [14C]Luseogliflozin[4]

| Tissues | Radioactivity (ng eq./g) | | | | | Tissue/Blood $AUC_{0-168}$ Ratio |
|---|---|---|---|---|---|---|
| | 1 h | 6 h | 24 h | 72 h | 168 h | |
| Plasma | 190 | 48.6 | 6.92 | 2.28 | ND | 1.58 |
| Blood | 115 | 29.4 | 4.45 | 1.50 | 0.47 | 1.00 |
| Brain | 4.3 | 1.82 | ND | ND | ND | 0.04 |
| Heart | 121 | 33.3 | 2.13 | ND | ND | 0.85 |
| Lungs | 123 | 38.4 | 2.72 | ND | ND | 0.94 |
| Liver | 925 | 466 | 71.8 | 34.5 | 13.5 | 14.2 |
| Kidneys | 1184 | 914 | 279 | 122 | 54.3 | 36.1 |
| Stomach | 1490 | 530 | 7.37 | ND | ND | 11.2 |
| Small intestine | 2113 | 1306 | 53.6 | 6.69 | 1.17 | 24.6 |

[4]  PMDA Database.   http://www.pmda.go.jp/drugs/2014/P201400033/index.html (accessed Mar 2016).
[9]  Yamamoto, K.; Uchida, S.; Kitano, K., et al. *Br. J. Pharmacol.* **2011**, *164*, 181-191.

# Metabolism

Table 13    Metabolites of [$^{14}$C]Luseogliflozin in Frozen Hepatocytes of Different Species[4]

| Conc. (μM) | Species | % of Radioactivity[a] | | | | | | | | | | | | | | |
| | | Luseogliflozin | M1 | M2 | M3 | M4 | M5, M7 | M8 | M9 | M10 | M11 | M12 | M14, M17 | M15 | M16 | Others |
|---|---|---|---|---|---|---|---|---|---|---|---|---|---|---|---|---|
| 5 | Rat | 4.5 | 2.4 | 1.0 | 0.3 | - | 0.5 | 18.2 | - | 6.0 | - | 13.3[b] | 4.1 | 7.7 | 19.7 | 19.1 |
| | Dog | 83.6 | 0.2 | 7.8 | 1.6 | - | - | 2.0 | 2.8 | - | - | - | - | - | - | 2.0 |
| | Monkey | 15.1 | - | 3.5 | 0.8 | 0.1 | 2.8 | 66.8 | - | - | 0.6 | 3.4 | 0.8[c] | - | - | 5.3 |
| | Human | 92.0 | 0.2 | 2.1 | 0.8 | 0.1 | 0.5 | 0.2 | - | - | - | - | 1.0[c] | - | - | 2.4 |
| 50 | Rat | 28.9 | 2.7 | 7.2 | 0.6 | - | 1.6 | 21.2 | - | 2.0 | - | 4.8[b] | 4.5 | 5.8 | 4.6 | 9.6 |
| | Dog | 87.5 | 0.3 | 4.1 | 0.9 | - | - | 2.7 | 2.0 | - | - | - | - | - | - | 2.5 |
| | Monkey | 47.7 | 0.6 | 7.4 | 0.7 | 1.8 | 4.2 | 26.0 | - | - | 0.8 | 2.5 | 0.6[c] | - | - | 4.7 |
| | Human | 94.5 | 0.2 | 1.3 | 0.5 | 0.2 | 0.3 | 0.5 | - | - | - | - | 0.8[c] | - | - | 1.4 |

[a] The incubation time was 4 h.   [b] Contain unknown structure metabolite.   [c] Only M17.

## Key Findings:

Metabolic enzyme identification using recombinant human CYPs and UGTs:[4]

❖ rhCYP (100 pmol/mL), luseogliflozin (10 μM), incubated for 60 min:
- CYP1A1, 3A4 and 3A5 were mainly responsible for biotransformation of luseogliflozin to M2, besides, others (CYP1B1, 2B6, 2C8, 2C9, 2C19, 2D6, 2J2, 4A11, 4F3A and 4F12) were involved.
- CYP4A11, 4F2, 4F3A and 4F3B were mainly responsible for luseogliflozin metabolizing to M3.

❖ rhUGTs (1 mg protein/mL), luseogliflozin (5 μM), incubated for 60 min:
- UGT1A1 was mainly responsible for luseogliflozin metabolizing to M8, besides, others (UGT1A3, 1A4, 1A8 and 1A9) were involved.

❖ rhUGTs (1 mg protein/mL), M2 (5 μM), incubated for 60 min:
- UGT1A1, 1A8 and 1A9 were mainly responsible for biotransformation of M2 to M12, besides, others (UGT1A3, 1A6, 1A7, 1A10, 2B15 and 2B17) were involved.

Table 14    In Vitro Metabolic Phenotype of Luseogliflozin Using Specific Chemical Inhibitors[4]

| Enzymes | Test System | Incubation Time (min) | Substrate | Inhibitor | %Inhibition |
|---|---|---|---|---|---|
| CYP3A | Human liver microsomes (0.5 mg protein/mL) | 15 | Luseogliflozin (10 μM) | Ketoconazole (0.3, 1 μM) | 67.1-77.1 |
| All CYPs | | | | 1-Amino-benzotrazole (500 μM) | >74.8 |
| CYP4 family | | | | 17-Octadecynoic acid (1, 10 μM) | 7.5-50.8 |
| CYP4A11 | | | | Lauric acid (100 μM) | 23.9 |
| ADH | Human liver cytosol (1 mg protein/mL) | 60 | M3 (5 μM) | 4-methylpyrazole(1, 10, 100 μM) | 32-78.6 |
| ALDH | | | | Disulfiram (10, 100, 1000 μM) | 28.3-90.5 |

[4] PMDA Database.   http://www.pmda.go.jp/drugs/2014/P201400033/index.html (accessed Mar 2016).

Table 15    Metabolites in Plasma, Urine and Feces in Rats, Dogs and Monkeys after Single Oral Dose of Luseogliflozin[4]

| Matrix | Species | Dose (mg/kg) | Time (h) | % of Radioactivity or % of Dose | | | | | | | | | |
|---|---|---|---|---|---|---|---|---|---|---|---|---|---|
| | | | | Parent | M1 | M2 | M3 | M4 | M8 | M9 | M10 | M13 | M14, M17 |
| Plasma | Rat (male) | 1 | 1 | 19.9 | 2.1 | - | - | - | 53.9 | - | - | - | - |
| | Dog (male) | 1 | 1 | 76.7 | - | 5.0 | 3.7 | - | 3.4 | - | - | - | 7.2[b] |
| | Monkey (male) | 1 | 1 | 0.9 | - | - | - | - | 87.4 | - | - | - | - |
| | Human (male)[a] | 5 | 0-∞ | 2060 | 17.9 | 497 | 33.5 | - | √ | √ | - | - | 185 |
| Kidneys | Rat (male) | 1 | 1 | 43.8 | 5.4 | 7.4 | 2.0 | - | 1.8 | - | 3.9 | - | 3.9 |
| Liver | Rat (male) | 1 | 1 | 31.4 | 6.5 | - | - | - | 19.8 | - | - | - | 8.3 |
| Urine | Rat (male) | 1 | 0-24 | 0.1 | 0.1 | 0.3 | - | - | - | - | 0.4 | - | 0.5 |
| | Dog (male) | 1 | 0-24 | 0.8 | - | 4.8 | - | - | 1.1 | - | - | - | 5.3 |
| | Monkey (male) | 1 | 0-24 | 0.9 | - | - | - | - | 52.0 | - | - | - | - |
| | Human (male) | 1 | 0-24 | 3.37 | - | 5.25 | 0.454 | √ | √ | √ | - | - | 3.16 |
| Bile | Rat (male) | 1 | 1 | - | - | - | - | - | 34.6 | 2.0 | - | - | - |
| Feces | Rat (male) | 1 | 1 | 18.8 | 1.2 | 2.0 | 1.8 | 1.7 | - | - | - | 10.9 | 1.0 |
| | Dog (male) | 1 | 0-48 | 9.0 | 1.8 | 14.3 | 5.5 | - | - | - | - | - | 16 |
| | Monkey (male) | 1 | 0-24 | 9.8 | 0.7 | 2.1 | - | - | - | - | - | - | 0.3[b] |

% of radioactivity for plasma, kidneys and liver.    % of dose for urine and feces.    [a] The values was AUC (ng·h/mL) for plasma in humans.    [b] Only M17.

[4]    PMDA Database.    http://www.pmda.go.jp/drugs/2014/P201400033/index.html (accessed Mar 2016).

Figure E    Proposed Pathways for *In Vivo* Biotransformation of [14C]Luseogliflozin in Rats, Dogs, Monkeys and Humans[4]

The red labels represent the major components in matrices.    P = Plasma, U = Urine, F = Feces, B = Bile, L = Liver, K = Kidneys and GA = Glucuronic acid.

[4]  PMDA Database.    http://www.pmda.go.jp/drugs/2014/P201400033/index.html (accessed Mar 2016).

## Excretion

Table 16    Excretion Profiles of [$^{14}$C]Luseogliflozin in Rats, Dogs, Monkeys and Humans after Single Oral and Intravenous Dose of Luseogliflozin[4]

| Species | State | Vehicle | Route | Dose (mg/kg) | Time (h) | Urine (% of dose) | Feces (% of dose) | Bile (% of dose) | Recovery (% of dose) |
|---|---|---|---|---|---|---|---|---|---|
| Rat (male) | Intact | 0.5% CMC-Na | p.o. | 1 | 0-168 | 5.7 ± 0.0 | 93.4 ± 0.8 | NA | 99.1 ± 0.8 |
| | | 22.5% HP$\beta$CD | i.v. | 1 | 0-168 | 9.9 ± 0.8 | 82.6 ± 0.1 | NA | 92.5 ± 0.7 |
| Rat (male) | BDC | 0.5% CMC-Na | p.o. | 1 | 0-168 | 3.4 ± 1.1 | 6.2 ± 4.8 | 76.6 ± 6.2 | 86.1 ± 8.8 |
| | | 22.5% HP$\beta$CD | i.v. | 1 | 0-168 | 15.7 ± 13.5 | 2.4 ± 0.6 | 75.8 ± 14.0 | 94.0 ± 0.8 |
| Dog (male) | Intact | 0.5% CMC-Na | p.o. | 1 | 0-168 | 35.2 ± 1.7 | 65.1 ± 1.7 | NA | 100.2 ± 0.0 |
| | | 22.5% HP$\beta$CD | i.v. | 1 | 0-168 | 34.5 ± 1.2 | 59.5 ± 2.4 | NA | 94.0 ± 1.2 |
| Monkey (male) | Intact | 0.5% CMC-Na | p.o. | 1 | 0-168 | 66.5 ± 5.9 | 24.7 ± 6.9 | NA | 91.2 ± 4.0 |
| | | 22.5% HP$\beta$CD | i.v. | 1 | 0-168 | 75.4 ± 5.9 | 17.2 ± 7.3 | NA | 92.6 ± 2.4 |
| Healthy human[a] (male) | Intact | Tablet | p.o. | 2.5 | 0-72 | 20 | NA | NA | NA |

[a] Final application formulation.    Urinary Excretion components included luseogliflozin and metabolites (M2, M3 and M17) in healthy humans.

## Drug and Drug Interaction

Table 17    *In Vitro* Evaluation of Luseogliflozin Hydrate as an Inhibitor and an Inducer of CYP450 Enzymes[4]

| Luseogliflozin as an Inhibitor | | Luseogliflozin as an Inducer | | | |
|---|---|---|---|---|---|
| CYPs | IC$_{50}$ ($\mu$M) | CYPs | Conc. ($\mu$M) | Induction Rate (%)[a] | %Positive Control |
| CYP1A2 | >100 | 1A2 | 0.1 | 100 ± 4.7 | 0.0 ± 0.0 |
| CYP2A6 | >100 | | 1 | 105 ± 6.3 | 0.0 ± 0.0 |
| CYP2B6 | >100 | | 10 | 119 ± 12.4 | 0.1 ± 0.0 |
| CYP2C8 | >100 | 2B6 | 0.1 | 95.8 ± 11.0 | -0.6 ± 1.3 |
| CYP2C9 | >100 | | 1 | 96.8 ± 8.5 | -0.2 ± 0.7 |
| CYP2C19 | 58.3 | | 10 | 136 ± 24.3 | 3.3 ± 2.7 |
| CYP2D6 | >100 | 3A4 | 0.1 | 122 ± 23.3 | 4.2 ± 5.0 |
| CYP2E1 | >100 | | 1 | 149 ± 43.0 | 9.2 ± 8.5 |
| CYP3A4 | >100 | | 10 | 346 ± 123.2 | 56.9 ± 5.1 |

Table 18    *In Vitro* Evaluation of Luseogliflozin Hydrate as a Substrate of P-gp and BCRP[4]

| Substrate | Conc. ($\mu$M) | Inhibitor (Conc.) | Efflux Ratio | | | Substrate | Conc. ($\mu$M) | Efflux Ratio | | |
|---|---|---|---|---|---|---|---|---|---|---|
| | | | Control Cell | P-gp Expressed Cell | Ratio | | | Control Cell | BCRP Expressed Cell | Ratio |
| Luseogliflozin hydrate | 1 | No | 1.0 | 10.7 | 10.7 | Luseogliflozin hydrate | 1 | 1.73 | 1.67 | 0.965 |
| | | Verapamil (30 $\mu$M) | 0.9 | 2.0 | 2.2 | | | | | |
| | | Cyclosporin A (10 $\mu$M) | 1.0 | 1.0 | 1.0 | | | | | |
| Digoxin | 1 | No | 1.0 | 26.4 | 26.4 | Prazosin | 5 | 1.33 | 10.7 | 8.05 |

[4]    PMDA Database.    http://www.pmda.go.jp/drugs/2014/P201400033/index.html (accessed Mar 2016).

Table 19   *In Vitro* Evaluation of Luseogliflozin Hydrate as an Inhibitor of Efflux Transporters[4]

| Conc. (μM) | Inhibition of P-gp by Luseogliflozin[a] | | | | Inhibition of BCRP by Luseogliflozin[b] | | | |
|---|---|---|---|---|---|---|---|---|
| | Efflux Ratio | | Ratio | % of Control | Efflux Ratio | | Ratio | % of Control |
| | Control | P-gp Expressed Cell | | | Control | BCRP Expressed Cell | | |
| 0 | 1.7 | 30.8 | 18.1 | 100 | 1.18 | 9.93 | 8.42 | 100.0 |
| 1 | 1.9 | 28.9 | 15.2 | 84.0 | 1.18 | 8.61 | 7.3 | 86.7 |
| 3 | 1.4 | 30.4 | 21.7 | 119.9 | 1.33 | 8.47 | 6.37 | 75.7 |
| 10 | 1.4 | 25.4 | 18.1 | 100.0 | 1.17 | 9.19 | 7.85 | 93.2 |
| 30 | 1.1 | 19.3 | 17.5 | 96.7 | 1.06 | 9.1 | 8.58 | 101.9 |
| 100 | 0.9 | 10.4 | 11.6 | 64.1 | 1.07 | 6.88 | 6.43 | 76.4 |
| Positive control | 0.9 | 1.3 | 1.4 | 7.7 | 1.11 | 1.01 | 0.91 | 10.8 |

[a] The substrate was [³H]digoxin.   [b] The substrate was [³H]prazosin.

Table 20   *In Vitro* Evaluation of Luseogliflozin Hydrate as an Inhibitor of Uptake Transporters[4]

| Transporter | OATP1B1 | OATP1B3 | OAT1 | OAT3 | OCT2 |
|---|---|---|---|---|---|
| IC$_{50}$ (μM) | >100 | 93.1 | >100 | >100 | >100 |

# 6   Non-Clinical Toxicology

## Summary

### Single-Dose Toxicity

❖ Luseogliflozin exhibited low acute toxicity by the oral route in both rodent and non-rodent species:
  • Rat ALD: >2000 mg/kg.
  • Dog ALD: >1500 mg/kg.

### Repeated-Dose Toxicity

❖ Sub- and chronic toxicological risk in rats (up to 26 weeks), dogs (up to 52 weeks) and monkeys (up to 13 weeks).
  • Pronounced side reactions were noted at non-lethal dose levels in all tested species, including erosion of glandular stomach/duodenum (rat), lower body weight (rat, dog), and loose stools/diarrhea (dog).
  • Based on the longest studies employed, safety margin in rodents was much closer to or even below 1.0, while in non-rodents it was far beyond, i.e., 4.5- to 5.5-fold for dogs, 20.7- to 25.5-fold for monkeys.

### Safety Pharmacology

❖ No much special concern on CNS, cardiovascular, respiratory and gastrointestinal tract functions.

### Genotoxicity

❖ Luseogliflozin, M2 and M17 got least potential for mutagenicity, clastogenicity, or direct DNA damage, based on the standard battery of genotoxicity studies plus unscheduled DNA synthesis assay.

### Reproductive and Developmental Toxicity

❖ Rat fertility and early embryonic development: NOAEL = 300 mg/kg (male) and 100 mg/kg (female).
❖ Embryo-fetal development: Rat NOAEL = 50 mg/kg, while rabbit NOAEL = 1000 mg/kg.
❖ Pre- and postnatal development: NOAEL was determined as 50 mg/kg.
❖ Luseogliflozin distributed to placenta and fetus in pregnant rats, and migrated radioactivity was less than 0.1%.
❖ Milk excretion of luseogliflozin was also found in lactating rats, milk/plasma ratio at 1-24 h post-dose ranged from 0.27 to 1.54.

### Carcinogenicity

❖ No potential.

### Special toxicity

❖ Got no stimulation of human vascular endothelial cell proliferation or risk of phototoxicity, however, might led to difference in calcium metabolism.

---

[4]  PMDA Database.   http://www.pmda.go.jp/drugs/2014/P201400033/index.html (accessed Mar 2016).

## Single-Dose Toxicity

Table 21    Single-Dose Toxicity Studies of Luseogliflozin Hydrate by Oral Administrations[4]

| Species | Dose (mg/kg) | ALD (mg/kg) | Finding |
|---|---|---|---|
| SD rat | 500, 1000, 2000 | >2000 | Gastrointestinal reaction at all doses, e.g., loose stool, diarrhea, etc., which recovered at 2 days post-dose. TK: Rapid absorption after administration, $C_{max}$ and $AUC_{0-24}$ increased less than dose proportional. |
| Beagle dog (male) | 60, 300, 1500 | >1500 | Gastrointestinal reaction at all doses, e.g., vomiting, loose stool, watery diarrhea, etc. TK: Reaching $C_{max}$ at 2-4 h post-dose, and still detectable at 24 h post-dose. |

Vehicle: 0.5% CMC-Na.

## Repeated-Dose Toxicity

Table 22    Repeated-Dose Toxicity Studies of Luseogliflozin Hydrate[4]

| Species | Duration (Week) | Dose (mg/kg/day) | NOAEL Dose (mg/kg/day) | NOAEL $AUC_{0-24}$ (ng·h/mL) | NOAEL Safety Margin (× MRHD) | Finding |
|---|---|---|---|---|---|---|
| SD rat | 4 | 0, 4, 20, 100, 500 | Male: 4 Female: 20 | Male: 732; Female: 6490 | Male: 0.4 Female: 3.5 | 500 mg/kg/day male: 1 death on Day 25 post-dose, diarrhea; Female: Loose stool, diarrhea, cecal mucosa hyperplasia and ulcer. ≥100 mg/kg/day male: Loose stool; female: ↑ Cecal weight, dark red point on gastric glandular and gastric erosion. ≥20 mg/kg/day male: ↓ Body weight, dark red point on gastric glandular and gastric erosion. |
| | 13 | 0, 4, 20, 100 | Male: 4 Female: 20 | Male: 633; Female: 7430 | Male: 0.3 Female: 4.0 | No death; 100 mg/kg/day male: ↓ Body weight, female: dark red point on gastric glandular and gastric erosion. ≥20 mg/kg/day male: Dark red point on gastric glandular and gastric erosion. |
| | 26 | 0, 4, 20, 100 | Male: 4 Female: 4 | Male: 884; Female: 1700 | Male: 0.5; Female: 0.8 | 100 mg/kg/day male: 1 death on Day 17 withdrawal (accident deaths in the urination disorder) and duodenal erosions. ≥20 mg/kg/day male: ↓ Body weight, female and male: dark red point on gastric glandular and gastric erosion. |
| Beagle dog | 4 | 0, 0.4, 2, 10, 50 | Male: 2 Female: 2 | Male: 10600; Female: 8400 | Male: 5.6; Female: 4.6 | No death. ≥10 mg/kg/day: Loose stool, watery stool and ↓ body weight. |
| | 13 | 0, 0.4, 2, 10, 50 | 2 | Male: 9060; Female: 7790 | Male: 4.8; Female: 4.1 | No death. 50 mg/kg/day: ↓ RBC. ≥10 mg/kg/day male: Loose stool and ↓ body weight. |
| | 52 | 0, 0.4, 2, 10, 50 | 2 | Male: 8540; Female: 10400 | Male: 4.5; Female: 5.5 | No death. ≥10 mg/kg/day: Loose stool and ↓ body weight. |
| Monkey | 2 | 0, 30, 100, 300 | 300 | Male: 82000; Female: 58500 | Male: 43.6; Female: 31.1 | No death or severe toxicity. |
| | 13 | 0, 10, 30, 100, 300 | 300 | Male: 39000; Female: 47900 | Male: 20.7; Female: 25.5 | No death or severe toxicity. |

Vehicle: 0.5% CMC-Na.    Safety Margin was calculated with exposure of the $7_{th}$ day at 5 mg human clinical dose, $AUC_\tau = 1880$ ng·h/mL.

[4]  PMDA Database.    http://www.pmda.go.jp/drugs/2014/P201400033/index.html (accessed Mar 2016).

## Safety Pharmacology

Table 23    Summary of Safety Pharmacology Studies of Luseogliflozin Hydrate[4]

| Study | System | Dose[a] | NOAEL | Finding |
|---|---|---|---|---|
| CNS safety | SD rat | 1, 10, 100 mg/kg, p.o. | 100 mg/kg | No effect on behavior, locomotor activity; 100 mg/kg: ↓ Body temperature at 8 h post-dose. |
| Cardiovascular safety | hERG transfected HEK293 cell | 0.0886, 0.973, 9.59 µM | 9.59 µM | 7.7% Inhibition of hERG potassium current at 9.59 µM. |
| | Papillary muscle cardiac action potential test | 0.0972, 0.945, 9.27 µM | 9.27 µM | Negative. |
| | Conscious Beagle dog | 1, 3, 10 mg/kg, p.o. | 10 mg/kg | No effect on blood pressure, heart rate and ECG. |
| Respiratory safety | SD rat (whole body plethysmograph) | 1, 10, 100 mg/kg, p.o. | 10 mg/kg | 100 mg/kg: increase in tidal volume at 8 h post-dose, and then disappear at 24 h post-dose. |
| Gastrointestinal tract function | SD rat | 1, 10, 100 mg/kg, p.o. | 100 mg/kg | Negative. |

Vehicle: 0.5% CMC-Na for *in vivo* studies, 0.1% DMSO in perfusion medium for *in vitro* studies.

## Genotoxicity

Table 24    Genetic Toxicity Studies of Luseogliflozin Hydrate and Metabolites[4]

| Assay | System | Compound | Metabolism Activity | Dose | Finding |
|---|---|---|---|---|---|
| *In vitro* bacterial reverse mutation assay | *S. typhimurium* TA98, TA100, TA1535, TA1537; *E. coli* WP2uvTA | Luseogliflozin hydrate | ±S9 | 0-5000 µg/plate | Negative. |
| | | M2 | -S9 | | |
| | | M17 | -S9 | | |
| *In vitro* mammalian cell chromosomal aberration | L5178Y t/k[+/-] 3.7.2C | Luseogliflozin hydrate | ±S9 | 0-260 µg/mL | Positive: +S9. |
| | | M2 | -S9 | 0-406 µg/mL | Negative. |
| | | M17 | -S9 | 0-465 µg/mL | Negative. |
| *In vivo* micronucleus test in rat | SD rat | Luseogliflozin hydrate | + | 0-2000 mg/kg | Negative. |
| *In vivo*/*In vitro* measurement of unscheduled DNA synthesis | SD rat | Luseogliflozin hydrate | + | 0-2000 mg/kg | Negative. |

## Reproductive and Developmental Toxicity

Table 25    Reproductive and Developmental Toxicology Studies of Luseogliflozin Hydrate[4]

| Study | Species | Dose (mg/kg/day) | Endpoint | NOAEL | | |
|---|---|---|---|---|---|---|
| | | | | Dose (mg/kg/day) | $AUC_{0-24}$ (ng·h/mL) | Safety Margin[a] (× MRHD) |
| Fertility and early embryonic development | SD rat | 30, 100, 300 | $F_0$ male (fertility) | 300 | 158100 | 84 |
| | | | $F_0$ female (fertility) | 100 | 50500 | 27 |
| | | | $F_1$ fetus | 300 | 151500 | 81 |
| Embryo-fetal development | SD rat | 50, 150, 500 | Maternal | 150 | 88400 | 47 |
| | | | Developmental | 50 | 28200 | 15 |
| | NZW rabbit | 500, 750, 1000 | Maternal | 500 | 18800 | 10 |
| | | | Developmental | 1000 | 60200 | 32 |
| Pre- and postnatal development | SD rat | 15, 50, 150 | $F_0$ | 150 | 75750 | 40 |
| | | | $F_1$ | 50 | 25250 | 13 |

Vehicle: 0.5% MC.    [a] Calculated with exposure of the $7_{th}$ day at 5 mg human clinical dose, $AUC_\tau$ = 1880 ng·h/mL.

[4]  PMDA Database.   http://www.pmda.go.jp/drugs/2014/P201400033/index.html (accessed Mar 2016).

## Carcinogenic Toxicity

Table 26    Carcinogenic Toxicity Studies of Luseogliflozin Hydrate[4]

| Species | Duration (Week) | Dose (mg/kg/day) | NOAEL (mg/kg/day) | Finding |
|---|---|---|---|---|
| Mouse B6C3F1/Crlj | 104 | 0, 10, 30, 30, 100 | 100 | No carcinogenic toxicity.    Non-carcinogenic dose: 100 mg/kg. |
| SD rat | 104 | 0, 4, 20, 100 | Male: 20 (6.1 × MRHD) Female: 100 (59 × MRHD) | 100 mg/kg/day male: Adrenal pheochromocytoma, interstitial cell tumor of the testis. |

Vehicle: 0.5% MC.    Safety Margin was calculated with exposure of the $7_{th}$ day at 5 mg human clinical dose, $AUC_\tau = 1880$ ng·h/mL.

## Special Toxicity

Table 27    Other Toxicity Studies of Luseogliflozin Hydrate[4]

| Experiment | Dose (mg/kg) | Finding |
|---|---|---|
| *In vivo* calcium metabolism | 500 | ↑ Calcium absorption from the intestinal tract, and ↑ calcium excretion from urine; No changes in calcium absorption rate. |
| *In vitro* human vascular endothelial cell proliferation | 6.25, 12.5, 25, 50, 100 μM | Negative. |
| *In vivo* phototoxicity test | 100 | Negative. |

[4]  PMDA Database.    http://www.pmda.go.jp/drugs/2014/P201400033/index.html (accessed Mar 2016).

# CHAPTER

## 17

---

## Naloxegol Oxalate

# Naloxegol Oxalate

## (Movantik®/Moventig®)

Research code: NKTR-118

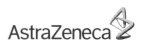

## 1 General Information

❖ Naloxegol is an opioid receptor antagonist, which was first approved in Sep 2014 by US FDA.

❖ Naloxegol was discovered by Nektar Therapeutics, developed and marketed by AstraZeneca.

❖ Naloxegol is a peripherally-acting μ-opioid receptor antagonist in the gastrointestinal tract with reduced CNS effects, thereby decreasing the constipating effects of opioids.

❖ Naloxegol is indicated for the treatment of opioid-induced constipation (OIC) in adult patients with chronic non-cancer pain.

❖ Available as tablet, with each containing 25 mg or 12.5 mg of naloxegol and the recommended dose is 25 mg once daily in the morning.

❖ The 2015 worldwide sale of Movantik®/Moventig® was 39 million US\$, referring to the financial reports of AstraZeneca and Daiichi-Sankyo.

### Key Approvals around the World*

|  | US (FDA) | EU (EMA) |
|---|---|---|
| First approval date | 09/16/2014 | 12/08/2014 |
| Application or approval No. | NDA 204760 | EMEA/H/C/002810 |
| Brand name | Movantik® | Moventig® |
| Indication | Opioid-induced constipation | Opioid-induced constipation |
| Authorisation holder | AstraZeneca | AstraZeneca |

*Till Mar 2016, it had not been approved by PMDA (Japan) and CFDA (China).

## Active Ingredient

*Molecular formula*: $C_{34}H_{53}NO_{11} \cdot C_2H_2O_4$
*Molecular weight*: 741.82
*CAS No.*: 854601-70-0 (Naloxegol)
1354744-91-4 (Naloxegol oxalate)
*Chemical name*: (5α,6α)-17-Allyl-6-(2,5,8,11,14,17, 20-heptaoxadocosan-22-yloxy)-4,5-epoxymorphinan-3, 14-diol oxalate

*Parameters of Lipinski's "Rule of 5"*

| MW[a] | $H_D$ | $H_A$ | FRB[b] | PSA[b] | cLogP[b] |
|---|---|---|---|---|---|
| 651.78 | 2 | 12 | 26 | 127Å$^2$ | -0.94 ± 0.85 |

[a] Molecular weight of naloxegol. [b] Calculated by ACD/Labs software V11.02.

## Drug Product*

*Dosage route*: Oral
*Strength*: 12.5 mg/25 mg (Naloxegol)
*Dosage form*: Tablet
*Inactive ingredient*: Mannitol, cellulose microcrystalline, croscarmellose sodium, magnesium stearate and propyl gallate, hypromellose, titanium dioxide, polyethylene glycol, iron oxide red and iron oxide black.
*Recommended dose*: 25 mg once daily; if not tolerated, reduce to 12.5 mg once daily.
Patients with renal impairment (CLcr <60 mL/min): 12.5 mg once daily; Increase to 25 mg once daily if tolerated and monitor for adverse reactions.

* Sourced from US FDA drug label information

## 2  Key Patents Information

### Summary

❖ Movantik® (Naloxegol oxalate) has got five-year NCE market exclusivity protection after it was initially approved by US FDA on Sep 16, 2014.

❖ Naloxegol was originally developed by Nektar Therapeutics and then licensed to AstraZeneca, and its compound patent application was filed as PCT application by Nektar Therapeutics in 1999.

❖ The compound patent will expire in 2019 foremost, which has been granted in the United States, Japan, Europe and China, successively.

Table 1    Naloxegol's Compound Patent Protection in Drug-Mainstream Country

| Country | Publication/Patent NO. | Application Date | Granted Date | Estimated Expiry Date |
|---------|------------------------|------------------|--------------|-----------------------|
| WO | WO2005058367A2 | 12/16/2004 | / | / |
| US | US7786133B2 | 12/16/2004 | 08/31/2010 | 12/19/2027[a] |
| EP | EP1694363B1 | 12/16/2004 | 01/22/2014 | 12/16/2024 |
| JP | JP4991312B2 | 12/16/2004 | 08/01/2012 | 12/16/2024 |
| CN | CN101805343B | 12/16/2004 | 04/16/2014 | 12/16/2024 |

[a] The term of this patent is extended by 1098 days.

Table 2    Originator's International Patent Application List (Patent Family)

| Publication NO. | Title | Applicant/Assignee/Owner | Publication Date |
|-----------------|-------|--------------------------|------------------|
| **Technical Subjects** | **Active Ingredient (Free Base)'s Formula or Structure and Preparation** | | |
| WO2005058367A2 | Chemically modified small molecules | Nektar Therapeutics | 06/30/2005 |
| **Technical Subjects** | **Salt, Crystal, Polymorphic, Solvate (Hydrate), Isomer, Derivative Etc. and Preparation** | | |
| WO2008057579A2 | Dosage forms and co-administration of an opioid agonist and an opioid antagonist | Nektar Therapeutics | 05/15/2008 |
| WO2012044243A1 | Crystalline naloxol-PEG conjugate | AstraZeneca | 04/05/2012 |
| **Technical Subjects** | **Indication or Methods for Medical Needs** | | |
| WO2009137086A1 | Oral administration of peripherally-acting opioid antagonists | Nektar Therapeutics | 11/12/2009 |

The data was updated until Jan 2016.

# 3　Chemistry

## Route 1:　Original Discovery Route

*Synthetic Route*:　In this original synthetic route, oxidation of thebaine **1** employing aqueous $H_2O_2$ in formic acid provided 14-hydroxy ketone **2** in 86% yield.　Next, selectively catalytic hydrogenation of unsaturated ketone **2** offered the corresponding saturated ketone **3** in 95% yield.　Quantitative acetylation of tertiary alcohol and the subsequent *N*-demethylation with BrCN in chloroform yielded the *N*-cyano derivative **5** in 93% yield.　*N*-cyano ketone **5** in refluxing 20% HBr went successively through deacetylation, hydrolysis of cyano, and decarboxylation to lead to the desired secondary amine **6** in 91% yield, which upon smooth *N*-allylation and saltification gave the key intermediate naloxone hydrochloride **8**, in which the free phenol was treated with methoxyethyl chloride in the presence of Huenig's base to give the protected ketone **9**.　Reduction of the ketone **9** with sodium borohydride exclusively provided the alcohol **10** in 92% yield over two steps.　Deprotonation of the alcohol with sodium hydride followed by alkylation with *m*PEG$_7$-Br **11** provided the pegylated intermediate **12**.　Acidic removal of the methoxyethyl ether protecting group followed by isolation *via* a silica gel column furnished a mixture of α- and β-epimers (3:7) of naloxegol in 56% yield over three steps.　The ultimate treatment with oxalic acid and succedent crystallization provided naloxegol oxalate in good yield.[1-8]

[1]　Aaslund, B. L.; Aurell, C.; Bohlin, M. H., et al. WO2012044243A1, **2012**.
[2]　Aaslund, B. L.; Aurell, C.; Bohlin, M. H., et al. US20150038524A1, **2015**.
[3]　Bentley, M. D.; Viegas, T. X.; Goodin, R. R., et al. WO2005058367A2, **2005**.
[4]　Bentley, M. D.; Viegas, T. X.; Goodin, R. R., et al. US7786133B2, **2010**.
[5]　Fishburn, C. S.; Lechuga-Ballesteros, D.; Viegas, T., et al. US20060182692A1, **2006**.
[6]　Fishburn, C. S.; Lechuga-Ballesteros, D.; Viegas, T., et al. US8067431B2, **2011**.
[7]　Qiu, Z.; Zheng, Y.; Lu, M., et al. CN101033228A, **2007**.
[8]　Zheng, Y.; Lu, M.; Wang, X., et al. *Fudan Univ. J. Med. Sci.* **2007**, *34*, 888-890.

# 4　Pharmacology

## Summary

*Mechanism of Action and In Vitro Efficacy*

❖ As a PEGylated derivative of naloxone, naloxegol binds to μ-opioid receptors in the gastrointestinal tract, thereby decreasing the constipating effects of opioid.

❖ Naloxegol acts as an antagonist of μ- ($K_i$ = 33.8 nM) and δ-opioid receptors ($K_i$ = 53.5 nM), as well as a weak partial agonist at κ-opioid receptors ($K_i$ = 186.5 nM).

❖ Naloxegol is a substrate of the P-gp transporter, which reduces its ability to cross the blood-brain barriers, resulting in reduction of CNS effects.[9]

❖ Naloxegol had no significant activity in radioligand binding and enzyme assays in a panel of 327 receptors, ion channels, transporters and enzymes at 10 μM or in a panel of 7 cardiac ion channels up to 100 μM, except μ-, δ- and κ- and other 7 receptors.[9, 10]

❖ *In vitro* antagonism at μ-opioid receptors expressed in cells:
  • In CHO-K1 cells: $pA_2$ = 7.95 and $IC_{50}$ = 11 nM.
  • In membranes from HEK293 cells:
    ◆ $pIC_{50}$ = 6.64 (DAMGO).
    ◆ $pIC_{50}$ = 7.25 (morphine).

❖ *In vitro* partial agonism at κ-opioid receptors:
  • Receptors expressed in HEK293 cells: $EC_{50}$ = 47 nM.
  • Contraction of rabbit vas deferens: No effect at 10 μM.

❖ *In vitro* antagonism at δ-opioid receptors expressed in CHO cells: $IC_{50}$ = 886 nM.

*In Vivo Efficacy*

❖ Morphine-induced charcoal meal delay in gastrointestinal transit model in rats:
  • Reversal of the morphine effect: $ED_{50}$ = 23.1 mg/kg and complete at 90 mg/kg.

❖ In an morphine-induced analgesia model in rats:
  • $ED_{50}$ = 55.4 nM and $ED_{50}$_Analgesia/$ED_{50}$_GI = 2.4.

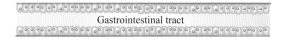
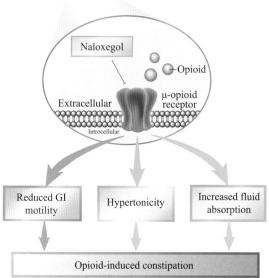

## Mechanism of Action and *In Vitro* Efficacy

Table 3　Binding Affinity of Naloxegol at Opioid Receptors Expressed in CHO Cells[9]

| Opioid Receptor | Source | Displacement probe | Naloxegol[a] $K_i$ (nM) | Naloxone | | MTNX | |
|---|---|---|---|---|---|---|---|
| | | | | $K_i$ (nM) | Naloxegol (fold change)[b] | $K_i$ (nM) | Naloxegol (fold change)[c] |
| Mu | Human recombinant | [³H]Naloxone | 33.8 | 1.7 | ↓ 20.1 | - | - |
| | | [³H]Naloxone | 77.3 | - | - | 8.46 | ↓ 9.1 |
| | | [³H]Diprenorphine | 7.42 | - | - | 22.1 | ↑ 3.0 |
| Kappa | Human recombinant | [³H]Naloxone | 186.5 | 4.0 | ↓ 46.6 | - | - |
| | | [³H]Naloxone | 230 | - | - | 130 | ↓ 1.8 |
| | Rat recombinant | [³H]U69593 | 203 | - | - | 1900 | ↑ 9.4 |
| Delta | Human recombinant | [³H]DPDPE | 53.5 | 10.3 | ↓ 5.2 | - | - |
| | | [³H]DPDPE | 52.1 | - | - | 247 | ↑ 4.7 |
| | | [³H]DADLE | 8.65 | - | - | 10.9 | ↑ 1.25 |

MTNX: (Methylnaltrexone), a marketed peripherally-acting μ-opioid receptor antagonist.　Diprenorphine: Opioid receptor antagonist.　U69593: κ-opioid receptor agonist.　DPDPE: A δ-opioid receptor agonist.　"-": Not detected.　[a] Values from different experiments.　[b] Fold change in affinity between naloxone and naloxegol, ↓ $K_i$_Naloxegol/$K_i$_Naloxone (or MTNX), ↑ $K_i$_ Naloxone (or MTNX)/$K_i$_Naloxegol.　[c] Fold change in affinity between MTNX and naloxegol.

[9]　U.S. Food and Drug Administration (FDA) Database.　http://www.accessdata.fda.gov/drugsatfda_docs/nda/2014/204760Orig1s000PharmR.pdf (accessed Mar 2016).

[10]　European Medicines Agency (EMA) Database.　http://www.ema.europa.eu/docs/en_GB/document_library/EPAR_-_Public_assessment_report/human/002810/WC500179077.pdf (accessed Mar 2016).

Table 4    *In Vitro* Function of Naloxegol at Human Opioid Receptors[9, 10]

| Opioid Receptor | System | Assay | Test Probe | Endpoint | Result Naloxegol | Control | Finding |
|---|---|---|---|---|---|---|---|
| Mu | CHO-K1 cells expressing receptors | [$^{35}$S]GTPγS binding assay | Agonist: morphine[a] | $pA_2$ | $7.95 \pm 0.11$ | $7.43 \pm 0.02$ | Control: MTX. 3.4-fold more potency. Effect: Antagonism. |
| | | | | $K_B$ (nM) | 11 | 37 | |
| | Membranes from HEK293 cells with transfected receptors | [$^{35}$S]GTPγS binding assay | DAMGO[b] | $pIC_{50}$ | $6.64 \pm 0.05$ | $7.30 \pm 0.08$ | Control: Naloxone. Effect: Full antagonism. |
| | | | Morphine[b] | $pIC_{50}$ | $7.25 \pm 0.15$ | $7.95 \pm 0.08$ | |
| Kappa | HEK293 cells expressing receptors | [$^{35}$S]GTPγS binding assay | NA[c] | $EC_{50}$ (nM) | 47 | - | Control: U69593. Effect: Partial agonist. |
| | | | | Max response | 39% | - | |
| | Rabbit vas deferens | Field-stimulated | Twitch contraction[d] | $IC_{50}$ (nM) | No effect at 10 μM | 33 | Control: U69593. Effect: No agonist activity. |
| Delta | CHO cells expressing receptors | [$^{35}$S]GTPγS binding assay | DPDPE[b] | $IC_{50}$ (nM) | 866 | - | Control: None. Effect: Antagonism. |

DAMGO: [D-Ala2, NMe-Phe4, Glyol5]-enkephalin.   [a] Antagonism of naloxegol on morphine binding to the receptor.   [b] Naloxegol inhibited test probe activity.   [c] Induced a concentration-dependent increase in the binding of [$^{35}$S]GTPγS.   [d] Decrease in the twitch contraction amplitude.

## *In Vivo* Efficacy

Table 5    *In Vivo* Efficacy of Naloxegol in Animal Models after a Single Administration[9, 10]

| Study | Animal model Animal | Test | Compound | Dose (mg/kg, p.o.) | Effect $ED_{50}$ (mg/kg) | Finding |
|---|---|---|---|---|---|---|
| Morphine-induced delay in gastrointestinal transit[a] (peripheral effects) | SD rat (male) | The meal travelled distance | Naloxegol | 10, 30, 90 | 23.1 | Complete inhibition of morphine effect at 90 mg/kg. |
| | | | Naloxone | 10 | 0.71 | Complete inhibition of morphine effect at 10 mg/kg. |
| Morphine-induced analgesia[b] (CNS effects) | SD rat (male) | Latency for hind paw withdrawal | Naloxegol | 10, 30, 90 | 55.4 | Partial reversal of analgesia at 90 mg/kg. $ED_{50}$_Analgesia/ $ED_{50}$_GI: 2.4. |
| | | | Naloxone | 1, 3, 10, 30 | 1.14 | Partial reversal of analgesia at 1 mg/kg, complete reverse at 10 mg/kg. $ED_{50}$_Analgesia/ $ED_{50}$_GI: 1.6. |

GI: Gastrointestinal.   [a] Rats were administered morphine (10 mg/kg, i.v.) 5 min prior to oral administration of compounds or saline.   A 1 mL charcoal meal suspension was given to rats by gavage 25 min later.   Rats were sacrificed at 30 min after the meal, and the charcoal meal travelled distance in GI tract and the total intestinal length were measured.   [b] Rats were administered morphine (5 mg/kg, i.v.) prior to oral administration of compounds or saline, hot plate stimulated hind paws 30 min later, and measured the latency for hind paw withdrawal.

[9]  FDA Database.   http://www.accessdata.fda.gov/drugsatfda_docs/nda/2014/204760Orig1s000PharmR.pdf (accessed Mar 2016).
[10]  EMA Database. http://www.ema.europa.eu/docs/en_GB/document_library/EPAR_-_Public_assessment_report/human/002810/WC500179077.pdf (accessed Mar 2016).

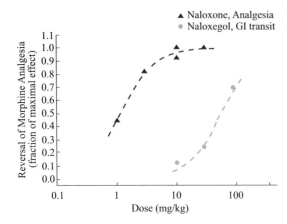

**Study:** Effects of naloxegol in rats of morphine-induced analgesia and gastrointestinal transit.

**Animal:** Sprague-Dawley rat, male.

**Model:** Morphine (10 mg/kg in GI transit and 5 mg/kg in analgesia, i.v.) prior to naloxegol administration; In GI transit, a charcoal meal given by gavage 25 min later; In analgesia, hot plate stimulus the hind paw 30 min later.

**Administration:** Naloxegol (10, 30, or 90 mg/kg) p.o., naloxone (10 mg/kg) in GI transit and (1, 3, 10, or 30 mg/kg) in analgesia p.o., vehicle (saline).

**Test:** Meal travelled distance in GI transit models and latency for hind paw withdrawal in analgesia models.

**Result:** There was only a limited separation of the desired antagonism of peripheral GI opioid receptors and undesired antagonism of CNS opioid receptors in rats.

Figure A    Dose-Response Relationship for Reversal of Morphine Effects in the GI tract and CNS for Naloxegol in Rats after a Single Admininstration[9]

# 5    ADME & Drug-Drug Interaction

## Summary

### Absorption of Naloxegol

❖ The increase in $AUC_{inf}$ appeared to be dose-proportional in humans in the dose range of 12.5 to 100 mg naloxegol, but $C_{max}$ was slightly more than dose-proportional after oral dose administration.

❖ Had low oral bioavailability in dogs (20.6%) and monkeys (2.26%).

❖ Was absorbed rapidly with the $T_{max}$ occurring 0.5 to 1 h in non-clinical species and humans.

❖ Showed a half-life ranging between 6.1-8 h in humans, shorter than that in dogs (9.58 h), but longer than that in monkeys (2.77 h) after oral administrations.

❖ Had high clearance in rats (2.65 L/h/kg), monkeys (1.46 L/h/kg) and dogs (2.65 L/h/kg), in contrast to liver blood flow, after intravenous administrations.   The clearance of naloxegol in humans was 158-174 L/h after oral administration.

❖ Exhibited an extensive tissue distribution in rats, dogs and monkeys, with apparent volumes of distribution at 3.14, 4.66 and 2.44 L/kg, respectively, after intravenous administrations.   The apparent volume of distribution in humans was 1550 L after oral administration.

❖ Showed a low permeability, with a $Papp_{(A \to B)}$ of $0.7 \times 10^{-6}$ cm/s in Caco-2 cell monolayer model, but exhibited moderate intestinal permeability.

### Distribution of Naloxegol Oxalate

❖ Exhibited low plasma protein binding in humans (4.2%), rats (14.1%), mice (20.8%), dogs (3.8%-53.3%) and monkeys (9.7%).

❖ Naloxegol had a low CNS penetration with a much lower uptake rate into the brain (4.1 pmol/g brain/sec).

❖ Pigmented male and albino female rats after single oral administrations:

• The drug was well distributed into most tissues except for the central nervous system (CNS) since the blood-brain barrier was crossed by a very small extent.

• Relatively higher concentration levels were observed in uveal tract, liver, kidneys and glandular tissues.

• In pigmented rats, the concentration of naloxegol in skin, eyes and uveal tract persisted up to 504 h, indicating naloxegol was likely bound to melanin.

• In albino females, radioactivity was widely distributed into all tissues including liver, kidneys, small intestine wall, placenta and uterus.

• A sex difference was observed in the female rats, i.e. an earlier $T_{max}$ and higher concentrations than males.

• By 48 h, the concentrations of radioactivity were low in the majority of tissues.

### Metabolism of Naloxegol Oxalate

❖ The metabolism of naloxegol was high in human and non-clinical hepatocytes.

❖ The major metabolites of naloxegol in human plasma were N-dealkylation (M1) and oxidative metabolism of the PEG chain (M7, M10, and M13), including partial cleavage but not complete removal of the chain.

[9] FDA Database.   http://www.accessdata.fda.gov/drugsatfda_docs/nda/2014/204760Orig1s000PharmR.pdf (accessed Mar 2016).

❖ All the metabolites found in humans could be found in other species. Glucuronide conjugation at the phenol hydroxyl was also a common process in animals and man but the naloxegol glucuronide showed very low concentrations in the human plasma.

❖ Naloxegol was predominantly metabolized by CYP3A4 with a minor contribution of CYP2D6.

## Excretion of Naloxegol Oxalate

❖ Was predominantly excreted in feces in all species, with parent as the major component in human and rat feces, but M10 in dog feces.

❖ About 66% of naloxegol was recovered *via* biliary excretion in bile duct-cannulated (BDC) rats, with M1 and M2 as the major components in rat bile.

## Drug-Drug Interaction

❖ Naloxegol was a weak inhibitor of CYP2D6 ($IC_{50}$ = 84.7 μM). Naloxegol had no inhibition for CYP1A2, 2C9 or 2C19.

❖ Time-dependent inhibition was observed at 50 μM for CYP3A4/5 (%inhibition = 24.3), but no time-dependent inhibition for CYP1A2, 2C9, 2C19 or 2D6.

❖ Naloxegol was not an inducer of CYP450 (CYP3A4, CYP2B6 or CYP1A2).

❖ Naloxegol was a substrate of P-gp and BCRP, but had no inhibition for P-gp or BCRP.

❖ Naloxegol was a substrate of OATP1B1, OATP1B3, but had no inhibition for OATP1B1, OATP1B3, OAT1, OAT3 or OCT2.

# Absorption

Table 6　*In Vivo* Pharmacokinetic Parameters of Naloxegol in Rats, Monkeys and Dogs after Single Intravenous and Oral Doses of Naloxegol[9]

| Species | Route | Dose (mg/kg) | $T_{max}$ (h) | $C_{max}$ (ng/mL) | $AUC_{inf}$ (ng·h/mL) | $T_{1/2}$ (h) | Cl (L/h/kg) | $V_{ss}$ (L/kg) | F (%) |
|---|---|---|---|---|---|---|---|---|---|
| SD rat (male) | i.v. | 10, 30, 100 | NA | NA | NA | 2.92 | 2.65 | 3.14 | NA |
| Beagle dog (male & female) | i.v. | 0.4 | NA | NA | NA | 5.7 | 2.65 | 4.66 | NA |
| | p.o. | 50 | 0.5 | 1530 | 3740 | 9.58 | NA | NA | 20.6 |
| Cynomolgus monkey (male) | i.v. | 1.0 | NA | NA | NA | 4.99 | 1.46 | 2.44 | NA |
| | p.o. | 5 | 0.69 | 41.6 | 78.1 | 2.77 | NA | NA | 2.26 |

Table 7　*In Vivo* Pharmacokinetic Parameters of Naloxegol in Humans after Single Oral Dose of Naloxegol[11]

| Species | Dose (mg) | $T_{max}$ (h) | $C_{max}$ (ng/mL) | $AUC_{inf}$ (ng·h/mL) | $T_{1/2}$ (h) | Cl/F (L/h) | $V_{ss}$/F (L) |
|---|---|---|---|---|---|---|---|
| Healthy human (male & female) | 25 | 1 (0.25-5.0) | 43 ± 18.6 | 178 ± 74 | 7.6 ± 6.2 | 163 ± 68 | 1550 ± 822 |
| | 12.5 | NA | 19 ± 5 | 86 ± 33 | 7.8 ± 3.14 | 158 ± 41 | NA |
| | 25 | NA | 46 ± 20 | 158 ± 42 | 7.7 ± 2.8 | 168 ± 43 | NA |
| | 50 | NA | 152 ± 94 | 371 ± 166 | 8.0 ± 3.7 | 174 ± 110 | NA |
| | 100 | NA | 375 ± 418 | 847 ± 483 | 6.1 ± 2.4 | 159 ± 93 | NA |

[9] FDA Database. http://www.accessdata.fda.gov/drugsatfda_docs/nda/2014/204760Orig1s000PharmR.pdf (accessed Mar 2016).
[11] FDA Database. http://www.accessdata.fda.gov/drugsatfda_docs/nda/2014/204760Orig1s000ClinPharm.pdf (accessed Mar 2016).

Table 8    *In Vitro* Permeability Study of Naloxegol in Caco-2 Cell Model and Jejunal Perfusion Model[9, 11]

| Compound | Caco-2 Cell Model | | | Jejunal Perfusion Model | | | |
|---|---|---|---|---|---|---|---|
| | Papp (1 × 10⁻⁶cm/s) | | Efflux Ratio | Conc. (mg/mL) | Peff (1× 10⁻⁴cm/s) | | Naloxegol/ Metoprolol |
| | A→B | B→A | | | Naloxegol | Metoprolol | |
| Naloxone | 27.3 | 25.0 | 0.91 | 2.0 | 0.143 ± 0.312 | 0.232 ± 0.323 | 0.420 |
| Naloxegol | 0.7 | 8.4 | 15.4 | 0.2 | 0.105 ± 0.180 | 0.303 ± 0.12 | 0.319 |
| Naloxegol + CsA | 1.8 | 1.8 | 1.0 | 0.02 | 0.065 ± 0.089 | 0.166 ± 0.076 | 0.471 |
| Naloxegol + Verapamil | 1.3 | 1.7 | 1.3 | | | | |
| Naloxegol + Elacridar | 2.3 | 2.5 | 1.1 | | | | |

Inhibitor: CsA (10 µM), verapamil (100 µM), and elacridar (0.5 µM).   Metoprolol perfusion concentration was 0.068 mg/mL.

## Distribution

Table 9    *In Vitro* Plasma Protein Binding of Naloxegol in Several Species[9-11]

| Conc. (µM) | %Bound | | | | |
|---|---|---|---|---|---|
| | SD Rat | CD1 Mouse | Beagle Dog | Cynomolgus Monkey | Human |
| 1.5, 15, 150 | 14.1 | 20.8 | 53.3, 29.5, 3.8[a] | 9.7 | 4.2 |

[a] Mean value from 15 to 150 µM.

Table 10    *In Vitro* Blood-Brain Permeability of Naloxegol Using an *In Situ* Brain Perfusion Technique in Rat[9]

| Compound | Naloxone | Naloxegol | Antipyrine (high permeability) | Atenolol (low permeability) |
|---|---|---|---|---|
| Mean brain uptake rate (pmol/g brain/sec) | 60.2 ± 13.7 | 4.1 ± 1.4 | 28.2 ± 14.3 | 5.2 ± 2.2 |

Table 11    *In Vivo* Tissue Distribution of [¹⁴C]Naloxegol in Pigmented Rats after Single Oral Dose of 50 mg/kg [¹⁴C]Naloxegol[9]

| Species | Pigmented Rat/Male | | | | | Pigmented Rat/Female | | | | |
|---|---|---|---|---|---|---|---|---|---|---|
| Tissue | Radioactivity (µg eq./g) | | | | | Tissue | Radioactivity (µg eq./g) | | | |
| | 0.5 h | 4 h | 24 h | 48 h | 504 h | | 0.5 h | 4 h | 24 h | 48 h |
| Blood | 3.03 | 2.14 | ND | ND | ND | Blood | 12.4 | 6.92 | ND | ND |
| Brain | 0.1 | 0.14 | ND | ND | ND | Brain | 0.34 | 0.28 | ND | ND |
| Kidneys | 31.6 | 27.6 | 1.44 | 1.13 | ND | Kidneys | 67.0 | 49.3 | 1.13 | 0.66 |
| Liver | 43.4 | 58.7 | 4.61 | 7.74 | ND | Liver | 68.7 | 58.8 | 4.42 | 2.68 |
| Uveal tract | 44.5 | 156 | 102 | 47.4 | 43.0 | Uveal tract | 15.3 | 17.4 | 2.94 | 1.16 |
| Skin (pigmented) | 1.80 | 6.20 | 7.88 | 3.92 | 2.11 | Skin | 3.41 | 5.37 | 0.29 | 0.14 |
| Eyes | 6.99 | 41.4 | 37.0 | 9.39 | 23.8 | Eyes | 2.46 | 4.17 | 0.77 | 0.23 |
| Small intestine wall | 9.59 | 31.1 | ND | ND | ND | Small intestine wall | 42.3 | 35.7 | ND | ND |
| Salivary gland | 28.6 | 9.51 | 0.30 | ND | ND | Placenta | 21.1 | 14.8 | 0.16 | 0.06 |
| Thyroid gland | 14.3 | 16.0 | 2.27 | 1.26 | ND | Uterus wall | 31.2 | 185 | 19.0 | 4.00 |

[9]  FDA Database.   http://www.accessdata.fda.gov/drugsatfda_docs/nda/2014/204760Orig1s000PharmR.pdf (accessed Mar 2016).
[10] EMA Database.   http://www.ema.europa.eu/docs/en_GB/document_library/EPAR_-_Public_assessment_report/human/002810/WC500179077.pdf (accessed Mar 2016).
[11] FDA Database.   http://www.accessdata.fda.gov/drugsatfda_docs/nda/2014/204760Orig1s000ClinPharm.pdf (accessed Mar 2016).

# Metabolism

Table 12   *In Vitro* Metabolic Stability of Naloxegol in Human CYP450 Isoforms[9]

| CYPs | Compound | $T_{1/2}$ (min) | % Parent Remaining | | | | | |
|------|----------|-----------------|--------|-------|--------|--------|--------|----------------|
| | | | 0-min | 5-min | 15-min | 30-min | 45-min | 45-min Control |
| 1A2 | Naloxegol | ND | 100 | 100 | 99.4 | 104 | 94.2 | 103 |
| | Naloxone | ND | 100 | 99.8 | 101 | 107 | 94.6 | 108 |
| 2C9 | Naloxegol | ND | 100 | 106 | 99.7 | 100 | 98.5 | 110 |
| | Naloxone | 145 | 100 | 97.7 | 86.8 | 81.3 | 82.0 | 103 |
| 2C19 | Naloxegol | ND | 100 | 101 | 98.8 | 98.7 | 99.6 | 99.3 |
| | Naloxone | 12.5 | 100 | 78 | 41.1 | 19.3 | 17.0 | 105 |
| 2D6 | Naloxegol | ND | 100 | 103 | 95.3 | 97.4 | 101 | 103 |
| | Naloxone | 229 | 100 | 96 | 90.0 | 90.4 | 85.7 | 96.8 |
| 3A4 | Naloxegol | 5.94 | 100 | 56.5 | 12.0 | 3.21 | 1.96 | 103 |
| | Naloxone | 53.9 | 100 | 92.6 | 80.5 | 69.5 | 55.0 | 102 |
| 2C8 | Naloxegol | ND | 100 | 101 | 102 | 99.1 | 101 | 104 |
| | Naloxone | 120 | 100 | 96.3 | 81.9 | 80.0 | 77.1 | 93.7 |

Table 13   Metabolites in the *In Vitro* Hepatocytes and *In Vivo* Plasma, Urine, Bile and Feces in Humans and Non-clinical Test Species after Single Oral Doses of Naloxegol[9-11]

| Matrix | Species | Route | Dose (mg/kg) | Time (h) | % of Dose | | | | | | | | | | | |
|--------|---------|-------|--------------|----------|------|------|------|------|------|------|------|------|------|------|------|------|
| | | | | | M0 | M1 | M2 | M4 | M6 | M7 | M10 | M12 | M13 | M25 | M26 | M47 |
| Hepat-ocyte[a] | Mouse | *In vitro* | 10 µM | 2 | NA | 15.1 | 28.9 | 5.3 | 17.3 | 9.0 | - | - | 5.7 | BLD | - | - |
| | Rat | | | 2 | NA | 31.3 | 31.5 | 2.9 | 11.8 | 6.5 | - | - | 3.6 | BLD | - | - |
| | Dog | | | 2 | NA | 3.9 | 70.8 | 0.8 | 1.83 | 3.1 | - | - | 0.19 | 2.5 | - | - |
| | Monkey | | | 2 | NA | 27.3 | 1.52 | 23.8 | 13.5 | 5.8 | - | - | 3.35 | BLD | - | - |
| | Human | | | 2 | NA | 21.8 | 0.97 | BLD | 17.4 | 16.4 | - | - | 13.5 | BLD | - | - |
| Plasma[b] | Rat | p.o. | 50 | 1-24 | 15.4 | √ | 5 | √ | - | √ | √ | √ | √ | - | - | - |
| | Dog | p.o. | 50 | 1 | 8.3 | √ | 62 | √ | - | √ | √ | √ | √ | - | 12 | 18 |
| | Human | p.o. | 25 mg | 4 | 64 | 5.5 | - | √ | - | 8.2 | 12 | - | 10 | - | - | - |
| Urine | Rat | p.o. | 50 | 0-72 | 7.4 | 0.3 | 2.4 | √ | - | √ | √ | √ | √ | - | - | - |
| | Dog | p.o. | 50 | 0-72 | 2.5 | - | 9.3 | - | - | - | - | - | - | - | 2.8 | 2.5 |
| | Human | p.o. | 25 mg | 0-24 | 9.9 | √ | - | √ | - | 0.7 | 1.5 | √ | 1.1 | - | - | - |
| Bile | Rat | p.o. | 50 | 0-72 | 1.5 | 10.1 | 7.7 | - | - | - | - | - | - | - | - | - |
| Feces | Rat | p.o. | 50 | 0-96 | 13.9 | 15.3 | 0.8 | 2.8 | - | - | - | - | - | - | - | - |
| | Dog | p.o. | 50 | 0-96 | 26 | 7.5 | - | - | - | 6.5 | 13 | - | - | - | - | - |
| | Human | p.o. | 25 mg | 0-96 | 16.2 | 13.7 | - | 3.8 | 6.5 | 10.9 | 9.1 | 4.5 | - | - | - | - |

BLD: Below the limit of detection.   [a] % of naloxegol peak by MS.   [b] % of chomatogram in plasma.

[9]  FDA Database.   http://www.accessdata.fda.gov/drugsatfda_docs/nda/2014/204760Orig1s000PharmR.pdf (accessed Mar 2016).
[10] EMA Database.   http://www.ema.europa.eu/docs/en_GB/document_library/EPAR_-_Public_assessment_report/human/002810/WC500179077.pdf (accessed Mar 2016).
[11] FDA Database.   http://www.accessdata.fda.gov/drugsatfda_docs/nda/2014/204760Orig1s000ClinPharm.pdf (accessed Mar 2016).

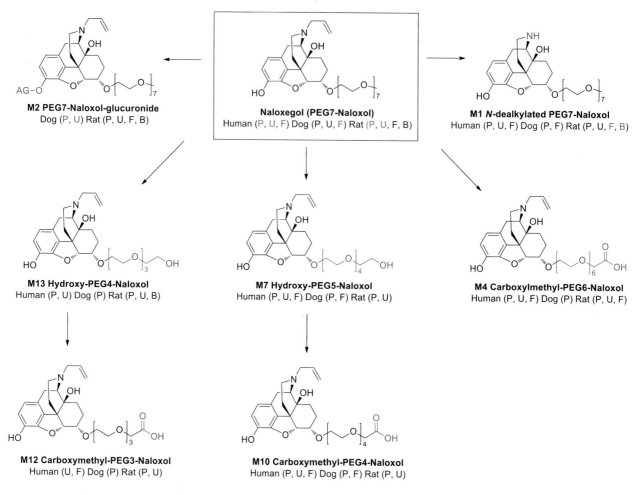

**Figure B    Proposed Pathways for *In Vivo* Biotransformation of Naloxegol in Rats, Dogs and Humans after Single Oral Dose of Naloxegol[9, 11]**

The red labels represent the major components in matrices.    R = Rat, D = Dog, P = Plasma, F = Feces, U = Urine and B = Bile.

## Metabolizing Enzyme Identification

❖ Naloxegol was predominantly metabolized by CYP3A4.    The only other enzyme identified *in vitro* in naloxegol metabolism appeared to be CYP2D6, the contribution of which to overall metabolism appeared to be minor and not likely to be of clinical relevance.

## Excretion

Table 15    Excretion Profiles of [14C]Naloxegol in Various Species after Single Oral Dose of Naloxegol[9, 11]

| Species | State | Route | Dose (mg/kg) | Time (h) | Bile (% of dose) | Urine (% of dose) | Feces (% of dose) | Cage Wash (% of dose) | Recovery (% of dose) |
|---|---|---|---|---|---|---|---|---|---|
| Rat (male) | BDC | p.o. | 50 | 0-168 | 66.0 | 13.2 | 15.0 | 0.7 | 94.9 |
| Rat (male) | Intact | p.o. | 50 | 0-72 | - | 18.8 | 78.9 | 0.7 | 98.4 |
| Rat (female) | Intact | p.o. | 50 | 0-168 | - | 30.2 | 66.4 | 1.4 | 98.0 |
| Dog (female) | Intact | p.o. | 50 | 0-168 | - | 25.2 | 63.4 | 4.5 | 93.1 |
| Human (male& female) | Intact | p.o. | 25 mg | 0-168 | - | <10 | 83 | - | <93 |

[9]  FDA Database.  http://www.accessdata.fda.gov/drugsatfda_docs/nda/2014/204760Orig1s000PharmR.pdf (accessed Mar 2016).
[11]  FDA Database.  http://www.accessdata.fda.gov/drugsatfda_docs/nda/2014/204760Orig1s000ClinPharm.pdf (accessed Mar 2016).

# Drug-Drug Interaction

Table 15  *In Vitro* Evaluation of Naloxegol as an Inhibitor and an Inducer of CYP Enzymes[9]

| Naloxegol as an Inhibitor | | | | Naloxegol as an Inducer | | | |
| --- | --- | --- | --- | --- | --- | --- | --- |
| Isoforms | Direct Inhibition | Time-Dependent Inhibition | | Isoforms | Fold Induction[a] | | |
| | $IC_{50}$ ($\mu$M) | Conc. ($\mu$M) | %Inhibition | | Conc. ($\mu$M) | Activity | mRNA Expression |
| CYP1A2 | >100 | 50 | <20 | CYP1A2 | 0.1 | 1.1 | 0.86 |
| CYP2C9 | >100 | 50 | <20 | | 16 | 0.82 | 0.81 |
| CYP2C19 | >100 | 50 | <20 | CYP2B6 | 0.1 | 1.27 | 0.92 |
| CYP2D6 | 84.7 | 50 | <20 | | 16 | 1.2 | 1.12 |
| CYP3A4[b] | >100 | 50 | <20 | CYP3A4 | 0.1 | 0.98 | 0.97 |
| CYP3A4[c] | >100 | 50 | 24.3 | | 16 | 0.30 | 1.35 |

[a] Mean induction.  [b] Testosterone as substrate.  [c] Midazolam as substrate.

Table 16  *In Vitro* Evaluation of Naloxegol as an Inhibitor and a Substrate of Transporters[9]

| Naloxegol as a Substrate | | | Naloxegol as an Inhibitor | |
| --- | --- | --- | --- | --- |
| Treatment | Conc.($\mu$M) | Net Uptake (pmol/min/cm$^2$) or Efflux Ratio | Transporter | $IC_{50}$ ($\mu$M) |
| OATP1B1 | 3 | 0.000637 ± 0.000168 | OCT2 | >100 |
| | 30 | 0.00293 ± 0.000851 | OAT1 | >100 |
| OATP1B3 | 3 | 0.000637 ± 0.000287 | OAT3 | >100 |
| | 30 | 0.00293 ± 0.000965 | OATP1B1 | >100 |
| BCRP | 3 | Efflux ratio: 13.6 | OATP1B3 | >100 |
| | 30 | Efflux ratio: 9.12 | P-gp | >100 |
| P-gp | 10 | Efflux ratio: 15.4 | BCRP | >100 |

**Key Findings:**
❖ Naloxgol was a substrate of human OATP1B1 and OATP1B3.[9]

# 6   Non-Clinical Toxicology

## Summary

### Single-Dose Toxicity

❖ Single-dose toxicity studies in mice (p.o.), rats (p.o. and i.v.) and dogs (p.o. and i.v.):
  • In mice, naloxegol was tolerated at up to 2000 mg/kg with in-life observation of intolerability (e.g., decreased motor activity and hunched posture).
  • In rats, naloxegol was tolerated at up to 2000 mg/kg with slight in-life observation of intolerability (e.g., decreased motor activity, hunched posture, pilo-erection and respiration changes).
  • In dogs, naloxegol was well tolerated despite of sporadic soft feces, although doses in these acute pharmacokinetic studies did not exceed 20 mg/kg.

### Repeated-Dose Toxicity

❖ Repeated-dose toxicity studies in mice (up to 3 months), rats (up to 6 months), and dogs (up to 9 months):
  • By the longest studies employed in each species, the NOAELs were <400/600 mg/kg/day (male/female) in mice (<49/135 × MRHD), 50 mg/kg/day in rats (143 × MRHD) and 200 mg/kg/day in dogs (169 × MRHD).

---

[9] FDA Database.  http://www.accessdata.fda.gov/drugsatfda_docs/nda/2014/204760Orig1s000PharmR.pdf (accessed Mar 2016).

- The most observed toxicities were generally limited to effects on body weight and food consumption as well as stress-related findings which occurred at dose levels above the NOAEL and generally at doses of or close to the MTD. A dose-related finding of soft stool/diarrhoea in the dog may reflect exaggerated pharmacological effect (inhibition of opioid receptor signaling). Some findings, such as ataxia, tremors and hypoactive behavior observed at HD (500 mg/kg/day) in the dog, were likely to be indicative of CNS exposure. It was not considered to be relevant for naloxegol at the intended clinical dose.

❖ The target organ of toxicity identified across all main toxicity species was the liver (weight increase and associated hypertrophy in rats, weight increase in dogs). But the findings were slight, adaptive and reversible, and occurred at exposures sufficiently above that of MRHD, so were hence to be considered of little relevance to clinical use.

Safety Pharmacology

❖ *In vitro* and *in vivo* safety pharmacology studies to evaluate effects on central nervous, cardiovascular, renal, gastrointestinal and respiratory system:

- No effect on central nervous and respiratory system.
- Cardiovascular effects: $IC_{50}$ of the hERG current was >300 μM considering the *in vitro* studies, suggestive of low potential for QT prolongation, and naloxegol was inactive at 7 cardiac ion channels, and had no effect on contractility parameters. However, in the conscious dog telemetry model, there were moderate decreases in ABP, LVSP, and indices of cardiac contractility and relaxation, the NOEL was considered to be 5 mg/kg, where $C_{max}$ was close to that of MRHD.
- Gastrointestinal effects: Striking increase of stomach weight, indicating decreased gastric emptying, and inhibited intestinal transport were noted in conscious rats, with NOEL of 30 mg/kg (15 × MRHD) and 300 mg/kg (113 × MRHD), respectively.
- Renal effects: Dose-related changes in clinical chemistry parameters were observed, but findings were not considered adverse for the overall low degree and 113 × MRHD $C_{max}$ of NOAEL.

Genotoxicity

❖ Genotoxicity in the *in vitro* Ames, MLA and the *in vivo* bone marrow micronucleus assay:

- Naloxegol was negative in MLA and bone marrow micronucleus assay, but was positive in Ames, likely due to its degradation to naloxone.

Reproductive and Developmental Toxicity

❖ Fertility and early embryonic development in rats:

- Naloxegol did not impair fertility in rats, and the NOAELs were ≥1000 mg/kg/day for males and females.

❖ Embryo-fetal development in rats and rabbits:

- The NOAELs for maternal and fetal development were 750 mg/kg/day in rats and 450 mg/kg/day in rabbits, sufficiently in excess of the MRHD.

❖ Pre- and postnatal development in rats:

- The NOAELs were 500 mg/kg/day for $F_0$ and $F_1$.

❖ Naloxegol was distributed into fetal brain, fetal liver, eye and uveal tract in pregnant rats.

❖ Naloxegol could efficiently transfer into milk.

Carcinogenicity

❖ 2-year carcinogenicity in mice and rats:

- For mice, there were no naloxegol-mediated clinical signs except for bodyweight changes and no neoplastic changes.
- For rats, there were no clinical signs except for bodyweight changes but increase of Leydig cell hyperplasia and adenoma.

Special Toxicity

❖ Non-clinical photoreactivity or photosafety test had not been conducted.

## Single-Dose Toxicity

Table 17    Single-Dose Toxicity Studies of Naloxegol by Intravenous and Oral Administration[9, 10]

| Species | Dose (mg/kg) | Finding |
|---|---|---|
| NMRI mouse | 500, 1000, 1500, 2000, p.o. | 2000 mg/kg: ↓ Motor activity, hunched posture, and pilo-erection. |
| SD rat | Free base: 500, 1000, 1500, 2000, p.o. Oxalate salt[a]: 500, 1000, p.o. | 2000 mg/kg free base: ↓ Motor activity, half-shut eyes, pilo-erection, and respiration changes. 1000 mg/kg oxalate salt: Half-shut eyes and pilo-erection in males. No drug-related gross necropsy finding. Generally similar exposure after dosing with 500 or 1000 mg/kg of free base or oxalate salt. |
| | 10, 30, 100, i.v. for 10 min | 100 and 30 mg/kg: Soft feces and associated urogenital staining. |
| Beagle dog | Free base: 0.4, 2, 10, 20, p.o. Free base: 0.4, i.v. | Sporadic soft feces. |

Vehicle: Water.    [a] Expressed as free base equivalent.

## Repeated-Dose Toxicity

Table 18    Repeated-Dose Toxicity Studies of Naloxegol by Oral Administration[9, 10]

| Species | Duration (Week) | Dose (mg/kg/day) | NOAEL Dose (mg/kg/day) | NOAEL AUC$_{0-24}$ (µg·h/mL) | NOAEL Safety Margin[a] (× MRHD) | Finding |
|---|---|---|---|---|---|---|
| Mouse | 13 | 50, 400, 600, 800 | Male/Female: <400/<600 | Male/Female: <16.3/<44.6 | Male/Female: <49/<135 | Based on toxicity, mortality, and body weight gain decreased (≥10%), the MTD in males appeared to be greater than 50, but less than 400 mg/kg/day, and in females the MTD appeared to be <600 mg/kg/day. |
| Rat | 1 | 100, 500, 1000 | 100[b] | Male/Female: 13.1/53.4 | 39.7/161.8 | No death or drug-related clinical sign. 1000 mg/kg: ↓ Body weight on Day 4, ↑ body weight on Day 7, ↓ blood urea nitrogen levels (female), ↑ cholesterol levels, ↑ adrenal weights, ↑ liver weights, ↑ diffuse hepatocellular hypertrophy (female). 500 mg/kg: ↓ Blood urea nitrogen levels (female), ↑ cholesterol levels, ↑ adrenal weights (male), and ↑ liver weights. |
| | 4 | 50, 150, 500 | 500 | Male/Female: 262.66/372.02 | 795.91/1127.3 | No death, drug-related clinical sign, change in bodyweight or food consumption, neurological effect, or ophthalmology finding. ↑ Cholesterol levels in both sexes at HD and in MD males, ↑ triglyceride levels in all drug-treated groups, but no longer present at the end of the 14-day recovery period. Exposure less than dose-proportional on Day 1, but greater than dose-proportional in males and approximately linear in females on Day 28.    Exposure was generally higher in females. |
| | 13 | 50, 400, 600, 800 | Male/Female: 600/800 | Male/Female: 337/580 | Male/Female: 1021/1758 | Based on the body weight decreased ≥10% male rats, the MTD in males was 600 mg/kg/day.    A MTD could not be defined in females, since there was no observed test article-related toxicity in female rats. |
| | 26 | 50, 200, 800 | 50 | 47.3 | 143 | 200 mg/kg: Excessive salivation, ↑ cholesterol, ↑ liver weight, carcinoma of mammary gland. 800 mg/kg: Colored and rough hair coats, minor skin lesions, hunched appearance.    Excessive salivation, ↓ bodyweight, ↑ cholesterol, ↑ liver weight, pancreatic atrophy, dilatation uterus, carcinoma of mammary gland, mandibular lymph node and tumor of brain. |

[9]  FDA Database.   http://www.accessdata.fda.gov/drugsatfda_docs/nda/2014/204760Orig1s000PharmR.pdf (accessed Mar 2016).
[10]  EMA Database.   http://www.ema.europa.eu/docs/en_GB/document_library/EPAR_-_Public_assessment_report/human/002810/WC500179077.pdf (accessed Mar 2016).

*Continued*

| Species | Duration (Week) | Dose (mg/kg/day) | NOAEL | | | Finding |
|---|---|---|---|---|---|---|
| | | | Dose (mg/kg/day) | AUC$_{0-24}$ ($\mu$g·h/mL) | Safety Margin[a] ($\times$ MRHD) | |
| Beagle dog | 2 | 25, 75, 200, 500 | 500 | Male/Female: 90.7/65.7 | 274.8/199.1 | 2 deaths, one 200 mg/kg, one 500 mg/kg. 200 mg/kg: Loose feces. 500 mg/kg: Loose feces, ↓ food consumption, ↓ bodyweight. |
| | 4 | 50, 150, 500 | 150 | Male/Female: 14.7/11.5 | 44.5/34.8 | No death. 150 mg/kg: Excessive salivation and emesis. 500 mg/kg: Excessive salivation and emesis, ↓ bodyweight, ↑ lymphocyte depletion. |
| | 39 | 20, 200, 500 | 200 | 55.9 | 169 | No death. 200 mg/kg: ↑ Emesis, ↑ cholesterol, excessive salivation. 500 mg/kg: Tremors, ataxia, hypoactive behavior, skin lesion, ↑ emesis, excessive salivation; ↑ cholesterol (male). |

[a] Human exposure at MRHD (25 mg/day): AUC = 330 ng·h/mL, $C_{max}$ = 80 ng/mL.   [b] NOEL: No observed effect level.   Average of male and female AUC was used when NOAEL for males and females was the same.

Table 19   Summary of Toxicokinetic Parameter of Naloxegol after Repeated-Dose Oral Administration to Mice, Rats and Dogs[9, 10]

| Species | Duration (Week) | Gender | Dose (mg/kg/day) | First Day | | Last Day | |
|---|---|---|---|---|---|---|---|
| | | | | AUC$_{0-24}$ ($\mu$g·h/mL) | $C_{max}$ ($\mu$g/mL) | AUC$_{0-24}$ ($\mu$g·h/mL) | $C_{max}$ ($\mu$g/mL) |
| Mouse[a] | 13 | Male | 50 | 1.60 | 0.849 | 1.73 | 0.945 |
| | | | 400 | 21.4 | 9.54 | 16.3 | 6.26 |
| | | | 600 | 25.1 | 11.5 | 60.2 | 28.5 |
| | | | 800 | 46.5 | 18.5 | 38.2 | 16.0 |
| | | Female | 50 | 1.39 | 0.802 | 1.84 | 0.701 |
| | | | 400 | 13.5 | 4.74 | 16.0 | 7.80 |
| | | | 600 | 29.0 | 14.1 | 44.6 | 21.1 |
| | | | 800 | 33.5 | 15.9 | 79.5 | 31.4 |
| Rat[b] | 13 | Male | 50 | 3.81 | 1.19 | 11.3 | 3.1 |
| | | | 400 | 53.7 | 11.8 | 252 | 31.3 |
| | | | 600 | 121 | 17.6 | 337 | 36.2 |
| | | | 800 | 161 | 22.2 | 478 | 54.6 |
| | | Female | 50 | 20.7 | 5.61 | 36.4 | 7.26 |
| | | | 400 | 245 | 31.1 | 367 | 31.9 |
| | | | 600 | 387 | 39.4 | 474 | 46.7 |
| | | | 800 | 656 | 42.5 | 580 | 56.6 |
| Rat[c] | 26 | Male | 50 | 4.48 | 1.21 | 9.17 | 2.82 |
| | | | 200 | 32.7 | 9.19 | 82.0 | 13.0 |
| | | | 800 | 169 | 17.7 | 389 | 36.9 |
| | | Female | 50 | 19.4 | 3.85 | 29.7 | 6.14 |
| | | | 200 | 117 | 16.4 | 127 | 15.1 |
| | | | 800 | 462 | 35.0 | 524 | 52.4 |

[9]  FDA Database.   http://www.accessdata.fda.gov/drugsatfda_docs/nda/2014/204760Orig1s000PharmR.pdf (accessed Mar 2016).
[10]  EMA Database.   http://www.ema.europa.eu/docs/en_GB/document_library/EPAR_-_Public_assessment_report/human/002810/WC500179077.pdf (accessed Mar 2016).

*Continued*

| Species | Duration (Week) | Gender | Dose (mg/kg/day) | First Day AUC$_{0-24}$ ($\mu$g·h/mL) | First Day C$_{max}$ ($\mu$g/mL) | Last Day AUC$_{0-24}$ ($\mu$g·h/mL) | Last Day C$_{max}$ ($\mu$g/mL) |
|---|---|---|---|---|---|---|---|
| Dog[d] | 39 | Male | 50 | 5.77 ± 1.53 | 3.42 ± 1.27 | 13.3 ± 3.32 | 6.60 ± 2.45 |
| | | | 200 | 36.0 ± 21.4 | 28.8 ± 20.0 | 54.4 ± 17.3 | 38.3 ± 15.6 |
| | | | 500 | 86.1 ± 14.2 | 58.7 ± 18.9 | 205 ± 46.9 | 138 ± 83.5 |
| | | Female | 50 | 6.93 ± 1.01 | 4.93 ± 1.76 | 6.12 ± 1.86 | 11.7 ± 3.54 |
| | | | 200 | 30.2 ± 4.04 | 16.9 ± 2.18 | 38.8 ± 24.5 | 57.4 ± 25.9 |
| | | | 500 | 88.0 ± 37.6 | 69.1 ± 51.5 | 106 ± 49.6 | 205 ± 46.9 |

[a] On Day 1 and 91.  [b] On Day 1 and 89.  [c] On Day 1 and 182.  [d] On Day 1 and 273.

## Safety Pharmacology

Table 20    Safety Pharmacological Studies of Naloxegol[9, 10]

| Study | Test System | Dose | NOAEL Dose (mg/kg) | NOAEL Safety Margin (× MRHD) | Finding |
|---|---|---|---|---|---|
| CNS effect | Wistar rat (male) | 30, 100, 300, 1000 mg/kg, p.o. | NA | NA | No proconvulsant or analgesic effect. No morphine-like discriminative effect. Mu-opioid antagonist-like effects at 30 and 300 mg/kg. No physical dependence liability. |
| Cardiovascular effect | HEK cell expressing hERG channel | 3, 30, 100, 300 $\mu$M | 100 $\mu$M | - | 300 $\mu$M: 13.3% inhibition. |
| | Telemetered conscious Beagle dog | Single p.o. 0, 5 mg/kg[a] | 5 | ≈1 | No effect. |
| Respiratory effect | Wistar rat (male) | Single p.o. 100, 300, 1000 mg/kg | 1000 | 347 | No effect.  Respiratory rate, tidal volume, expiration times, and peak inspiratory and expiratory flows. |
| Gastrointestinal effect | Wistar rat (male) | Single p.o. 100, 300, 1000 mg/kg | 30 for gastric 300 for intestinal transport | 15/113 | Stomach weight increased by 28%-78%. |
| Renal effect | Wistar rat (male) | 100, 300, 1000 mg/kg, p.o. | 300 | 113 | ↑ Urinary excretion of sodium, potassium, chloride and albumin. |

Vehicle: Sterile water *in vivo*.   Human exposure at MRHD (25 mg/day): AUC = 330 ng·h/mL, C$_{max}$ = 80 ng/mL.   [a] Single oral doses of 25, 75 and 200 mg/kg at 2 to 5-day dosing intervals in the first dosing phase, and 5 mg/kg at 2-day dosing intervals in the second dosing phase.

## Genotoxicity

Table 21    Genotoxicity Studies of Naloxegol[9, 10]

| Assay | Species/System | Metabolism Activity | Dose | Finding |
|---|---|---|---|---|
| *In vitro* bacterial reverse mutation assay (Ames) | *S. typhimurium* TA98, TA100, TA1535 and TA1537; *E. coli* WP2 *uvr*A | ±S9 | 49.1-5340 $\mu$g/plate | Positive (due to degradation product). |
| *In vitro* mouse lymphoma TK assay | L5178Y/t/k$^{+/-}$ | -S9, 4 h +S9, 24 h | 0-2600 $\mu$g/mL 0-2800 $\mu$g/mL | Negative. |
| *In vivo* mouse bone marrow micronucleus test | Mouse | + | 500, 1000, 2000 mg/kg | Negative. |

Vehicle: Deionized water.

[9] FDA Database.   http://www.accessdata.fda.gov/drugsatfda_docs/nda/2014/204760Orig1s000PharmR.pdf (accessed Mar 2016).
[10] EMA Database. http://www.ema.europa.eu/docs/en_GB/document_library/EPAR_-_Public_assessment_report/human/002810/WC500179077.pdf (accessed Mar 2016).

## Reproductive and Developmental Toxicity

Table 22   Reproductive and Development Toxicity Studies of Naloxegol[9, 10]

| Study | Species | Dose (mg/kg/day) | NOAEL | | | |
|---|---|---|---|---|---|---|
| | | | Endpoint | Dose (mg/kg/day) | AUC$_{0-24}$ (µg·hr/mL) | Safety Margin[a] (× MRHD) |
| Fertility and early embryonic development | Rat | 250, 500, 1000 | Female fertility | 1000 | NA | >1000[b] |
| | | | Male fertility | 1000 | NA | |
| Embryo-fetal development | Rat | 100, 300, 1000 | Maternal | 750 | 479 | 1452 |
| | | | Fetal development | 750 | 479 | 1452 |
| | NZW rabbit | 30, 150, 450 | Maternal | 450 | 135 | 409 |
| | | | Fetal development | 450 | 135 | 409 |
| Pre- and postnatal development | SD rat | 50, 250, 500 | F$_0$ | 500 | NA | 195[c] |
| | | | F$_1$ | 500 | NA | |

Vehicle: Water.   [a] Calculated with human AUC of 330 ng·h/mL at MRHD (25 mg/day) unless otherwise specified.   [b] Estimated based on TK data from the 3-month oral toxicity study in rats, in which the AUC values in the 800 mg/kg/day males and females were 399000 and 500000 ng·h/mL, respectively, on Day 29.   [c] Expressed based on BSA due to the absence of TK data.

Table 23   Rat Fetal and Maternal Tissue Concentration of Naloxegol after Single Oral Dose of 50 mg/kg Administration[9, 10]

| Organ | Radioactivity (µg eq./g) | | | | | | | | | AUC Ratio (fetal/maternal) |
|---|---|---|---|---|---|---|---|---|---|---|
| | Fetal | | | | Maternal | | | | | |
| | 0.5 h | 1 h | 4 h | 24 h | 0.5 h | 1 h | 4 h | 24 h | 48 h | |
| Brain | 0.47 | 0.40 | 0.41 | ND | 0.34 | 0.15 | 0.28 | ND | ND | 1.55 |
| Uveal tract | 4.95 | 3.53 | 5.41 | ND | 15.34 | 27.24 | 17.42 | 2.94 | 1.16 | 0.21 |
| Liver | 5.28 | 2.61 | 3.36 | ND | 68.67 | 56.01 | 58.78 | 4.42 | 2.68 | 0.05 |
| Eye | 3.23 | 2.17 | 3.92 | ND | 2.46 | 6.02 | 4.17 | 0.77 | 0.23 | 0.64 |

### Transfer of Naloxegol into Milk

❖ Measurements using a preliminary assay for naloxegol in rat milk showed high concentrations of naloxegol in milk, suggesting efficient transfer of naloxegol into milk.

[9]   FDA Database.   http://www.accessdata.fda.gov/drugsatfda_docs/nda/2014/204760Orig1s000PharmR.pdf (accessed Mar 2016).
[10]   EMA Database.   http://www.ema.europa.eu/docs/en_GB/document_library/EPAR_-_Public_assessment_report/human/002810/WC500179077.pdf (accessed Mar 2016).

# Carcinogenicity

Table 24    Carcinogenicity Studies of Naloxegol[9, 10]

| Dose (mg/kg/day) | Species | 0 | 40 | 120 | 400 |
|---|---|---|---|---|---|
| **104-Week Carcinogenic Study in Rat** | | | | | |
| Weight (%) | Male[a] | 100 | 92.8 | 99.4 | 82.7 |
| | Female[a] | 100 | 125.4 | 103.5 | 96.8 |
| Pituitary adenoma | Male | 65% | 55% | 61.7% | 51.7% |
| | Female | 88.3% | 81.7% | 76.7% | 75% |
| Mammary carcinoma | Female | 5% | 8.3% | 20% | 13.3% |
| Interstitial (Leydig) cell adenoma | Male | 0% | 0% | 6.7% | 11.7% |
| Interstitial (Leydig) cell hyperplasia | Male | 5% | 8.3% | 20% | 13.3% |

| Dose (ppm) | Species | 0 | 25/40 | 70/120 | 200/400 |
|---|---|---|---|---|---|
| **104-Week Carcinogenic Study in Mouse[a]** | | | | | |
| Weight (%) | Male | 100 | 126.7 | 100.9 | 127.6 |
| | Female | 100 | 94.5 | 93.8 | 75.2 |

Vehicle: Water.    [a] Different dosage design expressed as male/female.

[9]  FDA Database.    http://www.accessdata.fda.gov/drugsatfda_docs/nda/2014/204760Orig1s000PharmR.pdf (accessed Mar 2016).
[10]  EMA Database.    http://www.ema.europa.eu/docs/en_GB/document_library/EPAR_-_Public_assessment_report/human/002810/WC500179077.pdf (accessed Mar 2016).

# CHAPTER

## 18

---

## Nintedanib Esylate

# Nintedanib Esylate

(Ofev®/Vargatef®)

Research code: BIBF-1120

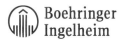

## 1 General Information

❖ Nintedanib is a tyrosine kinase inhibitor, which was first approved in Oct 2014 by US FDA.

❖ Nintedanib was discovered and marketed by Boehringer Ingelheim.

❖ Nintedanib is a small molecule that inhibits multiple receptor tyrosine kinases (RTKs) and non-receptor tyrosine kinases (nRTKs). Nintedanib competitively binds to these receptors, i.e. fibroblast growth factor receptor (FGFR), platelet derived growth factor receptor (PDGFR), and vascular endothelial growth factor receptor (VEGFR), and blocks the intracellular signaling which is crucial for the proliferation, migration, and transformation of fibroblasts representing essential mechanisms of the idiopathic pulmonary fibrosis (IPF) pathology. Based on its antiangiogenic action, nintedanib is expected to slow tumor growth.

❖ Nintedanib is indicated for the treatment of IPF approved by FDA, EMA and PMDA, and non-small cell lung cancer (NSCLC) approved by EMA.

❖ Available as oral capsule, with each containing 100, 150 mg of nintedanib and the recommended dose is 150 mg twice daily for IPF or 200 mg twice daily for non-small cell lung cancer taken with food.

❖ The sale of Ofev®/Vargatef® was not available up to Mar 2016.

### Key Approvals around the World*

| | US (FDA) | EU (EMA) | Japan (PMDA) |
|---|---|---|---|
| First approval date | 10/15/2014 | 11/21/2014; 01/15/2015 | 07/03/2015 |
| Application or approval No. | NDA 205832 | EMEA/H/C/002569; EMEA/H/C/003821 | 22700AMX 00693000; 22700AMX 00694000 |
| Brand name | Ofev® | Vargatef®/ Ofev® | Ofev® |
| Indication | IPF | NSCLC; IPF | IPF |
| Authorisation holder | Boehringer Ingelheim | Boehringer Ingelheim | Boehringer Ingelheim |

* Till Mar 2016, it had not been approved by CFDA (China).

## Active Ingredient

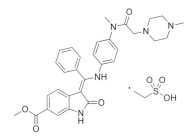

*Molecular formula*: $C_{31}H_{33}N_5O_4 \cdot C_2H_6O_3S$
*Molecular weight*: 649.76
*CAS No.*: 656247-17-5 (Nintedanib)
656247-18-6 (Nintedanib esylate)
*Chemical name*: Methyl (3Z)-3-[({4-[N-methyl-2-(4-methylpiperazin-1-yl)acetamido]phenyl}amino)(phenyl)methylidene]-2-oxo-2,3-dihydro-1H-indole-6-carboxylate monoethanesulfonate

*Parameters of Lipinski's "Rule of 5"*

| MWa | HD | HA | FRBb | PSAb | cLogPb |
|---|---|---|---|---|---|
| 539.62 | 2 | 9 | 8 | 94.2Å² | 2.38 ± 0.99 |

a Molecular weight of nintedanib.  b Calculated by ACD/Labs software V11.02.

## Drug Product*

*Dosage route*: Oral
*Strength*: 100 mg/150 mg (Nintedanib)
*Dosage form*: Capsule
*Inactive ingredient*: Triglycerides, hard fat, lecithin, gelatin, glycerol, titanium dioxide, red ferric oxide, yellow ferric oxide and black ink.
*Recommended dose*: The recommended dosage of nintedanib is 150 mg administered twice daily approximately 12 h apart taken with food for IPF.
Dosage adjustment to 100 mg twice daily with food, approximately 12 h apart for IPF.
The recommended dosage of nintedanib is 200 mg administered twice daily approximately 12 h apart taken with food for non-small cell lung cancer.

* Sourced from the US FDA and EMA drug label information

# 2   Key Patents Information

## Summary

❖ Ofev® (Nintedanib esylate) has got five-year NCE market exclusivity protection and seven-year orphan drug exclusivity after it was initially approved by US FDA on Oct 15, 2014.

❖ Nintedanib was originally developed by Boehringer Ingelheim, and its compound patent application was filed as PCT application by Boehringer Ingelheim in 2000.

❖ The compound patent will expire in 2020 foremost, which has been granted in the United States, Japan, China and Europe successively.

Table 1    Nintedanib's Compound Patent Protection in Drug-Mainstream Country

| Country | Publication/Patent NO. | Application Date | Granted Date | Estimated Expiry Date |
|---|---|---|---|---|
| WO | WO0127081A1 | 10/09/2000 | / | / |
| US | US6762180B1 | 10/03/2000 | 07/13/2004 | 12/10/2020[a] |
| EP | EP1224170B1 | 10/09/2000 | 08/12/2009 | 10/09/2020 |
| JP | JP4021664B2 | 10/09/2000 | 12/12/2007 | 10/09/2020 |
| CN | CN100455568C | 10/09/2000 | 01/28/2009 | 10/09/2020 |

[a] The term of this patent is extended by 68 days.

Table 2    Originator's International Patent Application List (Patent Family)

| Publication NO. | Title | Applicant/Assignee/Owner | Publication Date |
|---|---|---|---|
| **Technical Subjects** | **Active Ingredient (Free Base)'s Formula or Structure and Preparation** | | |
| WO0127081A1 | 6-Position substituted indoline, production and use thereof as a medicament | Boehringer Ingelheim | 04/19/2001 |
| **Technical Subjects** | **Salt, Crystal, Polymorphic, Solvate (Hydrate), Isomer, Derivative Etc. and Preparation** | | |
| WO2004013099A1 | 3-Z-[1-(4-(N-((4-methyl-piperazin-1-yl)-methylcarbonyl)-N-methyl-amino)anilino)-1-phenyl-methylene]-6-methoxycarbonyl-2-indolinone-monoethanesulphonate and the use thereof as a pharmaceutical composition | Boehringer Ingelheim | 02/12/2004 |
| WO2007141283A2 | New salts and crystalline salt forms of an indolinone derivative | Boehringer Ingelheim | 12/13/2007 |
| WO2009071523A1 | Process for the manufacture of an indolinone derivative | Boehringer Ingelheim | 06/11/2009 |
| **Technical Subjects** | **Formulation and Preparation** | | |
| WO2009147212A1 | Capsule pharmaceutical dosage form comprising a suspension formulation of an indolinone derivative | Boehringer Ingelheim | 12/10/2009 |
| WO2009147220A1 | Pharmaceutical dosage form for immediate release of an indolinone derivative | Boehringer Ingelheim | 12/10/2009 |
| **Technical Subjects** | **Indication or Methods for Medical Needs** | | |
| WO2004017948A2 | Use of Lck inhibitor for treatment of immunologic diseases | Boehringer Ingelheim | 03/04/2004 |
| WO2006067165A2 | Medicaments for the treatment or prevention of fibrotic diseases | Boehringer Ingelheim | 06/29/2006 |
| WO2007057397A1 | Treatment of cancer | Boehringer Ingelheim | 05/24/2007 |
| WO2010081817A1 | Method for treating colorectal cancer | Boehringer Ingelheim | 07/22/2010 |
| WO2010103058A1 | Method or system using biomarkers for the monitoring of a treatment | Boehringer Ingelheim | 09/16/2010 |
| WO2014180955A1 | Efficacious treatment of NSCLC and predictive clinical marker of the responsiveness of a tumor to a treatment | Boehringer Ingelheim | 11/13/2014 |
| **Technical Subjects** | **Combination Including at Least Two Active Ingredients** | | |
| WO2004096224A2 | Combinations for the treatment of diseases involving cell proliferation, migration or apoptosis of myeloma cells, or angiogenesis | Boehringer Ingelheim | 11/11/2004 |
| WO2006018182A1 | Combinations for the treatment of diseases involving cell proliferation | Boehringer Ingelheim | 02/23/2006 |

*Continued*

| Publication NO. | Title | Applicant/Assignee/Owner | Publication Date |
|---|---|---|---|
| WO2007054551A1 | Combination treatment of cancer comprising EGFR/HER2 inhibitors | Boehringer Ingelheim | 05/18/2007 |
| WO2009147218A1 | Pharmaceutical combination | Boehringer Ingelheim | 12/10/2009 |
| WO2010130757A1 | New combination therapy in treatment of oncological and fibrotic diseases | Boehringer Ingelheim | 11/18/2010 |
| WO2010130758A1 | New combination therapy in treatment of cancer and fibrotic diseases | Boehringer Ingelheim | 11/18/2010 |
| WO2011134898A1 | New combination therapy in treatment of oncological and fibrotic diseases | Boehringer Ingelheim | 11/03/2011 |
| WO2012095505A1 | Anticancer therapy with dual aurora kinase/MEK inhibitors | Boehringer Ingelheim | 07/19/2012 |
| WO2013144266A1 | Ang2-binding molecules | Boehringer Ingelheim | 10/03/2013 |
| WO2014009319A1 | Indolinone derivatives anticancer compounds | Boehringer Ingelheim | 01/16/2014 |
| WO2014009318A1 | 3-{3-[1-(4-Dimethylaminomethyl-phenylamino)-1-phenyl-meth-(Z)-ylidene]-2-oxo-2,3-dihydro-1H-indol-6-yll-propynoic acid ethylamide and its use in the treatment of cancer | Boehringer Ingelheim | 01/16/2014 |
| WO2014049099A1 | Pharmaceutical combinations comprising dual angiopoietin-2/DLL4 binders and anti-VEGF-R agents | Boehringer Ingelheim | 04/03/2014 |

The data was updated until Jan 2016.

# 3  Chemistry

## Route 1:  Original Discovery Route

*Synthesis Route*:  Electrophilic substitution of methyl 3-nitrobenzoate **1** by chloromethyl acetate **2** in 63% yield followed by reduction of the nitro group in acidic media with concomitant ring closure offered an easy approach for indolinone **4** in 98% yield.   73% N-acetylation of the indolinone **4** activated the 3-position for subsequent condensation with trimethyl orthobenzoate **6**.   Both steps could be combined in a practical one-pot sequence using acetic anhydride as a solvent.   For large-scale synthesis, a stepwise procedure was recommended, facilitating workup due to the cleaner reaction progress.   The amino side chain was introduced in the final step by addition and subsequent elimination of alcohol, followed by *in situ* acetyl cleavage to achieve nintedanib in 77% yield.   The double-bond geometry in the final compounds was locked in a *Z*-conformation due to an intramolecular hydrogen bond.[1-3]

[1]  Roth, G. J.; Heckel, A.; Colbatzky, F., et al. *J. Med. Chem.* **2009**, *52*, 4466-4480.
[2]  Roth, G. J.; Heckel, A.; Walter, R., et al. US6762180B1, **2004**.
[3]  Heckel, A.; Roth, G. J.; Walter, R., et al. WO200127081A1, **2001**.

## Route2

*Synthesis Route*:    The synthesis of indolinone **5** commenced with commecially available 4-chloro-3-nitrobenzoic acid **1**, esterification of which proceeded prior to displacement of the chloride by dimethyl malonate **3** in the presence of base generating nitrobenzene **4** in 77% yield from **1**.    Hydrogenation of **4** under acidic conditions furnished 6-methyoxycarbonyl-substituted oxindole **5** after thermal decarboxylative cyclization in 87% yield.    Acylation of indolinone **5** with chloroacetic anhydride **6** in refluxing toluene occurred prior to a condensation reaction with trimethyl orthobenzoate **8** resulting in indolone **9** which was isolated in 86% yield over the two-step sequence.    While these two steps could reportedly be combined into a one-pot protocol using acetic anhydride as the solvent, the stepwise procedure was found to be more amenable for large-scale synthesis due to fewer complications with undesired side products.    Subjection of **9** to methanolic potassium hydroxide prior to condensation with aniline fragment **11** in refluxing methanol and then exposure to aqueous ethanesulfonic acid **12** in methanol prior to recrystallization in IPA provided nintedanib esylate in 82% over the three-step sequence.

Aniline fragment **11** was prepared in 82% *via* a three-step sequence by initial acylation of *N*-methyl-4-nitroaniline **13** with chloro acetylchloride **14**, and then displacement of the amidochloride **15** with *N*-methylpiperazine **16**, finally hydrogenative reduction of the nitro group to furnish the desired aniline **11**.    The overall yield concerning the entire route was 38%.[4, 5]

[4]  Merten, J.; Linz, G.; Schnaubelt, J., et al. WO2009071523A1, **2009**.
[5]  Merten, J.; Linz, G.; Schnaubelt, J., et al. US8304541B2, **2012**.

# 4 Pharmacology

## Summary

### Mechanism of Action

❖ Nintedanib is a small molecule that inhibits multiple RTKs ($IC_{50}$ = 13-610 nM), including PDGFR$\alpha/\beta$ , FGFR1-3, VEGFR1-3 and Fms-like tyrosine kinase-3 (Flt-3) and nRTKs (Src family: Lck, Lyn, and Src, $IC_{50}$ = 16-195 nM).

❖ Nintedanib competitively binds to the adenosine triphosphate (ATP) binding pocket of the receptors, and blocks the intracellular signaling which is crucial for the proliferation, migrations and transformation of fibroblasts representing essential mechanism of the IPF pathology.

❖ Nintedanib inhibits mitogen-activated protein kinases and Akt signaling pathways in three cell types contributing to angiogenesis, resulting in inhibitions of cell proliferation and slowing tumor growth.

❖ Nintedanib inhibited the following receptors: PDGFR (PDGFR$\alpha$, $IC_{50}$ = 59 nM; PDGFR$\beta$, $IC_{50}$ = 65 nM), FGFRs ($IC_{50}$ = 37-610 nM), VEGFR ($IC_{50}$ = 13-34 nM), Flt-3 and Src.

❖ BIBF 1202 (M1), the main metabolite of nintedanib, inhibited VEGFR-2, FGFR-1 and PDGFR$\alpha$ ($IC_{50}$ = 62 nM, 240 nM and 433 nM, respectively).

❖ The non-specific bindings of nintedanib (5 μM) were detected in A3 receptors, NK2 receptors, $5HT_{1B}$ receptors and $Ca^{2+}$ channels (inhibition: 65%-102%).

### In Vitro Efficacy

❖ Inhibition of stimulus induced cell proliferation:
  • HUVEC: $IC_{50}$ = 9-3361 nM.
  • Human lung fibroblasts (IPF/N-HLF): $IC_{50}$ = <1-193 nM.
  • HSMEC/BRP/HUASMC: 7-79 nM.
  • FaDu/CuLa: $IC_{50}$ = 14-46 nM.

❖ Nintedanib inhibited the migration and proliferation of fibroblast:
  • Inhibited PDGF-induced autophosphate of N-HLF: $IC_{50}$ = 22-39 nM.
  • Inhibited PDGF-induced proliferation of IPF/N-HLF: $IC_{50}$ = 11/13 nM.
  • Inhibited bFGF-induced proliferation of IPF/N-HLF: $IC_{50}$ = 0.6-5.5 nM.
  • Inhibited VEGF-induced proliferation of IPF/N-HLF: $IC_{50}$ <1 nM.
  • Decreased migration of human lung fibroblast: $IC_{50}$ = 19-228 nM.
  • Inhibited TGF-beta-mediated transformation, from fibroblasts to myofibroblasts: $IC_{50}$ = 144 nM.

### In Vivo Efficacy

❖ Anti-tumor effects of nintedanib in tumor models:
  • Human FaDu xenografts nude mouse models: Tumor growth inhibition, T/C% = 46% at 25 mg/kg.
  • Caki-1 tumor xenografts：
    ◆ Good anti-tumor effect was observed at 50 mg/kg (T/C% = 25%).
    ◆ Reduction of tumor vessel density about 80% at 100 mg/kg/day.
  • Syngeneic GS9L rat model: Anti-tumor effect at 50 mg/kg (T/C% = 30%) and 25 mg/kg (T/C% = 45%).
  • Calu-6 NSCLC xenografts: Tumor growth inhibition, T/C% = 24% at 50 mg/kg.

❖ Nintedanib decreased the severity of lung fibrosis in animal models:
  • Bleomycin-induced lung fibrosis rat models:
    ◆ Prevented lung fibrosis at 50 mg/kg for 21 days.
    ◆ Dose-related decreased in the expression of both pro-collagen and TGF$\beta$1 genes at 10, 30, 50 mg/kg.

- Silica-induced lung fibrosis mouse models:
  - Decreased lung histology scores for granuloma, inflammation, and collagen deposition.
  - Decreased some inflammation markers at 30 and 100 mg/kg/day.
- Bleomycin-induced lung fibrosis mouse models: Effectively reduced lung fibrosis at 60 mg/kg/day.
- Rip1Tag2 transgenic mouse model: Nintedanib reduced tumor volume and improved survival.

## Mechanism of Action

Table 3    X-ray Crystallography of Nintedanib Binding Sites in FGFR-1[6, 7]

| Compound | Dose ($\mu$M) | $K_d$ (nM) | $K_{on}$ (1/Ms) | $T_{1/2}$ (s) | $K_{off}$ (1/s) | Finding |
|---|---|---|---|---|---|---|
| Nintedanib | 0.008-5 | 57 | $9.67 \times 10^5$ | 13.5 | $5.12 \times 10^{-2}$ | Nintedanib bound to the ATP-site in the cleft between $N$- and $C$-terminal lobes of the kinase domains. The binding site of nintedanib to immobilized FGFR-1 was the intracellular domain $AA_{456-765}$. |

Protein structures of the complexes were studied by X-ray crystallography.

Table 4    Potency and Selectivity of Nintedanib and Main Metabolites in Kinase Assays[6-9]

| Nintedanib | | | | BIBF 1202[a] | |
|---|---|---|---|---|---|
| Tyrosine Kinase | IC$_{50}$ (nM) | Tyrosine Kinase | IC$_{50}$ (nM) | Kinase | IC$_{50}$ (nM) |
| HuVEGFR-1 | 34 | Src | 156 | VEGFR-2 | 62 |
| HuVEGFR-2 | 21 | Lck | 16 | FGFR-1 | 240 |
| MuVEGFR-2 | 13 | Lyn | 195 | PDGFR$\alpha$ | 433 |
| VEGFR-3 | 13 | Abl | 41 | | |
| PDGFR$\alpha$ | 59 | InsR | >4000 | | |
| PDGFR$\beta$ | 65 | IGF1R | >1000 | | |
| FGFR-1 | 69 | EGFR | >50000 | | |
| FGFR-2 | 37 | HER2 | >50000 | | |
| FGFR-3 | 108 | CDK1 | >10000 | | |
| FGFR-4 | 610 | CDK2 | >10000 | | |
| Flt-3 | 26 | CDK4 | >10000 | | |

The *in vitro* activity of nintedanib was investigated in both enzymatic and cellular assays for VEGFR-2 inhibition.    The selectivity of this compound was tested with respect to inhibition of basic fibroblast growth factor (bFGF) mediated endothelial cell proliferation and inhibition of tumor cell lines proliferation.    Sf9-DELFIA assays were used to explore the inhibitory effect of BIBF 1120 on murine VEGFR-2 (flk-1), VEGFR-1 and VEGFR-3.    [a] BIBF 1202 was the main metabolite of nintedanib.

Table 5    The Non-Specific Binding of Nintedanib in a Battery of Receptors[6, 7]

| Receptors | Conc. ($\mu$M) | %Inhibition |
|---|---|---|
| A3 | 5 | 66 |
| NK2 | 5 | 84 |
| 5HT$_{1B}$ | 5 | 102 |
| Ca$^{2+}$ channels | 5 | 65 |

Using the CEREP screening package *in vitro*.

[6] Japan Pharmaceuticals and Medical Devices Agency (PMDA) Database.    http://www.pmda.go.jp/drugs/2015/P20150619001/index.html (accessed Mar 2016).

[7] U.S. Food and Drug Administration (FDA) Database.    http://www.accessdata.fda.gov/drugsatfda_docs/nda/2014/205832Orig1s000PharmR.pdf (accessed Mar 2016).

[8] Roth, G. J.; Binder, R.; Colbatzky, F., et al. *J. Med. Chem.* **2015**, *58*, 1053-1063.

[9] European Medicines Agency (EMA) Database.    http://www.ema.europa.eu/docs/en_GB/document_library/EPAR_-_Public_assessment_report/human/002569/WC500179972.pdf (accessed Mar 2016).

## *In Vitro* Efficacy

Table 6   Nintedanib and Metabolites Inhibited PDGFR Auto-Phosphorylation of RTKs in NHLF Cells[6, 7]

| Compound | Stimulator | Conc. of Stimulator(nM) | IC$_{50}$ (nM) | |
| --- | --- | --- | --- | --- |
| | | | PDGFR$\alpha$ | PDGFR$\beta$ |
| Nintedanib[a] | PDGF-BB | 50 | 21.6 | 38.7 |
| M1 | PDGF-BB | 50 | 5717 | 23510 |
| BIBF 1000 | PDGF-BB | 50 | 17.7 | 30.1 |
| Imatinib | PDGF-BB | 50 | 1168 | 718 |
| Pazopanib | PDGF-BB | 50 | 42.7 | 43.8 |

Normal human lung fibroblast (NHLF) cells were treated with various concentrations of nintedanib for 30 min.   The cells were then stimulated with 50 nM PDGF-BB 0 h to 11 days after nintedanib treatment.   The cells were lysed at the end of the PDGF-BB treatment.   Levels of phosphorylated PDGF receptors in the lysates were detected in ELISAs specific for human phospho-PDGFR$\alpha$ and phospho-PDGFR$\beta$, respectively.   [a] The respective inhibitions of PDGFR$\alpha$ and PDGFR$\beta$ were 36.3% and 18.9% on Day 4 in the transfer experiments, 8.6% and 16.2% at 24 h in the washout experiments.

Table 7   Inhibition of GF-Dependent Cell Proliferation by Nintedanib[7, 10]

| Cell Line | Cell Type | Stimulator | IC$_{50}$ (nM) |
| --- | --- | --- | --- |
| HUVEC[a] | Human umbilical vascular epithelial cell | VEGF | 9 ± 13 |
| | | bFGF | 290 ± 160, 80 ± 64, 3361 ± 1525 |
| | | VEGF-2 | 62 |
| | | VEGF-3 | 14.5 |
| | | PDGF$\alpha$ | 433 |
| N-HLF | Primary human lung fibroblasts from control donors | PDGF BB | 64 |
| | | PDGF BB | 1-10 |
| | | FGF2 | ~1 |
| | | VEGF | <1 |
| | | FBS | 13 |
| | | IL-1$\beta$ | 106 |
| IPF-HLF | Primary lung fibroblasts from patients with idiopathic pulmonary fibrosis | PDGF BB | ~10 |
| | | FGF2 | 1-10 |
| | | VEGF | <1 |
| | | IL-1$\beta$ | 193 |
| HSMEC | Human skin microvascular endothelial cell | VEGF | 7 ± 5 |
| BRP | Pericyte | PDGF BB | 79 ± 21 |
| HUASMC | Human umbilical artery smooth muscle cell | PDGF BB | 69 ± 29 |
| FaDu/CuLa | Endothelial cancer cell | VEGF-1 | 34 ± 15 |
| | | VEGF-2 | 14 ± 4 |
| | | VEGF-3 | 46 ± 9 |
| FaDu | Endothelial cancer cell | 10% FCS | >4500 |
| Calu-6 | Endothelial cancer cell | 10% FCS | >4500 |
| HeLa | Endothelial cancer cell | 10% FCS | >3500 |

[a] Cell proliferation was measured by the rate of [$^3$H-thymidine] incorporation.   Nintedanib inhibited proliferation of a number of cancer cells induced by FGF, PDGF and VEGF, but not by fetal calf serum (FCS) *in vitro*.   The IC$_{50}$s were approximately 8, 74 and 290 nM for VEGF, PDGF and FGF, respectively.

[6]   PMDA Database.   http://www.pmda.go.jp/drugs/2015/P20150619001/index.html (accessed Mar 2016).
[7]   FDA Database.   http://www.accessdata.fda.gov/drugsatfda_docs/nda/2014/205832Orig1s000PharmR.pdf (accessed Mar 2016).
[10]   Bonella, F.; Stowasser, S.; Wollin, L. *Drug Des. Devel. Ther.* **2015**, *9*, 6407-6419.

Table 8    Nintedanib Inhibited Fibroblast Migration, Proliferation and Transformation *In Vitro*[6, 7, 10]

| Study | Cell | Cell Type | Stimulus | Endpoint | IC$_{50}$ (nM) |
|---|---|---|---|---|---|
| Autophosphate | N-HLF | Primary human lung fibroblasts from control donors | PDGF BB | pPDGF$\alpha$ | 22 |
| | | | PDGF BB | pPDGF$\beta$ | 39 |
| Proliferation | K562 | Human chronic myelogenous leukemia | NA | Proliferation | 433 |
| | IPF-HLF[a] | Primary lung fibroblasts from patients with IPF | PDGF BB | Proliferation | 11 |
| | | | bFGF | Proliferation | 5.5 |
| | | | VEGF | Proliferation | <1 |
| | N-HLF[a] | Primary lung fibroblasts from patients with IPF | PDGF BB | Proliferation | 13 |
| | | | bFGF | Proliferation | 0.6 |
| | | | VEGF | Proliferation | <1 |
| Migration | IPF-HLF[b] | Primary lung fibroblasts from patients with IPF | PDGF BB | Coated membrane | 28 |
| | | | FGF2 | Coated membrane | 228 |
| | N-HLF[b] | Primary human lung fibroblasts from control donors | PDGF BB | Coated membrane | 19 |
| | | | FGF2 | Coated membrane | 86 |
| Transformation | IPF-HLF | Primary lung fibroblasts from patients with IPF | TGF-$\beta$ | $\alpha$-SMA mRNA expression | 144[c] |

[a] Fibroblasts were treated with nintedanib in the presence of GFs for 30 minutes (n = 4/group), cell proliferation was assessed by the number of cells at 48 h.   [b] The number of fibroblasts having crossed over a coated membrane within a 4 h period.   [c] Nintedanib inhibited TGF-$\beta$-induced transformation of fibroblasts to myofibroblasts, the expression of $\alpha$-smooth muscle actin was used as a marker for the cell transformation (fibroblast to myofibroblast).

## *In Vivo* Efficacy

Table 9    Anti-tumor Effect of Nintedanib in Cancer Models[6, 7, 9, 11, 12]

| Model | | | Dose (mg/kg, p.o.) | Duration (Day) | Results | |
|---|---|---|---|---|---|---|
| Cell Lines | Derivation | Animal | | | T/C Value [%][a] | Finding |
| FaDu | HNSCC | Nude mouse | 10 | QD × 21 | 82 | Significant anti-tumor effect was observed. |
| | | | 25 | QD × 21 | 46 | |
| | | | 50 | BID × 21 | 15 | |
| | | | 50 | QD × 21 | 14/27 | |
| | | | 100 | QD × 21 | 11 | |
| Caki-1 | Kidney | Nude mouse | 10 | QD × NA | 71 | Reduction of tumor vessel density of about 80% at 100 mg/kg/day. |
| | | | 50 | QD × NA | 25 | |
| | | | 100 | QD × NA | 16 | |
| GS-9L[b] | Glioma | Rat | 10 | QD × NA | 74 | Demonstrated anti-tumor efficacy was observed. |
| | | | 25 | QD × NA | 45 | |
| | | | 50 | QD × NA | 30 | |
| HT-29 | Colon | Nude mouse | 100 | QD × NA | 16 | Tumor growth inhibition. |
| SKOV-3 | Ovary | Nude mouse | 50 | QD × NA | 19 | |
| Calu-6 | NSCLC | Nude mouse | 50 | QD × NA | 24 | |
| PAC-120 | Prostate | Nude mouse | 100 | QD × NA | 34 | |

[a] Nude mice bearing established human xenografts tumor (0.05-0.1 cm³ volume) were treated once or twice daily with nintedanib p.o. (10-100 mg/kg) or vehicle control. For T/C values, the median tumor volume of each treatment group was compared to the median of the control group at the end of the experiment.   [b] GS-9L is a syngeneic rat tumor glioma model that has grown s.c..  HNSCC: Human head and neck squamous cell carcinoma.

[6]   PMDA Database.   http://www.pmda.go.jp/drugs/2015/P20150619001/index.html (accessed Mar 2016).

[7]   FDA Database.   http://www.accessdata.fda.gov/drugsatfda_docs/nda/2014/205832Orig1s000PharmR.pdf (accessed Mar 2016).

[9]   EMA Database.   http://www.ema.europa.eu/docs/en_GB/document_library/EPAR_-_Public_assessment_report/human/002569/WC500179972.pdf (accessed-Mar 2016).

[10]   Bonella, F.; Stowasser, S.; Wollin, L. *Drug Des. Devel. Ther.* **2015**, *9*, 6407-6419.

[11]   Hilberg, F.; Roth, G. J.; Krssak, M., et al. *Cancer Res.* **2008**, *68*, 4774-4782.

[12]   Roth, G. J.; Heckel, A.; Colbatzky, F., et al. *J. Med. Chem.* **2009**, *52*, 4466-4480.

Table 10    Efficacy in Animal Fibrotic Lung Models[7, 10, 13, 14]

| Animal Model | | Nintedanib Administration | | Effect | |
|---|---|---|---|---|---|
| Animal | Modeling | Dose (p.o., mg/kg) | Duration (Day) | ED (mg/kg) | Finding |
| Rat | Bleomycin  2.2 mg/kg, i.t. | 0, 10, 30, 50 | QD × 21[a] | 10 | Down-regulation of fibrosis scores and expressions of procollagen and TGFβ genes. |
| | Bleomycin  2.2 mg/kg, i.t. | 50 | QD × 11[b] | NA | Down-regulation of fibrosis scores and expressions of procollagen and TGFβ genes. |
| Mouse | Silica  2.5 mg/kg, intranasally | 0, 30, 100 | QD × 10-20[c] | 30 | Down-regulation of fibrosis scores and gene expressions of fibrotic and inflammatory markers. |
| | Bleomycin  3.0 mg/kg, intranasally | 0, 30, 60 | QD × 14[d] | 60 | Effective in reducing lung fibrosis. |
| Rip1Tag2 transgenic mouse | NA    NA | 0, 50 | QD × 21 | 50 | Reduced tumor volume and improved survival time. |

[a] Nintedanib treatment was started on the day of bleomycin dosing.    [b] Nintedanib treatment was started 10 days after bleomycin dosing.    [c] Nintedanib treatment was started 10 or 20 days after silica dosing.    [d] Nintedanib treatment was started 0 or 7 days after the bleomycin dosing.

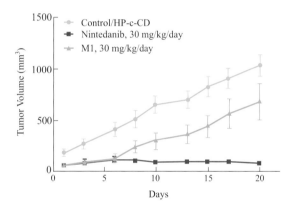

**Study:** Anti-tumor activities by nintedanib in human FaDu xenograft mouse model.

**Animal:** Nude mouse.

**Administration:** Nintedanib and M1, p.o., 30 mg/kg, QD for 20 days, respectively.

**Test:** The tumor volumes.

**Results:** Nintedanib inhibited tumor growth in this model, whereas M1 did not.

Figure A    Anti-tumor Efficacy of Nintedanib and M1 on FaDu Xenograft in Nude Mice[7]

[7]    FDA Database.    http://www.accessdata.fda.gov/drugsatfda_docs/nda/2014/205832Orig1s000PharmR.pdf (accessed Mar 2016).
[10]    Wollin, L.; Wex, E.; Pautsch, A., et al. *Eur. Respire. J.* **2015**, *45*, 1434-1445.
[13]    Wollin, L.; Maillet, I.; Quesniaux, V., et al. *J. Pharmacol. Exp. Ther.* **2014**, *349*, 209-220.
[14]    Bill, R.; Fagiani, E.; Zumsteg, A., et al. *Clin. Cancer. Res.* **2015**, *21*, 4856-4867.

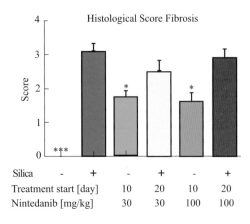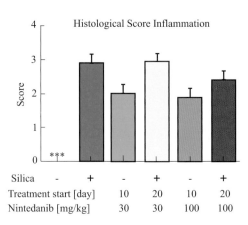

Figure B    Nintedanib Attenuated Silica-induced Lung Fibrosis in Mice[7]

**Study:** Effect on lung fibrosis and lung inflammation in mice fibrotic lung model.

**Animal:** BL6 mouse.

**Modeling:** Silica, intranasally 2.5 mg, induced lung fibrosis first.    Mice were sacrificed on Day 30 post silica instillation.

**Administration:** Nintedanib, p.o., 0, 30 or 100 mg/kg, treated 10 or 20 days.    Vehicle control: NA.

**Test:** BALF was examined for inflammation markers such as IL-1 and IL-6.

**Results**: Nintedanib was effective in reducing lung fibrosis scores and lung inflammation scores.

# 5    ADME & Drug-Drug Interaction

## Summary

### Absorption of Nintedanib

❖ Had low oral bioavailability in humans (4.7%), rats (11.9%), and cynomolgus monkeys (13.2%), and moderate in rhesus monkeys (23.8%).

❖ Was absorbed moderately with the $T_{max}$ occurring 2 to 3.98 h in humans.

❖ Showed a half-life ranging between 9 to 16 h in humans, longer than that in mice (5.15 h) after oral administrations.    The half-lives of nintedanib were 3.95 h in rats and 5.95-7.09 h in monkeys after intravenous administrations.

❖ Had high clearance in rats (202 mL/min/kg) and humans (18 mL/min/kg), but low in monkeys (30.2-37.5 mL/min/kg), in contrast to liver blood flow, after intravenous administrations.

❖ Exhibited an extensive distribution in tissues in humans, rats and monkeys, with apparent volumes of distribution at 13.6, 41.2 and 8-10 L/kg, respectively, after intravenous administrations.

### Distribution of Nintedanib

❖ Exhibited high plasma protein binding in humans (98%), rats (96%), mice (97%) and monkeys (91%-93%).    Note that nintedanib was mainly bound to HSA in human plasma.

❖ Had a $C_b$:$C_p$ ratio of 0.869 in humans, suggesting moderate penetration into red blood cells.

❖ Male rats after single intravenous and oral administration:

• After intravenous administration, most of the tissues took up radioactivity very rapidly.    Tissue drug levels were well above blood levels as early as 5 minutes after administration.

• After oral administration, the concentrations of radioactivity in most tissues followed a time course with maximum concentrations at 8 h post-dose.    Significant radioactivities were still present in the salivary gland, liver, spleen, and thymus at 48 h post-dose.

[7]    FDA Database.    http://www.accessdata.fda.gov/drugsatfda_docs/nda/2014/205832Orig1s000PharmR.pdf (accessed Mar 2016).

- In contrast, radioactivity showed an early peak in blood (0.5 h post-dose) and in liver (2 h post-dose). Rare radioactivity was found in the CNS tissues. Although the elimination was complete at 168 h post-dose, results suggested a long residual time for nintedanib in rats.
- ❖ Male rats after multiple oral administrations:
  - Nintedanib was rapidly and well distributed into most tissues including the central nervous system (CNS).
  - Relatively higher concentration tissues were observed in testes, kidneys, adrenals, liver, spleen, thymus, bone morrow, brine and heart. The accumulation factor was more than two in tissues after 13 days multiple administrations.
  - Statistically significant increases in tissues drug concentrations were observed in brain and heart.

## Metabolism of Nintedanib

- ❖ Nintedanib was extensively metabolized *in vitro* studies.
- ❖ The prevalent metabolic reaction was rapid hydrolytic cleavage by esterases resulting in BIBF1202. *In vitro* esterase and CYP3A4 hydrolyzed and desmethylated nintedanib to form BIBF1202. BIBF1202 was subsequently glucuronidated by UGT enzymes, namely UGT1A1, 1A7, 1A8 and 1A10 to BIBF1202 glucuronide.
- ❖ A minor extent of the biotransformation of nintedanib consisted of CYP pathways, predominantly CYP3A4 (oxidative *N*-demethylation).
- ❖ Overall, BIBF1202 (M1) represented the most abundant component in human plasma.
- ❖ All the metabolites found in humans could be found in rats and monkeys.
- ❖ The major metabolites were not active at clinically relevant concentrations.

## Excretion of Nintedanib

- ❖ Was predominantly excreted in feces of humans and animal species, with M1 as the most significant component in human and animal feces.
- ❖ Following intravenous administration, biliary excretion (61%) was the major contributing factor, however, following oral dose, the amount secreted in the bile (10%) was significantly less in rats.

## Drug-Drug Interaction

- ❖ Nintedanib, BIBF1202 and BIBF1202 glucuronide were not inhibitors or inducers of CYP pathways *in vitro* studies.
- ❖ Nintedanib inhibited UGT1A1 ($IC_{50}$ = 1.7 µM) *in vitro*.
- ❖ Nintedanib was a substrate of P-gp but not of BCRP and had weak inhibition for P-gp and BCRP.
- ❖ Nintedanib was a substrate of OCT1 and had strong inhibition for OCT1 *in vitro*.
- ❖ BIBF1202 was a substrate of OATP1B1 and OATP2B1 and had weak inhibition for transporters.
- ❖ BIBF1202 glucuronide was a substrate of MRP2 and BCRP and had no inhibition for transporters.

# Absorption

Table 11　*In Vivo* Pharmacokinetic Parameters of Nintedanib in Mice, Rats and Monkeys after Single Intravenous and Oral Dose of Nintedanib[7]

| Species | Route | Dose (mg/kg) | $C_{max}$ (ng/mL) | $AUC_{inf}$ (ng·h/mL) | $T_{1/2}$ (h) | Cl (mL/min/kg) | $V_d$ (L/kg) | F (%) |
|---|---|---|---|---|---|---|---|---|
| Mouse | p.o. | 50 | 547 | 2720 | 5.15 | - | - | - |
| Rat | i.v. | 2 | 124 | 181 | 3.95 | 202 | 41.2 | - |
| | p.o. | 50 | 105 | 375 | - | - | - | 11.9 |
| Cynomolgus monkey | i.v. | 5 | 1300 | 2260 | 5.95 | 37.5 | 8.64 | - |
| | p.o. | 40 | 175 | 2390 | - | - | - | 13.2 |
| Rhesus monkey | i.v. | 5 | 1090 | 2830 | 7.09 | 30.2 | 10.4 | - |
| | p.o. | 40 | 311 | 4440 | - | - | - | 23.8 |

[7] FDA Database. http://www.accessdata.fda.gov/drugsatfda_docs/nda/2014/205832Orig1s000PharmR.pdf (accessed Mar 2016).

Table 12 *In Vivo* Pharmacokinetic Parameters of Nintedanib and Metabolites in Humans after Single Dose of Nintedanib[7, 15]

| Species | Route | Dose (mg) | Analyte | $T_{max}$ (h) | $C_{max}$ (ng/mL) | $AUC_{inf}$ (ng·h/mL) | $T_{1/2}$ (h) | Cl or Cl/F (mL/min/kg) | $V_d$ or $V_d$/F (L/kg) | F (%) |
|---|---|---|---|---|---|---|---|---|---|---|
| Healthy human (male & female) | i.v. | 0.078 mg/kg | Nintedanib | NA | 12.3 | 71.9 | 17.9 | 18 | 13.6 | - |
| | p.o. | 1.29 mg/kg | Nintedanib | NA | 8.43 | 56.2 | 11.7 | - | - | 4.7 |
| Fasted healthy human (male)[a] | p.o. | 150 | Nintedanib | 2.0 (1.48-3.98) | 11.1 (60.3%) | 98.4 (33.0%) | 13.6 (15.2%) | 25400 (33.0%) mL/min | 29900 L (34.7%) | NA |
| Fed healthy human (female)[a] | p.o. | 150 | Nintedanib | 3.98 (1.5-6.05) | 13.2 (61.6%) | 119 (53.9%) | 16.2 (40.3%) | 20900 (53.9%) mL/min | 29400 L (47.0%) | NA |
| Patients with RCC (male & female) | p.o. | 200 | Nintedanib | 3.08 (0.883-12.0) | 0.159 (71.4%) | 1.33 (78.5%) | 9.18 (46.2%) | 12500 (78.5%) mL/min | 9970 L (72.2%) | NA |
| | p.o. | 200 | BIBF1202 | 3.92 (1.92-12.0) | 0.174 (117%) | 2.47 (186%) | 6.66 (29.2%) | NA | NA | NA |
| | p.o. | 200 | BIBF1202 glucuronide | 10.1 (4.08-13.0) | 0.21 (104%) | NC | 54.9 (76.0%) | NA | NA | NA |

[a] Vehicle was capsule.   $T_{max}$: Median (range).   NC: Not calculated as terminal phase not captured in the study.   RCC: Renal Cell Carcinoma.

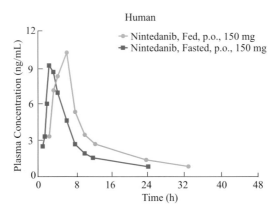

Human

Figure C   *In Vivo* Plasma Concentration-Time Profiles of Nintedanib in Humans after Single Dose of Nintedanib[15]

## Distribution

Table 13   *In Vitro* Plasma Protein Binding and Blood Partitioning of Nintedanib and Metabolites in Several Species[7, 15]

| Species | Plasma Protein Binding% | | | | | Blood Partitioning | |
|---|---|---|---|---|---|---|---|
| | Total Protein | | | HSA | AGP | $C_b:C_p$ | $C_c:C_p$ |
| | Nintedanib | BIBF1202 | BIBF1202-GA | Nintedanib | Nintedanib | Nintedanib | Nintedanib |
| Mouse | 97.2 | ND | ND | NA | NA | NA | NA |
| Rat | 95.8 | 77.2 | 96 | NA | NA | NA | NA |
| Cynomolgus monkey | 92.9 | ND | ND | NA | NA | NA | NA |
| Rhesus monkey | 91.4 | 55.0 | 84.0 | NA | NA | NA | NA |
| Human | 97.8 | 77.8 | 97.0 | 97.5 | 55.5-93.0[a] | 0.869 | 0.701 |

$C_b:C_p$: Blood to plasma concentration ratio.   $C_c:C_p$: Blood cell to plasma concentration ratio.   [a] The values were measured from 0.14 g/L AGP to 3.4 g/L AGP.

[7]   FDA Database.   http://www.accessdata.fda.gov/drugsatfda_docs/nda/2014/205832Orig1s000PharmR.pdf (accessed Mar 2016).
[15]   FDA Database.   http://www.accessdata.fda.gov/drugsatfda_docs/nda/2014/205832Orig1s000ClinPharmR.pdf (accessed Mar 2016).

## Tissue Distribution:[7]

❖ Male rats after single intravenous dose of 5 mg/kg and oral dose of 30 mg/kg nintedanib:
  • After intravenous administration, most of the tissues took up radioactivities very rapidly.　Tissue drug levels were well above blood levels as early as 5 minutes after administration.
  • After oral administration, the concentration of radioactivities in most tissues followed a time course with maximum concentrations at 8 h post-dose.　Significant radioactivities were still present in the salivary gland, liver, spleen, and thymus at 48 h post-dose.
  • In contrast, radioactivity showed an early peak in blood (0.5 h post-dose) and in liver (2 h post-dose).　Little radioactivity was found in the CNS tissues.　Although the elimination was complete at 168 h post-dose, results suggested a long residual time for nintedanib in rats.

Table 14　*In Vivo* Tissue Distribution in Albino and Pigmented Rats after Single Dose of Nintedanib[6]

| Tissue | Albino Rat/ p.o., 5 mg/kg | | | | | | Pigmented Rat/ p.o., 5 mg/kg | |
| | Radioactivity (ng eq./g tissue) | | | | | Tissue/Blood AUC$_{0-168}$ Ratio | Radioactivity (ng eq./g tissue) | |
| | 5 min | 2 h | 8 h | 48 h | 168 h | | 2 h | 168 h |
|---|---|---|---|---|---|---|---|---|
| Blood | 1529 | 277 | 58 | ND | ND | 1.0 | 366 | BLQ |
| Brain | 42 | BLQ | BLQ | BLQ | ND | 0.0 | BLQ | BLQ |
| Lungs | 10204 | 3832 | 488 | BLQ | ND | 9.2 | 2763 | 50 |
| Liver | 14526 | 4450 | 1388 | 264 | 53 | 19.0 | 7026 | 155 |
| Spleen | 12149 | 6475 | 1289 | 300 | 30 | 23.5 | 11801 | 272 |
| Adrenal gland | 36492 | 6479 | 864 | 50 | ND | 21.7 | 12302 | 124 |
| Kidneys | 33803 | 6388 | 1263 | 109 | BLQ | 24.5 | 11612 | 184 |
| Brown fat | 12898 | 2439 | 659 | 39 | ND | 10.3 | 5641 | 88 |
| Tongue | 11608 | 3386 | ND | ND | ND | 6.3 | 4098 | 30 |
| Pituitary | 9293 | 5484 | 4190 | 910 | ND | 50.6 | 12933 | 1154 |
| Eyes | 4380 | 3036 | 1371 | 307 | ND | 1.0 | 13246 | 582 |
| Skin (back) | 1341 | 1020 | 454 | 95 | ND | 0.0 | 1527 | 39 |

ND: Not determined.　BLQ: Below limit of quantification.

# Metabolism

Table 15　Correlation Analysis of U2, U3 and U4 Formation with Prototypical and Selective CYP Test Reactions for a Panel of 11 Individual Human Liver Microsomes[6]

| CYP | Correlation Coefficient | | |
| | U2 | U3 | U4 |
|---|---|---|---|
| 1A2 | 0.1996 | 0.0565 | 0.0000 |
| 2A6 | 0.2444 | 0.0292 | 0.0564 |
| 2B6 | 0.4946 | 0.2716 | 0.3079 |
| 2C8 | 0.0244 | 0.2865 | 0.3927 |
| 2C9 | 0.0477 | 0.1321 | 0.2538 |
| 2C19 | 0.1012 | 0.0353 | 0.1545 |
| 2D6 | 0.0287 | 0.0028 | 0.0028 |
| 2E1 | 0.0531 | 0.1279 | 0.0660 |
| 3A4/5 | 0.0446 | 0.7806 | 0.8747 |
| 4A11 | 0.0786 | 0.0659 | 0.0071 |
| Total | NA | 0.8499 | 0.7871 |

[6] PMDA Database.　http://www.pmda.go.jp/drugs/2015/P20150619001/index.html (accessed Mar 2016).
[7] FDA Database.　http://www.accessdata.fda.gov/drugsatfda_docs/nda/2014/205832Orig1s000PharmR.pdf (accessed Mar 2016).

Table 16    Enzyme Kinetic Parameters for Nintedanib Glucuronidation by Human Liver Microsomes and Expressed UGT1A1[6]

| Metabolite Formation | Microsome Sample | $V_{max}$ (pmoL/min/mg) | $K_m$ (µM) | $V_{max}/K_m$ (µL/min/mg) | Mean $V_{max}/K_m$ |
|---|---|---|---|---|---|
| M2 | Donor 23 (male) | 188 | 55.1 | 3.42 | 2.56 |
| | Donor 26 (male) | 71.3 | 44.3 | 1.61 | |
| | Donor 17 (male) | 188 | 71.0 | 2.64 | |
| | Donor 32 (female) | 337 | 64.1 | 5.26 | 2.90 |
| | Donor 70 (female) | 83.4 | 46.5 | 1.79 | |
| | Donor 71 (female) | 72.3 | 43.8 | 1.65 | |
| | UGT1A1 | 174 | 153 | 1.14 | - |
| | UGT1A7 | 21.8 | 30.5 | 1.4 | - |
| | UGT1A8 | 60.7 | 184 | 3.0 | - |
| | UGT1A10 | 112 | 87.9 | 0.8 | - |
| U3 | Human liver microsomes | 354 | 142 | 2.49 | - |
| U4 | CYP3A4 | 1278 | 22.3 | 57.3 | - |

## Metabolic Enzyme Identification:[15]

❖ Nintedanib was extensively metabolized, primarily through hydrolytic cleavage by esterases to BIBF1202.    BIBF1202 was subsequently glucuronidated by UGT enzymes, namely UGT1A1, UGT1A7, UGT1A8, and UGT1A10 to BIBF1202 glucuronide.

❖ A minor extent of the biotransformation of nintedanib consisted of CYP pathway, predominantly CYP3A4.

Table 17    Metabolites in Plasma, Urine and Feces in Humans and Non-clinical Species after Single Oral and Intravenous Dose of Nintedanib[6, 7, 15]

| Matrix | Species | Gender | Route | Dose (mg/kg) | Time (h) | % of Radioactivity or % of Dose | | | | | | | | |
|---|---|---|---|---|---|---|---|---|---|---|---|---|---|---|
| | | | | | | M0 | M1 | M2 | M3 | M4 | M5 | M9 | M13 | M14 |
| Plasma | Mouse | Male | p.o. | 30 | 1 | 20.6 | trace | 31.4 | 14.3 | trace | - | - | - | - |
| | | Female | p.o. | 30 | 1 | 31.3 | trace | 25.6 | trace | trace | - | - | - | - |
| | Rat | Male/Female | i.v. | 5 | 0.25 | 47.8 | 38.6 | 13.6 | - | - | - | - | - | - |
| | | | p.o. | 30 | 4 | 9.0 | 9.65 | 76.9 | - | 4.36 | - | - | - | - |
| | Rhesus monkey | Male/Female | i.v. | 5 | 1 | 87 | 12.1 | 1.79 | - | - | - | - | - | - |
| | | | p.o. | 20 | 3 | 35.8 | - | 55.1 | 7.6 | - | - | - | 10.6 | - |
| | Human | Male | p.o. | 100 mg | 2 | 34.5 | 38.7 | 15.3 | - | 11.6 | - | - | - | - |
| Urine[a] | Mouse | Male | p.o. | 30 | 0-48 | - | 1.3 | - | - | 0.6 | - | - | - | - |
| | Rat | Male/Female | i.v. | 5 | 0-24 | 0.29 | 3.23 | 0.37 | 0.1 | - | - | - | - | - |
| | | | p.o. | 30 | 0-24 | 0.11 | 0.66 | 0.73 | - | 0.12 | - | - | - | - |
| | Rhesus monkey | Male/Female | i.v. | 5 | 0-24 | 0.86 | 2.17 | 0.06 | 0.17 | 0.02 | 0.07 | - | 0.03 | 0.03 |
| | | | p.o. | 20 | 0-24 | 0.32 | 0.52 | 0.11 | 0.1 | 0.02 | 0.01 | 0.01 | - | - |
| | Human | Male | p.o. | 100 mg | 0-24 | 0.14 | 0.2 | 0.07 | 0.01 | 0.01 | 0.004 | 0.02 | 0.50 | 0.14 |
| Bile | Mouse | Male | p.o. | 30 | 0-6 | 0.8 | 4.4 | - | 2.1 | 1.8 | - | - | - | - |
| | Rat | Male/Female | i.v. | 5 | 0-6 | 16.0 | 20.2 | 5.23 | 19.5 | - | - | - | - | - |
| | | | p.o. | 30 | 0-6 | 2.8 | 4.4 | 1.8 | 0.98 | - | - | - | - | - |

[6]  PMDA Database.   http://www.pmda.go.jp/drugs/2015/P20150619001/index.html (accessed Mar 2016).
[7]  FDA Database.   http://www.accessdata.fda.gov/drugsatfda_docs/nda/2014/205832Orig1s000PharmR.pdf (accessed Mar 2016).
[15]  FDA Database.   http://www.accessdata.fda.gov/drugsatfda_docs/nda/2014/205832Orig1s000ClinPharmR.pdf (accessed Mar 2016).

*Continued*

| Matrix | Species | Gender | Route | Dose (mg/kg) | Time (h) | % of Radioactivity or % of Dose | | | | | | | | |
|---|---|---|---|---|---|---|---|---|---|---|---|---|---|---|
| | | | | | | M0 | M1 | M2 | M3 | M4 | M5 | M9 | M13 | M14 |
| Feces | Mouse | Male | p.o. | 30 | 0-48 | 14.4 | 49.3 | - | 9.4 | 26.2 | - | - | - | - |
| | Rat | Male/Female | i.v. | 5 | 0-24 | 10.9 | 50.2 | - | 11.0 | 5.8 | - | - | - | - |
| | | | p.o. | 30 | 0-24 | 15.6 | 47.3 | - | 1.96 | 2.17 | - | - | - | - |
| | Rhesus monkey | Male/Female | i.v. | 5 | 0-72 | 12.8 | 42.7 | - | 10.2 | 7.53 | 0.98 | 1.4 | - | - |
| | | | p.o. | 20 | 0-72 | 33.7 | 38.3 | - | 6.95 | 3.82 | 2.49 | 1.5 | - | 0.93 |
| | Human | Male | p.o. | 100 mg | 0-72 | 19.9 | 58.4 | 0.1 | 3.6 | 2.60 | 0.20 | - | - | - |

% of radioactivity for plasma, % of dose for urine, feces and bile.

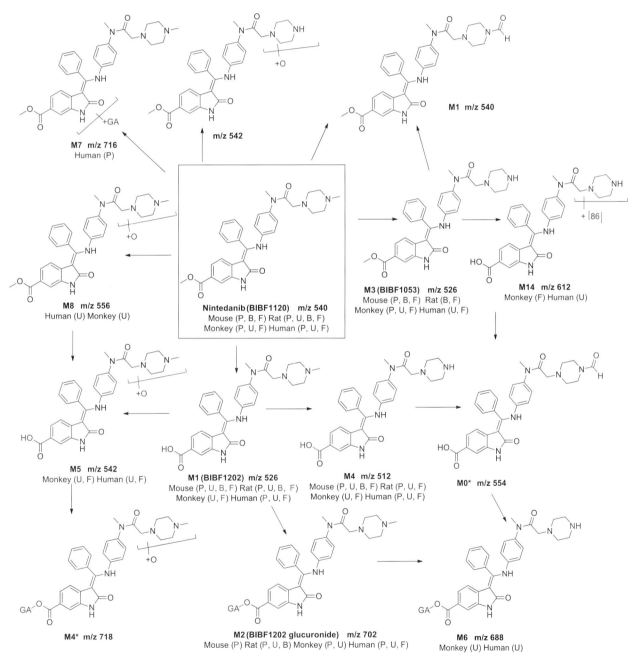

Figure D    Proposed Pathways for *In Vivo* Biotransformation of Nintedanib in Rats, Mice, Monkeys and Humans[6, 15]

The red labels represent the main comporents in matrices (p.o., male).    P = Plasma, U = Urine, F = Feces, B = Bile and GA = Glucuronic acid.

\* Co-elution minor/trace metabolite.

[6]  PMDA Database.   http://www.pmda.go.jp/drugs/2015/P20150619001/index.html (accessed Mar 2016).

[15]  FDA Database.   http://www.accessdata.fda.gov/drugsatfda_docs/nda/2014/205832Orig1s000ClinPharmR.pdf (accessed Mar 2016).

## Excretion

Table 18    Excretion Profiles of [$^{14}$C]Nintedanib in Various Species after Single Intravenous and Oral Dose of [$^{14}$C]Nintedanib[6, 7]

| Species | Route | Dose (mg/kg) | Bile (% of dose) | Urine (% of dose) | Feces (% of dose) |
|---|---|---|---|---|---|
| Mouse (male) | p.o. | 30 | 9.1 | 1.9 | 99.3 |
| Mouse (female) | p.o. | 30 | 19.5 | 0.8 | 90.7 |
| Rat (male) | i.v. | 5 | 61.0 | 4.0 | 77.9 |
| Rat (female) | p.o. | 30 | 10.0 | 1.6 | 67.0 |
| Monkey (male) | i.v. | 5 | - | 4.1 | 78.6 |
| Monkey (female) | p.o. | 20 | - | 1.2 | 87.7 |
| Human (male) | p.o. | 100 mg | - | 0.65 | 93.4 |

NE: Not examined.

## Drug-Drug Interaction

Table 19    *In Vitro* Evaluation Nintedanib and Metabolites (BIBF1202 and BIBF1202 glucuronide) as Inhibitors and Inducers of CYP/UGT Enzymes[6]

| Enzyme | IC$_{50}$ (µM) Nintedanib | BIBF1202 | BIBF1202 Glucuronide | Enzyme | Conc. (µM) | Fold Induction Activity | mRNA Expression |
|---|---|---|---|---|---|---|---|
| CYP1A2 | >100 | >100 | >100 | CYP1A2 | 0.02 | 0.91 | 0.97 |
| CYP2A6 | >100 | >100 | >100 | | 2 | 1.31 | 1.29 |
| CYP2B6 | >100 | >100 | >100 | CYP2B6 | 0.02 | 0.84 | 0.78 |
| CYP2C8 | >50 | >100 | >100 | | 2 | 1.12 | 1.66 |
| CYP2C9 | >100 | >100 | 85.5 | CYP2C8 | 0.02 | 1.51 | 0.97 |
| CYP2C19 | >100 | >100 | >100 | | 2 | 1.76 | 1.85 |
| CYP2D6 | >100 | >100 | >100 | CYP2C9 | 0.02 | 1.13 | 1.17 |
| CYP2E1 | >100 | >100 | >100 | | 2 | 1.18 | 1.10 |
| CYP3A4 | 70.1 | >100 | >100 | CYP2C19 | 0.02 | 0.79 | 0.55 |
| CYP4A11 | >100 | >100 | >100 | | 2 | 0.94 | 1.06 |
| UGT1A1 | 1.7 | >200 | NA | CYP3A4 | 0.02 | 0.91 | 0.90 |
| UGT2B7 | 77.6[a] | >200 | NA | | 2 | 0.91 | 1.04 |

[a] IC$_{50}$ for estradiol 17-glucuronidation.

[6]  PMDA Database.   http://www.pmda.go.jp/drugs/2015/P20150619001/index.html (accessed Mar 2016).
[7]  FDA Database.   http://www.accessdata.fda.gov/drugsatfda_docs/nda/2014/205832Orig1s000PharmR.pdf (accessed Mar 2016).

Table 20  *In Vitro* Evaluation of Nintedanib and Metabolites (BIBF1202 and BIBF1202 glucuronide) as Inhibitors and Substrates of Transporters[15]

| Transporter | | Nintedanib and Metabolites as Substrates | | | Nintedanib and Metabolites as Inhibitors | | |
| | | Substrate | | | Inhibitor/IC$_{50}$ (μM) | | |
| | | Nintedanib | BIBF1202 | BIBF1202 Glucuronide | Nintedanib | BIBF1202 | BIBF1202 Glucuronide |
|---|---|---|---|---|---|---|---|
| SLC | OATP1B1 | No | Yes | No | No/10 | 14 | No/100 |
| | OATP1B3 | No | No | No | No/10 | 79 | No/100 |
| | OATP2B1 | No | Yes | No | No/10 | 50 | ND |
| | OCT1 | Yes | No | No | 0.88 | 16 | ND |
| | OCT2 | No | No | ND | No/30 | No/100 | No/100 |
| | OAT1 | ND | ND | ND | ND | ND | No/100 |
| | OAT3 | ND | ND | ND | ND | ND | No/100 |
| ABC | P-gp | Yes | ND | ND | Weak/30[a] | No/30 | Weak/100 |
| | MRP2 | No | No | Yes | No/30 | No/30 | Weak/100 |
| | BCRP | No | No | Yes | Weak/30[a] | Weak/30 | No/100 |

[a] IC$_{50}$ was not determined and expected to be >30 μM.   ND: Not determined.

# 6   Non-Clinical Toxicology

## Summary

### Single-Dose Toxicity

❖  Single-dose oral or intravenous administration of nintedanib in rodents:
  • Mouse ALD: >2000 mg/kg (p.o.), and >40 mg/kg (i.v.).
  • Rat ALD: >2000 mg/kg (p.o.), and >40 mg/kg (i.v.).

### Repeated-Dose Toxicity

❖  Sub-acute, sub- and chronic toxicity by the oral route in mice (up to 13 weeks), rats (up to 26 weeks), dogs (up to 2 weeks), Cynomolgus monkeys (up to 13 weeks) and Rhesus monkeys (up to 52 weeks):
  • In view of the chronic rat and monkey studies, the identified NOAELs provided exposure margins of <1 to 2.6 folds (based on AUC) compared to the anticipated clinical exposure at the recommended dose.   Based on the indicated disease, these exposure margins were considered acceptable.
  • Target organs of toxicity: Bone (mice, rats, and monkeys), liver (mice and rats), kidneys (rats), ovaries (mice and rats), and the immune system (mice, rats, and monkeys).   The affected organs in the immune system included adrenal glands, bone marrow, spleen and thymus.

### Safety Pharmacology

❖  Safety pharmacology studies were conducted to evaluate the effects of nintedanib on the central nervous system, cardiovascular system, respiratory system, gastrointestinal tract, liver, kidney and locomotor activity.   No apparent toxicity was observed in the standard battery of safety pharmacology studies.

### Genotoxicity

❖  Nintedanib was negative in the *in vitro* bacterial gene mutation assay, the *in vitro* mouse lymphoma assay, and the *in vivo* micronucleus assay in rats.

### Reproductive and Developmental Toxicity

❖  Fertility and early embryonic development in rats:
  • Nintedanib had no effect on male fertility, nevertheless, it led to a reduction of female fertility, malformations in the vasculature, skeletal system and urogenital system, decreased post-natal viability of pups, and changes in the number and size of corpora lutea in the ovaries, which defined nintedanib as a potent reproductive toxicant.
❖  Embryo-fetal development in rats and rabbits:

---

[15]  FDA Database.   http://www.accessdata.fda.gov/drugsatfda_docs/nda/2014/205832Orig1s000ClinPharmR.pdf (accessed Mar 2016).

- Nintedanib tends to be a potent teratogen, embryo-fetal death and teratogenic effects emerged in both species at maternally nontoxic doses.   Malformations included abnormalities in the vasculature (e.g., missing or additional major blood vessels), skeletal system (e.g., hemivertebra, missing or asymmetrically ossified vertebra; bifid or fused ribs; fused, split, or unilaterally ossified sternebrae), and urogenital system (e.g., missing organs in some fetuses).
- A sex ratio change was also observed in rabbits (e.g., shift in female: male ratio to 71%:29%) at approximately 15 × MRHD in adults (on AUC basis at maternal oral dose of 60 mg/kg/day).
❖ Pre- and postnatal development in rats:
  - Nintedanib decreased postnatal viability during the first 4 postnatal days in rat pups when dams were exposed to less than the MRHD on AUC basis at maternal oral dose of 10 mg/kg/day.

Carcinogenicity

❖ Two-year oral carcinogenicity studies in mice and rats did not revealed any evidence of carcinogenic potential.

## Single-Dose Toxicity

Table 21    Single-Dose Toxicity Studies of Nintedanib by Oral and Intravenous Administration[9]

| Species | Dose (mg/kg) | ALD (mg/kg) | Finding |
|---|---|---|---|
| NMRI mouse | 2000, oral gavage | >2000 | No mortality. Body weights reduction, ataxia and drowsiness. No gross pathological lesion at the terminal necropsy. |
| | 40, i.v. infusion for 10 min | >40 | None noteworthy. |
| Wistar rat | 2000, oral gavage | >2000 | Sedation, staggered and diarrhea. |
| | 40, i.v. infusion for 10 min | >40 | None noteworthy. |

Vehicle: 0.5 % (w/v) HEC.

## Repeated-Dose Toxicity

Table 22    Repeated-Dose Toxicity Studies of Nintedanib by Oral gavage Administration[6]

| Species | Duration (Week) | Dose (mg/kg/day) | NOAEL Dose (mg/kg/day) | NOAEL $AUC_{0-24}^{a}$ (ng·h/mL) | Finding |
|---|---|---|---|---|---|
| CD-1 mouse | 13 | 0, 10, 30, 100 | <10 | 225/231 | Reduction of body weight gain was observed in all dose groups. Decreases of RBC, hemoglobin, MCV, reticulocytes, liver weights, and thickened epiphyseal plates, swelling of articular chondrocytes were observed at ≥30 mg/kg. Adenopathy, luteinized follicles, fewer mature corpora lutea were observed at 100 mg/kg. |
| Wistar rat | 4 | 0, 3, 20, 100 | 20 | 149/119 | Adenopathy was observed when dose ≥5 mg/kg. Decreases of RBC, PCV, hemoglobin and increases of MCV, MCHC, and hepatocellular hemosiderosis, swelling of articular chondrocytes were observed at ≥20 mg/kg. Reduction of body weight gain and organ weights (heart, lung, liver, kidneys, spleen), increases of the activity of ALT and AST were observed at ≥60 mg/kg. |
| | 13 | 0, 5, 20, 60 | <5 | 22.7/26.1 | 100 mg/kg: Reduction of bodyweight (recovery secondary to adenopathy) and organ weights (heart, lung, liver, kidneys, thymus), adenopathy, thickened epiphyseal plates were observed at ≥100 mg/kg. |
| | 13 | 0, 3, 20, 100 | 3 | 2.31/8.38 | Hepatocellular hemosiderosis in females at 20 mg/kg. Adenopathy, swelling of articular chondrocytes and cellular depletion (bone marrow) were observed at ≥20 mg/kg. At 100 mg/kg, 1 premature decedent, decreases of RBC, PCV, hemoglobin and increases of ALT, AST, GGT, thymus weights, and thickened epiphyseal plates, hepatocellular hemosiderosis, cellular depletion (spleen), corpora lutea reduced in size/increased in number were observed. |

[6]  PMDA Database.   http://www.pmda.go.jp/drugs/2015/P20150619001/index.html (accessed Mar 2016).
[9]  EMA Database.   http://www.ema.europa.eu/docs/en_GB/document_library/EPAR_-_Public_assessment_report/human/002569/WC500179972.pdf (accessed Mar 2016).

*Continued*

| Species | Duration (Week) | Dose (mg/kg/day) | NOAEL | | Finding |
|---------|-----------------|------------------|-------|--|---------|
| | | | Dose (mg/kg/day) | $AUC_{0-24}^{a}$ (ng·h/mL) | |
| Wistar rat | 26 | 0, 5, 20, 80 | 5 | 16.4/29.2 | Swelling of articular chondrocytes was observed at 20 mg/kg. |
| | | | | | Decreases of RBC, PCV, hemoglobin, organ weights (thymus, adrenals) and hepatocellular hemosiderosis, swelling of articular chondrocytes, corpora lutea reduced in size/increased in number were observed when dose ≥20 mg/kg. |
| | | | | | Premature decedents, the loss of bodyweight gain and increased ALT activity, adenopathy, thickened epiphyseal plates, cellular depletion (bone marrow, thymus, spleen) were observed at 80 mg/kg. |
| Beagle dog | 2 | 0, 3, 10, 30, 1000 | <3 | 233/782 | Loss of bodyweight/bodyweight gain, increase of cholesterol level, thickened epiphyseal plates were observed in all dose groups. |
| | | | | | Diarrhea, reduction of food consumption and large intestine goblet cell numbers were observed at ≥3 mg/kg. |
| | | | | | One animal was euthanized, and intestinal mucosa: erosions, villous atrophy, epithelial cell damage were observed at ≥10 mg/kg. |
| | | | | | At ≥30 mg/kg, all animals euthanized. Increases of ALT and AST activities, cellular depletion (bone marrow, lymphoid tissue), gall bladder inflammation, and some clinical signs included severe diarrhea, vomiting, salivation and paralysis/abnormal gait were observed. |
| Cynomolgus monkey | 4 | 0, 3, 15, 60 | 3 | 158/185 | Occasional diarrhea, vomitus was observed at 15 mg/kg. |
| | | | | | Diarrhea, vomitus, decreases of bodyweight, RBC, PCV and hemoglobin, increases of reticulocytes, platelets, ALT and AST activities, epithelial atrophy, villous atrophy (small intestine) and cellular depletion (thymus, lymph nodes, spleen, bone marrow) were observed at 60 mg/kg. |
| | 13 | 0, 3, 15, 30/20 | 3 | 305/345 | Loss of body weight gain and cellular depletion (bone marrow) were observed at ≥15 mg/kg. |
| | | | | | Reduction of thymic weights and cellular depletion (thymus, bone marrow) were observed at 30/20 mg/kg. |
| Rhesus monkey | 4 | 0, 10, 20, 40 | 10 | 357/529 | Yellow colored faces were observed at ≥10 mg/kg. |
| | | | | | Decreases of the levels of RBC and HB at 20 mg/kg. |
| | | | | | Loss of body weight, diarrhea, and vomitus, increases of activities of ALT, AST and GGT were observed at 60 mg/kg. |
| | 52 | 10, 20, 60/45/30 | 10 | 786/506 | Thickened epiphyseal plates were observed in all dose groups. Adrenal zona fasciculata atrophy was observed at 10 mg/kg of male group. |
| | | | | | Loss of body weight gain was observed in both sexes when dose ≥20 mg/kg, and special for females, loss of spleen weight was also observed. |
| | | | | | 60/45/30 mg/kg: one male and one female were euthanized and diarrhea, decreases of activities of albumin and total protein were observed. |

Vehicle: 0.5 % (w/v) HEC solution.    [a] Male/female.

## Safety Pharmacology

Table 23    Safety Pharmacology Studies of Nintedanib[7, 9]

| Study | System | Dose[a] | Finding |
|---|---|---|---|
| Neurobehavioral effect | NMRI mouse | p.o., 0, 50, 100, 300 mg/kg of nintedanib chloride | No effect in Irwin behavioral tests and nocturnal motility. |
| | Wistar rat | 0, 3, 20, 100 mg/kg | No effect in modified Irwin behavioral test. |
| Cardiovascular function | Isolated guinea pig papillary muscle | 0.1, 1, 3, 10 μM | Nintedanib had no effect on $APD_{90}$ in concentrations up to 10 μM, or any other measured parameters. No effect was observed on myocardial repolarization at human therapeutic plasma concentrations. |
| | HEK293-hERG cell | 0.1, 1, 3, 10 μM | Nintedanib had an $IC_{50}$ value of 4.0 μM on hERG-mediated potassium current in HEK293 cells. |
| | Cynomolgus monkey | p.o., 0, 3, 15, 60 mg/kg | No significant effect on cardiovascular parameters. |
| | Anaesthetized pig | i.v., 0, 3, 10, 30 mg/kg | Dose-related increases in heart rate, systolic and diastolic pressures. |
| Respiratory function | Wistar rat | p.o., 3, 20, 100 mg/kg | Negative. |
| | Conscious rat | p.o., 0, 10, 30, 100 mg/kg | Increased arterial blood pressure and respiratory rate at 100 mg/kg. |
| Liver function | Rat | 30, 100, 300 mg/kg | Dose-dependent inhibition of GI motility and gastric emptying time. |
| Renal and liver function | Conscious rat | 10, 30, 100 mg/kg | Modest increase (1.3-2.3) of ALT and $\beta$-NAG. |
| Gastrointestinal function | Rat | p.o., 0, 10, 30, 100 mg/kg of nintedanib chloride | The doses of 10 and 30 mg/kg induced no statistically significant effects on gastric emptying.   At 100 mg/kg a significant inhibition of gastric emptying was observed. No effect on gastric acid output, total acidity, gastric pH and volume were observed. No influence GI transit at 10 mg/kg, but does-dependently reduced intestinal transit at 30-100 mg/kg. |

Vehicle: 0.5 % (w/v) HEC.    [a] Single dose unless otherwise specified.

## Genotoxicity

Table 24    Genotoxicity Studies of Nintedanib[6, 9]

| Assay | Species | Metabolism | Dose | Finding |
|---|---|---|---|---|
| *In vitro* bacterial reverse mutation assay (Ames) | TA98, TA100, TA1535, TA1537, TA102 (*S. typhimurium*), WP2*uvr*A(*E. coli*) | ± S9 | 3-2500 μg/plate for nintedanib base; 50-500 μg/plate for nintedanib chloride | Negative. |
| *In vitro* gene mutation assay in mammalian cell | Mouse lymphoma L5178Y (t/k[+/-]) cell | ± S9 | 5-50 μg/mL for nintedanib chloride | Negative. |
| *In vivo* chromosomal aberration study in cultured mammalian cell | SD rat | + | NA | Negative. |

Vehicle: 0.5 % (w/v) HEC solution *in vivo* tests, while DMSO for *in vitro* tests.

[6]  PMDA Database.   http://www.pmda.go.jp/drugs/2015/P20150619001/index.html (accessed Mar 2016).
[7]  FDA Database.   http://www.accessdata.fda.gov/drugsatfda_docs/nda/2014/205832Orig1s000PharmR.pdf (accessed Mar 2016).
[9]  EMA Database.   http://www.ema.europa.eu/docs/en_GB/document_library/EPAR_-_Public_assessment_report/human/002569/WC500179972.pdf (accessed Mar 2016).

## Reproductive and Developmental Toxicity

Table 25   Reproductive and Developmental Toxicology Studies of Nintedanib by Oral Administration[6, 7, 9]

| Study | Species | Daily Dose of Free Base (mg/kg) | Endpoint | NOAEL Dose (mg/kg/day) | NOAEL AUC$_{0-24}$ (ng·h/mL) | NOAEL Safety Margin (× MRHD) | Finding |
|---|---|---|---|---|---|---|---|
| Fertility and early embryonic development | SD rat | 0, 3, 20, 100 | Male fertility | 100 | NA | NA | None. |
| | | | Female fertility | 20 | 116 | 0.4 | ↑ Resorptions at ≥ MD. |
| | | | Embryo development | 3 | NA | NA | |
| Embryo-fetal development | SD rat | 0, 2.5, 5, 10 | Maternal | 10 | 34.2 | 0.1 | ↑ Number of variations and malformations at ≥ LD. |
| | | | Development | <2.5 | NA | NA | |
| | NZW rabbit | 0, 15, 30, 60 | Maternal | 60 | 5340 | 17.6 | ↓ Sex ratio (male: female) & numerical. |
| | | | Development | <15 | <1920 | <6.3 | ↑ Malformations at LD. |
| Pre- and postnatal development | Wistar rat | 0, 2.5, 5, 10 | F$_0$ | 5 | 16.5 | 0.05 | ↓ F$_1$ fetal weight & number of live pup at HD. |
| | | | F$_1$ | 5 | | | |
| | | | F$_2$ | NA | | | |

Vehicle: 0.5 % (w/v) HEC solution.   Safety margin was calculated based on exposure of 304 ng·h/mL at MRHD (150 mg, BID).

Table 26   Milk Excretion of [$^{14}$C]Nintedanib by Single-Dose Oral Administration of 30 mg/kg to Lactating Rat on 12 Days after Delivery[6, 7]

| Time (h) | Radioactivity Converted Conc. (ng eq./mL) Plasma | Radioactivity Converted Conc. (ng eq./mL) Milk | Parameter | Pharmacokinetics Property Plasma | Pharmacokinetics Property Milk |
|---|---|---|---|---|---|
| 1 | 2260 | 269 | $C_{max}$ (ng eq./mL) | NA | NA |
| 6 | 478 | 1060 | $T_{max}$ (h) | NA | NA |
| 24 | 7.92 | 106 | $T_{1/2}$ (h) | 3.3 | 5.5 |
| | | | AUC$_{0-24}$ (ng eq.·h/mL) | 12400 | 14000 |

Vehicle: 0.5 % (w/v) HEC.

## Carcinogenicity

Table 27   Carcinogenicity Toxicity Studies of Nintedanib by Oral Administrations[6, 7]

| Species | Duration$^a$ (Week) | Dose (mg/kg/day) | AUC$_{0-24}$ at HD$^a$ (ng·h/mL) | Fold of MRHD | Finding |
|---|---|---|---|---|---|
| CD-1 mouse | 102/103 | 0, 5, 15, 30 | 1090/1580 | 4 | No statistically significant tumor finding. Higher mortality in all female groups, but not dose dependent. Treatment-related non-neoplastic findings included in the gallbladder (fibrosis and ulceration), skin (dermal inflammation, epidermal ulceration and hyperplasia, edema, and scabs), uterus (arteritis/periarteritis/vascular mural fibrinoid necrosis), and adipose tissue (inflammation and necrosis). |
| Wistar rat | 104 | 0, 2.5, 5, 10 | 82.95 | 0.25 | No non-neoplastic finding. |

Vehicle: 0.5 % (w/v) HEC.   Safety margin was calculated based on exposure of 327 ng·h/mL at MRHD (150 mg, BID).   $^a$ Male/Female.

[6]  PMDA Database.   http://www.pmda.go.jp/drugs/2015/P20150619001/index.html (accessed Mar 2016).
[7]  FDA Database.   http://www.accessdata.fda.gov/drugsatfda_docs/nda/2014/205832Orig1s000PharmR.pdf (accessed Mar 2016).
[9]  EMA Database.   http://www.ema.europa.eu/docs/en_GB/document_library/EPAR_-_Public_assessment_report/human/002569/WC500179972.pdf (accessed Mar 2016).

# CHAPTER

## 19

---

## Olaparib

# Olaparib

## (Lynparza®)

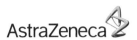

## 1   General Information

❖ Olaparib is a poly (ADP-ribose) polymerase (PARP) inhibitor, which was first approved in Dec 2014 by EMA.

❖ Olaparib was discovered by Kudos Pharmaceuticals, developed and marketed by AstraZeneca.

❖ Olaparib is an inhibitor of PARP enzymes which are required for the efficient repair of DNA single strand breaks. Olaparib leads to DNA double strand breaks (DSBs) and genomic instability in the absence of functional BRCA 1/2, resulting in cancer cell death.

❖ Olaparib is indicated for the treatment of patients with deleterious or suspected deleterious germline BRCA mutated advanced ovarian cancer.

❖ Available as oral capsule, with each containing 50 mg of olaparib and the recommended dose is 400 mg twice daily.

❖ The 2015 worldwide sale of Lynparza® was 94 million US$, referring to the financial reports of AstraZeneca.

## Key Approvals around the World*

|  | EU (EMA) | US (FDA) |
|---|---|---|
| **First approval date** | 12/16/2014 | 12/19/2014 |
| **Application or approval No.** | EMA/H/C/003726 | NDA 206162 |
| **Brand name** | Lynparza® | Lynparza® |
| **Indication** | Ovarian neoplasms | gBRCA-mutated advanced ovarian cancer |
| **Authorisation holder** | AstraZeneca | AstraZeneca |

* Till Mar 2016, it had not been approved by PMDA (Japan) and CFDA (China).

## Active Ingredient

*Molecular formula*:   $C_{24}H_{23}FN_4O_3$
*Molecular weight*:   434.46
*CAS No.*:   763113-22-0 (Olaparib)
*Chemical name*:   4-[(3-{[4-(Cyclopropylcarbonyl) piperazin-1-yl]carbonyl}-4-fluorophenyl)methyl] phthalazin-1(2*H*)-one

*Parameters of Lipinski's "Rule of 5"*

| MW | $H_D$ | $H_A$ | FRB[a] | PSA[a] | cLogP[a] |
|---|---|---|---|---|---|
| 434.46 | 1 | 7 | 4 | 82.1Å$^2$ | 1.45 ± 0.77 |

[a] Calculated by ACD/Labs software V11.02.

## Drug Product*

*Dosage route*:   Oral
*Strength*:   50 mg (Olaparib)
*Dosage form*:   Capsule
*Inactive ingredient*:   Lauroyl polyoxylglycerides, hypromellose, titanium dioxide, gellan gum, potassium acetate, shellac and ferrosoferric oxide.
*Recommended dose*: The recommended starting dose is 400 mg twice daily.
   Dosage adjustment to 200 mg twice daily, in patients with adverse reactions.

* Sourced from US FDA drug label information

## 2 Key Patents Information

## Summary

❖ Lynparza® (Olaparib) has got five-year NCE market exclusivity protection and seven-year orphan drug exclusivity after it was initially approved by US FDA on Dec 19, 2014.

❖ Olaparib was originally discovered by Kudos Pharmaceuticals and then developed by AstraZeneca, and its compound patent application was filed as PCT application by Kudos Pharmaceuticals in 2004.

❖ The compound patent will expire in 2024 foremost, which has been granted in Japan, the United States, China and Europe successively.

Table 1    Olaparib's Compound Patent Protection in Drug-Mainstream Country

| Country | Publication/Patent NO. | Application Date | Granted Date | Estimated Expiry Date |
|---------|------------------------|------------------|--------------|-----------------------|
| WO | WO2004080976A1 | 03/12/2004 | / | / |
| US | US7449464B2 | 03/12/2004 | 2008/11/11 | 10/11/2024[a] |
| US | US7981889B2 | 03/12/2004 | 2011/07/19 | 10/11/2024[b] |
| EP | EP1633724B1 | 03/12/2004 | 2011/05/04 | 03/12/2024 |
| JP | JP4027406B2 | 03/12/2004 | 2007/12/26 | 03/12/2024 |
| JP | JP4268651B2 | 03/12/2004 | 2009/05/27 | 03/12/2024 |
| CN | CN1788000B | 03/12/2004 | 2010/07/28 | 03/12/2024 |

[a] The term of this patent is extended by 213 days.    [b] The term of this patent is extended by 316 days (TD).

Table 2    Originator's International Patent Application List (Patent Family)

| Publication NO. | Title | Applicant/Assignee/Owner | Publication Date |
|-----------------|-------|--------------------------|------------------|
| Technical Subjects | Active Ingredient (Free Base)'s Formula or Structure and Preparation | | |
| WO2004080976A1 | Phthalazinone derivatives | Kudos | 09/23/2004 |
| Technical Subjects | Salt, Crystal, Polymorphic, Solvate (Hydrate), Isomer, Derivative Etc. and Preparation | | |
| WO2008047082A2 | Phthalazinone derivative | Kudos | 04/24/2008 |
| WO2009050469A1 | 4-[3-(4-Cyclopropanecarbonyl-piperazine-1-carbonyl)-4-fluoro-benzyl]-2*H*-phthalazin-1-one | Kudos | 04/23/2009 |
| Technical Subjects | Formulation and Preparation | | |
| WO2010041051A1 | Pharmaceutical formulation 514 | AstraZeneca | 04/15/2010 |
| Technical Subjects | Indication or Methods for Medical Needs | | |
| WO2005053662A1 | DNA damage repair inhibitors for treatment of cancer | Kudos | 06/16/2005 |
| WO2008020180A2 | Methods of increasing the sensitivity of cancer cells to DNA damage | Kudos | 02/21/2008 |
| Technical Subjects | Combination Including at Least Two Active Ingredients | | |
| WO2008146035A1 | Combination of CHK and PARP inhibitors for the treatment of cancers | AstraZeneca | 12/04/2008 |
| WO2015170081A1 | Imidazo[4,5-c]quinolin-2-one compounds and their use in treating cancer | AstraZeneca | 11/12/2015 |
| Technical Subjects | Others | | |
| WO2011058367A2 | Diagnostic test for predicting responsiveness to treatment with poly(ADP-ribose) polymerase (PARP) inhibitor | AstraZeneca | 05/19/2011 |

The data was updated until Jan 2016.

# 3 Chemistry

## Route 1: Original Discovery Route

HBTU: 2-(1H-Benzotriazole-1-yl)-1,1,3,3-tetramethyluronium hexafluorophosphate
IMS: Industrial methylated spirits

*Synthetic Route*: An optimized synthesis process derived from original route began with displacement of commercially available dimethyl phosphite **2** to *o*-phthalaldehydic acid **1** to generate the corresponding phosphonate **3** in 95% yield. Addition of aldehyde **4** to this phosphonate **3** led to the formation of olefins **5** in 96% yield as a 1:1 mixture of *E/Z* isomers. From olefins **5**, a one-pot, three-step sequence was furtherly performed to provide access to dihydrophthalazinyl acid **6**. First, lactone ring-opening and cyano hydrolysis were facilitated by reaction with aqueous sodium hydroxide under an elevated temperature, allowing for subsequent *in situ* formation of the corresponding dihydrophthalazine intermediate **6** after addition of hydrazine hydrate. Acidification and precipitation of this product with 2M HCl led to isolation of the desired material in 77% yield and 96% purity after filtration. Further coupling of carboxylic acid **6** with Boc-piperazine **7** and subsequent removal of the carbamate with HCl/EtOH provided intermediate **9** in 46% yield from **6**, relying on a pH-controlled workup procedure to enable isolation of material in high purity (94%) without requiring chromatography. The final step of the olaparib synthesis was completed *via* treatment of piperazine **9** with cyclopropane carbonyl chloride **10** and triethylamine, leading to olaparib in 83% yield and 99.3% purity. The overall yield was 27%.[1-4]

[1] Menear, K. A.; Ottridge, A. P.; Londesbrough, D. J., et al. WO2008047082A2, **2008**.
[2] Menear, K. A.; Ottridge, A. P.; Londesbrough, D. J., et al. US20080146575A1, **2008**.
[3] Martin, N. M. B.; Smith, G. C. M.; Jackson, S. P., et al. WO2004080976A1, **2004**.
[4] Martin, N. M. B.; Smith, G. C. M.; Jackson, S. P., et al. US20050059663A1, **2005**.

## Route 2

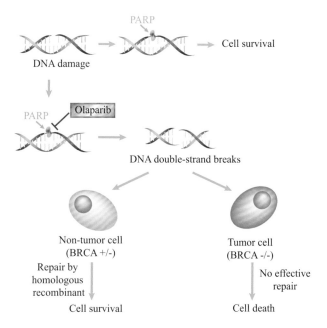

HBTU: 2-(1*H*-Benzotriazole-1-yl)-1,1,3,3-tetramethyluronium hexafluorophosphate

*Synthetic Route*:　Differentiate from the nucleophilic addition of 3*H*-isobenzofuran-1-one **1** to 3-formylbenzonitrile proceeding in refluxing methanol using sodium methoxide as base, as for the corresponding fluoro analog of 3-formylbenzonitrile **2**, in which the fluoro was ortho to the nitrile group was labile to nucleophilic displacement, an alternative milder condition starting from 3-dimethoxyphosphosphoryl-3*H*-2-benzofuran-1-one, which was prepared from addition of **1** to dimethylphosphite by means of sodium *t*-amylate, was required.　Thus, the freshly prepared phosphonate was coupled to **2**, along with the following mesylation and successive immediate elimination in TEA, generating 2-fluoro-5(3-oxo-3*H*-isobenzofuran-1-ylidene methyl)benzonitrile **3** in 65% yield over two steps.　Without separation, a mixture of *E* and *Z* isomers was treated with hydrazine hydrate to construct the phthalazinone core.　Base hydrolysis of the pendant nitrile provided the key carboxylic acid intermediate **5**.　The functionalized amine **6** was then coupled to the acid **5** with HBTU to give the target amide olaparib in 62% yield with 34% overall yield.[1, 2, 5]

## 4　Pharmacology

## Summary

Mechanism of Action

❖　Olaparib is an orally inhibitor of human PARPs (PARP-1, PARP-2 and PARP-3, $IC_{50}$ = 1-5 nM), which are required for the efficient repair of DNA single strand breaks.

❖　In replicating cells, PARPs inhibition by olaparib leads to DSBs, which cannot be repaired *via* homologous recombination repair (HRR) in the absence of functional BRCA1 or 2.　It can reach insupportable levels of genomic instability and result in cancer cell death, as cancer cells have a high DNA damage load relative to normal cells.

❖　Olaparib showed no significant activity in a panel of 239 in the *in vitro* radioligand binding and enzyme assays at 10 μM, which covered a diverse panel of molecular targets including enzymes, receptors, transporters and ion channels.

[1]　Menear, K. A.; Ottridge, A. P.; Londesbrough, D. J.; et al. WO2008047082A2, **2008**.
[2]　Menear, K. A.; Ottridge, A. P.; Londesbrough, D. J.; et al. US20080146575A1, **2008**.
[5]　Menear, K. A.; Adcock, C.; Boulter, R.; et al. *J. Med. Chem.* **2008**, *51*, 6581-6591.

*In Vitro* Efficacy

❖ The inhibition of colony formation in breast cancer cell lines:
  • Olaparib: $IC_{50}$ = 18-8280 nM.
❖ Change of methanemethylsulfate (MMS) activities on cell proliferation in SW620:
  • Olaparib increased MMS-induced decrease in cell death.
❖ Olaparib inhibited colony formation in cell lines:
  • In BRCA1/2 WT cells: $IC_{50}$ = 110-1463 nM (except 59M/NCI-H1838/HCC 1187 cell lines, $IC_{50}$ = 21-86 nM).
  • In BRCA1/2 mutation cells: $IC_{50}$ = 18-32 nM (except SUM149PT cells, $IC_{50}$ = 125 nM).

*In Vivo* Efficacy

❖ HBCx-10 xenograft models after an oral administration of olaparib:
  • Tumor decreased at ≥50-100 mg/kg.
❖ Combination of cisplatin in patient-derived tumor triple negative breast cancer (TNBC) and NSCLC xenograft models:
  • HBCx-10, 17 and Lu7433: Anti-tumor growth activity.
  • HBCx-9 and Lu7414: No significant inhibition.

## Mechanism of Action

Table 3    Activity of Olaparib against PARP Enzymes[6, 7]

| Enzyme | Resource | $IC_{50}$ (nM) | $IC_{90}$ (nM) |
|--------|----------|----------------|----------------|
| PARP-1 | Purified PARP enzyme | 5 | NA |
| PARP-2 | Purified PARP enzyme | 1 | NA |
| PARP-3 | PARP-3-meiated PAR expression | 4 | NA |
| PARP | Expressed in SW620 cells | 5.438 | 60.08 |

SW620 was first treated with 0, 1, 3, 10, 30 or 300 nM olaparib 1 h prior to treatment with 0, 3, 5, 7, 10, 12 or 15 μg/mL MMS.   Following 4-day incubation, cell viability was analyzed using a sulphorhodamine-B (SRB) dye-based assay.

## *In Vitro* Efficacy

Table 4    Chemotherapeutic Agents Activity across the Breast Cancer Cell Lines[6]

| Cell Line | $IC_{50}$ (nM) | | | | |
|-----------|-----------|--------------|-------------|------------|------------|
| | Olaparib | Camptothecin | Carboplatin | Doxorubicin | Paclitaxel |
| MDA-MB-436 | 18 | 0.047 | 66 | 4.443 | 2.804 |
| HCC 1395 | 20 | 0.788 | 396 | 18.95 | 4.795 |
| HCC 1187 | 79 | 1.761 | 391 | 3.474 | 0.407 |
| SUM1315MO2 | 32 | 1.092 | 100 | 7.331 | 0.594 |
| SUM 149PT | 125 | 1.353 | 328 | 5.566 | 0.967 |
| MDA-MB-468 | 896 | 4.833 | 709 | 14.726 | 1.614 |
| MCF7 | 1790 | 1.846 | 2903 | 16.330 | 0.231 |
| HCC 1937 | 2820 | 11.598 | 483 | 16.809 | 1.251 |
| T47D | 3024 | 6.194 | 3361 | 4.835 | 1.739 |
| BT549 | 4505 | 5.355 | 1915 | 8.013 | 1.305 |
| MDA-MB-231 | 8280 | 25.920 | 29730 | 100 | 0.782 |

The objective of this study was to evaluate the growth inhibitory activity of olaparib (as well as carboplatin, camptothecin, doxorubicin, and paclitaxel) in a panel of 95 cancer cell lines using the colony formation assay.

[6]  U.S. Food and Drug Adminstration (FDA) Database.   http://www.accessdata.fda.gov/drugsatfda_docs/nda/2014/206162Orig1s000PharmR.pdf (accessed Mar 2016).
[7]  European Medicines Agency (EMA) Database.    http://www.ema.europa.eu/docs/en_GB/document_library/EPAR_-_Public_assessment_report/human/003726/WC500180154. pdf (accessed Mar 2016).

Table 5    Combination of DNA-damaging Chemotherapeutic Agents Methanemethylsulfate (MMS) and Olaparib in SW620[6]

| Cell Line | Cell Type | Olaparib (nM) | MMS IC$_{50}$ (µg/mL) | MMS PF$_{50}$ |
|---|---|---|---|---|
| SW620 | Human colorectal adenocarcinoma | 0 | 4.395/4.349 | 1.000 |
| | | 1 | 3.814 | 1.152 |
| | | 3 | 2.919 | 1.506 |
| | | 10 | 2.023 | 2.172 |
| | | 30 | 1.563 | 2.783 |
| | | 100 | 1.232 | 3.530 |
| | | 300 | 1.339 | 3.248 |

SW620 was first treated with 0, 1, 3, 10, 30 or 300 nM olaparib one hour prior to treatment with 0, 3, 5, 7, 10, 12, or 15 µg/mL MMS.    Following 4-day incubation, cell viability was analyzed using a sulphorhodamine-B (SRB) dye-based assay.    PF$_{50}$ (potentiation factor at 50% cell viability) was defined as the ratio of the IC$_{50}$ for MMS alone vs MMS in combination with a single concentration of olaparib.

Table 6    Olaparib Activity and HRD Classification across Cancer Cell Line Panel[6]

| Tumor Type | Cell Line | IC$_{50}$ (nM) | HR Deficiency (HRD) | | Putative Resistance Gene Expression | |
|---|---|---|---|---|---|---|
| | | | BRCA1/2 Mutation | Low BRCA1/2 Expression | Low PARP1 | High ABCB1 (P-gp) |
| Breast | MDA-MB-436 | 18 | BRCA1 (5396 + 1G >A) | NA | NA | Low |
| | HCC 1395 | 20 | BRCA1 (R1751X) | BRCA1 | High | NA |
| | SUM1315MO2 | 32 | BRCA1 (185 delAG) | NA | NA | Low |
| | HCC 1187 | 79 | NA | NA | NA | Low |
| | SUM 149PT | 125 | BRCA1 (2288 delT) | NA | High | NA |
| | MDA-MB-453 | 399 | NA | BRCA1 | High | NA |
| | HCC 1569 | 574 | NA | BRCA2 | NA | NA |
| | MDA-MB-468 | 896 | NA | NA | NA | Low |
| | BT-20 | 920 | NA | NA | NA | NA |
| | MDA-MB-361 | 1156 | NA | NA | NA | NA |
| Ovarian | 59M | 21 | NA | NA | NA | NA |
| | OVCAR-3 | 221 | NA | NA | NA | NA |
| | IGROV-1 | 391 | NA | BRCA1 | Low | Moderate |
| | TOV-21G | 568 | NA | NA | Low | Low |
| | OAW28 | 596 | NA | NA | NA | NA |
| | A2780 | 629 | NA | NA | High | NA |
| | OV90 | 687 | NA | NA | NA | Low |
| Pancreatic | CAPAN-1 | 24 | BRCA2 (6174 delT) | NA | NA | NA |
| | T3M4 | 1463 | NA | NA | NA | Moderate |
| Non-small lung cell | NCI-H1838 | 86 | NA | NA | NA | Low |
| | HOP-92 | 110 | NA | BRCA2 | NA | Low |
| | NCI-H23 | 626 | NA | NA | NA | Low |
| | NCI-H1755 | 801 | NA | NA | NA | High |
| | DMS 114 | 908 | NA | NA | High | Low |

[6]   FDA Database.   http://www.accessdata.fda.gov/drugsatfda_docs/nda/2014/206162Orig1s000PharmR.pdf (accessed Mar 2016).

*Continued*

| Tumor Type | Cell Line | IC₅₀ (nM) | HR Deficiency (HRD) | | Putative Resistance Gene Expression | |
|---|---|---|---|---|---|---|
| | | | BRCA1/2 Mutation | Low BRCA1/2 Expression | Low PARP1 | High ABCB1 (P-gp) |
| Colorectal | SKCO1 | 157 | NA | NA | NA | Low |
| | HCT 116 | 198 | NA | BRCA1, 2 | NA | Moderate |
| | LS 180 | 731 | NA | NA | NA | High |
| | HCA7 | 736 | NA | BRCA1 | NA | NA |
| | LOVO | 1030 | NA | BRCA2 | NA | High |
| | SW620 | 1305 | NA | NA | NA | High |
| Head & neck SCC | PE/CA-PJ41 | 385 | NA | NA | NA | NA |
| | RPMI2650 | 472 | NA | NA | NA | NA |
| | KYSE-30 | 519 | NA | NA | NA | Low |
| | Hs840.T | 533 | NA | BRCA1, 2 | Low | High |
| | PE/CA-PJ34 | 1121 | NA | NA | NA | Low |
| | Detroit 562 | 1243 | NA | NA | NA | NA |
| | FaDu | 1323 | NA | NA | NA | Low |
| | CAL27 | 1432 | NA | BRCA2 | Low | NA |

Cell lines were incubated in 10% (v/v) DMSO (vehicle control) or 0.123, 0.370, 1.111, 3.333, 10.00 μM olaparib at 37 °C until >50 colonies had formed (6-28 days). Cell viability was determined using the colony formation assay by counting Giemsa-stained colonies using colcount software (Oxford Optronix). Gene and protein expression for a number of DNA damage response genes such as BRCA1, BRCA2 were also determined by qRT-PCR and western blotting.

## *In Vivo* Efficacy

Table 7   *In Vivo* Correlation of Olaparib and Platinum Response in Patient-derived Mice Tumor Models[6, 7]

| Xenograft System | | | Dose (mg/kg, i.p.) | Duration (Day) | Effect | |
|---|---|---|---|---|---|---|
| Cell Type | Tumor Model | Mutation | | | ED (mg/kg) | Finding |
| Breast ductal adenocarcinomaᵃ | HBCx-10 | BRCA2, TP53 | Olaparib: 2.5, 10, 25, 50, 100 | QD × 30 (2.5, 10, 25); QD × 64 (50, 100) | 50 | Tumor decreased at 50-100 mg/kg. |
| | HBCx-10 | BRCA2, TP53 | Olaparib: 50; | QD × >90 | 50 | Significant tumor inhibition. Increased anti-tumor effect by combination. |
| | | | Cisplatin: NA; | QD × >60 | | |
| | | | Olaparib + Cisplatin | QD × >90 | | |
| | HBCx-17 | BRCA2, TP53 | Olaparib: 50; | QD × ~56 | 50 | Inhibited tumor growth by single dose or combination. |
| | | | Cisplatin: NA; | QD × 50 | | |
| | | | Olaparib + Cisplatin | QD × >80 | | |
| | HBCx-9 | TP53 | Olaparib: 50; | QD × 30 | NA | No significant effect. |
| | | | Cisplatin: NA; | QD × ~40 | | |
| | | | Olaparib + Cisplatin | QD × ~40 | | |
| Lung squamous cell carcinoma | Lu7433 | TP53, EGFR | Olaparib: 50; | QD × ~54 | 50 | Anti-tumor growth after single dose or combination. |
| | | | Cisplatin: NA; | QD × ~54 | | |
| | | | Olaparib + Cisplatin | QD × ~54 | | |
| | Lu7414 | NA | Olaparib: 50; | QD × ~30 | NA | No significant effect. |
| | | | Cisplatin: NA; | QD × ~30 | | |
| | | | Olaparib + Cisplatin | QD × ~30 | | |

Anti-tumor activity was evaluated in patient derived tumor mice models of NSCLC and triple negative breast cancer.   HBCx: Human breast cancer xenograft.
ᵃ patient-derived tumor xenograft (PTX) models derived from triple negative breast cancer (TNBC) patients.

[6] FDA Database.   http://www.accessdata.fda.gov/drugsatfda_docs/nda/2014/206162Orig1s000PharmR.pdf (accessed Mar 2016).
[7] EMA Database.   http://www.ema.europa.eu/docs/en_GB/document_library/EPAR_-_Public_assessment_report/ human/003726/WC500180154.pdf (accessed Mar 2016).

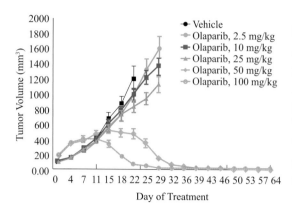

Figure A    Anti-tumor Activities of Olaparib in the TNBC PTX *In Vivo* HBCx-10 Model[6]

**Study:** Anti-tumor activities of olaparib in HBCx-10 mouse xenograft model.

**Animal:** Athymic mouse.

**Model:** HBCx-10 patient-derived tumor xenograft into mice.

**Administration:** Treated once daily, Olaparib: 2.5, 10, 25, 50, 100 mg/kg/day, i.p. for 30 days (2.5, 10, 25 mg/kg/day), i.p. for 64 days (50, 100 mg/kg/days); Vehicle control: NA.

**Test:** Tumor volume.

**Result:** Treatment with olaparib caused significant tumor growth delay at 50-100 mg/kg/day and some regression in dose dependent manner.

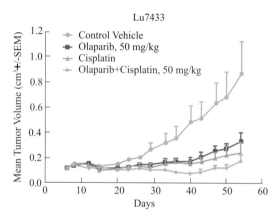

Figure B    Anti-tumor Activities of Olaparib in the NSCLC PTX *In Vivo* Lu7433 Model[6]

**Study:** Anti-tumor activities of olaparib in Lu7433 xenograft mouse model.

**Animal:** Athymic mouse.

**Model:** Lu7433 tumors from patients with TP53 and EGFR mutation were implanted into mice s.c..

**Administration:** Treated once daily, i.p. for ~54 days, Olaparib 50 mg/kg/day; Cisplatin: NA; Olaparib 50 mg/kg/day + Cisplatin NA; Vehicle control: NA.

**Test:** Tumor volume.

**Result:** Treatment with olaparib, cisplatin or co-treatment of both drugs caused significant tumor growth delay.

# 5   ADME & Drug-Drug Interaction

## Summary

### Absorption of Olaparib

❖ Exhibited a non-linear pharmacokinetics in humans following oral administration.    The increases in $C_{max}$ and $AUC_{inf}$ appeared to be less than dose-proportional in the dose range of 50-400 mg olaparib.

❖ Had low oral bioavailability in rats (17.2% for males and 19.2% for females), but high in mice (55.4% for males & 59.9% for females) and dogs (78.9% for males).

❖ Was absorbed rapidly to moderately with the $T_{max}$ occurring at 0.3-3 h in non-clinical species and humans.

❖ Showed a half-life ranging between 5.5-12 h in humans, much longer than those in mice (1.74-2.12 h), rats (2.5-3.0 h) and dogs (4.61 h), after oral administrations.

❖ Had low clearance in male mice (1.34 L/h/kg) and dogs (0.39 L/h/kg), in contrast to liver blood flow, after intravenous administrations.    The clearance in humans was 3.0-12 L/h after oral administration.

❖ Exhibited an extensive tissue distribution in dogs, but low in mice, with apparent volumes of distribution at 0.93 and 0.36 L/kg, respectively, after intravenous administration.    The apparent volume of distribution was 26-167 L in humans after oral administration.

### Distribution of Olaparib

❖ Exhibited moderate plasma protein binding in humans (81.9%-91.2%), rats (72.7%-73.5%), mice (69.4%-71.6%) and dogs (54.7%-61.9%).

❖ Had a $C_b$:$C_p$ ratio of 0.60-0.74 in humans, suggesting rare penetration into red blood cells.

❖ Tumor-bearing mice after single oral administration:
  • Relatively higher concentration levels were observed in the gastrointestinal tract and liver at 6 h post-dose.    At 96 h, radioactivity was detected only in the gastrointestinal contents, liver and tumor tissues.

[6] FDA Database.    http://www.accessdata.fda.gov/drugsatfda_docs/nda/2014/206162Orig1s000PharmR.pdf (accessed Mar 2016).

- The apparent tissue half-lives were 25.7 h in the liver and 36.0 h in the tumor.
❖ Rats after single oral administration:
  - The drug was rapidly and well distributed into most tissues except for the central nervous system (CNS) since the blood-brain barrier was crossed by a very small extent.
  - Relatively higher concentration levels were observed in the liver, uveal tract, kidneys, stomach, small intestine, large intestine, cecum, and urinary bladder at 1 h post-dose.
  - Radioactivity was below the limit of quantification in spinal cord and below the concentration in blood in many tissues.
  - By 7 days post-dose, radioactivity was detectable at low levels in only liver and uveal tract. Radioactivity was undetectable in any tissues by 28 days after dosing although very low levels were detected in whole eyes.
  - Similar tissue distribution of olaparib was noted in male and female animals.

## Metabolism of Olaparib

❖ CYP3A5 played a role in the formation of the major metabolites of olaparib incubated in human liver microsomes. CYP2A6 and CYP1A1 also formed the major metabolites but to a lesser extent.
❖ Overall, the parent drug represented the most abundant component in human plasma, with M18 as the major metabolite. Dehydrogenation and oxidation were identified as the major metabolic pathways. The three metabolites M12, M15 and M18 in human plasma accounted for approximate 10% of the radioactivity (M12 at 9.3%, M15 at 10.3% and M18 at 13.7%).
❖ No unique human metabolite was identified.
❖ However, the pharmacological activity of the metabolites had not been assessed.

## Excretion of Olaparib

❖ Was predominantly excreted in feces (41.8%) and urine (44.1%) in humans, and approximately 15% of the dose was parent in urine and 6% in feces.
❖ 18 metabolites were observed in the human urine, 20 moieties were identified in the human feces.
❖ About 75.7% (male) and 18.2% (female) of olaparib were recovered *via* biliary excretion in bile duct-cannulated (BDC) rats.

## Drug-Drug Interaction

❖ Olaparib was not an inhibitor of CYP450 enzymes.
❖ Olaparib was an inducer of CYP2B6, but had no induction for CYP1A2, CYP2C9, CYP2C19 or CYP3A.
❖ Olaparib was a substrate of P-gp but not a substrate of BCRP, and had no inhibition for P-gp but had inhibition for BCRP.
❖ Olaparib was a substrate of OATs but not a substrate of MRP2, and had inhibition for OATP1B1 ($IC_{50}$ = 20.3 μM), OCT1 ($IC_{50}$ = 37.9 μM), OCT2 ($IC_{50}$ = 19.9 μM), OAT1 ($IC_{50}$ = 13.5 μM), OAT3 ($IC_{50}$ = 18.4 μM), MATE1 ($IC_{50}$ = 5.5 μM) and MATE2K ($IC_{50}$ = 47.1 μM) *in vitro*.

# Absorption

Table 8    *In Vivo* Pharmacokinetic Parameters of Olaparib in Mice, Rats and Dogs after Single Intravenous and Oral Dose of Olaparib[6, 7]

| Species | Gender | Route | Dose (mg/kg) | $T_{max}$ (h) | $C_{max}$ (μg/mL) | $AUC_{inf}$ (μg·h/mL) | $AUC_{last}$ (μg·h/mL) | $T_{1/2}$ (h) | Cl (L/h/kg) | $V_{ss}$ (L/kg) | F (%) |
|---|---|---|---|---|---|---|---|---|---|---|---|
| Mouse[a] | Male | i.v. | 20 | NA | NA | 14.9 | 14.9 | 0.648 | 1.34 | 0.356 | - |
| | | p.o. | 80 | 0.5 | 28.6 | 33.0 | 33.1 | 1.74 | NA | NA | 55.4 |
| | Female | i.v. | 20 | NA | NA | 12.0 | 12.0 | 0.969 | 1.66 | 0.428 | - |
| | | p.o. | 80 | 0.33 | 29.0 | 28.6 | 28.9 | 2.12 | NA | NA | 59.9 |
| Rat | Male | i.v. | 1 | 0.5 | 1.08 | 0.59 | NA | 0.8 | NC | NC | - |
| | | p.o. | 5 | 1.0 | 0.162 | 0.494 | NA | 2.5 | NC | NC | 17.2 |
| | Female | i.v. | 1 | 0.25 | 1.34 | 2.52 | NA | 8.9 | NC | NC | - |
| | | p.o. | 5 | 2.0 | 0.408 | 2.38 | NA | 3.0 | NC | NC | 19.2 |
| Dog[b] | Male | i.v. | 1 | 0.083 | 1.41 ± 0.39 | 2.75 ± 0.79 | NA | 1.71 ± 0.30 | 0.39 ± 0.13 | 0.93 ± 0.14 | - |
| | | p.o. | 5 | 1.0 | 2.13 ± 0.18 | 10.3 ± 2.01 | NA | 4.61 ± 1.66 | NC | NC | 78.9 ± 11.5 |

Pharmacokinetic parameters for rats were determined from composite profiles based on animals/sex/timepoint. [a] The units of AUC and $C_{max}$ for mice were μM·h/L and μM/L. [b] Values were Mean ± SD.

[6] FDA Database. http://www.accessdata.fda.gov/drugsatfda_docs/nda/2014/206162Orig1s000PharmR.pdf (accessed Mar 2016).
[7] EMA Database. http://www.ema.europa.eu/docs/en_GB/document_library/EPAR_-_Public_assessment_report/human/003726/WC500180154. pdf (accessed Mar 2016).

Table 9    *In Vivo* Pharmacokinetic Parameters of Olaparib in Humans after Single
Oral Dose of Olaparib[8]

| Species | Route | Dose (mg) | $T_{max}$ (h) | $C_{max}$ (µg/mL) | $AUC_{inf}$[a] (µg·h/mL) | $AUC_{0-t}$[b] (µg·h/mL) | $T_{1/2}$ (h) | Cl/F (L/h) | $V_d$/F (L) |
|---|---|---|---|---|---|---|---|---|---|
| Healthy human (male & female) | p.o. | 50 | 1.5 (1.0-3.0) | 1.8 (26) | 10 (45) | 9.9 (43) | 7.9 ± 1.7 | 5.4 ± 2.4 | 61 ± 31 |
| | p.o. | 100 | 1.3 (1.0-2.0) | 2.9 (23) | 17 (32) | 17 (33) | 8.4 ± 2.9 | 6.2 ± 2.1 | 81 ± 50 |
| | p.o. | 400 | 1.3 (1.0-8.0) | 5.7 (47) | 58 (78) | 54.7 (79) | 12 ± 4.8 | 8.6 ± 7.1 | 167 ± 196 |
| Japanese patient with cancer (male & female) | p.o. | 100 | 1.0 (0.5-1.4) | 2.3 ± 0.9 (39) | 17 ± 12 (69) | 11 ± 5.3 (48) | 7.8 ± 6.5 | 9.3 ± 7.8 | 59 ± 17 |
| | p.o. | 200 | 2.1 (1.5-3.0) | 3.5 ± 0.7 (19) | 21 ± 6.6 (32) | 16 ± 3.3 (21) | 6.9 ± 3.8 | 10 ± 3.4 | 75 ± 9.9 |
| | p.o. | 400 | 2.4 (1.6-4.2) | 4.9 ± 0.7 (15) | 39 ± 12 (30) | 28 ± 7.3 (26) | 11 ± 5.3 | 12 ± 4.9 | 112 ± 37 |
| Patient with cancer | p.o. | 10 | 2.0 (0.5-2.0) | 0.4 ± 0.1 (30) | 1.3 ± 0.5 (37) | 1.5 ± 0.6 (40) | 6.7 ± 0.3 | 7.0 ± 2.4 | 67 ± 26 |
| | p.o. | 20 | 1.5 (1.0-1.5) | 1.2 ± 0.6 (54) | 4.0 ± 1.9 (47) | 5.1 ± 2.4 (46) | 6.1 ± 0.5 | 4.2 ± 1.6 | 38 ± 16 |
| | p.o. | 40 | 1.5 (1.0-4.0) | 2.0 ± 0.5 (23) | 10 ± 2.2 (22) | 14 ± 4.2 (31) | 6.1 ± 0.5 | 3.0 ± 0.9 | 26 ± 6.7 |
| | p.o. | 60 | 2.3 (0.5-3.0) | 2.7 ± 0.9 (33) | 9.5 ± 2.1 (22) | NC | NC | NC | NC |
| | p.o. | 80 | 1.5 (1.5-1.5) | 3.5 ± 0.7 (20) | 14 ± 6.1 (43) | 18 ± 10 (55) | 5.5 ± 0.3 | 5.1 ± 2.4 | 40 ± 17 |
| | p.o. | 100 | 1.0 (1.0-3.0) | 3.6 ± 1.6 (45) | 19 ± 13 (66) | NC | NC | NC | NC |
| | p.o. | 200 | 1.5 (1.0-4.0) | 5.3 ± 2.9 (55) | 26 ± 17 (64) | NC | NC | NC | NC |
| | p.o. | 400 | 1.75 (1.5-8.0) | 6.2 ± 1.2 (19) | 33 ± 11 (35) | NC | NC | NC | NC |
| | p.o. | 600 | 3.0 (2.0-4.0) | 11 ± 3.5 (32) | 67 ± 26 (39) | NC | NC | NC | NC |

Median (range) for $T_{max}$ and geometrical mean (CV%) for other parameters.    $AUC_{0-t}$ for Japanese patients with cancer was the area under the plasma concentration-time curve from time zero up to 12 h post-dose.    [a] $AUC_{0-10}$ for patients with cancer.    [b] $AUC_{0-24}$ for patients with cancer.

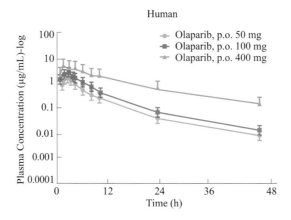

Figure C    *In Vivo* Plasma Concentration-Time Profiles in Plasma of Olaparib in Humans after Single
Oral Dose of Olaparib[8]

## Distribution

Table 10    *In Vitro* Plasma Protein Binding and Blood Partitioning of [$^{14}$C]Olaparib in Several Species[6-8]

| Plasma Protein Binding | | | Blood Partitioning | | | | |
|---|---|---|---|---|---|---|---|
| Species | Conc. (µM) | %Bound | Species | Conc. (µM) | $C_b$:$C_p$ | Partition Coefficient (%) | Blood Cell Association (%) |
| Mouse | 0.023-23 | 69.4-71.6 | CD1 mouse | 0.023-23 | 0.67 | 75.0-75.9 | 24.1-25.0 |
| Rat | 0.023-23 | 72.7-73.5 | Han Wistar rat | 0.023-23 | 0.71 | 75.8-76.1 | 23.9-24.2 |
| Dog | 0.023-23 | 54.7-61.9 | Beagle dog | 0.023-23 | 0.79-0.92 | 56.3-66.0 | 34.0-43.7 |
| Human | 0.023-23 | 81.9-91.2 | Human | 0.023-23 | 0.60-0.74 | 70.4-87.8 | 12.2-29.6 |

$C_b$:$C_p$: Blood to plasma concentration ratio.    Mouse and rat data generated using pooled blood.    Dog and human data was mean of three individual assays.

[6] FDA Database.    http://www.accessdata.fda.gov/drugsatfda_docs/nda/2014/206162Orig1s000PharmR.pdf (accessed Mar 2016).
[7] EMA Database.    http://www.ema.europa.eu/docs/en_GB/document_library/EPAR_-_Public_assessment_report/human/003726/WC500180154. pdf (accessed Mar 2016).
[8] FDA Database.    http://www.accessdata.fda.gov/drugsatfda_docs/nda/2014/206162Orig1s000ClinPharmR.pdf (accessed Mar 2016).

Table 11    *In Vivo* Tissue Distribution of [$^{14}$C]Olaparib in Tumor Bearing Mice after Single
Oral Dose of 30 mg/kg [$^{14}$C]Olaparib[6, 7]

| Tissue | Radioactivity (ng eq./g) | | | | | Tissue/Blood AUC$_{0-96}$ Ratio |
|---|---|---|---|---|---|---|
| | 6 h | 24 h | 48 h | 72 h | 96 h | |
| Blood | 0.053 | 0.052 | BLQ | BLQ | BLQ | 1.0 |
| Brain | BLQ | BLQ | BLQ | BLQ | BLQ | - |
| Liver | 12.9 | 8.33 | 4.57 | 1.51 | 1.34 | 445 |
| Large intestine contents | 274 | 70.7 | 5.30 | NS | 4.16 | 5063 |
| Large intestine mucosa | 7.99 | 9.41 | 0.595 | NS | BLQ | 315 |
| Small intestine contents | 167 | 35.1 | 0.803 | 0.926 | 0.768 | 2529 |
| Small intestine mucosa | 14.4 | 3.93 | 0.455 | BLQ | BLQ | 266 |
| Stomach contents | 193 | 23.5 | 0.883 | 0.428 | 0.501 | 2579 |
| Stomach mucosa | 15.8 | 1.46 | 1.98 | BLQ | BLQ | 268 |
| Tumor | 0.339 | 0.208 | 0.116 | 0.103 | 0.053 | 13.0 |

The value upper limit of quantification (139 g eq./g) was extrapolated.    NS: Sample was not sectioned.    BLQ: Below limit of quantification.

## Key Findings:[6-8]

❖ Tumor bearing mice after single oral administration:
  • The highest concentrations of radioactivity were observed in the gastrointestinal tract and liver at 6 h post-dose.    At 96 h, radioactivity was detected only in the gastrointestinal contents, liver and tumor tissues.
  • The apparent tissue half-lives were 25.7 h in the liver and 36.0 h in the tumor.
❖ Rats after single oral administration:
  • Olaparib was rapidly and well distributed into most tissues.    Maximal concentrations were measured in many tissues at 1 h post-dose.
  • The highest levels of radioactivity were observed in the liver, uveal tract and kidneys, stomach, small intestine, large intestine, cecum and urinary bladder at 1 h post-dose.
  • Radioactivity was below the limit of quantification in the brain and spinal cord, and below the concentration in blood in many tissues.
  • By 4 h post-dose, concentrations of radioactivity had decreased in most tissues although the uveal tract (2.49-3.07), prostate (1.54-7.34) and seminal vesicles were notable exceptions.    Concentrations of radioactivity also increased in parts of the GI tract at this time although they decreased in liver (48.7-21.4) and kidneys (10.2-4.2).
  • By one day post-dose, radioactivity was below the limit of quantification in the majority of tissues although it was still detectable at low levels in a small number of tissues including parts of the GI tract, excretory organs, pigmented skin and uveal tract.
  • By 7 days post-dose, radioactivity was detectable by QWBA at low levels only in liver and uveal tract.    Radioactivity was undetectable by QWBA in any tissues by 28 days post-dose although very low levels were detected in whole eyes by LSC.
  • Similar tissue distribution of olaparib was noted in male and female animals.

[6]  FDA Database.    http://www.accessdata.fda.gov/drugsatfda_docs/nda/2014/206162Orig1s000PharmR.pdf (accessed Mar 2016).
[7]  EMA Database.    http://www.ema.europa.eu/docs/en_GB/document_library/EPAR_-_Public_assessment_report/human/003726/WC500180154. pdf (accessed Mar 2016).
[8]  FDA Database.    http://www.accessdata.fda.gov/drugsatfda_docs/nda/2014/206162Orig1s000ClinPharmR.pdf (accessed Mar 2016).

## Metabolism

Table 12    Metabolites in Plasma, Urine and Feces of Humans and Non-clinical Test Species after Single Oral and Intravenous Dose of Olaparib[6, 7]

| Matrix | Species | Route | Dose (mg/kg) | Time (h) | % of Radioactivity | | | |
|---|---|---|---|---|---|---|---|---|
| | | | | | M0 | M12 | M15 | M18 |
| Plasma | Rat (male) | p.o. | 5 | Pool | 70.4 | 12.3 | 9.4 | 7.9 |
| | Rat (female) | p.o. | 5 | Pool | 100 | √ | √ | √ |
| | Dog (male) | i.v. | 1 | 1 | 86.6 | NI | NI | NI |
| | Dog (male) | p.o. | 5 | 1 | 90.9 | NI | NI | NI |
| | Human (female) | p.o. | 100 mg | NA | 70.0 | 9.3 | 10.3 | 13.7 |
| Urine[a] | Human | p.o. | 100 mg | NA | 15 | NA | 6 | NA |
| Feces[a] | Human | p.o. | 100 mg | NA | 6 | NA | 5 | NA |

NI: Not identified (no quantitative or qualitative identification completed).    [a] % of dose.

### Key Findings:[6-8]

❖ Main Metabolites:
- Dehydrogenation and oxidation were identified as the major metabolic pathways. 18 metabolites were observed in the urine, and 20 moieties were identified in the feces.
- The M12 was identified as a ring-opened hydroxyl-cyclopropyl moiety, M15 as a mono-oxygenated metabolite and M18 as a dehydrogenated piperazine.

❖ Metabolic phenotyping identification:
- CYP3A5 played a role in the formation of the three metabolites of olaparib incubated in human liver microsomes.
- The three metabolites were M11a/b (a monooxygenated, dehydrogenated piperazine metabolite and a monooxygenated, fluorophenol metabolite), M15/M16 (a fluorophenol metabolite, and an *N,N*-desethyl piperazine metabolite) and M18/M39 (a dehydrogenated piperazine metabolite and a monooxygenated metabolite).
- CYP2A6 and CYP1A1 also formed the three metabolites but to a lesser extent.

## Excretion

Table 13    Excretion Profiles of [14C]Olaparib in Rats, Dogs and Humans after Single Oral and Intravenous Dose of Olaparib[6, 7]

| Species | State | Route | Dose (mg/kg) | Time (h) | Bile (% of dose) | Urine (% of dose) | Feces (% of dose) | Cage Wash (% of dose) | Recovery (% of dose) |
|---|---|---|---|---|---|---|---|---|---|
| Rat (male) | Intact | p.o. | 5 | 0-120 | - | 7.8 | 88.7 | 0.6 | 97.1 |
| Rat (female) | Intact | p.o. | 5 | 0-120 | - | 23.2 | 72.8 | 2.0 | 98.2 |
| Rat (male) | BDC | i.v. | 1 | 0-48 | 75.7 | 17.1 | 8.8 | 2.2 | 105 |
| Rat (female) | BDC | i.v. | 1 | 0-48 | 18.2 | 41.0 | 28.6 | 10.6 | 101 |
| Dog (male) | Intact | i.v. | 1 | 0-168 | - | 23.4 | 77.8 | 1.9 | 101 |
| Dog (male) | Intact | p.o. | 5 | 0-168 | - | 14.9 | 78.5 | 1.8 | 93.4 |
| Human | Intact | p.o. | 140 mg | 0-168 | - | 44.1 ± 6.71 | 41.8 ± 21.6 | - | 85.8 ± 18.1 |

[6] FDA Database. http://www.accessdata.fda.gov/drugsatfda_docs/nda/2014/206162Orig1s000PharmR.pdf (accessed Mar 2016).
[7] EMA Database. http://www.ema.europa.eu/docs/en_GB/document_library/EPAR_-_Public_assessment_report/human/003726/WC500180154. pdf (accessed Mar 2016).
[8] FDA Database. http://www.accessdata.fda.gov/drugsatfda_docs/nda/2014/206162Orig1s000ClinPharmR.pdf (accessed Mar 2016).

## Drug-Drug Interaction

Table 14   *In Vitro* Evaluation of Olaparib as an Inhibitor and an Inducer of Enzymes in Human Liver Microsomes[6-8]

| | Olaparib as an Inhibitor | | | Olaparib as an Inducer | |
|---|---|---|---|---|---|
| Enzyme | Conc. (μM) | %Inhibition | IC50 (μM) | Conc. (μM) | Fold Induction |
| CYP1A2 | 0.1-100 | <10 | >100 | 0.3-30 | No induction |
| CYP2A6 | 0.1-100 | <10 | >100 | NA | NA |
| CYP2B6 | 0.1-100 | <10 | >100 | 0.3-30 | 1.5-3.2 |
| CYP2C8 | 0.1-100 | <10 | >100 | NA | NA |
| CYP2C9 | 0.1-100 | <10 | >100 | 0.3-30 | No induction |
| CYP2C19 | 0.1-100 | <10 | >100 | 0.3-30 | No induction |
| CYP2D6 | 0.1-100 | <10 | >100 | NA | NA |
| CYP2E1 | 0.1-100 | <10 | >100 | NA | NA |
| CYP3A | 30 | 30 | >100 | 0.3-30 | No induction |

Table 15   *In Vitro* Evaluation of Olaparib as an Inhibitor and a Substrate of Uptake Transporters and Efflux Transporters[6-8]

| Olaparib as a Substrate, Efflux Ratio | | | | | Olaparib as an Inhibitor, IC50 (μM) | | | | | | | | |
|---|---|---|---|---|---|---|---|---|---|---|---|---|---|
| Conc. (μM) | BCRP | P-gp | MRP2 | OATs | P-gp | BCRP | OATP1B1 | OCT1 | OCT2 | OAT1 | OAT3 | MATE1 | MATE2K |
| 1-10 | No | 6-7.5 | 0.7-0.9 | Yes | No | Yes | 20.3 | 37.9 | 19.9 | 13.5[a] | 18.4 | 5.5 | 47.1 |

[a] 13.5% inhibition at 100 μM.

## 6   Non-Clinical Toxicology

### Summary

Single-Dose Toxicity
- ❖ Unnecessary to support this NDA, so not reviewed (FDA).
- ❖ According to the assessment by EMA, oral and intravenous studies had been performed in two rodent species:
  - Mouse MTD: 300 mg/kg (p.o.); 70 mg/kg (i.v.).
  - Rat MTD: 240 mg/kg (p.o.); 70 mg/kg (i.v.).

Repeated-Dose Toxicity
- ❖ Repeat-dose toxicity were evaluated by the oral route for up to 26 weeks in rats and dogs:
  - By the longest studies employed, the NOAELs in rats were 30 and 5 mg/kg/day for males and females, which equated to 0.06 and 0.04 × MRHD, respectively.   In dogs, the NOAELs were 3 mg/kg/day for both sexes, approximately 0.05 × MRHD.
  - The major target organ across species was hematopoietic system, e.g. reduced RBC and leukocyte population, associated with histopathology findings in the bone marrow (atrophy, reduced hematopoiesis), thymus (atrophy, involution), spleen (pigmented macrophages) and liver (hemosiderin pigmented cells).   Generally, the system was fully or partially recovered by the end of the non-dosing period.
  - Toxicokinetics parameters indicated no apparent accumulation in both species.

Safety Pharmacology
- ❖ Standard studies to investigate effects on central nervous, cardiovascular and respiratory system:
  - No effect was observed on the CNS and the respiratory system.
  - Olaparib inhibited the hERG tail current with an IC50 of 226 μM, making a low potency or ineffective blocker. Consistently, there was no evidence for QT prolongation in the dog study.

[6] FDA Database.   http://www.accessdata.fda.gov/drugsatfda_docs/nda/2014/206162Orig1s000PharmR.pdf (accessed Mar 2016).
[7] EMA Database.   http://www.ema.europa.eu/docs/en_GB/document_library/EPAR_-_Public_assessment_report/human/003726/WC500180154. pdf (accessed Mar 2016).
[8] FDA Database.   http://www.accessdata.fda.gov/drugsatfda_docs/nda/2014/206162Orig1s000ClinPharmR.pdf (accessed Mar 2016).

Genotoxicity

❖ Consistent with the mechanism of action, olaparib was not mutagenic in the *in vitro* bacterial reverse mutation (Ames) assay, but was clastogenic in the *in vitro* mammalian cell chromosomal aberration assay and *in vivo* rat bone marrow micronucleus assay.

Reproductive and Developmental Toxicity

❖ Fertility and early embryonic development in rats:
  • There were no treatment-related effects on mating/fertility at HDs (40 and 15 mg/kg/day in males and females, and equate to 7% and 11% of human AUC at the recommended clinical dose, respectively).

❖ Embryo-fetal development in rats:
  • Olaparib was embryotoxic and teratogenic when administered to pregnant rats during the period of organogenesis.
  • Major fetal malformations of the eyes, vertebra/ribs, skull and diaphragm, as well as minor skeletal and visceral abnormalities were observed at doses ≤0.5 mg/kg/day (≤0.3% of human AUC at the recommended clinical dose).

❖ Pre- and postnatal development studies had not been conducted.

Carcinogenicity

❖ According to the current ICH S9 guidance, carcinogenicity studies were not warranted to support approval of an NDA in the intended patient population.

## Single-Dose Toxicity

Table 16    Single-Dose Toxicity Studies of Olaparib[6]

| Species | Route | Doses (mg/kg)[a] | Finding |
|---|---|---|---|
| ICR mouse | p.o. | Preliminary phase: 50, 100, 200, 300 main test: 300 | Preliminary and main phases: 50, 100, 200, 300 mg/kg: No mortality or adverse sign.    All mice gained weight over the course of the study. 300 mg/kg: No macroscopic abnormality at necropsy (on Day 8 or Day 15). |
| | i.v. | Preliminary phase: 25, 50, 70, 100, 140, 200 main test: 100, 140 | Preliminary phase: 200 mg/kg: Both animals died immediately post-dose. 140 mg/kg: Male and female have prone posture within 2 min of dosing but recovered at 15 min post-dose. 100 and 70 mg: Only males have prone posture within 2 min of dosing but recovered at 15 min post-dose.    No macroscopic change observed in any animal at necropsy. Main test: 140 mg/kg: 4 males and 3 females died immediately post-dose; Prone posture and dyspnoea; Ataxia, palpebral closure, hunched posture and/or ↓ activity with lethargy. 100 mg/kg: 1 male and 1 female died at 5 min post-dose; Prone posture and dyspnoea; Ataxia, palpebral closure, hunched posture and/or ↓ activity with lethargy.    No macroscopic changes seen in any animal at necropsy. |

---

[6]  FDA Database.   http://www.accessdata.fda.gov/drugsatfda_docs/nda/2014/206162Orig1s000PharmR.pdf (accessed Mar 2016).

*Continued*

| Species | Route | Doses (mg/kg)<sup>a</sup> | Finding |
|---|---|---|---|
| Wistar rat | p.o. | Preliminary phase: 50, 100, 200, 240, 300 main test: 240 | Preliminary phase:<br>300 mg/kg: Both animals found dead on Day 2 or 3.   Palpebral closure, ↓ activity, hypothermia, tremors, salivation, piloerection and lachrymation.<br>50, 100, 200 and 240 mg/kg: Well tolerated, with no mortality.   No macroscopic change related to treatment at necropsy.<br>Main test:<br>240 mg/kg: Well tolerated, with no mortality. |
| | p.o. | Preliminary phase: 240, 300 main test: 240, 300 | Preliminary phase:<br>300 mg/kg: Female dosed at 300 mg/kg found dead on Day 2.   Salivation, lachrymation, hypothermia, ↓ activity, hunched posture and palpebral closure.   Macroscopic examination revealed severe darkening to all lobes of the lungs.   Well tolerated in the male; Adverse signs in animals included red extremities on Day 1 and/or 2.<br>240 mg/kg: Well tolerated in both sexes; adverse signs in animals included red extremities on Day 1 and/or 2.<br>Main test:<br>300 mg/kg: One male at 300 mg/kg found dead on Day 1; No macroscopic changes were observed at necropsy.   Salivation and red extremities on Day 1, with diarrhea and discoloured feces and anogenital soiling from Day 2. |
| | i.v. | Preliminary phase: 25, 50, 70, 100 main test: 70 | Preliminary phase:<br>100 mg/kg: Both animals died immediately post-dose.<br>70 mg/kg: ↓ Activity observed for both animals from approximately 15 min post-dosing, with recovery at 2 h post-dose.   No macroscopic changes at necropsy for animals that died on Day 1 or were killed on Day 8.<br>Main test:<br>70 mg/kg: Well tolerated, with no mortality.   Clinical signs limited to palpebral closure, observed from approximately 15 min post-dosing on Day 1, with recovery by 2 h post-dose.   All animals gained weight during the observation period and there were no macroscopic changes at necropsy on Day 15. |

Vehicles: 10% DMSO, 10% HPβCD in PBS.   <sup>a</sup> Well tolerated up to doses underlined.

## Repeated-Dose Toxicity

Table 17   Repeated-Dose Toxicity Studies of Olaparib by Oral (Gavage) Administration[6, 7]

| Species | Duration (Week) | Dose (mg/kg/day) | NOAEL | | | Finding |
|---|---|---|---|---|---|---|
| | | | Dose (mg/kg/day) | AUC$_{0-24}$<sup>a</sup> (ng·h/mL) | Safety Margin<sup>a</sup> (× MRHD<sup>b</sup>) | |
| Wistar rat | 4 | 0, 5, 15, 40 | 15 | 1057/6267 | 0.01/0.08 | 40 mg/kg: ↓ Peripheral RBCs and WBCs, primarily in female rats, elevated reticulocyte and platelet counts correlated with microscopic findings of bone marrow and splenic hematopoiesis, indicative of regenerative response.<br>The major target organs: Bone marrow, spleen, thymus, liver and kidneys.<br>No remarkable finding at the end of recovery.<br>$C_{max}$ and AUC increased dose-proportionally with ascending dose levels in males, while greater than dose-proportionally from 5-15 mg/kg and approximately proportionally from 15-40 mg/kg in females, 3-8 folds higher in females compared to males.   No apparent accumulation, peak plasma concentrations at 0.5-2 h post-dose. |

[6] FDA Database.   http://www.accessdata.fda.gov/drugsatfda_docs/nda/2014/206162Orig1s000PharmR.pdf (accessed Mar 2016).
[7] EMA Database.   http://www.ema.europa.eu/docs/en_GB/document_library/EPAR_-_Public_assessment_report/human/003726/WC500180154. pdf (accessed Mar 2016).

*Continued*

| Species | Duration (Week) | Dose (mg/kg/day) | NOAEL Dose (mg/kg/day) | AUC$_{0-24}$[a] (ng·h/mL) | Safety Margin[a] (× MRHD[b]) | Finding |
|---------|-----------------|------------------|-------------------------|---------------------------|------------------------------|---------|
| Wistar rat | 26 | Male: 0, 5, 15, 30 Female:0, 1, 5, 15 | 30/5 | 4230/3150 | 0.06/0.04 | No test article-related early mortality. Female rats at the 15 mg/kg dose level experienced a 10% decrease in body weight and 21% decrease in body weight gain, consistent with higher olaparib exposure. The major target organ was hematopoietic system. $C_{max}$ and AUC increased greater than dose proportionally. No apparent accumulation, significantly higher systemic exposure in females (up to 14-fold). $T_{max}$ at 1 to 4 h on Day 1 and 0.25 to 2 h after repeat-dosing, $T_{1/2}$ ranged from 1.4 to 5.5 h. |
| Beagle dog | 4 | 0, 2.5, 5, 15 | 5 | 5559/ 6519 | 0.07/0.09 | All animals survived to scheduled necropsy. The major target organ was the hematopoietic system. Olaparib caused a dose-dependent decrease in reticulo-cytes, platelets, total leukocytes, and lymphocytes at ≥2.5 mg/kg, corresponding to microscopic findings of bone marrow atrophy and delays in erythroid cell development. Minimal or slight microscopic findings were also observed in the spleen, GI tract, kidneys, urinary bladder, parathyroid, and prostate, primarily at ≥ 5 mg/kg. $C_{max}$ and AUC increased generally less than dose proportionally across the tested dose range. $T_{max}$ at 1.0 to 5.8 on Day 1 and 1 to 2.8 h in Week 4, systemic exposure in Week 4 comparable to Day 1, $C_{max}$ and AUC ~2-fold higher in females than males at HD, but not at LD and MD. |
| Beagle dog | 26 | 0, 1, 3, 10 | 3 | 3830/3600 | 0.05/0.05 | There were no test article-related early mortality. The major target organ was the hematopoietic system. Dogs given ≥3 mg/kg olaparib had a reduction in red cell mass, reticulocytes, platelets and leukocyte counts. Minimal to slight inflammation was noted in the stomach and prostate gland at ≥3 mg/kg, and pigmented macrophages and Kupffer cells were observed in the liver at 1 and 10 mg/kg with no apparent effect on liver function. $C_{max}$ increased less than dose proportionally, while AUC less than dose proportionally from 1 to 3 mg/kg and greater than dose proportional from 3 to 10 mg/kg. Systemic exposure in Week 13 and Week 26 comparable to Day 1, $T_{max}$ ranged from 1 to 6 h, $T_{1/2}$ ranged from 2.3 to 12.4 h, no apparent gender difference. |

Vehicle: 1% (v/v) DMSO and 10% HP$\beta$CD in PBS pH 7.4 for rat studies, 1% (w/v) MC in purified water for dog studies.   [a] Male/Female.   [b] Estimated mean total steady state AUC$_{0-24}$ after dosing at 400 mg BID (~6.67 mg/kg BID) in humans (76.6 µg·h/mL).   Human dose of 400 mg BID = 800 mg/day, equivalent to 6.67 mg/kg BID (for 60 kg human).   Human exposure data pooled from studies D0810C00002, D0810C00008, D0810C00009, D0810C00012 and D0810C00024.   AUC$_{0-12}$ was calculated from samples taken over 12 h after dosing; AUC$_{0-24}$ was estimated by doubling the AUC$_{0-12}$ values.

# Safety Pharmacology

Table 18    Safety Pharmacology Studies of Olaparib[6, 7]

| Study | System | Dose | Finding |
|-------|--------|------|---------|
| Central nervous system | Wistar rat (Irwin's method) | 0, 20, 115, 250 mg/kg, p.o. | No test article-related behavioral, autonomic, and motor change. |
| Cardiovascular system | CHO cell expressing hERG channel | 1, 3, 10, 30, 100, 300 μM | $IC_{50}$ of hERG tail current: 226 μM. |
| | Anaesthetised Beagle dog | 0, 1.5, 5, 15 mg/kg Single i.v. infusion over 10 min | No statistically significant change in cardiovascular parameters at LD and MD. Slight ↑ HR and dP/dtmax at HD without statistical significance. ↓ PR interval at 10 min post-dose at HD. |
| Respiratory system | Anaesthetised Beagle dog | 0, 1.5, 5, 15 mg/kg Single i.v. infusion over 10 min | No noticeable effect on respiratory parameters. |

Vehicle: 10% DMSO and 10% (w/v) HPBC in pH 7.4 PBS for *in vivo* test.

# Genotoxicity

Table 19    Genotoxicity Studies of Olaparib[6, 7]

| Assay | Species/System | Metabolism Activity | Dose | Finding |
|-------|----------------|---------------------|------|---------|
| *In vitro* bacterial reverse mutation assay (Ames) | *S. typhimurium* TA1535, TA1537, TA98, TA100; *E. coli* WP2PuvrA | ±S9 | Up to 5000 μg/plate | Negative. |
| *In vitro* mammalian cell cytogenetic test | CHO | ±S9 | Up to 2500 μg/mL | Positive. |
| *In vivo* rodent micronucleus assay | CD rat | + | 100, 200, 400 mg/kg/day, QD × 2 | Positive. |

Vehicle: DMSO for *in vitro* tests, 10% DMSO and 10% HPβCD in PBS for *in vivo* test.

# Reproductive and Developmental Toxicity

Table 20    Reproductive and Developmental Toxicology Studies of Olaparib by Oral (Gavage) Administration[6, 7]

| Studies | Species | Dose (mg/kg/day) | Finding |
|---------|---------|------------------|---------|
| Fertility and early embryonic development | Wistar rat (female) | 0, 0.05, 0.5, 15 | Minimal maternal toxicity was noted at the 15 mg/kg dose level (↓ 4%-6% body weight). A higher incidence of extended estrus (9/34 females) was observed at the 15 mg/kg dose level but had no effect on mating and fertility. There was a statistically significant increase in pre-implantation loss, early intrauterine deaths, and post-implantation loss in the 15 mg/kg dose group (11% of human AUC at the recommended clinical dose). Following a 4-week recovery period, 15 mg/kg female rats showed no treatment-related effect on mating, fertility, or embryo-fetal survival. NOEL = 0.5 mg/kg/day ($AUC_{0-24}$ = 257 ng·h/mL). |
| | Wistar rat (male) | 0, 5, 15, 40 | At 40 mg/kg, males experienced reduced body weight and body weight gain as well as clinical signs of salivation and hair loss. There were no test article-related effects on mating and fertility rates at doses up to 40 mg/kg/day compared to controls (approximately 7% of human AUC at the recommended clinical dose based on TK analysis in 4-week repeat-dose study). NOEL = 40 mg/kg/day ($AUC_{0-24}$ = 25842 ng·h/mL). |
| Embryo-fetal development | Wistar rat (female) | 0, 0.05, 0.5 | A slight increase in early intrauterine deaths was reported at the 0.5 mg/kg dose level, resulting in a reduced number of viable offspring compared to controls. Major fetal malformations (eye, vertebra/ribs, skull and diaphragm) and minor skeletal and visceral abnormalities were noted at 0.05 and 0.5 mg/kg ($AUC_{0-24}$ = 209 ng·h/mL) dose levels (≤0.3% of human AUC at the recommended clinical dose; AUC could not be calculated for the low dose level). |

Vehicle: 10% DMSO and 10% (w/v) HPBC in PBS (pH 7.4).    Human AUC at recommended clinical dose: 38.3 μg·h/mL.

[6] FDA Database.    http://www.accessdata.fda.gov/drugsatfda_docs/nda/2014/206162Orig1s000PharmR.pdf (accessed Mar 2016).
[7] EMA Database.    http://www.ema.europa.eu/docs/en_GB/document_library/EPAR_-_Public_assessment_report/human/003726/WC500180154. pdf (accessed Mar 2016).

# CHAPTER

20

## Oritavancin Diphosphate

# Oritavancin Diphosphate

## (Orbactiv®)

The
Medicines
Company

Research code: LY-333328

## 1  General Information

❖ Oritavancin diphosphate is a semi-synthetic, lipoglyco-peptide antibacterial drug, which was first approved in Aug 2014 by US FDA.

❖ Oritavancin diphosphate was originally discovered by Eli Lilly, discovered and marketed by The Medicines Company.

❖ Oritavancin diphosphate, as a lipoglycopeptide antibacterial drug, inhibits cell wall biosynthesis and disrupts bacterial membrane integrity leading to depolarization, permeabilization and bacterial cell death.

❖ Oritavancin diphosphate is indicated for the treatment of adult patients with acute bacterial skin and skin structure infections (ABSSSI) caused by susceptible isolates of designated Gram-positive microorganisms.

❖ Available as lyophilized powder, containing 400 mg of free oritavancin and the recommended dosage is 1200 mg administered as a single dose by intravenous (i.v.) infusion over 3 h in patients 18 years and older.

❖ Sales of Orbactiv® were 0.8 and 9.1 million US$ in 2014 and 2015, respectively, according to the financial reports of The Medicines Company.

### Key Approvals around the World[*]

|  | US (FDA) | EU (EMA) |
|---|---|---|
| First approval date | 08/06/2014 | 03/19/2015 |
| Application or approval No. | NDA 206334 | EMEA/H/C/003785 |
| Brand name | Orbactiv® | Orbactiv® |
| Indication | Acute bacterial skin and skin structure infections (ABSSSI) | Acute bacterial skin and skin structure infections (ABSSSI) |
| Authorisation holder | The Medicines Company | The Medicines Company |

[*] Till Mar 2016, it had not been approved by PMDA (Japan) and CFDA (China).

## Active Ingredient

· 2 $H_3PO_4$

Molecular formula: $C_{86}H_{97}N_{10}O_{26}Cl_3 \cdot 2H_3PO_4$
Molecular weight: 1989.09
CAS No.: 171099-57-3 (Oritavancin)
192564-14-0 (Oritavancin diphosphate)
Chemical name: [4″ R]-22-O-(3-amino-2,3,6-trideoxy-3-C-methyl-α-L-arabinohexopyranosyl)-N3″-[(4′-chloro[1,1′-biphenyl]-4-yl)methyl]vancomycin phosphate [1:2] [salt]

### Parameters of Lipinski's "Rule of 5"

| MW[a] | $H_D$ | $H_A$ | FRB[b] | PSA[b] | cLogP[b] |
|---|---|---|---|---|---|
| 1793.10 | 22 | 36 | 29 | 561Å² | 3.84 ± 1.49 |

[a] Molecular weight of oritavancin.　[b] Calculated by ACD/Labs software V11.02.

## Drug Product[*]

Dosage route: Intravenous injection
Strength: 400 mg (Oritavancin)
Dosage form: White to offwhite lyophilized powder
Inactive ingredient: Mannitol and phosphoric acid (to adjust pH 3.1 to 4.3).
Recommended dose: The recommended dosage of oritavancin diphosphate is 1200 mg administered as an intravenous infusion over 3 h in patients 18 years and older.

[*] Sourced from US FDA drug label information

# 2 Key Patents Information

## Summary

❖ Orbactiv® (Oritavancin diphosphate) has got five-year NCE market exclusivity protection after it was initially approved by US FDA on Aug 06, 2014.

❖ Oritavancin was originally discovered by Eli Lilly and then acquired by Targanta Therapeutics in 2005. In 2009, the development rights were acquired by The Medicines Company.

❖ The compound patent application of oritavancin was originally filed by Eli Lilly in 1996.

❖ The compound patent expired in 2015, which had been granted in the United States, China, Europe and Japan successively.

Table 1    Oritavancin's Compound Patent Protection in Drug-Mainstream Country

| Country | Publication/Patent NO. | Application Date | Granted Date | Estimated Expiry Date |
|---------|------------------------|-----------------|--------------|----------------------|
| WO | WO9630401A1 | 03/14/1996 | / | / |
| US | US5840684A | 01/28/1994 | 11/24/1998 | 11/24/2016[a] |
| EP | EP0667353B1 | 01/25/1995 | 10/29/2003 | 01/25/2015 |
| JP | JP3756539B2 | 01/27/1995 | 03/15/2006 | 01/27/2015 |
| CN | CN1071334C | 01/27/1995 | 09/19/2001 | 01/27/2015 |

[a] The term of this patent is extended by 1 year.

Table 2    Originator's International Patent Application List (Patent Family)

| Publication NO. | Title | Applicant/Assignee/Owner | Publication Date |
|-----------------|-------|--------------------------|------------------|
| Technical Subjects | Active Ingredient (Free Base)'s Formula or Structure and Preparation | | |
| WO9630401A1 | Glycopeptide antibiotic derivatives | Eli Lilly | 10/03/1996 |
| Technical Subjects | Salt, Crystal, Polymorphic, Solvate (Hydrate), Isomer, Derivative Etc. and Preparation | | |
| WO9821952A1 | Reducing agent for reductive alkylation of glycopeptide antibiotics | Eli Lilly | 05/28/1998 |
| WO9822121A1 | Reductive alkylation of glycopeptide antibiotics | Eli Lilly | 05/28/1998 |
| WO2008077241A1 | Phosphonated glycopeptide and lipoglycopeptide antibiotics and uses thereof for the prevention and treatment of bone and joint infections | Targanta | 07/03/2008 |
| WO2008118784A1 | Glycopeptide and lipoglycopeptide antibiotics with improved solubility | Targanta | 10/02/2008 |
| WO2011019839A2 | Glycopeptide and lipoglycopeptide antibiotics with improved solubility | The Medicines | 02/17/2011 |
| Technical Subjects | Formulation and Preparation | | |
| WO2013016529A2 | Disk diffusion assay for oritavancin | The Medicines | 01/31/2013 |
| Technical Subjects | Indication or Methods for Medical Needs | | |
| WO2008097364A2 | Use of oritavancin for prevention and treatment of anthrax | Targanta | 08/14/2008 |
| WO2009036121A1 | Method of inhibiting clostridium difficile by administration of oritavancin | Targanta | 03/19/2009 |
| WO2009126502A2 | Methods of inhibiting and treating biofilms using glycopeptide antibiotics | Targanta | 10/15/2009 |
| WO2010025438A2 | Methods of treatment using single dose of oritavancin | Targanta | 03/04/2010 |
| WO2010129233A2 | Methods of treating bacterial infections using oritavancin | Targanta | 11/11/2010 |
| WO2014176068A2 | Treatment and prevention of bacterial skin infections using oritavancin | The Medicines | 10/30/2014 |
| WO2015031313A2 | Methods for treating bacteremia and osteomyelitis using oritavancin | The Medicines | 03/05/2015 |
| Technical Subjects | Combination Including at Least Two Active Ingredients | | |
| WO2010019511A2 | Phosphonated rifamycins and uses thereof for the prevention and treatment of bone and joint infections | Targanta | 02/18/2010 |
| WO2015031579A2 | Methods for treating bacterial infections using oritavancin and polymyxins | The Medicines | 03/05/2015 |

The data was updated until Jan 2016.

# 3   Chemistry

## Route 1:   Original Discovery Route

*Synthesis Route*: Commercial eremomycin **1** was treated with 4'-chlorobiphenylcarboxaldehyde **2** followed by sodium cyanoborohydride in refluxing methanol to give oritavancin. Interestingly, there are three amino groups within eremomycin that can undergo reductive alkylation and this chemistry preferentially occurs at the disaccharide amino group. The reaction is reported to occur in 69.3% crude yield and giving 18% yield of oritavancin after HPLC purification.[1-3]

# 4  Pharmacology

## Summary

### Mechanism of Action

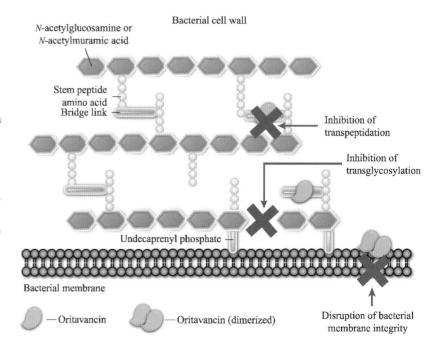

❖ Oritavancin is a semi-synthetic lipoglycopeptide antibacterial drug with a structure resembles vancomycin.

❖ Oritavancin exerts its action via three mechanisms: i) inhibition of the transglycosylation (polymerization) step of cell wall biosynthesis; ii) inhibition of transpeptidation (cross-linking) step of cell wall biosynthesis; iii) disruption of bacterial membrane integrity, leading to depolarization, permeabilization and cell death.

❖ Oritavancin has two cell wall binding sites, the peptidoglycan D-Ala-D-Ala pentapeptide stem terminus of lipid II and the peptide bridging segment.

❖ Oritavancin showed inhibition of radioligand binding at dopaminergic $D_1$ ($K_i$ = 2.25 µM) and $D_2$ ($K_i$ = 3.46 µM) receptors in rat brain homogenates. Oritavancin exhibited a slight inhibition on the force of acetylcholine-induced contractions of guinea pig ileum tissue.[4, 5]

### In Vitro Efficacy

❖ Antibacterial activity against *staphylcocci*, *streptococci*, and *enterococci* isolates:
  • MIC range = 0.001-0.5 µg/mL.
  • $MIC_{50}$ = 0.008-0.06 µg/mL.
❖ Antibacterial activity against resistant *S. aureus* and *E. faecalis*:
  • *E. faecalis*: MIC = 0.008-0.12 µg/mL (except ID1058946, MIC = 0.5 µg/mL).
  • MRSA and MSSA: MIC = 0.03-0.12 µg/mL.
  • VISA and VRSA: MIC = 0.25-1 µg/mL.
❖ Oritavancin was a better and faster bactericidal agent against *S. aureus* and *enterococci* than vancomycin, teicoplanin, linezolid or dapatomycin.[4]

### In Vivo Efficacy

❖ Granuloma pouch infection model with *S. aureus* (ATCC 13709):
  • Oritavancin: Delayed regrowth for at least 72 h at 30 mg/kg.
  • Vancomycin: Regrowth began at 24 h post-dose at 100 mg/kg.
❖ Bacteremia in MSSA mouse model: Reduced the bacterial burden in blood by 1.7 $log_{10}$ at 100 mg by 72 h.
❖ Central venous catheter (CVC) rat model with *S. aureus*: Reduced bacterial counts significantly at 20 mg/kg.
❖ Endocarditis in different models:
  • MRSA rabbit model:
    ✦ Reduced the bacterial burden in the vegetations by 6 $log_{10}$ CFU.
    ✦ Reduced the bacterial burden in the kidneys and spleen by >4 $log_{10}$ CFU.
  • MSSA rat model: Reduced the bacterial burden in the vegetations by 5 $log_{10}$ CFU.
  • Glycopeptied-susceptible *E. faecalis* and Glycopeptied-resistant *E. faecalis* models with VanA or VanB phenotypes: Reduced the bacterial burden in the vegetations by 1.8-2.8 $log_{10}$ CFU.

[1] Cooper, R. D. G.; Snyder, N. J.; Zweifel, M. J., et al. *J. Antibiot.* **1996**, *49*, 575-581.
[2] Cooper, R. D. G.; Huff, B. E.; Nicas, T. I., et al. WO9630401A1, **1996**.
[3] Cooper, R. D. G.; Huff, B. E.; Nicas, T. I., et al. US5840684A, **1998**.
[4] U.S. Food and Drug Administration (FDA) Database. http://www.accessdata.fda.gov/drugsatfda_docs/nda/2014/206334Orig1s000MicroR.pdf (accessed Mar 2016).
[5] Patti, G. J.; Kim, S. J.; Yu, T. Y., et al. *J. Mol. Biol.* **2009**, *392*, 1178-1191.

❖ Pneumonia infection (MRSA) in mouse and rat models:
  • Penicillin-susceptible *S. pneumonia* model: Reduced bacterial counts in lungs at ≥6.5 mg/kg.
  • MRSA model: Reduced the bacterial burden in lungs by 3.5 $\log_{10}$ CFU.
❖ Biofilm infection in MSSA model: Oritavancin and oxacillin significantly decreased *S. aureus* densities.
❖ Meningitis in models:
  • Penicillin susceptible *S. pneumonia* model:
    ✦ Decreased the bacterial burden: $0.51 \pm 0.54 \log_{10}$ CFU/mL in CSF.
    ✦ Ceftriaxone decreased the bacterial burden: $0.34 \pm 0.15 \log_{10}$ CFU/mL in CSF.
  • Cephalosporin-resistant *S. pneumoniae* model: Reduced the bacterial density: CFU = 3.0 to 5.2 $\log_{10}$/mL.
❖ Inhalational anthrax in *B. anthracis* models:
  • Post-exposure prophylaxis: Protected 70% and 100% of lethally-challenged mice at 15 or 50 mg/kg.
  • Post-exposure treatment: Protected 56% of lethally-challenged mice at 50 mg/kg.
  • Pre-exposure prophylaxis: Protected 90% of mice to the 34 days post-challenge endpoint at 50 mg/kg.

## Mechanism of Action

Table 3   Distribution of D-Ala or Tripeptides in Peptidoglycan of *E. faecium* (Mid-exponential Growth) by Oritavancin[5]

| Compound | Dose (μg/mL) | D-Ala (%) | | | Stem-linked (%) | Tripeptides (%) |
|---|---|---|---|---|---|---|
| | | D-Ala-D-Asp | D-Ala-D-Ala | D-Ala | | |
| Vancomycin | 0 | 76 | 24 | 0 | 60 | 40 |
| | 15 | 48 | 47 | 5 | 65 | 35 |
| | 25 | 45 | 48 | 7 | 65 | 35 |
| Oritavancin | 0 | 76 | 24 | 0 | 63 | 37 |
| | 15 | 83 | 17 | 0 | 37 | 63 |
| | 25 | 89 | 11 | 0 | 31 | 69 |

Each drug was added to cultures in mid-exponential growth phase (OD$_{660}$ ≈ 0.4), and the cells were harvested for analysis approximately 45 min later.

Table 4   Effects of Oritavancin on Cell-wall Cross-links per Unit Peptidoglycan[6]

| Control | Vancomycin | Oritavancin | Penicillin |
|---|---|---|---|
| 1.00 | 0.87 | 0.64 | 0.42 |

Drugs were added to *S. aureus* in exponential growth.   The cross-links were determined from the 175-ppm 8-T$_r$ $^{13}$C{$^{15}$N} REDOR difference (ΔS) for whole cells labeled by D-[1-$^{13}$C]alanine and [$^{15}$N]glycine in the presence of a racemase inhibitor.   The cross-links were measured relative to the total of mature and immature peptidoglycan as determined by the intensities of the 70-ppm $^{13}$C full-echo (S0) sugar peaks.

## *In Vitro* Efficacy

Table 5   Antimicrobial Spectrum of Oritavancin[4, 7-9]

| Organism | Type | Strain number | MIC (μg/mL) | | |
|---|---|---|---|---|---|
| | | | MIC Ranging | MIC$_{50}$ | MIC$_{90}$ |
| *Staphylococci* | MSSA | 2186 | ≤0.002-0.5 | 0.03 | 0.06 |
| | MRSA | 1604 | ≤0.002-0.25 | 0.03 | 0.06 |
| | ATCC 29213[a] | 10 | 0.015-0.12 | NA | NA |
| | MSCoNS | 233 | 0.004-0.25 | 0.03 | 0.12 |
| | MRCoNS | 353 | 0.004-0.25 | 0.06 | 0.12 |

[4] FDA Database.   http://www.accessdata.fda.gov/drugsatfda_docs/nda/2014/206334Orig1s000MicroR.pdf (accessed Mar 2016).
[5] Patti, G. J.; Kim, S. J.; Yu, T. Y., et al. *J. Mol. Biol.* **2009**, *392*, 1178-1191.
[6] Kim, S. J.; Cegelski, L.; Stueber, D., et al. *J. Mol. Biol.* **2008**, *377*, 281-293.
[7] European Medicines Agency (EMA) Database.   http://www.ema.europa.eu/docs/en_GB/document_library/EPAR_-_Public_assessment_report/human/003785/WC500186347.pdf (accessed Mar 2016).
[8] Biedenbach, D. J.; Arhin, F. F.; Moeck, G., et al. *Int. J. Antimicrob. Agents* **2015**, *46*, 674-681.
[9] Vaudaux, P.; Huggler, E.; Arhin, F. F., et al. *Int. J. Antimicrob. Agents* **2009**, *34*, 540-543.

*Continued*

| Organism | Type | Strain Number | MIC (µg/mL) | | |
|---|---|---|---|---|---|
| | | | MIC Ranging | MIC$_{50}$ | MIC$_{90}$ |
| Enterococci | VSEfa, VREfa | 635 | 0.002-0.25 | 0.015 | 0.06 |
| | *Enterococcus faecalis* ATCC 29212[a] | 243 | 0.008-0.03 | NA | NA |
| Streptococci | *S. pneumoniae* | 4349 | 0.008-0.12 | <0.008 | 0.015 |
| | *S. pneumonia* ATCC49619[a] | NA | 0.001-0.004 | NA | NA |
| | Beta-Hemolytic *Streptococci* (*S. pyogenes, S. agalactiae*) | 1061 | ≤0.002-0.5 | 0.03-0.06 | 0.25 |
| | Viridans Group *Streptococci* | 835 | ≤0.002-0.12 | <0.008 | 0.06 |
| | *S. anginosus* group | 102 | ≤0.008-0.12 | <0.008 | 0.0015 |
| | *S. dysgalactiae* | 34 | ≤0.008-0.25 | 0.06 | 0.25 |

MIC: Minimum inhibitory concentrations.   MSSA: Methicillin-susceptible *S. aureus*.   MRSA: Methicillin-resistant *S. aureus*.   MSCoNS: Methicillin-susceptible coagulase-negative *staphylococci*.   MRCoNS: Methicillin-resistant coagulase-negative *staphylococci*.   VSEfa: Vancomycin-susceptible *E. faecalis*.   VREfa: Vancomycin-resistant *E. faecalis*.   [a] Quality control, determined by broth microdilution with 0.002% polysorbate-80.

Table 6    Antibacterial Activity of by Oritavancin against *S. aureus* and *Enterococcus* Strains[10]

| Strain | Phenotype | MIC (µg/mL) | | | | |
|---|---|---|---|---|---|---|
| | | Oritavancin | Vancomycin | Teicoplanin | Linezolid | Daptomycin |
| *S. aureus* ATCC 29213 | MSSA | 0.06 | 1 | 0.5 | 2 | 0.5 |
| *S. aureus* ATCC 700699 | VISA | 1 | 8 | 4 | 1 | 2 |
| *S. aureus* NRS 121 | LZD-NS MRSA | 0.03 | 2 | 0.5 | 64 | 0.5 |
| *S. aureus* NRS 123 | CA-MRSA | 0.12 | 2 | 1 | 2 | 0.5 |
| *S. aureus* NRS 402 | VISA | 1 | 4 | 8 | 1 | 4 |
| *S. aureus* VRS 5 | VRSA | 0.25 | 256 | 32 | 2 | 0.5 |
| *E. faecalis* ATCC 29212 | VSE | 0.03 | 4 | 0.12 | 2 | 8 |
| *E. faecalis* ATCC 51299 | VRE | 0.008 | 128 | 2 | 1 | 8 |
| *E. faecalis* ID1058946 | VRE | 0.5 | 2048 | 256 | 2 | 2 |
| *E. faecalis* ATCC 51559 | VRE | 0.12 | >1024 | >128 | 1 | 16 |
| *E. faecalis* ID1058946 | VRE | 0.015 | 512 | 0.25 | 2 | 4 |

Following CLSI-recommended guidelines and including 0.002% polysorbate-80 for oritavancin (M7-A7; M100-S18).   MIC: Minimum inhibitory concentrations. MSSA: Methicillin-susceptible *S. aureus*.   LZD-NS: Linezolid-non-susceptible.   MRSA: Methicillin-resistant *S. aureus*.   VISA: Vancomycin-intermediate *S. aureus*. VRSA: Vancomycin-resistant *S. aureus*.   VSE: Vancomycin-susceptible *Enterococcus*.   VRE: Vancomycin-resistant *Enterococcus*.

[10]   McKay, G. A.; Beaulieu, S.; Sarmiento, I., et al. *J. Antimicrob. Chemother.* **2009**, *63*, 1191-1199.

## *In Vivo* Efficacy

Table 7   Effects of Oritavancin in the Animal Infection Models[4, 5, 10, 11]

| Infection Model | | | | Drug | Dose (mg/kg) | Route & Duration (Day) | Finding |
|---|---|---|---|---|---|---|---|
| Study | Strain | CFU | Animal | | | | |
| Granuloma pouch infection | *S. aureus* ATCC 13709 | $10^5$ | Rat | Oritavancin | 0.25-30 | i.v., single dose | 30 mg/kg: Delayed regrowth for $\geq$72 h. |
| | | | | Vancomycin | 100 | s.c., single dose | Regrowth began 24 h. |
| Bacteremia | *S. aureus* | $10^7$ | Mouse | Oritavancin | 100, 400, 800 mg[a] | i.v., QD × 3 | Reduced the bacterial burden in blood by 1.7 $\log_{10}$ at 100 mg by 72 h. |
| | | | | Oritavancin | 1200 mg | i.v., single dose | Reduced the bacterial burden to the limit of detection or by approximately 2.8 $\log_{10}$ CFU. |
| Central venous catheter (CVC) infection | *S. aureus* | $10^5$ | Rat | Oritavancin | 2.5/12 h, 5/24 h, 10/48 h, or 20/96 h, total dose: 20 mg/kg over 96 h | i.v. | Reduced bacterial counts in 20 mg/kg dose group. Higher doses and less frequently: More effective. |
| | *E. faecium* | 625 | Rat | Oritavancin | 20 | i.v., single dose | None of eight animals developed CVC infection. |
| Endocarditis | MRSA | $10^6$ | Rabbit | Oritavancin | 25 | i.v., QD × 4 | Oritavancin and vancomycin each reduced the bacterial burden ~6 $\log_{10}$ CFU in the vegetation, and >4 $\log_{10}$ CFU in the kidneys and spleen. |
| | | | | Vancomycin | 25 | i.v., TID × 4 | |
| | MSSA | $10^6$ | Rat | Oritavancin | 80 | i.v., QD × 4 | Oritavncin, daptomycin and oxacillin: A 5 $\log_{10}$ reduction in CFUs in the vegetation. Vancomycin: 3 $\log_{10}$ decrease in CFUs. All agents equally in reducing CFUs in the kidney and spleen: 2.5 to 3.5 $\log_{10}$ CFU. |
| | | | | Vancomycin | 120 | i.v., BID × 4 | |
| | | | | Daptomycin | 10 | i.v., QD × 4 | |
| | | | | Oxacillin | 200 | i.v., TID × 4 | |
| | Glycopeptied-susceptible, or resistant *E. faecalis* with VanA or VanB phenotypes | NA | Rabbit | Oritavancin | NA | NA | Reduced the bacterial density of vegetations by 1.8 to 2.8 $\log_{10}$ CFU/g. |
| | | | | Oritavancin | 20 | NA | Limited activity, CFU/g: 7.9 to 8.1 $\log_{10}$. |
| | | | | Oritavancin + gentamicin | NA | NA | Active against all tested strains, CFU/g: 6.1 to 6.8 $\log_{10}$. |
| Pneumonia infection | Penicillin-susceptible *S. pneumoniae* | $10^6$ | Mouse | Oritavancin | 0.25-32 | i.v., single dose | Reduced bacterial counts in lungs to the limit of detection at $\geq$6.5 mg/kg. |
| | MRSA | $10^{3.5}$ | Rat | Oritavancin | 50 | i.v., QD × 6 | Reduced the bacterial burden in lungs by 3.5 $\log_{10}$ CFU. |
| Biofilm infection[b] | MSSA | $10^5$ | Mouse | Oritavancin | 80 | i.v., QD × 4 | Oritavancin and oxacillin significantly decreased *S. aureus* densities. |
| | | | | Vancomycin | 120 | s.c., BID × 4 | |
| | | | | Daptomycin | 10 | i.v., QD × 4 | |
| | | | | Oxacillin | 200 | i.m., TID × 4 | |
| | | | | Rifampin | 30 | i.p., BID × 4 | |
| Meningitis | Penicillin susceptible *S. pneumoniae* | $10^6$ | Rabbit | Oritavancin | 1, 2.5, 10, 40 | i.v., single dose | 40 mg/kg: Decreased the bacterial burden by 0.51 ± 0.54 $\log_{10}$ CFU/mL in CSF. |
| | | | | Ceftriaxone | 20 mg/kg bolus, followed by 10 mg/kg/h i.v. infusion | i.v., single dose | Decreased the bacterial burden by 0.34 ± 0.15 $\log_{10}$ CFU/mL in CSF. |
| | Cephalosporin-resistant *S. pneumoniae* | NA | Rabbit | Oritavancin | 10 | i.v., single dose | Reduced the bacterial density by 3.0 to 5.2 $\log_{10}$ CFU/mL. |

[4]  FDA Database.   http://www.accessdata.fda.gov/drugsatfda_docs/nda/2014/206334Orig1s000MicroR.pdf (accessed Mar 2016).
[5]  EMA Database.   http://www.ema.europa.eu/docs/en_GB/document_library/EPAR_-_Public_assessment_report/human/003785/WC500186347.pdf (accessed Mar 2016).
[10]  McKay, G. A.; Beaulieu, S.; Sarmiento, I., et al. *J. Antimicrob. Chemother.* **2009**, *63*, 1191-1199.
[11]  Heine, H. S.; Bassett, J.; Miller, L., et al. *Antimicrob. Agents. Chemother.* **2008**, *52*, 3350-3357.

*Continued*

| | Infection Model | | | Drug | Dose (mg/kg) | Route & Duration (Day) | Finding |
|---|---|---|---|---|---|---|---|
| Study | Strain | CFU | Animal | | | | |
| Inhalational anthrax | *B. anthracis* | NA | Mouse | Oritavancin | 15 or 50 | i.v., single dose | Post-exposure prophylaxis: Protected 70% and 100% of lethally-challenged mice, respectively. |
| | | | | | 50 | i.v., single dose | Post-exposure treatment: Protected 56% of lethally-challenged mice. |
| | | | | | 50 | i.v., single dose | Pre-exposure prophylaxis: Protected 90% of mice to the 34 days post-challenge endpoint. |

MSSA: Methicillin susceptible *S. aureus*.　MRSA: Methicillin-resistant *Staphylococcus aureus*.　CFU: Colony forming units.　QD: Once daily.　BID: Twice daily. TID: Three times daily.　i.v.: Intravenous injection.　s.c.: Subcutaneous injection.　NA. Not available.　[a] Mice treated i.v. with oritavancin simulating human doses of 100, 400 and 800 mg daily.　[b] Monitored by real-time bioluminescence.

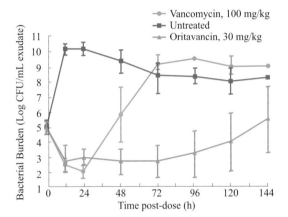

**Study:** Bacterial burden in rats with granuloma pouch infection of *S. aureus*.

**Animal:** Non-neutropenic rat.

**Model:** Granuloma pouches were induced in non-neutropenic rats then inoculated with approximately $1 \times 10^5$ CFU of *S. aureus* ATCC 13709.

**Administration:** 2 h post-inoculation.　Oritavancin: single i.v., 0.25 to 30 mg/kg; Vancomycin: single s.c., 100 mg/kg.

**Test:** Bacterial burden post-dose.

**Results:** Oritavancin at 30 mg/kg delayed regrowth of the infecting *S. aureus* strain for at least 72 h, whereas regrowth began 24 h after a single dose of vancomycin at 100 mg/kg.　Oritavancin efficacy *in vivo* was sustained for 72 h under these experimental conditions, following administration of a single dose.

Figure A　The Antibacterial Activity of Oritavancin in a Rat Granuloma Pouch Infection Model[4]

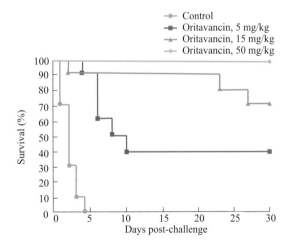

**Study:** Efficacy of oritavancin in the mouse inhalation anthrax model.

**Animal:** Mouse.

**Model:** NA.

**Administration:** Oritavancin, single i.v., 5-50 mg/kg.　Oritavancin concentrations were maintained above 1 mg/mL during dissolution and filtration before dilution and administration.

**Test:** Proportional survival.

**Results:** 15 or 50 mg/kg oritavancin protected 70% and 100% of lethally-challenged mice.

Figure B　Proportional Survival from Oritavancin Treatment in the Post-exposure Prophylaxis Model of Inhalation Anthrax[11]

[4]　FDA Database.　http://www.accessdata.fda.gov/drugsatfda_docs/nda/2014/206334Orig1s000MicroR.pdf (accessed Mar 2016).
[11]　Heine, H. S.; Bassett, J.; Miller, L., et al. *Antimicrob. Agents. Chemother*. **2008**, *52*, 3350-3357.

# 5 ADME & Drug-Drug Interaction

## Summary

### Absorption of Oritavancin Diphosphate

❖ Exhibited a linear pharmacokinetics in humans and rabbits after intravenous dosing. The increases of $C_{max}$ and AUC appeared to be dose-proportional in the dose range of 0.5-3 mg/kg in humans and 10-40 mg/kg in rabbits.
❖ Was absorbed rapidly in humans with $T_{max} = 0.5$ h post-dose.
❖ Showed half-lives of 8-33 h in mice, 4-14 h in rats, 66.9 h in dogs, 62.4 h in rabbits and 245 h in humans, which might be attributed to the difference in sampling time point.
❖ The central volume of distribution ($V_c$) in humans was 5.9 L, which was similar to plasma volume, but the total volume of distribution was approximately 100 L.

### Distribution of Oritavancin Diphosphate

❖ Exhibited moderate serum protein binding in mice (85.3%), rats (82.4%), dogs (87.1%) and humans (81.9%). Most binding of oritavancin in serum was bound to albumin.
❖ Rats after single intravenous administration:
  • The drug was distributed to most tissues with peak levels attained within 1-6 h of intravenous administration.
  • Relatively higher radioactivity levels were observed in liver and intestinal, and moderate levels in the adrenal gland, bone marrow, cecal wall, kidneys, lungs, salivary gland and spleen, and low or background levels in brain, eyes and testes.
  • $T_{1/2}$ ranged between 100 to 200 h in the majority of tissues.
❖ In dogs, mostly accumulated in liver.

### Metabolism of Oritavancin Diphosphate

❖ There was not appeared to have any evidence of metabolism from *in vitro* or *in vivo* animal models (mice, rats, dogs and monkeys).
❖ *In vitro* human liver microsomes study demonstrated no metabolism by the human cytochrome P450 system.

### Excretion of Oritavancin Diphosphate

❖ Oritavancin was excreted unchanged primarily *via* the bile into the feces in mice, rats and dogs.
❖ In contrast to animals where feces was as the primary route of excretion, in humans the majority of recovered dose was in urine (~5%) and the rest in feces (<1%).

### Drug-Drug Interaction

❖ Oritavancin showed weak inhibitory activity to CYPs in human liver microsomes, including CYP3A4, CYP2D6, CYP2C9, CYP2C19, CYP2B6 and CYP1A2.
❖ In human hepatocytes, oritavancin at concentrations ≤50 μM did not induce CYP1A2, CYP2A6, CYP2C9, CYP2C19 or CYP2D6 activities. At 50 μM oritavancin slightly increased CYP2E1 activity. At 2.5 μM oritavancin slightly increased CYP3A4 activity, but at higher concentrations inhibited CYP3A4 activity.
❖ Neither a substrate or an inhibitor of the efflux transporter P-glycoprotein (P-gp), nor transporter protein studies with oritavancin were reported.

## Absorption

Table 8   *In Vivo* Pharmacokinetic Parameters of Oritavancin in Rabbits after Single Intravenous Dose of Oritavancin[12]

| Species | Dose (mg/kg) | $T_{max}$ (h) | $C_{max}$ (μg/mL) | $T_{1/2}$ (h) | $AUC_{0-24}$ (μg·h/mL) | Cl (mL/h/kg) |
|---------|------|------|------|------|------|------|
| Rabbit | 20[a] | 0.2 | 219 | 62.4 | 1672[b] | 12.0 |
| | 10 | NA | 71.8 ± 11.0 | NA | 450 ± 46.9 | NA |
| | 15 | NA | 113 ± 13.1 | NA | 786 ± 84.0 | NA |
| | 20 | NA | 148 ± 12.0 | NA | 966 ± 48.8 | NA |
| | 40 | NA | 252 ± 38.4 | NA | 1835 ± 88.2 | NA |

[a] Oritavancin concentration in serum.   [b] $AUC_{0-168}$.

[12] Lehoux, D.; Ostiguy, V.; Cadieux, C., et al. *Antimicrob. Agents Chemother.* **2015**, *59*, 6501-6505.

## Key Findings:

❖ Terminal plasma half-life ranged from 8 h to 33 h in mice, from 4 h to14 h in rats, 66.9 h in dogs and 245 h in humans, which might be attributed to the difference in sampling time point.[4]

❖ The central volume of distribution ($V_c$) in humans was 5.9 L, which was similar to plasma volume, but the total volume of distribution was approximately 100 L.[5]

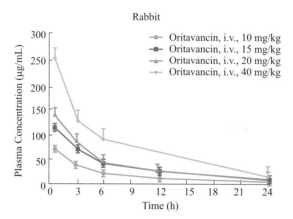

Figure C    *In Vivo* Plasma Concentration-Time Profiles of Oritavancin in Rabbits after Single Intravenous Dose of Oritavancin[12]

Table 9    *In Vivo* Pharmacokinetic Parameters of Oritavancin in Humans after Single Intravenous Doses[5]

| Dose (mg/kg) | $T_{max}$ (h) | $C_{max}$ (µg/mL) | $T_{1/2}$ (h) | $AUC_{inf}$ (µg·h/mL) | Cl (L/h) | $V_{ss}$ (L) |
|---|---|---|---|---|---|---|
| 0.5 | 0.50 | 5.29 ± 0.46 | 240 ± 29.7 | 101 ± 11.0 | 0.306 ± 0.019 | 78.8 ± 12.4 |
| 1.0 | 0.50 | 11.0 ± 1.19 | 178 ± 55.9 | 179 ± 26.5 | 0.340 ± 0.060 | 53.7 ± 13.7 |
| 2.0 | 0.50 | 25.7 ± 2.57 | 285 ± 45.0 | 448 ± 67.9 | 0.299 ± 0.044 | 66.7 ± 9.56 |
| 3.0 | 0.50 | 37.7 ± 6.11 | 322 ± 58.4 | 650 ± 118 | 0.282 ± 0.066 | 61.4 ± 17.9 |

Mean ± SD.

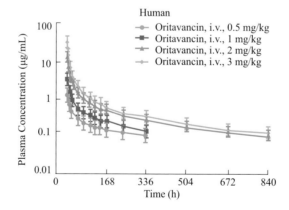

Figure D    *In Vivo* Plasma Concentration-Time Profiles of Oritavancin in Humans after Single Intravenous Dose of Oritavancin (n = 5)[13]

[4]  FDA Database.   http://www.accessdata.fda.gov/drugsatfda_docs/nda/2014/206334Orig1s000MicroR.pdf (accessed Mar 2016).

[5]  EMA Database.   http://www.ema.europa.eu/docs/en_GB/document_library/EPAR_-_Public_assessment_report/human/003785/WC500186347.pdf (accessed Mar 2016).

[12]  Lehoux, D.; Ostiguy, V.; Cadieux, C., et al. *Antimicrob. Agents Chemother.* **2015**, *59*, 6501-6505.

[13]  FDA Database.   http://www.accessdata.fda.gov/drugsatfda_docs/nda/2014/206334Orig1s000PharmR.pdf (accessed Mar 2016).

# Distribution

Table 10    *In Vitro* Plasma Protein Binding of Oritavancin in Humans[4, 14]

| Species | Human | | | Mouse | Rat | Dog | |
|---------|-------|---|---|-------|-----|-----|---|
| Matrix | Plasma | Albumin | Serum | Serum | Plasma | Serum | Serum |
| %Bound | 87.5 | 79 ± 0.2 | 81.9 | 85.3 | >80 | 82.4 | 87.1 |

# Key Findings:

❖ Rats after single intravenous Dose of Oritavancin:[13]
  • The drug was distributed into most tissues with peak levels attained within 1-6 h of intravenous administration.
  • Relatively higher radioactivity levels were observed in liver and intestinal, and moderate levels in the adrenal gland, bone marrow, cecal wall, kidneys, lungs, salivary gland and spleen, and low or background levels in brain, eyes and testes.
  • $T_{1/2}$ ranged between 100 to 200 h in the majority of tissues.

# Metabolism

❖ *In vitro* monkey hepatic microsomal metabolism studies did not show any evidence to suggest that oritavancin was metabolized by the CYP system.    There was no metabolite peak observed and no depletion of oritavancin over time.[5]

❖ Comparison of plasma concentrations of oritavancin to plasma radio-equivalent concentrations of [$^{14}$C]oritavancin suggested that there was no circulating metabolite of oritavancin in the plasma.    Furthermore, analysis of plasma and bile from mice, rats and dogs administered single intravenous doses of [$^{14}$C]oritavancin did not indicate the presence of any metabolite of oritavancin.[5]

# Excretion

❖ In rats and dogs, oritavancin was excreted unchanged primarily *via* the bile into the feces.    After 14 days of administration to rats, approximately 50% of the dose was eliminated in the feces, approximately 5% in the urine and the remaining dose was still in the carcass, reflective of the long tissue retention time.[5]

❖ Dogs showed a similar pattern of excretion.    However, by 14 days approximately 10% of the dose was recovered in feces, 6% in the urine and the remaining dose was still in the carcass.    The long retention time in animals was consistent with observations in humans where <5% of the administered dose was recovered in urine and feces after 14 days of dose administration.[5]

❖ In contrast to animals in which feces was the primary route of excretion, in humans the majority of recovered dose was in urine (~5%) and the rest in feces (<1%).[4]

# Drug-Drug Interaction

## CYP Enzymes-Based DDI[5]

❖ Using midazolam (5 μM), there was 39% inhibition of CYP3A-mediated metabolism.
❖ Using diclofenac (2.5 μM), there was <10% inhibition of CYP2C9-mediated metabolism.
❖ Conversion of phenacetin (12.5 μM) to acetaminophen by CYP1A2 was slightly inhibited (21%).
❖ Modelling the data to conventional enzyme inhibition relationships, the form-selective biotransformation for CYP2D6 (1′-hydroxylation of bufuralol) was non-competitively inhibited by oritavancin yielding a $K_i$ of 12.6 ± 1.3′-hydroxylation.
❖ The order of potential inhibition by oritavancin of the metabolism of co-administered drugs by the cytochrome P450 isoforms was determined to be CYP2D6 > CYP3A4 > CYP1A2 > CYP2C9.

[4]  FDA Database.    http://www.accessdata.fda.gov/drugsatfda_docs/nda/2014/206334Orig1s000MicroR.pdf (accessed Mar 2016).
[5]  EMA Database.    http://www.ema.europa.eu/docs/en_GB/document_library/EPAR_-_Public_assessment_report/human/003785/WC500186347.pdf (accessed Mar 2016).
[13]  FDA Database.    http://www.accessdata.fda.gov/drugsatfda_docs/nda/2014/206334Orig1s000PharmR.pdf (accessed Mar 2016).
[14]  Arhin, F. F.; Belley, A.; Mckay, G., et al. *Antimicrob. Agents Chemother.* **2010**, *54*, 3481-3483.

❖ When HLMs were pre-incubated with oritavancin (2.5 to 50 µM), the known substrates for CYP2D6 (dextromethorphan) and 3A4 (testosterone), CYP2D6 and CYP3A4 were inhibited in a concentration-dependent manner.

❖ In human hepatocytes, oritavancin at concentrations ≤50 µM did not induce CYP1A2, CYP2A6, CYP2C9, CYP2C19 or CYP2D6 activities. At 50 µM oritavancin slightly increased CYP2E1 activity. At 2.5 µM oritavancin slightly increased CYP3A4 activity but at higher concentrations inhibited CYP3A4 activity.

Table 11   *In Vitro* Evaluation of Oritavancin as an Inhibitor and Inducer of Enzymes[5]

| Oritavancin as an Inhibitor | | | | Oritavancin as an Inducer | | | |
|---|---|---|---|---|---|---|---|
| CYP Isoform | IC$_{50}$ (µM) | C$_{max}$$^a$/IC$_{50}$ -200 mg Daily | C$_{max}$$^b$/IC$_{50}$ -1200 mg Single Dose | CYP Isoform | % of Vehicle Control | | |
| | | | | | 2.5 µM | 25 µM | 50 µM |
| CYP1A2 | 40.5 | 0.34 | 1.71 | CYP1A2 | - | - | - |
| CYP2B6 | 31.0 | 0.44 | 2.24 | CYP2A6 | - | - | - |
| CYP2C9 | 16.7 | 0.82 | 4.15 | CYP2C9 | - | - | - |
| CYP2C19 | 40.3 | 0.34 | 1.72 | CYP2C19 | - | - | - |
| CYP2D6 | 18.5 | 0.74 | 3.75 | CYP2D6 | - | - | - |
| CYP3A | 16.1 | 0.85 | 4.30 | CYP2E1 | - | 111 | 150$^c$ |
| | | | | CYP3A4 | 117 | - | - |

$^a$ Oritavancin mean ± SD C$_{max}$ of 27.3 ± 12.1 µg/mL (equivalent to 13.7 µM) based on population PK analysis of 200 mg once daily dosing.   $^b$ Oritavancin mean ± SD C$_{max}$ of 138 ± 31.7 µg/mL (equivalent to 69.3 µM) based on population PK analysis of single 1200 mg dosing.   $^c$ Statistically significant.

**Transporter-Based DDI**

❖ Neither a substrate or an inhibitor of the efflux transporter P-glycoprotein (P-gp), nor transporter protein studies with oritavancin were reported.[5]

# 6   Non-Clinical Toxicology

## Summary

### Single-Dose Toxicity

❖ Single-dose toxicity studies by intravenous administrations in mice and rats: MNLDs were 40 mg/kg both in mice and rats, but accompanying with histamine-like infusion reactions.

### Repeated-Dose Toxicity

❖ Repeated-dose toxicity studies by the intravenous route for up to 13 weeks in rats and dogs:
- In view of the 13-week studies, both rats and dogs showed remarkably similar pathology with the major finding of histiocytosis in the kidneys, liver, lymph nodes, spleen, thymus, bone marrow, and injection site, along with significant reductions in RBC number (and associated parameters).
- The NOAEL in dogs was 5 mg/kg/day, approximately 3-fold exposure of MRHD. NOAEL in rats was not established.

### Safety Pharmacology

❖ Studies of core battery plus renal and GI performance:
- No significant change was tested article-related in behavior, autonomic and motor in rats at 50 mg/kg.
- Ion channel current IC$_{50}$s ranged from 0.5 µM for Na$^+$ channel to 22 µM for K$^+$ channel, suggesting weak potential for QT prolongation but higher possibility to induce prolongation of the QRS or PR interval. However, *in vivo* studies exhibited significant histaminic changes without any ECG irregularity.
- Renal effects were considered mild, based on the slight decrease of creatinine and sodium clearance in the *in vivo* rat studies.
- No change in GI transit time was noted in mice after 50 mg/kg i.v. of oritavancin.

### Genotoxicity

❖ There was no gene mutation or chromosomal damage observed in any of the genotoxicity studies conducted with oritavancin.

---

[5] EMA Database.  http://www.ema.europa.eu/docs/en_GB/document_library/EPAR_-_Public_assessment_report/human/003785/WC500186347.pdf (accessed Mar 2016).

Reproductive and Developmental Toxicity

❖ Fertility and early embryonic development in rats:
  • There was no treatment-related effect on mating/fertility up to 30 mg/kg/day in either sex.
❖ Embryo-fetal development in rats and rabbits:
  • Oritavancin diphosphate was not embryotoxic and teratogenic when administered to pregnant rats and rabbits up to 30 or 15 mg/kg/day during the period of organogenesis.
❖ Pre- and postnatal development in rats:
  • Maternal toxicity was evident at 30 mg/kg, e.g., reduced body weight gains, as reductions in offspring ($F_1$) birth weight associated.
❖ Juvenile toxicity studies in rats and dogs:
  • Similar to that in adult animals, juvenile toxicity included: Increased body weight, liver and spleen weights, and decreased red blood cell count and hematocrit in rats; Increased body weight in dogs.

Carcinogenicity

❖ Carcinogenicity study was not performed.   In view of the results of the genotoxicity studies conducted and the proposed short duration of clinical treatment with oritavancin, carcinogenicity studies were not required in compliance with ICH guidelines.

# Single-Dose Toxicity

Table 12   Single-Dose Toxicity Studies of Oritavancin Diphosphate by i.v. Administrations[4, 13]

| Species | Dose (mg/kg) | MNLD (mg/kg) | Finding |
|---|---|---|---|
| SD rat | 40, 80, 120 | 40 | Mortality at MD and HD.<br>Clinical signs, including ↓ activity, hunched posture, severely swollen, dark-blue tongues, intermittent tremors, red soiling of perineal and muzzle areas, ataxia, red lacrimation and/or ↓ feces. |
| | Phase A: 0ª, 60;<br>Phase B: 0ª, 28, 60 | NA | In Phase A, minimal ↓ erythrocyte parameters and minimal ↑ AST/ALT on Day 2. ↑ Reticulocytes on Day 8, indicative of a regenerative response.<br>In Phase B, death of undetermined reasons at HD.   Clinical findings consisted of red skin discoloration of the tail for all lots, and rigid, black and/or purple discoloration of the tail, clear and/or red discharge from the injection site, and swelling of the nose/muzzle.<br>Adverse microscopic findings locally at the infusion site at HD. |
| Mouse | 5, 15, 20 | NA | 50 mg/kg: Led reduction in writing and a transient reduction of 1.1 °C in body temperature. |

NA: Not applicable.   ª Vehicle was 5% Dextrose, vehicle and test were administered to all groups as a single 1h intravenous infusion into the tail vein.

# Repeated-Dose Toxicity

Table 13   Repeated-Dose Toxicity Studies of Oritavancin Diphosphate by i.v. Administrations[4]

| Species | Duration (Week) | Dose (mg/kg/day) | NOAEL (mg/kg/day) | Finding |
|---|---|---|---|---|
| Rat | 2 | 1, 5, 15 | 1 | ↓ RBC, BW, ↑ AST/ALT.   Eosinophilic granules in renal cortical epithelium, Kupffer cells, and granules in macrophages of spleen, thymus and LN. |
| | 2 | 1, 5, 15 | 5 | ↓ RBC, WBC, ↑ AST/ALT.   Eosinophilic granules in Kupffer cells, LN, bone marrow at all doses. |
| | 2ª | 5, 30, 60 | 30 | ↓ BW, food consumption, ↑ AST/ALT, liver weight, hepatocellular necrosis and inflammation.   Heart: myocardial degeneration and inflammation; gross changes in spleen, kidney, LN. |
| | 2 | 1, 5, 15 | 5 | ↓ RBC, ↑ AST/ALT, Kupffer cell degeneration, PAS+ material in hepatocytes/Kupffer cells and spleen, lymph nodes, marrow. |
| | 4 | 5, 10, 15, 30, 40 | 5 | ↓ BW, ↓ RBC, ↑ AST/ALT/ALP, BUN; Liver, spleen, thymus, LN: eosinophilic granules in macrophages. |

[4]  FDA Database.   http://www.accessdata.fda.gov/drugsatfda_docs/nda/2014/206334Orig1s000MicroR.pdf (accessed Mar 2016).
[13]  FDA Database.   http://www.accessdata.fda.gov/drugsatfda_docs/nda/2014/206334Orig1s000PharmR.pdf (accessed Mar 2016).

*Continued*

| Species | Duration (Week) | Dose (mg/kg/day) | NOAEL (mg/kg/day) | Finding |
|---------|-----------------|------------------|-------------------|---------|
| Rat | 4[b] | 5, 10, 15 | 5 | ↑ AST/ALT, periportal liver degeneration, injection site inflammation and fibrosis, lymphoid hyperplasia in lymph nodes, spleen (also congestion). |
| | 13 | 5, 15, 45/30 | NA | Deaths in 15 C, 30 L, 25 M, and 39 H; Signs = swellings, masses, paralysis, limp; ↓ BW, food consumption, ↑ AST/ALT/ALP; Hepatic necrosis, inflammation, accumulation of histiocytes with eosinophilic granules in liver, spleen, lymph nodes, thymus, lung catheter site, and ovaries; masses at injection site. |
| Dog | 2 | 1, 5, 15 | 5 | ↑ Histamine, face reddened, loose stools, emesis; ↑ BUN, AST/ALT, eosinophilic granules in hepatocytes, renal cortical cells and macrophages. |
| | 2[a] | 5, 30, 60 | 30 | ↓ BW, food consumption; ↑ AST/ALT, hepatocellular degeneration and necrosis, renal tubular degeneration and mineralization, macrophages with cytoplasmic acidophilic granules near sinusoid spaces. |
| | 4 | 5, 10, 30 | 5 | Signs: redness, welts, emesis, stool changes, ↑ APTT, BUN, AST/ALT eosinophilic granules in liver, kidneys, lymph nodes, spleen. |
| | 13 | 5, 15, 45 | 5 | Emesis, stool changes; ↓ BW; ↑ AST/ALT, BUN, APTT, ↑ organ weight of liver, spleen, kidneys, eosinophilic histiocytes in sinusoids of liver, lymph nodes, alveoli, submucosa of kidney and injection site. |

$AUC_{0-t}$ exposure levels for oritavancin at the NOAELs were ranged from 2.4 to 11.9 folds higher than human exposure levels and sufficiently high to qualify impurities in the drug substance.    [a] 1 h infusion instead of 30 min.    [b] Spiked with new impurities.

## Safety Pharmacology

Table 14    Safety Pharmacology Studies of Oritavancin Diphosphate by i.v. Administrations[4]

| Study | System | Dose (mg/kg) | Finding |
|-------|--------|--------------|---------|
| Neurological effect | Mouse | up to 50 | Slight ↑ hexobarbital sleep time, ↓ body temperature. No change in activity was noted. |
| Cardiovascular effect | Human myocyte | NA | $IC_{50}$: 0.5 μM (1.0 μg/mL) for the $Na^+$ channel; 22 μM (43 μg/mL) for the $K^+$ channel. |
| | Conscious dog | 5, 10, 25, i.v. for 1 h | No change in ECG. Significant histaminic responses at HD, including ↑ BP and HR. |
| Renal effect | Female rat | up to 50 | A slight decrease in creatinine and sodium clearance were noted at the highest dose tested. |
| Gastrointestinal effect | Mouse | up to 50 | No change in gastrointestinal transit time was noted in mice after dose. |

NA: Not applicable.

## Genotoxicity

### Key Finding:

❖ *In vitro* (Ames, mouse lymphoma, chromosomal aberrations) and *in vivo* (mouse micronucleus) genetic toxicity testing had been adequately conducted.    Results of all the studies were negative.[4]

❖ No mutagenicity or clastogenicity was observed in studies conducted with oritavancin spiked with 4.7% alkylated Factor A.    Therefore, neither oritavancin nor the impurities in the drug substance was shown to be genotoxic.[13]

Table 15    Genotoxicity Studies of Oritavancin Diphosphate[5]

| Specie | Gender | Dose (mg/kg) | Finding |
|--------|--------|--------------|---------|
| Rat | Male | Up to 30, single dose for ≥4 weeks | Oritavancin did not affect the fertility or reproductive performance. |
| | Female | Up to 30, single dose for ≥2 weeks | Oritavancin did not affect the fertility or reproductive performance. |

Higher doses were not evaluated in nonclinical fertility studies.

[4]  FDA Database.   http://www.accessdata.fda.gov/drugsatfda_docs/nda/2014/206334Orig1s000MicroR.pdf (accessed Mar 2016).

[5]  EMA Database.   http://www.ema.europa.eu/docs/en_GB/document_library/EPAR_-_Public_assessment_report/human/003785/WC500186347.pdf (accessed Mar 2016).

[13]  FDA Database.   http://www.accessdata.fda.gov/drugsatfda_docs/nda/2014/206334Orig1s000PharmR.pdf (accessed Mar 2016).

# Reproductive and Developmental Toxicity

Table 16    Reproductive and Developmental Toxicology Studies of Oritavancin Diphosphate[4, 13]

| Study | Species | Dose (mg/kg/day) | NOAEL | | Finding |
| | | | Dose (mg/kg/day) | AUC (μg·h/mL) | |
| --- | --- | --- | --- | --- | --- |
| Fertility and early embryonic development | Rat/Male | 0, 5, 15, 30, i.v. infusion over 1 h | 30 | 407 | ↓ Body weight and food consumption, red colored urine, ↑ urinary volume, and changes in serum or urinary clinical chemistry parameters at all dose levels.<br>Pale liver at 15 and 30 mg/kg/day and enlarged spleen at 30 mg/kg/day.<br>There were also test item-related microscopic lesions of the kidney at 15 and 30 mg/kg/day comprising eosinophilic inclusions and cell degeneration in the cortical tubular epithelium, nuclear pyknosis/tubular basophilia of the renal medulla, as well as cellular cast(s) and/or multifocal tubular dilatation secondary to the corticotubular changes. |
| | Rat/Female | 0, 5, 15, 30, i.v. infusion over 1h | 30 | 343 | ↓ Body weight gain in the 30 mg/kg/day group during gestation Days 0-8 only, followed by a recovery.    ↓ Food consumption in a dose-related manner in the mid and high dose groups during the gestation period only.<br>The percentage of post-implantation loss and the mean live litter size were comparable in all groups.    Pre-implantation loss was greater in the low- and mid-dose groups than in the control or high-dose groups.<br>The mean ovarian weights were slightly higher in all treated groups than in the control group.<br>There was no adverse effect of treatment in any group on mating performance, gonadal function, fertility or early gestation. |
| Embryo-fetal development | Rat | 0, 5, 15, 30 | 30 | 522 | No embryo-fetal developmental effect was observed in rats administered ≤30 mg/kg oritavancin on GD 6 to 17. |
| | Rabbit | 0, 1, 5, 15 | 15 | NA | No embryo-fetal developmental effect was observed in rabbits administered ≤15 mg/kg oritavancin on GD 7 to 19. |
| Pre- and post-natal development | Rat | 0, 5, 15, 30 | 30 | NA | $F_0$ maternal body weight and food consumption were decreased after oritavancin administration in the 30 mg/kg group during the postnatal period.    There was no adverse effect on pregnancy, parturition or lactation.<br>Offspring ($F_1$) of animals in the 30 mg/kg dose group had lower body weights during the study intervals although not during the post-weaning period (PND 8 to 57), but had normal physical development.    $F_1$ neuro-behavioral and reproductive functions were not affected by oritavancin administration at any dose. |
| Juvenile toxicity | Rat | Up to 45/30 | 5 | NA | ≥15 mg/kg resulted in increased body weight, liver and spleen weights and decreased red blood cell count and haematocrit. Mortalities occurred in the 45/30 mg/kg/day dose group. |
| | Dog | 45 | 5 | NA | At doses of 15 and 45 mg/kg; associated with clinical observations, decreased the mean body weights and body weight gains. Macroscopic and microscopic findings were associated with the injection sites, liver, and lymph nodes in the 45 mg/kg dose group.<br>Juvenile dogs administered i.v. doses of 45 mg/kg for 30 days, showed vacuoles within hepatocyte cytoplasm that was suggestive of diffuse glycogen accumulation. |

Oritavancin did not affect fertility in the rats, fetal development in the rats and rabbits, or pre-and postnatal development in rats.    Given a human plasma AUC after a 200 mg dose of 139 μg·h/mL, and plasma AUCs in the rat of 340 to 520 μg·h/mL, a margin of safety of approximately 2.4 to 3.7 was observed.    Vehicle: 5% Dextrose injection.    NA: Not applicable.

[4]  FDA Database.    http://www.accessdata.fda.gov/drugsatfda_docs/nda/2014/206334Orig1s000MicroR.pdf (accessed Mar 2016).
[13]  FDA Database.    http://www.accessdata.fda.gov/drugsatfda_docs/nda/2014/206334Orig1s000PharmR.pdf (accessed Mar 2016).

# CHAPTER

## 21

## Phenothrin (JAN, r-INN)

# Phenothrin (JAN, r-INN)

## (Sumithrin®)

Research code: KC-1001

## 1 General Information

- ❖ Phenothrin, a synthetic type-I non-cyano pyrethroid insecticide, which was first approved in Mar 2014 by PMDA of Japan.

- ❖ Phenothrin was discovered by Sumitomo, developed and marketed by Kracie.

- ❖ Phenothrin showed an insecticidal effect by blocking the repetitive depolarization or nerve conduction.

- ❖ Phenothrin is indicated for the treatment of keratinocytes type scabies and nail scabies.

- ❖ Available as lotion, containing 5% of phenothrin and the recommended starting dose is 30 g of the lotion once weekly to the skin of neck below and plantar.

- ❖ The sale of Sumithrin® was not available up to Mar 2016.

### Key Approvals around the World[*]

|  | Japan (PMDA) |
| --- | --- |
| First approval date | 03/24/2014 |
| Application or approval No. | 22600AMX00559000 |
| Brand name | Sumithrin® |
| Indication | Keratinocytes type scabies/Nail scabies |
| Authorisation holder | Kracie |

[*] Till Mar 2016, it has not been approved by FDA (US), EMA (EU) and CFDA (China).

## Active Ingredient

| Molecular formula: | $C_{23}H_{26}O_3$ |
| Molecular weight: | 350.45 |
| CAS No.: | 26002-80-2 (Phenothrin) |
| Chemical name: | 3-Phenoxybenzyl (1$RS$,3$RS$;1$RS$,3$SR$)-2,2-dimethyl-3-(2-methylprop-1-enyl) cyclopropanecarboxylate |

*Parameters of Lipinski's "Rule of 5"*

| MW | $H_D$ | $H_A$ | FRB[a] | PSA[a] | cLogP[a] |
| --- | --- | --- | --- | --- | --- |
| 350.45 | 0 | 3 | 7 | 35.5Å$^2$ | 7.68 ± 0.44 |

[a] Calculated by ACD/Labs software V11.02.

## Drug Product[*]

| Dosage route: | Topical |
| Strength: | 5% (Phenothrin) |
| Dosage form: | Lotion |

*Inactive ingredient*: Isopropyl myristate, liquid paraffin, glycerin, polyoxyethylene cetyl ether, glyceryl monostearate, dibutylhydroxytoluene, methyl *p*-benzoic acid, carboxy vinyl polymer, sodium hydroxide and purified water.

*Recommended dose*: Phenothrin lotion is smeared to the topical skin.

Apply 30 g of the lotion once weekly to the skin of neck below and plantar, then remove it after more than 12 h.

[*] Sourced from Japan PMDA drug label information

## 2   Key Patents Information

### Summary

❖  Sumithrin® (Phenothrin) was approved by PMDA of Japan on Mar 24, 2014.

❖  Phenothrin was originally discovered by Sumitomo and then developed by Kracie, and its compound patent application was filed by Sumitomo in 1969.

❖  The compound patent expired in 1989 which had only been granted in Great Britain.

Table 1   Apremilast's Compound Patent Protection in Drug-Mainstream Country

| Country | Publication/Patent NO. | Application Date | Granted Date | Estimated Expiry Date |
|---------|------------------------|------------------|--------------|-----------------------|
| WO | NA | / | / | / |
| US | NA | / | / | / |
| EP | GB1243858A | 05/29/1969 | 08/25/1971 | 05/29/1989 |
| JP | NA | / | / | / |
| CN | NA | / | / | / |

The data was updated until Jan 2016.

## 3   Chemistry

### Route 1:   Original Discovery Route

*Synthetic Route*:   Commercially available chrysanthemic acid **1** was converted to the corresponding acyl chloride **2** in 99% yield, which was further condensed with 3-phenoxyphenyl methanol **3** in pyridine to provide phenothrin in 96% yield and the overall yield of 95% from **1**.[1-4]

### Route 2

[1]  Ma, Z.; Wang, G.; Han, G. *J. hyg. Res.* **2001**, *30*, 367-368.

[2]  Itaya, N.; Kamoshita, K.; Kitamura, S., et al. GB1243858A, **1971**.

[3]  Coelho, P. S.; Brustad, E. M.; Arnold, F. H., et al. WO2014058744A2, **2014**.

[4]  Coelho, P. S.; Brustad, E. M.; Arnold, F. H., et al. US8993262B2, **2015**.

*Synthetic Route*: Adhering the identical activation manner to starting material chrysanthemic acid **1** as previous routes, the target phenothrin was synthesized *via* a step-wise procedure from acyl chloride **2** that was distinguished from the second step in route **1**. Esterification of acyl chloride in pyridine provided **4** in 96% yield over two steps from chrysanthemic acid **1**. Diphenyl ether could be prepared by Ullmann reaction in alkaline medium at an elevated temperature in the presence of heavy metal (copper). Thus, under the standard conditions, phenothrin was generated in 87% yield by heating aryl bromide **4** with an alkali phenolate. The overall yield was 84%.[5]

## Route 3

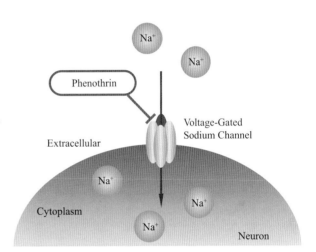

1          2          Phenothrin

*Synthetic Route*: A neat addition of vinyl 2,2-dimethyl-3-(2-methyl-1-propenyl) cyclopropanecarboxylate **1** and 3-phenoxy-benzyl alcohol **2** in a schlenk-type tube in the presence of catalytic triisopropoxylanthanum (III) at 80 °C provided phenothrin in 97% GC yield.[6]

## 4   Pharmacology

### Summary

#### Mechanism of Action

❖ Phenothrin, a synthetic type-I non-cyano pyrethroid insecticide, killed insects by disrupting the transmission of nerve impulses along axons and the elongated parts of nerve cells.

❖ Phenothrin enhanced the permeability of $Na^+$ by delaying the obstruction, thereby causing a depolarization after potential and repeat excitement. Thereafter, phenothrin showed an insecticidal effect by blocking the repetitive depolarization or nerve conduction.

#### *In Vitro* Efficacy

❖ The $LD_{50}$ of farinae and tyrophagus with Phenothrin:
  • Farinae: $LD_{50} <0.01$ μg/cm$^2$.
  • Tyrophagus: $LD_{50} = 0.46$ μg/cm$^2$.
❖ Effects of phenothrin on killing ticks and tyrophagus at 1-4 weeks:
  • Ticks:
    ◆ 0.1% concentration: Inhibition = 90.2%-100%.
    ◆ 0.01% concentration: Inhibition = 72.4%-97.2%.
  • Tyrophagus: 0.001% concentration: Inhibition = 98.8%-99.9%.
❖ The effect of phenothrin on insecticidal:
  • Musca domestica, micro spot method: $LD_{50} = 0.022$-0.056 μg/fly.
  • Musca domestica, turntable method: $LC_{50} = 20.2$-34.5 mg/100 mL.
  • Culex pipiens pallens, micro spot method: $LD_{50} = 0.0075$ μg/insect.
  • Blattella germanica, micro spot method: $LD_{50} = 0.89$ μg/insect.
  • Blattella germanica, direct spray method: $LC_{50} = 66$ mg/100 mL.

[5]  Gergely, H.; Dezso, K.; Endre, P. GB2169293A, **1986**.
[6]  Oda Y.; Yako M. US6531626B1, **2003**.

## *In Vitro* Efficacy

Table 2    Insecticidal Effects of Phenothrin on Fariniae and Tyrophagus[7]

| Compound | $LD_{50}$ (µg/cm$^2$) | |
| --- | --- | --- |
| | Farinae | Tyrophagus |
| Phenothrin | <0.01 | 0.46 |
| Permethrin | 0.045 | 1.9 |
| Ivermectin | <0.01 | >100 |

$LD_{50}$: Lethal dose, 50%.    The effect of phenothrin, permethrin and ivermectin were measured by dry film method.    The tests were repeated three times.

Table 3    The Growth Inhibitory Effect of Phenothrin on Killing Ticks and Tyrophagus[7]

| Drug | Conc. (%) | Inhibition of Ticks (%) | | | | Inhibition of Tyrophagus (%) | | | |
| --- | --- | --- | --- | --- | --- | --- | --- | --- | --- |
| | | 1 Week | 2 Weeks | 3 Weeks | 4 Weeks | 1 Week | 2 Weeks | 3 Weeks | 4 Weeks |
| Phenothrin | 1 | 99.7 | 100 | 100 | 100 | 100 | 100 | 100 | 100 |
| | 0.1 | 90.2 | 96.8 | 99.6 | 100 | 100 | 100 | 100 | 100 |
| | 0.01 | 72.4 | 87.1 | 93.7 | 97.2 | 100 | 100 | 100 | 100 |
| | 0.001 | 30.7 | 48.6 | 59.9 | 73.4 | 98.8 | 99.7 | 99.9 | 99.8 |
| Permethrin | 1 | 98.9 | 99.9 | 100 | 100 | 97.9 | 100 | 100 | 100 |
| | 0.1 | 83.4 | 96.7 | 99.6 | 99.7 | 96.3 | 100 | 100 | 100 |
| | 0.01 | 57.7 | 77.1 | 94.4 | 98.3 | 93.3 | 100 | 99.9 | 99.9 |
| | 0.001 | 39.9 | 47.2 | 66.6 | 79.4 | 66.3 | 68.5 | 84.6 | 65.3 |
| Ivermectin | 1 | 96.6 | 99.4 | 100 | 100 | 100 | 100 | 100 | 100 |
| | 0.1 | 95.9 | 99.5 | 99.9 | 100 | 100 | 100 | 100 | 100 |
| | 0.01 | 94.6 | 97.9 | 99.6 | 99.9 | 99.2 | 100 | 100 | 100 |
| | 0.001 | 85.1 | 94.8 | 97.3 | 99.3 | 94.2 | 99.8 | 100 | 100 |

The long-term growth inhibition of phenothrin, permethrin and ivermectin on ticks and tyrophagus were examined by incorporation method.    After growth with drugs for 1, 2, 3 and 4 weeks, observed the number of surviving ticks or tyrophagus.    Each was repeated twice or more times.

Table 4    Effects of Phenothrin on Insecticidal[7]

| Species | Test | Breed | Insecticidal Effect (Relative Activities)[a] | | |
| --- | --- | --- | --- | --- | --- |
| | | | Phenothrin | Resmethrin | Pyrethrin |
| Musca domestica | Micro spot method ($LD_{50}$ µg/fly) | SK | 0.022 (10.1) | 0.020 (11.2) | 0.223 (1.0) |
| | | CSMA | 0.022 (16.8) | 0.015 (24.6) | 0.370 (1.0) |
| | | Lab-em-7-em | 0.050 (20.0) | 0.028 (35.7) | 1.0 (1.0) |
| | | NAIDM | 0.056 (15.9) | 0.034 (26.2) | 0.89 (1.0) |
| Musca domestica | Turntable method ($LC_{50}$ mg/100 mL) | Lab-em-7-em | 34.5 (8.7) | 22.0 (13.6) | 300 (1.0) |
| | | NAIDM | 20.2 (8.5) | 16.5 (10.4) | 172 (1.0) |
| Culex pipiens pallens | Micro spot method ($LD_{50}$ µg/insect) | NA | 0.0075 (2.9) | 0.0125 (1.8) | 0.022 (1.0) |
| Blattella germanica | Micro spot method ($LD_{50}$ µg/insect) | NA | 0.89 (1.3) | 0.80 (1.4) | 1.15 (1.0) |
| | Direct spray method ($LC_{50}$ mg/100 mL) | NA | 66 (1.3) | 80 (1.1) | 88 (1.0) |

$LD_{50}$: Lethal dose, 50%.    $LC_{50}$: Lethal concentration 50.    [a] Relative insecticidal effect of pyrethrins was 1.0, the date showed in brackets.

[7]  Japan Pharmaceuticals and Medical Devices Agency (PMDA) Database.    http://www.pmda.go.jp/drugs/2014/P201400043/index.html (accessed Mar 2016).

# 5 ADME & Drug-Drug Interaction

## Summary

### Absorption of Phenothrin

❖ Phenothrin was absorbed slowly with the $T_{max}$ occurring 4 to 48 h in rats and humans after topical administrations.

❖ The absorption rates of phenothrin in different formulations in rats were different after topical administration: Emulsion (8.4%-16.8%), powder (3.4%-6.6%) and lotion (9.5%-12.5%).

### Distribution of Phenothrin

❖ *Cis*-phenothrin, *trans*-phenothrin (1-100 ng/mL) and 3-phenoxybenzoic acid (5-5000 ng/mL) exhibited high plasma protein binding in humans.

❖ Male SD rats after single topical administration:
  • The highest concentration tissue was the administrated skin, and the radioactivity in other tissues was very low. So phenothrin had a limited distribution in tissues after topical administration.

### Metabolism of Phenothrin

❖ Phenothrin was metabolized primarily in the liver.

❖ The primary metabolic pathways of phenothrin involved esterification reaction and hydrolysis reaction.

❖ 3-Phenoxybenzoic acid was the predominant metabolite.

### Excretion of Phenthrin

❖ *Cis*-phenothrin was predominantly excreted in feces, but *trans*-phenothrin was predominantly excreted in urine in rats, after oral administration.

### Drug-Drug Interaction

❖ *Cis*-phenothrin and *trans*-phenothrin were less likely to cause inhibition of any of the CYP enzymes evaluated (CYP1A2, 2A6, 2B6, 2C8, 2C9, 2C19, 2D6, 2E1 or 3A4) at concentrations of 0.001-0.3 μM. Metabolite 3-phenoxybenzoic acid did not inhibit CYPs at 0.1-30 μM.

❖ *Cis*-phenothrin, *trans*-phenothrin and metabolite 3-phenoxybenzoic acid did not induce CYP1A2, 2B6 or 3A4 neither in enzyme activities nor mRNA level.

# Absorption

Table 5   *In Vivo* Pharmacokinetic Parameters of Phenothrin in Rats and Rabbits after Single Topical and Oral Dose of Phenothrin[7]

| Species | Route | Dose (mg/kg) | Formulation | Analyte | Male $T_{max}$ (h) | Male $C_{max}$ (ng/mL) | Male $AUC_{0-72}$ (ng·h/mL) | Female $T_{max}$ (h) | Female $C_{max}$ (ng/mL) | Female $AUC_{0-72}$ (ng·h/mL) |
|---|---|---|---|---|---|---|---|---|---|---|
| SD Rat | Topical | 50 | Emulsion | *Cis*-phenothrin | 4 | 0.830 | 19.4 | 8 | 1.53 | 39.9 |
| | | | | *Trans*-phenothrin | 4 | 0.796 | 7.91 | 4 | 2.18 | 48.0 |
| | | | | 3-Phenoxybenzoic acid | 4 | 113 | 3360 | 8 | 143 | 4790 |
| | | | | 3-(4'-hydroxy) Phenoxybenzoic acid | 12 | 3.04 | 104 | 8 | 9.98 | 355 |
| | Topical | 100 | Emulsion | *Cis*-phenothrin | 12 | 0.759 | 27.5 | 12 | 2.26 | 68.9 |
| | | | | *Trans*-phenothrin | 8 | 0.726 | 18.2 | 12 | 2.73 | 74.4 |
| | | | | 3-Phenoxybenzoic acid | 8 | 143 | 3790 | 4 | 266 | 7960 |
| | | | | 3-(4'-hydroxy) Phenoxybenzoic acid | 8 | 1.97 | 92.5 | 12 | 7.31 | 279 |
| | Topical | 200 | Emulsion | *Cis*-phenothrin | 48 | 2.24 | 115 | 12 | 4.12 | 154 |
| | | | | *Trans*-phenothrin | 48 | 2.04 | 89.4 | 12 | 5.63 | 176 |
| | | | | 3-Phenoxybenzoic acid | 4 | 270 | 7020 | 4 | 385 | 13500 |
| | | | | 3-(4'-hydroxy) Phenoxybenzoic acid | 4 | 3.96 | 105 | 8 | 13.3 | 459 |
| SD Rat | p.o. | 50 | Suspension | *Cis*-phenothrin | 8 | 182 | 2130 | 8 | 166 | 1460 |
| | | | | *Trans*-phenothrin | 8 | 247 | 2710 | 8 | 321 | 2300 |
| | | | | 3-Phenoxybenzoic acid | 12 | 19200 | 268000 | 8 | 19100 | 208000 |
| | | | | 3-(4'-hydroxy) Phenoxybenzoic acid | 8 | 295 | 4780 | 8 | 830 | 10900 |
| | p.o. | 100 | Suspension | *Cis*-phenothrin | 8 | 331 | 3580 | 8 | 279 | 3350 |
| | | | | *Trans*-phenothrin | 8 | 490 | 5010 | 8 | 497 | 4730 |
| | | | | 3-Phenoxybenzoic acid | 8 | 14000 | 189000 | 12 | 18800 | 305000 |
| | | | | 3-(4'-hydroxy) Phenoxybenzoic acid | 8 | 582 | 8290 | 8 | 987 | 16900 |
| | p.o. | 200 | Suspension | *Cis*-phenothrin | 8 | 622 | 9130 | 12 | 435 | 6340 |
| | | | | *Trans*-phenothrin | 4 | 1000 | 11800 | 12 | 677 | 10300 |
| | | | | 3-Phenoxybenzoic acid | 12 | 41200 | 708000 | 12 | 38300 | 678000 |
| | | | | 3-(4'-hydroxy) Phenoxybenzoic acid | 12 | 1920 | 26300 | 12 | 4160 | 60200 |
| | p.o. | 1000 | Suspension | *Cis*-phenothrin | 4 | 1690 | 26000 | 12 | 618 | 10400 |
| | | | | *Trans*-phenothrin | 4 | 3130 | 45200 | 12 | 1290 | 18100 |
| | | | | 3-Phenoxybenzoic acid | 8 | 142000 | 3510000 | 12 | 156000 | 4730000 |
| | | | | 3-(4'-hydroxy) Phenoxybenzoic acid | 4 | 5590 | 107000 | 24 | 19100 | 565000 |
| NZW Rabbit | p.o. | 500 | 0.5% MC | Phenothrin | NA | NA | NA | 3 | 256 | 4877 |
| | | | | 3-Phenoxybenzoic acid | NA | NA | NA | 10 | 111000 | 2498000 |
| | p.o. | 500 | Corn oil | Phenothrin | NA | NA | NA | 8 | 352 | 4920 |
| | | | | 3-Phenoxybenzoic acid | NA | NA | NA | 10 | 101000 | 2571000 |

NA: Not available.

[7]  PMDA Database.   http://www.pmda.go.jp/drugs/2014/P201400043/index.html (accessed Mar 2016).

Table 6    *In Vivo* Pharmacokinetic Parameters of Phenothrin in Male SD Rats after Single Dose of Phenothrin[7]

| Formulation | Emulsion | | | | Powder | | | | Lotion | |
|---|---|---|---|---|---|---|---|---|---|---|
| Analyte | [14C]1R-*trans* Phenothrin | | [14C]1R-*cis* Phenothrin | | [14C]1R-*trans* Phenothrin | | [14C]1R-*cis* Phenothrin | | [14C] 1R-*trans* Phenothrin | [14C]1R-*cis* Phenothrin |
| Dose (mg/body) | 0.2 | 2 | 0.2 | 2 | 0.2 | 2 | 0.2 | 2 | 0.18 | 0.18 |
| $K$ (h$^{-1}$) | 0.363 | 0.238 | NA | NA | 0.068 | 0.067 | NA | NA | 0.693 | 0.277 |
| $T_{1/2}$ (h) | 53 | 74 | NA | NA | 24 | 22 | NA | NA | NA | NA |
| Absorption (%) | 10.9 | 8.4 | 16.8 | 16.3 | 3.7 | 3.4 | 6.6 | 4.5 | 12.5 | 9.5 |

NA: Not available.

Table 7    *In Vivo* Pharmacokinetic Parameters of Phenothrin in Humans after Topical Dose of Phenothrin[7]

| Species | Route | Analyte | $T_{max}$ (h) | $C_{max}$ (ng/mL) | $AUC_{0-168}$ (ng·h/mL) |
|---|---|---|---|---|---|
| Healthy human (male) | Topical | *Cis*-phenothrin | $24.0 \pm 0.0$ | $1.58 \pm 1.39$ | $42.4 \pm 44.8$ |
| | Topical | *Trans*-phenothrin | $14.3 \pm 19.0$ | $1.99 \pm 2.47$ | $50.2 \pm 71.0$ |
| | Topical | 3-phenoxybenzoic acid | $24.0 \pm 0.0$ | $161 \pm 51.3$ | $6807 \pm 2181$ |

Mean ± SD for $T_{max}$, $C_{max}$ and $AUC_{0-168}$.

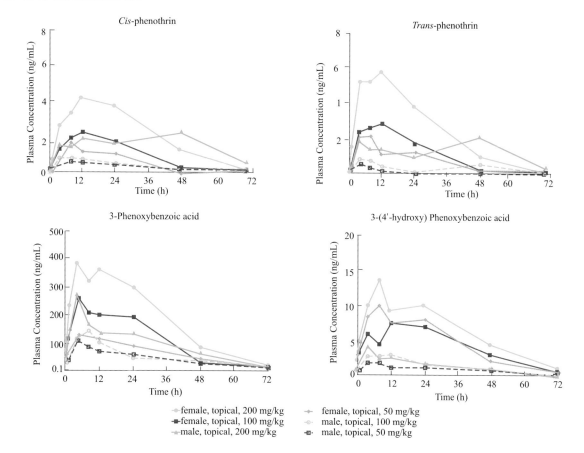

Figure A    *In Vivo* Plasma Concentration-Time Profiles of *cis*-Phenothrin, *trans*-Phenothrin, 3-Phenoxybenzoic and 3-(4'-hydroxy)Phenoxybenzoic Acid in Rats after Single Topical Dose of Phenothrin[7]

[7]    PMDA Database.    http://www.pmda.go.jp/drugs/2014/P201400043/index.html (accessed Mar 2016).

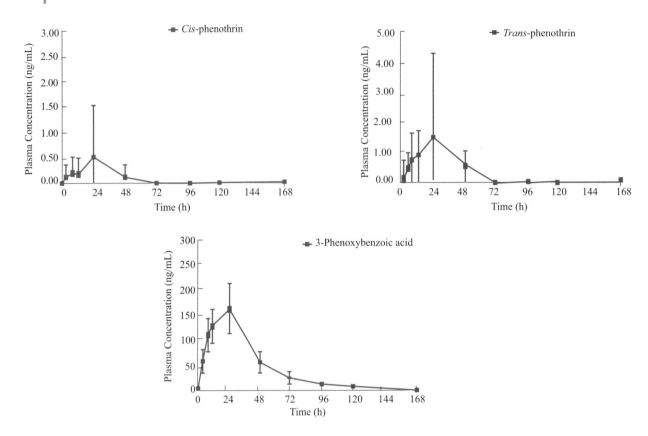

Figure B    *In Vivo* Plasma Concentration-Time Profiles of *cis*-Phenothrin, *trans*-Phenothrin and 3-Phenoxybenzoic in Healthy Humans after Single Topical Dose of Phenothrin[7]

## Distribution

Table 8    *In Vitro* Plasma Protein Binding of [14C]Phenothrin and Metabolite in Humans[7]

| Analyte | Conc. (ng/mL) | %Bound |
|---|---|---|
| *Cis*-[14C]phenothrin | 0.1 | >30.6 |
| | 1 | >93.2 |
| | 10 | 97.4 |
| | 100 | 97.6 |
| *Trans*-[14C]phenothrin | 0.1 | >27.5 |
| | 1 | >93.2 |
| | 10 | 98.6 |
| | 100 | 98.5 |
| [14C]3-Phenoxybenzoic acid | 5 | >98.3 |
| | 50 | >99.8 |
| | 500 | 99.96 |
| | 5000 | 99.94 |

[7]  PMDA Database.   http://www.pmda.go.jp/drugs/2014/P201400043/index.html (accessed Mar 2016).

Table 9    *In Vivo* Tissue Distribution of [$^{14}$C]Phenothrin in Male SD Rats after Single Topical Dose of [$^{14}$C]Phenothrin[7]

| Formulation | Emulsion | | | | Powder | | | |
| --- | --- | --- | --- | --- | --- | --- | --- | --- |
| Analyte | [$^{14}$C]1*R-trans*-Phenothrin | | [$^{14}$C]1*R-cis*-Phenothrin | | [$^{14}$C]1*R-trans*-Phenothrin | | [$^{14}$C]1*R-cis*-Phenothrin | |
| Dose (mg/body) | **0.2** | **2** | **0.2** | **2** | **0.2** | **2** | **0.2** | **2** |
| Tissue | Radioactivity (μg eq./g) | | | | | | | |
| Blood | <0.006 | 0.014 | 0.023 | 0.039 | <0.006 | 0.009 | 0.023 | 0.029 |
| Brain | <0.006 | <0.008 | <0.006 | <0.006 | <0.006 | <0.008 | <0.006 | <0.006 |
| Adrenal gland | <0.006 | <0.023 | <0.006 | <0.014 | <0.006 | <0.008 | <0.006 | <0.006 |
| Cecum | NA | NA | 0.010 | 0.103 | NA | NA | <0.006 | <0.006 |
| Fat | <0.006 | 0.022 | 0.040 | 0.585 | <0.006 | <0.008 | 0.014 | 0.038 |
| Heart | <0.006 | <0.008 | <0.006 | 0.010 | <0.006 | <0.008 | <0.006 | <0.006 |
| Intestine | NA | NA | 0.012 | 0.053 | NA | NA | <0.006 | <0.006 |
| Kidneys | <0.006 | 0.036 | 0.007 | 0.031 | <0.006 | 0.008 | <0.006 | 0.008 |
| Liver | <0.006 | 0.030 | <0.006 | 0.042 | <0.006 | <0.008 | <0.006 | <0.006 |
| Lungs | <0.006 | 0.010 | <0.006 | 0.011 | <0.006 | <0.008 | <0.006 | <0.006 |
| Non treatment skin | 0.036 | 0.034 | 0.029 | 0.584 | 0.006 | 0.052 | <0.006 | 0.033 |
| Treatment skin | 0.460 | 6.69 | 0.582 | 3.94 | 0.047 | 0.388 | 0.113 | 0.429 |
| Stomach | <0.006 | 0.050 | <0.006 | 0.011 | <0.006 | <0.008 | <0.006 | <0.006 |

NA: Not available.

# Metabolism

Table 10    Metabolism of Phenothrin in Rat and Human Plasma, Liver S9 and Skin S9[7]

| Species | Matrix | Isomer | Metabolism Ratio of Phenothrin or Formation Rate of Metabolites (pmol/min/mg protein) | | | | |
| --- | --- | --- | --- | --- | --- | --- | --- |
| | | | Phenothrin | 3-Phenoxybenzyl Alchol | 3-Phenoxy-benzoic Acid | 3-(4'-hydroxy) Phenoxybenzoic Acid | UK-2 |
| Rat | Plasma | *Cis*-phenothrin | 7.35 | 7.29 | NE | NA | - |
| | | *Trans*-phenothrin | 7.58 | 7.53 | NE | NE | - |
| | Liver S9 | *Cis*-phenothrin | 13.4 | 1.25 | 0.417[a] | NE | 6.88 |
| | | *Trans*-phenothrin | 22.0 | 10.7 | 4.92[a] | 0.0417 | 4.50 |
| | Skin S9 | *Cis*-phenothrin | 0.750 | 0.125 | NE | NE | - |
| | | *Trans*-phenothrin | 0.333 | 0.292 | NE | NE | - |
| Human | Plasma | *Cis*-phenothrin | 0.0917 | 0.0167 | NE | NE | - |
| | | *Trans*-phenothrin | 0.0417 | 0.0167 | NE | NE | - |
| | Liver S9 | *Cis*-phenothrin | 5.13 | 1.08 | 1.63[a] | NE | 1.46 |
| | | *Trans*-phenothrin | 17.1 | 6.21 | 9.88[a] | 0.00 | 0.667 |
| | Skin S9 | *Cis*-phenothrin | 0.792 | 0.0833 | NE | NE | - |
| | | *Trans*-Phenothrin | 0.0417 | 0.0417 | NE | NE | - |

NE: Not estimated.    UK-2: Phenothrin·H$_2$O.    [a] Including the UK-1.

[7]  PMDA Database.   http://www.pmda.go.jp/drugs/2014/P201400043/index.html (accessed Mar 2016).

Table 11    Metabolites in SD Rats Urine and Feces after Topical Dose of Phenothrin[7]

| Formulation | Emulsion | | | | Powder | | | |
|---|---|---|---|---|---|---|---|---|
| **Dose** | 2 (mg/body) | | | | 2 (mg/body) | | | |
| **Isomer** | [14C]1R-trans-Phenothrin | | [14C]1R-cis-Phenothrin | | [14C]1R-trans-Phenothrin | | [14C]1R-cis-Phenothrin | |
| **Matrix** | Urine | Feces | Urine | Feces | Urine | Feces | Urine | Feces |
| Metabolite | | | | | | | | |
| 3-Phenoxybenzoicacid free | 0.3 | 0.1 | 0.2 | - | 0.2 | <0.1 | 0.1 | - |
| 3-Phenoxybenzoicacid gly | 0.1 | - | - | - | <0.1 | - | - | - |
| 3-(4'-OH)-PB acid free | 0.2 | 0.3 | 1.2 | - | 0.7 | 0.2 | 0.5 | - |
| 3-(4'-OH)-PB acid sul | 1.6 | | 0.2 | - | 0.5 | - | <0.1 | - |
| *Trans*-phenothrin (*t*-phen) | - | - | - | - | - | <0.1 | - | - |
| *Cis*-phenothrin(c-phen) | - | - | - | 0.1 | - | - | - | <0.1 |
| ω*t*-Acid-c-phenothrin | - | - | - | 0.2 | - | - | - | 0.1 |
| ω*c*-Alc-c-phenothrin | - | - | - | 0.1 | - | - | - | <0.1 |
| ω*t*-Alc-c-phenothrin | - | - | - | <0.1 | - | - | - | <0.1 |
| 4'-OH-ω*c*-alc-c-phenothrin | - | - | - | <0.1 | - | - | - | <0.1 |
| 4'-OH-ω*t*-alc-c-phenothrin | - | - | - | <0.1 | - | - | - | <0.1 |
| 4'-OH-*c*-acid-c-phenothrin | - | - | - | <0.1 | - | - | - | <0.1 |
| 4'-OH-*t*-acid-c-phenothrin | - | - | - | 0.1 | - | - | - | <0.1 |
| ω*t*-Acid-2-OH(*t*)-c-phenothrin | - | - | - | 0.1 | - | - | - | <0.1 |
| 4'-OH-ω*t*-acid-2-OH(*t*)-c-phenothrin | - | - | - | 0.2 | - | - | - | 0.1 |
| Unknown | 1.2 | 0.1 | 0.2 | 0.2 | 0.3 | 0.1 | <0.1 | 0.2 |

Gly: Glycine conjugate.    Sul: Sulfate conjugate.    "-": Not detected.

Table 12    *In Vitro* Metabolites in Liver Supernatant[7]

| Species | Analytes | NADPH (+/-) | Metabolites (% of Radioactivity) | | | |
|---|---|---|---|---|---|---|
| | | | Parent | 3-Phenoxybenzyl Alcohol | 3-Phenoxybenzoic Acid | 3-(4'-hydroxy) Phenoxybenzoic Acid |
| Mouse | 1R-trans-phenothrin | - | 78.9 | 10.9 | 1.2 | 0.3 |
| | | + | 76.9 | 1.9 | 6.6 | 3.5 |
| Rat | 1R-trans-phenothrin | - | 75.1 | 13.9 | 2.5 | 0.3 |
| | | + | 73.4 | 6.6 | 6.8 | 1.7 |
| | 1R-cis-phenothrin | - | 93.1 | 0.5 | 0.4 | 0.0 |
| | | + | 76.2 | 0.8 | 0.4 | 3.1 |
| Guinea pig | 1R-trans-phenothrin | - | 60.8 | 26.8 | 1.3 | 0.2 |
| | | + | 63.1 | 1.9 | 21.9 | 1.8 |
| Rabbit | 1R-trans-phenothrin | - | 68.3 | 16.3 | 8.1 | 0.7 |
| | | + | 67.0 | 0.4 | 21.9 | 1.7 |
| Dog | 1R-trans-phenothrin | - | 66.1 | 24.9 | 3.5 | 0.3 |
| | | + | 55.3 | 17.4 | 6.3 | 0.7 |

[7]  PMDA Database.    http://www.pmda.go.jp/drugs/2014/P201400043/index.html (accessed Mar 2016).

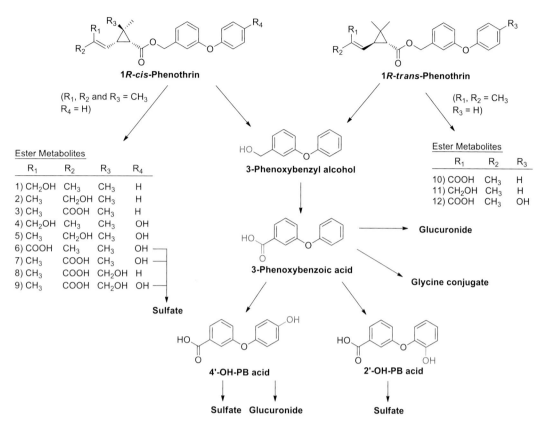

Figure A    Proposed Pathways for *In Vivo* and *In Vitro* Biotransformation of Phenothrin in Rats[7]

## Excretion

Table 13    Excretion Profiles of [$^{14}$C]Phenothrin in SD Rats after Topical and Oral Dose of Phenothrin[7]

| Species | Formulation | Analyte | Route | Dose (mg/ body) | Time (h) | Urine (% of dose) | Feces (% of dose) | Skin Washing Liquid (% of dose) | Gauze | Recovery (% of dose) |
|---|---|---|---|---|---|---|---|---|---|---|
| SD rat (male) | Emulsion | [$^{14}$C]1*R-trans*-phenothrin | Topical | 0.2 | 0-24 | 8.7 | 2.2 | 85.3 | - | 96.2 |
| | | | | 2 | 0-24 | 6.6 | 1.8 | 85.4 | - | 93.8 |
| | | [$^{14}$C]1*R-cis*-phenothrin | Topical | 0.2 | 0-24 | 4.5 | 12.3 | 80.8 | - | 97.6 |
| | | | | 2 | 0-24 | 4.8 | 11.5 | 77.7 | - | 94.0 |
| | Powder | [$^{14}$C]1*R-trans*-phenothrin | Topical | 0.2 | 0-24 | 2.6 | 1.1 | 16.7 | 72.6 | 93.0 |
| | | | | 2 | 0-24 | 2.8 | 0.6 | 20.4 | 65.6 | 89.4 |
| | | [$^{14}$C]1*R-cis*-phenothrin | Topical | 0.2 | 0-24 | 2.6 | 4.0 | 24.9 | 66.1 | 97.6 |
| | | | | 2 | 0-24 | 1.5 | 3.0 | 17.0 | 76.6 | 98.1 |
| | Oral | [$^{14}$C]1*R-trans*-phenothrin | p.o. | 2 | - | 75.1 | 20.9 | - | - | 96.0 |
| | | [$^{14}$C]1*R-cis*-phenothrin | p.o. | 2 | - | 22.4 | 73.5 | - | - | 95.9 |

[7]  PMDA Database.   http://www.pmda.go.jp/drugs/2014/P201400043/index.html (accessed Mar 2016).

## Drug-Drug Interaction

Table 14   *In Vitro* Evaluation of Phenothrin as an Inhibitor and an Inducer of Enzymes[7]

| Phenothrin as an Inhibitor | | | | Phenothrin as an Inducer | | | | | |
|---|---|---|---|---|---|---|---|---|---|
| Enzyme | IC50 (μM) | | | Enzyme | Conc. (μM) | Fold Induction | | | |
| | | | | | | Cis-Phenothrin | Trans-Phenothrin | 3-Phenoxy-benzoic Acid | |
| | Cis-Phenothrin | Trans-Phenothrin | 3-Phenoxy-benzoic Acid | | | 0.01-1.0 | 0.02-2.0 | 1-100 | |
| CYP1A2 | >0.3 | >0.3 | >30 | CYP1A2 | Enzyme activities | 0.9-1.1 | 1.0-1.1 | 1.2-1.5 | |
| CYP2A6 | >0.3 | >0.3 | >30 | | mRNA level | 1.1-1.2 | 1.0-1.3 | 1.2-1.8 | |
| CYP2B6 | >0.3 | >0.3 | >30 | | | | | | |
| CYP2C8 | >0.3 | >0.3 | >30 | CYP2B6 | Enzyme activities | 1.0-1.1 | 1.1-1.1 | 1.2-1.4 | |
| CYP2C9 | >0.3 | >0.3 | >30 | | mRNA level | 1.1-1.3 | 1.3-1.4 | 1.3-1.9 | |
| CYP2C19 | >0.3 | >0.3 | >30 | | | | | | |
| CYP2D6 | >0.3 | >0.3 | >30 | CYP3A4 | Enzyme activities | 1.0-1.0 | 1.0-1.1 | 1.1-1.2 | |
| CYP2E1 | >0.3 | >0.3 | >30 | | mRNA level | 1.0-1.6 | 0.9-1.1 | 1.1-1.5 | |
| CYP3A4 | >0.3 | >0.3 | >30 | | | | | | |
| CYP3A4 | >0.3 | >0.3 | >30 | | | | | | |

## 6   Non-Clinical Toxicology

## Summary

### Single-Dose Toxicity

❖ Single-dose toxicity, concurrent with toxicokinetic research, by the dermal manner in rats with intact or artificially damaged skin:
- Overall, phenothrin led to no drug-related adverse effect.
- $AUC_{0-72}$ indicated that phenothrin and its main metabolites (3-phenoxybenzoic acid and 3-(4'-hydroxy)phenoxybenzoic acid) tended to increase in a dose-dependent manner, and that systemic exposure was much higher in artificial stratum corneum damage model (~2-fold), and exhibited sex differences (female > male).

### Repeated-Dose Toxicity

❖ Sub- and chronic toxicity studies, concurrent with toxicokinetic research, by the dermal or the oral manner in rats (up to 4 weeks) and dogs (up to 1 year):
- Major target organs of toxicity by oral consistently included liver and kidneys yet phenothrin exhibited no drug-related effects by dermal.
- Exposure indicated no accumulation but sex difference (female > male).

### Safety Pharmacology

❖ Safety pharmacology to evaluate effects on central nervous and cardiovascular system:
- Neither neurological nor cardiovascular function was affected.

### Genotoxicity

❖ Both *in vitro* and *in vivo* genotoxicity assays with phenothrin: Phenothrin was not mutagenic or clastogenic in any tests.

### Reproductive and Developmental Toxicity

❖ Embryo-fetal development in rats and rabbits:

---

[7]  PMDA Database.   http://www.pmda.go.jp/drugs/2014/P201400043/200738000/index.html (accessed Mar 2016).

- Maternal toxicities were founded, e.g. decreased body weight and food consumption at HD (rats: 3000 mg/kg, rabbits: 500 mg/kg); There were no malformations in any groups, but resorption and lower fetal weight were identified at HD.
- ❖ Pre- and postnatal development in rats:
  - $F_0$ maternal toxicity was demonstrated by reducing premating and gestational body weight.
  - $F_1$ generation toxicity was showed by decreasing litter size, reducing survival ratio, diminishing birth and wean weight, dysontogenesis postpartum until adulthood and abnormalities in reproductive organ, yet there was no maternal toxicity observed.
  - $F_2$ generation toxicity exhibited lower birth and wean weight.

Carcinogenicity

- ❖ Two-year carcinogenicity bioassays were conducted in rats: Neoplasms in liver were identified in rats at 20000 ppm.

Special Toxicity

- ❖ Not conducted.

## Single-Dose Toxicity

Table 15    Single-Dose Toxicity Studies of Phenothrin by the Dermal Route[7]

| Species/Strain | Dose (mg/kg) | Finding |
|---|---|---|
| SD Rat | 0, 50, 100, 200 | None drug-related. |
| | 0, 100[a] | None drug-related. |

Sham operation group: Retaining with sterile gauze and non-irritating tape.    [a] Artificial stratum corneum damage.

## Repeated-Dose Toxicity

Table 16    Repeated-Dose Toxicity Studies of Phenothrin[7]

| Species/Strain | Duration | Dosage (mg/kg/day) | NOAEL (mg/kg/day) | Finding |
|---|---|---|---|---|
| SD rat | 28 days | 0, 25, 50, 100 (dermal) | 100 | None drug-related. |
| | 21 days | 0, 100, 300 1000 (dermal) | 1000 | None drug-related. |

Vehicle: Corn oil.

## Safety Pharmacology

Table 17    Safety Pharmacological Studies of Phenothrin[7]

| Study | System | Dosage (mg/kg) | Finding |
|---|---|---|---|
| CNS effect | WIST rat | 200, 600, 2000 (oral gavage) | None specific. |
| | WIST rat | 1000, 3000, 10000, 20000 ppm/day for 13 weeks (dietary) | NOAEL = 20000 ppm/day (1456 mg/kg/day in males and 1502 mg/kg/day in females). |
| Cardiovascular effect | Beagle dog (male, telemetry) | Single ascending dose: 500, 2000 (oral gavage) | None. |

## Genotoxicity

Table 18    Genotoxicity Studies of Phenothrin[7]

| Assay | Species/Strain | Dosage | Finding |
|---|---|---|---|
| *In vitro* microbial reverse mutation assay | *S. typhimurium*/TA98, TA100, TA1535, TA1537; *E. coli*/WP2 *uvr*A | 313-5000 µg/plate (±S9) | Negative. |
| *In vitro* chromosome aberration assay in mammalian cells | CHO-WBL | 101, 151, 202, 252 µg/mL (-S9 for 20 h); 202, 303, 404, 505 µg/mL (+S9 for 2 h, 20 h in total); 202, 303, 404, 505 µg/mL (+S9 for 2 h, 30 h in total); | Negative. |
| *In vivo* bone marrow cell chromosome aberration assay | ICR mouse | 2500, 5000, 10000 mg/kg for 4 h, i.p. | Negative. |

Vehicle: DMSO for *in vitro* studies.

---

[7]    PMDA Database.    http://www.pmda.go.jp/drugs/2014/P201400043/index.html (accessed Mar 2016).

## Reproductive and Developmental Toxicity

Table 19    Reproductive and Developmental Toxicology Studies of Phenothrin[7]

| Studies | Species/Strain | Dose (mg/kg/day) | NOAEL | | Finding |
|---|---|---|---|---|---|
| | | | Endpoint | Dose (mg/kg/day) | |
| Embryo-fetal development | SD rat | 300 ,1000 , 3000 | Maternal/Fetal | 300 | Maternal toxicity: ↓ BW and food consumption at HD; ↓ Water consumption at MD and HD. Embryo-fetal toxicity: No malformations in any groups;↓ Fetal weight at HD. |
| | NZW rabbit | 30 ,100, 300 ,500 (oral gavage) 750 (stomach tube) | Maternal/Fetal teratogenic | 300 | Maternal toxicity: ↓ BW and food consumption at HD. Embryo-fetal toxicity: Aborted litters; Slight ↓ Fetal weight; ↑ Malformation/ variation rates; Slightly delayed ossification, esp. pelvis at HD. |
| Pre- and postnatal development | SD rat | 1000, 3000, 10000 ppm (dietary) | $F_0$ | 1000 ppm | $F_0$: ↓ Premating and gestational BW and food consumption in MDF and 2HD; ↑ BW on lactation in all females; ↑ Liver weight in MDF and HDF. |
| | | | $F_1$ development | 1000 ppm | $F_1$: ↓ Fetal litter size and survival ratio; ↓ Birth and wean weight. ↓ BW throughout lactation and into adulthood at 2MD and 2HD; ↑ Brain, liver, seminal vesicle and left testicle weight in 2HD; ↓ Ovary weight in HDF. |
| | | | $F_1$ fertility | 10000 ppm | No maternal toxicity. $F_2$: ↓ Birth and wean weight. |

Vehicle: Corn oil for rat studies.    0.5% CMC for rabbit study.

## Carcinogenicity

Table 20    104-week Carcinogenicity Studies of Phenothrin[7]

| Species | Dose (ppm) | NOAEL | Finding |
|---|---|---|---|
| F344 rat | 0, 1000,10000, 20000 | Combined:1000 ppm, namely 51 mg/kg/day in males, 63 mg/kg/day in females | ↑ Kidney, thyroid, and liver weight, ↓ spleen weight. Liver neoplasia at HD, testicular subcapsular reservoir in HD males, abnormal kidney shape in HD females. |

[7]  PMDA Database.    http://www.pmda.go.jp/drugs/2014/P201400043/index.html (accessed Mar 2016).

# CHAPTER

22

# Ripasudil Hydrochloride Hydrate

# Ripasudil Hydrochloride Hydrate

## (Glanatec®)

Research code: K-115

## 1  General Information

❖ Ripasudil hydrochloride hydrate is a small moleculer Rho-associated coiled coil-containing protein kinase (ROCK) inhibitor, which was first approved in Sep 2014 by PMDA of Japan.

❖ Ripasudil hydrochloride hydrate was discovered by D. Western Therapeutics Institute, developed and marketed by Kowa Company.

❖ Ripasudil hydrochloride hydrate reduced intraocular pressure (IOP) by directly acting on the trabecular meshwork via increasing conventional outflow through the Schlemm's canal.

❖ Ripasudil is indicated for the treatment of patients with glaucoma and ocular hypertension.

❖ Available as ophthalmic solution, containing 0.4% ripasudil and the recommended dose is one drop in the affected eye, twice daily.

❖ The sale of Glanatec® ophthalmic solution 0.4% was not available up to Mar 2016.

### Key Approvals around the World*

|  | Japan (PMDA) |
| --- | --- |
| First approval date | 09/26/2014 |
| Application or approval No. | 22600AMX01307 |
| Brand name | Glanatec®ophthalmic solution 0.4% (グラナテック®点眼液 0.4% ) |
| Indication | Glaucoma & Ocular hypertension |
| Authorisation holder | Kowa Company |

* Till Mar 2016, it had not been approved by FDA (US), EMA (EU) and CFDA (China).

## Active Ingredient

*Molecular formula*:  $C_{15}H_{18}FN_3O_2S \cdot HCl \cdot 2H_2O$
*Molecular weight*:  395.88
*CAS No.*:  223645-67-8 (Ripasudil)
  887375-67-9 (Ripasudil hydrochloride dihydrate)
*Chemical name*:  4-Fluoro-5-{[(2*S*)-2-methyl-1,4-diazepan-1-yl]sulfonyl}isoquinoline monohydrochloride dihydrate

*Parameters of Lipinski's "Rule of 5"*

| MW[a] | H$_D$ | H$_A$ | FRB[b] | PSA[b] | cLogP[b] |
| --- | --- | --- | --- | --- | --- |
| 323.39 | 1 | 5 | 2 | 70.7Å$^2$ | 2.47 ± 1.07 |

[a] Molecular weight of ripasudil.  [b] Calculated by ACD/Labs software V11.02.

## Drug Product*

*Dosage route*:  Ophthalmic/Topical instillation
*Strength*:  0.4% (Ripasudil)
*Dosage form*:  Sterile aqueous ophthalmic solution
*Inactive ingredient*:  Anhydrous sodium dihydrogen phosphate, glycerin, sodium hydroxide and 50% concentrated benzalkonium chloride solution.
*Recommended dose*: The recommended starting dose is one drop in the affected eye, twice daily.

* Sourced from Japan PMDA drug label information

# 2 Key Patents Information

## Summary

❖ Glanatec® (Ripasudil hydrochloride hydrate) was approved by PMDA of Japan on Sep 26, 2014.

❖ Ripasudil was originally discovered by D. Western Therapeutics Institute and then developed by Kowa Company, but its compound patent application was filed as PCT application by Nippon Shinyaku in 1998.

❖ The compound patent will expire in 2023, which has only been granted in Japan.

Table 1    Ripasudil's Compound Patent Protection in Drug-Mainstream Country

| Country | Publication/Patent NO. | Application Date | Granted Date | Estimated Expiry Date |
|---|---|---|---|---|
| WO | WO9920620A1 | 10/22/1998 | / | / |
| US | NA | / | / | / |
| EP | NA | / | / | / |
| JP | JP4316794B2 | 10/22/1998 | 08/19/2009 | 10/22/2023[a] |
| CN | NA | / | / | / |

[a] The term of this patent is extended by 5 years.

Table 2    Originator's International Patent Application List (Patent Family)

| Publication NO. | Title | Applicant/Assignee/Owner | Publication Date |
|---|---|---|---|
| Technical Subjects | Active Ingredient (Free Base)'s Formula or Structure and Preparation | | |
| WO9920620A1 | Isoquinoline derivative and drug | Nippon Shinyaku | 04/29/1999 |
| Technical Subjects | Salt, Crystal, Polymorphic, Solvate (Hydrate), Isomer, Derivative Etc. and Preparation | | |
| WO2006057397A1 | (S)-(-)-1-(4-fluoroisoquinolin-5-yl)sulfonyl-2-methyl-1,4-homopiperazine hydrochloride dihydrate | Kowa | 06/01/2006 |
| WO2006115247A1 | Highly selective Rho-kinase inhibitor | D. Western Therapeutics Institute | 11/02/2006 |
| WO2012026529A1 | Novel production method for isoquinoline derivatives and salts thereof | Kowa | 03/01/2012 |
| Technical Subjects | Indication or Methods for Medical Needs | | |
| WO2006068208A1 | Preventive or therapeutic agent for glaucoma | Kowa | 06/29/2006 |
| WO2014174747A1 | Therapeutic agent for eyeground disease | Kowa | 10/30/2014 |
| Technical Subjects | Combination Including at Least Two Active Ingredients | | |
| WO2007007737A1 | Agent for prevention or treatment of glaucoma | Kowa | 01/18/2007 |
| WO2006137368A1 | Preventive or remedy for glaucoma | Kowa | 12/28/2006 |
| WO2012105674A1 | Drug therapy for preventing or treating glaucoma | Kowa | 08/09/2012 |

The data was updated until Jan 2016.

# 3 Chemistry

## Route 1: Original Discovery Route

*Synthetic Route*: While the early synthetic route to ripasudil was carried out through a stepwise functionalization of 4-fluoroisoquinoline-5-sulfonyl chloride **9**, a more recent report described an efficient approach to ripasudil employing a late stage-coupling of Boc-diazepane **8** with **9**, enabling the synthesis on multi-kilogram scale with high purity. This optimized route to ripasudil started with 2-nitrobenzene sulfonyl chloride (NsCl)-mediated protection of (*S*)-2-amino-1-propanol **1** in 82% yield. In this case, use of the NaHCO₃/THF/H₂O condition was essential for preventing bis-nosylation. Alcohol activation with MsCl/NMM took place smoothly to give the corresponding mesylate **3** in 91% yield. Direct mesylate displacement with 3-aminopropanol **4** and subsequent amine protection in a one-pot fashion provided the corresponding Boc-amino propanol product **6** in 95% yield over two steps. With the acyclic diazepane precursor **6** in hand, employment of the intramolecular Fukuyama-Mitsunobu *N*-alkyl cyclization allowed generation of the diazepane **7** in 75% yield. Nosyl group cleavage with thiophenol/K₂CO₃ provided the Boc-diazepane **8** in 86% yield. Sulfonyl chloride **9** enabled the coupling with diazepane **8** to access the ripasudil framework in quantitative yield. Synthesis of the final target by deprotection with 4M HCl in ethyl acetate followed by neutralization with aqueous sodium hydroxide provided ripasudil in 93% yield and with 99.9% *ee*. The overall yield concerning this route was 43%.[1-4]

[1] Gomi, N.; Ohgiya, T.; Shibuya, K., et al. WO2012026529A1, **2012**.
[2] Gomi, N.; Ohgiya, T.; Shibuya, K., et al. US20150087824A1, **2015**.
[3] Hidaka, H.; Matsuura, A. WO9920620A1, **1999**.
[4] Gomi, N.; Kouketsu, A.; Ohgiya, T., et al. *Synthesis* **2012**, *44*, 3171-3178.

## Route 2

*Synthetic Route:* In the procedure involving a multi-kilogram scale preparation, the $HSO_4^-$ salt of isoquinoline **2** was easier for handling than free base **1** in the sulfonylation reaction. The regioselective of 5-sulfonyl chloride **3** and 8-sulfonyl chloride was 1.8:1. The approach to satisfyingly pure **3** was achieved by crystallization to provide the hydrochloride salt **3** in 39% yield, while the byproduct 8-sulfonyl chloride could be simply removed by filtration. Sulfonylamidation of **3** with (*S*)-2-aminopropanol **4** under mild condition gave the corresponding sulfonylamide **5** in 84% yield. Mesylation of **5** led to a mixture of the mesylate and the aziridine intermediate. *N*-Alkylation was carried out *in situ*, and the mixture was directly treated with 3-aminopropanol **6** and salification to afford the desired oxalate **7** in 73% yield over two steps. After basifying of **7** to afford the free amine, the intramolecular cyclization was conducted under Mitsunobu conditions. The reaction proceeded smoothly to provide the desired product with 95% purity. Finally, the purification of ripasudil was accomplished by the crystallization as the HCl salt in 73% yield over three steps with >99.9% *ee*. The API was sufficiently pure for clinical use.[3, 5-7]

## 4   Pharmacology

### Summary

Mechanism of Action

❖ Ripasudil hydrochloride hydrate is a selective ROCK inhibitor (ROCK-1: $IC_{50}$ = 0.051 μM, $K_i$ = 0.023 μM; ROCK-2: $IC_{50}$ = 0.019 μM, $K_i$ = 0.037 μM), of which the important downstream effector is Rho guanosine triphosphates (GTP), playing a critical, calcium-independent role in the regulation of the contractile tone of smooth muscle tissues.

❖ Ripasudil hydrochloride hydrate is an "out-flow" drug, which reduces IOP by stimulating aqueous humor drainage through the trabecular meshwork.

❖ Ripasudil hydrochloride hydrate showed no binding affinity for adrenergic receptors, angiotensin II receptors, endothelin receptors, glutamate receptors, histamine receptors, muscarinic receptors, prostanoid receptors, serotonin receptors, $Ca^{2+}$ and $K^+$ channels, carbonic anhydrase and HMG-CoA reductase at 1 μM.[8]

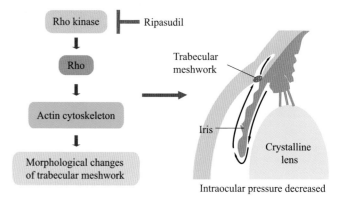

[3]  Hidaka, H.; Matsuura, A. WO9920620A1, **1999**.

[5]  Gomi, N.; Ohgiya, T.; Shibuya, K., et al. *Heterocycles* **2011**, *83*, 1771-1781.

[6]  Ohshima, T.; Hidaka, H.; Shiratsuchi, M., et al. WO2006057397A1, **2006**.

[7]  Ohshima, T.; Hidaka, H.; Shiratsuchi, M., et al. US7858615B2, **2010**.

[8]  Japan Pharmaceuticals and Medical Devices Agency (PMDA) Database.   http://www.pmda.go.jp/drugs/2014/P201400129/index.html (accessed Mar 2016).

*In Vitro* Efficacy

❖ In monkey TM cells:
  • Induced retraction and rounding.
  • Reduced actin bundles.
❖ In the barrier function of monkey SCE cell monolayers:
  • Reduced TEER.
  • In the SCE cells: Decreased ZO-1 immunostaining areas.

*In Vivo* Efficacy

❖ IOP-lowering effects in animals:
  • In normal IOP rabbits:
    ◆ Reduced IOP in a dose-dependent manner at 0.0625%.
    ◆ The maximum IOP reduction at 1 h after instillation.
  • In high IOP rabbits:
    ◆ Reduced IOP in a dose-dependent manner at 0.4%.
    ◆ The maximum IOP reduction at 2 h after instillation.
  • In monkeys:
    ◆ Reduced IOP in a dose-dependent manner.
    ◆ The maximum IOP reduction at 2 h after instillation.
❖ Aqueous humor dynamics in rabbits:
  • No effect on aqueous flow rate or uveoscleral outflow.
  • Significantly increased outflow facility vs. vehicle by 2.2-fold, and reduced IOP.

# Mechanism of Action

Table 3　Inhibition of Ripasudil Hydrochloride Hydrate against ROCKs[8]

| Enzyme | $IC_{50}$ (µM)[a] | | | | | | $K_i$ (µM) |
|--------|------------------------------------|------|------|------|----------------|-----------------|------------------------------------|
|        | Ripasudil Hydrochloride Hydrate | M1 | M2 | M6 | Y-27632[b] | HA-1077[b] | Ripasudil Hydrochloride Hydrate |
| ROCK-1 | 0.051 | 0.32 | 1.4 | 20 | 0.11 | 0.29 | 0.023 |
| ROCK-2 | 0.019 | 0.17 | 0.47 | 7.1 | 0.17 | 0.35 | 0.037 |
| PKACα | 2.1 | NA | NA | NA | 50 | 1.1 | NA |
| PKC | 27 | NA | NA | NA | 32 | 17 | NA |
| CaMK2α | 0.37 | NA | NA | NA | 8.1 | 2.9 | NA |

PKACα: Protein kinase A catalytic α.　PKC: Protein kinase C.　CaMK2α: Calmodulin-dependent protein kinase 2α.　M1, M2 and M6 were the metabolites.
[a] $P < 0.05$.　[b] Rho kinase inhibitors.

# *In Vitro* Efficacy

Table 4　*In Vitro* Pharmacodynamics of Ripasudil Hydrochloride Hydrate in Cells[9]

| Study | Cell Line | Dose (µM) | Test | Results |
|-------|-----------|-----------|------|---------|
| Morphology | TM cell | 1, 10 | Morphology | Induced retraction and rounding. Reduced actin bundles in majority of cells. |
| Barrier function | SEC cell | 1, 5, 25 | TEER | Significant reduction in TEER at 1 µM (60-min) and 5 µM (30-min). |
| Cell-cell contraction | SEC cell | 1, 5, 25 | Associated molecules | Decreased ZO-1, pan-cadherin and β-Catenin at 25 µM. |

TEER: Trans-epithelial electrical resistance.　TM cell: Monkey trabecular meshwork cell.　SEC cell: Schlemm's canal endothelial cell.　ZO-1: Zonula occludens-1.

[8] PMDA Database.　http://www.pmda.go.jp/drugs/2014/P201400129/index.html (accessed Mar 2016).
[9] Kaneko, Y.; Ohta, M.; Inoue, T., et al. *Scientific reports* **2016**, *6*, 19640-19649.

## *In Vivo* Efficacy

Table 5    *In Vivo* Effects of Topical Ripasudil Hydrochloride Hydrate on IOP[8, 10]

| Model | Animal | Dose (Instillation)[a] | Efficacy Time of Maximum IOP Reduction after Instillation (h) | Efficacy Maximum IOP Reduction (mmHg) (Mean ± SE)[b] | Finding |
|---|---|---|---|---|---|
| High IOP model | Rabbit | 0.4% | 1 | NA | Significant IOP-lowering effects in a dose-dependent manner for 1 to 4 h after instillation. |
| Normal IOP model | Rabbit | 0.0625% | 1 | 2.90 ± 0.71 ($P$ <0.05) | Significant dose-dependent IOP-lowering effects for up to 5 h after instillation. |
| | | 0.125% | 1 | 3.60 ± 0.68 ($P$ <0.05) | |
| | | 0.25% | 1 | 7.80 ± 1.88 ($P$ <0.001) | |
| | | 0.5% | 1 | 8.55 ± 1.09 ($P$ <0.001) | |
| | | Ripasudil hydrochloride hydrate: 0.4% + Nipradilol: 0.25% | 1 | ~10.0 ($P$ <0.001) | Significantly enhanced IOP-lowering effects with combined administration. Combination effect. |
| | | Ripasudil hydrochloride hydrate: 0.4% + Carbonic anhydrase inhibitor: 1% | 1 | ~10.0 ($P$ <0.001) | |
| | | 0.4% M1 | 2 | ~2.80 | Significant IOP-lowering effects. |
| | Cynomolgus monkey | 0.1% | 2 | 2.29 ± 0.24 ($P$ <0.05) | Ocular hypotensive duration in a dose-dependent manner. Significant IOP-lowering effects. |
| | | 0.2% | 2 | 3.28 ± 0.28 ($P$ <0.01) | |
| | | 0.4% | 2 | 4.36 ± 0.32 ($P$ <0.001) | |
| | | Latanoprost: 0.005% | 4 | 2.50 ± 0.16 ($P$ <0.01) | Increased the effect of lowering IOP after 2 h of instillation by combined administration. Combination effect. |
| | | Ripasudil hydrochloride hydrate: 0.4% + Latanoprost: 0.005% | 4 | ~6.00 ($P$ <0.01) | |

IOP was monitored using a pneumatonometer, and M1 was the main metabolite.    [a] Single instillation.    [b] The IOPs were compared with the results on the instillation side at pre-dose and at each time point after instillation of ripasudil hydrochloride hydrate, and were compared with the results for ripasudil and untreated eye(s) at each time point.

Table 6    Effects of Topical Ripasudil Hydrochloride Hydrate on Aqueous Humor Dynamics in Rabbits[8-10]

| Group | Dose | Aqueous Flow Rate (µL/min)[a] Pre-dose | Aqueous Flow Rate (µL/min)[a] Post-dose | Uveoscleral Outflow (µL/min)[b] | Outflow Facility (µL/min/mmHg)[b] |
|---|---|---|---|---|---|
| Vehicle | NA | 1.69 ± 0.18 | 1.54 ± 0.23 | 0.134 ± 0.026 | 0.086 ± 0.021 |
| Ripasudil hydrochloride hydrate | 0.4% | 1.97 ± 0.23 | 1.88 ± 0.35 | 0.155 ± 0.023 | 0.193 ± 0.038 |

[a] Determined by fluorophotometry.    Pre- and post-dose: For 2 h prior to dosing and for 2 h after dosing, respectively.    [b] Measured by two-level constant pressure and perfusion technique using fluorescrein isothiocyanate-dextran.    All data were mean ± SE (n = 6-8).

[8]  PMDA Database.    http://www.pmda.go.jp/drugs/2014/P201400129/index.html (accessed Mar 2016).
[9]  Kaneko, Y.; Ohta, M.; Inoue, T., et al. *Scientific reports* **2016**, *6*, 19640-19649.
[10]  Isobe, T.; Mizuno, K.; Kaneko, Y., et al. *Curr. Eye Res.* **2014**, *39*, 813-822.

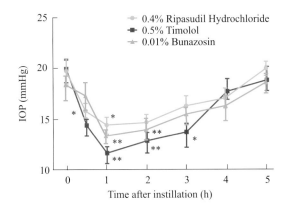

**Study:** Effects of ripasudil hydrochloride hydrate on intraocular pressure in rabbits.

**Animal:** Male albino rabbit (n = 9).

**Administration:** Ripasudil hydrochloride hydrate: 0.4%; Timolol: 0.5%; Bunazosin: 0.01%, 50 μL, instillation into one eye.

**Test:** The contralateral eye was not treated. IOP was measured in both eyes prior to the experiment and at 0.5, 1, 2, 3, 4 and 5 h after instillation.

**Results:** 0.4% ripasudil hydrochloride hydrate ophthalmic solution showed a significant IOP-lowering effect. Similar effects were observed by other glaucoma therapeutic agents. $^{*}P < 0.05$, $^{**}P < 0.01$, compared with preinstillation values (Dunnett's multiple comparison test).

Figure A    Intraocular Pressure (IOP)-lowering Effects of Topical Ripasudil Hydrochloride Hydrate in Rabbits[8, 9]

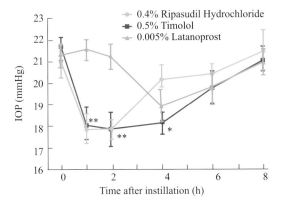

**Study:** Effects of ripasudil hydrochloride hydrate on intraocular pressure in monkeys.

**Animal:** Male cynomolgus monkey (n = 5-6).

**Administration:** Ripasudil hydrochloride hydrate: 0.4%; Timolol: 0.5%; Latanoprost: 0.005%, 20 μL, instillation into one eye.

**Test:** IOP was measured using pneumotonometers prior to experiments and at 1, 2, 4, 6 and 8 h after instillation.

**Results:** 0.4% ripasudil hydrochloride hydrate ophthalmic solution showed a significant IOP-lowering effect. Additionally, an IOP-lowering effect of 0.4% ripasudil hydrochloride hydrate was similar to existing agents. $^{*}P < 0.05$, $^{**}P < 0.01$, compared with preinstillation values (Dunnett's multiple comparison test).

Figure B    Intraocular Pressure (IOP)-lowering Effects of Topical Ripasudil Hydrochloride Hydrate in Monkeys[8, 9]

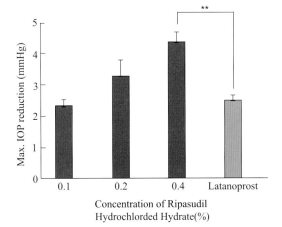

**Study:** Effects of ripasudil hydrochloride hydrate on intraocular pressure in monkeys.

**Animal:** Male cynomolgus monkey (n = 8).

**Administration:** Ripasudil hydrochloride hydrate: 0.1%, 0.2%, 0.4%; Latanoprost: 0.005%, 20 μL, instillation into the eye.

**Test:** The maximum IOP reduction monitored using a pneumatonometer and evaluated by Dunnett's multiple comparison.

**Results:** 0.2% and 0.4% of ripasudil hydrochloride hydrate showed strong and rapid ocular hypotensive effects compared with 0.005% latanoprost. $^{**}P < 0.01$, compared with 0.005% latanoprost (Dunnett's test).

Figure C    Effects of Topical Ripasudil Hydrochloride Hydrate on Intraocular Pressure (IOP) in Monkeys[8, 10]

[8]   PMDA Database.   http://www.pmda.go.jp/drugs/2014/P201400129/index.html (accessed Mar 2016).
[9]   Kaneko, Y.; Ohta, M.; Inoue, T., et al. *Scientific reports* **2016**, *6*, 19640-19649.
[10]   Isobe, T.; Mizuno, K.; Kaneko, Y., et al. *Curr. Eye Res.* **2014**, *39*, 813-822.

# 5   ADME & Drug-Drug Interaction

## Summary

### Absorption of Ripasudil

❖ Exhibited a linear pharmacokinetics in rats after oral administrations.    The increases in $C_{max}$ and AUC appeared to be dose-proportional in the dose range of 1 to 10 mg/kg ripasudil.

❖ Had high ophthalmic bioavailability in rabbits (95.8%) and low to high in rats (11.7%, 29.2% and 108%, respectively) from low to high dose.

❖ Was absorbed rapidly ($T_{max}$ = 14.9-25.5 min) in rats after oral administrations, and also rapidly in rabbits ($T_{max}$ = 6.26 min) and humans ($T_{max}$ = 0.137-0.301 h) after ophthalmic administrations.

❖ Showed a half-life ranging between 0.49-0.73 h in humans, longer than those in rabbits (24.9 min) after ophthalmic administrations.

❖ Had high clearance in rabbits (64.4-109 mL/min/kg) and moderate in rats (35.0 mL/min/kg), in contrast to liver blood flow, after intravenous administrations.

❖ Exhibited an extensive tissue distribution in all species, with apparent volumes of distribution in rats (1620 mL/kg) and rabbits (2800-3130 mL/kg), respectively, after intravenous administrations.

### Distribution of Ripasudil

❖ Exhibited moderate plasma protein binding in humans (56.4%-57.5%), but low in dogs (41.8%-43.1%), rabbits (41.2%-41.9%) and rats (35.3%-36.7%).

❖ The blood cell partition was less than 50% in most species, suggesting low penetration into red blood cells.    After a single oral dose of 3 mg/kg to male rats, blood cell partition increased in a time-dependent manner.[8]

❖ After single oral administration of [$^{14}$C]ripasudil hydrochloride (3 mg/kg) to male rats:
- The drug was widely distributed into most tissues with high levels of the drug observed in the liver, kidneys, urine in bladder, but the radioactivity in the brain was low.
- Radioactivity concentrations were declined to below measureable levels in most tissues at 168 h post-dose.
- No accumulation was observed.

❖ After single ophthalmic administration of [$^{14}$C]ripasudil hydrochloride (1.0%) to male rabbits:
- The highest concentration of [$^{14}$C]ripasudil radioactivity was found at 0.25 h post-dose, and the highest levels of the drug observed in the iris-ciliary body, kidneys, tear retina and choroid.
- Radioactivity concentrations were declined to below measurable levels in most tissues at 366 h post-dose.

### Metabolism of Ripasudil

❖ The major metabolite was hydroxylation derivative M1 in human plasma, rabbit cornea, aqueous humor and crystalline lens, but the major metabolites were M5 and M3 in rat plasma.    All the metabolites identified in humans could be found in other species.

❖ Aldehyde oxidase was involved in the formation of M1.    Ripasudil was metabolized to M2 by CYP3A5 and 3A4, and M4 by CYP3A5, 3A4 and 2C8.

❖ M1 was an active metabolite.

### Excretion of Ripasudil

❖ Was predominantly excreted through urine in rats and humans, with M5 as the major significant compound in rat urine.

❖ The radioactivity in bile was 38.9% of dose in BDC rats.

### Drug-Drug Interaction

❖ Ripasudil exhibited inhibitory effect on CYP2D6 with the $IC_{50}$ = 5.1 μM (without pre-incubation) and 3.8 μM (with pre-incubation).    In addition, ripasudil showed inhibitory effect on CYP3A4/5 in the pre-incubation group ($IC_{50}$ = 14 μM). Ripasudil showed aldehyde oxidase inhibitory activity ($IC_{50}$ = 1.4 μM).

❖ Ripasudil was not an inducer of CYP1A2, 2A6, 2C8, 2C9, 2C19 or 2D6.

---

[8]   PMDA Database.    http://www.pmda.go.jp/drugs/2014/P201400129/index.html (accessed Mar 2016).

# Absorption

Table 7 *In Vivo* Pharmacokinetic Parameters of Ripasudil in Rats and Rabbits after Single Intravenous, Oral and Ophthalmic Dose of Ripasudil[8]

| Species | Route | Dose (mg/kg) | $T_{max}$ (min) | $C_{max}$ (μg/mL) | $AUC_{0-t}$ (μg·min/mL) | $AUC_{inf}$ (μg·min/mL) | $T_{1/2}$ (min) | Cl (mL/min/kg) | $V_{ss}$ (mL/kg) | F (%) |
|---|---|---|---|---|---|---|---|---|---|---|
| SD rat (male) | i.v.[a] | 1 | NA | NA | NA | 28.7 ± 2.2 | $\alpha = 10.4 \pm 3.7$ $\beta = 47.1 \pm 10.3$ | 35.0 ± 2.6 | 1620 ± 228 | - |
| | p.o. | 1 | 14.9 ± 0.1 | 0.073 ± 0.018 | 3.01 ± 0.99 | 3.37 ± 0.99 | 30.9 ± 9.0 | NA | NA | 11.7 |
| | p.o. | 3 | 15.0 ± 0.1 | 0.487 ± 0.155 | 24.5 ± 10.9 | 25.1 ± 10.6 | 38.4 ± 6.4 | NA | NA | 29.2 |
| | p.o. | 10 | 25.5 ± 9.0 | 2.850 ± 0.811 | 305 ± 65 | 309 ± 69 | 54.2 ± 17.7 | NA | NA | 108 |
| Japanese white rabbit (male) | o.s. or o.d. | 1.0%[b] | 6.26 ± 2.03 | 0.064 ± 0.017 | 2.08 ± 0.95 | 2.18 ± 0.95 | 24.9 ± 5.9 | NA | NA | 95.8 ± 41.4[c] |
| | i.v. | 1 | 6.00 | NA | NA | 9.35 ± 1.63 | $\alpha = 9.81 \pm 3.89$ $\beta = 32.2 \pm 5.5$ | 109 ± 18 | 3130 ± 802 | - |
| | i.v. | 3 | 5.02 | NA | NA | 35.4 ± 8.0 | $\alpha = 15.4 \pm 2.2$ $\beta = 44.7 \pm 8.0$ | 87.7 ± 19.4 | 2800 ± 785 | - |
| | i.v. | 10 | 5.29 | NA | NA | 165 | $\alpha = 27.6$ $\beta = 88.5$ | 64.4 | 2850 | - |

Vehicle: Saline for i.v., water for p.o., ophthalmic solution for o.s. or o.d..  o.u.: Both eyes administration.  o.s. or o.d: Single eye administration.  [a] In male.  [b] The volume of administration was 50 μL/eye.  [c] Based on AUC at 1 mg/kg after i.v. administration.

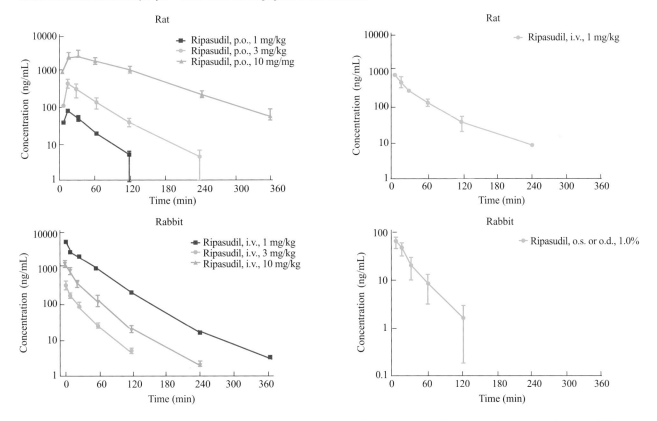

Figure D   *In Vivo* Plasma Concentration-Time Profiles of Ripasudil in Rats and Rabbits after Single Dose of Ripasudil[8]

[8]  PMDA Database.   http://www.pmda.go.jp/drugs/2014/P201400129/index.html (accessed Mar 2016).

Table 8    *In Vivo* Pharmacokinetic Parameters of Ripasudil and Metabolite M1 in Healthy Humans after Single Ophthalmic Dose of Ripasudil[8]

| Species | Analyte | Dose | Route | $T_{max}$ (h) | $C_{max}$ (ng/mL) | $AUC_{0-t}$ (ng·h/mL) | $T_{1/2}$ (h) |
|---|---|---|---|---|---|---|---|
| Healthy human (male) | Ripasudil | 0.05% | o.u. | NC | $0.000 \pm 0.000$ | $0.000 \pm 0.000$ | NC |
| | | 0.1% | o.u. | $0.137 \pm 0.088$ | $0.115 \pm 0.076$ | $0.018 \pm 0.015$ | NC |
| | | 0.2% | o.u. | $0.144 \pm 0.088$ | $0.456 \pm 0.186$ | $0.168 \pm 0.066$ | 0.730 |
| | | 0.4% | o.u. | $0.301 \pm 0.293$ | $0.656 \pm 0.354$ | $0.390 \pm 0.169$ | $0.620 \pm 0.212$ |
| | | 0.8% | o.u. | $0.165 \pm 0.091$ | $0.880 \pm 0.413$ | $0.470 \pm 0.231$ | $0.495 \pm 0.148$ |
| | M1 | 0.05% | o.u. | $0.714 \pm 0.267$ | $0.169 \pm 0.093$ | $0.275 \pm 0.240$ | NC |
| | | 0.1% | o.u. | $0.750 \pm 0.267$ | $0.404 \pm 0.088$ | $1.10 \pm 0.43$ | $2.30 \pm 0.26$ |
| | | 0.2% | o.u. | $0.750 \pm 0.267$ | $1.25 \pm 0.14$ | $3.80 \pm 0.55$ | $2.06 \pm 0.22$ |
| | | 0.4% | o.u. | $1.000 \pm 0.463$ | $2.35 \pm 0.75$ | $8.61 \pm 2.26$ | $2.66 \pm 0.48$ |
| | | 0.8% | o.u. | $0.813 \pm 0.259$ | $3.01 \pm 0.99$ | $10.6 \pm 4.2$ | $2.44 \pm 0.37$ |

The vehicle was ophthalmic solution.    The volume of administration was 50 μL/eye.    NC: Below the lower limit of quantitation.    o.u.: Both eyes administration.
M1: Hydroxylation metabolite.

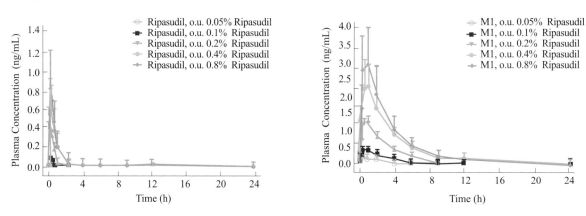

Figure E    *In Vivo* Plasma Concentration-Time Profiles of Ripasudil and M1 in Healthy Humans after Single Dose of Ripasudil (n = 8)[8]

## Distribution

Table 9    *In Vitro* Plasma Protein Binding and Blood Partitioning of [$^{14}$C]Ripasudil in Several Species[8]

| Species | Plasma Protein Binding (%) | | | Blood Cell Partitioning (%) | | | Isolated Human Protein Binding (%) | | | |
|---|---|---|---|---|---|---|---|---|---|---|
| | 10 ng/mL | 100 ng/mL | 1000 ng/mL | 10 ng/mL | 100 ng/mL | 1000 ng/mL | Protein | 10 ng/mL | 100 ng/mL | 1000 ng/mL |
| SD rat | $35.3 \pm 0.8$ | $36.7 \pm 0.1$ | $35.9 \pm 1.6$ | $48.9 \pm 1.9$ | $49.4 \pm 1.6$ | $48.0 \pm 1.0$ | 4% HSA | $22.7 \pm 0.8$ | $19.7 \pm 0.7$ | $20.3 \pm 0.3$ |
| Beagle dog | $43.1 \pm 0.9$ | $42.5 \pm 1.4$ | $41.8 \pm 0.6$ | $47.5 \pm 6.7$ | $50.3 \pm 3.1$ | $52.2 \pm 2.5$ | | | | |
| Japanese white rabbit | $41.9 \pm 1.9$ | $41.3 \pm 1.3$ | $41.2 \pm 0.6$ | $50.9 \pm 2.8$ | $48.4 \pm 1.0$ | $47.6 \pm 0.5$ | 0.1% $\alpha_1$-AGP | $30.4 \pm 2.4$ | $30.3 \pm 0.4$ | $27.6 \pm 0.8$ |
| Human | 57.5 | 56.4 | 56.4 | 40.9 | 41.1 | 40.8 | | | | |

HSA: Human serum albumin.    $\alpha_1$-AGP: $\alpha_1$-acid glycoprotein.

[8]  PMDA Database.    http://www.pmda.go.jp/drugs/2014/P201400129/index.html (accessed Mar 2016).

Table 10　*In Vivo* Tissue Distribution of Ripasudil in SD Rats and Dutch Rabbits after Single Dose of [$^{14}$C]Ripasudil Hydrochloride[8]

| Species | SD Rat/Male | | | Dutch Rabbit/Male | | | |
|---|---|---|---|---|---|---|---|
| Administration | 3 mg/kg p.o. | | | 1.0% o.u.[a] | | | |
| Tissue | Radioactivity (μg eq./g or mL) | | Tissue/Blood AUC$_{0-168}$ Ratio | Tissue | Radioactivity (μg eq./g or mL) | | Tissue/Blood AUC$_{0-336}$ Ratio |
| | 0.25 h | 168 h | | | 0.25 h | 336 h | |
| Blood | 0.947 ± 0.125 | 0.012 ± 0.002 | 1.00 | Blood | 0.276 ± 0.053 | 0.0032 | 1.00 |
| Brain | 0.256 ± 0.022 | 0.006 ± 0.001 | 0.30 | Cornea | 42.5 ± 10.7 | 0.0788 ± 0.0436 | 71.3 |
| Eyes | 0.270 ± 0.054 | 0.003 ± 0.001 | 0.33 | Aqueous humor | 5.19 ± 0.76 | 0.0057 | 6.06 |
| Kidneys | 10.6 ± 2.6 | 0.070 ± 0.009 | 10.53 | Iris-ciliary body | 40.3 ± 22.3 | 6.55 ± 1.99 | 1908 |
| Urine in bladder | 4.68 ± 1.86 | 0.009 ± 0.001 | 4.52 | Crystalline lens | 0.206 ± 0.171 | 0.0026 ± 0.0012 | 3.80 |
| Liver | 14.3 ± 2.1 | 0.179 ± 0.014 | 29.21 | Retina, choroid | 5.62 ± 3.10 | 1.81 ± 0.16 | 303 |
| Brown fat | 1.17 ± 0.42 | 0.025 ± 0.006 | 1.87 | Tear | 41.5 ± 24.4 | 0.529 | 309 |

Sample time for rats: 0.25 h, 4 h, 24 h, 72 h, 168 h and sample time for rabbits: 0.25 h, 1 h, 6 h, 24 h, 72 h, 168 h and 336 h.　Vehicle: Water for rats and ophthalmic solution for rabbits.　[a] The volume of administration was 50 μL/eye.　o.u.: Both eyes administration.

Table 11　*In Vitro* Cornea Permeability of Ripasudil of Different Species[8]

| Species | Eye Ball | $K_p$ (1 × 10$^{-6}$ cm/s) | Lag-time (min) |
|---|---|---|---|
| Human | DMEM, 5 days, 4 °C | 6.81 | 40.5 |
| Cynomolgus monkey | Fresh | 6.44 ± 1.21 | 51.4 ± 3.6 |
| Beagle dog | Fresh | 2.91 ± 0.20 | 52.6 ± 2.6 |
| NZW rabbit | Fresh | 5.96 ± 1.83 | 37.7 ± 0.8 |

DMEM: Dulbecco's Modified Eagle's Medium.

Table 12　*In Vitro* Lens Binding of Ripasudil of Different Species[8]

| Species | Eye Ball | Conc.(ng/mL) | Lens Binding% |
|---|---|---|---|
| Human | DMEM, 5 days, 4 °C | 100 | 27.9 |
| Cynomolgus monkey | Fresh | 100 | 23.6 |
| Beagle dog | Fresh | 10-1000 | 20.3-25.6 |
| NZW rabbit | Fresh | 10-1000 | 17.9-23.8 |
| Dutch rabbit | Fresh | 10-1000 | 17.6-24.4 |

[8]　PMDA Database.　http://www.pmda.go.jp/drugs/2014/P201400129/index.html (accessed Mar 2016).

## Metabolism

Table 13   *In Vitro* the Formation of Metabolites and the Depletion of [14C]Ripasudil Hydrochloride in S9 and Cryopreserved Hepatocytes of Several Species[8]

| Analyte | %Remaining or %Formation | | | | | | | | | |
| | Cryopreserved Hepatocyte | | | | | S9[a] | | | | |
| | Rat[b] | Dog[b] | Rabbit[b] | Monkey[b] | Human[b] | Rat[c] | Dog[c] | Rabbit[c] | Monkey[c] | Human[c] |
|---|---|---|---|---|---|---|---|---|---|---|
| Ripasudil | 41.6 | 33.9 | - | - | 19.7 | 48.4/92.6 | 66.0/95.3 | 1.5/77.0 | 7.6/13.7 | 8.9/14.3 |
| M1 | 3.3 | 1.2 | 4.5 | 39.0 | 66.3 | 3.0/- | 1.3/- | 4.2/17.5 | 44.8/82.2 | 84.0/80.9 |
| M2 | 16.0 | 25.3 | 3.6 | - | 2.23 | 5.5/1.3 | 2.0/- | 22.4/- | 12.1/- | 1.6/1.5 |
| M3 | 8.3 | 1.1 | 26.4 | 2.8 | 4.83 | 6.1/- | -/- | 19.9/- | 1.6/- | -/- |
| M4 | 7.4 | 15.2 | - | - | 0.33 | 14.2/- | 16.7/- | 13.8/- | 6.5/- | 1.6/- |
| M5 | 7.8 | - | 1.4 | 5.7 | - | 8.0/- | -/- | -/- | 1.7/- | -/- |
| M6 | - | - | 22.5 | 36.1 | 1.83 | -/- | 1.1/- | 9.3/- | 12.8/1.1 | 1.4/1.4 |

[a] The value presented as with NADPH-regenerating system v.s. without NADPH-regenerating system in the incubation for 60 min.   [b] 5 μM [14C]ripasudil hydrochloride was added in cryopreserved hepatocytes of several species and incubated for 4 h.   [c] 3 μM [14C]ripasudil hydrochloride was added in S9 of several species and incubated for 1 h.

Table 14   *In Vitro* the Intrinsic Clearance of [14C]Ripasudil Hydrochloride in S9 and Cryopreserved Hepatocytes of Several Species[8]

| Species | $Cl_{int}$ (μL/min/mg protein) | | $Cl_{int}$ (μL/min/10^6 cell) |
| | S9[a] | | |
| | +NRS | -NRS | Cryopreserved Hepatocyte[b] |
|---|---|---|---|
| Human | 38.0 | 30.3 | 63.6/4.19/17.0[c] |
| Monkey | 42.1 | 32.4 | 45.3 |
| Dog | 6.35 | - | 7.11 |
| Rabbit | 67.7 | 3.31 | 46.7 |
| Rat | 10.6 | - | 5.86 |

NRS: NADPH-regenerating system.   [a] 3 μM [14C]ripasudil hydrochloride was added in liver S9 fraction (1 mg protein/mL) of several species.   [b] 5 μM [14C]ripasudil hydrochloride was added in cryopreserved hepatocytes (1.5 × 10^5 cells/0.25mL) of several species.   [c] Data for male/male/female humans.

Table 15   *In Vitro* Metabolic Phenotype of Ripasudil Hydrochloride and Metabolites in S9 and Recombinant Human CYPs[8]

| System | S9[a] | | | | Recombinant Human CYPs[b] | | | | | | | |
| Species | Inhibitor | % of Radioactivity | | | Enzyme | $Cl_{int}$ (μL/min/pmoL CYP) | | | | | | |
| | | Ripasudil | M1 | M2 | M6 | | Ripasudil | M1 | M2 | M3 | M4 | M5 | M6 |
|---|---|---|---|---|---|---|---|---|---|---|---|---|---|
| Human | Control | 23.1 | 71.6 | 1.8 | - | CYP1A2 | - | 0.0131 | - | - | - | - | - |
| | Allopurinol | 26.3 | 68.4 | 1.9 | - | CYP2B6 | 0.0286 | - | - | - | - | - | - |
| | Menadione | 76.6 | 19.7 | - | - | CYP2C8 | 0.0384 | 0.0258 | - | - | - | - | - |
| | Raloxifene | 96.8 | - | - | - | CYP2C9 | - | - | - | - | - | - | - |
| Monkey | Control | 23.5 | 71.9 | - | - | CYP2C19 | 0.0354 | 0.0174 | 0.032 | - | - | - | - |
| | Allopurinol | 35.2 | 61.2 | - | - | | | | | | | | |
| | Menadione | 80.2 | 16.4 | - | - | CYP2D6 | 0.0634 | 0.0284 | - | - | - | - | - |
| | Raloxifene | 81.5 | 15.7 | - | 1.1 | | | | | | | | |

[8]   PMDA Database.   http://www.pmda.go.jp/drugs/2014/P201400129/index.html (accessed Mar 2016).

*Continued*

| System | S9[a] | | | | Recombinant Human CYPs[b] | | | | | | | |
|---|---|---|---|---|---|---|---|---|---|---|---|---|
| Species | Inhibitor | % of Radioactivity | | | | Enzyme | Cl$_{int}$ (µL/min/pmoL CYP) | | | | | | |
| | | Ripasudil | M1 | M2 | M6 | | Ripasudil | M1 | M2 | M3 | M4 | M5 | M6 |
| Rabbit | Control | 82.6 | 13.6 | - | - | CYP3A4 | 0.135 | 0.108 | 0.402 | 0.0414 | 0.0676 | - | - |
| | Allopurinol | 85.2 | 11.5 | - | - | | | | | | | | |
| | Menadione | 96.2 | - | - | - | CYP3A5 | 0.250 | 0.0386 | 0.214 | 0.0248 | 0.132 | 0.0338 | 0.0332 |
| | Raloxifene | 95.5 | 1.8 | - | - | | | | | | | | |

Control: No inhibitor.   Allopurinol: Xanthine oxidase inhibitor.   Menadione: Aldehyde oxidase (AO) inhibitor.   Raloxifene: Potent AO inhibitor.
[a] 3 µM [$^{14}$C]ripasudil hydrochloride was added in liver S9 fraction of several species and incubated for 1 h, and the concentration of the inhibitors was 100 µM.
[b] 3 µM [$^{14}$C]ripasudil hydrochloride and metabolites were added in recombinant human CYPs and incubated for 20 min.

Table 16   Metabolites in Urine and Feces of Humans and Rats after Single Oral and Ophthalmic Dose[8]

| Matrix | Species | Route | Dose (mg/kg) | Time (h) | % of Radioactivity | | | | | | |
|---|---|---|---|---|---|---|---|---|---|---|---|
| | | | | | Ripasudil | M1 | M2 | M3 | M4 | M5 | M6 |
| Plasma | Rat | p.o. | 3[a] | 0.5 | 11.3 | 1.6 | 6.6 | 14.9 | 7.7 | 19.5 | 6.2[b] |
| | Human | o.u. | 0.8%[c] | 0-4 | √ | Major | - | - | - | - | √ |
| Urine | Rat | p.o. | 3[a] | 0-24 | 5.23 | 9.53 | 3.60 | 22.0 | 4.83 | 25.3 | 4.13 |
| | Human | o.u. | 0.4%[c] | 0-48 | 1.34 | 48.7 | - | - | - | - | √ |
| Feces | Rat | p.o. | 3[a] | 0-24 | 5.20 | 9.07 | 7.57 | 1.60 | - | - | 5.53 |

"√": Be observed.   [a] Vehicle: Water.   [b] Combination of the adjacent unidentified metabolites.   [c] Vehicle: Ophthalmic solution.

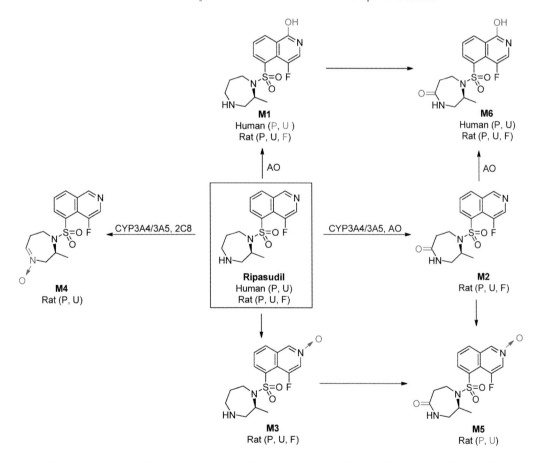

Figure F   Proposed Pathways for *In Vivo* Biotransformation of Ripasudil in Rats and Humans[8]
The red labels represent the major components in matrices.   P = Plasma, F = Feces, U = Urine and AO = Aldehyde Oxidase.

[8]   PMDA Database.   http://www.pmda.go.jp/drugs/2014/P201400129/index.html (accessed Mar 2016).

# Excretion

Table 17    Excretion Profiles of Ripasudil in Rats and Humans after Single Oral Dose[8]

| Species | Analyte | Route | State | Dose (mg/kg) | Time (h) | Bile (% of dose) | Urine (% of dose) | Feces (% of dose) | Recovery (% of dose) |
|---|---|---|---|---|---|---|---|---|---|
| SD rat (male) | Ripasudil | p.o. | Intact | 1 | 0-72 | - | 0.570 ± 0.160 | 0.324 ± 0.076 | 0.89 |
| | | p.o. | Intact | 3 | 0-72 | - | 2.32 ± 0.16 | 0.378 ± 0.201 | 2.70 |
| | | p.o. | Intact | 10 | 0-72 | - | 3.55 ± 1.05 | 0.693 ± 0.158 | 4.24 |
| SD rat (female) | | p.o. | Intact | 1 | 0-72 | - | 3.92 ± 1.94 | 0.190 ± 0.043 | 4.11 |
| | | p.o. | Intact | 3 | 0-72 | - | 4.35 ± 1.15 | 0.246 ± 0.177 | 4.60 |
| | | p.o. | Intact | 10 | 0-72 | - | 3.91 ± 1.11 | 0.218 ± 0.103 | 4.13 |
| SD rat (male) | Radioactivity | p.o. | Intact | 3 | 0-168 | - | 43.8 ± 12.7 | 42.1 ± 5.3 | 85.9 |
| SD rat (male) | Radioactivity | p.o. | BDC | 3 | 0-48 | 38.9 ± 5.3 | 46.0 ± 3.3 | 9.84 ± 1.55 | 94.7 |
| Human (male) | Ripasudil & M1 | o.u. | Intact | - | 0-48 | - | Major | NA | NA |

Vehicle: Water.    BDC: Bile duct-cannulated.

# Drug-Drug Interaction

Table 18    *In Vitro* Evaluation of Ripasudil Hydrochloride as an Inhibitor of Enzymes[8]

| Enzyme | Reaction | IC$_{50}$ without Pre-incubation (µM) | | IC$_{50}$ with Pre-incubation (µM) | |
|---|---|---|---|---|---|
| | | Ripasudil[a] | M1[a] | Ripasudil[a] | M1[a] |
| CYP1A2 | Phenacetin O-deethylation | >25 | >25 | >25 | >25 |
| CYP2C8 | Paclitaxel 6α-hydroxylase | >25 | >25 | >25 | >25 |
| CYP2C9 | Diclofenac 4'-hydroxylation | >25 | >25 | >25 | >25 |
| CYP2C19 | S-mephenytoin 4'-hydroxylation | >25 | >25 | >25 | >25 |
| CYP2D6 | Dextromethorphan O-demethylation | 5.1 | >25 | 3.8 | >25 |
| CYP3A4/5[a] | Testosterone 6β-hydroxylation | >25 | >25 | 14 | >25 |
| CYP3A4/5[b] | Midazolam 1'-hydroxylation | >25 | >25 | >25 | >25 |
| Aldehyde oxidase | - | 1.4[b] | - | - | - |

[a] The concentrations were 0.04, 0.2, 1, 5 and 25 µM.    [b] In this study, the concentration of ripasudil was 0.00064-10 µM.

[8]   PMDA Database.    http://www.pmda.go.jp/drugs/2014/P201400129/index.html (accessed Mar 2016).

Table 19 *In Vitro* Evaluation of Ripasudil Hydrochloride Hydrate as an Inducer of
CYP Enzymes in Human Cryopreserved Hepatocytes[8]

| Enzyme | Determination | Lot. | Fold Induction | | | | | | Positive Control |
| | | | Ripasudil Hydrochloride Hydrate | | | | | | |
| | | | 0.0032 μM | 0.016 μM | 0.08 μM | 0.4 μM | 2 μM | 10 μM | |
|---|---|---|---|---|---|---|---|---|---|
| CYP1A2 | Phenacetin *O*-deethylation | IPH | 0.98 ± 0.00 | 0.94 ± 0.11 | 1.07 ± 0.03 | 1.09 ± 0.08 | 1.12 ± 0.08 | 1.42 ± 0.07 | 6.98 ± 0.77 |
| | | VRS | 1.01 ± 0.04 | 1.04 ± 0.06 | 1.02 ± 0.12 | 1.01 ± 0.11 | 1.25 ± 0.10 | 1.48 ± 0.08 | 21.0 ± 0.8 |
| | | IZT | 0.99 ± 0.11 | 0.98 ± 0.03 | 0.88 ± 0.09 | 0.80 ± 0.12 | 0.92 ± 0.08 | 0.89 ± 0.08 | 12.6 ± 1.3 |
| CYP2B6 | Bupropion hydroxylation | IPH | 1.06 ± 0.05 | 0.98 ± 0.07 | 1.05 ± 0.13 | 1.01 ± 0.17 | 0.99 ± 0.03 | 1.10 ± 0.05 | 7.63 ± 0.61 |
| | | VRS | 1.30 ± 0.15 | 1.27 ± 0.05 | 1.19 ± 0.13 | 1.30 ± 0.14 | 1.32 ± 0.09 | 1.08 ± 0.08 | 28.3 ± 4.9 |
| | | IZT | 0.97 ± 0.13 | 1.01 ± 0.08 | 1.12 ± 0.07 | 1.24 ± 0.03 | 1.32 ± 0.03 | 1.36 ± 0.17 | 5.95 ± 0.08 |
| CYP3A4 | Testosterone 6β-hydroxylation | IPH | 1.09 ± 0.06 | 1.09 ± 0.05 | 1.09 ± 0.04 | 0.95 ± 0.06 | 0.90 ± 0.01 | 0.96 ± 0.10 | 12.8 ± 1.4 |
| | | VRS | 1.01 ± 0.02 | 0.93 ± 0.06 | 0.91 ± 0.04 | 0.84 ± 0.04 | 0.84 ± 0.06 | 0.75 ± 0.10 | 20.8 ± 0.9 |
| | | IZT | 0.94 ± 0.07 | 0.98 ± 0.06 | 0.90 ± 0.03 | 0.87 ± 0.05 | 0.75 ± 0.01 | 0.57 ± 0.04 | 6.16 ± 0.29 |
| | mRNA | IPH | 1.47 ± 0.22 | 1.01 ± 0.05 | 1.61 ± 0.35 | 1.70 ± 0.42 | 2.28 ± 0.36 | 5.57 ± 0.59 | 90.8 ± 21.8 |
| | | VRS | 0.97 ± 0.14 | 1.24 ± 0.26 | 0.93 ± 0.32 | 1.18 ± 0.21 | 1.20 ± 0.04 | 1.99 ± 0.10 | 16.7 ± 2.7 |
| | | IZT | 1.27 ± 0.23 | 1.21 ± 0.29 | 0.94 ± 0.35 | 1.18 ± 0.26 | 1.58 ± 0.28 | 1.68 ± 0.49 | 61.1 ± 6.0 |

# 5　Non-Clinical Toxicology

## Summary

### Single-Dose Toxicity
❖ Single-dose toxicity by the oral or intravenous route in mice, rats and dogs:
- Mouse ALD: 122 mg/kg (p.o.) and ≥20.4 mg/kg (i.v.).
- Rat ALD: 81.7 mg/kg (p.o.) and 20.4 mg/kg (i.v.).
- Dog MTD: <25 mg/kg in males and 18 mg/kg in females.

### Repeated-Dose Toxicity
❖ Repeated-dose toxicity studies by the eye-instillation or oral route in rabbits (26 weeks), dogs (up to 13 weeks), monkeys (52 weeks) and rats (4 weeks):
- For rabbits: The NOAEL was 1.0% (BID, o.l.), determined by the 26-week study.　There was no mortality at all doses after ocular instillation, and clinical signs included hyperemia of the bulbar and palpebral conjunctiva, and white spots of the lens.
- For dogs: The NOAEL was 2.0% (QID, o.l.) and 7.5 mg/kg/day (p.o.), determined by the 13-week study.　There was no mortality after oral administration or ocular instillation, and clinical signs mainly included hyperemia of the bulbar and palpebral conjunctiva and exposure of nictitating membranes.
- For monkeys: The NOAEL was 2.0% (QID, o.l.), determined by the 52-week study.　There were mortalities observed.
- For rats: The NOAEL was 10 and 30 mg/kg/day (p.o.) for males and females, determined by the 4-week study.　There were mortalities at oral administration of 90 mg/kg/day, and clinical signs including hyperplasia of bile duct, increased BW, and prolonged PT.

### Safety Pharmacology
❖ Both *in vitro* and *in vivo* safety pharmacology studies to assess the effects on neurological, cardiovascular and respiratory system:
- Neurological function: No effect was observed on general behavior or locomotor activity, but redness of the pinna and limbs in 3/4 cases and a transient and mild hypothermia were observed.
- Cardiovascular function: ↑ $APD_{50}$ (>0.82 μM); ↑ $APD_{70}$ and ↑ $APD_{90}$ (>8.2 μM); Significant reduction on the maximum rate of repolarization (82 μM).　The $IC_{50}$ of hERG potassium current inhibition was 39.5 μM.
- Respiratory function: No effects on respiratory function.

---

[8] PMDA Database.　http://www.pmda.go.jp/drugs/2014/P201400129/index.html (accessed Mar 2016).

Genotoxicity
* Ripasudil demonstrated no genotoxicity in all assays employed, i.e., Ames, *in vitro* chromosomal aberration, *in vivo* rat micronucleus or UDS assay.

Reproductive and Developmental Toxicity
* Fertility and early embryonic development in rats: No effects.
* Embryo-fetal development in rats and rabbits:
  * For rats: For the maternal: ↑ BWG and ↓ food consumption.    For the fetal: ↓ Live fetus, ↑ resorptions and post implantation loss, ↓ fetal weights, and high incidence of incompletely ossifications/delayed fetal ossification.
  * For rabbits: Continuous convulsions, tachypnea, ↓ locomotor activity, partly closed eyes, spasms, salivation, ↑ BW, ↓ food consumption.    There was no effect on fetal development.
* Pre- and postnatal development in rats:
  * For $F_0$: ↓ BWG and ↓ food consumption, related effect on fertility, ↓ birth rate, ↑ gestation period, no delivery signs and no mortalities in childbirth.
  * For $F_1$: Low fetal survival rate and suppressed postnatal development.
* Ripasudil could be excreted to milk in lactating rats.

Carcinogenicity
* Conventional carcinogenicity studies were not carried out, but ripasudil was convinced of no carcinogenic potential based on the following evidences:[8]
  * Ripasudil and M1 had a profile of rapid transition and elimination through systemic circulation, which indicated no accumulation in tissues.
  * Qualitative structure-activity relationship (QSAR, DEREK™) models gave no structural alert.
  * The negative results of *in vivo* genotoxicity studies got ripasudil less carcinogenic concern, so did no proliferative or precancerous lesion in the 52-week chronic toxicity study.
  * Ophthalmic solution of ripasudil hydrochloride hydrate did not cause inflammatory changes around the eyes.

Special toxicity
* Local irritation test: Conjunctival redness.
* No evidence on skin sensitization and phototoxicity.
* Local optic toxicity:
  * In rabbits, 2 HD (2.0%) females got opacity under the lens cortex shallow layer.    NOAEL: 2.0/1.0% BID (male/female).
  * In monkeys, no significant change.    NOAEL: 2.0% BID.

## Single-Dose Toxicity

Table 20    Single-Dose Toxicity Studies of Ripasudil Hydrochloride Hydrate[8]

| Species | Dosage (mg/kg) | ALD (mg/kg) | | Finding |
| --- | --- | --- | --- | --- |
| | | Male | Female | |
| CD-1 mouse | 122, p.o. | 122 | 122 | 122 mg/kg: Mortality (1 male and 1 female). |
| | 20.4, i.v. | 20.4 | >20.4 | 20.4 mg/kg: Mortality (1 male). Clinical sign (i.v.): Decreased locomotor activity, tachypnea, incomplete eye opening, piloerection, tremors, spasms and hypothermia. |
| SD rat | 0, 40.85, 81.70, 101.96, p.o. | 102 | 102 | 102 mg/kg: Mortality (3 males and 1 female). |
| | 20.4, i.v. | 20.4 | 20.4 | 20.4 mg/kg: Mortality in both sexes. Clinical signs: Red skin, crouching, piloerection, decreased locomotion activity, incomplete eye opening, tachypnea, abnormal gait, convulsions and spasms. |
| Beagle dog | Male: 25 (2 days) Female: 6.25 (3 days), 12.5 (4 days), 18 (4 days), p.o. | - | - | 25 mg/kg/day: Mortality (1 male and 1 female), ankylosing walk, convulsions, MTD: <25 mg/kg. |
| | | - | - | 12.5 and 18 mg/kg in females: Decreased locomotion activity and ankylosing walk, MTD: 18 mg/kg. |

[8]  PMDA Database.    http://www.pmda.go.jp/drugs/2014/P201400129/index.html (accessed Mar 2016).

## Repeated-Dose Toxicity

Table 21   Repeated-Dose Toxicity Studies of Ripasudil Hydrochloride Hydrate[8]

| Species | Duration (Week) | Daily Dose | NOAEL | Finding |
|---|---|---|---|---|
| Dutch rabbit | 26[a] | 0, 1.0%, 2.0%, QID, o.l. | NA | >1.0%: No mortality, hyperemia of the bulbar and palpebral conjunctiva, and white spots of the lens. |
| | 26[b] | 0, 0.5%, 1.0%, BID, o.l. | 1.0% | >0.5%: No mortality, hyperemia of the bulbar and palpebral conjunctiva. |
| Beagle dog | 4[d] | 2.0%, QID, o.d. | 2.0% | Hyperemia and exposure of nictitating membranes. |
| | 4 | 0, 3.75, 7.5, 15 mg/kg/day, p.o. | 3.75/7.5[c] | 3.75 mg/kg/day: Hyperemia of the bulbar and palpebral conjunctiva and exposure of nictitating membranes. 15 mg/kg/day: Severe spasms, tremors, decreased locomotion activity, ankylosing walk, staggering gait and tachypnea. |
| | 13[e] | 0, 1.0%, 2.0%, QID, o.l. | 2.0% | >1.0%: Hyperemia of the bulbar and palpebral conjunctiva. |
| | 13 | 3.75, 7.5 mg/kg/day, p.o. | 7.5 | None. |
| Cynomolgus monkey | 52[f] | 0 (QID), 1.0% (BID), 2.0% (BID), 2.0% (QID), o.l. | 2.0%, QID | 1.0%: Unclear boundaries and various sizes in corneal endothelium cells. 2.0% (BID): Mortality (1 female). 2.0% (QID): Mortality (1 female), hyperemia of the bulbar and palpebral conjunctiva. |
| SD rat | 4 | 0, 10, 30, 90 mg/kg/day, p.o. | 10/30[c] mg/kg/day | 10 mg/kg/day: Redness of the extremities. 30 mg/kg/day: Hypertrophy of centrilobular hepatocellular. 90 mg/kg/day: 3 deaths (male), hyperplasia of bile duct, increased BW, and prolonged PT. |

o.l.: Oculus laevus.   o.d.: Oculus dexter.   [a] 50 μL/eye/time in 2 h intervals.   [b] 50 μL/eye/time in 7-8 h intervals.   [c] Male/Female.   [d] 100 μL/eye/time in 4 h intervals.
[e] 100 μL/eye/time in 2 h intervals.   [f] 20 μL/eye/time twice per day in 7-8 h intervals, and four times per day in 2-3 h intervals.

## Safety Pharmacology

Table 22   Safety Pharmacology Studies of Ripasudil Hydrochloride Hydrate[8]

| Study | System | Dose | Finding |
|---|---|---|---|
| Cardiovascular effect | Beagle dog | 0.03, 0.3, 3 mg/kg, p.o. | No cardiovascular effect. |
| | Rabbit isolated purkinje fiber | 0.82-100 μM | >0.82 μM: ↑ $APD_{50}$. >8.2 μM: ↑ $APD_{70}$ and ↑ $APD_{90}$. 82 μM: Significant reduction on the maximum rate of rise. |
| | HEK293 cell expressing hERG | 1-1000 μM | $IC_{50}$ of hERG potassium current: 39.5 μM. |
| Respiratory effect | SD rat (male) | 0.3, 3, 30 mg/kg, p.o. | No effect on respiratory function. |
| Neurological effect | SD rat (male) | 0.3, 3, 30 mg/kg, p.o. | 30 mg/kg: No effect was observed on general behavior, locomotion activity, or redness of the pinna and limbs were observed in 3/4 cases. A transient and mild hypothermia after 90 and 150 min of administration. |

$APD_{50}$, $APD_{70}$ and $APD_{90}$: APD at 50%, 70% and 90% repolarization.

[8]   PMDA Database.   http://www.pmda.go.jp/drugs/2014/P201400129/index.html (accessed Mar 2016).

# Genotoxicity

Table 23    Genotoxicity Studies of Ripasudil Hydrochloride Hydrate[8]

| Assay | Species/System | Metabolism Activity | Dose | Finding |
|---|---|---|---|---|
| In vitro bacterial reverse mutation assay (Ames) | S. typhimurium TA98, TA100, TA1535, TA1537; E. coli WP2 uvrA | ±S9 | 4-4080 μg/plate | Negative. |
| In vitro mammalian cell chromosome aberration assay | HPBL | ±S9 | -S9: 36.5, 73, 146 μg/mL +S9: 292, 584, 1168 μg/mL | Negative. |
| In vivo rodent micronucleus assay | SD rat | + | 0, 25, 50, 100 mg/kg/day, p.o. for 2 days | Negative. |
| In vivo UDS test | Corneal epithelial cell in JW Rabbit | - | Single, 0, 1.0%, 2.0%, o.u. | Negative. |

Vehicle: DMSO for in vivo assays.    o.u.: Oculus uterque.    UDS: Unscheduled DNA Synthesis.

# Reproductive and Developmental Toxicity

Table 24    Reproductive and Developmental Toxicology Studies of Ripasudil Hydrochloride Hydrate by Oral Administration[8]

| Study | Species | Dose (mg/kg/day) | NOAEL Endpoint | NOAEL (mg/kg/day) | $AUC_{0-24}$ (ng·h/mL) | Safety Margin[a] (× MRHD) | Finding |
|---|---|---|---|---|---|---|---|
| Fertility and early embryonic development | SD rat | 0, 3, 10, 30 | Male/Female fertility | 30 | NA | NA | No effect on fertility (in both sexes) up to 30 mg/kg/day. |
| | | | Early embryo | 30 | NA | NA | No effect on early embryonic development up to 30 mg/kg/day. |
| Embryo-fetal development | SD rat | 0, 3, 10, 30 | Maternal/Fetal | 10 | 1170 | 2303 | $F_0$: ↑ BWG and ↓ food consumption at HD. $F_1$: ↓ Live fetus, ↑ resorptions and post implantation loss, ↓ fetal weights, and high incidence of incomplete/delayed fetal ossification at HD. |
| | NZW rabbit | 0, 3, 10, 30 | Maternal | 10 | 276 | 543 | $F_0$: Continuous convulsions, tachypnea, ↓ locomotion activity, partly closed eyes, spasms, salivation, ↑ BW, ↓ food consumption at HD. $F_1$: No effects on fetal development. |
| | | | Fetal | 30 | 2770 | 5453 | |
| Pre- and postnatal development | SD rat | 0, 3, 10, 30 | $F_0/F_1$ | 10 | 1170 | 2303 | $F_0$: ↓ BWG and ↓ food consumption, related effect on fertility, ↓ birth rate, ↑ gestation period, no delivery signs, deaths in childbirth at HD. $F_1$: ↓ Average birth number, ↓ birth rate and ↓ BW at HD. |

[a] Safety margins were based on human exposure of 0.508 μg·h/mL at 0.4% (BID) of ripasudil HCl after instillation.

Table 25    Transfer to Milk After Oral Administration of 3 mg/kg [$^{14}$C]Ripasudil Hydrochloride to Lactating Rats[8]

| Parameter | Analyte | %Radioactivity | | | |
|---|---|---|---|---|---|
| | | 0.25 h | 1 h | 3 h | 6 h |
| Milk | Ripasudil HCl | 68.1 | 26.9 | 10.4 | 16.9 |
| | M1 | 3.11 | 10.4 | 9.43 | 10.1 |
| | M2 | 16.9 | 27.8 | 17.2 | 6.70 |
| Plasma | Ripasudil HCl | 38.9 | 26.8 | 18.7 | 19.2 |
| | M1 | 2.99 | 3.68 | 3.70 | 7.06 |
| | M2 | 19.9 | 25.0 | 25.3 | 20.9 |

M1 and M2: The major metabolites.

[8]  PMDA Database.   http://www.pmda.go.jp/drugs/2014/P201400129/index.html (accessed Mar 2016).

# Special Toxicity

Table 26    Local Irritation Tests of Ripasudil Hydrochloride Hydrate[8]

| Study | Species | Duration | Dose/Route | Finding |
|---|---|---|---|---|
| Primary rabbit eye mucous membrane irritation test | Rabbit | 1 day | 2.0% o.d. 50 μL × 8 times/day, instillation | A mild irritation, conjunctival redness. |
| Rabbit eye mucosa cumulative irritation test | Rabbit | 2 weeks | 2.0% o.d., 50 μL × QID, instillation | Redness of the conjunctiva, and no confirmed cumulative irritation. |

Table 27    Skin Sensitization Tests of Ripasudil Hydrochloride Hydrate[8]

| Study | Species | Test Article | Dose (w/v%) | Dpm/node[c] | SI | Result |
|---|---|---|---|---|---|---|
| Local lymph node proliferation test | Mouse | Dimethylformamide[a] | 0 | 114 | NA | - |
| | | Ripasudil hydrochloride hydrate | 0.82 | 196 | 1.7 | Negative. |
| | | | 4.08 | 250 | 2.2 | Negative. |
| | | | 8.17 | 202 | 1.8 | Negative. |
| | | Hexyl cinnamic aldehyde[b] | 25 | 2551 | 22.4 | Positive. |

[a] Negative control.    [b] Positive control.    [c] One minute of radioactive decay of 3HTdR per lymph node.    SI: Stimulation index.

Table 28    Phototoxicity Studies of Ripasudil Hydrochloride Hydrate[8]

| Study | Species | Test Article | Dose (w/v%) | UV Irradiation | Dpm/node[c] | SI | Result |
|---|---|---|---|---|---|---|---|
| Lymph node proliferation test under local light irradiation | Mouse | Dimethylformamide[a] | 0 | No | 114 | NA | - |
| | | Ripasudil hydrochloride hydrate | 8.17 | No | 280 | 2.1 | Negative. |
| | | Tetrachlorosalicylanilide[b] | 1.0 | No | 5859 | 43.8 | Positive. |
| | | Dimethylformamide[a] | 0 | Yes | 235 | NA | - |
| | | Ripasudil hydrochloride hydrate | 0.82 | Yes | 247 | 1.1 | Negative. |
| | | | 4.08 | Yes | 276 | 1.2 | Negative. |
| | | | 8.17 | Yes | 323 | 1.4 | Negative. |
| | | Tetrachlorosalicylanilide[b] | 1.0 | Yes | 13962 | 59.5 | Positive. |

[a] Negative control.    [b] Positive control.    [c] One minute of radioactive decay of 3HTdR per lymph node.    SI: Stimulation index.

Table 29    Local Optic Toxicity of Ripasudil Hydrochloride Hydrate[8]

| Species | Duration (week) | Dose/Route | Finding |
|---|---|---|---|
| Rabbit | 13 | 0, 0.5 %, 1.0 %, 2.0 %, BID, instillation | 2 females at 2.0% (BID) observed opacity under the lens cortex shallow layer. NOAEL: 2.0/1.0% BID (male/female). |
| Monkey | 13 | 0, 0.5 %, 1.0 %, 2.0 %, BID, instillation | No significant change. NOAEL: 2.0% BID. |

[8]    PMDA Database.    http://www.pmda.go.jp/drugs/2014/P201400129/index.html (accessed Mar 2016).

# CHAPTER

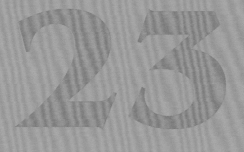

## Suvorexant

# Suvorexant

## (Belsomra®)

Research code: MK-4305

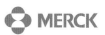

## 1 General Information

❖ Suvorexant is an orexin receptor (OXR) antagonist, which was first approved in Aug 2014 by FDA of US.

❖ Suvorexant was discovered, developed and marketed by Merck & Co.

❖ Suvorexant is an orexin receptor antagonist which is thought to suppress wake drive, blocking the binding of wake-promoting neuropeptides orexin A and orexin B to OX1R and OX2R.

❖ Suvorexant is indicated for the treatment of insomnia, characterized by difficulties with sleep onset and/or sleep maintenance.

❖ Available as tablet, with each containing 5, 10, 15 or 20 mg of suvorexant and the recommended dose is 10 mg per night.

❖ The sale of Belsomra® was not available up to Mar 2016.

### Key Approvals around the World*

|  | US (FDA) | Japan (PMDA) |
|---|---|---|
| First approval date | 08/13/2014 | 09/26/2014 |
| Application or approval No. | NDA 204569 | 22600AMX01302000; 22600AMX01303000 |
| Brand name | Belsomra® | Belsomra® |
| Indication | Insomnia | Insomnia |
| Authorisation holder | Merck & Co. | Merck & Co. |

* Till Mar 2016, it had not been approved by EMA (EU) and CFDA (China).

## Active Ingredient

*Molecular formula*: $C_{23}H_{23}ClN_6O_2$
*Molecular weight*: 450.92
*CAS No.*: 1030377-33-3 (Suvorexant)
*Chemical name*: [(7R)-4-(5-chloro-2-benzoxazolyl) hexahydro-7-methyl-1H-1,4-diazepin-1-yl][5-methyl-2-(2H-1,2,3-triazol-2-yl)phenyl]methanone

*Parameters of Lipinski's "Rule of 5"*

| MW | $H_D$ | $H_A$ | FRB[a] | PSA[a] | cLogP[a] |
|---|---|---|---|---|---|
| 450.92 | 0 | 8 | 3 | 80.3Å² | 3.27 ± 0.74 |

[a] Calculated by ACD/Labs software V11.02.

## Drug Product*

*Dosage route*: Oral
*Strength*: 5 mg/10 mg/15 mg/20 mg (Suvorexant)
*Dosage form*: Film-coated tablet
*Inactive ingredient*: Polyvinylpyrrolidone/vinyl acetate copolymer (copovidone), microcrystalline cellulose, lactose monohydrate, croscarmellose sodium, magnesium stearate, hypromellose, titanium dioxide, iron oxide (5 mg) and triacetin.
*Recommended dose*: The recommended dose of suvorexant is 10 mg, taken no more than once per night and within 30 mins of going to bed, with at least 7 h remaining before the planned time of awakening. If the 10 mg dose is well-tolerated but not effective, the dose can be increased. The maximum recommended dose is 20 mg once daily.

* Sourced from US FDA drug label information

# 2 Key Patents Information

## Summary

❖ Belsomra® (Suvorexant) has got five-year NCE market exclusivity protection after it was initially approved by US FDA on Aug 13, 2014.

❖ Suvorexant was originally discovered by Merck & Co., and its compound patent application was filed as PCT application by Merck & Co. in 2007.

❖ The compound patent will expire in 2027 foremost, which has been granted in the United States, Europe, China and Japan successively.

Table 1    Suvorexant's Compound Patent Protection in Drug-Mainstream Country

| Country | Publication/Patent NO. | Application Date | Granted Date | Estimated Expiry Date |
|---------|------------------------|------------------|--------------|-----------------------|
| WO | WO2008069997A1 | 11/30/2007 | / | / |
| US | US7951797B2 | 11/30/2007 | 05/31/2011 | 11/20/2029[a] |
| EP | EP2089382B1 | 11/30/2007 | 10/24/2012 | 11/30/2027 |
| JP | JP4675427B2 | 11/30/2007 | 11/06/2013 | 07/21/2031[b] |
| CN | CN101627028B | 11/30/2007 | 03/27/2013 | 11/30/2027 |
| | CN101880276B | 11/30/2007 | 06/19/2013 | 11/30/2027 |

[a] The term of this patent is extended by 721 days.    [b] The term of this patent is extended by 1329 days.

Table 2    Originator's International Patent Application List (Patent Family)

| Publication NO. | Title | Applicant/Assignee/Owner | Publication Date |
|-----------------|-------|--------------------------|------------------|
| **Technical Subjects** | **Active Ingredient (Free Base)'s Formula or Structure and Preparation** | | |
| WO2008069997A1 | Substituted diazepan compounds as orexin receptor antagonists | Merck & Co. | 06/12/2008 |
| **Technical Subjects** | **Salt, Crystal, Polymorphic, Solvate (Hydrate), Isomer, Derivative Etc. and Preparation** | | |
| WO2012148553A1 | Process for the preparation of an orexin receptor antagonist | Merck & Co. | 11/01/2012 |
| WO2013169610A1 | Process for the preparation of an intermediate for an orexin receptor antagonist | Merck & Co. | 11/14/2013 |
| WO2015164160A1 | Pharmaceutical salts of an orexin receptor antagonist | Merck & Co. | 10/29/2015 |
| **Technical Subjects** | **Formulation and Preparation** | | |
| WO2013181174A2 | Solid dosage formulations of an orexin receptor antagonist | Merck & Co. | 12/05/2013 |
| WO2015120014A1 | Novel disintegration systems for pharmaceutical dosage forms | Merck & Co. | 08/13/2015 |

The data was updated until Jan 2016.

# 3 Chemistry

## Route 1: Original Discovery Route

DEA: Diethylamine

*Synthesis Route*: As illustrated in top scheme, this modified route provided a related strategy utilizing the commercially available *N*-Boc-1,2-diaminoethane **1** as a surrogate for the azide. Conjugate addition of the monoprotected diamine to methyl vinyl ketone **2** followed by *in situ* trapping with benzyl chloroformate provided ketone **3**. Boc-deprotection and subsequent intramolecular reductive amination with NaBH(OAc)₃ constructed the diazepane ring. A Boc group was reinstalled to simplify purification, resulting in a 38% overall yield of **5** for the four steps from methyl vinyl ketone. Significantly, this chemistry could be carried out on a large scale to provide access to quantities of **5** for analogue synthesis and *in vivo* evaluation of leading compounds. A chiral stationary phase HPLC resolution was then introduced to racemic **5** to provide the desired (*R*)-enantiomer **6** as the first eluting isomer with >98% *ee*. Boc deprotection followed by amide coupling to 2-(2*H*-1,2,3-triazol-2-yl)-5-methylbenzoic acid **8** provided amide **9** in 87% yield. Removal of the benzyl carbamate followed by reaction with 2,5-dichlorobenzoxazole **11**, was required for the final generation of suvorexant.[1-4]

During this, 2-iodo-5-methylbenzoic acid **12** and 1,2,3-triazole **13** went through modified Buchwald-Hartwig coupling reaction to generate benzoic acid **8**.[1-4]

[1] Bergman, J. M.; Breslin; M. J.; Coleman, P. J., et al. WO2008069997A1, **2008**.
[2] Bergman, J. M.; Breslin; M. J.; Coleman, P. J., et al. US20080132490A1, **2008**.
[3] Cox, C. D.; Breslin, M. J.; Whitman D. B., et al. *J. Med. Chem.* **2010**, *53*, 5320-5332.
[4] Baxter, C. A.; Cleator, E.; Krska, S. W., et al. WO2012148553A1, **2012**.

## Route 2

DMEAD: Bis(2-methoxyethyl) azodicarboxylate

*Synthesis Route*:    This chiral controlled synthesis began with the preparation of β-amino ester **3** derived from conjugate addition of (*R*)-*N*-benzyl-1-phenylethanamine **1** to (*E*)-methyl but-2-enoate **2** with 85% yield and 95% *de*, which was then converted to amide **5** under thermal conditions in 81% yield.    Reduction of the amide **3** followed by treatment of the resultant amine with Boc₂O gave rise to the alcohol **6** with a two-step yield of 73%.    Global deprotection of both benzyl and phenethyl protective groups with Pearlman's catalyst afforded the corresponding amine, which was transformed into sulfonamide **7** in 79% yield over two steps.    After screening of the condensation agents under the Mitsunobu reaction conditions, the authors found in the case of DMEAD, a clean reaction proceeded and resulted in the desired (*R*)-1,4-diazepane **8** in good yield (96%). Removal of the nosyl group on **8** afforded the secondary amine **9**, which was treated with 2-(2*H*-1,2,3-triazol-2-yl)-5-methyl-benzoic acid **10** under coupling conditions to give rise to amide **11**.    Finally, general Boc deprotection conditions and condensation with 2,5-dihalobenzoxazole **12** furnished the titled compound with the yield of 81% across two steps and the overall yield of 26%.[5-7]

[5]  Minehira, D.; Takahara, S.; Adachi, I., et al. *Tetrahedron Lett.* **2014**, *55*, 5778-5780.
[6]  Davies, S. G.; Icbibara, O. *Tetrahedron: Assymetr.* **1991**, *2*, 183-186.
[7]  Chen, Y.; Zhou, Y.; Li, J., et al. *Chin. Chem. Lett.* **2015**, *26*, 103-107.

# Route 3

*Synthesis Route:* For the preparation of the diazepine-containing portion of suvorexant, the synthesis commenced with the condensation of commercial 2-amino-4-chlorophenol **1** with thiophosgene **2** to furnish benzoxazole **3** in 90% yield. Next, thiol **3** was converted to the corresponding chloride **4** prior to exposure to Boc-protected ethylenediamine **5** under basic conditions, and this was followed by a Michael addition of the resultant aminobenzoxazole **6** and methyl vinyl ketone **7**. The result of this sequence of reactions delivered aminobenzoxazole ketone **8** in 75% yield over three steps. Next, subjection of the carbamate **8** to methanesulfonic acid removed the Boc functionality and was followed by an intramolecular reductive amination sequence to construct the diazaepine ring. Acid-base workup ultimately provided the racemic diazepine **10** in 92% yield from **8**. Furtherly, resolution with a benzoyl tartaric acid **11** and subsequent recrystallization using isopropyl acetate and methanol at ambient temperature afforded the tartrate salt **12** in poor yield (27%) but excellent enantiomeric excess (96% *ee*). Salt **12** was freebased using sodium hydroxide prior to exposure to the crude acyl chloride under basic conditions to ultimately deliver suvorexant in 95% yield and with 98.5% *ee* across the two-step sequence.[8-10]

# 4 Pharmacology

# Summary

## Mechanism of Action

❖ Suvorexant is a proposed selective and potent orexin receptor (OXR) antagonist, which had high binding affinity for human OX1R ($K_i$ = 0.55 nM, IC$_{50}$ = 50 nM) and OX2R ($K_i$ = 0.35 nM, IC$_{50}$ = 55 nM), broadly expressed in cortical, thalamic and hypothalamic brain areas. Suvorexant blocks the binding of wake-promoting neuropeptides orexin A and orexin B to receptors OX1R and OX2R, which is thought to suppress wake drive.

❖ The metabolites of suvorexant were found to bind to human OX1R (M9, $K_i$ = 4.1 nM; M16, $K_i$ = 54.7 nM; M17, $K_i$ = 355 nM) and OX2R (M9, $K_i$ = 2.2 nM; M16, $K_i$ = 4.5 nM; M17, $K_i$ = 46.5 nM).

❖ Suvorexant had affinities for a number of targets at the monoamine transporter ($K_i$ = 4.2 μM), A3 receptor ($K_i$ = 3.9 μM), and the dopamine transporter ($K_i$ = 3.8 μM) in a panel of *in vitro* radioligand binding assays for 170 GPCRs, transporters, ion channels and enzymes.

[8]  Baxter, C. A.; Cleator, E.; Brands, K. M. J., et al. *Org. Process Res. Dev.* **2011**, *15*, 367-375.
[9]  Fleitz, F.; Mangion, I.; Yin, J., et al. WO2013169610A1, **2013**.
[10] Mangion, I. K.; Sherry, B. D.; Yin, J., et al. *Org. Lett.* **2012**, *14*, 3458-3461.

*In Vivo* Efficacy
- ❖ Orexin receptor occupancy in brain:
  - OX2R was dose-dependent occupancy in the brain of transgenic rats.
  - 90% receptor occupancy:
    - ◆ Plasma: Conc. = 1228 nM.
    - ◆ Brain: Conc. = 1291 nM.
- ❖ Locomotor activity in rat:
  - 30 mg/kg: Reduced 28% cumulative locomotor activity (plasma conc. = 5.6 µM).
  - 60 mg/kg: Reduced 44% cumulative locomotor activity (plasma conc. = 9.5 µM).
- ❖ Electroencephalography (EEG):
  - In rats:
    - ◆ Significantly increased the delta sleep and REM sleep in a dose-dependent manner.
    - ◆ Significantly decreased the length of the active awakening and shallow sleep.
  - In dogs:
    - ◆ Reduced the awake time.
    - ◆ Increased delta sleep, SWS sleep I and REM sleep.
  - In monkeys:
    - ◆ Reduced the awake time.
    - ◆ Increased delta sleep and REM sleep.

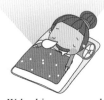

Wake drive suppressed

## Mechanism of Action

Table 3    The Binding Affinity and Inhibition of Suvorexant at Orexin Receptors[11, 12]

| Receptor | Resource | Binding and Efficacy | | | | |
|---|---|---|---|---|---|---|
| | | $K_{on}$ (M$^{-1}$·min$^{-1}$) | $K_{off}$ (min$^{-1}$) | $K_i$ (nM) | $K_b$ (nM) | IC$_{50}$ (nM) |
| OX1R | Human[a] | $4.9 \times 10^7$ | 0.0085 | 0.55 ± 0.095 | 65 ± 8.2 | 49.9 ± 2.6 |
| | Rat | NA | NA | 0.56 ± 0.08 | 61 ± 8.3 | 35.1 ± 2.1 |
| | Dog | NA | NA | 0.41 ± 0.05 | 86 ± 9.4 | NA |
| | Mouse | NA | NA | 0.62 ± 0.10 | 53 ± 10.1 | NA |
| | Rabbit | NA | NA | 1.2 ± 0.11 | 76 ± 9 | NA |
| | Rhesus monkey | NA | NA | 2.1 ± 0.22 | 51 ± 6.7 | NA |
| OX2R | Human[a] | $7.63 \times 10^6$ | 0.007784 | 0.35 ± 0.057 | 41 ± 1.3 | 54.8 ± 4.2 |
| | Rat | NA | NA | 0.36 ± 0.03 | 96 ± 6.5 | 38.1 ± 2.2 |
| | Dog | NA | NA | 0.48 ± 0.06 | 68 ± 10.3 | NA |
| | Mouse | NA | NA | 0.65 ± 0.05 | 38 ± 12.8 | NA |
| | Rabbit | NA | NA | 0.32 ± 0.04 | 93 ± 15.9 | NA |
| | Rhesus monkey | NA | NA | 0.68 ± 0.07 | 80 ± 14.6 | NA |

$K_b$ = [antagonist]/(($EC_{50}$ + antagonist/$EC_{50}$)-1).    [a] Data from stably transfected CHO line and expressed as mean ± SEM.

[11] Japan Pharmaceuticals and Medical Devices Agency (PMDA) Database.   http://www.pmda.go.jp/drugs/2014/P201400117/index.html (accessed Mar 2016).
[12] U.S. Food and Drug Administration (FDA) Database.   http://www.accessdata.fda.gov/drugsatfda_docs/nda/2014/204569Orig1s000PharmR.pdf. (accessed Mar 2016).

Table 4    Inhibition of the Metabolites of Suvorexant against Orexin Receptors[11]

| Receptor | Resource | $K_i$ (nM) | | | IC$_{50}$ (nM) | | |
|---|---|---|---|---|---|---|---|
| | | M9 | M16 | M17 | M9 | M16 | M17 |
| OX1R | Human | 4.1 | 54.7 | 355 | 35.0 | 59.8 | 233 |
| | Rat | NA | NA | NA | 36.4 | 43.5 | 127 |
| OX2R | Human | 2.2 | 4.5 | 46.5 | 79.2 | 45.7 | 232 |
| | Rat | NA | NA | NA | 34.9 | 37.8 | 152 |

M9, M16 and M17 were the metabolites.    n = 6 for all assays not noted above.

Table 5    The Off Targets Activity of Suvorexant in Radioligand Binding Assays[11, 12]

| Target | IC$_{50}$ (μM) | Target | IC$_{50}$ (μM) |
|---|---|---|---|
| Monoamine transporter | 4.2 | Na$^+$ channel | 7 |
| A3 receptor | 3.9 | hERG | 5.5 |
| Dopamine transporter | 3.8 | | |

Suvorexant was evaluated in a panel of *in vitro* radioligand binding assays for 170 GPCRs, transporters, ion channels and enzymes.

## *In Vivo* Efficacy

Table 6    *In Vivo* Effects of Suvorexant[11, 12]

| Study | Model Animal | Model Vehicle | Dose (mg/kg/day) | Route & Duration (Day) | Finding |
|---|---|---|---|---|---|
| Orexin receptor occupancy of brain | Rat | NA | NA | i.v., single dose (continuous 30 min) | Dose-dependent OX2R occupancy in the brain of transgenic rats. 90% receptor occupancy: Plasma: Conc. = 1228 nM. Brain: Conc. = 1291 nM. |
| Locomotor activity | SD rat | PEG200 | 10, 20, 30, 60 | i.p., single dose | Reduced cumulative locomotor activity after 1 h: 28% at 30 mg/kg (plasma conc. = 5.6 μM). 44% at 60 mg/kg (plasma conc. = 9.5 μM). Significant inhibition on spontaneous momentum of rats in a dose-dependent manner (reversible). |
| EEG | Rat | 20% TPGS | 10, 30, 100 | p.o., 18[a] | Significantly increased the delta sleep and REM sleep in a dose-dependent manner. Significantly decreased the length of the active awakening and shallow sleep at the same time. |
| | | PEG200 | 30 mg/kg | p.o., 7 or 3 | Significantly sleep-promoting effect in front of the dark or dark period. |
| | | | 60 mg/kg | i.p., 7 or 3 | |
| | Dog | PEG400 | 1, 3 | p.o., QD × 5 or 7 | Decreased the overall activity arousal time (30% by 3 mg/kg, 22% by 1 mg/kg). Increased SWS sleep I (96% by 3 mg/kg, 61% by 1 mg/kg). Increased delta sleep (150% by 3 mg/kg, 67% by 1 mg/kg). Increased REM sleep (47% by 3 mg/kg, 19% by 1 mg/kg). |
| | Monkey | 0.5% Methylcellulose, PEG200, DMSO | 10, 30 | p.o., QD × 7 | Reduced the awake time. Increased delta sleep and REM sleep. |
| | | | 0.5 | i.v., QD × 2 | |

EEG: Electroencephalography.    SWS: Slow wave sleep.    REM: Rapid eye movement.    [a] 18 days for a total that 2 days with no administration, 2 days with medium, and 7 days of replacing the drug-media administration.

[11]  PMDA Database.    http://www.pmda.go.jp/drugs/2014/P201400117/index.html (accessed Mar 2016).
[12]  FDA Database.    http://www.accessdata.fda.gov/drugsatfda_docs/nda/2014/204569Orig1s000PharmR.pdf (accessed Mar 2016).

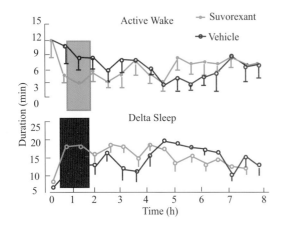

Figure A    The Effect of Suvorexant on Wake Time in Rats[12]

**Study:** The effect of suvorexant on active time and delta sleep.

**Animal:** Rat.

**Administration:** Suvorexant, single i.p. for 60 mg/kg.    Vehicle: PEG200.

**Test:** The duration of active time and delta sleep post-dose.

**Results:** Suvorexant reduced the awake time and increased delta sleep, 1 h before the normal active period.

# 5    ADME & Drug-Drug Interaction

## Summary

### Absorption of Suvorexant

❖ Exhibited a non-linear pharmacokinetics in humans following oral dosing.    The increase in $AUC_{inf}$ appeared to be less than dose-proportional in the dose range of 10 to 80 mg suvorexant.

❖ Had moderate oral bioavailability in dogs (33.9%) and rats (48.2%).

❖ Was absorbed moderately in humans ($T_{max}$ = 1.0-2 h), but rapidly in rats (0.4 h) and dogs (0.7 h), after oral administrations.

❖ Showed a half-life ranging between 8.9-13.5 h in humans, much longer than that in rats (0.8 h) and dogs (3.8 h), after intravenous administrations.

❖ Had moderate system clearance in humans (48.6-80.6 mL/min) and rats (35.3 mL/min/kg), but low in dogs (3.5 mL/min/kg), in contrast to liver blood flow, after intravenous administrations.

❖ Exhibited an extensive distribution in humans, rats and dogs, with apparent volumes of distribution at 36.5-57.3 L, 1.9 L/kg and 1.3 L/kg, respectively, after intravenous administrations.

❖ Showed a high permeability, with a $Papp_{(A→B)}$ of $(22.8-25.9) × 10^{-6}$ cm/s at 0.5-5 μM in LLC-PK1 cell monolayer model.

### Distribution of Suvorexant

❖ Exhibited high plasma protein binding with unbound fraction 0.3%-4.4% in mice, rats, rabbits, dogs and humans.    The metabolites M9 and M17 were also bounded highly to plasma proteins in animals and humans.    Note that suvorexant was highly bound to both human serum albumin and $α_1$-acid glycoprotein.

❖ Had a $C_b$:$C_p$ ratio of 0.59-0.68 in humans, suggesting low penetration into red blood cells.    The metabolite M9 had a similar distribution to red blood cells in humans.

❖ Sprague-Dawley rats and Long-Evans rats following single oral administrations:
  • Suvorexant was widely distributed into tissues in rats, except for central nervous system.
  • Relatively higher concentration levels were observed in adrenal gland, bile, liver, urine, cecum intestine contents, large intestine contents, small intestine contents, renal medulla and renal cortex of the male.    It was similar between Sprague-Dawley rats and Long-Evans rats.    No apparent retention in pigmented tissues (eyes and skin).
  • In addition to the liver, elimination was complete in the majority of tissues at 168 h post-dose.
  • Some accumulation was observed in the liver.

### Metabolism of Suvorexant

❖ Three major metabolites (M8, M9 and M10a) were generated in rat, dog and human liver microsomes.    In human hepatocytes, the major metabolites were M4, M7b and M9.

❖ Suvorexant was eliminated almost entirely through metabolism in humans, primarily by CYP3A, with less extent by CYP2C19.

❖ The major components were M9 and parent in human plasma.    The major metabolic pathways of suvorexant in humans included oxidation and glucuronidation.

❖ M9 did not penetrate into the brain.    M9 was not expected to be active *in vivo* based on results from *in vitro* and EEG studies in dogs.

---

[12]    FDA Database.    http://www.accessdata.fda.gov/drugsatfda_docs/nda/2014/204569Orig1s000PharmR.pdf. (accessed Mar 2016).

❖ All of the human circulating metabolites were also detected in the plasma of preclinical species including mice, rats, rabbits, dogs and monkeys, except for M17 which was not present in rat plasma.

## Excretion of Suvorexant

❖ Was predominantly excreted in feces in humans after oral administrations.

❖ In Sprague-Dawley rats, oral administered of [$^{14}$C]suvorexant resulted in 84% excreted in the bile, and approximately 10% excreted in urine and feces.

❖ In Beagle dogs, oral administration of [$^{14}$C]suvorexant resulted in 33% excreted in the bile, 10% in the urine, and 42% in the feces.

## Drug-Drug Interaction

❖ In human liver microsomes, suvorexant was a moderate inhibitor of CYPs 3A4 (IC$_{50}$ = 4.0 μM) and 2C19 (IC$_{50}$ = 5.3 μM), and a weak inhibitor of CYPs 1A2, 2B6, 2C8, 2C9 and 2D6 (IC$_{50}$ ≥15 μM).

❖ M9 was a moderate inhibitor of CYP3A4 (IC$_{50}$ = 11 μM for testosterone and 26 μM for midazolam), and a weak inhibitor of CYPs 1A2, 2B6, 2C8, 2C9, 2C19 and 2D6 (IC$_{50}$ ≥35 μM).

❖ M17 was a weak inhibitor of CYPs 2C9, 2D6 and 3A4 (IC$_{50}$ ≥28 μM).

❖ In cryopreserved human hepatocytes, suvorexant increased CYPs 3A4, 1A2 and 2B6 mRNA levels, showing that suvorexant can induce these CYPs.

❖ Suvorexant was not a substrate of P-gp. However, the metabolites M9 was a P-gp substrate. Suvorexant inhibited P-gp with an IC$_{50}$ of 18.7 μM.

❖ Suvorexant inhibited OCT2 with an IC$_{50}$ of 1.3 μM. Suvorexant and M9 had IC$_{50}$ values >10 μM at the human transporters OATP1B1 and BCRP.

# Absorption

Table 7    *In Vivo* Pharmacokinetic Parameters of Suvorexant in Rats and Dogs
after Single Intravenous and Oral Dose of Suvorexant[11, 12]

| Species | Route | Dose (mg/kg) | Vehicle | T$_{max}$ (h) | C$_{max}$ (μM) | AUC$_{inf}$ (μM·h) | T$_{1/2}$ (h) | Cl (mL/min/kg) | V$_{ss}$ (L/kg) | F (%) |
|---|---|---|---|---|---|---|---|---|---|---|
| SD rat (male) | i.v. | 3 | DMSO | NA | NA | 4.9 ± 4.4 | 0.8 ± 0.2 | 35.3 ± 21.2 | 1.9 ± 1.1 | - |
| | p.o. | 10 | 20% Vitamin E-TPGS | 0.4 | 2.3 | 7.9 | NA | NA | NA | 48.2 |
| Beagle dog (male) | i.v. | 2 | DMSO | NA | NA | 26.3 ± 16.7 | 3.8 ± 1.1 | 3.5 ± 1.7 | 1.3 ± 0.5 | - |
| | p.o. | 5 | 20% Vitamin E-TPGS | 0.7 ± 0.3 | 3.2 ± 0.7 | 22.3 ± 4.0 | NA | NA | NA | 33.9 ± 6.0 |

Mean ± SD.    DMSO: Dimethylsulfoxide.    Vitamin E-TPGS: Vitamin E polyethylene glycol succinate.

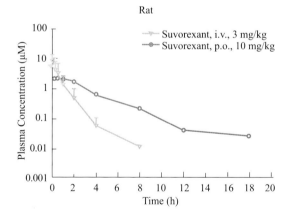
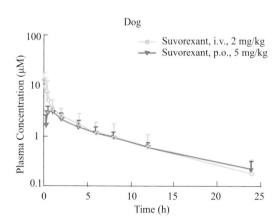

Figure B    *In Vivo* Plasma Concentration-Time Profiles of Suvorexant in Rats (n = 5) and
Dogs (n = 6) after Single Intravenous and Oral Dose of Suvorexant[12]

[11]  PMDA Database.   http://www.pmda.go.jp/drugs/2014/P201400117/index.html (accessed Mar 2016).
[12]  FDA Database.   http://www.accessdata.fda.gov/drugsatfda_docs/nda/2014/204569Orig1s000PharmR.pdf (accessed Mar 2016).

Table 8 *In Vivo* Pharmacokinetic Parameters of Suvorexant in Healthy Male and Female Humans after Single Intravenous and Oral Dose of Suvorexant[13]

| Route | Dose (mg) | $T_{max}$[a] (h) | $C_{eoi}$ or $C_{max}$[a, b] (μM) | $AUC_{inf}$[a] (μM·h) | $T_{1/2}$[c] (h) | Cl[a] (mL/min) | $V_{ss}$[a] (L) |
|---|---|---|---|---|---|---|---|
| i.v. | 5 | NA | 0.543 (0.470-0.627) | 3.46 (2.78-4.32) | 9.2 (3.4) | 52.3 (42.0-65.1) | 36.5 (31.2-42.7) |
| | 10 | NA | 1.04 (0.904-1.21) | 6.92 (5.54-8.63) | 9.9 (5.2) | 52.7 (42.4-65.6) | 42.5 (36.3-49.7) |
| | 20 | NA | 1.75 (1.52-2.02) | 15.1 (12.1-18.8) | 13.5 (5.0) | 48.6 (39.0-60.5) | 57.1 (48.8-66.8) |
| | 30[d] | NA | 1.90 (1.64-2.19) | 13.7 (11.0-17.1) | 8.9 (1.7) | 80.6 (64.8-100) | 57.3 (49.0-67.1) |
| p.o. | 10 | 1.5 (1.0-4.0) | 0.456 (0.403-0.516) | 5.32 (4.55-6.23) | 12.1 (1.8) | NA | NA |
| | 20 | 1.0 (1.0-4.0) | 0.646 (0.572-0.731) | 9.51 (8.12-11.1) | 12.5 (2.6) | NA | NA |
| | 40 | 2.0 (1.0-4.0) | 0.956 (0.845-1.08) | 16.2 (13.8-19.0) | 12.6 (2.5) | NA | NA |
| | 80 | 2.0 (0.5-6.0) | 1.52 (1.34-1.72) | 27.3 (23.3-31.9) | 13.6 (2.9) | NA | NA |

$C_{eoi}$: Concentration at the end of the infusion. [a] Back-transformed least squares mean and 95% confidence interval from fixed effects model performed on natural log-transformed values. [b] The values of i.v was $C_{eoi}$, the values of p.o. was $C_{max}$. [c] Harmonic mean, jack-knife SD. [d] Infusion time for 30 mg was 1.5 h, compared to the 1 h infusion time for 5, 10 and 20 mg.

Table 9 *In Vitro* Permeability of Suvorexant in LLC-PK1 Cell Monolayer Model[11, 14]

| Compound | Conc. (μM) | Papp ($1 \times 10^{-6}$ cm/s) | Permeability Class |
|---|---|---|---|
| Suvorexant | 0.5-5 | 22.8-25.9 | High |
| M9 | 0.1-1 | 26.7-30.8 | High |
| M17 | 0.1-1 | 3.9-4.0 | Moderate |

## Distribution

Table 10 *In Vitro* Plasma Protein Binding and Blood Partitioning of Suvorexant[12, 13]

| Unbound Fraction in Total Plasma% | | | | | Unbound Fraction in Isolated Human Plasma Protein (%) | | Blood Partitioning ($C_b$:$C_p$) | | | |
|---|---|---|---|---|---|---|---|---|---|---|
| Species | 1 μM | 5 μM | 10 μM | 25 μM | | | Species | 1 μM | 10 μM | 25 μM |
| Human | 0.3 ± 0.0 | 0.5 ± 0.1 | ND | 0.5 ± 0.1 | HSA (40 mg/mL) | 2.80 ± 0.05 | Human | 0.59 | 0.68 | 0.61 |
| Rat | 1.1 ± 0.1 | 1.4 ± 0.1 | ND | 1.7 ± 0.2 | | | Rat | 0.60 | 0.60 | 0.60 |
| Dog | 0.9 ± 0.1 | 1.0 ± 0.0 | ND | 1.7 ± 0.1 | | | Dog | 0.51 | 0.54 | 0.57 |
| Monkey | 1.0 ± 0.0 | 1.4 ± 0.1 | ND | 1.9 ± 0.0 | | | | | | |
| Mouse | ND | 1.8 ± 0.1 | ND | ND | $\alpha_1$-AGP (1 mg/mL) | 0.40 ± 0.07 | Monkey | 0.55 | 0.54 | 0.64 |
| Rabbit | 3.7 ± 0.2 | ND | 4.4 ± 0.2 | ND | | | | | | |

$C_b$:$C_p$: Blood to plasma concentration ratio. HSA: Human serum albumin. $\alpha_1$-AGP: $\alpha_1$-acid glycoprotein.

Table 11 *In Vitro* Plasma Protein Binding and Blood Partitioning of Metabolites M9 and M17 in Several Species[12, 13]

| Species | Unbound Fraction in Plasma% | | | | Blood Partitioning ($C_b$:$C_p$) | |
|---|---|---|---|---|---|---|
| | M9 (L-002015883) | | | M17 (L-002440877) | M9 | |
| | 1 μM | 5 μM | 10 μM | 2.5 μM | Species | 1 μM |
| Human | ND | 0.2 ± 0.0 | ND | 0.2 ± 0.0 | Human | 0.60 |
| Rat | ND | 2.9 ± 0.2 | ND | 6.2 ± 0.5 | Rat | ND |
| Dog | ND | 1.9 ± 0.2 | ND | NA | Dog | ND |
| Monkey | ND | 4.9 ± 0.2 | ND | NA | | |
| Mouse | ND | 1.8 ± 0.1 | ND | NA | Monkey | ND |
| Rabbit[a] | 7.8 | ND | 10.4 | NA | | |

$C_b$:$C_p$: Blood to plasma concentration ratio. [a] For M9, rabbit plasma protein binding values represented an average of n = 2.

[11] PMDA Database. http://www.pmda.go.jp/drugs/2014/P201400117/index.html (accessed Mar 2016).
[12] FDA Database. http://www.accessdata.fda.gov/drugsatfda_docs/nda/2014/204569Orig1s000PharmR.pdf (accessed Mar 2016).
[13] FDA Database. http://www.accessdata.fda.gov/drugsatfda_docs/nda/2014/204569Orig1s000ClinPharmR.pdf (accessed Mar 2016).
[14] Cui, D.; Cabalu, T.; Yee, K. L., et al. *Xenobiotica* **2016**, published online.

Table 12  *In Vivo* Tissue Distribution of Suvorexant in Sprague-Dawley (SD) and Long-Evans (LE) Rats after Single Oral Dose of 20 mg/kg [$^{14}$C]Suvorexant[12]

| Species | SD Rat/Male | | | | | LE Rat/Male | | | | |
| Tissues | $T_{max}$ (h) | $C_{max}$ (ng eq./g) | $T_{1/2}$ (h) | $AUC_{0-t}$ (ng eq.·h/g) | Tissue/Blood $AUC_{0-t}$ Ratio | $T_{max}$ (h) | $C_{max}$ (ng eq./g) | $T_{1/2}$ (h) | $AUC_{0-t}$ (ng eq.·h/g) | Tissue/Blood $AUC_{0-t}$ Ratio |
|---|---|---|---|---|---|---|---|---|---|---|
| Adrenal gland | 0.50 | 5740 | 2.69 | 24700 | 1.2 | 1.00 | 3390 | NC | NC | - |
| Blood | 1.00 | 1590 | 2.69 | 7580 | 0.4 | 1.00 | 1710 | NC | NC | - |
| Blood (LSC) | 1.00 | 1770 | 69.7 | 21300 | 1.0 | 1.00 | 1400 | 237 | 48000 | 1 |
| Bile | 0.50 | 156000 | 6.20 | 1080000 | 50.7 | 1.00 | 98100 | NC | NC | - |
| Cecum content | 8.00 | 569000 | NC | 6710000 | 315 | 24.0 | 8670 | NC | 104000 | 2.2 |
| Cerebrum | 0.50 | 279 | 8.62 | 207 | 0.01 | 1.00 | 199 | NC | NC | - |
| Plasma (LSC) | 1.00 | 2830 | 14.7 | 22800 | 1.1 | 1.00 | 2220 | 4.86 | 27600 | 0.6 |
| Kidneys | 1.00 | 4350 | 16.0 | 28800 | 1.4 | 1.00 | 3330 | 5.18 | 41700 | 0.9 |
| Large intestine content | 8.00 | 473000 | 4.42 | 5750000 | 270 | 24.0 | 25600 | NC | 294000 | 0.2 |
| Liver | 1.00 | 52200 | 44.1 | 480000 | 22.5 | 1.00 | 47500 | 61.9 | 814000 | 17.0 |
| Lungs | 1.00 | 1290 | 2.48 | 6110 | 0.3 | 1.00 | 1380 | NC | NC | - |
| Non-pigmented skin | 1.00 | 765 | NC | 500 | 0.02 | 1.00 | 631 | NC | NC | - |
| Pigmented skin | - | - | - | - | - | 1.00 | 765 | NC | NC | - |
| Renal cortex | 0.50 | 3770 | 19.7 | 28000 | 1.3 | 1.00 | 3220 | 5.48 | 40700 | 0.9 |
| Renal medulla | 1.00 | 5820 | 16.1 | 28800 | 1.4 | 1.00 | 3170 | NC | NC | - |
| Small intestine content | 1.00 | 857000 | 13.4 | 4510000 | 212 | 1.00 | 613000 | 3.09 | 7400000 | 154 |
| Urine | 1.00 | 36100 | NC | 161000 | 7.6 | 1.00 | 24900 | NC | NC | - |

Vehicles: 20% vitamin E-TPGS.   SD rats: 0.5, 1, 8, 24, 72 and 168 h.   LE rats: 1, 24, 168 and 672 h.   NC: Not calculated.

Table 13  *In Vivo* Distribution of Metabolites M9 in Central Nervous System[11]

| System | Route | Dose (mg/kg) | Time (h) | Conc. (µM) | | |
| | | | | Plasma | Brain | Cerebrospinal Fluid |
|---|---|---|---|---|---|---|
| CF-1 (+/+) mouse | i.v. | 3 | 0.25 | 4.15 ± 0.72 | 0.27 ± 0.15 | 0.03 |
| | | | 0.5 | 2.13 ± 0.40 | 0.14 ± 0.05 | 0.01 |
| | | | 1 | 0.62 ± 0.33 | 0.05 ± 0.03 | BLQ |
| CF-1 (-/-) mouse | i.v. | 3 | 0.25 | 4.00 ± 0.45 | 2.96 ± 0.86 | 0.08 |
| | | | 0.5 | 1.51 ± 0.81 | 1.44 ± 0.57 | 0.02 |
| | | | 1 | 0.61 ± 0.10 | 0.66 ± 0.11 | 0.01 |

CF (+/+): Wild (P-gp), CF (-/-): P-gp knockout.   Vechile: DMSO/PEG400 (50/50).   BLQ: Below limit of quantification.

[11]  PMDA Database.   http://www.pmda.go.jp/drugs/2014/P201400117/index.html (accessed Mar 2016).
[12]  FDA Database.   http://www.accessdata.fda.gov/drugsatfda_docs/nda/2014/204569Orig1s000PharmR.pdf (accessed Mar 2016).

# Metabolism

Table 14  *In Vitro* Metabolites Formed in Liver Microsomes and Hepatocytes[11, 13]

| Analyte | Liver Microsomes | | | | | Hepatocytes[a] | | |
| | Mouse | Rabbit | SD Rat (n = 68) | Beagle Dog (n = 8) | Human (n = 150) | SD Rat (n = 14) | Beagle Dog (n = 3) | Human (n = 10) |
|---|---|---|---|---|---|---|---|---|
| Suvorexant | NA | NA | NA | NA | 33% | NA | NA | 48% |
| M3 | - | - | - | - | - | - | √ | 3% |
| M4 | √ | √ | √ | - | 6% | √ | √ | 12% |
| M6a | √ | - | √ | - | - | √ | - | - |
| M6b | √ | - | - | - | - | - | - | - |
| M6c | √ | √ | - | √ | 4% | √ | - | - |
| M7a | - | √ | - | √ | 4% | - | - | - |
| M7b | √ | √ | √ | √ | 3% | - | √ | 9% |
| M7c | √ | √ | - | - | - | - | - | - |
| M8 | √ | √ | √ | √ | 8% | - | - | - |
| M9 | √ | √ | √ | √ | 22% | √ | √ | 20% |
| M10a | √ | √ | √ | √ | 2% | √ | √ | 3% |
| M10b | √ | - | √ | - | - | - | - | - |
| M11 | - | - | - | - | - | - | √ | - |
| M12 | - | - | - | - | - | √ | √ | 3% |
| M13b | - | - | √ | - | - | √ | - | - |
| M16 | Trace | √ | √ | √ | - | - | - | - |
| M17 | Trace | √ | - | √ | √ | - | - | - |
| M20 | - | - | - | - | - | √ | - | - |

√: Be observed.   Trace: Detected only in MS.   NA: Not available.   [a] The concentration of [$^{14}$C]suvorexant was 10 μM.

Table 15  *In Vitro* Metabolic Phenotype of Suvorexant with Human Liver Microsomes[13]

| | Immuno-Inhibition | | | | | Specific Chemical Inhibitors | | | |
| Inhibitory Antibody | Suvorexant | %Inhibition (%Control ± SD) | | | Chemical Inhibitor | Suvorexant | %Inhibition (%Control ± SD) | |
| | Conc. (μM) | M8 | M9 | M10a | | Conc. (μM) | M9 | M10a |
|---|---|---|---|---|---|---|---|---|
| Anti-CYP1A2 | 2 | NI | 6 ± 1 | 10 ± 9 | Ketoconazole | 2 | 82 ± 4 | 85 ± 2 |
| | 20 | NI | NI | NI | | | | |
| Anti-CYP2C | 2 | NI | NI | 11 ± 9 | | 20 | 70 ± 4 | 74 ± 3 |
| | 20 | 8 ± 10 | 31 ± 9 | 13 ± 22 | | | | |
| Anti-CYP2D6 | 2 | NI | NI | NI | N-3-benzyl-phenobarbital | 2 | NI | NI |
| | 20 | NI | NI | NI | | | | |
| Anti-CYP3A | 2 | 100 ± 0 | 80 ± 4 | 92 ± 7 | | 20 | 28 ± 4 | 20 ± 3 |
| | 20 | 82 ± 11 | 65 ± 6 | 92± 5 | | | | |

NI: No inhibition.

[11]  PMDA Database.   http://www.pmda.go.jp/drugs/2014/P201400117/index.html (accessed Mar 2016).
[13]  FDA Database.   http://www.accessdata.fda.gov/drugsatfda_docs/nda/2014/204569Orig1s000ClinPharmR.pdf (accessed Mar 2016).

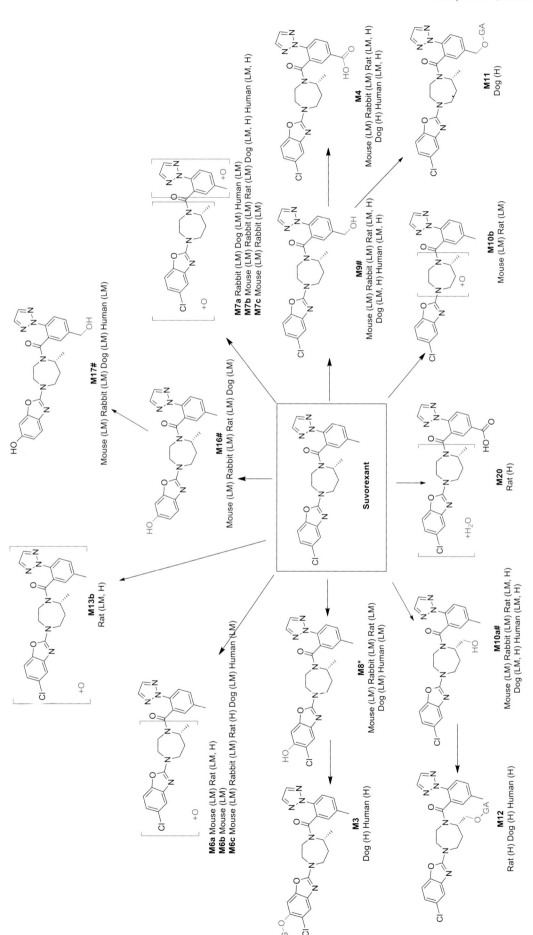

Figure C   Proposed Pathways for *In Vitro* Biotransformation of [$^{14}$C]Suvorexant in Liver Microsomes and Hepatocytes[12]
LM = liver microsomes and H = hepatocytes.   * Structure of M8 confirmed by NMR.   # Synthetic standards of M9, M10a, M16 and M17 were available.

[12]   FDA Database.   http://www.accessdata.fda.gov/drugsatfda_docs/nda/2014/204569Orig1s000PharmR.pdf (accessed Mar 2016).

Table 16    Metabolites in Plasma, Urine, Bile and Feces in Humans and Non-clinical Species
after Oral Dose of Suvorexant[11, 13, 14]

| Matrix | Plasma (% of radioactivity) | | | | | Bile (% of dose) | | Urine (% of dose) | | | | Feces (% of dose) | | | |
|---|---|---|---|---|---|---|---|---|---|---|---|---|---|---|---|
| Species | Mouse | Rat | Rabbit | Dog | Human | Rat | Dog | Mouse | Rabbit | Dog | Human | Mouse | Rabbit | Dog | Human |
| Dose (mg/kg) | 30 | 20 | 100 mg/kg/day[a] | 5 | 50 mg | 20 | 5 | 30 | 20 | 5 | 50 mg | 30 | 20 | 5 | 50 mg |
| Parent | √ | √ | √ | √ | 30.1 | - | - | - | - | - | - | √ | - | √ | Trace |
| M3 | - | - | √ | √ | - | √ | √ | √ | √ | √ | 3.8 | - | - | - | - |
| M4 | √ | √ | √ | √ | 1.5 | √ | √ | √ | √ | √ | 4.1 | √ | √ | √ | 17.0 |
| M6a | - | - | - | √ | - | - | - | - | - | - | - | √ | - | √ | - |
| M6b | - | - | - | - | - | √ | √ | - | - | √ | ND | √ | √ | - | 2.6 |
| M6c | - | - | - | - | - | √ | √ | - | - | √ | ND | √ | √ | - | 2.0 |
| M7a | - | - | √ | √ | 3.4 | - | - | - | - | √ | - | - | √ | √ | √ |
| M7b | - | - | - | - | - | - | - | - | - | - | - | √ | √ | √ | - |
| M7c | - | - | - | - | - | - | - | √ | - | - | - | √ | - | - | - |
| M8 | - | √ | √ | √ | 6.0 | - | - | √ | - | - | - | √ | √ | √ | Trace |
| M9 | √ | √ | √ | √ | 36.5 | - | - | √ | - | - | - | √ | √ | √ | 9.5 |
| M10a | - | √ | √ | √ | 2.3 | - | √ | √ | - | √ | - | √ | √ | √ | 9.2 |
| M11 | - | - | √ | √ | - | √ | √ | √ | √ | √ | 1.4 | - | - | - | - |
| M12 | - | √ | √ | √ | 12.2 | √ | √ | √ | √ | √ | 2.7 | - | - | - | - |
| M13a | - | - | - | - | - | - | - | - | - | √ | - | - | √ | √ | 2.2 |
| M13b | - | - | - | - | - | - | - | - | - | √ | - | - | √ | - | 0.3 |
| M13c | - | - | - | - | - | - | - | - | - | √ | - | - | √ | - | 5.4 |
| M14a | - | - | - | - | - | √ | √ | - | √ | √ | - | - | - | - | - |
| M14b | - | - | - | √ | - | √ | √ | - | √ | √ | - | - | - | - | - |
| M14c | - | - | - | - | - | √ | √ | - | √ | √ | - | - | - | - | - |
| M14d | - | - | - | - | - | - | - | - | - | √ | - | - | - | - | - |
| M14e | - | - | - | - | - | - | - | - | - | √ | - | - | - | - | - |
| M15a | - | - | - | - | - | √ | - | √ | - | - | - | - | - | - | - |
| M15b | - | - | - | - | - | √ | - | - | - | - | - | - | - | - | - |
| M15c | - | - | - | - | - | - | - | √ | - | - | - | - | - | - | - |
| M16 | √ | √ | √ | √ | 4.8 | - | √ | - | - | - | - | - | √ | - | 2.6 |
| M17 | √ | - | √ | √ | 3.3 | - | - | - | - | √ | - | - | √ | - | Trace |
| M18 | - | - | - | - | - | - | - | - | - | √ | - | - | √ | - | 10.6 |
| M18b | - | - | - | - | - | - | - | - | - | - | - | - | √ | - | - |
| M19 | - | - | - | - | - | - | - | - | - | √ | 5.3 | - | - | - | - |
| M21 | - | - | - | - | - | - | - | - | √ | - | - | - | - | - | - |

√: Be observed.    Trace: Detected only in MS.    [a] 100 mg/kg/day, once daily from gestation Day 7 to Day 15.

[11]  PMDA Database.   http://www.pmda.go.jp/drugs/2014/P201400117/index.html (accessed Mar 2016).
[13]  FDA Database.   http://www.accessdata.fda.gov/drugsatfda_docs/nda/2014/204569Orig1s000ClinPharmR.pdf (accessed Mar 2016).
[14]  Cui, D.; Cabalu, T.; Yee, K. L., et al. *Xenobiotica* **2016**, published online.

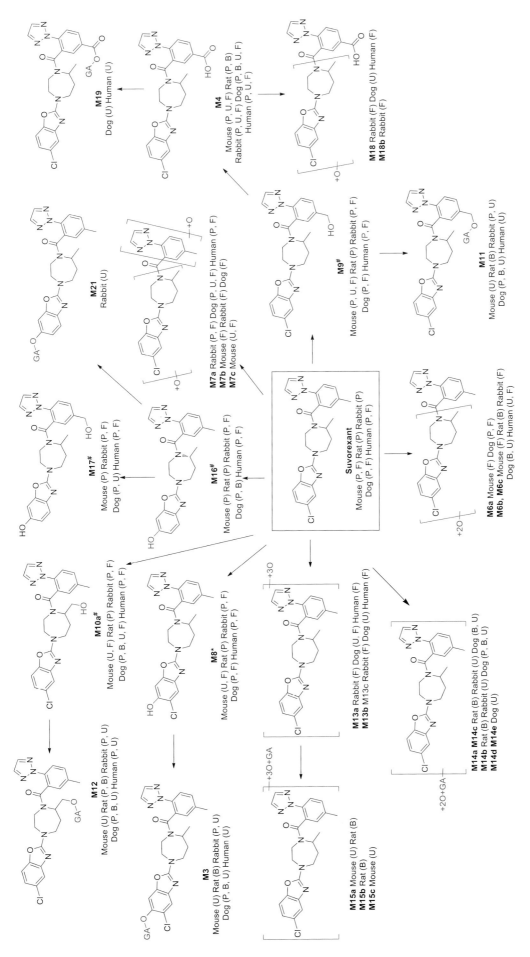

Figure D　Proposed Pathways for *In Vivo* Biotransformation of [¹⁴C]Suvorexant in Mice, Rabbits, Rats, Dogs and Humans[12]

The red labels represent the major metabolic compounds in the matrices.　P = Plasma, U = Urine, F = Feces, B = Bile and GA = Glucuronic acid.
\* Synthetic standards of M9, M10a, M16 and M17 were available.　# Structure of M8 confirmed by NMR.

[12]　FDA Database.　http://www.accessdata.fda.gov/drugsatfda_docs/nda/2014/204569Orig1s000PharmR.pdf (accessed Mar 2016).

# Excretion

Table 17    Excretion Profiles of [$^{14}$C]Suvorexant in Various Species after Single Intravenous and Oral Dose of [$^{14}$C]Suvorexant[11]

| Species | Route | State | Vehicle | Dose (mg/kg) | Time (h) | Bile (% of dose) | Urine (% of dose) | Feces (% of dose) | Recovery (% of dose) |
|---|---|---|---|---|---|---|---|---|---|
| SD rat (male) | p.o. | BDC | 20% Vitamin E-TPGS | 20 | 0-72 | 83.5 ± 1.2 | 1.8 ± 0.4 | 8.6 ± 1.3 | 94.1 ± 0.5 |
| | i.v. | BDC | DMSO | 5 | 0-72 | 90.0 ± 1.5 | 5.4 ± 2.5 | NA | 95.4 ± 4.0 |
| Beagle dog (male) | p.o. | BDC | 20% Vitamin E-TPGS | 5 | 0-72 | 32.8 | 10.2 | 41.7 | 84.7 |
| | i.v. | BDC | DMSO | 1 | 0-72 | 91.1 | 5.5 | NA | 96.6 |
| Dutch Belted rabbit (female) | p.o. | Intact | 0.5% Methylcellulose (MC)/ 5 mM hydrochloride | 20 | 0-72 | NA | 27.5 | 44.5 | 85.8[a] |
| Human (male) | p.o. | Intact | Capsule | 50 mg | 0-336 | NA | 23.0 ± 6.3 | 66.4 ± 5.5 | 89.7 ± 6.0 |

BDC: Bile duct-cannulated.    NA: Not available.    [a] Containing wash liquid.

# Drug-Drug Interaction

Table 18    *In Vitro* Evaluation of Suvorexant and Metabolites as Inhibitors of CYP Enzymes in Human Liver Microsomes[11, 13]

| Enzymes Isoform | IC$_{50}$ (μM)[a] | | | $K_i$ (μM) | | Time-dependent Inhibition | |
|---|---|---|---|---|---|---|---|
| | Suvorexant | M9 | M17 | Suvorexant | M9 | Suvorexant[d] | M9[e] |
| CYP1A2 | 74 | >100 | NA | NA | NA | NA | NA |
| CYP2B6 | 64 | 44 | NA | NA | NA | NA | NA |
| CYP2C8 | 15 | 37 | NA | NA | NA | NA | NA |
| CYP2C9 | 15 | 47 | >50 | NA | NA | NA | NA |
| CYP2C19 | 5.3 | 35 | NA | NA | NA | NA | NA |
| CYP2D6 | 17 | 39 | >50 | NA | NA | NA | NA |
| CYP3A4[b] | 4.0 | 11 | 28 | 11.6 ± 1.9 | NC | Yes | Yes |
| CYP3A4[c] | NA | 26 | NA | NA | NA | NA | NA |

[a] IC$_{50}$ values represented the average value from duplicate determinations.    [b] The substrate was testosterone.    [c] The substrate was midazolam.    [d] The concentration was 2, 5, 10, 20, 30, 50, 100 μM, and suvorexant was the time dependent inhibitor of CYP3A4.    [e] The concentration was 10, 50 μM, and M9 was the time dependent inhibitor of CYP3A4.

Table 19    *In Vitro* Evaluation of Suvorexant as an Inducer of Enzymes in Cryopreserved Human Hepatocytes[11, 12]

| Conc. (μM) | CYP3A4 | | CYP2B6 | | CYP1A2 | |
|---|---|---|---|---|---|---|
| | mRNA | Activity | mRNA | Activity | mRNA | Activity |
| | Fold Induction | Fold Induction | Fold Induction | Fold Induction | Fold Induction | Fold Induction |
| 0.1 | 1.6 ± 0.4 | 0.8 ± 0.2 | 0.8 ± 0.2 | 1.0 ± 0.2 | 0.8 ± 0.0 | 0.9 ± 0.1 |
| 0.5 | 3.3 ± 1.8 | 0.7 ± 0.2 | 0.9 ± 0.1 | 1.1 ± 0.1 | 1.0 ± 0.2 | 1.2 ± 0.2 |
| 1 | 10.3 ± 13.3 | 0.6 ± 0.3 | 1.2 ± 0.4 | 1.5 ± 0.4 | 2.2 ± 0.1 | 1.2 ± 0.3 |
| 5 | 22.0 ± 10.9 | 0.4 ± 0.3 | 2.4 ± 0.6 | 2.3 ± 1.4 | 4.8 ± 0.5 | 2.3 ± 0.7 |
| 10 | 13.9 ± 7.0 | 0.3 ± 0.1 | 2.0 ± 1.1 | 1.7 ± 1.1 | 4.5 ± 0.7 | 2.7 ± 1.4 |
| 20 | 9.3 ± 8.1 | 0.4 ± 0.1 | 0.2 ± 0.2 | 0.0[a] | 3.8 ± 2.3 | 2.7 ± 1.7 |

Average from n = 3 donors.    Mean ± SD.    [a] Value represented average of two values, or only one value because at least one donor was reported as NR.    NR: Not reported since response was less than vehicle control.

[11]  PMDA Database.   http://www.pmda.go.jp/drugs/2014/P201400117/index.html (accessed Mar 2016).
[12]  FDA Database.   http://www.accessdata.fda.gov/drugsatfda_docs/nda/2014/204569Orig1s000PharmR.pdf (accessed Mar 2016).
[13]  FDA Database.   http://www.accessdata.fda.gov/drugsatfda_docs/nda/2014/204569Orig1s000ClinPharmR.pdf (accessed Mar 2016).

Table 20    *In Vitro* Evaluation of Suvorexant and M9 as Inhibitors and Substrates of Transporters[11-13]

| Treatment | Suvorexant as a Substrate of P-gp | | | Suvorexant and M9 as Inhibitors | | | |
|---|---|---|---|---|---|---|---|
| | Substrate | Conc. (µM) | Efflux Ratio | Transporter | Substrate | IC50 (µM) | |
| | | | | | | Suvorexant | M9 |
| Suvorexant | No | 0.5-5 | 1.0-1.6 | P-gp | Digoxin | $18.7 \pm 3.3$ | $73 \pm 16$ |
| | | | | BCRP | Methotrexate | 10-15 | ~15 |
| M9 | Yes | 0.1-1 | 3.2-4.3 | OATP1B1 | Pitavastatin | ~10 | >15 |
| | | | | OCT2 | Metformin | $1.3 \pm 0.3$ | >15 |

~: Approximately.

# 6    Non-Clinical Toxicology

## Summary

### Repeated-Dose Toxicity

❖ Sub- and chronic toxicity with two different formulations by the oral route in rats (up to 6 months) and dogs (up to 9 months):
  • Determined by the longest studies conducted, the NOAEL in rats were 100 (male) and 25 (female) mg/kg/day, approximately 23 (female) and 19 (male) × MRHD exposure, and that in dogs were 5 (male) and 25 (female) mg/kg/day, approximately 45 × MRHD exposure.
  • The major target organs in both species were thyroid glands, liver and CNS.

### Safety Pharmacology

❖ Core battery of safety pharmacology studies to investigate the effects on cardiovascular, central nervous and respiratory system:
  • Neurological effects: No drug-related behavior, autonomic and motor changes in rats at 80 mg/kg.
  • Cardiovascular effects: The hERG tail current was inhibited with an IC50 of 2.6 µM, indicative of potential for QT prolongation, yet no statistically significant changes were observed in dog studies at doses up to 3 mg/kg (i.p.).
  • Respiratory effects: No statistically significant changes in SD rats at doses up to 1200 mg/kg.

### Genotoxicity

❖ Suvorexant was neither mutagenic nor clastogenic, in view of the standard battery of genotoxicity assays carried out.

### Reproductive and Developmental Toxicity

❖ Fertility and early embryonic development in rats using two formulations:
  • There were no treatment-related effect on mating/fertility at 80 mg/kg/day in females and >1200 mg/kg/day in males.
❖ Embryo-fetal development studies in rats and rabbits using two formulations:
  • Suvorexant was embryotoxic and teratogenic when administered to pregnant rats at the >150 mg/kg/day during the period of organogenesis.
  • Major fetal malformations of ectrodactyly, fetal skeletal malformations and omphalocele were observed at doses >100 mg/kg/day.
❖ Pre- and postnatal development in rats using spray dried formulation (SDF):
  • Maternal toxicity was evident at 200 mg/kg/day (HD) and included reduced body weight gains.    This dose associated with reductions in offspring birth weight and preputial separation in HD $F_1$ males.

### Carcinogenicity

❖ The carcinogenic potential in a 26-week Tg.rasH2 mouse study and 2-year rat study:
  • No evidence of suvorexant-induced neoplasm at oral doses up to 650 mg/kg/day in mice.
  • Thyroid follicular cell adenomas, as well as combined adenomas and carcinomas were significantly increased in male rats at 325 mg/kg/day (7 × MRHD).

### Special Toxicology

❖ Suvorexant was not phototoxic under the *in vivo* conditions tested.

[11]  PMDA Database.    http://www.pmda.go.jp/drugs/2014/P201400117/index.html (accessed Mar 2016).
[12]  FDA Database.    http://www.accessdata.fda.gov/drugsatfda_docs/nda/2014/204569Orig1s000PharmR.pdf (accessed Mar 2016).
[13]  FDA Database.    http://www.accessdata.fda.gov/drugsatfda_docs/nda/2014/204569Orig1s000ClinPharmR.pdf (accessed Mar 2016).

## Repeated-Dose Toxicity

Table 21  Repeated-Dose Toxicity Studies of Suvorexant by Oral (Gavage) Administration[11, 12]

| Species | Dura-tion | Dose (mg/kg/day) | NOAEL | | | Finding |
|---------|-----------|------------------|-------|-------|------------------------|---------|
| | | | Dose (mg/kg/day) | AUC$_{0-24}$ (µM·h) | Safety Margin[a] (× MRHD) | |
| SD rat | 3 days | Vehicle: SDF Female: 15, 50, 100, 325; Male: 30, 50, 100, 325 | NA | Parent NA | NA | One LD female died on Day 1, the death was attributed to the collection procedure. Plasma exposure to suvorexant was greater in females than males. Plasma exposure was generally greater than dose-proportional at the lower doses. |
| | 1 month | Vehicle: PEG 400 and 0.5% MC 100, 300, 1200 | 300 | Parent Male: 75.2; Female: 298 | NA | Increased in cholesterol and globulin at 300 or 1000 mg/kg/day in females. |
| | 1 month | Vehicle: SDF 0, 80, 160, 325, Vehicle: TPGS 1200 | 325 | M9 Female: 45; Male: 55 | NA | The main histopathological findings were thyroid follicular cell and hepatocellular hypertrophy that increased with an increase in dose. Follicular cell and hepatocellular hypertrophy were observed at >160 mg/kg/day, respectively. |
| | | | | Parent Male:434; Female:760 | NA | |
| | 6 months | Vehicle: TPGS Female: 0, 25, 75, 1200; Male: 0, 100, 300, 1200 | Male: 100; Female: 25 | Parent Male: 69.2 ± 7.53[b]; Female: 45.5 ± 4.33[b] | NA | The main histopathological findings were an increased in incidence and severity of thyroid follicular cell and hepatocellular at the MD and HD in males and females; these changes corresponded to an increase in thyroid and liver weights. Follicular cell and hepatocellular hypertrophy was observed at ≥75 and ≥300 mg/kg/day in females and males, respectively. |
| | 6 months | Vehicle: SDF Female: 0, 30, 80, 325; Male: 0, 80, 160, 325 | Female: 80; Male:160 | M9 Female: 14.3; Male: 30.8 | Female: 1.1; Male: 2.4 | One HD female was sacrificed on Day 2 due to signs of lateral recumbency, unsteady gait, decreased activity, impaired righting reflex, labored breathing, urine/fecal staining, cool to touch, and hunched posture. Dose-dependent increases in liver and thyroid gland weights occurred in females and males at all doses. Microscopic finding of hypertrophy of thyroid gland follicular cell and hepatocytes were observed at MD and HD, and erosion of the stomach glandular mucosa was observed at HD. |
| | | | | Parent Female: 212; Male: 178 | Female: 23; Male: 19 | |
| Beagle dog | 7 days | Vehicle: TPGS 25, 400, 800, 1125 | NA | Parent NA | NA | No major suvorexant related change was observed at any dose after 1 week of treatment. |
| | 1 month | Vehicle: TPGS 0, 10, 30, 400 | 400 | M9 Male: 228; Female: 168 | NA | Decreased prostatic weights/prostatic atrophy at MD and HD in males. Slight decreased in erythrocyte parameters in females at HD. None of these findings were considered toxicologically significant by this reviewer. |
| | | | | Parent Male: 319; Female: 402 | NA | |

[11] PMDA Database.  http://www.pmda.go.jp/drugs/2014/P201400117/index.html (accessed Mar 2016).
[12] FDA Database.  http://www.accessdata.fda.gov/drugsatfda_docs/nda/2014/204569Orig1s000PharmR.pdf (accessed Mar 2016).

*Continued*

| Species | Duration | Dose (mg/kg/day) | NOAEL | | | Finding |
|---|---|---|---|---|---|---|
| | | | Dose (mg/kg/day) | AUC$_{0-24}$ (μM·h) | Safety Margin[a] (× MRHD) | |
| Beagle dog | 1 month | Vehicle: SDF 0, 60, 125, 250; vehicle: TPGS 800 | 125 | M9 Male: 660; Female:622 | NA | One Group (4 males) was sacrificed in Week 2 with signs that included decreased activity, unsteady gait, intermittent whole body trembling, and thin appearance; the dog had also lost 1.0 kg of body weight and was not eating food satisfactorily. Histopathological changes included hepatocellular hypertrophy. An increase in mean liver weight occurred in Groups (2-4 females and males) and histopathological findings included hepatocellular hypertrophy that generally increased in severity with an increase in dose. Plasma exposure to suvorexant was approximately equivalent between the SDF formulation at 60 mg/kg/day and the TPGS formulation at 800 mg/kg/day and was approximately 2-fold higher with 250 mg/kg/day (SDF formulation). |
| | | | | Parent Male: 701; Female: 798 | NA | |
| | 9 months | Vehicle: TPGS 0, 5, 25, 800 | 25 | Parent Male:186; Female: 161 | NA | One HD male had intermittent head trembling in weeks 1 and 11, at approximately T$_{max}$. An increase in liver weight was observed at all doses in females and in HD males. Hepatocellular hypetrophy was observed in all HD females and 1 HD male at the interim sacrifice at 6 months but was not observed at the end of treatment. |
| | 9 months | Vehicle: SDF 0, 10, 50, 125 | 50 | M9 Male: 253; Female: 290 | 21 | Incidences of salivation occurred dose-dependently at all doses. During the study, 1 MD male suffered from an injury that resulted in a swollen hindlimb that became non-weight bearing. An increase in ALP was observed that was dose-dependent and became more severe with the duration of the study. An increase in liver weight was observed. Hepatocellular hypertrophy was observed in 1 HD male at the interim sacrifice and at the end of treatment in 1 LD female, 1 MD female and 1 HD female. |
| | | | | Parent Male: 388, Female: 440 | 45 | |

SDF: Formulation in 0.5% MC with 5 mM HCl in deionized water.    TPGS: D-alpha-tocopheryl PEG 1000 succinate.    [a] Calculated with the clinical recommended dose of 20 mg daily: suvorexant, AUC$_{0-24}$ was 9.2 μM·h; M9, AUC$_{0-24}$ = 12.8 μM·h.

## Safety Pharmacology

Table 22    Safety Pharmacology Studies of Suvorexant[11, 12]

| Study | System | Dose | Finding |
|---|---|---|---|
| Neurological effect | Rat | Vehicle: SDF 80, 160, 325 mg/kg Vehicle: TPGS 1200 mg/kg p.o. | A decrease in mean body temperature was observed in 1 rat at 160 mg/kg. At 160 and 325 mg/kg 1 or 4 h after administration: Decreased muscle tone, flattened posture, unsteady gait, hunched posture and abnormal gait. At 1200 mg/kg 4 or 8 h after administration: Hunched posture, unsteady gait, slow righting reflex and a decrease in mean body temperature. |
| Cardiovascular effect | CHO cell expressing hERG channel | 0.3, 1, 3, 10 µM | Affinity for the hEGR potassium channel, with a $K_i$ value of 5.5 µM. Dose-dependently inhibited hEGR, $IC_{50}$ = 2.6 µM, $IC_{20}$ = 0.66 µM. |
| | Anesthetized Mongrel dog (female) | 1, 2, 3 mg/kg, i.v. | No cardiovascular effect.    At 3 mg/kg, $C_{max}$ = 23.8 µM. |
| | Male Beagle dog (telemetry) | Vehicle: TPGS 10, 30, 400 mg/kg, p.o. | No cardiovascular effect.    At 400 mg/kg, $C_{max}$ = 16.7 µM, $AUC_{0-24}$ = 248 µM. |
| Pulmonary effect | SD rat (male) | Vehicle: TPGS 100, 300, 1200 mg/kg, p.o. | No adverse effects on respiratory parameters were reported after single oral dose up to 1200 mg/kg. |

SDF: Formulation in 0.5% methylcellulose with 5 mM HCl in deionized water.    TPGS: D-alpha-tocopheryl polyethylene glycol-1000 succinate.

## Genotoxicity

Table 23    Genotoxicity Studies of Suvorexant[11, 12]

| Assay | Species/System | Metabolism | Dose | Finding |
|---|---|---|---|---|
| In vitro reverse mutation assay in bacterial cells (Ames) | S. typhimurium TA1535, TA97a, TA98, TA100; E. coli WP2PuvrA | ±S9 | 30-6000 µg/plate | Negative. |
| In vitro mammalian cell cytogenetic test | CHO | ±S9 | ~150 µg/mL | Negative at concentrations up to 90 µM with S9, and up to 105 µM and 60 µM without S9 (3 and 20 h treatment). |
| In vitro alkaline elution rat hepatocyte assay | Rat hepatocytes | NA | 0, 35, 70, 100, 150 µM | Negative. |
| In vivo clastogenicity assay in rodent (Micronucleus assay) | Rat | +S9 | 0, 100, 300, 1200 mg/kg/day, for 1 month | Negative. |

[11]  PMDA Database.   http://www.pmda.go.jp/drugs/2014/P201400117/index.html (accessed Mar 2016).
[12]  FDA Database.   http://www.accessdata.fda.gov/drugsatfda_docs/nda/2014/204569Orig1s000PharmR.pdf (accessed Mar 2016).

## Reproductive and Developmental Toxicity

Table 24    Reproductive and Developmental Toxicology Studies of Suvorexant[11, 12]

| Studies | Species | Dosage (mg/kg/day) | NOAEL | | | | Finding |
|---------|---------|--------------------|---------|------|------|------|---------|
| | | | Endpoint | Dose (mg/kg/day) | AUC (μM·h) | Safety Margin[a] (× MRHD) | |
| Fertility and early embryonic development | SD rat | Female: 25, 75, 1200; Male: 100, 300, 1200; (In TPGS) | Male FED | >1200 | 405 | 44.0 | Body weight gain was decreased in females at all doses (during gestation), and increased in males. Food consumption was decreased in HD females. Resorptions/implants were increased in LD, MD and HD females; Corpora lutea/dam and implants/dam were decreased at HD; Percent of pre-implantation loss was increased in HD females and in untreated females mated with HD males. |
| | | | Female FED | 75 | 227 | 24.7 | |
| | | Female: 30, 80, 325; Male: 80, 160, 325; (In SDF) | Male FED | 325 | 396 | 43.0 | Body weight gain was decreased in females (during gestation), and increased in males. Food consumption was decreased in HD females. Resorptions/implants were increased in LD, MD and HD females, and untreated females mated with HD males; Corpora lutea/dam and implants/dam were decreased at the HD; Percent of pre-implantation loss was increased in LD and HD females, and untreated females mated with HD males. For fertility female, as HD females had a decrease in mean number of implants/pregnant females and increase in resorptions that resulted in a decrease in liver fetuses/pregnant females. |
| | | | Female FED | 325 | 695 | 75.5 | |
| Embryo-fetal development | SD rat | 30, 150, 1000 (In TPGS) | Maternal | 30 | 30.9 | 3.4 | MD dams had an initial decrease in mean body weight gain and HD dams had an initial body weight loss. Fetal weight was decreased in HD fetuses of both sexes. Skeletal changes included hypoplastic ribs in MD and HD fetuses, increased cervical and supernumerary ribs in MD and HD fetuses, and an increase in incomplete ossification of the sternebra in LD and MD fetuses. |
| | | | Fetal | 150 | 279 | 30.3 | |
| | | 30, 80, 325 (In SDF) | Maternal | 30 | 76.8 | 8.3 | One HD dam was found laterally recumbent and was sacrificed. A decrease in mean body weight gain was observed in HD dams. Fetal weight was decreased in HD fetuses of both sexes. |
| | | | Fetal | 80 | 230 | 25.0 | |
| | Dutch Belted rabbit | 40, 100, 300 (In TPGS) | Maternal | 100 | 95.7 | 10.4 | One HD dam was sacrificed early on GD 15. HD dams had an initial decrease in body weight gain. Skeletal changes included an increase in incomplete ossification in fetuses at the HD. Omphalocele was observed in 1 MD fetus, a vestigial tail in 1 HD fetus, and palate dysplasis and thoraco-schisis in 1 HD fetus. |
| | | | Fetal | 300 | 255 | 27.7 | |

[11]   PMDA Database.   http://www.pmda.go.jp/drugs/2014/P201400117/index.html (accessed Mar 2016).
[12]   FDA Database.   http://www.accessdata.fda.gov/drugsatfda_docs/nda/2014/204569Orig1s000PharmR.pdf (accessed Mar 2016).

*Continued*

| Studies | Species | Dosage (mg/kg/day) | NOAEL | | | | Finding |
|---|---|---|---|---|---|---|---|
| | | | Endpoint | Dose (mg/kg/day) | AUC (µM·h) | Safety Margin[a] (× MRHD) | |
| Embryo-fetal development | Dutch Belted rabbit | 50, 150, 325 (In SDF) | Maternal | 50 | 46.6 | 5.1 | HD dams were sacrificed early between GD 11-15, with no developmental data generated. MD dams had an initial decrease in mean body weight gain and HD dams had an initial body weight loss. Skeletal ossification in the metacarpal. In addition, ectrodactyly (malformation) was observed in 2 MD fetuses from the same litter. |
| | | | Fetal | 150 | 361 | 39.2 | |
| Pre- and post-natal development | SD rat | 30, 80, 200 (In SDF) | $F_0$, $F_1$ | 80 | 230 | 25.0 | In HD $F_0$ dams, an initial (GD 6-8) decrease in mean body weight was observed resulting in a decrease in mean body weight gain during gestation (GD 6-21). During lactation, mean body weight gain was decreased between days 7-14. In HD $F_1$ pups, a decrease in mean body weight gain was observed on PNDs 7, 14 and 21. Post-weaning, a decrease in mean body weight gain (>8%) was observed in $F_1$ female at all doses, until mating occurred in Week 12. Preputial separation occurred later in HD $F_1$ males than control $F_1$ males, by 1.2 days. |

SDF: Formulation in 0.5% methylcellulose with 5 mM HCl in deionized water.   TPGS: D-alpha-tocopheryl polyethylene glycol-1000 succinate.   [a] Calculated with the clinical recommended dose $AUC_{0-24}$ of 9.2 µM·h in human at the proposed recommended daily dose of 20 mg.

# Carcinogenicity

Table 25   Carcinogenic Toxicity Studies of Suvorexant[11, 12]

| Test | Species | Dose (mg/kg/day) | | | | |
|---|---|---|---|---|---|---|
| **6-Month Carcinogenic Study in Tg.rasH2 Mice** | | | | | | |
| | | 0[a] | 25 | 50 | 200 | 650 |
| Plasma conc. (0.5 h after administration) | Male | NA | 8.43 | 28.5 | 50.2 | 105 |
| | Female | NA | 10.9 | 25.6 | 65.1 | 69.2 |
| Malignant neoplasms (number) | Male | 1, 6 | 1 | 1 | 2 | 0 |
| | Female | 0, 0 | 2 | 3 | 2 | 4 |
| Benign neoplasms (number) | Male | 0, 1 | 2 | 3 | 1 | 3 |
| | Female | 0, 2 | 3 | 1 | 1 | 0 |
| Neoplasms (number) | Male | 1, 7 | 3 | 4 | 3 | 3 |
| | Female | 0, 2 | 5 | 4 | 3 | 4 |

| Test | Species | Dose (mg/kg/day) | | | |
|---|---|---|---|---|---|
| **2-Year Carcinogenic Study in SD Rats** | | | | | |
| | | 0[a] | 40 (M)/80 (F) | 80 (M)/160 (F) | 325 |
| Survival (%) | Male | 60, 48 | 52 | 72 | 58 |
| | Female | 68, 54 | 66 | 72 | 70 |
| Adenoma (number) | Male | 0, 0 | 2 | 1 | 1 |
| | Female | 6, 4 | 5 | 5 | 0 |

[11]  PMDA Database.   http://www.pmda.go.jp/drugs/2014/P201400117/index.html (accessed Mar 2016).
[12]  FDA Database.   http://www.accessdata.fda.gov/drugsatfda_docs/nda/2014/204569Orig1s000PharmR.pdf (accessed Mar 2016).

*Continued*

| | | 2-Year Carcinogenic Study in SD Rats | | | |
|---|---|---|---|---|---|
| **Test** | **Species** | **Dose (mg/kg/day)** | | | |
| | | **0[a]** | **40 (M)/80 (F)** | **80 (M)/160 (F)** | **325** |
| Carcinoma (number) | Male | 0, 0 | 0 | 1 | 1 |
| | Female | 1, 1 | 0 | 0 | 2 |
| Benign phenochromocytoma (number) | Male | 0, 2 | 2 | 0 | 1 |
| | Female | 1, 0 | 0 | 1 | 0 |
| Malignant phenochromocytoma (number) | Male | 0, 0 | 0 | 1 | 0 |
| | Female | 0, 0 | 0 | 0 | 1 |
| Benign ganglioneuroma (number) | Male | 0, 0 | 0 | 0 | 0 |
| | Female | 0, 1 | 0 | 0 | 0 |
| Finding | No effect on mortality in suvorexant treated groups in either females or males.<br>Decrease in mean body weight gain was observed in HD females and HD males in week 102.<br>The incidences of thyroid follicular cell adenomas and combined adenomas and carcinomas was significantly increased in MD males and HD.<br>Non-neoplastic histopathological findings include liver hepatocellular hypertrophy, eosinophilic cellular alteration, cystic degeneration and Kupffer cell pigmentation, thyroid gland follicular cell hypertrophy and hyperplasia, retinal atrophy, and chronic progressive nephropathy in the kidneys. | | | | |

M: Male.　F: Female.　NA: Not applicable.　[a] Two groups of dose 0 mg/kg/day.

## Special Toxicology

Table 26　Special Toxicology Studies of Suvorexant[11, 12]

| Study | Species | Finding |
|---|---|---|
| Phototoxicity assay | Murine (Pigmented rat) | Exposure to UVR did not result any skin reactions or ocular changes.<br>The NOEL for phototoxicity was greater than 325 mg/kg/day. |

Before UVR exposure, hair was shaved from the backs of all rats.　A UVR dose equivalent to 0.5 instrumental MED (a UVR dose adequate to elicit a barely perceptible response in skin) was delivered to each rat skin and eyes over a period of 30 ± 5 min.

[11]　PMDA Database.　http://www.pmda.go.jp/drugs/2014/P201400117/index.html (accessed Mar 2016).
[12]　FDA Database.　http://www.accessdata.fda.gov/drugsatfda_docs/nda/2014/204569Orig1s000PharmR.pdf (accessed Mar 2016).

# CHAPTER

## 24

## Tasimelteon

# Tasimelteon

## (Hetlioz®)

Research code: VEC-162

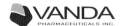

## 1   General Information

❖ Tasimelteon is a melatonin receptor agonist, which was first approved in Jan 2014 by US FDA.

❖ Tasimelteon was discovered by Bristol-Myers Squibb, developed and marketed by Vanda.

❖ The activities of tasimelteon at the $MT_1$ and $MT_2$ receptors are believed to contribute to its sleep-promoting properties, as these receptors, acted upon by endogenous melatonin, are thought to be involved in the maintenance of the circadian rhythm underlying the normal sleep-wake cycle.

❖ Tasimelteon is indicated for the treatment of Non-24-Hour Sleep-Wake Disorder.

❖ Available as capsule, with each containing 20 mg of tasimelteon and the recommended dose is 20 mg orally once daily until disease progression or unacceptable toxicity.

❖ Sales of Hetlioz® were 12.8 and 44.3 million US$ in 2014 and 2015, respectively, referring to the financial reports of Vanda.

## Key Approvals around the World*

|  | US (FDA) | EU (EMA) |
|---|---|---|
| First approval date | 01/31/2014 | 07/03/2015 |
| Application or approval No. | NDA 205677 | EMEA/H/C/003870 |
| Brand name | Hetlioz® | Hetlioz® |
| Indication | Non-24-Hour Sleep-Wake Disorder | Non-24-Hour Sleep-Wake Disorder |
| Authorisation holder | Vanda | Vanda |

* Till Mar 2016, it had not been approved by PMDA (Japan) and CFDA (China).

## Active Ingredient

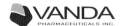

*Molecular formula*:   $C_{15}H_{19}NO_2$
*Molecular weight*:   245.32
*CAS No.*:   609799-22-6 (Tasimelteon)
*Chemical name*:   (1*R*,2*R*)-*N*-[2-(2,3-dihydrobenzofuran-4-yl)cyclopropylmethyl]propanamide

*Parameters of Lipinski's "Rule of 5"*

| MW | $H_D$ | $H_A$ | FRB[a] | PSA[a] | cLogP[a] |
|---|---|---|---|---|---|
| 245.32 | 1 | 3 | 4 | 38.3Å² | 1.86 ± 0.38 |

[a] Calculated by ACD/Labs software V11.02.

## Drug Product*

*Dosage route*:   Oral
*Strength*:   20 mg (Tasimelteon)
*Dosage form*:   Capsule
*Inactive ingredient*:   Lactose anhydrous, microcrystalline cellulose, croscarmellose sodium, colloidal silicon dioxide, magnesium stearate, gelatin, titanium dioxide, FD&C Blue #1, FD&C Red #3 and FD&C Yellow #6.
*Recommended dose*:   The recommended starting dose is 20 mg orally once daily prior to bedtime without food, at same time every night.
Because of individual differences in circadian rhythms, drug effect may not occur for weeks or months.

* Sourced from US FDA drug label information

## 2   Key Patents Information

### Summary

❖ Hetlioz® (Tasimelteon) has got five-year NCE market exclusivity protection and seven-year orphan drug exclusivity protection after it was initially approved by US FDA on Jan 31, 2014.

❖ Tasimelteon was originally discovered by Bristol-Myers Squibb and then developed by Vanda Pharmaceuticals, and its compound patent application was filed as PCT application by Bristol-Myers Squibb in 1997.

❖ The compound patent will expire in 2017 foremost, which has been granted in the United States, China, Europe and Japan successively.

Table 1   Tasimelteon's Compound Patent Protection in Drug-Mainstream Country

| Country | Publication/Patent NO. | Application Date | Granted Date | Estimated Expiry Date |
|---|---|---|---|---|
| WO | WO9825606A1 | 12/09/1997 | / | / |
| US | US5856529A | 12/09/1997 | 01/05/1999 | 12/09/2017 |
| EP | EP1027043B1 | 12/09/1997 | 11/10/2004 | 12/09/2017 |
| JP | JP4290765B2 | 12/09/1997 | 07/08/2009 | 12/09/2017 |
| CN | CN1152679C | 12/09/1997 | 06/09/2004 | 12/09/2017 |

Table 2   Originator's International Patent Application List (Patent Family)

| Publication NO. | Title | Applicant/Assignee/Owner | Publication Date |
|---|---|---|---|
| Technical Subjects | Active Ingredient (Free Base)'s Formula or Structure and Preparation | | |
| WO9825606A1 | Benzodioxole, benzofuran, dihydrobenzofuran, and benzodioxane melatonergic agents | Bristol-Myers Squibb | 06/18/1998 |
| Technical Subjects | Salt, Crystal, Polymorphic, Solvate (Hydrate), Isomer, Derivative Etc. and Preparation | | |
| WO2013173707A1 | Metabolites of (1R-trans)-N-[[2-(2,3-dihydro-4-benzofuranyl) cyclopropyl]methyl]propanamide | Vanda | 11/21/2013 |
| WO2015123389A1 | Highly purified pharmaceutical grade tasimelteon | Vanda | 08/20/2015 |
| Technical Subjects | Indication or Methods for Medical Needs | | |
| WO2007137244A1 | Melatonin agonist treatment | Vanda | 11/29/2007 |
| WO2007137247A2 | Treatment for depressive disorders | Vanda | 11/29/2007 |
| WO2011009102A1 | Use of a melatonin agonist for the treatment of sleep disorders including primary insomnia | Vanda | 01/20/2011 |
| WO2013112949A2 | Treatment of circadian rhythm disorders | Vanda | 08/01/2013 |
| WO2013112951A2 | Treatment of circadian rhythm disorders | Vanda | 08/01/2013 |
| WO2015108728A1 | Administration of tasimelteon under fasted conditions | Vanda | 07/23/2015 |
| Technical Subjects | Combination Including at Least Two Active Ingredients | | |
| WO2007016203A1 | Method of improving wakefulness | Vanda | 02/08/2007 |
| WO2007137227A1 | Treatment for depressive disorders | Vanda | 11/29/2007 |
| WO2014100292A1 | Treatment of circadian rhythm disorders | Vanda | 06/26/2014 |
| WO2015117048A1 | Treatment of circadian rhythm disorders | Vanda | 08/06/2015 |
| Technical Subjects | Others | | |
| WO2009036257A1 | Prediction of sleep parameter and response to sleep-inducing compound based on PER3 VNTR genotype | Vanda | 03/19/2009 |

The data was updated until Jan 2016.

# 3 Chemistry

## Route 1: Original Discovery Route

MNNG: 1-Methyl-3-nitro-1-nitrosoguanidine

*Synthetic Route:* In this synthetic route, the target tasimelteon was synthesized from methyl 3-(allyloxy)benzoate **1** through 16 steps. Successively, thermal Claisen rearrangement of allyl ether **1**, oxidative cleavage of terminal vinyl group in **2**, dehydration of hemiacetal **3**, and then hydrolysis of methyl ester **4** provided the key intermediate benzofuran-4-carboxylic acid **5** in 22% yield over four steps. Catalytic hydrogenation of **5** provided 2,3-dihydrobenzofuran **6**, which was reduced with LAH and then suffered from Swern oxidation produced aldehyde **8** with the yield of 73% across three steps. Subjection of **8** with malonic acid **9** afforded propenoic acid derivative **10** in nearly quantitative yield, along with chlorination using thionyl chloride and condensation with chiral auxiliary (-)-2,10-camphorsultam **12** to supply asymmetric amide **13** in 90% yield over two steps. Pd(II)-catalyzed cyclopropanation using diazomethane *in situ* generated from MNNG gave rise to optically active cyclopropane **14** with the yield of 67%. Afterwards, release the free alcohol by general reduction and upon succedent Swern oxidation led to the cyclopropane carboxaldehyde **16** in excellent yield over two steps, which was transformed to tasimelteon *via* condensation with hydroxylamine, reduction and acylation in a three-step sequence with 43% yield. The overall yield was 5%.[1-3]

[1]  Catt, J. D.; Johnson, G.; Keavy, D. J., et al. WO9825606A1, **1998**.
[2]  Catt, J. D.; Johnson, G.; Keavy, D. J., et al. US5856529A, **1999**.
[3]  Eissenstat, M. A.; Bell, M. R.; D'Ambra, T. E., et al. *J. Med. Chem.* **1995**, *38*, 3094-3105.

## Route 2

(DHQ)₂PHAL: Hydroquinine 1,4-phthalazinediyl diether
TMOA: Trimethylorthoacetate

*Synthetic Route*:    Sharpless asymmetric dihydroxylation of olefin **1** delivered diol **2** in 86% yield and impressive enantiose-lectivity (99.4% *ee*).    After this diol was activated with trimethylsilyl chloride and then treated with base, epoxide **3** was generated in 89% yield with 98.2% *ee*.    Next, a modified Horner-Wadsworth-Emmons reaction involving triethylphosphonoacetate (TEPA, **4**) was employed to convert epoxide **3** to cyclopropane **5**.    The reaction presumably proceeded through removal of the acidic TEPA proton followed by nucleophilic attack at the terminal epoxide carbon.    The resulting alkoxide underwent an intramolecular phosphoryl transfer reaction resulting in an enolate which then attacked the newly formed phosphonate ester in an $S_N2$ fashion resulting in the trans-cyclopropane ester **5**, which was ultimately saponified and reacidified to furnish cyclopropane acid **6** in 88% yield across a two-step sequence.    Conversion of this acid to the corresponding primary amide **8** preceded carbonyl reduction with sodium borohydride, and the resulting amine **9** was acylated with propionyl chloride **10** to furnish tasimelteon as the final product in 68% yield across the four-step sequence with the overall yield of 46%.[4-8]

## Route 3

[4]   Prasad, J. S.; Vu, T.; Totleben, M. J., et al. *Org. Process Res. Dev.* **2003**, *7*, 821-827.
[5]   Singh, A. K.; Rao, M. N.; Simpson, J. H., et al. *Org. Process Res. Dev.* **2002**, *6*, 618-620.
[6]   Liu, Y.; Zhang, H.; Liu J. CN102675268A, **2012**.
[7]   Liu, Y.; Zhang, H.; Liu J. CN103113177A, **2013**.
[8]   Liu, Y.; Zhang, H.; Liu J. CN103087019A, **2013**.

*Synthetic Route*:    In this synthetic route, EDC-condensation of *trans*-2-(2,3-dihydrobenzofuran-4-yl)cyclopropanecarboxylic acid **1** with the chiral auxillary 1-[(*R*)-amino(phenyl)methyl]naphthalen-2-ol **2**, followed by separation of the obtained mixture of diastereomers from recrystallization in Hexane/DCM, gave chiral amide **3** in 85% yield, which upon acidic removal of chiral auxillary afforded the key (1*R*,2*R*)-2-(2,3-dihydrobenzofuran-4-yl)cyclopropanecarboxylic acid **4**.    Amination after activation of acid **4** as its acyl chloride yielded amide **5**, which went through borane reduction and acidic quench to produce amine hydrochloride **6** with 76% yield from acid **4**, in which the free amine group was subjected to propionyl chloride **7** in basic conditions to generate the titled compound in 82% yield.    The overall yield was 44%.[9-11]

## Route 4

TBAH: Tetrabutylammonium hydroxide
BTBSC: (*R*,*R*)-(-)-*N*,*N'*-Bis(3,5-*di-tert*-butylsalicylidene)-1,2-cyclohexanediamine
(+)-DAA: (+)-Dehydroabietylamine

*Synthetic Route*:    This process represented an industrial scale production of tasimelteon illustrated in top scheme.    An initial reaction mixture was prepared by slowly adding oxalyl chloride to a solution of DMF in $CH_3CN$ to complete the formation of Vilsmeier reagent (*N*,*N*-dimethylchloromethyleneiminium chloride) *in situ*, which exposure to firstly triol **1** in portions and then a solution of TEA in $CH_3CN$.    When the addition was complete, the mixture was heated at elevated temperature to lead to dihydrobenzofuran **3** used directly into the next step.    Vinyl-dihydrobenzofuran **4** was synthesized from TBAH-facilitated elimination.    Next, a chiral Ru catalyst was prepared from BTBSC and a fresh prepared LDA solution, and then **4** was subjected to the preceding catalytic system followed by the addition of ethyl diazoacetate ready for Ru-catalyzed cyclopropanation, upon which the key intermediate (1*R*,2*R*)-2-(2,3-dihydrobenzofuran-4-yl)cyclopropanecarboxylic acid ethyl ester **6** was produced in a kg scale used straightway along with saponification and acidic quench to afford carboxylic acid **7**.    Further purification was achieved by the resolution of **7** with (+)-DAA, which was prior to the activation with thionyl chloride and succedent amination.    Next, amide **9** was suffered from LAH reduction and acidic workup to supply the free amine of tasimelteon **10** as a hydrochloride salt.    Finally, condensation with propionyl chloride **11** in basic conditions produced tasimelteon after recrystallization in $EtOH/H_2O$.[12-14]

[9]   Xu, X. CN104327022A, **2015**.
[10]   Sun, L. Q.; Takaki, K.; Chen, J., et al. *Bioorg. Med. Chem. Lett.* **2004**, *14*, 5157-5160.
[11]   Sun, L. Q.; Takaki, K.; Chen, J., et al. *Bioorg. Med. Chem. Lett.* **2005**, *15*, 1345-1349.
[12]   Phadke, D.; Platt, N. M. WO2015123389A1, **2015**.
[13]   Pereira, D. E.; Aumiller, W.; Dagger, R. US7754902B2, **2010**.
[14]   Pereira, D. E.; Aumiller, W.; Dagger, R. US20070270593A1, **2007**.

## 4   Pharmacology

## Summary

Mechanism of Action

❖ Tasimelteon is a full agonist at melatonin receptors $MT_1$ ($K_i = 0.304$ nM, $IC_{50} = 0.586$ nM) and $MT_2$ ($K_i = 0.0692$ nM, $IC_{50} = 0.133$ nM).

❖ Tasimelteon demonstrated potent, concentration-dependent inhibition of forskolin-stimulated cAMP accumulation ($MT_1$, $EC_{50} = 0.74$ nM; $MT_2$, $EC_{50} = 0.1$ nM).

❖ The metabolite of tasimelteon showed nanomolar affinity at human melatonin receptor $MT_1$ (M13, $IC_{50} = 7.69$ nM) and melatonin receptor $MT_2$ (M11, $IC_{50} = 6.63$ nM; M12, $IC_{50} = 20.8$ nM; M13, $IC_{50} = 1.78$ nM; M14, $IC_{50} = 8.42$ nM).

❖ Tasimelteon showed no significant binding affinity for 63 and 170 different targets in two separate screens at 10 and 100 µM.[15, 16]

❖ Binding affinity of tasimelteon at the human melatonin receptors:
- In NIH-3T3 cell lines containing melatonin receptors:
  ❖ Human $MT_1$ receptor: $K_i = 0.35$ nM.
  ❖ Human $MT_2$ receptor: $K_i = 0.17$ nM.
- In CHO-K1 cell lines containing melatonin receptors:
  ❖ $MT_1$ receptor: $K_i = 0.304$ nM.
  ❖ $MT_2$ receptor: $K_i = 0.0692$ nM.

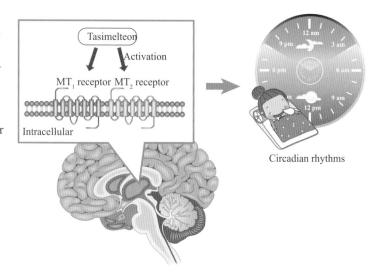

Circadian rhythms

*In Vivo* Efficacy

❖ The *ex vivo* study of brain slices taken from rats: Suprachiasmatic nucleus (SCN) electrical activity rhythms shifted significantly faster than those in slices from the vehicle-treated animals.

❖ The model of acute phase shifting of locomotor activity in rats: Advanced the onset of running-wheel activity in rats.

❖ The model of entrainment of "free-running" activity rhythms in rats: The onset of activity coincided with the injection time, $ED_{50} = 0.21$ mg/kg.

## Mechanism of Action

Table 3   Comparative Affinity of Tasimelteon and Its Metabolites for the Human Melatonin Receptors $MT_1$ and $MT_2$[15-17]

| Compound | MT₁ | | | | MT₂ | | | |
|---|---|---|---|---|---|---|---|---|
| | Conc. (µM) | %Inhibition | $K_i$ (nM) | $IC_{50}$ (nM) | Conc. (µM) | %Inhibition | $K_i$ (nM) | $IC_{50}$ (nM) |
| Tasimelteon | 0.001 | 57 | $0.304 \pm 0.013$ | $0.586 \pm 0.025$ | 0.0003 | 60 | $0.0692 \pm 0.007$ | $0.133 \pm 0.014$ |
| M3 | 10 | 52 | 1750 | 3370 | 1 | 61 | 180 | 360 |
| M9 | 3 | 50 | $1180 \pm 179$ | $2260 \pm 346$ | 0.3 | 61 | $71.9 \pm 3$ | $139 \pm 5$ |
| M11 | 1 | 62 | $250 \pm 24$ | $481 \pm 47$ | 0.01 | 55 | $3.44 \pm 0.66$ | $6.63 \pm 1.28$ |
| M12 | 1 | 70 | 136 | 261 | 0.1 | 74 | 10.8 | 20.8 |
| M13 | 0.01 | 52 | $4 \pm 0.216$ | $7.69 \pm 0.42$ | 0.003 | 54 | $0.922 \pm 0.224$ | $1.78 \pm 0.43$ |
| M14 | 1 | 77 | 103 | 198 | 0.01 | 53 | 4.37 | 8.42 |

Tasimelteon showed potent inhibition of 2-[$^{125}$I]iodomelatonin binding at the $MT_1$ and $MT_2$ receptors in radioligand binding studies.

[15] U.S. Food and Drug Administration (FDA) Datadase.   http://www.accessdata.fda.gov/drugsatfda_docs/nda/2014/205677Orig1s000PharmR.pdf (accessed Mar 2016).
[16] European Medicines Agency (EMA) Database.   http://www.ema.europa.eu/docs/en_GB/document_library/EPAR_-_Public_assessment_report/human/003870/WC500190309.pdf (accessed Mar 2016).
[17] Lavedan, C.; Forsberg, M.; Gentile, A. J. *Neuropharmacology* **2015**, *91*, 142-147.

Table 4    *In Vitro* Binding Affinity of Tasimelteon against the Human Melatonin Receptors in Cells[17]

| Cell Line | EC$_{50}$ (nM) | | E$_{max}$ (%) | | K$_i$ (nM) | | K$_i$ Ratio |
|---|---|---|---|---|---|---|---|
| | MT$_1$ | MT$_2$ | MT$_1$ | MT$_2$ | MT$_1$ | MT$_2$ | MT$_1$/MT$_2$ |
| NIH-3T3 | 0.74 | 0.1[a] | 59 ± 1 | 60 ± 3 | 0.35 | 0.17 | 2.1 |
| CHO-K1 | NA | NA | NA | NA | 0.304 | 0.0692 | 4.4 |

Two cell lines of NIH-3T3 cells and CHO-K1 cells were used; the first expressed the human MT$_1$ receptor while the second expressed the human MT$_2$ receptor.    Data were analyzed by a 4-parameter logistic, non-linear least squares regression to yield IC$_{50}$ values (concentration producing 50% of the maximal effect), which were converted to dissociation constant for the inhibitor (K$_i$) values.    [a] In FDA the value was 1 nM.

## *In Vivo* Efficacy

Table 5    *In Vivo* Efficacy of Tasimelteon in Rat Models[15, 16]

| Models | Animal | Administration | | Effect | |
|---|---|---|---|---|---|
| | | Dose (mg/kg/day) | Duration & Route (Day) | ED$_{50}$[a] (mg/kg) | Finding |
| Light-dark cycle[b] | Brain slices in rat | Melatonin: 1.0 Tasimelteon: 1.0, 5.0 | s.c., single dose | NA | SCN electrical activity rhythms shifted significantly faster in the slices taken from melatonin-tasimelteon-treated animals than those in slices from the vehicle-treated animals. |
| Constant darkness, acute phase shifting of locomotor activity | Rat | Melatonin: 0.1, 1.0 Tasimelteon: 1.0, 5.0 | s.c. | NA | Melatonin and tasimelteon advanced the onset of running-wheel activity in rats. |
| Entrainment of "free-running" activity rhythms | Rat | Melatonin: 1.0 Tasimelteon: 1.0, 5.0 | s.c. QD × 66 | 0.21 | Melatonin and tasimelteon were reported to "synchronize" the "free-running" locomotor rhythms so that the onset of activity coincided with the injection time. |

SCN: Suprachiasmatic nuclei.    [a] ED$_{50}$ was analyzed with tasimelteon.    [b] *Ex vivo* study, light-dark cycle: Light onset delayed by 12 h.

# 5    ADME & Drug-Drug Interaction

## Summary

### Absorption of Tasimelteon

❖ Exhibited a linear pharmacokinetics in humans following oral dosing.    The increases in C$_{max}$ and AUC appeared to be dose-proportional in the dose range of 1-300 mg tasimelteon.

❖ Had good bioavailability in rats (58.5%) and humans (50%), but poor in monkeys (11.7%), after oral administrations.

❖ Was absorbed quickly (T$_{max}$ = 0.25-1.25 h) in humans, female rats and monkeys.

❖ Showed a half-life of 1.02 h in humans, shorter than those in rats and monkeys (2.1 h), after intravenous administrations.

❖ Had high clearance in rats (5.3 L/h/kg), but moderate in monkeys (1.6 L/h/kg) and humans (505 mL/min), in contrast to liver blood flow, after intravenous administrations.

❖ Exhibited an extensive tissue distribution in rats, monkeys and humans, with apparent volumes of distribution at 3.8, 1.4 L/kg and 42.7 L, respectively, after intravenous administrations.

❖ Showed a high permeability, with the Papp$_{(A→B)}$ = (19.4–63.9) × 10$^{-6}$ cm/s in Caco-2 cells monolayer model.

### Distribution of Tasimelteon

❖ Exhibited moderate plasma protein binding in humans (85.8%-90.3%), mice (73.5%-77.6%), rats (76.8%-84.8%) and monkeys (69.0%-79.7%).

❖ Rats after oral administration:
  • The drug was widely distributed into tissues, and had a relatively short half-life.
  • Relatively higher drug concentration levels (in order) were observed in stomach, small intestine, liver, kidneys, plasma, large intestine, blood and adrenals.
  • Based on the long half-life of radioactivity in the eyes (126 h) and pigmented versus non-pigmented skin (15.4 vs. 7.6 h) following dosing of [$^{14}$C]tasimelteon, binding of tasimelteon to melanin was suggested.

[15]  FDA Datadase.    http://www.accessdata.fda.gov/drugsatfda_docs/nda/2014/205677Orig1s000PharmR.pdf (accessed Mar 2016).
[16]  EMA Database.    http://www.ema.europa.eu/docs/en_GB/document_library/EPAR_-_Public_assessment_report/human/003870/WC500190309.pdf (accessed Mar 2016).
[17]  Lavedan, C.; Forsberg, M.; Gentile, A. J. *Neuropharmacology* **2015**, *91*, 142-147.

- The half-life of elimination of the radioactivity from brain was approximately 1 h.   The tissues still showing radioactivity after 168 h were eyes, liver, thyroid, lungs and kidneys.

## Metabolism of Tasimelteon

❖ Tasimelteon was extensively metabolized by CYP enzymes in the liver primarily by CYP1A2 and CYP3A4, and to a lesser extent by CYP1A1, CYP2D6, CYP2C19 and CYP2C9.

❖ The major metabolic routes of tasimelteon in humans were oxidation at multiple sites and oxidative dealkylation resulting in opening of the furan ring (O-dealkylation), followed by further oxidation to give carboxylic acid.   Phenolic glucuronidation was the major phase II metabolic route.

❖ M9 represented the most abundant component in human plasma, with M12, M13, M9, M11 and M14 as the major metabolites.   However, metabolites M12, M14 and M9 were inactive.

❖ Total of eight metabolites were identified in plasma, urine and feces of humans.

❖ Human metabolite M11 was not detected in rats.

## Excretion of Tasimelteon

❖ Was predominantly excreted in urine of humans and monkeys, with M9 as the major significant component in human urine.

## Drug-Drug Interaction

❖ Tasimelteon and the major metabolites (M9, M12 and M13) had no direct inhibition or time-dependent inhibition of CYP enzymes evaluated (CYP1A2, CYP2B6, CYP2C8, CYP2C9 or CYP2D6) *in vitro*.   Tasimelteon and M12 had weak inhibition for CYP3A4 and CYP2C19 *in vitro*.

❖ Tasimelteon induced CYP2C8 (up to 60.3%) and CYP3A4 (up to 83.2%) *in vitro,* but tasimelteon and its metabolites (M9, M12 and M13) did not induce CYP1A2 or CYP2B6.

❖ Tasimelteon was not a substrate of P-gp, OATP1B1 or OATP1B3.

❖ Tasimelteon had no inhibition for OATP1B1, OATP1B3, OAT1, P-gp or BCRT, but had weak inhibition for OAT3 and OCT2 *in vitro*.

# Absorption

Table 6   *In Vivo* Pharmacokinetic Parameters of Tasimelteon in Rats and Monkeys after Single Intravenous and Oral Dose of Tasimelteon[15, 16, 18]

| Species | Route | Dose (mg/kg) | $T_{max}$ (h) | $C_{max}$ (ng/mL) | $AUC_{0-24}$ (ng·h/mL) | $T_{1/2}$ (h) | Cl (L/h/kg) | $V_{ss}$ (L/kg) | F (%) |
|---|---|---|---|---|---|---|---|---|---|
| Rat | i.v. | 1.0 | NA | NA | NA | $2.1 \pm 1.0$ | $5.3 \pm 1.3$ | $3.8 \pm 1.6$ | - |
| | p.o. | 1.0 | 0.25 | $51 \pm 24$ | NA | NA | NA | NA | 58.5 |
| Monkey | i.v. | 1.0 | NA | NA | NA | $2.1 \pm 0.3$ | $1.6 \pm 0.1$ | $1.4 \pm 0.1$ | - |
| | p.o. | 1.0 | 0.67 | $54.2 \pm 41$ | NA | NA | NA | NA | $11.7 \pm 8.2$ |
| Rat (male) | p.o. | 25 | $4^a$ | $4140 \pm 760$ | $21700 \pm 6810$ | 1.0 | NA | NA | NA |
| | p.o. | 100 | $8^a$ | $11300 \pm 5600$ | $95900 \pm 23000$ | NA | NA | NA | NA |
| | p.o. | 250 | $6^a$ | $16000 \pm 4400$ | $182000 \pm 29000$ | 2.8 | NA | NA | NA |
| | p.o. | 500 | $0.5^a$ | $23300 \pm 2200$ | $207000 \pm 2300$ | NA | NA | NA | NA |
| Rat (female) | p.o. | 25 | $0.5^a$ | $6990 \pm 2800$ | $20400 \pm 3400$ | NA | NA | NA | NA |
| | p.o. | 100 | $0.5^a$ | $13700 \pm 3500$ | $105000 \pm 1000$ | 4.5 | NA | NA | NA |
| | p.o. | 250 | $0.5^a$ | $24000 \pm 12300$ | $191000 \pm 8500$ | NA | NA | NA | NA |
| | p.o. | 500 | $0.5^a$ | $21900 \pm 4500$ | $159000 \pm 31000$ | NA | NA | NA | NA |

NA: Not available.   $^a$ Median for $T_{max}$.

[15]  FDA Database.   http://www.accessdata.fda.gov/drugsatfda_docs/nda/2014/205677Orig1s000PharmR.pdf (accessed Mar 2016).
[16]  EMA Database.   http://www.ema.europa.eu/docs/en_GB/document_library/EPAR_-_Public_assessment_report/human/003870/WC500190309.pdf (accessed Mar 2016).
[18]  Vachharajani, N. N.; Yeleswaram, K.; Boulton, D. W. *J. Pharm. Sci.* **2003**, *92*, 760-772.

Table 7  *In Vivo* Pharmacokinetic Parameters of Tasimelteon in Humans after
Single Intravenous and Oral Dose of Tasimelteon[19]

| Species | Route | Dose (mg) | $C_{max}$ (ng/mL) | $T_{1/2}$ (h) | $AUC_{inf}$ (ng·h/mL) | $T_{max}$ (h) | Cl or Cl/F (mL/min) | $V_{ss}$ (L) | F (%) |
|---|---|---|---|---|---|---|---|---|---|
| | i.v. | 2 | 82.2 ± 20.5 | 1.02 ± 0.23 | 71.6 ± 23.9 | 0.28 | 505 ± 135 | 42.7 ± 7.0 | - |
| | p.o. | 20 | 260 ± 189 | 1.06 ± 0.23 | 358 ± 271 | 0.50 | 2241 ± 3592 | 178 ± 261 | 50 |
| Healthy human | | 1 | 8.3 | 1.11 | 14.0 | 0.50 | NA | NA | NA |
| | | 3 | 15.6 | 1.48 | 20.8 | 0.63 | NA | NA | NA |
| | p.o. | 10 | 66.6 | 1.95 | 111 | 0.75 | NA | NA | NA |
| | | 30 | 104 | 1.95 | 189 | 0.75 | NA | NA | NA |
| | | 100 | 313 | 4.8 | 935 | 1.25 | NA | NA | NA |
| | | 300 | 901 | 5.07 | 2943 | 1.00 | NA | NA | NA |

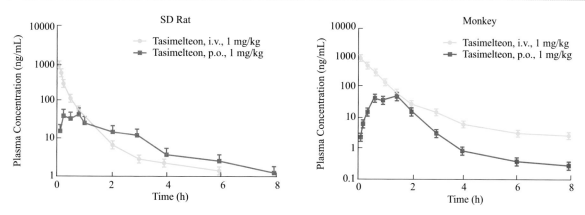

Figure A  *In Vivo* Plasma Concentration-Time Profiles of Tasimelteon in Male Rats and Male Monkeys after Single
Intravenous and Oral Dose of Tasimelteon[18]

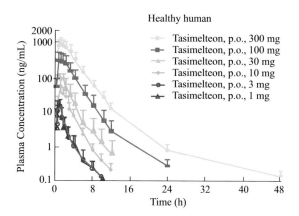

Figure B  *In Vivo* Plasma Concentration-Time Profiles of Tasimelteon in Healthy Humans after
Single Oral Dose of Tasimelteon (n = 8)[19]

[18]  Vachharajani, N. N.; Yeleswaram, K.; Boulton, D. W. *J. Pharm. Sci.* **2003**, *92*, 760-772.
[19]  FDA Datadase.  http://www.accessdata.fda.gov/drugsatfda_docs/nda/2014/205677Orig1s000ClinPharmR.pdf (accessed Mar 2016).

Table 8    *In Vitro* Permeability of Tasimelteon in Caco-2 Cell Monolayer Model[19]

| Test Article | Conc. (µM) | Papp$_{(A \to B)}$ ($1 \times 10^{-6}$ cm/s) | Permeability Class |
|---|---|---|---|
| Tasimelteon | 0.6 | $32.6 \pm 21$ | High |
| | 6 | $19.4 \pm 2.7$ | High |
| | 60 | 63.9 | High |

Mean ± SD for Papp.

## Distribution

Table 9    *In Vitro* Plasma Protein Binding of Tasimelteon in Several Species[15, 19]

| Species | Conc. (ng/mL) | %Bound |
|---|---|---|
| Mouse | 200-20000 | 73.5-77.6 |
| Rat | 200-20000 | 76.8-84.8 |
| Monkey | 200-20000 | 69.0-79.7 |
| Human | 10-2000 | 85.8-90.3 |

### Key Findings:[15]

❖ Orally administered tasimelteon was widely distributed, and had a relatively short half-life.

❖ The tissues with the highest mean concentrations (in order) were stomach, small intestine, liver, kidneys, plasma, large intestine, blood and adrenals.

❖ Based on the long half-life of radioactivity in the eyes (126 h) and pigmented versus non-pigmented skin (15.4 vs. 7.6 h) following dosing of [$^{14}$C]tasimelteon, binding of tasimelteon to melanin was suggested.

❖ Following oral administration of [$^{14}$C]tasimelteon to rats, plasma levels of radioactivity declined through 120 h and were not detected by 168 h post-dose.

❖ Terminal half-life of the radioactivity was also extended in lungs (66 h), kidneys (49 h), liver (47 h), adrenal (40 h) and stomach (22 h).

❖ The half-life of elimination of the radioactivity from brain was approximately 1 h.   The tissues still showing radioactivity after 168 h were eyes, liver, thyroid, lungs and kidneys.

## Metabolism

Table 10    *In Vitro* Metabolic Phenotype of Tasimelteon[19]

| Methods | Specific Chemical Inhibitor, HLM, 0.25 mg/mL, Tasimelteon 100 µM | | | | | Recombinant Enzyme, 50 pmol/mL, Tasimelteon 100 µM | | | | |
|---|---|---|---|---|---|---|---|---|---|---|
| Parameter | %Inhibition[a] | | | | | Formation of Metabolites[b] | | | | |
| Analyte | M9 | M11 | M12 | M13 | M14 | M9 | M11 | M12 | M13 | M14 |
| CYP1A2 | 42.9 | 40.9 | 47.3 | 69.3 | 67.6 | 487 (high) | 540 (high) | 171(high) | 434 (high) | ND |
| CYP2B6 | 30.0 | 1.44 | 49.3 | NA | 58.8 | 23 (very low)[c] | NA | NA | 42 (low)[d] | ND |
| CYP2C8 | 83.1 | 45.5 | NA | 37.6 | NA | 5 (very low)[c] | NA | NA | 6 (very low)[c] | ND |
| CYP2C9 | 80.8 | 4.38 | 29.4 | NA | 46.0 | 15 (very low)[c] | NA | NA | 46 (low)[d] | ND |
| CYP2C19 | 41.9 | 21.2 | 4.50 | 17.6 | 32.1 | 117 (high) | 130 (high) | NA | 283 (high) | ND |
| CYP2D6 | 13.5 | NA | 2.39 | 11.9 | 43.4 | 98 (high) | 149 (high) | NA | 571 (high) | ND |
| CYP2E1 | 48.9 | 35.2 | 52.3 | 12.9 | 87.0 | NA | NA | NA | NA | ND |
| CYP3A4 | 44.2 | NA | 74.3 | 7.28 | 99.0 | 7 (very low) | 0 | 287 (high) | NA | 226 (high) |

NA: Not available.   ND: Not detected.   [a] Percent inhibition of formation of tasimelteon metabolites by isoform-selective chemical inhibitor compared to no inhibitor control in human liver microsomes.   [b] Formation of tasimelteon metabolites by recombinant human cytochrome P450 isoform.   [c] Formation of metabolite ≤5% of the highest value.   [d] Formation of metabolite ≤10% of the highest value.

[15]  FDA Database.   http://www.accessdata.fda.gov/drugsatfda_docs/nda/2014/205677Orig1s000PharmR.pdf (accessed Mar 2016).
[19]  FDA Datadase.   http://www.accessdata.fda.gov/drugsatfda_docs/nda/2014/205677Orig1s000ClinPharmR.pdf (accessed Mar 2016).

Table 11 Metabolites in Plasma, Urine and Feces of Rats, Monkeys and Humans after Single Oral Dose of Tasimelteon[15, 19]

| Species | Matrix | Gender | Dose (mg/kg) | Time (h) | Percent of Total Radioactivity (% AUC or % Dose) | | | | | | | | |
|---------|--------|--------|--------------|----------|--------|------|-------|------|------|------|------|------|------|
| | | | | | Parent | M1 | M3 | M8 | M9 | M11 | M12 | M13 | M14 |
| Plasma | Rat | Male | 25 | 0-8 | 15.7 | NA | 3.8 | NA | 4.16 | NA | 48.4 | 0.57 | 1.58 |
| | Monkey | Male | 25 | 0-12 | 8.91 | 1.43 | 4.18 | 3.98 | 10.3 | 1.76 | 3.72 | 4.12 | 2.61 |
| | | Female | 25 | 0-12 | 17.7 | 1.2 | 3.94 | 4.12 | 6.72 | 1.35 | 10.0 | 2.47 | 4.36 |
| | Human | Male | 100 mg | - | 8.22 | 3.24 | 7.80 | 3.46 | 19.8 | 3.56 | 3.94 | 14.6 | 7.13 |
| Urine | Human | Male | 100 mg | 0-72 | ND | 3.69 | 12.53 | 4.87 | 29.69 | ND | ND | ND | ND |
| Feces | Human | Male | 100 mg | 0-120 | 0.04 | ND | ND | ND | 0.85 | ND | ND | ND | ND |

ND: Not detected.    %AUC for plasma.

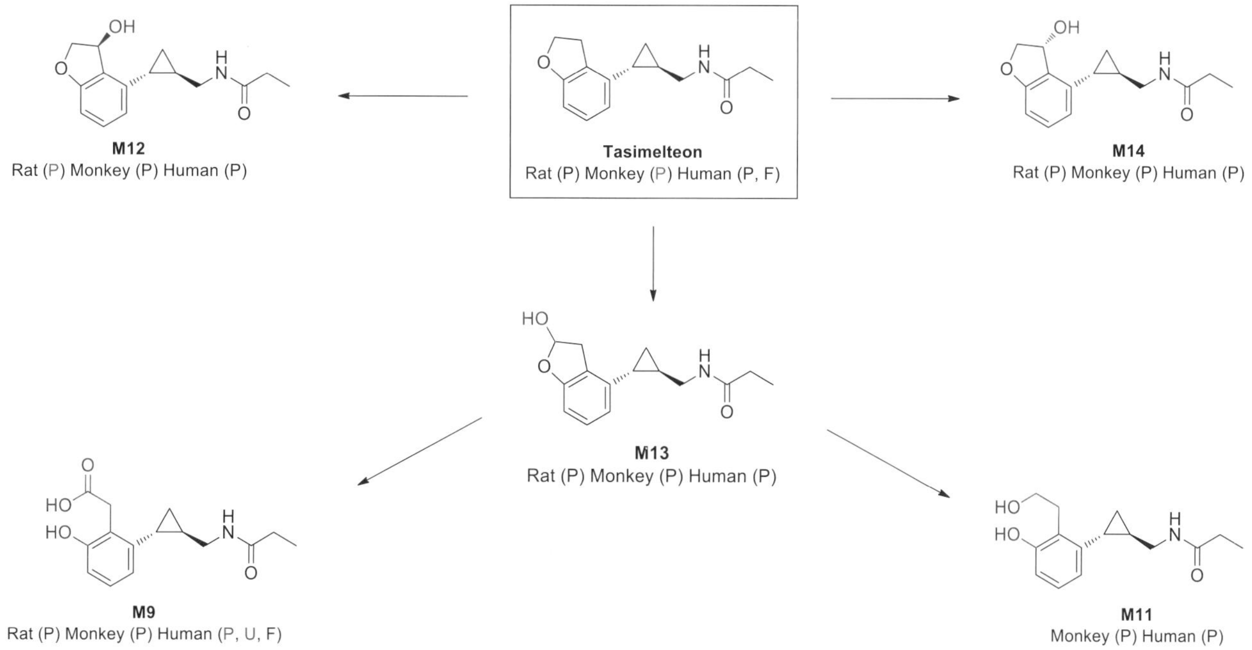

**M12**
Rat (P) Monkey (P) Human (P)

**Tasimelteon**
Rat (P) Monkey (P) Human (P, F)

**M14**
Rat (P) Monkey (P) Human (P)

**M13**
Rat (P) Monkey (P) Human (P)

**M9**
Rat (P) Monkey (P) Human (P, U, F)

**M11**
Monkey (P) Human (P)

Figure C    Proposed Pathways for *In Vivo* Biotransformation of Tasimelteon in Rats, Monkeys and Humans[15, 19]
The red labels represent the major components in the matrices.    P = Plasma, U = Urine and F = Feces.

# Excretion

Table 12    Excretion Profiles of [14C]Tasimelteon in Humans after Single Oral Dose of Tasimelteon[15, 19]

| Species | State | Route | Dose (mg) | Time (h) | Urine (% of dose) | Feces (% of dose) | Recovery (% of dose) |
|---------|-------|-------|-----------|----------|-------------------|-------------------|----------------------|
| Monkey (male & female) | Intact | p.o. | 25 | 0-24 | 80 | 5 | 85 |
| Human (male) | Intact | p.o. | 100 | 0-192 | 80.4 | 3.72 | 84.1 |

[15] FDA Database.   http://www.accessdata.fda.gov/drugsatfda_docs/nda/2014/205677Orig1s000PharmR.pdf (accessed Mar 2016).
[19] FDA Datadase.   http://www.accessdata.fda.gov/drugsatfda_docs/nda/2014/205677Orig1s000ClinPharmR.pdf (accessed Mar 2016).

## Drug-Drug Interaction

Table 13    *In Vitro* Evaluation of Tasimelteon and Major Metabolites as Inhibitors of Enzymes[15, 19]

| Pre-incubation | Tasimelteon as an Inhibitor | | | | Metabolites as Inhibitors | | | | | |
| | Direct Inhibition | | Metabolism-dependent Inhibition | | M9 | | M12 | | M13 | |
| | 0-min[a] | | 30-min[b] | | 0-min[a] | 30-min[b] | 0-min[a] | 30-min[b] | 0-min[a] | 30-min[b] |
| Enzyme | IC$_{50}$ (µM) | Inhibition at 100 µM (%) | IC$_{50}$ (µM) | Inhibition at 100 µM (%) | IC$_{50}$ (µM) | | IC$_{50}$ (µM) | | IC$_{50}$ (µM) | |
|---|---|---|---|---|---|---|---|---|---|---|
| CYP1A2 | >100 | 30 | >100 | 29 | >100 | >100 | >100 | >100 | >100 | >100 |
| CYP2C8 | >100 | 28 | >100 | 13 | >100 | >100 | >100 | >100 | >100 | >100 |
| CYP2C9 | >100 | 12 | >100 | 26 | >100 | >100 | >100 | 85[c], >100[d] | >100 | >100 |
| CYP2C19 | 80 ± 24 | 55 | 68 ± 25 | 61 | >100 | >100 | >100 | 24[c], 92[d] | >100 | >100 |
| CYP2D6 | >100 | 17 | >100 | 1.2 | >100 | >100 | >100 | >100 | >100 | >100 |
| CYP3A4/5[e] | >100 | 34 | >100 | 35 | NA | NA | NA | NA | NA | NA |
| CYP3A4/5[f] | >100 | 32 | >100 | 38 | NA | NA | NA | NA | NA | NA |
| CYP3A4/5[g] | >100 | 28 | >100 | 34 | >100 | >100 | 84 | 61 | >100 | >100 |
| CYP2B6 | 550 ± 150 | NA | 150 ± 20[h] | NA | NA | NA | NA | NA | NA | NA |

[a] 0-min pre-incubation.   [b] 30-min pre-incubation.   [c] Result as determined using the initial lot of M12 received.   [d] Result as determined using a second, purer batch of M12.   [e] Testosterone 6β-hydroxylation.   [f] Testosterone 6β-hydroxylation repeat.   [g] Midazolam 1'-hydroxylation.   [h] 30-min pre-incubation plus NADPH(value ± standard error).

Table 14    *In Vitro* Evaluation of Tasimelteon and Major Metabolites as Inducers of Enzymes[15, 19]

| CYP Enzyme | Conc. (µM) | Tasimelteon as an Inducer | | | Metabolites as Inducers | | | | | |
| | | Enzyme Activity | | mRNA Level | M9 | | M12 | | M13 | |
| | | | | | Enzyme Activity | mRNA Level | Enzyme Activity | mRNA Level | Enzyme Activity | mRNA Level |
| | | Fold Induction | % of Positive Control | Fold Induction | Fold Induction | Fold Induction | Fold Induction | Fold Induction | Fold Induction | Fold Induction |
|---|---|---|---|---|---|---|---|---|---|---|
| 1A2 | 1, 10, 100 | No | NA | No | <2 | <2 | <2 | 2.29 | <2 | <2 |
| 2B6 | 1, 10, 100 | 100 µM: 6-fold | NA | 100 µM: 21-fold | NA | NA | 100 µM: 10-fold | 100 µM: 16-fold | 100 µM: 5-fold | 100 µM: 6-fold |
| 2C8 | 1, 10, 100 | 4.43 | 60.3 | NA | NA | NA | NA | NA | NA | NA |
| 2C9 | 1, 10, 100 | Decreased | NA | NA | NA | NA | NA | NA | NA | NA |
| 2C19 | 1, 10, 100 | Decreased | NA | NA | NA | NA | NA | NA | NA | NA |
| 3A4/5 | 1, 10, 100 | 2.27 | 83.2 | NA | NA | NA | NA | NA | NA | NA |

NA: Not available.

[15]  FDA Database.   http://www.accessdata.fda.gov/drugsatfda_docs/nda/2014/205677Orig1s000PharmR.pdf (accessed Mar 2016).
[19]  FDA Datadase.   http://www.accessdata.fda.gov/drugsatfda_docs/nda/2014/205677Orig1s000ClinPharmR.pdf (accessed Mar 2016).

Table 15   *In Vitro* Evaluation of Tasimelteon and Major Metabolites as Inhibitors and Substrates of P-gp[19]

| Tasimelteon as a P-gp Substrate | | | | | Tasimelteon and Metabolites as Inhibitors | | | |
|---|---|---|---|---|---|---|---|---|
| Treatment | Conc. (µM) | Papp(A→B) (1 × 10⁻⁶ cm/s) | Papp(B→A) (1 × 10⁻⁶ cm/s) | Efflux Ratio | Treatment | Papp(A→B) (1 × 10⁻⁶ cm/s) | Papp(B→A) (1 × 10⁻⁶ cm/s) | Efflux Ratio |
| Tasimelteon | 0.6 | 32.6 ± 21 | 29.3 ± 5.0 | 0.897 | 10 µM Digoxin + 326 µM tasimelteon | 1.26 ± 0.33 | 14.4 ± 1.0 | 11.4 |
|  |  |  |  |  | 10 µM Digoxin + 5 µM M9 | 0.426 ± 0.03 | 15.6 ± 3.0 | 36.6 |
| Tasimelteon | 6 | 19.4 ± 2.7 | 28.8 ± 4.4 | 1.48 | 10 µM Digoxin + 5 µM M11 | 0.404 | 25.2 ± 5.0 | 62.5 |
|  |  |  |  |  | 10 µM Digoxin | 0.811 ± 0.07 | 14.8 ± 1.1 | 18.3 |
| Tasimelteon | 60 | 63.9 | 28.9 ± 1.1 | 0.452 | 10 µM Digoxin + 5 µM M13 | 0.697 ± 0.05 | 16.8 ± 3.5 | 24.1 |
|  |  |  |  |  | 10 µM Digoxin | 0.546 ± 0.21 | 17.5 ± 0.62 | 32.0 |

Mean ± SD for Papp.

Table 16   *In Vitro* Evaluation of Tasimelteon and Major Metabolites as Inhibitors and Substrates of Uptake Transporters and Efflux Transporters[15, 19]

| Transporter | Tasimelteon and Metabolites as Inhibitors | | | | Tasimelteon and Metabolites as Substrates | | | |
|---|---|---|---|---|---|---|---|---|
|  | IC₅₀ (µM) | | | | Tasimelteon | M9 | M12 | M13 |
|  | Tasimelteon | M9 | M12 | M13 | | | | |
| OATP1B1 | >100 | >100 | >100 | >100 | No | No | No | No |
| OATP1B3 | >100 | >100 | >100 | >100 | No | No | No | No |
| OCT2 | 60.1 | >100 | 41.3 | 75.2 | - | - | - | - |
| OAT1 | >100 | >100 | >100 | 72.3 | - | - | - | - |
| OAT3 | 34.5 | 6.80 | >100 | 37.2 | - | - | - | - |
| BCRP | No inhibition | 18.1 | NA | No inhibition | - | - | - | - |

# 6   Non-Clinical Toxicology

## Summary

### Single-Dose Toxicity

❖ Single-dose toxicity in rats, mice and monkeys:
  • Generally, single doses up to 400 mg/kg in rats and mice, as well as 200 mg/kg in monkeys were tolerated.
  • Rat MNLD was considered at 1750 mg/kg, yet the tests showed CNS signs, labored respiration and BW reductions.
  • In mice, 1750 mg/kg resulted in mortality, in addition to the signs previously noted in rats at the same dose.

### Repeated-Dose Toxicity

❖ Sub- and chronic toxicity studies by the oral route in mice (up to 13 weeks), rats (up to 6 months) and monkeys (up to 12 months):
  • Major target organs of toxicity consistently in all species included the CNS, liver, kidneys and reproductive organs. Some changes were observed in the hematologic and endocrine systems, and related organs as well.
  • Exposure indicated accumulation and sex difference.

[15]   FDA Database.   http://www.accessdata.fda.gov/drugsatfda_docs/nda/2014/205677Orig1s000PharmR.pdf (accessed Mar 2016).
[19]   FDA Datadase.   http://www.accessdata.fda.gov/drugsatfda_docs/nda/2014/205677Orig1s000ClinPharmR.pdf (accessed Mar 2016).

Safety Pharmacology

❖ The core battery of safety pharmacology studies were not performed, except for *in vitro* and *in vivo* (dog) cardiovascular studies.
  • CNS and respiratory effects were not studied, thereby not determinate.
  • The major cardiovascular findings were reductions in BP and HR, and shortened APD in anesthetized dogs.   Besides, tasimelteon seemed vasoconstrictive.

Genotoxicity

❖ *In vitro* and *in vivo* genotoxicity on tasimelteon and M11 (a non-major human circulating metabolite that had poor coverage in the animal species):
  • Tasimelteon was neither mutagenic in an Ames assay nor clastogenic in an *in vivo* rat micronucleus assay, however, an *in vitro* chromosomal aberration assay presented equivocal/positive clastogenic effects.
  • Metabolite M11 was not mutagenic, but was clastogenic in an *in vitro* chromosomal aberration assay in CHO cells.

Reproductive and Developmental Toxicity

❖ Fertility and early embryonic development in rats:
  • Irregular estrus cycles, slightly increased infertile pairings, and slight reductions in fertility parameters were observed in females.
❖ Embryo-fetal development in rats and rabbits:
  • Slight delays in development and decreased fetal BWs were observed at MD and HD in rats (50 and 500 mg/kg/day) and rabbits (30 and 200 mg/kg/day), and some maternal toxicities were observed at HD in the dams and does.
❖ Pre- and postnatal development in rats:
  • Limited $F_0$ maternal toxicity was demonstrated; Clear toxicity in the $F_1$ generation was demonstrated particularly as developmental delays and a reduced growth rate postpartum and into adulthood, and meanwhile exposure through milk to tasimelteon, M9, M12 and M14 were identified; In the adult female $F_1$ generation, there were some evidences for maternal toxicities and reductions in fertility at 450 mg/kg/day.

Carcinogenicity

❖ Two-year carcinogenicity bioassays in rats and mice 450 mg/kg/day:
  • Neoplasms in liver, uterus and cervix were drug-related in rats, yet which were not identified in mice.

Special Toxicity

❖ Phototoxicity of tasimelteon and metabolites:[16]
  • Tasimelteon absorbed light at 290 nm.   However, it was shown to have a Molar Extinction Coefficient (MEC) of 689.41 L/mol/cm, less than 1000 L/mol/cm, which were deemed less of a photosafety risk since this low level of light absorption was unlikely to prove harmful.
  • Metabolites M3, M12 and M14 were reported to have MEC values that exceeded 1000 L/mol/cm at the absorption wavelength of 290 nm.   In the single dose distribution study, a long half-life of radioactivity in the eyes (126 h) and longer half-life in pigmented skin (15.4 h) versus non-pigmented skin (7.6 h) were reported (suggesting binding of [$^{14}$C]tasimelteon associated activity to melanin).
  • CHMP had recommended that phototoxic concern will be investigated as a post-approval measure (PAM).

## Single-Dose Toxicity

Table 17    Single-Dose Toxicity Studies of Tasimelteon by the Oral Route[15, 16]

| Species/Strain | Dose (mg/kg) | Finding |
|---|---|---|
| Rat | 400, 1750[a], etc. | None mortality. <br> 1750 mg/kg: Ataxia, ptosis, and hypoactivity on Day 1.   Loss of righting reflex and prostration on Day 2 and 3. <br> 400 mg/kg: Tolerated. <br> MNLD: 1750 mg/kg. |
| Mouse | 400, 1750[a], etc. | 1750 mg/kg: Mortality.   Tonic convulsions, inappropriate locomotion, disequilibrium, and signs previously noted in rats at the same dose. <br> 400 mg/kg: Tolerated. |
| Monkey | 200, etc. | 200 mg/kg: Tolerated. |

[a] Higher doses could not be tested because of the toxicity of PEG 400 and the drug's solubility limit.

[15]  FDA Database.   http://www.accessdata.fda.gov/drugsatfda_docs/nda/2014/205677Orig1s000PharmR.pdf (accessed Mar 2016).
[16]  EMA Database.   http://www.ema.europa.eu/docs/en_GB/document_library/EPAR_-_Public_assessment_report/human/003870/WC500190309.pdf (accessed Mar 2016).

## Repeated-Dose Toxicity

Table 18   Repeated-Dose Toxicity Studies of Tasimelteon by the Oral Route[15, 16]

| Species | Duration | Dose (mg/kg/day) | NOAEL | | | Finding |
|---------|----------|------------------|-------|---|---|---------|
| | | | Dose (mg/kg/day) | AUC[a] (ng·h/mL) | Safety Margin[a] (× MRHD) | |
| Mouse | 13 weeks | 25, 100, 400, 600, 800 | 100 | 26892/32698 | NA | Mortality in 9 mice at 800 mg/kg (2 test, 9 TK). Clinical signs: Labored breathing, prostration at ≥400 mg/kg. Clinical pathology: Minimal ↑ total protein and albumin, males at ≥400 mg/kg. Necropsy: Dose related ↑ liver weights at ≥400 mg/kg. Histopathology: Hepatocellular hypertrophy at ≥400 mg/kg. TK: Greater than proportional increase in systemic exposures (AUC).   No gender difference. |
| SD rat | 2 weeks | 50, 100, 200, 400 | 50 | 1178/4083 | NA | No mortality/clinical sign. ↑ Cholesterol at ≥100 mg/kg, ↑ serum glucose, triglycerides at ≥200 mg/kg.   ↑ Total protein, globulins and ↓ albumin/globulin ratio, ↑ calcium, ↓ sodium at 400 mg/kg. Necropsy: ↑ Liver weights at ≥100 mg/kg, ↑ liver size at ≥200 mg/kg. Histopathology: Hepatocellular hypertrophy at ≥100 mg/kg, ↑ Hepatocellular mitoses at 400 mg/kg, hyaline droplet accumulation proximal renal tubules (male) at ≥100 mg/kg. TK: Exposure at each dose was verified. |
| | 1 month | 25, 100, 400 | 25 | 2468/10196 | 6/28 | Mortality: 400 mg/day female euthanized moribund, signs of dehydration. Clinical signs: Hypoactivity, ptosis, ↓ food consumption in 400 mg/kg females. Clinical pathology: ↑ Reticulocyte (female), ↑ absolute neutrophils in males at 400 mg/kg.   ↑ Cholesterol ≥25 mg/kg (female), ↑ triglycerides ≥100 mg/kg (female).   ↑ Total protein, albumin, globulins, ALT, calcium, potassium, ↓ urea nitrogen and creatinine, ↑ urine volume, ↓ urine specific gravity in males and/or females at 400 mg/kg. Necropsy: ↑ Liver weight and/or size at ≥100 mg/kg.   ↑ Kidney weight (male), adrenal and heart weights (female) at 400 mg/kg. Histopathology: Hepatocellular hypertrophy at ≥100 mg/kg. Increased severity hyaline droplets in renal tubules. |
| | 26 weeks | 5, 50, 500 | 5 | 670/1458 | 2/4 | Mortality: 1 Female, Day 3 given 500 mg/kg. Clinical signs: Convulsions, hypoactivity, laboured respiration, ataxia, loss of righting reflex, extension of the limbs, recumbency, tremors; More severe in HD females.   ↓ BWG in males overall.   ↑ BWG in HD females. Clinical pathology: ↓ RBC indices, ↑ neutrophils/WBCs, ↑ PLT, effects on coagulation parameters, changes in liver and kidney serum chemistry, ↑ triglycerides, cholesterol, and glucose, ↓ sodium and chloride, ↑ calcium, ↑ total protein from ↑ albumin and globulins, ↑ urine volume and protein, ↓ specific gravity at MD and HD. Necropsy: Large livers and increased liver weights at MD and HD.   ↑ Kidney, heart, adrenal and spleen weights mainly at HD. Histopathology: 500 or 50 mg/kg.   Centrilobular hepatocellular hypertrophy, increased incidence and/or severity of chronic progressive nephropathy in males and females, increased hemosiderosis and extramedullary hematopoiesis in females at MD and HD. TK: Systemic exposure increased in dose-related manner and greater in females.   Exposures decreased with repeated dosing at MD and HD. |

[15]  FDA Datadase.   http://www.accessdata.fda.gov/drugsatfda_docs/nda/2014/205677Orig1s000PharmR.pdf (accessed Mar 2016).
[16]  EMA Database.   http://www.ema.europa.eu/docs/en_GB/document_library/EPAR_-_Public_assessment_report/human/003870/WC500190309.pdf (accessed Mar 2016).

*Continued*

| Species | Duration | Dose (mg/kg/day) | NOAEL | | | Finding |
|---------|----------|------------------|-------|---|---|---------|
| | | | Dose (mg/kg/day) | AUC[a] (ng·h/mL) | Safety Margin[a] (× MRHD) | |
| Cynomolgus monkey | 1 week | 50, 100, 175 | 50 | NA | NA | Mortality: None.<br>Clinical signs: Emesis, salivation, ↓ food consumption, BW loss at HD.<br>Clinical pathology: ↓ Serum chloride, ↑ glucose, ↑ alanine aminotransferase at ≥100 mg/kg.  ↑ Triglycerides, ↓ phosphorus, ↓ sodium, ↑ fibrinogen at HD. |
| | 1 month | 15, 45, 125 | 15 | 5968/3504 | 16/10 | Mortality: None.<br>Clinical signs: None.<br>Clinical pathology: None.<br>Necropsy: ↑ Liver size, ↓ spleen weight at HD; ↑ Liver weights at MD.<br>Histopathology: None.<br>TK: Systemic exposures $AUC_{tau}$ increased in a greater than dose proportional manner.  Generally greater exposures in males (1.2 to 1.9 folds). |
| | 12 months | 3, 20, 150 | 3 | 384/352 | 1/1 | Mortality: None drug-related.<br>Clinical signs: ↓ Appetite and ↑ salivation at ≥20 mg/kg; ↓ BWG, ↓ activity, ↑ emesis, and convulsions at HD.  One male prostration, ataxia at 3 mg/kg.<br>Clinical pathology: ↓ Erythron mass parameters, ↑ ALT, GGT at HD.<br>Necropsy: ↑ Liver size and weights at HD.<br>Histopathology: Possible ↓ in ovarian CLs at HD.<br>TK: Dose-related greater than proportional systemic exposures, no gender differences, decreased exposures with multiple doses. |

Vehicle: PEG 400.  [a] Present as male/female, data were directly provided in EMA assessment report, but it's not clear about the referred human AUC exposure.  For reference, sponsor-provided human AUC plasma exposures to tasimelteon at the RHD of 20 mg in FDA official documents was 411.4 ng·h/mL.

## Safety Pharmacology

Table 19   Safety Pharmacological Studies of Tasimelteon[15, 16]

| Study | Species/Strain | Treatment | Finding |
|-------|----------------|-----------|---------|
| Cardiovascular | Anesthetized/Conscious dog | 0.1-3.0 mg/kg, i.v. | In anesthetized dogs: ↓ MABP (14%); Steady ↓ in HR (Max 17%) at 3.0 mg/kg.<br>In conscious dogs: No change in MABP, HR or ECG (including QT). |
| | HEK 293 cell expressing hERG channel | Up to 100 μM | 100 μM: Inhibited hERG current by 14.0 ± 2.2%.<br>$IC_{50}$ not calculated. |
| | Rabbit cardiac purkinje fiber | 1, 10, 100 μM | 100 μM: ↓ $APD_{90}$ at 1 and 0.5 second basic cycle lengths; No statistically significant change in resting membrane potential, action potential amplitude, or the maximum rate of depolarization. |
| | Rat anterior cerebral artery (ACA) and isolated rat caudal artery (CA) | NA | With lower potency than melatonin, vasoconstrictive in pressurized (60 mmHg, constant) ACA and CA in a concentration-dependent manner ($EC_{50}$ estimated to be 500 nM and 180 nM, respectively). |

[15]  FDA Datadase.   http://www.accessdata.fda.gov/drugsatfda_docs/nda/2014/205677Orig1s000PharmR.pdf (accessed Mar 2016).

[16]  EMA Database.   http://www.ema.europa.eu/docs/en_GB/document_library/EPAR_-_Public_assessment_report/human/003870/WC500190309.pdf (accessed Mar 2016).

# Genotoxicity

Table 20    Genotoxicity Studies of Tasimelteon or M11[15, 16]

| Assay | Species/Strain | Metabolism Activity | Treatment | Finding |
|---|---|---|---|---|
| *In vitro* chromosome aberration assay in mammalian cells (Tasimelteon) | HPBL | ±S9 | 0, 100, 200, 400, and 800 µg/mL (+S9, 5 h) 0, 25, 50, 100, and 200 µg/mL (-S9, 24 h) | Increased aberrations in the presence of cytotoxicity. |
| *In vivo* rat micronucleus assay as part of the 1-month toxicity study (Tasimelteon) | Rat | + | Up to 400 mg/kg/day | Negative. |
| *In vitro* microbial reverse mutation assay (M11) | *S. typhimurium* TA98, TA100, TA1535, TA1537; *E. coli* WP2 *uvr*A | ±S9 | 8, 40, 200, 1000, or 5000 µg/plate (TA1537 at 1. 6, 8, 40, 200, 1000, 5000 µg/plate) | Negative. |
| *In vitro* chromosome aberration assay in mammalian cell (M11) | CHO | ±S9 | 0, 10, 200, and 1000 µg/mL (+S9, 3 h) 0, 10, 200, and 1000 µg/mL (+S9, 3 h) 0, 50, 1000, and 1500 µg/mL (-S9, 15 h) | Positive (+S9). Negative (-S9). |

Vehicle: DMSO for *in vitro* assays.

# Reproductive and Developmental Toxicity

Table 21    Reproductive and Developmental Toxicology Studies of Tasimelteon by the Oral Route[15, 16]

| Study | Species | Dose (mg/kg/day) | NOAEL Endpoint | NOAEL Dose (mg/kg/day) | Finding |
|---|---|---|---|---|---|
| Fertility and early embryonic development | SD rat | 0, 5, 50, 500 | Male fertility | 500 | ↑ Irregular estrus cycles in MDF and HDF. Slight ↑ infertile mating & ↓ fertility parameter at MD & HD, not attributed to males. |
| | | | Female fertility | 50 | |
| | | | $F_1$ | 500 | |
| Embryo-fetal development | SD rat | 0, 5 ,50 , 500 | Maternal | 50 | Maternal toxicity: Mortality, ↓ BW and food consumption at HD. Embryo-fetal toxicity: No malformations in any groups; incomplete ossification at MD and HD; ↓ Fetal weight at HD. |
| | | | Fetal | 500 | |
| | NZW rabbit | 0, 5 ,30 , 200 | Maternal | 30 | Maternal toxicity: Clinical signs, ↓ BW and food consumption at HD. Embryo-fetal toxicity: Aborted litters; Slightly ↓ fetal weight; ↑ Malformation/variation rates; Slightly delayed ossification, especially pelvis at HD. |
| | | | Fetal | 30 | |
| Pre- and postnatal developement | SD rat | 0, 50 ,150 , 450 | $F_0$ maternal | 150 | $F_0$ dams: Slight ↓ BW at MD and/or HD during gestation and in all dams during lactation; Slight ↑ gestation period; Slight ↓ live birth index at HD. $F_1$: ↑ Incidence of underactive, swollen area on the abdomen, and small build; Reduced (~15%) BW throughout lactation and into adulthood; Sexual maturation at a lower BW in males (similar PND) but delayed in females; Other delayed developmental milestones (e.g., righting responses); Clear deficits in Morris Water maze test (i.e., trial times, sector entries, failed trials) in males; ↓ BW in females during gestation; ↓ Fertility parameters (e.g., corpora lutea, implantations, late resorptions, post-implantation loss %, and live births) at HD; Exposure to tasimelteon, M9, M12 and M14 (much lesser than $F_0$ dams). |
| | | | $F_1$ | 150 | |

Vehicle: PEG400

[15]  FDA Datadase.   http://www.accessdata.fda.gov/drugsatfda_docs/nda/2014/205677Orig1s000PharmR.pdf (accessed Mar 2016).
[16]  EMA Database.   http://www.ema.europa.eu/docs/en_GB/document_library/EPAR_-_Public_assessment_report/human/003870/WC500190309.pdf (accessed Mar 2016).

# Carcinogenicity

Table 22    104-Week Carcinogenicity Studies of Tasimelteon by the Oral Route[15, 16]

| Species | Dose (mg/kg/day) | NOAEL (mg/kg/day) | Finding |
|---|---|---|---|
| SD rat | 0, 20,100, 250 | 20 | Neoplastic:<br>Dose-related ↑ hepatocellular adenoma; Isolated hepatocellular carcinoma 100 mg/kg (male); ↑ Endometrial adenocarcinoma and squamous cell carcinoma in uterus at HD.<br>Non-neoplastic:<br>Centrilobular hepatocyte hypertrophy ≥20mg/kg; Bile duct hyperplasia ≥100 mg/kg; Regenerative hyperplasia, cystic degeneration; Centrilobular hepatocyte vacuolation in male ≥100 mg/kg; Pigment in hepatocytes and ↓ incidence of basophilic foci in female ≥100 mg/kg; Renal cortical tubular pigments (female); ↑ Ovarian cysts ≥100 mg/kg, ↑ epithelial hyperplasia/keratinisation at HD. |
| CD-1 mouse | 0, 30, 100, 300 | 100 | No treatment-related neoplastic finding.<br>Non-neoplastic:<br>↑ Hepatocyte hypertrophy ≥100 mg/kg males, 300 mg/kg females. |

Vehicle: PEG400.

[15]  FDA Datadase.   http://www.accessdata.fda.gov/drugsatfda_docs/nda/2014/205677Orig1s000PharmR.pdf (accessed Mar 2016).
[16]  EMA Database.   http://www.ema.europa.eu/docs/en_GB/document_library/EPAR_-_Public_assessment_report/human/003870/WC500190309.pdf (accessed Mar 2016).

# CHAPTER

## 25

---

## Tavaborole

# Tavaborole

## (Kerydin®)

Research code: AN-2690

## 1 General Information

❖ Tavaborole was an oxaborole antifungal drug, which was first approved in Jul 2014 by US FDA.

❖ Tavaborole was originally discovered, developed and marketed by Anacor Pharmaceuticals.

❖ Tavaborole is an oxaborole antifungal, which inhibits fungal protein synthesis by inhibition of aminoacyl-transfer ribonucleic acid (tRNA) synthetase (AARS).

❖ Tavaborole is indicated for the treatment of onychomycosis of the toenails due to *Trichophyton rubrum* or *Trichophyton mentagrophytes*.

❖ Available as topical solution, containing 5% of tevaborole and the recommended dose is once daily for 48 weeks.

❖ The sale of Kerydin® was not available up to Mar 2016.

### Active Ingredient

| | |
|---|---|
| *Molecular formula*: | $C_7H_6BFO_2$ |
| *Molecular weight*: | 151.93 |
| *CAS No.*: | 174671-46-6 (Tavaborole) |
| *Chemical name*: | 5-Fluoro-1,3-dihydro-1-hydroxy-2, 1-benzoxaborole |

*Parameters of Lipinski's "Rule of 5"*

| MW | $H_D$ | $H_A$ | FRB[a] | PSA[a] | cLogP[a] |
|---|---|---|---|---|---|
| 151.93 | 1 | 2 | 1 | 29.5Å$^2$ | NA |

[a] Calculated by ACD/Labs software V11.02.

### Key Approvals around the World[*]

| | US (FDA) |
|---|---|
| First approval date | 07/07/2014 |
| Application or approval No. | NDA 204427 |
| Brand name | Kerydin® |
| Indication | Onychomycosis |
| Authorisation holder | Anacor Pharmaceuticals |

[*] Till Mar 2016, it has not been approved by EMA (EU), PMDA (Japan) and CFDA (China).

### Drug Product[*]

| | |
|---|---|
| *Dosage route*: | Topical |
| *Strength*: | 5% (Tavaborole) |
| *Dosage form*: | Solution |
| *Inactive ingredient*: | Alcohol, edetate calcium disodium and propylene glycol. |
| *Recommended dose*: | Apply to the affected toenails once daily for 48 weeks. |

[*] Sourced from US FDA drug label information

# 2　Key Patents Information

## Summary

❖ Kerydin® (Tavaborole) has got five-year NCE market exclusivity protection after it was approved by US FDA on Jul 07, 2014.

❖ Tavaborole was discovered by Anacor Pharmaceuticals, and has no compound patent application.

Table 1　Originator's International Patent Application List (Patent Family)

| Publication NO. | Titlet | Applicant/Assignee/Owner | Publication Date |
|---|---|---|---|
| **Technical Subjects** | **Salt, Crystal, Polymorphic, Solvate (Hydrate), Isomer, Derivative Etc. and Preparation** | | |
| WO2006089067A2 | Boron-containing small molecules | Anacor | 08/24/2006 |
| WO2007078340A2 | Boron-containing small molecules | Anacor | 07/12/2007 |
| WO2007131072A2 | Hydrolytically-resistant boron-containing therapeutics and methods of use | Anacor | 11/15/2007 |
| **Technical Subjects** | **Indication or Methods for Medical Needs** | | |
| WO2007095638A2 | Boron-containing small molecules as anti-inflammatory agents | Anacor | 08/23/2007 |
| WO2007146965A2 | Compounds for the treatment of periodontal disease | Anacor | 12/21/2007 |
| WO2015171186A1 | Compounds and nail polish | Anacor | 11/12/2015 |
| **Technial Subjects** | **Others** | | |
| WO2008070257A2 | Crystal structure of a tRNA synthetase | Anacor | 06/12/2008 |

The data was updated until Jan 2016.

# 3　Chemistry

## Route 1:　Original Discovery Route

*Synthetic Route*:　3-Fluorobenzaldehyde **1** was condensed with *p*-toluenesulfonylhydrazide **2** to give the corresponding *N*-tosyl hydrazide **3**.　Subsequent reaction of **3** with boron tribromide in the presence of anhydrous ferric chloride, followed by refluxing in 2N NaOH and quenching with 1N HCl, led to the title compound.[1-3]

[1]　Austin, P. W.; Kneale, C. J.; Crowley, P. J., et al. WO9533754A1, **1995**.
[2]　Austin, P. W.; Kneale, C. J.; Crowley, P. J., et al. US5880188A, **1999**.
[3]　Revill, P.; Bolos, J.; Serradell, N. *Drug Future* **2006**, *31*, 667-669.

## Route 2

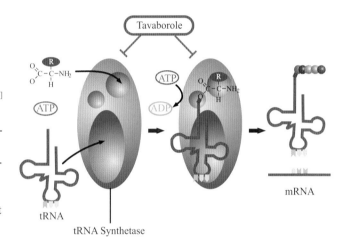

*Synthetic Route*:    The 26.9 g scale approach was started with the reduction of 2-bromo-5-fluorobenzaldehyde **1**.    The resultant benzyl alcohol was condensed with chloro(methoxy)methane **2** to produce *o*-bromobenzyl alcohol derivative **3** quantitively, which was borated with triisopropylborate after lithiated by *n*-butyllithium in THF and then an one-pot deprotection and spontaneous cyclization to deliver tavaborole in 60% yield over four steps and with the overall yield of 60%.[3-6]

## 4   Pharmacology

### Summary

Mechanism of Action

❖ Tavaborole is an oxaborole antifungal, which inhibits fungal protein synthesis by inhibition of tRNA synthetase ($K_i$ = ~2 μM), acting as a low tight-binding inhibitor.[7]

❖ Tavaborole formed an adduct with the leucine-specific tRNA (tRNA$^{Leu}$) in the editing site of leucyl-tRNA synthetase, thus inhibiting synthesis of tRNA$^{Leu}$.

❖ Tavaborole had no significant radioligand binding inhibition on a panel of 50 transmembrane and soluble receptors, ion channels, mono-amino transporters, and 5 human recombinant CYP 450 isoforms in the off-target activity assay at 10 μM.[8]

*In Vitro* Efficacy

❖ Antifungal activity:

- Broad-spectrum antifungal activity against 19 test strains of fungi: MIC = 0.25-2 μg/mL.
- *Trichophyton* strains: MIC = 1-16 μg/mL.
- *Trichophyton rubrum* from clinical isolates:
  - ♦ MIC$_{90}$ = 8.0 μg/mL and MIC = 1.0-8.0 μg/mL.
  - ♦ MFC$_{90}$ = 64 μg/mL and MFC = 8.0-128 μg/mL.
- *Trichophyton mentagrophytes* from clinical isolates:
  - ♦ MIC$_{90}$ = 8.0 μg/mL and MIC = 4.0-8.0 μg/mL.
  - ♦ MFC$_{90}$ = 64 μg/mL and MFC = 16->128 μg/mL.

❖ Tavaborole resistant mutants in *S. cerevisiae* or *C. Albicans*:

- *S. Cerevisiae* wild type: MIC = 0.125 μg/mL.
- Tavaborole resistant mutants *S. Cerevisiae*: MIC = 4-32 μg/mL (mutations in CDC60).
- *C. Albicans* wild type: MIC = 1 μg/mL.
- *Tavaborole* resistant mutants *C. Albicans*: MIC ≥64 μg/mL (T321I or K510E in CDC60).

❖ Antibacterial activity against 12 strains of bacterial: MIC = 4->64 μg/mL.

*In Vivo* Efficacy

❖ In the *Candida albicans* systemic infection mouse model:

- Ineffective at preventing mortality in mice caused by an injection of *C. albicans*.
- No significant decrease of the *C. albicans* CFUs in the kidneys.

[3] Revill, P.; Bolos, J.; Serradell, N. *Drug Future* **2006**, *31*, 667-669.
[4] Baker, S. J.; Zhang, Y.; Akama, T., et al. *J. Med. Chem.* **2006**, *49*, 4447-4450.
[5] Hinklin, R. J.; Wallace, O. B. WO2004009578A2, **2004**.
[6] Hinklin, R. J.; Wallace, O. B. US2005261277A1, **2005**.
[7] FDA Datadase.   http://www.accessdata.fda.gov/drugsatfda_docs/nda/2014/204427Orig1s000PharmR.pdf (accessed Mar 2016).
[8] U.S. Food and Drug Adminstration (FDA) Datadase.   http://www.accessdata.fda.gov/drugsatfda_docs/nda/2014/204427Orig1s000MicroR.pdf (accessed Mar 2016).

## Mechanism of Action

Table 2    The Inhibition of Tavaborole[9]

| Compound | Incubated (min) | Test | $K_i$ (μM) | $IC_{50}$ (μM) |
|---|---|---|---|---|
| Tavaborole | NA | Aminoacylation inhibition | · NA | 2.1 |
| | 2 | tRNA | 31.4 ± 2.8 | NA |
| | 20 | tRNA | 1.85 ± 0.1 | NA |

All reactions were performed in triplicate, and the mean values were used to determine a median inhibitory concentration ($IC_{50}$) with Prism 4.

## *In Vitro* Efficacy

Table 3    Antifungal Spectrum of Tavaborole[7]

| Species | Culture Medium | MIC or MFC (μg/mL) | | | | |
|---|---|---|---|---|---|---|
| | | Tavaborole | Ciclopirox | Terbinafine | Fluconazole | Itraconazole |
| *Aspergillus fumigatus* ATCC 13073 | RPMI | 0.25 | NT | NT | >64 | 0.25 |
| *Candida albicans* ATCC 90028 | RPMI | 1 | 0.5 | NT | 0.25 | ≤0.12 |
| *C. albicans* F 56 | RPMI | 0.5 | NT | NT | >64 | 0.25 |
| *Candida glabrata* ATCC 90030 | RPMI + MOPS | ≤0.5 | ≤0.5 | 64 | NT | ≤0.5 |
| *Candida krusei* ATCC 44507 | RPMI + MOPS | 1 | ≤0.5 | 64 | NT | ≤0.5 |
| *Cryptococcus neoformans* F 285 | RPMI | 0.25 | NT | NT | 2 | ≤0.12 |
| *Candida parapsilosis* ATCC 22019 | RPMI + MOPS | ≤0.5 | ≤0.5 | ≤0.5 | NT | ≤0.5 |
| *Candida tropicalis* ATCC 13803 | RPMI + MOPS | ≤0.5 | ≤0.5 | 256 | NT | 1 |
| *Epidermophyton floccosum* ATCC 52066 | RPMI + MOPS | ≤0.5 | ≤0.5 | ≤0.5 | NT | ≤0.5 |
| *Fusarium solani* ATCC36031 | RPMI + MOPS | ≤0.5 | 4 | 64 | NT | >256 |
| *Malassezia furfur* ATCC 44344 | Urea | 1 | ≤0.5 | 2 | NT | ≤0.5 |
| *Malassezia pachydermatis* ATCC 96746 | Urea | 1 | ≤0.5 | ≤0.5 | NT | ≤0.5 |
| *Malassezia sympodialis* ATCC 44031 | Urea | 1 | ≤0.5 | ≤0.5 | NT | ≤0.5 |
| *Microsporum audouinii* ATCC 42558 | RPMI + MOPS | 2 | 1 | ≤0.5 | NT | ≤0.5 |
| *Microsporum canis* ATCC 10214 | RPMI + MOPS | 2 | ≤0.5 | ≤0.5 | NT | ≤0.5 |
| *Mucrisoirym gypseum* ATCC 24103 | RPMI + MOPS | 2 | ≤0.5 | ≤0.5 | NT | ≤0.5 |
| *Trichophyton mentagrophytes* F 311 | RPMI + MOPS | 1 | 0.5 | ≤0.5 | 32 | ≤0.12 |
| *Trichophyton rubrum* F 296 | RPMI/MOPS | 1 | 1 | ≤0.5 | 1 | ≤0.12 |
| *T. rubrum* F 296 | RPMI/MOPS + 5% keratin powder | 2 | 1 | NT | 1 | NT |
| *Trichophyton tonsurans* ATCC 28942 | RPMI/MOPS | 2 | ≤0.5 | ≤0.5 | NT | ≤0.5 |
| *T. rubrum* F 296[a] | RPMI/MOPS | 8 | 2 | ≤0.5 | NT | 4 |
| *T. mentagrophytes* F 311[a] | RPMI/MOPS | 16 | 1 | ≤0.5 | NT | 4 |

MOPS: 3-(*N*-morpholino) propanesulfonic acid.    NT: Not tested.    MIC: Minimal inhibitory concentraton.    MFC: Minimal fungicidal concentration.    [a] MFC value.

[7]    FDA Database.    http://www.accessdata.fda.gov/drugsatfda_docs/nda/2014/204427Orig1s000MicroR.pdf (accessed Mar 2016).
[9]    Rock, F. L.; Mao, W.; Yaremchuk, A., et al. *Science* **2007**, *316*, 1759-1761.

Table 4　Antifungal Efficacy of Tavaborole against Clinical Isolates[7]

| Species | Compound | MIC (μg/mL) | | | MFC (μg/mL) | | |
|---|---|---|---|---|---|---|---|
| | | $MIC_{50}$ | $MIC_{90}$ | MIC Range | $MFC_{50}$ | $MFC_{90}$ | MFC Range |
| *Trichophyton rubrum* | Tavaborole | 4.0 | 8.0 | 1.0-8.0 | 64 | 64 | 8.0-128 |
| | Ciclopirox | 0.25 | 0.5 | 0.06-1.0 | >16 | >16 | 0.5->16 |
| | Terbinafine | 0.008 | 0.016 | 0.002-0.03 | NA | NA | NA |
| | United States (n = 129) | 4 | 16 | 2-16 | >32 | >32 | 2->32 |
| | Mexico (n = 93) | 16 | 16 | 2-32 | >32 | >32 | 4->32 |
| *Trichophyton mentagrophytes* | Tavaborole | 4.0 | 8.0 | 4.0-8.0 | >16 | >16 | 16->128 |
| | Ciclopirox | 0.25 | 0.5 | 0.125-0.5 | >16 | >16 | 1.0->16 |
| | Terbinafine | 0.004 | 0.008 | 0.002-2.0 | NA | NA | NA |
| | United States (n = 129) | ND | ND | 4-8 | ND | ND | 32->32 |
| | Mexico (n = 93) | ND | ND | 8-32 | ND | ND | >32 |

MIC: Minimal inhibitory concentration.　$MIC_{50}$: Minimum inhibitory concentration required to inhibit the growth of 50% of isolates tested.　$MIC_{90}$: Minimum inhibitory concentration required to inhibit the growth of 90% of isolates tested.　MFC: Minimal fungicidal concentration.　$MFC_{50}$: Minimum fungicidal concentration required to kill (defined at a >99.9% reduction in colony count from the original inoculum) 50% of the strains tested.　$MFC_{90}$: Minimum fungicidal concentration required to kill (defined at a >99.9% reduction in colony count from the original inoculum) 90% of the strains tested.

Table 5　Tavaborole Resistant Mutants in *S. Cerevisiae* or *C. Albicans*[7]

| *S. Cerevisiae* | Mutation in CDC60 | MIC (μg/mL) | *C. Albicans* | Mutation in CDC60 | MIC (μg/mL) |
|---|---|---|---|---|---|
| ATCC201388 | None | 0.125 | Wild type | None | 1 |
| ANA320 | N415D | 4 | | | |
| ANA321 | R316I | 16 | Mutant-1 | T321I | >64 |
| ANA322 | C326F | 16 | | | |
| ANA323 | G405V | 16 | Mutant-2 | T321I | >64 |
| ANA324 | C326R | 16 | | | |
| ANA326 | L315V | 16 | Mutant-3 | T321I | >64 |
| ANA327 | T314M | 32 | | | |
| ANA358 | S416L | 32 | Mutant-4 | K510E | 64 |
| ANA360 | T319I | 32 | | | |

The mutants ANA320-327 were selected spontaneously, ANA358 and 360 were induced by ethyl methanesulfonate (EMS).

[7]　FDA Datadase.　http://www.accessdata.fda.gov/drugsatfda_docs/nda/2014/204427Orig1s000MicroR.pdf (accessed Mar 2016).

Table 6    Antibacterial Spectrum of Tavaborole[7]

| Species | MIC (µg/mL) | |
| --- | --- | --- |
| | Tavaborole | Ciprofloxacin |
| *Staphylococcus aureus* ATCC 29213 (MSSA) | 32 | 0.25 |
| *Staphylococcus aureus* ATCC 33591 (MRSA) | 64 | ≤0.12 |
| *Staphylococcus epidermidis* ATCC 12228 | 8 | ≤0.12 |
| *Staphylococcus pyogenes* ATCC 19615 | 16 | 0.25 |
| *Propionibacterium acnes* ATCC 11827 | 32 | 0.5 |
| *Pseudomonas aeruginosa* ATCC 27853 | >64 | ≤0.12 |
| *Enterococcus faecalis* ATCC 29212 | >64 | 0.5 |
| *Enterococcus faecium* CT-26 | >64 | >64 |
| *Streptococcus mutans* ATCC 25175 | 64 | 1 |
| *Escherichia coli* ATCC 25922 | 4 | ≤0.12 |
| *Haemophilus actinomycetemcomitans* ATCC 29523 | 16 | ≤0.12 |
| *Porphyromonas gingivalis* ATCC 33277 | 4 | 0.5 |

MIC: Minimal inhibitory concentration.

## *In Vivo* Efficacy

Table 7    Effects of Tavaborole in Systemic *Candida Albicans* Infection Mouse Models[7]

| Systemic Infection Model | | | Dose (mg/kg) | Route & Duration (Day) | Effect | |
| --- | --- | --- | --- | --- | --- | --- |
| Study | Animal | Compound | | | %Survival | Finding |
| Survival of post infection | Mouse | Vehicle | 0 | p.o., BID × 8 | 20 | NA. |
| | | Fluconazole | 1 | p.o., BID × 8 | 100 | The positive control fluconazole completely protected the mice. |
| | | Tavaborole | 30 | p.o., BID × 8 | 0 | Ineffective at preventing mortality in mice caused by an injection of *Candida albicans*. |
| | | | 30 | s.c. BID × 8 | 20 | |
| | | | 30ª | s.c. BID × 8 | 100 | |
| The therapeutic activity and safety | Mouse | Fluconazole | 30 | p.o., QD × 12 | NA | Fluconazole significantly protected the mice at any dose. |
| | | | 30 or 100 | p.o., BID × 12 | NA | |
| | | Tavaborole | 30 or 100 | p.o., BID × 12 | NA | Tavaborole did not prevent the death of the mice induced by the lethal injection of *C. albicans* at any dose. Tavaborole did not significantly decrease the *C. albicans* CFUs in kidneys. |

Vehicle: 1% CMC.   All treatments were given orally in 0.1 mL and were formulated using 1% CMC.   All surviving animals were euthanatized and the CFU remaining in the kidneys were determined by quantitative plating of organ homogenates.   CMC: Carboxymethylcellulose (diluent control).   ª For safety evaluation of tavaborole, animals were not infected in this group.   Using kidney *C. albicans* CFU and mouse survival as endpoint.

[7]   FDA Datadase.   http://www.accessdata.fda.gov/drugsatfda_docs/nda/2014/204427Orig1s000MicroR.pdf (accessed Mar 2016).

# 5 ADME & Drug-Drug Interaction

## Summary

### Absorption of Tavaborole

❖ Was absorbed rapidly in rats and dogs following oral administrations, but slowly in humans ($T_{max}$ = 12 h) following topical administration.

❖ Systemic exposure was extremely low, even below the level of quantitation, following s.c. and topical administrations to rats and minipigs.

❖ The ratio of $C_{max}$ for plasma tavaborole/plasma total radioactivity was approximately 0.146, and the systemic exposure to tavaborole was approximately 15% of the exposure to plasma total radioactivity in healthy adult male humans.

❖ Showed a half-life of 7.68 h in humans after topical administration.

### Distribution of Tavacorole

❖ Exhibited low to moderate plasma protein binding in humans (45.8%-76.9%), rats (40.7%-59.3%), rabbits (46.4%-62.3%), dogs (38.7%-66.3%) and minipigs (55.0%-80.2%), but lower in mice (26.9%-48.7%).

❖ After single oral administration, [$^{14}$C]tavaborole was rapidly and incompletely absorbed in pigmented mice and widely distributed to tissues. Concentrations of [$^{14}$C]tavaborole were below quantifiable limits in all tissues at 168 h (7 days) post-dose.

### Metabolism of Tavacorole

❖ Tavaborole was metabolically stable in mouse, rat, minipig and human liver fractions.

❖ CYP3A5 and CYP2C18 were the major metabolizing enzymes for tavaborole, with CYP2C19 and CYP3A4 responsible for a minor role and flavin monooxygenases (FMO3 and FMO5) involved in the formation of the major metabolite M6 (AN3019).

❖ Tavaborole underwent extensive metabolism in humans. Trace levels of M5 and M6a were detected at steady-state in plasma.

❖ In mice after dermal administration, the prominent circulating drug-derived components in plasma were the parent drug, M5, M2, M6 and M6a.

❖ In rats after oral administration, the major drug-related components in plasma were M5, M6a, M6, M2, M3 and M7, while M6-glucuronide (M4) as a minor metabolite.

### Excretion of Tavacorole

❖ Was excreted in urine (17.9%) in humans after topical administration, with M5 sulfate-conjugate as the most significant component in human urine.

❖ Was predominantly excreted in urine in rats and mice after dermal administration, with M5 as the most significant component in mouse urine.

### Drug-Drug Interaction

❖ Tavaborole did not directly inhibit the activity of CYP1A2, CYP2A6, CYP2B6, CYP2C8, CYP2C9, CYP2C19, CYP2D6, CYP2E1 or CYP3A4/5 ($IC_{50}$ >100 µM), but had time-dependent inhibitions for CYP2A6 and CYP2E1.

❖ Tavaborole did not induce the activity of CYP1A2, CYP2B6, CYP2C8, CYP2C9, CYP2C19 or CYP3A4/5.

## Absorption

Table 8   *In Vivo* Pharmacokinetic Parameters of Tavaborole in Humans after Single Topical Dose of 5% Tavaborole Solution[10]

| Species | Route | Dose (µL) | $T_{max}$ (h) | $C_{max}$ (ng/mL) | $AUC_{last}$ (ng·h/mL) | $T_{1/2}$ (h) |
|---------|-------|-----------|---------------|-------------------|------------------------|----------------|
| Patient | Topical | 200 | 12.0 (4.03-23.9) | 3.54 ± 2.26 | 44.4 ± 25.5 | 7.68 |

Median (range) for $T_{max}$.   Mean ± SD for $C_{max}$ and AUC.   $AUC_{last}$ = Area under the concentration-time curve from time 0 to the time of the final measurable sample.

[10]  FDA Datadase.   http://www.accessdata.fda.gov/drugsatfda_docs/nda/2014/204427Orig1s000ClinPharmR.pdf (accessed Mar 2016).

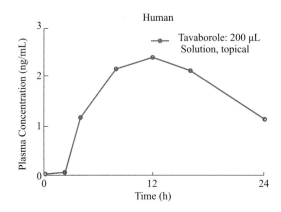

Figure A    *In Vivo* Plasma Concentration-Time Profiles of Tavaborole in Humans after Single Topical Dose of Tavaborole[10]

## Key Findings:[8]

❖ After single dermal dose, [14C]tavaborole was rapidly and incompletely absorbed, then widely distributed to tissues. Concentrations of [14C]tavaborole were below quantifiable limits in all tissues at 168 h (7 days) post-dose.

## Distribution

Table 9    *In Vitro* Plasma Protein Binding of [3H]Tavaborole in Several Species[8]

| Species | Human | Rat | Mouse | Dog | Minipig | Rabbit |
|---|---|---|---|---|---|---|
| %Bound | 45.8-76.9 | 40.7-59.3 | 26.9-48.7 | 38.7-66.3 | 55.0-80.2 | 46.4-62.3 |

## Metabolism

❖ Tavaborole was metabolically stable in mouse, rat, minipig and human liver fractions.[8]

❖ *In vitro*, the human cytochrome P450 enzymes mainly responsible for the metabolism of tavaborole were CYP3A5 and CYP2C18.   CYP2C19 and CYP3A4 had a minor role in the formation of the major metabolite M6 (AN3019).   Flavin monooxygenases (FMO3 and FMO5) were involved in the formation of the intermediate metabolite M6.[8]

❖ Biotransformation of tavaborole after dermal administration to mice involved oxidative oxaborole ring cleavage followed by sulfation or glucuronidation.[8]

❖ In male and female mice dosed with a dermal application of radiolabeled tavaborole, the prominent circulating drug-derived components in plasma were the parent drug, sulfate-conjugate metabolite (M5), glucuronide-conjugate metabolite (M2), benzyl alcohol metabolite (M6) and benzoic acid metabolite (M6a).[8]

Table 10    Metabolites in Plasma, Urine and Feces of Several Species after Single Intravenous, Oral and Topical Dose of Tavaborole[8, 10]

| Matrix | Species | Route | % of Dose | | | | | | | |
|---|---|---|---|---|---|---|---|---|---|---|
| | | | M0 | M2 | M3 | M4 | M5 | M6 | M6a | M7 |
| Plasma | Mouse | i.v. | √ | √ | - | - | √ | √ | √ | - |
| | Rat | p.o. | Minor | Minor | Minor | Minor | 62 | Minor | Minor | Minor |
| | Human | Topical | NA | NA | NA | NA | Trace | NA | Trace | NA |
| Urine | Mouse | Dermal | NA | NA | NA | NA | 31-35 | NA | NA | NA |
| | Rat | p.o. | - | √ | √ | √ | - | - | √ | √ |
| | Human | Topical | - | - | - | - | 14.6 | - | - | - |
| Feces | Human | Topical | NA | NA | NA | NA | NA | NA | NA | NA |

√: Detected.   M2: Glucuronide-conjugate.   M3: Boronic acid-glucuronide metabolite.   M4: M6-glucuronide.   M5: Sulfate-conjugate.   M6a: Benzoic acid metabolite. M6: Benzyl alcohol metabolite.   M7: Cysteine-conjugate metabolite.

[8]   FDA Datadase.   http://www.accessdata.fda.gov/drugsatfda_docs/nda/2014/204427Orig1s000PharmR.pdf (accessed Mar 2016).
[10]   FDA Datadase.   http://www.accessdata.fda.gov/drugsatfda_docs/nda/2014/204427Orig1s000ClinPharmR.pdf (accessed Mar 2016).

Figure B    Proposed Pathways for *In Vivo* Biotransformation of Tavaborole in Rats, Mice and Humans after Single Dose of Tavaborole[10]

The red labels represent the main components in the matrices.    P = Plasma, U = Urine and GA = Glucuronic acid.

## Excretion

Table 11    Excretion Profiles of [$^{14}$C]Tavaborole in Various Species after Single Dermal and Topical Dose of Tavaborole[8, 10]

| Species | Route | Dose (μL) | Time (h) | Urine (% of dose) | Feces (% of dose) |
|---|---|---|---|---|---|
| Rat | Dermal | - | - | ≥33.5 | ≤1.71 |
| Mouse | Dermal | - | - | ≥81.2 | ≤2.87 |
| Human | Topical | 200 | 0-240 | 17.9 (16) | - |

## Drug-Drug Interaction

Table 12    *In Vitro* Evaluation of Tavaborole as an Inhibitor and an Inducer of Enzymes[10]

| Enzyme | Direct Inhibition | | Time-dependent Inhibition | | | CYP Induction | | | | | |
|---|---|---|---|---|---|---|---|---|---|---|---|
| | 0-min Pre-incubation | | 30-min Pre-incubation | | | | | | | | |
| | IC$_{50}$ (μM)[a] | Maximum Inhibition at 100 μM (%)[b] | IC$_{50}$ (μM)[a] | Maximum Inhibition at 100 μM (%)[b] | Potential for TDI[c] | Enzyme | Conc. (μM) | Fold Induction[e] | Enzyme | Conc. (μM) | Fold Induction[e] |
| CYP1A2 | >100 | 1.5 | >100 | 5.5 | No | | 0.126 | 1.06 ± 0.14 | | 0.126 | 1.01 ± 0.15 |
| CYP2A6 | >100 | 4.3 | >100 | 41 | Yes[d] | CYP1A2 | 1.26 | 0.926 ± 0.183 | CYP2C9 | 1.26 | 0.899 ± 0.084 |
| CYP2B6 | >100 | NA | >100 | 0.5 | No | | 12.6 | 1.06 ± 0.21 | | 12.6 | 0.972 ± 0.182 |
| CYP2C8 | >100 | 9.5 | >100 | 7.1 | No | | 0.126 | 0.944 ± 0.044 | | 0.126 | 1.09 ± 0.10 |
| CYP2C9 | >100 | NA | >100 | NA | No | CYP2B6 | 1.26 | 0.940 ± 0.175 | CYP2C19 | 1.26 | 1.06 ± 0.15 |
| CYP2C19 | >100 | 11 | >100 | 5.5 | No | | 12.6 | 0.855 ± 0.144 | | 12.6 | 1.06 ± 0.13 |

[8]   FDA Datadase.   http://www.accessdata.fda.gov/drugsatfda_docs/nda/2014/204427Orig1s000PharmR.pdf (accessed Mar 2016).
[10]   FDA Datadase.   http://www.accessdata.fda.gov/drugsatfda_docs/nda/2014/204427Orig1s000ClinPharmR.pdf (accessed Mar 2016).

*Continued*

| Enzyme | Direct Inhibition | | Time-dependent Inhibition | | | CYP Induction | | | | | |
| | 0-min Pre-incubation | | 30-min Pre-incubation | | Potential for TDI[c] | Enzyme | Conc. (μM) | Fold Induction[e] | Enzyme | Conc. (μM) | Fold Induction[e] |
| | IC$_{50}$ (μM)[a] | Maximum Inhibition at 100 μM (%)[b] | IC$_{50}$ (μM)[a] | Maximum Inhibition at 100 μM (%)[b] | | | | | | | |
| CYP2D6 | >100 | 14 | >100 | 8.5 | No | | 0.126 | $1.06 \pm 0.15$ | | 0.126 | $1.09 \pm 0.10$ |
| CYP2E1 | >100 | 42 | 57 | 73 | Yes[d] | CYP2C8 | 1.26 | $0.98 \pm 0.27$ | CYP3A4/5 | 1.26 | $0.932 \pm 0.167$ |
| CYP3A4/5 | >100 | 5.7 | >100 | 4.3 | No | | 12.6 | $1.00 \pm 0.20$ | | 12.6 | $1.04 \pm 0.14$ |
| CYP3A4/5 | >100 | NA | >100 | 1.2 | No | | | | | | |

[a] Average data (i.e., percent of control activity) obtained from duplicate samples for each test article concentration were used to calculated IC$_{50}$ values. IC$_{50}$ values were calculated with XLFit. [b] Maximum inhibition (%) was calculated with the following formula and data for the highest concentration of test article evaluated (results were rounded to two significant figures): Maximum inhibition (%) = 100%-Percent solvent control. [c] TDI: Time-dependent inhibition, was determined by comparison of IC$_{50}$ values with and without pre-incubation, by comparison of maximum inhibition (%) with and without pre-incubation and by visual inspection of the IC$_{50}$ plot. [d] Time-dependent inhibition was found to be at least partially dependent upon the presence of NADPH-generating system. [e] Values were the mean ± SD of three determinations (human hepatocyte preparations H920, H921 and H923).

# 6 Non-Clinical Toxicology

## Summary

Single-Dose Toxicity
❖ Not conducted.

Repeated-Dose Toxicity
❖ Toxicities of repeated oral dosage for up to 6 months in rats, and those of repeated dermal dosage for up to 9 months in minipigs:
  • In the 6-month rat study, the NOAEL was 30 mg/kg/day, approximately 3 times higher than the mean human AUC$_{tau}$ of 75.8 ng·h/mL. The target organ of toxicity identified was the non-glandular stomach which presented as epithelial hyperplasia and hyperkeratosis.
  • In the 9-month minipig study, the systemic NOAEL was 3%, approximately 10 times higher than the mean human AUC$_{tau}$. The identified target organ of toxicity was the skin at the site of administration.

Safety Pharmacology
❖ Central nervous system: No effect on the function in rats.
❖ Cardiovascular system: As a low-potency hERG-channel blocker (less than 25% inhibition), tavaborole may have less probability of QT prolongation. In dogs, NOEL was 30 mg/kg. Tavaborole caused a dose-related, reversible, mild to marked hypotension and variable, transient increases in heart and pulse rates at doses of 100 and 200 mg/kg in dogs.

Genotoxicity
❖ Tavaborole was not genotoxic in the Ames test, the human lymphoma assay or the rat micronucleus assay.

Reproductive and Developmental Toxicity
❖ Fertility and early embryonic development in rats:
  • The NOAEL for paternal toxicity was 100 mg/kg/day, based on one male death, decreased body weight gains and thickening and discoloration of the non-glandular stomach in males at 300 mg/kg/day. The NOAEL for fertility and reproductive performance was 300 mg/kg/day, based on no treatment related effect on fertility at oral doses up to 300 mg/kg/day; the exposure (AUC) was approximately 107 times higher than the mean human AUC$_{tau}$.
❖ Embryo-fetal development in rats and rabbits:
  • Rats: The NOAEL for maternal and fetal developmental toxicity was 100 mg/kg/day, based on an increase in embryo-fetal resorption and/or embryo-fetal death at 300 mg/kg/day. The NOAEL for drug related malformations was 100 mg/kg/day, based on the skeletal malformations and variations at 300 mg/kg/day; the AUC$_{0-4}$ on GD 19 was approximately 29 times higher than the mean human AUC$_{tau}$.
  • Rabbits: In the dermal embryo-fetal development study, the NOAEL for malformations was 10% tavaborole solution, based on no drug-related malformations at 10% tavaborole solution; the AUC$_{0-4}$ on GD 28 was approximately 36 times higher than the mean human AUC$_{tau}$. The NOAEL for maternal and fetal developmental toxicity was 5% tavaborole

solution, based on decreased fetal body weight at 10% tavaborole solution; the $AUC_{0-4}$ on GD 28 was approximately 26 times higher than the mean human $AUC_{tau}$.
- Rabbits: In the oral embryo-fetal development study, the NOAEL for malformations was 150 mg/kg/day; the $AUC_{0-4}$ was 155 times higher than the mean human $AUC_{tau}$. The NOAEL for maternal and embyo-fetal toxicity was 50 mg/kg/day, based on an increase in mortality, body weight loss and post-implantation loss and decreased live fetuses; the $AUC_{0-4}$ was 16 times higher than the mean human $AUC_{tau}$.

❖ Pre- and postnatal development in rats:
- $F_0$ maternal toxicity: The NOAEL was 60 mg/kg/day, based on decreased motor activity and excess salivation at 100 mg/kg/day.
- $F_1$ and $F_2$ offspring toxicity: The NOAEL was 100 mg/kg/day, based on no treatment related effects; The $AUC_{0-4}$ was approximately 29 times higher than the mean human $AUC_{tau}$.

Carcinogenicity
❖ An oral carcinogenicity study in rats and a dermal one in mice:
- No drug-related increase in the incidence of neoplasms was noted in either study.

# Repeated-Dose Toxicity

Table 13　Repeated-Dose Toxicity Studies of Tavaborole[8]

| Species | Duration | Dose (mg/kg/day) | NOAEL | | | Finding |
| | | | Dose (mg/kg/day) | AUC (ng·h/mL) | Safety Margin (× MRHD) | |
|---|---|---|---|---|---|---|
| SD rat | 4 weeks | 100, 200, 500, 1000, p.o. | 100 | NA | NA | 200 mg/kg/day: A significant decrease in serum cholesterol. 500 mg/kg/day: 6% mortality. Body weight gains was decreased and body temperature was routinely 2-3 °C lower than the control group. 1000 mg/kg/day: 100% mortality. |
| | 4 weeks | 30, 50, 100, 200, p.o. | Not established | NA | NA | Microscopic findings were noted in the non-glandular stomach in all dose groups. |
| | 6 months | 30, 50, 100, 200, p.o. | 30 | 225 | 3 | A decrease in body weight was noted in high dose animals (males: ↓ 12%; females: ↓ 5%). Microscopic findings: A dose-dependent increase in severity and incidence were noted for the epithelial hyperplasia and hyperkertaosis in the non-glandular stomach in mid-low, mid-high and high dose groups. Histopathological findings: Very minimal effects were noted in the non-glandular stomach in low dose group. |
| Gottingen minipig[a] | 4 weeks | 0.9, 6.4, 9.2, 13.8, dermal | Systemic: 13.8 Dermal: 0.9 | NA | NA | The only treatment-related toxicity was a dose-dependent increase in dermal irritation at the treatment site. |
| | 3 months | 1.0, 2.8, 4.7, 9.6, dermal | Systemic: 9.6 Dermal: 1.0 | NA | NA | The only treatment-related toxicity was a dose-dependent increase in dermal irritation at the treatment site. |
| | 6 months | 0.9, 2.8, 4.7, 9.2, dermal | Systemic: 9.2 Dermal: 0.9 | NA | NA | The only treatment-related toxicity was a dose-dependent increase in dermal irritation at the treatment site. |
| | 9 months | 0.3%, 1%, 3% , 3% (+ degradants), dermal | Systemic: 3% Dermal: Not established | 753 | 10 | The only treatment-related toxicity was a dose-dependent increase in the incidence and severity of dermal effects at the treatment site. Systemic exposure was only noted in the 3% tavaborole solution group. |

Vehicle: 1% CMC for oral studies and 20% (v/v) PEG in ethanol for dermal studies.　[a] Based on mean human $AUC_{tau}$ under maximal use conditions = 75.8 ng·h/mL.

[8]　FDA Datadase.　http://www.accessdata.fda.gov/drugsatfda_docs/nda/2014/204427Orig1s000PharmR.pdf (accessed Mar 2016).

## Safety Pharmacology

Table 14    Safety Pharmacology Studies of Tavaborole[8]

| Study | System | Dose | Finding |
|---|---|---|---|
| Neurological effect | SD rat | 0, 30, 100, 200 mg/kg, p.o. | No eliciting any neurological effect at doses up to 200 mg/kg. |
| Cardiovascular effect | HEK293 cell expressing hERG channel | NA | The mean percent inhibition of tail current amplitude: 22.6%, which defined tavaborole as a low-potency hERG-channel blocker (less than 25% inhibition). |
| | Telemetered Beagle dog | 0, 30, 100, 200 mg/kg, p.o. | NOEL: 30 mg/kg. No treatment-related effect on the pattern of the P-QRS-T complexes, PR, QT and QTc intervals and the duration of the QRS complex were noted at doses up to 200 mg/kg. 100 and 200 mg/kg: A dose-related, reversible, mild to marked hypotension, in parallel with variable, transient increases in heart and pulse rates shortly after administration. |

Vehicle: 1% CMC.

## Genotoxicity

Table 15    Genotoxicity Studies of Tavaborole[8]

| Assay | Species/System | Metabolism | Dose | Finding |
|---|---|---|---|---|
| In vitro reverse mutation assay in bacterial cells (Ames) | S. typhimurium TA98, TA100, TA1535, TA1537; E. coli WP2 uvrA | ±S9 | 0.5, 1.5, 5.0, 15, 50, 150 µg/plate for TA98 and TA1537 (±S9) and TA1535 (-S9) 1.5, 5.0, 15, 50, 150 and 500 µg/plate for all other possible test conditions | Negative. |
| In vitro mammalian cell chromosome aberration assay | HPBL | ±S9 | 1.25, 2.5, 5, 10, 15, 20, 25 µg/mL | Negative. |
| In vivo rodent micronucleus assay | SD rat | + | 0, 250, 500, 1000 mg/kg | Negative. |

## Reproductive and Developmental Toxicity

Table 16    Reproductive and Developmental Toxicology Studies of Tavaborole[8]

| Study | Species | Dose (mg/kg/day) | NOAEL Endpoint | NOAEL Dose (mg/kg/day) | NOAEL AUC (ng·h/mL) | NOAEL Safety Margin[a] (× MRHD) | Finding |
|---|---|---|---|---|---|---|---|
| Fertility and early embryonic development | SD rat | 30, 100, 300, p.o. | Fertility | 300 | 8077[b] | 107 | No effect on reproductive organs, fertility or pregnancy indices, or uterine implantation parameters in all tested animals. |
| Embryo-fetal development | SD rat | 30, 100, 300 | Maternal/Fetal | 100 | 2199 | 29 | All limited to the HD, including ↑ resorbing fetuses, ↓ mean gravid uterine weight (34%), ↓ mean fetal weight (38%) and delay in ossification. No treatment-related effect on fetal sex ratio, fetal external malformations, variations of visceral malformations or variation. |
| | NZW rabbit | 1% (0.33), 5% (1.65), 10% (3.3), dermal | Malformation | 10% | 2766 | 36 | No treatment-related effects on maternal mortality, clinical observations, BW/BWG, food consumption or uterine implantation. |
| | | | Maternal/fetal development | 5% | 1977 | 26 | Dermal irritation being sporadic at MD, achieving severe erythema near the end of the dosing period at HD. No drug related malformation. |

[8]  FDA Datadase.  http://www.accessdata.fda.gov/drugsatfda_docs/nda/2014/204427Orig1s000PharmR.pdf (accessed Mar 2016).

*Continued*

| Study | Species | Dose (mg/kg/day) | NOAEL | | | | Finding |
|---|---|---|---|---|---|---|---|
| | | | Endpoint | Dose (mg/kg/day) | AUC (ng·h/mL) | Safety Margin[a] (× MRHD) | |
| Embryo-fetal development | NZW rabbit | 15, 50, 150, p.o. | Malformation | 150 | 11800 | 155 | All limited to the HD, including ↑ mortality and body weight loss, ↑ post-implantation loss (81.1%) mainly due to ↑ early resorption. |
| | | | Maternal/ embryofetal | 50 | 1220 | 16 | No treatment-related effect on fetal external malformations or variations, fetal visceral malformations or variations or fetal skeletal malformations or variations. |
| Pre- and postnatal development | SD rat 15, 60, 100, p.o. | | $F_0$ | 60 | NA | NA | Treatment-related effects on clinical signs, limited to HD $F_0$ dams, including ↓ motor activity and excess salivation (slight to moderate). |
| | | | | | | | No treatment-related effect on the evaluated physical and behavioral development parameters in $F_1$ animals. |
| | | | $F_1/F_2$ | 100 | 2199 | 29 | No treatment-related effect on viability, BW, clinical signs or macroscopic parameters in $F_2$ pups. |

Vehicle: 1% CMC and 0.4% MC for oral studies in rats and rabbits, respectively; 20% PEG in ethanol for dermal studies in rabbits. [a] Mean human $AUC_{tau}$ under maximal use conditions = 75.8 ng·h/mL. [b] Based on a linear extrapolation of the 200 mg/kg/day AUC value for male and female rats combined after 3 months of treatment in the 6 months oral rat toxicity study.

## Carcinogenicity

Table 17    104-Week Carcinogenic Toxicity Studies of Tavaborole[8]

| Species | Dose (mg/kg/day) | NOAEL | | | Finding |
|---|---|---|---|---|---|
| | | Dose (mg/kg/day) | $AUC_{0-24}$ (nM·h) | Safety Margin[a] (× MRHD) | |
| SD rat | 12.5, 25, 50, p.o. | 50 | 1090 | 14 | No treatment-related neoplastic finding. Treatment-related increased incidence of hyperplasia of the non-glandular stomach at HD, but whose clinical significance is unclear given the absence of non-glandular stomach. |
| CD-1 mouse | 50 (5%), 100 (10%), 150 (15%), dermal | 15% | 6740 | 89 | No treatment-related neoplastic finding. Treatment-related increased incidence/severity of epidermal hyperplasia, hyperkeratosis and inflammation in treated skin, correlated with treatment-related dermal irritation noted at the treatment site. |

[a] Based on mean human $AUC_{tau}$ under maximal use conditions = 75.8 ng·h/mL.

# CHAPTER

26

## Tedizolid Phosphate

# Tedizolid Phosphate

## (Sivextro®)

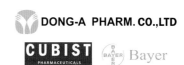

Research code: TR-701 FA; TR-701; DA-7218

## 1    General Information

- ❖ Tedizolid phosphate belongs to the oxazolidinone class of antibacterial drugs, which was approved in Jun 2014 by US FDA.

- ❖ Tedizolid phosphate was discovered by Dong-A, developed and marketed by Cubist.

- ❖ Tedizolid phosphate is a novel oxazolidinone prodrug antibiotic which is converted *in vivo* by phosphatases to the microbiologically active moiety tedizolid.  Tedizolid is a protein synthesis inhibitor that interacts with bacterial ribosome and prevents translation.

- ❖ Tedizolid phosphate is indicated in adults for the treatment of acute bacterial skin and skin structure infections (ABSSSI) caused by designated susceptible bacteria.

- ❖ Available as oral tablet or intravenous (i.v.) injection powder, containing 200 mg of tedizolid phosphate and the recommended dose is 200 mg once daily orally or as an intravenous (i.v.) infusion over 1 h for six days.

- ❖ The sale of Sivextro® was not available up to Mar 2016.

### Key Approvals around the World[*]

|  | US (FDA) | EU (EMA) |
|---|---|---|
| First approval date | 06/20/2014 | 03/23/2015 |
| Application or approval No. | NDA 205435; NDA 205436 | EMEA/H/C/002846 |
| Brand name | Sivextro® | Sivextro® |
| Indication | Acute bacterial skin and skin structure infections (ABSSSI) | |
| Authorisation holder | Cubist (acquired by Merck & Co.) | |

[*] Till Mar 2016, it has not been approved by PMDA (Japan) and CFDA (China).

## Active Ingredient

| Molecular formula: | C$_{17}$H$_{16}$FN$_6$O$_6$P |
|---|---|
| Molecular weight: | 450.32 |
| CAS No.: | 856866-72-3 (Tedizolid) |
|  | 856867-55-5 (Tedizolid phosphate) |
| Chemical name: | [(5R)-(3-{3-fluoro-4-[6-(2-methyl-2H-tetrazol-5-yl)pyridin-3-yl]phenyl}-2-oxooxazolidin-5-yl] methyl hydrogen phosphate |

*Parameters of Lipinski's "Rule of 5"*

| MW | H$_D$ | H$_A$ | FRB[a] | PSA[a] | cLogP[a] |
|---|---|---|---|---|---|
| 450.32 | 2 | 12 | 6 | 163Å$^2$ | -0.39 ± 0.71 |

[a] Calculated by ACD/Labs software V11.02.

## Drug Product[*]

| Dosage route: | Oral and intravenous infusion |
|---|---|
| Strength: | 200 mg (Tedizolid phosphate) |
| Dosage form: | Tablet and powder |

*Inactive ingredient (Tablet):*    Microcrystalline cellulose, mannitol, crospovidone, povidone, magnesium stearate, polyvinyl alcohol, titanium dioxide, polyethylene glycol/macrogol, talc and yellow iron oxide.

*Inactive ingredient (Injection):* Mannitol (105 mg), sodium hydroxide and hydrochloric acid, which is used in minimal quantities for pH adjustment.

*Recommended dose:* The recommended dosage is 200 mg administered once daily for six days either orally (with or without food) or as an intravenous infusion in patients 18 years of age or older.

No dosage adjustment is necessary when changing from intravenous to oral.

[*] Sourced from US FDA drug label information

## 2 Key Patents Information

### Summary

❖ Sivextro® (Tedizolid phosphate) has got five-year NCE market exclusivity protection after it was initially approved by US FDA on Jun 20, 2014.

❖ Tedizolid was originally discovered by Dong-A and then licensed to Trius Therapeutics (now belonging to Cubist), and its compound patent application was filed as PCT application by Dong-A in 2004.

❖ The compound patent will expire in 2024 foremost, which has been granted in Europe, Japan, China and the United States successively.

Table 1  Tedizolid Phosphate's Compound Patent Protection in Drug-Mainstream Country

| Country | Publication/Patent NO. | Application Date | Granted Date | Estimated Expiry Date |
|---|---|---|---|---|
| WO | WO2005058886A1 | 12/17/2004 | / | / |
| US | US8420676B2 | 12/17/2004 | 04/16/2013 | 02/23/2028[a] |
| EP | EP1699784B1 | 12/17/2004 | 06/29/2011 | 12/17/2024 |
| JP | JP4739229B2 | 12/17/2004 | 08/03/2011 | 12/17/2024 |
| CN | CN101982468B | 12/17/2004 | 02/08/2012 | 12/17/2024 |

[a] The term of this patent is extended by 1208 days (TD).

Table 2  Originator's International Patent Application List (Patent Family)

| Publication NO. | Title | Applicant/Assignee/Owner | Publication Date |
|---|---|---|---|
| **Technical Subjects** | **Active Ingredient (Free Base)'s Formula or Structure and Preparation** | | |
| WO2005058886A1 | Novel oxazolidinone derivatives | Dong-A | 06/30/2005 |
| **Technical Subjects** | **Salt, Crystal, Polymorphic, Solvate (Hydrate), Isomer, Derivative Etc. and Preparation** | | |
| WO2010042887A2 | Methods for preparing oxazolidinones and compositions containing them | Trius Therapeutics | 04/15/2010 |
| WO2010091131A1 | Crystalline form of (R)-3-(4-(2-(2-methyltetrazol-5-yl) pyridin-5-yl)-3-fluorophenyl)-5-hydroxymethyl oxazolidin-2-one dihydrogen phosphate | Trius Therapeutics | 08/12/2010 |
| **Technical Subjects** | **Formulation and Preparation** | | |
| WO2010138649A1 | Oxazolidinone containing dimer compounds, compositions and methods to make and use | Trius Therapeutics | 12/02/2010 |
| **Technical Subjects** | **Indication or Methods for Medical Needs** | | |
| WO2015054246A1 | Methods of treating subjects with renal impairment using tedizolid | Trius Therapeutics | 04/16/2015 |
| **Technical Subjects** | **Combination Including at Least Two Active Ingredients** | | |
| WO2013059610A1 | Therapeutic combination of daptomycin and protein synthesis inhibitor antibiotic, and methods of use | Trius Therapeutics | 04/25/2013 |

The data was updated until Jan 2016.

# 3 Chemistry

## Route 1: Original Discovery Route

*Synthetic Route*: The synthetic strategy utilized a convergent approach where an organo-tin phenyl oxazolidinone **6** was coupled to a heterocyclic-bromopyridine **7** using a Stille reaction. For the synthesis of the organotin phenyl oxazolidinone, the phenyloxazolidinone **4** was synthesized using a one-step process to convert the carbobenzyloxy (Cbz)-protected fluoroaniline **2** directly into a 5-hydroxymethyl oxazolidinone **4** in 70% yield. Iodination followed by the palladium-catalyzed exchange reaction provided the tributyltin derivative **6** in 61% yield. The corresponding heterocyclic-bromopyridine **7** was synthesized from a 2,5-dibromopyridine **9**, substituted by cyanide ion using copper cyanide and sodium cyanide as co-reagent under refluxing DMF in 70% yield. The tetrazole ring of 2-(tetrazol-5-yl)-5-bromopyridine **11** was made with sodium azide under elevated temperature in 85% yield. The addition of iodomethane to the solution of **11** in DMF produced a mixture of 1-methyltetrazolyl pyridine and 2-methyltetrazolyl pyridine at room temperature, which was separated by silica-gel column chromatography to give the desired 2-methyltetrazyl pyridine **7** in 45% yield. Finally, Stille coupling reaction of **6** with **7** provided the desired tetrazolyl 5-hydroxymethyl oxazolidinone **8** in 26% yield, which upon phosphorylation and hydrolysis of the resultant phosphoryl ester through workup with $H_2O$ provided tedizolid phosphate in 67% yield and the overall yield of 1%.[1-3]

[1] Im, W. B.; Choi, S. H.; Park, J. Y., et al. *Eur. J. Med. Chem.* **2011**, *46*, 1027-1039.
[2] Rhee, J. K.; Im, W. B.; Cho, C. H. WO2005058886A1, **2005**.
[3] Rhee, J. K.; Im, W. B.; Cho, C. H. US7816379B2, **2010**.

## Route 2

*Synthetic Route*: Synthesis of free acid of tedizolid phosphate using 1-iodo-2-fluoro-4-isocyanatobenzene **1** as starting materials was described here. The process involved Suzuki coupling as a key step. Cyclocondensation of isocyanates **1** with (*R*)-glycidyl tosylate **2** in the presence of LiI in refluxing THF yielded oxazolidine derivative **3**, in which the tosylate group upon acidic deprotection afforded primary alcohol **4**. Afterwards, phosphorylation of alcohol **4** with POCl₃ in PO(OEt)₃, prior to hydrolysis of the resultant chloride *via* aqueous workup provided phosphonic acid derivative **5** in 64% yield over three steps, correspondingly. Suzuki coupling of aryl iodide **5** with pyridinyl boronic acid **6** smoothly produced tedizolid phosphate in 85% yield.[4]

Synthesis of boronic acid **6** was completed in a one-pot manner: Metalation of commercially ready 5-bromo-2-(2-methyl-2*H*-tetrazol-5-yl)pyridine **7** prior to the subjection of resultant Grignard reagent to trimethyl borate led to borate **8**, which underwent acidic hydrolysis to produce **6** after recrystallized in water as a white solid with 78% yield across two steps. The overall yield hereof was 42%.[4]

[4] Xu, X. CN104327119A, **2015**.

## Route 3

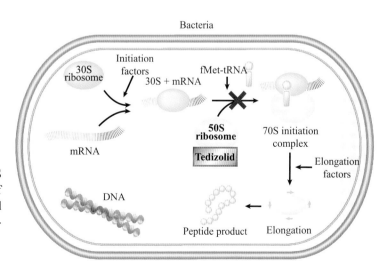

*Synthetic Route*: Commercial 5-bromo-2-cyanopyridine **8** was treated with sodium azide and ammonium chloride in DMF to produce tetrazole **9**, which was isolated by precipitation of the tetrazole ammonium salt. Subsequent methylation with methyl iodide in THF/DMF (3:1) afforded a 3.85:1 mixture of **4** accompanying with the corresponding *N*1-regioisomer. Acidification followed by treatment with aqueous NaOH (to pH 10.6) enabled isolation of **4** in 96% isomeric purity; crude **4** was further purified by recrystallization from isopropyl acetate in 33% yield from **9**. A Suzuki reaction of **4** with boronic acid **3** provided intermediate **5** in 85% yield. Recrystallization from ethyl acetate reduced the level of palladium in the product to 6 ppm. Boronic acid **3** was synthesized in two steps and 61% yield from commercial 4-bromo-3-fluoroaniline **1**, *via* Cbz protection and lithiation/borylation. Deprotonation of the carbamate in **5** using LiHMDS followed by reaction with *R*-(-)-glycidyl butyrate **6** in the presence of DMPU generated tedizolide **7** in 89% yield. Reaction with POCl$_3$ in the presence of TEA at 1-2 °C followed by subjection to sodium hydroxide and then subsequent acidification furnished tedizolid phosphate in 96% yield with the overall yield of 12%.[5, 6]

## 4    Pharmacology

### Summary

Mechanism of Action

❖ Tedizolid phosphate is a novel oxazolidinone prodrug antibiotic that is rapidly converted *in vivo* by phosphatases to the microbiologically active moiety tedizolid.

❖ Tedizolid is a protein synthesis inhibitor (IC$_{50}$ = 957 nM) that interacts with the bacterial 23S rRNA bacterial ribosome which is a subunit of 50S bacterial ribosome containing the peptidyl transferase center, thereby preventing the initiation of translation by inhibiting formation of the initiation complex.

[5] Costello, C. A.; Simson, J. A.; Duguid, R. J., et al. WO2010042887A2, **2010**.
[6] Ware, J. A.; Costello, C. A.; Duguid, R. J., et al. US8604209B2, **2013**.

❖ The off target profile of tedizolid was tested in a panel of 147 biochemical assays and 30 enzyme assays using concentrations of tedizolid of up to 20 μM.   In this *in vitro* assessment of the potential secondary pharmacological activity of tedizolid carried out with biochemical, enzyme and radioligand binding assays, the only noteworthy finding was a weak and reversible inhibition of MAO-A and MAO-B.   This lack of activity *in vivo* is predicted by low circulating peak tedizolid plasma concentrations relative to the $IC_{50}$ for MAO inhibition.[7]

*In Vitro* Efficacy

❖ The antibacterial activity of tedizolid:
  • *Staphylococci*: $MIC_{50}$ = 0.25-0.5 μg/mL (LRSA: 1-4 μg/mL), MIC ranging: 0.06-16 μg/mL.
  • *Streptococci*: $MIC_{50}$ = 0.12-0.25 μg/mL, MIC ranging: 0.03-1 μg/mL.
  • *Enterococci*: $MIC_{50}$ = 0.25-0.5 μg/mL (Linezolid-resistant: 1-4 μg/mL), MIC ranging: 0.03-1 μg/mL.
❖ Susceptibilities of gram-positive organisms to tedizolid:
  • MIC ranging: 0.06-1 μg/mL, $MIC_{50}$ = 0.25-0.5 μg/mL, $MIC_{90}$ = 0.25-1 μg/mL.
❖ Bactericidal activity for *Staphylococcus*:
  • $MBC_{50}$ = 2-16 μg/mL, $MBC_{90}$ = 16-32 μg/mL.

*In Vivo* Efficacy

❖ Systematic infection in mice:
  • *Staphylococcal* systemic infection model: MIC = 0.25-0.5 μg/mL, $ED_{50}$ = 0.46-7.6 mg/kg.
  • Systemic *enterococcal* infection model: $ED_{50}$ = 2.2-11.3 mg/kg.
  • *Streptococcal* systemic infection model: MIC = 0.125 μg/mL, $ED_{50}$ = 3.19-11.53 mg/kg.
  • *Streptococcus pneumoniae* pneumonia model: $ED_{50}$ = 2.8 mg/kg.
❖ Animal infection models:
  • Skin and soft tissue infections (MRSA in mice and rats): 1.4-5.42 $\log_{10}$ CFU/mL .
  • Lung infections epithelial lining fluid (MRSA in mice): 0.76-1.4 $\log_{10}$ CFU in thigh.
  • Neutropenic mouse model (*S. aureus* in mice): 3.93 $\log_{10}$ CFU in lung.
  • Heat valve infection (MRSA in rabbits): 2.5-6.0 $\log_{10}$ CFU in tissue.

## Mechanism of Action

Table 3    Prokaryotic and Eukaryotic Protein Synthesis Inhibition of Test Compounds[8]

| Test | Drug | $IC_{50}$ (nM) |
|---|---|---|
| | Tedizolid | 957 |
| | Tedizolid phosphate | 3496 |
| Coupled transcription-translation assay | Linezolid | 3296 |
| | Choramphenicol | 1266 |
| | Ampicillin | >20000 |

The inhibition of protein synthesis was evaluated in a coupled transcription-translation assay that use pBEST circular plasmid DNA encoding for luciferase reporter gene and an *E. coli* according to methods provided by manufacturer.

## *In Vitro* Efficacy

Table 4    Antibacterial Spectrum of Tedizolid[8]

| Gram-positive Organism | Type | MIC (μg/mL) | | |
|---|---|---|---|---|
| | | MIC Ranging | $MIC_{50}$ | $MIC_{90}$ |
| *Staphylococci* | Methicillin-susceptible *S. aureus* (MSSA) | 0.06-2 | 0.25-0.5 | 0.25-0.5 |
| | Methicillin-resistant *S. aureus* (MRSA) | 0.06-2 | 0.25-0.5 | 0.25-0.5 |

[7]  Europen Medicines Agency (EMA) Datadase.   http://www.ema.europa.eu/docs/en_GB/document_library/EPAR_-_Public_assessment_report/human/002846/WC500184803.pdf (accessed Mar 2016).
[8]  U.S. Food and Drug Adminstration (FDA) Datadase.   http://www.accessdata.fda.gov/drugsatfda_docs/nda/2014/205436Orig1s000MicroR.pdf (accessed Mar 2016).

*Continued*

| Gram-positive Organism | Type | MIC (μg/mL) | | |
|---|---|---|---|---|
| | | MIC Ranging | MIC$_{50}$ | MIC$_{90}$ |
| Staphylococci | Vancomycin-intermediate *S. aureus* (VISA) | 0.12-1 | 0.25 | 1 |
| | Vancomycin-resistant *S. aureus* (VRSA) | 0.25-1 | 0.25 | - |
| | Linezolid-resistant *S. aureus* (LRSA) | 0.25-16 | 1-4 | 4-8 |
| | Methicillin-susceptible coagulase-negative *staphylococci* (MSCoNS) | 0.06-1 | 0.25-0.5 | 0.25-0.5 |
| | Methicillin-resistant coagulase-negative *staphylococci* (MRCoNS) | 0.03-4 | 0.25-0.5 | 0.25-0.5 |
| Enterococci | Vancomycin-susceptible *E. faecalis* (VSEfa) | 0.12-1 | 0.25-0.5 | 0.5-1 |
| | Vancomycin-resistant *E. faecalis* (VREfa) | 0.25-1 | 0.25-0.5 | 0.5 |
| | Vancomycin-susceptible *E. faecium* (VSEfm) | 0.03-1 | 0.25-0.5 | 0.25-0.5 |
| | Vancomycin-resistant *E. faecium* (VSEfm) | 0.06-4 | 0.25-0.5 | 0.25-0.5 |
| | Linezolid-resistant strains | 0.5-16 | 1-4 | 2-4 |
| Streptococci | Penicillin-susceptible *S. pneumoniae* (PSSP) | 0.03-0.5 | 0.25 | 0.25 |
| | Penicillin-intermediate *S. pneumoniae* (PISP) | 0.06-0.5 | 0.25 | 0.25-0.5 |
| | Penicillin-resistant *S. pneumoniae* (PRSP) | 0.06-0.5 | 0.25 | 0.25 |
| | *Streptococcus pyogenes* | 0.06-0.5 | 0.12-0.25 | 0.25-0.5 |
| | *Streptococcus agalactiae* | 0.06-1 | 0.12-0.25 | 0.25-0.5 |
| | Viridans group *streptococci* | 0.06-0.5 | 0.25 | 0.25 |

MIC: Minimum inhibitory concentrations.

Table 5    Susceptibilities of Gram-positive Organisms to Tedizolid[8, 9]

| Strain | Strain Number | Antimicrobial Agent (μg/mL) | | |
|---|---|---|---|---|
| | | Range | MIC$_{50}$ | MIC$_{90}$ |
| MSSA | 95 | 0.25-1 | 0.5 | 0.5 |
| MRSA | 103 | 0.25-1 | 0.5 | 0.5 |
| CA-MRSA | 100 | 0.25-1 | 0.5 | 0.5 |
| MSSE | 48 | 0.12-1 | 0.25 | 0.5 |
| MRSE | 72 | 0.12-1 | 0.25 | 0.5 |
| VS *Enterococcus faecalis* | 73 | 0.25-1 | 0.5 | 1 |
| VR *E. faecalis* | 49 | 0.25-1 | 0.5 | 0.5 |
| VS Enterococcus faecium | 53 | 0.25-2 | 0.5 | 1 |
| VR *E. faecium* | 51 | 0.12-1 | 0.5 | 0.5 |
| PSSP | 38 | 0.06-0.5 | 0.25 | 0.25 |
| PISP | 37 | 0.06-0.5 | 0.25 | 0.25 |
| PRSP | 35 | 0.06-0.5 | 0.25 | 0.25 |
| *Streptococcus pyogenes* | 102 | 0.06-0.5 | 0.25 | 0.25 |
| *Streptococcus agalactiae* | 52 | 0.06-1 | 0.25 | 0.5 |

MIC: Minimum inhibitory concentrations.    MRSA: Methicillin-resistant *S. aureus*.    CA-MRSA: Community-acquired methicillin-resistant *S. aureus*.    MRSE: Methicillin-resistant *S. epidermidis*.    MSSA: Methicillin-susceptible *S. aureus*.    MSSE: Methicillin-susceptible *S. epidermidis*.    PISP: Penicillin-intermediate *S. pneumonia*.    PRSP: Penicillin-resistant *S. pneumonia*.    PSSP: Penicillin-susceptible *S. pneumonia*.    VR: Vancomycin-resistant.    VS: Vancomycin-susceptible.

[8]  FDA Datadase.    http://www.accessdata.fda.gov/drugsatfda_docs/nda/2014/205436Orig1s000MicroR.pdf (accessed Mar 2016).
[9]  Kanafani, Z. A.; Corey, G. R. *Expert Opin. Invest. Drugs* **2012**, *21*, 515-522.

Table 6    Bactericidal Activity of Tedizolid and Linezolid against *Staphylococci*[8]

| Organism | Type | Drug | MBC (μg/mL) | | |
|---|---|---|---|---|---|
| | | | MIC Ranging | MBC$_{50}$ | MBC$_{90}$ |
| *Staphylococci aureus* | All | Tedizolid | 0.5->32 | 4 | 16 |
| | | Linezolid | 2->8 | >8 | >8 |
| | Methicillin-susceptible | Tedizolid | 1-32 | 16 | 32 |
| | | Linezolid | 4->8 | >8 | >8 |
| | Methicillin-resistant | Tedizolid | 0.5->32 | 2 | 16 |
| | | Linezolid | 2->8 | 8 | >8 |
| *Coagulase-negative staphylococci* | All | Tedizolid | 2->32 | 16 | 32 |
| | | Linezolid | 2->8 | >8 | >8 |
| | Methicillin-susceptible | Tedizolid | 2->32 | 16 | 32 |
| | | Linezolid | 2->8 | >8 | >8 |
| | Methicillin-resistant | Tedizolid | 2->32 | 16 | 32 |
| | | Linezolid | 8->8 | >8 | >8 |

MBC: Minimum bactericidal concentrations.

Table 7    Antibacterial Activity of Tedizolid and Its Metabolites[8]

| Specie | Strain | MIC (μg/mL) | | | |
|---|---|---|---|---|---|
| | | Tedizolid | Desmethyl-Tedizolid (M1) | Sulfate-Tedizolid (M3) | Carboxy-Tedizolid (M2) |
| *Staphylocoocci aureus* | ATCC 33591 | 0.5 | 8 | 16 | >128 |
| *S. aureus* | ATCC 13709 | 0.5 | 8 | 16 | >128 |
| | ATCC 13709 + serum | 0.5 | 16 | 16 | >128 |
| | RN4220 | 0.25 | 8 | 16 | >128 |
| *Staphylococcus epidermidis* | ATCC 12228 | 0.25 | 8 | 8 | >128 |
| *Enterococcus faecalis* | ATCC 29212 | 1 | 16 | 32 | >128 |
| *Enterococcus faecium* | ATCC 19434 | 0.5 | 16 | 16 | >128 |
| *E. faecium* | ATCC 700221 | 0.5 | 8 | 16 | >128 |
| *Streptococcus pneumoniae* | ATCC 49619 | 0.25 | 4 | 8 | >128 |
| *S. pneumoniae* | ATCC 51916 | 0.25 | 8 | 16 | >128 |
| *Streptococcus pyogenes* | ATCC 19615 | 0.25 | 2 | 8 | >128 |
| *Haemophilus influenza* | ATCC 49247 | 32 | 32 | 128 | >128 |
| *Escherichia coli* | ATCC 25922 | >32 | >128 | >128 | >128 |

The carboxy analog was inactive (MIC values >128 μg/mL).    The desmethyl metabolite exhibited a very low level of activity (MIC values 8- to 32-fold higher than tedizolid).    The sulfate sample contained 7% tedizolid parent molecule.    MIC: Minimum inhibitory concentrations.

[8]    FDA Datadase.    http://www.accessdata.fda.gov/drugsatfda_docs/nda/2014/205436Orig1s000MicroR.pdf (accessed Mar 2016).

Table 8　Resistant Development During Serial Passages[7, 8]

| Organism | Strain | Compound | MIC Range (μg/mL) | MIC Increase Fold | Mutation (23S rRNA) |
|---|---|---|---|---|---|
| *Staphylocoocci aureus* | MRSA | Tedizolid | 0.25-2 | 8 | T2571C/G2576T |
| | | Linezolid | 1-32 | 32 | G2576T/L4[a] |
| | MSSA | Tedizolid | NA | No change | None |
| | | Linezolid | 2-128 | 64 | G2447T/L3[a] |
| *Enterococcus faecalis* | VSEF | Tedizolid | NA | 16 | T2504A |
| | | Linezolid | NA | 64 | G2576T |
| | VREF | Tedizolid | NA | 4 | G2576T |
| | | Linezolid | NA | 16 | G2576T |
| *Streptococcus pyogenes* *Streptococcus agalactiae* | | Tedizolid | NA | No change | None |
| | | Linezolid | NA | No change | None |

[a] L4 and L3 were the ribosomal proteins.

## *In Vivo* Efficacy

Table 9　*In Vivo* Systematic Infection in Mice[7, 8]

| Organism | Strain | Drug | Dose (mg/kg) | Route & Duration (Day) | Effect MIC (μg/mL) | Effect $ED_{50}$ (mg/kg) |
|---|---|---|---|---|---|---|
| *Staphylococcal* | MSSA, MRSA | Tedizolid phosphate | 1.1-30 | i.v., QD × 7 | NA | 1.5-4.3 |
| | | | | p.o., QD × 7 | NA | 3.2-7.6 |
| | | Linezolid | 1.1-30 | i.v., QD × 7 | NA | 7.7-29.1 |
| | | | 3.3-30 | p.o., QD × 7 | NA | 9.6-21.4 |
| | MRSA LZD-R (*cfr* +) | Tedizolid phosphate | 1, 5, 10, 20 | p.o., QD × 1 | 0.5 | NA |
| | | Linezolid | 5, 10, 20, 50 | p.o., QD × 1 | 8 | NA |
| | CoNSMR | Tedizolid phosphate | 1.1-30 or 1.48-40 | i.v., QD × 7 | 0.25-0.5 | 0.46-1.29 |
| | | | | p.o., QD × 7 | 0.25-0.5 | 2.01-3.25 |
| | | Linezolid | 1.1-30 or 3.3-30 | i.v., QD × 7 | 1-2 | 1.8-6.56 |
| | | | | p.o., QD × 7 | 1-2 | 2.41-7.48 |
| *Enterococcal* | Vancomycin-susceptible or vancomycin-resistant enterococci | Tedizolid phosphate | 1.1-30 or 2.5-40 | i.v., QD × 7 | NA | 2.2-9.1 |
| | | | | p.o., QD × 7 | NA | 4.3-11.3 |
| | | Linezolid | 1.1-30 or 5.0-40 | i.v., QD × 7 | NA | 11.1->40 |
| | | | | p.o., QD × 7 | NA | 17.6-25.9 |
| *Streptococcal* | Penicillin-resistant streptococcal | Tedizolid phosphate | 1.48, 4.44, 13.33, 40 | i.v., QD × 7 | 0.125 | 3.52-10.2 |
| | | | | p.o., QD × 7 | 0.125 | 3.19-11.5 |
| | | Linezolid | 1.48, 4.44, 13.33, 40 | i.v., QD × 7 | 0.5 | 17.6-39.5 |
| | | | | p.o., QD × 7 | 0.5 | 6.38-14.8 |
| *Streptococcus pneumoniae* | PSSP | Tedizolid phosphate | 2.5, 5, 10, 20 | p.o., QD × 2 | NA | 2.8 |
| | | Linezolid | 2.5, 5, 10, 20 | p.o., QD × 2 | NA | 8.09 |

[7] EMA Datadase. http://www.ema.europa.eu/docs/en_GB/document_library/EPAR_-_Public_assessment_report/human/002846/WC500184803.pdf (accessed Mar 2016).

[8] FDA Datadase. http://www.accessdata.fda.gov/drugsatfda_docs/nda/2014/205436Orig1s000MicroR.pdf (accessed Mar 2016).

Table 10    Effects of Tedizolid Phosphate in the Animal Infections Models[7, 8]

| Study | Type | Animal | Drug | Does (mg/kg) | Route & Duration (Day) | Colony Count (× CFU) |
|---|---|---|---|---|---|---|
| Skin and soft tissue infection | MRSA | Mouse | Tedizolid phosphate | 5 | p.o., QD × 2 | 5.21/9.07 (thigh/air pouch, $\log_{10}$/mL) |
| | | | | | p.o., BID × 2 | 5.42/5.00 (thigh/air pouch, $\log_{10}$/mL) |
| | | | | 10 | p.o., QD × 2 | 4.60/2.44 (thigh/air pouch, $\log_{10}$/mL) |
| | | | | | p.o., BID × 2 | 3.51/3.25 (thigh/air pouch, $\log_{10}$/mL) |
| | | | | 20 | p.o., QD × 2 | 3.16/2.33 (thigh/air pouch, $\log_{10}$/mL) |
| | | | | | p.o., BID × 2 | 3.17/2.84 (thigh/air pouch, $\log_{10}$/mL) |
| | | Mouse | Linezolid | 5 | p.o., QD × 2 | 6.07/8.49 (thigh/air pouch, $\log_{10}$/mL) |
| | | | | | p.o., BID × 2 | 5.62/7.12 (thigh/air pouch, $\log_{10}$/mL) |
| | | | | 10 | p.o., QD × 2 | 5.47/5.40 (thigh/air pouch, $\log_{10}$/mL) |
| | | | | | p.o., BID × 2 | 7.44/8.41 (thigh/air pouch, $\log_{10}$/mL) |
| | | | | 20 | p.o., QD × 2 | 6.04/8.29 (thigh/air pouch, $\log_{10}$/mL) |
| | | | | | p.o., BID × 2 | 4.69/3.60 (thigh/air pouch, $\log_{10}$/mL) |
| | | Rat | Tedizolid phosphate | 5, 10, 20, 50 | p.o., QD × 1 | 1.4-2.56 ($\log_{10}$/g, thigh) |
| | | | Linezolid | 5, 10, 20, 50 | p.o., QD × 1 | 1-1.3 (($\log_{10}$/g, thigh) |
| Lung infections epithelial lining fluid (ELF) | MRSA | Mouse | Tedizolid phosphate | 20 | i.p., QD × 1 | 0.76-1.4 ($\log_{10}$/g, lung) |
| | | | Linezolid | 120 | s.c., BID × 1 | 1.2-2.0 ($\log_{10}$/g, lung) |
| | | | Vancomycin | 25 | s.c., BID × 1 | NA |
| Neutropenic mouse model | S. aureus | Mouse | Tedizolid phosphate | 0.625-160 | p.o., BID × 1 | 3.93 ($\log_{10}$/g, lung) |
| | | | Linezolid | 1.25-80 | p.o., BID × 1 | 3.27 ($\log_{10}$/g, lung) |
| Heat valve infections[a] | MRSA | Rabbit | Tedizolid phosphate | 15 | i.v., BID × 4 | 2.5-6.0 ($\log_{10}$/g, tissue) |
| | | | Vancomycin | 30 | i.v., BID × 4 | 2.6-5.5 ($\log_{10}$/g, tissue) |
| | | | Daptomycin | 18 | i.v., BID × 4 | 2.2-3.5 ($\log_{10}$/g, tissue) |

MRSA: Methicillin-resistant *Staphylococcus aureus*.    CFU: Colony Forming Units.    Air pouches were induced in male ICR mice by injecting 5 mL of sterile filtered air into loose connective dorsal tissue.    QD: Once daily.    BID: Twice daily.    p.o.: Oral.    i.p.: Intraperitoneal injection.    s.c.: Subcutaneous injection.    i.v.: Intravenous injection.    [a] The test of CFU tissues were vegetations, spleen and kidney.

[7]  EMA  Datadase.    http://www.ema.europa.eu/docs/en_GB/document_library/EPAR_-_Public_assessment_report/human/002846/WC500184803.pdf (accessed Mar 2016).
[8]  FDA  Datadase.    http://www.accessdata.fda.gov/drugsatfda_docs/nda/2014/205436Orig1s000MicroR.pdf  (accessed Mar 2016).

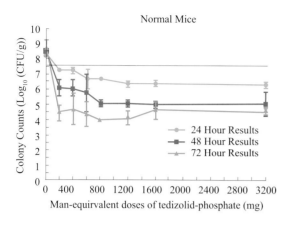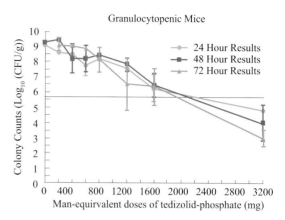

Figure A    Impact of Granulocytes on the Antibacterial Effect of Tedizolid Phosphate in a Mouse Thigh Infection Model[8]

**Study:** Colony counts over 72 h of *S. Aureus* in the thighs of granulocytopenic mouse.

**Animal:** Female Swiss Webster mouse.

**Model:** Granulocytopenic mice induced by cyclophosphamide, i.p. 150 mg/kg on Day 4 and 100 mg/kg on Day 1.    MRSA (strain ATCC335911), non-granulocytopenic mice: $1 \times 10^7$ CFU/thigh, granulocytopenic mice: $5 \times 10^5$ CFU in thigh.

**Administration:** i.p., QD for 3 days, tedizolid phosphate: equivalent to human oral dose of 200, 400, 600, 800, 1200, 1600 or 3200 mg.

**Test:** MRSA viable counts in thigh muscle at 24, 48 and 72 h.

**Results:** Granulocytopenic mice doses were slightly less than the human-equivalent doses of 2300 mg/day at 24 h, 2100 mg/day at 48 h, and 2000 mg/day at 72 h.    In normal mice, stasis was achieved at human-equivalent dose of slightly greater than 100 mg/day at 24 h and less than 100 mg/day at 48 and 72 h.    The majority of bacterial killing was attributable to the effects of tedizolid mediated through granulocytes.

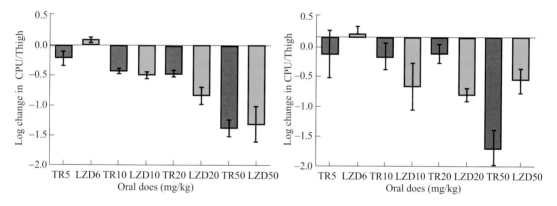

Figure B    Efficacy of Tedizolid against MRSA in the Skin and Soft Tissue Infection Rat Model[8]

**Study:** Skin and soft tissue infection rat model.

**Animal:** Male Sprague-Dawley rat.

**Model:** Cyclophosphamide, i.p. 150 mg/kg on Day 4 and 100 mg/kg on Day 1 relative to inoculation.    MRSA strain ATCC 33591 intramuscular i.m. $1 \times 10^7$ CFU in thigh.

**Administration:** Tedizolid phosphate or linezolid: 5, 10, 20, 50 mg/kg, p.o., QD for 1 day.    Vehicle: Water.

**Test:** Cultured bacterial counts in right thigh.

**Results:** Both tedizolid phosphate and linezolid produced a clear antibacterial response relative to untreated controls at the 50 mg/kg dose. Tedizolid phosphate was slightly more effective at this dose in both experiments, providing a 1.4 to 2.56 $\log_{10}$ CFU reduction in bacterial count, whereas linezolid produced a 1 to 1.3 $\log_{10}$ CFU reduction.

[8]  FDA Datadase.    http://www.accessdata.fda.gov/drugsatfda_docs/nda/2014/205436Orig1s000MicroR.pdf (accessed Mar 2016).

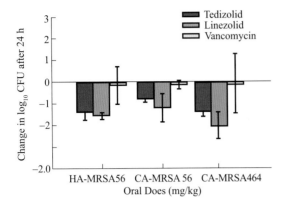

**Study:** Lung infections epithelial lining fluid mouse model.

**Animal:** Female Balb/c mouse.

**Model:** MRSA *via* oral instillation into the lungs, 0.05 mL of $1 \times 10^9$ CFU/mL.

**Administration:** Tedizolid phosphate: 20 mg/kg, i.p., QD for 1 day; Linezolid: 120 mg/kg, s.c., BID for 1 day; Vancomycin: 25 mg/kg, s.c., BID for 1 day.

**Test:** Collecting of bronchoalveolar lavage (BAL) fluid, 12 to 24 h after dose intervals, counting $\log_{10}$ CFU/lung at 24 h.

**Results:** Antibacterial efficacy was similar for tedizolid phosphate and linezolid, vancomycin was less effective than either of the oxazolidinones in terms of efficacy and reduction in mortality in this model.

Figure C    The Antibacterial Activity and Epithelial Lining Fluid Exposures of Tedizolid, Linezolid and Vancomycin[8]

## 5   ADME & Drug-Drug Interaction

### Summary

Absorption of Tedizolid

❖ Exhibited a non-linear pharmacokinetics in humans following oral administration.   The increase in AUC of tedizolid was dose-proportional, but in $C_{max}$ was less than dose-proportional in the dose range of 200 to 1200 mg tedizolid phosphate.

❖ Had high oral bioavailability in humans (91%) and mice (89.5%-92.9%).

❖ Was absorbed moderately to slowly in humans ($T_{max}$ = 2.5-4.0 h) and rats ($T_{max}$ = 0.13-5.1 h), rapidly to moderately in mice ($T_{max}$ = 0.5-2 h) and dogs ($T_{max}$ = 0.83-1.67 h).

❖ Showed a half-life ranging between 11 to 13.4 h in humans, much longer than those in mice (3.05-3.42 h), rats (1.44-1.92 h), and dogs (0.58-0.90 h) after intravenous administration of tedizolid phosphate.

❖ Had high clearance in dogs (26.9-39.2 mL/min/kg) but low in mice (3.11-3.98 mL/min/kg), in contrast to liver blood flow, after intravenous administration of tedizolid phosphate.

❖ Exhibited a moderate tissue distribution in mice, but extensive in dogs, with appearance distribution volumes at 0.918-0.949 and 1.66-1.93 L/kg, respectively, after intravenous administration of tedizolid phosphate.   The mean steady state volume of distribution of tedizolid in healthy adults after single intravenous dose of 200 mg tedizolid phosphate was 67.1 L.

❖ Showed a high permeability with the $P_{app(A \to B)}$ = 18.5-29.1 $\times 10^{-6}$ cm/s in Caco-2 cell monolayer model.

Distribution of Tedizolid

❖ Exhibited moderate plasma protein binding in humans (84.6%), and dogs (78%), but high in rats (97.7%) and mice (92.6%).

❖ In SD and Long-Evans rats after single oral administration of tedizolid phosphate:
  • Tedizolid was distributed from blood into many tissues.
  • Relatively higher drug concentration levels were observed in liver, adrenal gland, intestine and stomach.   The tissues with the lowest concentrations were eyes and brain.
  • Concentrations were approximately 3-20 folds increased in Long-Evans rats compared to SD rats, and the half-life was greatly increased by 10 folds to approximately 40 h suggesting melanin binding.
  • In almost all tissues, radioactive levels decreased to below the lowest level of quantification by 72 h post-dose in SD rats.

❖ In Beagle dogs after single oral administration of tedizolid phosphate:
  • Relatively higher drug concentration levels were observed in large and small intestine, liver, eye solids and kidneys. The lowest measured concentrations were exhibited in brain, eye vitreous, bone and fat.
  • In most tissues, radioactivity was below the lower limit of quantification (LLOQ) by 24 h post-dose.

Metabolism of Tedizolid Phosphate

❖ Tedizolid phosphate and tedizolid were both stable in rat, dog, monkey and human liver microsomes.   But the metabolisms of tedizolid phosphate were high in mouse, dog and human plasma (conversion to tedizolid).

[8]  FDA Datadase.   http://www.accessdata.fda.gov/drugsatfda_docs/nda/2014/205436Orig1s000MicroR.pdf (accessed Mar 2016).

❖ Tedizolid phosphate was rapidly and extensively converted by phosphatases to tedizolid (TR-700). Transformation of tedizolid phosphate was not mainly *via* phase I hepatic metabolism.

❖ Total eight metabolites were identified in plasma, urine and feces of rats, dogs and humans.

❖ Only the active metabolite tedizolid (TR700) was detected in human, mouse, rat and dog plasma. No parent compound was present in plasma, urine and feces.

❖ The metabolisms of tedizolid phosphate were similar in rats, dogs and humans.

## Excretion of Tedizolid Phosphate

❖ Was predominantly excreted in feces in humans and tested animals, with tedizolid sulfate (M4) as the most significant component in mouse, rat, dog and human feces.

❖ Minimal biliary excretion was observed in rats.

❖ No gender differences were observed.

## Drug-Drug Interaction

❖ Tedizolid phosphate and tedizolid were not inhibitors ($IC_{50}$ >50 µM) or inducers of major CYP enzymes (CYP 1A2, 2B6, 2C8, 2C9, 2C19, 2D6 or 3A4).

❖ Tedizolid was not a substrate or an inhibitor of major membrane transporters (OAT1, OAT3, OATP1B1, OATP1B3, OCT1, OCT2 or P-gp), but inhibited BCRP with an $IC_{50}$ of 51.1 µM.

# Absorption

Table 11    *In Vivo* Pharmacokinetic Parameters of Tedizolid Phosphate and Tedizolid in Mice, Rats and Dogs after Single Dose[10]

| Species | Route | Dose (mg/kg) | Administration Article | Analyte | $T_{max}$ (h) | $C_{max}$ (µg/mL) | $AUC_{inf}$ (µg·h/mL) | $T_{1/2}$ (h) | Cl or Cl/F (mL/min/kg) | $V_{ss}$ (L/kg) | F (%) |
|---|---|---|---|---|---|---|---|---|---|---|---|
| Mouse (male) | i.v. | 10 | Tedizolid | Tedizolid | NA | NA | 103 | 3.49 | 1.61 | 0.512 | - |
| | p.o. | 10 | | | 2 | 4.62 | 50.2 | 3.12 | NA | NA | 48.5 |
| Mouse (male) | i.v. | 10 | Tedizolid phosphate | Tedizolid | 0.0167 | 8.81 | 53.6 | 3.42 | 3.11 | 0.918 | - |
| | p.o. | 10 | | | 0.5 | 8.37 | 49.8 | 3.82 | NA | NA | 92.9 |
| Mouse (female) | i.v. | 10 | Tedizolid phosphate | Tedizolid | 0.0167 | 9.51 | 41.9 | 3.05 | 3.98 | 0.949 | - |
| | p.o. | 10 | | | 0.5 | 6.99 | 37.5 | 2.83 | NA | NA | 89.5 |
| Mouse | p.o. | 1.33 | Tedizolid phosphate | Tedizolid | 0.5 | 0.73 | 6.90 | 6.04 | 2.42 | NA | NA |
| | p.o. | 2.67 | | | 0.5 | 1.07 | 12.3 | 5.50 | 2.71 | NA | NA |
| | p.o. | 5.33 | | | 0.5 | 2.19 | 23.2 | 6.22 | 2.88 | NA | NA |
| | p.o. | 10.7 | | | 0.5 | 4.61 | 43.4 | 5.57 | 3.07 | NA | NA |
| | p.o. | 21.3 | | | 0.5 | 9.37 | 99.0 | 5.21 | 2.69 | NA | NA |
| | p.o. | 85.3 | | | 1 | 44.5 | 471 | 7.57 | 2.26 | NA | NA |
| | p.o. | 341 | | | 2 | 71.2 | NA | NA | NA | NA | NA |
| Rat (male) | i.v. | 10 | Tedizolid | Tedizolid | NA | NA | 53.1 | 2.15 | 3.15 | 0.274 | - |
| | p.o. | 10 | | | 5.00 | 1.87 | 15.8 | 3.59 | NA | NA | 29.8 |
| Rat (female) | i.v. | 10 | Tedizolid | Tedizolid | NA | NA | 149 | 3.98 | 1.13 | 0.343 | - |
| | p.o. | 10 | | | 5.10 | 3.04 | 40.8 | 6.75 | NA | NA | 27.4 |
| Rat (male) | i.v. | 5 | Tedizolid phosphate | Tedizolid | 0.20 | 12.5 | 15.1 | 1.44 | NA | NA | - |
| | i.v. | 10 | | | 0.13 | 20.8 | 29.6 | 1.86 | NA | NA | - |
| | i.v. | 20 | | | 0.18 | 45.4 | 67.8 | 1.92 | NA | NA | - |
| | i.v. | 5 | | Tedizolid phosphate | NA | NA | 5.22 | 0.230 | 16.0 | 0.085 | - |
| | i.v. | 10 | | | NA | NA | 11.0 | 0.375 | 15.1 | 0.073 | - |
| | i.v. | 20 | | | NA | NA | 21.7 | 0.908 | 15.3 | 0.117 | - |

[10]  FDA Datadase.   http://www.accessdata.fda.gov/drugsatfda_docs/nda/2014/205435Orig1s000PharmR.pdf (accessed Mar 2016).

*Continued*

| Species | Route | Dose (mg/kg) | Test Article | Analyte | $T_{max}$ (h) | $C_{max}$ (µg/mL) | $AUC_{inf}$ (µg·h/mL) | $T_{1/2}$ (h) | Cl or Cl/F (mL/min/kg) | $V_{ss}$ (L/kg) | F (%) |
|---|---|---|---|---|---|---|---|---|---|---|---|
| Rat (male) | p.o. | 20 | Tedizolid phosphate | Tedizolid | 0.43 | 14.7 | 49.2 | 2.76 | NA | NA | NA |
| | p.o. | 50 | | | 0.75 | 21.3 | 140.0 | 5.35 | NA | NA | NA |
| | p.o. | 100 | | | 0.75 | 34.6 | 295 | 6.52 | NA | NA | NA |
| | p.o. | 20 | | Tedizolid phosphate | 0.73 | 0.23 | 0.75 | 1.38 | NA | NA | NA |
| | p.o. | 50 | | | 1.36 | 0.29 | 1.33 | 2.73 | NA | NA | NA |
| | p.o. | 100 | | | 2.00 | 0.43 | 2.83 | 2.91 | NA | NA | NA |
| Long-Evans rat (male) | p.o. | 10 | Tedizolid phosphate | Tedizolid | 1 | 6.18 | 24.6[a] | 3.3 | NA | NA | NA |
| | p.o. | 30 | | | 1 | 15.7 | 134[a] | 2.1 | NA | NA | NA |
| | p.o. | 100 | | | 8 | 35.3 | 500[a] | 2.8 | NA | NA | NA |
| Long-Evans rat (female) | p.o. | 5 | Tedizolid phosphate | Tedizolid | 1 | 7.24 | 61.3[a] | 4.3 | NA | NA | NA |
| | p.o. | 15 | | | 1 | 21.5 | 219[a] | 3.5 | NA | NA | NA |
| | p.o. | 50 | | | 4 | 40.2 | 581[a] | 5.1 | NA | NA | NA |
| Dog (male) | i.v. | 10 | Tedizolid phosphate | Tedizolid | 0.08 | 5.37 | 4.42 | 0.58 | 39.2 | 1.66 | - |
| | i.v. | 30 | | | 0.19 | 17.4 | 18.6 | 0.90 | 26.9 | 1.93 | - |
| | i.v | 10 | | Tedizolid phosphate | NA | NA | 10.0 | 0.05 | 17.0 | 0.031 | - |
| | i.v. | 30 | | | NA | NA | 17.2 | 0.05 | 29.1 | 0.077 | - |
| | p.o. | 10 | Tedizolid phosphate | Tedizolid | 1.67 | 1.38 | 2.78 | 0.64 | NA | NA | NA |
| | p.o | 30 | | | 0.83 | 5.85 | 14.2 | 0.94 | NA | NA | NA |

[a] $AUC_{0-last}$.

Table 12 *In Vivo* Pharmacokinetic Parameters of Tedizolid Phosphate and Tedizolid in Humans after Single Oral and Intravenous Dose of Tedizolid Phosphate[11]

| Species | Route | Dose (mg) | Test Article | Analyte | $C_{max}$ (µg/mL) | $T_{1/2}$ (h) | $AUC_{inf}$ (µg·h/mL) | $T_{max}$ (h) | $V_{ss}$ (L) | Cl or Cl/F (L/h) |
|---|---|---|---|---|---|---|---|---|---|---|
| Healthy human | p.o. | 200 | Tedizolid phosphate | Tedizolid | 2.0 (0.7) | NA | 23.8 (6.8) | 2.5 (1.0-8.0) | NA | 6.9 (1.7) |
| | i.v. | 200 | | | 2.3 (0.6) | NA | 26.6 (5.2) | 1.1 (0.9-1.5) | NA | 6.4 (1.2) |
| Healthy human | p.o. | 200 | Tedizolid phosphate | Tedizolid | 1.99 | 11.2 | 25.4 | 3.01 | NA | 6.08 |
| | p.o. | 400 | | | 3.77 | 10.8 | 56.1 | 3.50 | NA | 5.58 |
| | p.o. | 600 | | | 5.21 | 11.4 | 79.3 | 2.50 | NA | 6.58 |
| | p.o. | 800 | | | 5.52 | 10.6 | 91.8 | 4.00 | NA | 6.65 |
| | p.o. | 1200 | | | 9.49 | 10.4 | 123 | 4.00 | NA | 7.77 |
| | i.v. | 100 | | | 1.16 | 13.4 | 17.4 | 1.92 | 74.5 | 4.77 |
| | i.v. | 200 | | | 2.62 | 11.0 | 32.6 | 2.17 | 67.1 | 5.41 |
| | i.v. | 400 | Tedizolid phosphate | | 5.13 | 11.3 | 58.7 | 2.10 | 67.5 | 5.79 |
| | i.v. | 100 | | Tedizolid phosphate | 0.579 | 0.102 | 0.778 | 0.917 | 11.5 | 132 |
| | i.v | 200 | | | 1.01 | 0.121 | 1.29 | 0.500 | 9.79 | 161 |
| | i.v | 400 | | | 2.46 | 0.682 | 3.08 | 0.500 | 10.6 | 133 |

## Key Findings:[11]

❖ The absolute bioavailability was approximately 91% in humans. The mean steady state volume of distribution of tedizolid in healthy adults following a single intravenous dose of 200 mg tedizolid phosphate was 67.1 L.

[11] FDA Datadase. http://www.accessdata.fda.gov/drugsatfda_docs/nda/2014/205435Orig1s000ClinPharmR.pdf (accessed Mar 2016).

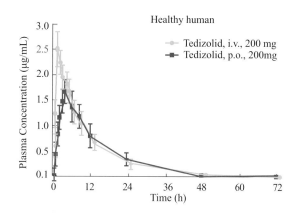

Figure D  *In Vivo* Plasma Concentration-Time Profiles of Tedizolid in Healthy Humans after Single Intravenous and Oral Dose of Tedizolid Phosphate[11]

Table 13  *In Vitro* Permeability of Tedizolid in Caco-2 Cell Monolayer Model[11]

| Test Article | pH | Conc. (µM) | $Papp_{(A \to B)}$ ($1 \times 10^{-6}$cm/s) | $Papp_{(B \to A)}$ ($1 \times 10^{-6}$cm/s) | Efflux Ratio | Permeability Class |
|---|---|---|---|---|---|---|
| Tedizolid | 7.4 | 1 | 21.3 | 40.2 | 1.9 | High |
| | | 10 | 18.5 | 29.8 | 1.6 | High |
| | | 100 | 29.1 | 24.6 | 0.8 | High |

## Distribution

Table 14  *In Vitro* Plasma Protein Binding of Tedizolid Phosphate and Tedizolid in Several Species[10]

| Species | Conc. (µg /mL) | %Bound | |
|---|---|---|---|
| | | Tedizolid Phosphate | Tedizolid |
| Mouse | 0.1-50 | 74.8 | 92.6 |
| Rat | 0.1-50 | 97.2 | 97.7 |
| Dog | 0.1-50 | 85.1 | 78.0 |
| Human | 0.1-50 | 86.6 | 84.6 |

Table 15  *In Vivo* Tissue Distribution of [$^{14}$C ]Tedizolid Phosphate in Male Beagle Dogs and Male Sprague-Dawley Rats after Single Oral Dose of 25 mg/kg [$^{14}$C]Tedizolid Phosphate[10]

| Species | Beagle Dog | | | | SD Rat | | | |
|---|---|---|---|---|---|---|---|---|
| Tissue | $C_{max}$ (µg/g) | $T_{1/2}$ (h) | $AUC_{inf}$ (µg·h/g) | Tissue/Plasma $AUC_{inf}$ Ratio | $C_{max}$ (µg eq./g) | $T_{1/2}$ (h) | $AUC_{inf}$ (µg eq.·h/g) | Tissue/Plasma $AUC_{inf}$ Ratio |
| Plasma | 3.30 | 1.33 | 10.9 | 1.00 | 17.8 | 3.3 | 120 | 1.0 |
| Brain | 1.20 | NC | 2.41 | 0.23 | 0.96 | 13.0 | 14.34 | 0.0 |
| Adrenal gland | 9.52 | 1.50 | 24.8 | 2.23 | 13.1 | 3.1 | 106 | 0.9 |
| Epididymis | 7.13 | 1.64 | 23.2 | 2.07 | NC | NC | NC | NC |
| Eyes (solids) | 7.51 | 6.01 | 66.9 | 3.38 | 0.35 | 76.8 | 36.9 | 0.1 |
| Kidneys | 17.0 | 12.2 | 56.6 | 5.15 | 15.2 | 3.0 | 108 | 0.9 |
| Large intestine | 17.5 | 19.6 | 400 | 21.2 | 52.1 | NC | NC | 3.0 |
| Liver | 32.4 | 4.33 | 119 | 11.0 | 27.6 | 3.1 | 221 | 1.8 |
| Pancreas | 7.68 | 1.49 | 25.7 | 2.32 | 8.87 | 7.3 | 91.6 | 0.4 |

[10] FDA Datadase.  http://www.accessdata.fda.gov/drugsatfda_docs/nda/2014/205435Orig1s000PharmR.pdf (accessed Mar 2016).
[11] FDA Datadase.  http://www.accessdata.fda.gov/drugsatfda_docs/nda/2014/205435Orig1s000ClinPharmR.pdf (accessed Mar 2016).

*Continued*

| Species | Beagle Dog | | | | Sprague-Dawley Rat | | | |
|---|---|---|---|---|---|---|---|---|
| Tissue | $C_{max}$ (μg/g) | $T_{1/2}$ (h) | $AUC_{inf}$ (μg·h/g) | Tissue/Plasma $AUC_{inf}$ Ratio | $C_{max}$ (μg eq./g) | $T_{1/2}$ (h) | $AUC_{inf}$ (μg eq.·h/g) | Tissue/Plasma $AUC_{inf}$ Ratio |
| Small intestine | 29.5 | 3.16 | 102 | 9.55 | 16.8 | 3.0 | 122 | 1.0 |
| Stomach | 9.10 | 1.43 | 27.6 | 2.50 | 15.8 | NC | NC | 2.0 |
| Submaxillary glands | 6.03 | 28.3 | 27.8 | 2.05 | NC | NC | NC | NC |
| Testes | 7.84 | 2.05 | 27.8 | 2.34 | 4.19 | 25.4 | 114 | 0.2 |

NC: Not calculated.

Table 16   *In Vivo* Tissue Distribution of [$^{14}$C]Tedizolid Phosphate in Male Long-Evans Rats after Single Oral Dose of 25 mg/kg [$^{14}$C]Tedizolid Phosphate[10]

| Tissues | $C_{max}$ (μg eq./g) | $T_{1/2}$ (h) | $AUC_{inf}$ (μg eq.·h/g) | Tissue/Plasma $AUC_{inf}$ Ratio |
|---|---|---|---|---|
| Plasma | 21.9 | 2.8 | 163 | 1.0 |
| Blood | 13.0 | 2.9 | 100 | 0.6 |
| Eyes | 0.478 | NC | NC | 0.0 |
| Fat | 3.46 | 7.1 | 33.1 | 0.1 |
| Skin | 6.94 | NC | NC | 0.3 |
| Uveal Tract | 166 | 44 | 3991 | 23 |

NC: Not calculated.

# Metabolism

Table 17   *In Vitro* Metabolic Stability of Tedizolid Phosphate and Tedizolid in Liver Microsomes and Plasma[11, 12]

| | % Tedizolid or Tedizolid Phosphate Remaining | | | | |
|---|---|---|---|---|---|
| Metabolic System | Liver Microsomes | | Plasma | | |
| Species | Tedizolid | Tedizolid Phosphate | Species | Tedizolid Phosphate | |
| | 10 μM, 2 h | 10 μM, 2 h | | 2 μg/mL, 2 h | |
| Rat | 91.7 | 87.1 | Mouse | 4.1 | |
| Dog | 105 | 92.7 | Rat | 29.6 | |
| Monkey | 123 | 83.7 | Dog | 3.4 | |
| Human | 116 | 88.7 | Human | 8.5 | |

## Key Findings:[11]

❖ Tedizolid phosphate was a prodrug that was rapidly and extensively converted by phosphatases to tedizolid.

❖ *In vitro*, neither tedizolid phosphate nor tedizolid was shown to be a substrate of major cytochrome P450 enzymes (CYP1A2, CYP2B6, CYP2D6, CYP2C8, CYP2C9, CYP2C19 and CYP3A4).

[10]   FDA Datadase.   http://www.accessdata.fda.gov/drugsatfda_docs/nda/2014/205435Orig1s000PharmR.pdf (accessed Mar 2016).
[11]   FDA Datadase.   http://www.accessdata.fda.gov/drugsatfda_docs/nda/2014/205435Orig1s000ClinPharmR.pdf (accessed Mar 2016).
[12]   Ong, V.; Flanagan, S.; Fang, E.; et al. *Drug Metab. Dispos.* **2014**, *42*, 1275-1284, 1210 pp.

Table 18    Metabolites in Plasma, Urine and Feces of Humans and Non-clinical Species after Oral and Intravenous Dose of Tedizolid Phosphate[10, 11]

| Matrix | Species | Gender | Route | Dose (mg/kg) | Time (h) | % of Total Radioactivity | | | | | | |
| --- | --- | --- | --- | --- | --- | --- | --- | --- | --- | --- | --- | --- |
| | | | | | | M1 | M2 | M3 | M4 | M5 | M6 | M7 |
| Plasma | Rat | Male | p.o. | 25 | 4 | NA | NA | NA | NA | 100.0 | NA | NA |
| | | Female | p.o. | 25 | 2 | NA | NA | NA | NA | 100.0 | NA | NA |
| | | Male | i.v. | 10 | 2 | NA | NA | NA | NA | 100.0 | NA | NA |
| | | Female | i.v. | 10 | 2 | NA | NA | NA | NA | 100.0 | NA | NA |
| | Dog | Male | i.v. | 10 | 10 min | NA | NA | NA | NA | 100.0ᵃ | NA | NA |
| | Human | Male | p.o. | 200 mg | 168 | NA | NA | NA | <1 | 94.5-98.2 | NA | NA |
| Urine | Rat | Male | p.o. | 25 | 6 | <1ᵃ | 7.8 | <1ᵃ | 62.3 | 2.3 | 2.4 | 24.5 |
| | | Female | p.o. | 25 | 6 | 11.8 | 9.2 | 1.0 | 67.8 | 6.0 | 3.3 | <1ᵃ |
| | | Male | i.v. | 10 | 6 | 1.6 | 7.5 | <1 | 65.0 | 2.6 | 1.5 | 21.3 |
| | | Female | i.v. | 10 | 6 | 14.0 | 8.3 | <1ᵃ | 65.0 | 8.3 | 3.3 | <1ᵃ |
| | Dog | Male | p.o. | 25 | 12 | 39.6 | 1.1ᵃ | NA | 57.6 | <1ᵃ | 1.0ᵃ | NA |
| | | Female | p.o. | 25 | 6 | 55.5 | 1.5 | <1ᵃ | 37.4 | <1ᵃ | 1.6 | 2.5 |
| | | Male | i.v. | 10 | 6 | 65.6 | 2.6ᵃ | NA | 27.7 | 1.5ᵃ | NA | 1.8ᵃ |
| | | Female | i.v. | 10 | 6 | 56.5 | <1ᵃ | NA | 41.8 | 1.5ᵃ | NA | NA |
| | Human | Male | p.o. | 200 mg | 168 | 0.53-2.38 | 2.54-4.68 | NA | 56.8-79.5 | 0.438-1.62 | NA | NA |
| Feces | Rat | Male | p.o. | 25 | 24 | NA | 1.4ᵃ | NA | 96.7 | 1.9ᵃ | NA | NA |
| | | Female | p.o. | 25 | 24 | NA | NA | NA | 90.0 | 8.7ᵃ | NA | NA |
| | | Male | i.v. | 10 | 24 | NA | 1.9ᵃ | NA | 97.6 | <1ᵃ | NA | NA |
| | | Female | i.v. | 10 | 24 | NA | NA | NA | 87.1 | 12.9 | NA | NA |
| | Dog | Male | p.o. | 25 | 12 | 2.3ᵃ | NA | NA | 87.9 | 2.6ᵃ | NA | NA |
| | | Female | p.o. | 25 | 12 | 3.1 | <1ᵃ | NA | 68.9 | 16.8 | NA | NA |
| | | Male | i.v. | 10 | 12 | 2.0ᵃ | NA | NA | 78.5 | 5.5ᵃ | NA | NA |
| | | Female | i.v. | 10 | 12 | 1.1ᵃ | NA | NA | 84.9 | 1.1ᵃ | NA | NA |
| | Human | Male | p.o. | 200 mg | 168 | NA | <6 | NA | 86.8-95.6 | <3 | NA | NA |

M1: Dimethyl tedizolid.    M2: Carboxyl tedizolid.    M3: Hydroxyl tedizolid.    M4: Tedizolid sulfate.    M5: Tedizolid (TR700).    M6: Unknown.    M7: Demethyl tedizolid sulfate.    ᵃ Indicated that the radioactive peak height had a S/N ratio that was less than 3.

[10]  FDA Datadase.   http://www.accessdata.fda.gov/drugsatfda_docs/nda/2014/205435Orig1s000PharmR.pdf (accessed Mar 2016).
[11]  FDA Datadase.   http://www.accessdata.fda.gov/drugsatfda_docs/nda/2014/205435Orig1s000ClinPharmR.pdf (accessed Mar 2016).

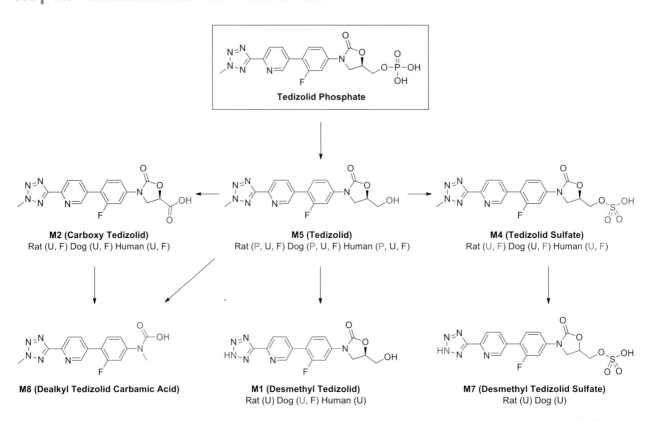

Figure E    Proposed Pathways for *In Vivo* Biotransformation of Tedizolid Phosphate in Rats, Dogs and Humans[10, 11]

The red labels represent the major components in the matrices.    P = Plasma, U = Urine and F = Feces.

## Excretion

Table 19    Excretion Profiles of [$^{14}$C]Tedizolid Phosphate in Rats and Dogs
after Oral and Intravenous Dose of [$^{14}$C]Tedizolid Phosphate[10]

| Species | State | Route | Dose (mg/kg) | Time (h) | Bile (% of dose) | Urine (% of dose) | Feces (% of dose) | Recovery[a] (% of dose) |
|---|---|---|---|---|---|---|---|---|
| SD rat (male) | Intact | p.o. | 25 | 0-168 | - | 8.69 | 89.4 | 98.1 |
| | | i.v. | 10 | 0-168 | - | 11.3 | 87.8 | 99.1 |
| SD rat (female) | Intact | p.o. | 25 | 0-168 | - | 10.7 | 83.2 | 93.9 |
| | | i.v. | 10 | 0-168 | - | 9.92 | 86.0 | 95.9 |
| Dog (male) | Intact | p.o. | 25 | 0-72 | - | 10.9 | 90.7 | 102 |
| | | i.v. | 10 | 0-72 | - | 10.1 | 81.4 | 91.5 |
| Dog (female) | Intact | p.o. | 25 | 0-72 | - | 8.06 | 84.3 | 92.7 |
| | | i.v. | 10 | 0-72 | - | 10.4 | 102 | 113 |
| SD rat (male) | BDC | i.v. | 13.3 | 0-4 | 1.76 | NA | NA | NA |
| Human (male) | Intact | p.o. | 204 mg | 0-228 | - | 18.0 | 81.5 | 99.5 |

BDC: Bile duct-cannulated.    [a] These figures included radioactivity recovered in cage washing and cage debris.

[10]    FDA Datadase.    http://www.accessdata.fda.gov/drugsatfda_docs/nda/2014/205435Orig1s000PharmR.pdf (accessed Mar 2016).
[11]    FDA Datadase.    http://www.accessdata.fda.gov/drugsatfda_docs/nda/2014/205435Orig1s000ClinPharmR.pdf (accessed Mar 2016).

## Drug-Drug Interaction

Table 20　*In Vitro* Evaluation of Tedizolid Phosphate and Tedizolid as an Inhibitor and an Inducer of Enzymes[11]

| Tedizolid Phosphate and Tedizolid as Inhibitors | | | Tedizolid as an Inducer | | | |
|---|---|---|---|---|---|---|
| Enzyme | $IC_{50}$ (μM) | | Enzyme | % of Positive Control[a] | | |
| | Tedizolid Phosphate | Tedizolid | | 0.1 μM | 1 μM | 10 μM |
| CYP3A4 | >50 | >50 | CYP1A2 | 0.70/-0.57/-1.2 | 5.7/-1.3/-0.93 | 0.34/-1.7/-0.30 |
| CYP2D6 | >50 | >50 | CYP2B6 | -0.58/1.0/0.55 | -0.30/-0.44/-0.97 | 1.0/0.78/-0.31 |
| CYP2C9 | >50 | >50 | CYP2C8 | -4.9/0.72/-7.4 | -8.1/5.0/-6.4 | -7.4/16/-8.4 |
| CYP1A2 | >50 | >50 | CYP2C9 | -12/-13/-1.5 | -5.3/-19/1.2 | -9.2/-9.2/14 |
| CYP2C19 | >50 | >50 | CYP2C19 | 3.8/0.34/4.9 | 0.4/4.7/2.0 | 21/-1.2/-4.1 |
| CYP2A6 | >50 | >50 | CYP3A4 | 0.04/-0.49/1.7 | 0.11/-0.30/0.82 | 0.07/0.10/2.1 |
| CYP2C8 | >50 | >50 | | | | |

[a] Data obtained from 3 donors.

Table 21　*In Vitro* Evaluation of Tedizolid as an Inhibitor and a Substrate of Uptake Transporters and Efflux Transporters[11]

| Transporter | ABC | | SLC | | | | | |
|---|---|---|---|---|---|---|---|---|
| | BCRP | P-gp | OCT1 | OCT2 | OAT1 | OAT3 | OATP1B1 | OATP1B3 |
| %Inhibition at 30 μM | 27.9 ± 8.82 | 8.42 ± 1.29 | 23.6 ± 4.43 | 4.72 ± 9.94 | 3.88 ± 8.04 | 25.1 ± 9.62 | 29.0 ± 11.9 | 13.2 ± 7.04 |
| $IC_{50}$ (μM) | 51.1 | NA | NA | NA | NA | NA | NA | NA |
| Substrare (Efflux Ratio) | No | 0.8-1.9 (1-100 μM) | No | No | No | No | No | No |

Mean ± SD for % inhibition.

# 6　Non-Clinical Toxicology

## Summary

### Single-Dose Toxicity
❖ Acute toxicity in mice (p.o.) and rats (i.v.):
  • Mouse NOAEL: 500 mg/kg/day.
  • Rat NOAEL: 62 mg/kg/day.

### Repeated-Dose Toxicity
❖ Repeated-dose toxicity studies in rats (p.o., up to 9 months; i.v., 4 weeks) and dogs (p.o., up to 3 months; i.v., 14 days):
  • In rats: The oral and intravenous toxicities primarily targeted GI tract, hematologic system and immune system, which were dose- and duration-dependent, but as with the oral route, the effects showed evidence of reversibility.　By the 9-month study, NOAELs were 30 mg/kg/day in males and 10 mg/kg/day in females, approximately 7-8 folds of exposure produced by the human clinical dose.
  • In dogs: Dose-dependent GI tract effects, clinical signs associated with histopathology, occurred in all the oral and intravenous treatment groups.　By the 3-month study, the NOAEL was 400 mg/kg/day, with about 5.5-fold (male) and 8.9-fold (female) exposure of MRHD.
  • Severe injection site reactions occurred predominantly in dogs, and the rats did not exhibit similar effects.

### Safety Pharmacology
❖ Safety pharmacology studies to investigate effects on neurological, cardiovascular, pulmonary, renal and GI function:
  • Significantly reduced spontaneous locomoter activity after dosing with 30 and 100 mg/kg/day and increased in hexobarbital-induced sleep time in 100 mg/kg/day.
  • Tedizolid phospate was not likely to prolong QT interval, considering no inhibition of hERG tail current up to 10 μM.
  • On pulmonary function, tedizolid phosphate did not alter any of the parameters relative to the control group.
  • Urinary sodium and chloride were reduced in the rats after administered 30 and 100 mg/kg/day compared to that in the control group.

[11]　FDA Datadase.　http://www.accessdata.fda.gov/drugsatfda_docs/nda/2014/205435Orig1s000ClinPharmR.pdf (accessed Mar 2016).

- Mean gastric volume and mean total acidity were reduced approximately 40%-50% in high dose animals (100 mg/kg).

## Genotoxicity

❖ In view of the *in vitro* and *in vivo* studies conducted, tedizolid phospate and tedizolid were negative for mutagenicity, clastogenesis and direct DNA damage, except that chromosome aberration frequency was significantly increased after 6 h incubation either with or without S9 metabolism activation at concentrations not associated with precipitation or >50% cytotoxicity.

❖ The weight of evidence from these studies as a whole indicated that neither tedizolid phospate nor tedizolid presented substantial genotoxic risks in humans.

## Reproductive and Developmental Toxicity

❖ Fertility and early embryonic development in rats:
  - Mating/fertility NOAELs were 50 mg/kg/day in males and 15 mg/kg/day in females, respectively, with over 4-5 times greater exposure than those at the 200 mg/day clinical dose, suggesting the least potential to affect fertility in humans.

❖ Embryo-fetal development studies in mice, rats and rabbits:
  - Drug-related maternal toxicity and fetus-developmental malformations or variations were consistently observed in all tested species, with exposures of NOAEL approximately equal to or 25-fold less than the expected clinical exposure, considering which as a sign of caution for usage in pregnant women.

❖ Pre- and postnatal development in rats:
  - No adverse effect was observed on offspring growth, maturation, or measures of behavior or reproductive function at all doses tested, with exposure of the HD (3.75 mg/kg/day) approximately equal to that produced by a 200 mg/day clinical dose.
  - Concentrations of tedizolid in maternal milk were at approximating maternal plasma levels, and mean plasma fetal concentrations were approximately 24%-37% of the maternal plasma concentration at 2 h post-dose.

## Carcinogenicity

❖ Carcinogenicity studies were not performed or required based on the limited duration of clinical administration.

## Special Toxicology

❖ Immunotoxicity: Significantly reduced total spleen cell counts in high dose groups in SD rats.

❖ Local irritation: Slightly more severe signs of local irritation including hemorrhage, and focal muscle degeneration with histocyte infiltration were observed compared to vehicle injections.

# Single-Dose Toxicity

Table 22   Single-Dose Toxicity Studies of Tedizolid Phosphate[10]

| Species | Dose (mg/kg) | NOAEL (mg/kg/day) | Finding |
|---------|--------------|-------------------|---------|
| Mouse | 0, 500, 1000, 2000, p.o. | 500 | Rough fur, loss of fur, ptosis and ↓ locomotor activity at MD and HD. |
| | 0, 62, 125, 250, i.v. | NI | At HD: 2 males and 1 female deaths at HD, ↓ locomotor activity and dyspnea (HD males, MD females), dilation of cecum in MD males, and HD females, decreased/suppressed body weight gain at all doses. |
| Rat | 0, 500, 1000, 2000, p.o. | NI | 2 females deaths at HD, rough fur, loss of fur, ↓ locomotor activity, weakening, diarrhea, ↓ body weight, cecal dilation, splenic atrophy, thymus atrophy, reddish spots on stomach, marked cecal blood vessels, ↓ body weight at all doses. |
| | 0, 62, 125, 250, i.v. | 62 | 3 males and 3 females deaths, dyspnea in all HD animals, ↓ body weight in MD males and HD females, dilation of cecum in all males and females at MD and HD, marked blood vessels in cecum in MD females. |

NI: Data not identified.

[10] FDA Datadase.   http://www.accessdata.fda.gov/drugsatfda_docs/nda/2014/205435Orig1s000PharmR.pdf (accessed Mar 2016).

# Repeated-Dose Toxicity

Table 23    Repeated-Dose Toxicity Studies of Tedizolid Phosphate by Oral or Intravenous Administration[10]

| Species | Duration | Dose (mg/kg/day) | NOAEL Dose (mg/kg/day) | NOAEL Safety Margin[a] (× MRHD) | Finding |
|---------|----------|------------------|------------------------|----------------------------------|---------|
| Rat | 4 weeks | 0, 10, 30, 100 p.o. | Male: 30; Female: 10. | Male: 3.2; Female: 2.1 | Gender differences in toxicity associated with greater systemic exposure in females. Substantial mortality in females with a total of 13 animals found dead or euthanized in extremis at HD. Target organs for toxicity in females: Blood cells (↓ WBC, reticulocyte and neutrophil percentages) mesenteric lymph nodes (atrophy), spleen (atrophy), thymus (atrophy, ↓ weights), bone marrow (atrophy), liver (↑ ALT and ALP, hepatocellular hypertrophy), and GI tract (enlarged cecums, stomach erosion, duodenal inflammation, erosion). ↓ RBCs, ↑ BUN, enlarged cecums, and ↓ thymus and liver weights in HD males, yet without histopathology in males. |
|  | 3 months | M: 0, 10, 30, 100 F: 0, 3, 10, 30 p.o. | Male: 30; Female: 10 | Male: 6.3; Female: 4.8 | Four high-dose males and one high-dose female died early or were euthanized early due to drug-related toxicity. At the early termination in Week 5, high-dose male and female body weights were reduced 27.1% and 15.7%, respectively, compared to the control group. After the recovery period, partial weight gain occurred for high-dose animals compared to controls. Hematology changes including significantly lower platelets and reticulocytes in high-dose males correlated with bone marrow atrophy and demonstrated reversal during the recovery period. Serum chemistry changes including increased liver enzymes (ALT, AST and SDH) in high-dose males correlated with hepatocellular degeneration and atrophy. Histopathology mainly occurring in early death animals included bone marrow hypocellularity, small and large intestine degeneration and atrophy, hepatic degeneration and atrophy, and in early death males, seminiferous tubule degeneration and testicular hemorrhage. |
|  | 9 months | M: 0, 7.5, 15, 30; F: 0, 2.5, 5, 10, p.o. | Male: 30; Female: 10 | Male: 8.7; Female: 7.4 | Body weights were reduced in high-dose with greater reductions occurring with the duration of dosing. No gross pathology or histopathology was noted for a battery of examined neural tissues, the eyes or skeletal muscle.    No drug-related ophthalmic lesions were observed. |
|  | 4 weeks | M: 0, 10, 30, 90; F: 0, 5, 15, 45, i.v. | Male: 30; Female: 15. | Male: 5.0; Female: 3.3 | No drug-related death was observed.    Clinical signs included: soft and/or mucoid feces primarily in high-dose males and females, and labored and shallow respiration, hyporeactivity, pale extremities, and muscle rigidity in several high-dose males. Body weights for high-dose males were reduced by 8% compared to controls at the end of dosing. Serum potassium, total protein and globulin were reduced and the albumin/globulin ratio was increased in a dose-dependent manner in mid- and high-dose males and females.    These serum chemistry changes may have occurred in association with soft and mucoid feces and demonstrated total or partial reversal in recovery animals. No drug-related gross pathology or histopathology findings was reported. |

[10]  FDA Datadase.   http://www.accessdata.fda.gov/drugsatfda_docs/nda/2014/205435Orig1s000PharmR.pdf (accessed Mar 2016).

*Continued*

| Species | Duration | Dose (mg/kg/day) | NOAEL Dose (mg/kg/day) | NOAEL Safety Margin[a] (× MRHD) | Finding |
|---------|----------|------------------|-------------------------|----------------------------------|---------|
| Beagle dog | 4 weeks | 0, 100, 200, 400, p.o. | 400 | Male: 7.9; Female: 2.6 | Dose-dependent vomiting and salivation in all treatment groups. No other adverse finding in body weight, food consumption, clinical pathology or histopathology. Similar toxicokinetics values for both genders. |
| | 3 months | 0, 100, 200, 400, p.o. | 400 | Male: 5.5; Female: 8.9 | No drug-related death occurred. The primary clinical signs were abnormal feces and emesis occurring 1-2 h after dosing for all drug treatment groups. Other than emesis, no other toxicity clearly related to tedizolid phosphate administration was observed. |
| | 14 days | 0, 25, 50, 100, i.v. | 50 | Male: 1.1; Female: 0.8 | The primary clinical signs were severe injection-site reactions primarily in high-dose (200 mg/kg/day) males and females, with lesser incidence in mid-dose animals. Emesis occurred in individual animals in all drug treatment groups with incidence and severity increasing with dose. Because of severe injection-site reactions, all high-dose (200 mg/kg/day) males and females were euthanized early on Day 8 or 9. Body weights for high-dose males and females were approximately 10% lower than for control animals. In mid-dose animals hematology changes including increased WBC, absolute neutrophils, and monocytes may have been secondary to the injection-site reactions. Thymic atrophy which was demonstrated in a dose-dependent manner in all groups and much of the drug-related gross pathology and histopathology in the low- and mid-dose groups may have been related to stress secondary to the injection-site reactions. Bone marrow hypocellularity occurred in 2/3 high-dose females euthanized early. |

[a] The mean tedizolid plasma steady state $AUC_{0-24}$ associated with multiple doses of the clinical daily dose (200 mg/kg/day) has been determined to be 25.6 µg·h/mL.

## Safety Pharmacology

Table 24    Safety Pharmacology Studies of Tedizolid Phosphate[10]

| Study | System | Parameter | Dose (mg/kg) | Finding |
|-------|--------|-----------|--------------|---------|
| Neurological effect | Rat | General behavior | 0, 10, 30, 100, p.o. | No tedizolid phosphate-related change in any evaluated parameter. |
| | Mouse | Spontaneous locomotor activity | 0, 10, 30, 100, p.o. | Significantly reduced spontaneous locomotor activity 30 min after dosing with 30 and 100 mg/kg tedizolid phosphate. Compared to baseline, the mean locomotor activity at 30 and 100 mg/kg decreased 16.7 counts/5 min and 30.6 counts/5 min at 30 min after dosing, respectively, whereas activity decreased 0.2 counts/5 min in the vehicle control group and 25.6 counts/5 min in the positive control group receiving 10 mg/kg diazepam. |
| | | Hexobarbital-induced sleep[a] | 0, 10, 30, 100, p.o. | The high dose produced a significant increase in hexobarbital-induced sleep time (51.5 min) compared to vehicle control animals (41.8 min). The positive control, 6 mg/kg chlorpromazine significantly increased hexobarbital-induced sleep time to 72.6 min. |
| | | Strychnine-induced convulsions[b] | 0, 10, 30, 100, p.o. | None of the doses changed the clonic convulsion response or mortality compared to vehicle. |
| | | Analgesia[c] | 0, 10, 30, 100, p.o. | None of the doses affected the writhing response compared to the control treatment. |

[10]  FDA Datadase.  http://www.accessdata.fda.gov/drugsatfda_docs/nda/2014/205435Orig1s000PharmR.pdf (accessed Mar 2016).

*Continued*

| Study | System | Test | Dose (mg/kg) | Finding |
|---|---|---|---|---|
| Neurological effect | Mouse | Analgesia by hot plate | 0, 10, 30, 100, p.o. | None of the doses affected the licking response to hot-plate exposure compared to the control treatment. |
| | | Pentylenetetrazole-induced convulsions[d] | 0, 10, 30, 100, p.o. | Was not observed any changes of the clonic convulsion response or mortality rate compared to the vehicle control group. |
| | | Electric-shock induced convulsion | 0, 10, 30, 100, p.o. | No change of tonic convulsion response or mortality compared to vehicle. |
| | Mouse | Body temperature | 0, 10, 30, 100, p.o. | Produced a small but significant decrease in body temperature 60 to 120 min after dosing. |
| | Guinea pig ileum | Autonomic nervous system | 0.1, 1, 10 µM | Did not block the contractile responses at any of the tested concentrations. |
| Cardiovascular effect | Dog | Blood pressure, heart rate and ECG | 20, 60, 200 | None of the measured parameters was affected by any of the tedizolid phosphate dose. |
| | HEK cell | hERG channel tail currents | 1, 10 µM | No significant effect on hERG channel K$^+$ current amplitude compared to pretreatment valves. |
| | Rat heart | Cardiac function | 1, 10 µM | No effect on measured parameters in isolated perfused rat hearts. |
| Pulmonary function | Rat | Respiration rate and volume | 10, 30, 100 | Did not alter any of the parameters relative to the control group. |
| Renal effect | Rat | Renal function | 10, 30, 100 | 100 mg/kg produced significant reductions in urinary sodium and chloride concentrations of approximately 30% and 35%, respectively, compared to the vehicle control group. Urinary sodium and chloride were also reduced by approximately 20% and 32%, respectively, in the rats administered 30 mg/kg compared to the control group, but the changes were not statistically significant. Urine volume was increased but not significantly in the 30 and 100 mg/kg groups by approximately 76% and 73%, respectively, compared to the control group. |
| Gastroinestinal effect | Mouse | Gastrointestinal transport | 10, 30, 100 | Did not affect intestinal transport compared to the control group. |
| | Rat | Gastric secretion | 10, 30, 100 | The high-dose significantly reduced mean gastric volume by approximately 40% compared to control animals. Also mean total acidity was lowered in high-dose animals by approximately 48% compared to control animals but the reduction was not statistically significant. Stomach juice pH was not changed compared to the control group. |

[a] Administered single oral doses of tedizolid phosphate or vehicle followed 30 min later by intraperitoneal hexobarbital (70 mg/kg). [b] Treated intraperioneal stychine (1 mg/kg) to induce convulsions after 30 min post-dose of tedizolid phosphate. [c] Injected acetic acid to induce a writhing-pain response after single dose. [d] Using a single intraperitoneal dose of pentylenetetrazole (100 mg/kg) to induce clonic convulsions.

## Genotoxicity

Table 25  Genotoxicity Studies of Tedizolid Phosphate (TR-701) and Tedizolid (TR-700)[10]

| Assay | Specie/System | Metabolism | Dose | Finding |
|---|---|---|---|---|
| *In vitro* bacterial reverse mutation assay (Ames) | *S. typhimurium* TA98, TA100, TA1535, TA1537; *E. coli* WP2 uvrA | ±S9 | TR-701: 9.8-5000 µg/plate TR-700: 0.313-80 µg/plate | Negative. |
| *In vitro* mammalian cell chromosome abberation assay | CHL cell | ±S9 | TR-701: 19.5-625 µg/mL TR-700: 12.5-400 µg/mL | Negative. |
| *In vitro* mouse lymphoma cell mutation assay | L5178Y cell | ±S9 | TR-700: 1.75-224.6 µg/mL | Negative. |
| *In vivo* mammalian erythrocyte micronucleus test | Male and female ICR mouse | + | TR-701: 500-2000 mg/kg/day TR-700: 500-2000 mg/kg/day | Negative. |
| *In vivo* unscheduled DNA synthesis test | Male SD rat | + | TR-701: 600, 2000 mg/kg/day | Negative. |

[10] FDA Datadase.  http://www.accessdata.fda.gov/drugsatfda_docs/nda/2014/205435Orig1s000PharmR.pdf (accessed Mar 2016).

## Reproductive and Developmental Toxicity

Table 26   Reproductive and Developmental Toxicology Studies of Tedizolid Phosphate[10]

| Study | Species | Dose (mg/kg/day) | NOAEL | | | Finding |
|---|---|---|---|---|---|---|
| | | | Dose (mg/kg/day) | AUC (µg·h/mL) | Safety Margin[a] (× MRHD) | |
| Fertility and early embryonic development | SD rat | 0, 5, 15, 50 | Male: 50; Female: 15 | Male: 130; Female: 104 | Male: 5.08 Female: 4.06 | Parameters of reproductive performance including mating index, fertility index, copulation index (males only), mean estrus cycle length (females only) or mean pre-coital interval (female only) were minimally affected by daily oral doses of tedizolid ≤50 mg/kg/day for males or ≤15 mg/kg/day for females compared to the vehicle control group. Mean testicular sperm numbers, sperm production rate, sperm motility, and morphology for male rats administered 50 mg/kg/day were not significantly different compared to the control group values. In the high-dose male rats, epididymal sperm numbers and epididymal weights (significant only for the L. cauda epididymis) were reduced compared to the concurrent control values. However, because male fertility parameters were not significantly altered, these findings were not considered toxicologically significant. No drug-related gross pathology or histopathogy findings was noted for males or females. None of the intrauterine parameters was significantly altered in gravid female rats by ≤15 mg/kg/day compared to control values. |
| Embryo-fetal development | SD rat | 0, 2.5, 5, 15 | Maternal/Fetal: 2.5 | 30.2 | 1.18 | No drug-related maternal mortality or clinical signs was noted, but dose-related reductions in maternal food consumption and mean body weight gains were observed throughout the treatment period for all the doses. |
| | Mouse | 0, 1, 5, 25 | Maternal: 25 Fetal: 5 | Maternal: 95.7 Fetal: 17.6 | Male: 3.74 Female: 0.69 | Mean fetal weights for both genders were significantly reduced by 25 mg/kg/day. Not significantly increased numbers of malformations occurred in fetuses born to high-dose dams compared to control dams. |
| | Rabbit | 0, 1, 2,5, 5 | Maternal/Fetal: 1.0 | 1.09 | 0.04 | Drug-related maternal toxicity manifest as mortality, morbidity and/or abortions and dose-dependent weight loss accompanied by corresponding reductions in food intake. Mean fetal weights in the 2.5 and 5 mg/kg/day were 23.5% and 19.8% lower than control group. No drug-related developmental malformation or variations was noted. |
| Pre- and postnatal development | Rat | 0, 1.25, 2.5, 3.75 | 3.75 | 30.2 | 1.18 | At doses of ≤3.75 to pregnant dams did not produce clinical signs. Oral administration of tedizolid phosphate to pregnant $F_0$ rats resulted in tedizolid exposure to fetuses in utero and the presence of tedizolid in milk. Developmental landmarks in the $F_1$ generation were unaffected by $F_0$ maternal exposure to tedizolid phosphate at all dosage levels. No drug-related effect was noted in the $F_1$ or $F_2$ generation. |

[a] The mean tedizolid plasma steady state $AUC_{0-24}$ associated with multiple doses of the clinical daily dose (200 mg/kg/day) has been determined to be 25.6 µg·h/mL.

[10]   FDA Datadase.   http://www.accessdata.fda.gov/drugsatfda_docs/nda/2014/205435Orig1s000PharmR.pdf (accessed Mar 2016).

# Special Toxicology

Table 27    Special Toxicology Studies of Tedizolid Phosphate[10]

| Study | Species | Dose (mg/kg/day) | Finding |
|-------|---------|------------------|---------|
| Oral immunotoxicity study | SD rat | Male: 0, 10, 30, 100 <br> Female: 0, 3, 10, 30 | Total spleen cell counts were significantly reduced by 40% in high-dose males and nonsignificantly by 20% in high dose females. <br><br> High dose males had significantly decreased T cells (-17%), B cells (-25%) and double positive T cells (CD4$^+$/CD8$^+$; -40%) in spleen cell populations. Spleen T cells were reduced 13% in high dose females. <br><br> Mean IgG titers were significantly decreased in the mid- and high-dose males by 61% in both groups and non-significantly in the low-dose males (-43%). IgG titers were also significantly decreased in high dose females by 76%. |
| Acute perivascular, intramuscular and subcutaneous irritation study | Rabbit | 200 (PV$^a$, IM$^b$ or SC$^c$) | One day and four days after tedizolid phosphate administration in single doses by PV, IM and SC injections, slightly more severe signs of local irritation including hemorrhage, focal muscle degeneration with histocyte infiltration were observed compared to vehicle injections. |

[a] Administered by single bolus injection (0.3 mL) into the perivascular space around the marginal ear vein of the right ear and vehicle was injected into the left ear in the same manner of the same animals.    [b] Was administered by single IM injection (0.5 mL) at a site in the *M. vastus lateralis* muscle of the right leg of each animal, and vehicle was injected in the same manner in the *M. vastus laterailis* in the left leg of the same animals.    [c] Single SC injection (1.0 mL) at a shave site located to the right of the midline of the back of each animal and vehicle was injected in the same manner at a site to the left of the midline of the back of the same animals.    PV: Perivascular. IM: Intramuscular.    SC: Subcutaneous.

[10]  FDA Datadase.    http://www.accessdata.fda.gov/drugsatfda_docs/nda/2014/205435Orig1s000PharmR.pdf (accessed Mar 2016).

# CHAPTER

27

## Tofogliflozin Hydrate

# Tofogliflozin Hydrate

## (Deberza®)

Research code: CSG-452

## 1 General Information

❖ Tofogliflozin is a sodium-glucose cotransporter 2 (SGLT2) inhibitor, which was approved in Mar 2014 by PMDA of Japan.

❖ Tofogliflozin was discovered by Chugai, co-developed and co-marketed by Chugai, Sanofi and Kowa.

❖ Tofogliflozin is a selective inhibitor of SGLT2, which is the major transporter involved in the reabsorption of glucose in kidneys, thereby reducing blood glucose.

❖ Tofogliflozin is indicated for the treatment of type 2 diabetic mellitus.

❖ Available as tablet, with each containing 20 mg of tofogliflozin and the recommended dose is 20 mg once daily before or after breakfast.

❖ The sale of Deberza® was not available up to Mar 2016.

### Key Approvals around the World*

|  | Japan (PMDA) |
| --- | --- |
| First approval date | 03/24/2014 |
| Application or approval No. | 22600AMX00548 |
| Brand name | Deberza® |
| Indication | Type 2 diabetes mellitus |
| Authorisation holder | Chugai (Roche)/Kowa/Sanofi |

* Till Mar 2016, it had not been approved by FDA (US), EMA (EU) or CFDA (China).

### Active Ingredient

*Molecular formula*: $C_{22}H_{26}O_6 \cdot H_2O$
*Molecular weight*: 404.45
*CAS No.*: 903565-83-3 (Tofogliflozin)
1201913-82-7 (Tofogliflozin hydrate)
*Chemical name*: (1*S*,3'*R*,4'*S*,5'*S*,6'*R*)-6-[(4-ethylphenyl)methyl]-6'-(hydroxymethyl)-3',4',5',6'-tetrahydro-3*H*-spiro[2-benzofuran-1,2'-pyran]-3',4',5'-triol monohydrate

*Parameters of Lipinski's "Rule of 5"*

| MW[a] | $H_D$ | $H_A$ | FRB[b] | PSA[b] | cLogP[b] |
| --- | --- | --- | --- | --- | --- |
| 386.44 | 4 | 6 | 8 | 99.4Å² | 2.27 ± 0.70 |

[a] Molecular weight of tofogliflozin. [b] Calculated by ACD/Labs software V11.02.

### Drug Product*

*Dosage route*: Oral
*Strength*: 20 mg (Tofogliflozin)
*Dosage form*: Tablet
*Inactive ingredient*: Lactose hydrate, microcrystalline cellulose, croscarmellose sodium, hydrogenated oil, magnesium stearate, hypromellose, titanium oxide, macrogol 6000, talc and yellow ferric oxide.
*Recommended dose*: The recommended starting dose for adults is 20 mg once daily, taken before or after breakfast.

* Sourced from Japan PMDA drug label information

# 2 Key Patents Information

## Summary

❖ Deberza® (Tofogliflozin hydrate) was approved by PMDA of Japan on Mar 24, 2014.

❖ Tofogliflozin was originally discovered by Chugai, co-developed and co-marketed by Chugai, Sanofi and Kowa.

❖ The compound patent application was filed as PCT application by Chugai in 2006.

❖ The compound patent will expire in 2026 foremost, which has been granted in Japan, the United States, and China successively.

Table 1    Tofogliflozin's Compound Patent Protection in Drug-Mainstream Country

| Country | Publication/Patent NO. | Application Date | Granted Date | Estimated Expiry Date |
|---------|------------------------|------------------|--------------|-----------------------|
| WO | WO2006080421A1 | 01/27/2006 | / | / |
| US | US7767651B2 | 01/27/2006 | 08/03/2010 | 01/31/2027[a] |
| EP | EP1852439A1 | 01/27/2006 | Examination | / |
| JP | JP4093587B2 | 01/27/2006 | 06/04/2008 | 01/27/2026 |
| CN | CN101111508B | 01/27/2006 | 03/30/2011 | 01/27/2026 |

[a] The term of this patent is extended by 369 days.

Table 2    Originator's International Patent Application List (Patent Family)

| Publication NO. | Title | Applicant/Assignee/Owner | Publication Date |
|-----------------|-------|--------------------------|------------------|
| Technical Subjects | Active Ingredient (Free Base)'s Formula or Structure and Preparation | | |
| WO2006080421A1 | Spiroketal derivative and use thereof as diabetic medicine | Chugai | 08/03/2006 |
| Technical Subjects | Salt, Crystal, Polymorphic, Solvate (Hydrate), Isomer, Derivative Etc. and Preparation | | |
| WO2009154276A1 | Crystal of spiroketal derivative, and process for production thereof | Chugai | 12/23/2009 |
| WO2011074675A1 | Process for preparation of spiroketal derivative | Chugai | 06/23/2011 |
| WO2012115249A1 | Crystal of spiroketal derivative | Chugai | 08/30/2012 |
| Technical Subjects | Formulation and Preparation | | |
| WO2015099139A1 | Solid preparation comprising tofogliflozin and method for producing same | Chugai | 07/02/2015 |
| Technical Subjects | Combination Including at Least Two Active Ingredients | | |
| WO2014056938A1 | Pyrrolidinone derivatives as GPR119 modulators for the treatment of diabetes, obesity, dyslipidemia and related disorders | Sanofi | 04/17/2014 |
| WO2015150563A1 | Substituted indanone compounds as GPR119 modulators for the treatment of diabetes, obesity, dyslipidemia and related disorders | Sanofi | 10/08/2015 |
| WO2015150564A1 | Substituted fused heterocycles as GPR119 modulators for the treatment of diabetes, obesity, dyslipidemia and related disorders | Sanofi | 10/08/2015 |
| WO2015150565A1 | Isoindolinone compounds as GPR119 modulators for the treatment of diabetes, obesity, dyslipidemia and related disorders | Sanofi | 10/08/2015 |

The data was updated until Jan 2016.

# 3 Chemistry

## Route 1: Original Discovery Route

*Synthetic Route*: The synthetic route was established with reference[1-3] to the methods of the key intermediates of antibiotic papulacandins, involving a complex intermediate **6**. Reduction of two carboxyl groups of commercially available 2-bromote-rephtalic acid **1** provided diol **2** in 92% yield, followed by protection of these two hydroxyl groups with triphenylmethyl, afforded **3** in merely 18% yield. **5** was obtained by adding the tetra benzyl-protected gluconolactone **4** to the aryl lithium prepared *in situ* by treatment of **3** with *sec*-butyllithium. Deprotection with concomitant spirocyclization of **5** using triethylsilane and boron trifluoride-diethyl etherate gave the benzyl alcohol **6** in 56% yield. Diphenylmethanol **9** was synthesized from the aldehyde **7**, which was obtained by Dess-Martin oxidation of **6** and exposed to Grignard reagent **8** to afford **9** in 80% yield. The efficient reduction furnished methylene dibenzyl derivative **10** in 83% yield, whose benzyl groups upon global removal *via* catalytic hydrogenation generated to fogliflozin in 99% yield and the overall yield of 2%.[1-3]

[1]  Kobayashi, T.; Sato, T.; Nishimoto, M. WO2006080421A1, **2006**.
[2]  Kobayashi, T.; Sato, T.; Nishimoto, M. US7767651B2, **2010**.
[3]  Ohtake, Y.; Sato, T.; Kobayashi, T., et al. *J. Med. Chem.* **2012**, *55*, 7828-7840.

## Route 2

*Synthetic Route*: Reduction of commercially available 2-bromoterephtalic acid **1** through the use of trimethoxyborane and borane-THF proceeded well in 89% yield to afford diol **2**. Subjection of this intermediate to 2-methoxypropene **3** under acidic conditions generated bis-acetonide **4**. The bromide **4** then underwent lithium-halogen exchange and was furtherly activated by magnesium bromide etherate prior to exposure to lactone **5**. This mixture was then worked up with aqueous ammonium chloride and upon treatment with *p*-TsOH in methanol resulted in spiroacetal **6** with 50% yield over three steps. Next, global protection of all alcohol functionalities within **6** was affected by reaction with methylchloroformate and DMAP in acetonitrile. Then, the benzyl carbonate within spiroacetal **7** was selectively connected *via* Suzuki coupling with 4-ethyl-phenylboronic acid **8** to afford methylene dibenzyl derivative **9** in 77% yield over two steps. Saponification of **9** followed by crystallization from acetone and water (1:6) furnished tofogliflozin hydrate in 75% yield and overall yield of 26%.[4-7]

## 4 Pharmacology

### Summary

Mechanism of Action

❖ As an inhibitor of SGLT2, tofogliflozin selectively inhibited human SGLT2 ($K_i = 2.9$ nM, $IC_{50} = 2.9$ nM, selectivity for SGLT1: 2069-fold) in kidneys, which resulted in decrease of renal glucose reabsorption, thereby increasing urinary glucose excretion (UGE) and lowering plasma glucose in type 2 diabetes patients.

❖ The metabolites had pharmacological profiles similar to tofogliflozin on inhibiting SGLT2 with less potent (M6, $IC_{50} = 4.6$ nM; M4, $IC_{50} = 4.9$ nM; M5, $IC_{50} = 16$ nM).

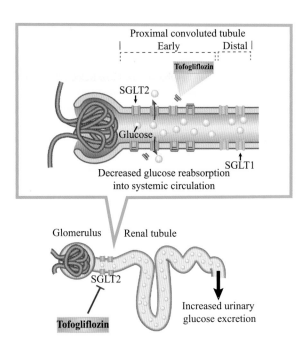

[4] Murakata, M.; Ikeda, T.; Kawase, A., et al. WO2011074675A1, **2011**.
[5] Murakata, M.; Ikeda, T.; Kawase, A., et al. CN102656177A, **2012**.
[6] Murakata, M.; Ikeda, T.; Kimura, N., et al. WO2009154276A1, **2009**.
[7] Murakata, M.; Ikeda, T.; Kimura, N., et al. US8569520B2, **2013**.

❖ Tofogliflozin showed no binding inhibition activity at 10 µM in a panel of receptors or ion channels, except SGLT2 and the secondary hydroxide epimer 2 (64%).[8]

*In Vivo* Efficacy

❖ Increased urinary glucose excretion (UGE):
  - *db/db* diabetic mouse: MED = 0.005%.
  - ZDF diabetic rat: MED = 3 mg/kg.
  - DIO non-diabetic rat: Increased UGE at 0.05%.
  - SD non-diabetic rat: MED = 1 mg/kg for $AUC_{0-6}$.
❖ Decreased blood glucose concentration and blood glucose AUC:
  - *db/db* diabetic mouse:
    ◆ Dose-dependently reduced the level and $AUC_{0-12}$ of blood glucose at ≥0.1 mg/kg.
    ◆ In OGTT: Dose-dependently reduced glucose concentration and blood glucose $AUC_{0-4}$ at ≥3 mg/kg.
  - ZDF diabetic rat: Dose-dependently reduced the level and $AUC_{0-12}$ of blood glucose at ≥0.1 mg/kg.
  - Wistar non-diabetic rat: No significant difference at 24 h.
  - GK non-fatty diabetic rat: Significantly reduced glucose concentration and blood glucose $AUC_{0-4}$ at ≥1 mg/kg.
  - KKAy diabetic with obesity mouse: Decreased plasma glucose level at 0.015% in diets.
❖ Increased insulin levels at 3 mg/kg in *db/db* diabetic mouse.
❖ Attenuated body weight gain: At 0.05% in diets in DIO non-diabetic rat and at 0.015% in KKAy mouse.

## Mechanism of Action

Table 3    *In Vitro* Binding Affinity and Inhibition of Tofogliflozin on SGLT2[8-11]

| System | Compound | $K_i$ (nM) | | | $IC_{50}$ (nM) | | |
|---|---|---|---|---|---|---|---|
| | | SGLT2 | SGLT1 | Fold[a] | SGLT2 | SGLT1 | Fold[a] |
| Human recombinant protein | Tofogliflozin | 2.9 | 6000 | 2069 | NA | NA | NA |
| | Phlorizin | 14 | 150 | 11 | NA | NA | NA |
| Mouse recombinant protein | Tofogliflozin | 6.4 | 1200 | 188 | 5.0 | 1800 | 360 |
| | Phlorizin | 14 | 270 | 19 | 17 | 310 | 19 |
| Monkey recombinant protein | Tofogliflozin | NA | NA | NA | 8.9 | 8875 | 997 |
| | Phlorizin | NA | NA | NA | 35.8 | 309 | 8.6 |
| Rat recombinant protein[b] | Tofogliflozin | 18 | 30000 | 1700 | 14.5 | 8200 | 566 |
| | Phlorizin | 250 | 67 | 0.3 | 48.2 | 970 | 20 |

[a] Fold: Selectivity of SGLT1/SGLT2.    [b] $K_i$: *In vivo* parameter.

Table 4    *In Vitro* Selectivity of Tofogliflozin on Human SGLT2 and Other Targets[9]

| Inhibitor | $IC_{50}$ (nM) | SGLT2 Selectivity (Fold) | | | | | | |
|---|---|---|---|---|---|---|---|---|
| | hSGLT2 | hSGLT2 | hSGLT1 | hSGLT3 | hSGLT4 | hSGLT5 | hSGLT6 | hSMIT1 |
| Tofogliflozin | 2.9 ± 0.7 | 1 | 2900 | 19000 | 1500 | 540 | 6200 | 28000 |
| Dapagliflozin | 1.3 ± 0.2 | 1 | 610 | 190000 | 3000 | 210 | 1300 | 22000 |
| Canagliflozin | 6.7 ± 2.9 | 1 | 290 | 52000 | 2800 | 180 | 200 | 5600 |
| Ipragliflozin | 2.8 ± 0.5 | 1 | 860 | 7700 | 4500 | 87 | 3500 | 21000 |
| Empagliflozin | 3.6 ± 1.6 | 1 | 1100 | 62000 | 2200 | 110 | 1100 | 8300 |
| Luseogliflozin | 3.1 ± 0.1 | 1 | 1600 | 8100 | 9800 | 280 | 220 | 7800 |
| Phlorizin | 16.4 ± 5.2 | 1 | 11 | 1300 | 490 | 36 | 1000 | 25000 |

The inhibitory activities of tofogliflozin and other SGLT inhibitors against the seven human SGLTs (hSGLT1, hSGLT2, hSGLT3, hSGLT4, hSGLT5, hSGLT6 and hSMIT1) were compared in SGLT-overexpressing cells (CHO, HEK293 or COS-7) by measuring sodium-dependent sugar (AMG, fructose or MI) uptake.

[8]   Japan Pharmaceuticals and Medical Devices Agency (PMDA) Database.    http://www.pmda.go.jp/drugs/2014/P201400036/index.html (accessed Mar 2016).
[9]   Suzuki, M.; Honda, K.; Fukazawa, M., et al. *J. Pharmacol. Exp. Ther.* **2012**, *341*, 692-701.
[10]  Yamaguchi, K.; Kato, M.; Suzuki, M., et al. *J. Pharmacol. Exp. Ther.* **2013**, *345*, 52-61.
[11]  Nagata, T.; Suzuki, M.; Fukazawa, M., et al. *Am. J. Physiol. Renal Physiol.* **2014**, *306*, F1520-1533.

Table 5  *In Vitro* Inhibition of Tofogliflozin and Its Major Metabolites on Human Recombinant SGLT2[8]

| Compound | | $IC_{50}$ (nM) | | $IC_{50}$ Ratio to Tofogliflozin | |
|---|---|---|---|---|---|
| | | hSGLT2 | hSGLT1 | hSGLT2 | hSGLT1 |
| Tofogliflozin | | 3.9 | 13000 | 1 | 1 |
| Phlorizin | | 15 | 200 | 3.7 | 0.016 |
| Metabolites of tofogliflozin | CH5086516 | 4.6 | 6600 | 1.2 | 0.51 |
| | CH5098291 | 16 | 44000 | 4.1 | 3.4 |
| | CH5106786 | 15 | 42000 | 3.8 | 3.3 |
| | CH5106787 | 14 | 45000 | 3.5 | 3.5 |
| | CH5108987 | 4.9 | 17000 | 1.3 | 1.3 |
| | CH5234447 | 2700 | >200000 | 700 | >15 |

CH5086516 (M6): Dehydrogenation body.　CH5098291 (M5): Ketone body.　CH5106786: Secondary hydroxylated epimer 1.　CH5106787: Secondary hydroxylated epimer 2.　CH5108987 (M4): Primary hydroxylated.　CH5234447 (M1): Carboxylate form.

## *In Vivo* Efficacy

Table 6  *In Vivo* Effects of Tofogliflozin in Non-clinical Pharmacology Studies[8, 9, 12-15]

| Study | System | | Dose (p.o.) | Duration (Weeks) | Effect | |
|---|---|---|---|---|---|---|
| | Animal | Type | | | MED (mg/kg) | Finding |
| Urinary glucose excretion (UGE) | *db/db* mouse | Diabetic | 0.005%, 0.015%, 0.045% in diets | 8 | 0.005% | Dose-dependently increased UGE. |
| | ZDF rat | Diabetic | 0.1, 0.3, 1, 3, 10 mg/kg | Single dose | 3 | Significantly increased UGE at 3 and 10 mg/kg in a dose-dependent manner. |
| | DIO rat | Obesity | 0.05%[a] in diets | 9 | 0.05% | Increased UGE. |
| | SD rat | Normal | 1, 3, 10 mg/kg | 1 (0-6 h) 3 (6-12 h) 10 (12-24 h) | Significantly increased UGE (1: 0-6 h; 3: 0-12 h; 10: 0-24 h post-dose) in a dose dependent manner. |
| Blood glucose | *db/db* mouse | Diabetic | 0.005%, 0.015%, 0.045% in diets | 8 | 0.005% | Reduced blood glucose levels at 0.005% and 0.015%, while no improvement at 0.045%. |
| | | | 0.1, 0.3, 1, 3, 10 mg/kg | Single dose | 0.1 | Dose-dependently reduced blood glucose level and blood glucose $AUC_{0-12}$. |
| | | Diabetic | 0.1, 0.3, 1, 3, 10 mg/kg | QD × 4 | 3 | Dose-dependently reduced blood glucose levels and $AUC_{0-4}$ at ≥3 mg/kg following OGTT 4 days after final treatment. Significantly decreased glycated hemoglobin level at 0.3 mg/kg after 4 weeks treatment. |
| | ZDF rat | Diabetic | 0.1, 0.3, 1, 3, 10 mg/kg | Single dose | 0.1 | Dose-dependently reduced blood glucose level and $AUC_{0-12}$. |
| | Wistar rat | Normal | 0.1, 0.3, 1, 3, 10 mg/kg | Single dose | NA | No significant difference in blood glucose changed. |
| | GK rat | Non-fatty diabetic | 1, 3, 10 mg/kg. | Single dose | 1 | Significantly reduced the area under the curve of blood glucose level $AUC_{0-4}$ at ≥1 mg/kg after feed. |
| | KKAy mouse | Diabetic with obesity | CE-2 or CE-2/TOFO (0.015%) | 3 or 5 | 0.015% | Decreased plasma glucose level. |

[8]  PMDA Database.　http://www.pmda.go.jp/drugs/2014/P201400036/index.html (accessed Mar 2016).
[9]  Suzuki, M.; Honda, K.; Fukazawa, M., et al. *J. Pharmacol. Exp. Ther.* **2012**, *341*, 692-701.
[12]  Pafili, K.; Papanas, N. *Expert Opin. Pharmacother.* **2014**, *15*, 1197-1201.
[13]  Ohtake, Y.; Sato, T.; Kobayashi, T., et al. *J. Med. Chem.* **2012**, *55*, 7828-7840.
[14]  Suzuki, M.; Takeda, M.; Kito, A., et al. *Nutr. Diabetes.* **2014**, *4*, e125.
[15]  Nagata, T.; Fukuzawa, T.; Takeda, M., et al. *Br. J. Pharmacol.* **2013**, *170*, 519-531.

*Continued*

| Study | System | | Administration | | | Effect |
| | Animal | Type | Dose (p.o.) | Duration (Weeks) | MED (mg/kg) | Finding |
|---|---|---|---|---|---|---|
| Insulin secretion | *db/db* mouse | Diabetic | 0.1, 0.3, 1, 3, 10 mg/kg/day | QD × 4 | 3 | Significantly increased insulin levels at ≥3 mg/kg. |
| Body weight gain | DIO rat | Obesity | 0.05%[a] | 9 | 0.05% | Body weight gain attenuated. |
| | KKAy mouse | Diabetic | CE-2 or CE-2/TOFO (0.015%) | 3 or 5 | NA | Body weight gain decreased. |

[a] The normal diet (ND) and HFD groups were fed for 13 weeks. The TOFO group was fed HFD for 4 weeks and HFD/TOFO for additional 9 weeks. DIO: Diet-induced obese. KKAy mouse: A mouse model of diabetes with obesity. CE-2: Rodent diet (Clea Japan, Tokyo, Japan). CE-2/TOFO: CE-2 containing 0.015 or 0.0015% tofogliflozin. MED: Minimum effective dose.

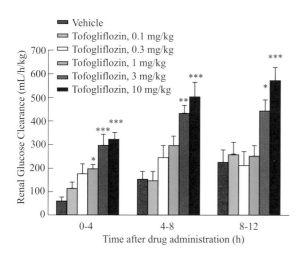

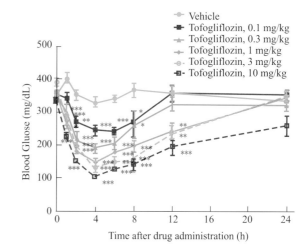

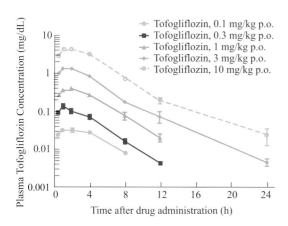

**Study:** Renal glucose clearance, blood glucose-lowering effects and plasma tofogliflozin concentration in ZDF diabetic rat.

**Animal:** Zucker diabetic fatty rat.

**Administration:** p.o., single dose, tofogliflozin: 0.1, 0.3, 1, 3 or 10 mg/kg, vehicle: 0.5% CMC, 5 mL/kg.

**Test:** Urine glucose, plasma tofogliflozin concentration and blood glucose before administration (0 h) and at 1, 2, 4, 6, 8, 10, 12, and 24 h after administration.

**Result:** Tofogliflozin dose-dependently increased renal glucose clearance, and significantly increased in renal glucose clearance in the period of 8 to 12 h at 3 and 10 mg/kg. Tofogliflozin reduced blood glucose levels transiently from 1 to 12 h after administration in a dose-dependent manner.

Figure A   Effects of Single Oral Administration on Renal Glucose Clearance, Blood Glucose Level and Plasma Tofogliflozin Concentration in ZDF Rat[9]

[9]  Suzuki, M.; Honda, K.; Fukazawa, M., et al. *J. Pharmacol. Exp. Ther.* **2012**, *341*, 692-701.

# 5 ADME & Drug-Drug Interaction

## Summary

### Absorption of Tofogliflozin

❖ Had high oral bioavailability in rats (75%), monkeys (58.6%) and humans (97.5%).

❖ Was absorbed rapidly ($T_{max}$ = 0.75-1.92 h) in rats, monkeys and humans.

❖ Showed a half-life of 5.02 h in monkeys, longer than that in humans (4.65 h) and rats (1.15 h), after intravenous administrations.

❖ Had moderate clearance in rats (19.4 mL/kg/min) and humans (9.96 L/h), but low in monkeys (3.65 mL/kg/min), in contrast to liver blood flow, after intravenous administrations.

❖ Exhibited an extensive tissue distribution in rats, monkeys and humans, with apparent volumes of distribution at 1.15, 0.919 L/kg and 50.6 L, respectively, after intravenous administrations.

### Distribution of Tofogliflozin

❖ Exhibited moderate plasma protein binding in mice (77.3%-78.2%), rats (83.0%-83.8%), monkeys (76.2%-76.9%) and humans (82.3%-82.6%).

❖ Had a blood cell association of 24.8%-29.1% in humans.

❖ SD and Long-Evans male rats after single oral administration:
  • The drug was rapidly and well distributed into most tissues including the central nervous system *via* going through the blood-brain barrier.
  • Relatively higher concentration levels were observed in liver, kidneys, stomach, small intestine and adrenal gland. The lowest concentration level was observed in cerebrum.
  • The radioactivity elimination was completed at 168 h post-dose.

### Metabolite of Tofogliflozin

❖ The major metabolites were M2, M3 (CH5098293, hydroxide) and M5 (CH5098291, ketone) in rat plasma. The parent drug and the two major metabolites accounted for 80%-100% of the total radioactivity in rat plasma, kidneys, liver, urine and feces.

❖ The major metabolite in human plasma was M1 (CH5234447, carboxylic metabolite).

❖ CYP2C18, 4A11 and 4F3B were found to be primarily responsible for the first hydroxylated metabolite (M4). CYP2C18, 3A4 and 3A5 were responsible for secondary hydroxylated metabolite (M2, M3) and ADH for the carboxylic metabolite (M1).

### Excretion of Tofogliflozin

❖ Was predominantly excreted in urine in humans, with M1 as the most significant component in human urine.

❖ Urinary and feces excretion were 44.6% and 52.7%, respectively, and the total excretion was 97.4% after administration at 168 h in rats.

❖ Biliary excretion generally accounted for 28.2% of the balance of drug equivalents in monkeys.

### Drug-Drug Interaction

❖ Tofogliflozin didn't inhibit major human CYP450 enzymes at the expected human dose. The carboxylic metabolite showed the limited potential to inhibit CYP2C19 ($IC_{50}$ = 27.1 μM). Tofogliflozin didn't induce CYP450 enzymes (CYP1A2, CYP3A4 or CYP2B6).

❖ Tofogliflozin was a substrate of P-gp but not the inhibitor of it. M1 was not the substrate or inhibitor of P-gp.

❖ Tofogliflozin was not a substrate of transporters OCT2, OAT1, OAT3, OATP1B1 or OATP1B3.

❖ Tofogliflozin and M1 were not inhibitors of OCT2, OAT1 or OAT1B1.

# Absorption

Table 7  *In Vivo* Pharmacokinetic Parameters of Tofogliflozin in Different Species after Single Intravenous and Oral Dose of Tofogliflozin[8]

| Species | Route | Dose (mg/kg) | $C_{max}$ (ng/mL) | $T_{max}$ (h) | $AUC_{inf}$ (ng·h/mL) | $T_{1/2}$ (h) | Cl (mL/kg/min) | $V_{ss}$ (L/kg) | F (%) |
|---|---|---|---|---|---|---|---|---|---|
| Wistar rat (male) | i.v. | 1 | 1060 ± 99.7 | 0.083[a] | 869 ± 125 | 1.15 ± 0.06 | 19.4 ± 2.6 | 1.15 ± 0.06 | - |
| | p.o. | 1 | 221 ± 49 | 1 ± 0 | 807 ± 445 | 2.56 ± 0.64 | - | - | 75.0 ± 32.3[b] |
| Cynomolgus monkey (male) | i.v. | 1 | 2170 ± 507 | 0.083[a] | 4690 ± 920 | 5.02 ± 0.87 | 3.65 ± 0.68 | 0.919 ± 0.201 | - |
| | p.o. | 1 | 550 ± 94 | 1 ± 0 | 2750 ± 230 | 10.5 ± 4.4 | - | - | 58.6 ± 12.5 |

The vehicle for p.o. administration was 20% PEG400 in saline and the vehicle for i.v. administration was 0.2 w/v% HCO-60 solution containing 0.5 w/v% CMC.
[a] First sampling time.   [b] Calculated using $AUC_{0-7}$.

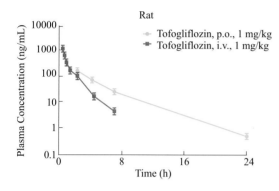
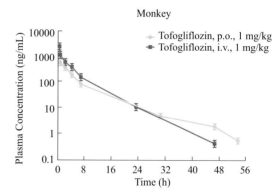

Figure B  *In Vivo* Plasma Concentration-Time Profiles of Tofogliflozin in Rats and Monkeys after Intravenous and Oral Dose of Tofogliflozin[8]

Table 8  *In Vivo* Pharmacokinetic Parameters of Tofogliflozin in Humans after Single Intravenous and Oral Dose of Tofogliflozin[8]

| Species | Route | Dose (mg) | $C_{max}$ (ng/mL) | $T_{max}$ (h) | $AUC_{inf}$ (ng·h/mL) | $T_{1/2}$ (h) | Cl or Cl/F (L/h) | $V_{ss}$ (L) | F (%) |
|---|---|---|---|---|---|---|---|---|---|
| Healthy human (male) | i.v. | 0.1 | 4.47 ± 0.753 | 0.250 ± 0.00 | 9.57 ± 1.26 | 4.65 ± 0.836 | 9.96 ± 1.25 | 50.6 ± 6.74 | - |
| | p.o. | 20 | 489 ± 78.8 | 0.75 | 1970 ± 496 | 6.33 ± 1.99 | 10.4 ± 2.31 | 92.6 ± 30.4 | 97.5 ± 12.3 |
| Japanese (male) | p.o. | 10 | 310 ± 63.7 | 1.00 ± 0.316 | 1330 ± 444 | 5.71 ± 0.682 | NA | NA | NA |
| | p.o. | 20 | 506 ± 61.4 | 1.00 ± 0.00 | 1900 ± 264 | 5.29 ± 0.508 | NA | NA | NA |
| | p.o. | 40 | 1210 ± 133 | 1.00 ± 0.00 | 5640 ± 1170 | 5.77 ± 0.600 | NA | NA | NA |
| | p.o. | 80 | 1930 ± 420 | 1.00 ± 0.316 | 8830 ± 1670 | 5.73 ± 0.701 | NA | NA | NA |
| | p.o. | 160 | 3710 ± 1240 | 1.00 ± 0.00 | 21800 ± 5580 | 5.63 ± 0.522 | NA | NA | NA |
| | p.o. | 320 | 6740 ± 598 | 1.25 ± 0.418 | 38100 ± 7680 | 5.53 ± 0.357 | NA | NA | NA |
| | p.o. | 640 | 11900 ± 1130 | 1.92 ± 0.665 | 99100 ± 26800 | 6.06 ± 0.666 | NA | NA | NA |

In human, subjects received 20 mg [$^{12}$C/$^{14}$C]tofogliflozin orally as a solution (100 μL ethanolic stock solution in 20 mL water) and a concomitant microdose of 0.1 mg [$^{13}$C]tofogliflozin (5 mL isotonic sodium chloride) intravenously 45 min after oral administration as an intravenous constant rate infusion over 15 min.

[8]  PMDA Database.   http://www.pmda.go.jp/drugs/2014/P201400036/index.html (accessed Mar 2016).

## Distribution

Table 9    *In Vitro* Plasma Protein Binding and Blood Partitioning of [$^{14}$C]Tofogliflozin in Several Species[8]

| Conc. (µg/mL) | Plasma Protein Binding (%) | | | | Blood Cells Association (%) | | | |
|---|---|---|---|---|---|---|---|---|
| | Mouse | Rat | Monkey | Human | Mouse | Rat | Monkey | Human |
| 0.1 | 78.1 ± 0.2 | 83.0 ± 0.3 | 76.9 ± 0.3 | 82.3 ± 0.1 | 55.7 ± 1.4 | 42.7 ± 1.2 | 30.4 ± 0.5 | 24.8 ± 2.8 |
| 1 | 78.2 ± 0.2 | 83.8 ± 0.1 | 76.8 ± 0.2 | 82.6 ± 0.2 | 55.8 ± 0.5 | 43.0 ± 2.9 | 31.2 ± 1.6 | 27.6 ± 4.7 |
| 10 | 77.3 ± 0.3 | 83.8 ± 0.2 | 76.2 ± 0.2 | 82.5 ± 0.1 | 55.0 ± 1.5 | 43.7 ± 1.0 | 32.7 ± 1.6 | 29.1 ± 2.6 |

Table 10    *In Vivo* Tissue Distribution of [$^{14}$C]Tofogliflozin in Male Rats after Single Oral Dose of [$^{14}$C]Tofogliflozin[8]

| Tissue | SD Rat Radioactivity Conc. (ng eq./g tissue)[a] | | | | | | | Long-Evans Rat Radioactivity Conc. (ng eq./g tissue) | | | | |
|---|---|---|---|---|---|---|---|---|---|---|---|---|
| | 30 min | 2 h | 8 h | 24 h | 48 h | 168 h | Tissue/Plasma AUC$_{0-168}$ Ratio | 30 min | 8 h | 24 h | 48 h | Tissue/Plasma AUC$_{0-48}$ Ratio |
| Adrenal gland | 1180 | 583 | 56 | 3 | ND | ND | 1.88 | 1312 | 65 | NS | NS | 1.76 |
| Cerebrum | 12 | 12 | 6 | 1 | ND | ND | 0.07 | 12 | BLQ | NS | NS | 0.01 |
| Eyeballs | 72 | 61 | 9 | 2 | 1 | ND | 0.24 | 65 | 15 | 6 | NS | 0.16 |
| Kidneys | 2516 | 1874 | 621 | 70 | 14 | 1 | 8.78 | 2634 | 572 | 47 | NS | 5.33 |
| Liver | 5809 | 2529 | 207 | 13 | 8 | 3 | 8.66 | 3717 | 221 | NS | NS | 5.11 |
| Small intestine | 2662 | 738 | 59 | 4 | 1 | ND | 2.88 | 505 | NS | NS | NS | 0.59 |
| Stomach | 2209 | 440 | 32 | 2 | 1 | ND | 2.01 | 753 | NS | NS | NS | 0.88 |

ND: Not detected.    NS: Not specified.    [a] 1 mg/kg/0.2 w/v% HCO-60 solution containing 1 v/v% ethanol and 0.5 w/v% CMC.

## Metabolism

Table 11    *In Vitro* Metabolism of [$^{14}$C]Tofogliflozin in Hepatocytes[8]

| Species | Conc. (µM) | Incubation Time (h) | % of Total Peak Area | | | | | | | | | | %Radioactivity | | | | |
|---|---|---|---|---|---|---|---|---|---|---|---|---|---|---|---|---|---|
| | | | HM1 | HM2 | HM3 | Hydroxylated Metabolites | M5 | HM4 | HM5 | HM6 | HM7 | Tofogliflozin | Tofogliflozin | M2, M3 | M4 | M5 | M1 |
| Mouse | 10 | 8 | ND | ND | ND | ND | ND | 6.8 | 0.5 | ND | ND | 91.5 | NA | NA | NA | NA | NA |
| Rat | 10 | 8 | ND | ND | ND | 11.4 | 26.5 | 2.1 | ND | ND | 2.6 | 55.2 | NA | NA | NA | NA | NA |
| Dog | 10 | 8 | 3.1 | ND | ND | 3.3 | 1.4 | ND | ND | 1.3 | ND | 90.7 | NA | NA | NA | NA | NA |
| Monkey | 10 | 8 | 2.6 | 1.7 | 1.6 | 3.7 | 6.3 | ND | 8.4 | 9.1 | ND | 65.1 | NA | NA | NA | NA | NA |
| Human | 10 | 8 | 4.8 | ND | ND | 0.7 | 4.8 | ND | ND | ND | ND | 89.3 | NA | NA | NA | NA | NA |
| Human | 1 | 5 | NA | NA | NA | NA | NA | NA | NA | NA | NA | NA | 62.7 | 0.6 | 1.1 | 3.7 | 30.9 |

M2, M3 (CH5098293): Secondary hydroxylated metabolite.    M4 (CH5108987): First hydroxylated metabolite.    M5 (CH5098291): Ketone body.    M1 (CH5234447): Carboxylate metabolite.    ND: Less than 0.5%.    HM4: Glucuronide of tofogliflozin.

[8]  PMDA Database.    http://www.pmda.go.jp/drugs/2014/P201400036/index.html (accessed Mar 2016).

Table 12  Metabolites in Plasma, Urine, Bile and Feces in Humans and Animal Species after Single Oral
Dose of [$^{14}$C]Tofogliflozin[8]

| Matrix | Species | Dose (mg/kg) | Time (h) | % of Radioactivity | | | | | | | | | |
|--------|---------|-------------|----------|--------|----------|-------|--------|------|-------|-----------|--------|------|------|
| | | | | Parent | M2, M3-GA | M1-GA | M4-glu | M1 | M5-GA | Parent-GA | M2, M3 | M5 | M4 |
| Plasma | Rat | 1 | 8 | 38.7 | NA | NA | NA | NA | NA | NA | 33.4 | 27.9 | NA |
| | Monkey | 10.8 | 0-24 | 64.4 | 10.9 | 1.3 | 2.0 | 2.6 | 2.7 | 8.5 | 3.2 | 1.0 | - |
| | Human | 20 | 0-24 | 42 | NA | 2.6 | NA | 52 | NA | NA | 5.2 | 3.2 | NA |
| Urine | Rat | 1 | 0-24 | 22.0 | NA | NA | NA | NA | NA | NA | 24.9 | 42.9 | NA |
| | Monkey | 10.8 | 0-48 | 33.3 | 11.1 | 2.8 | 3.4 | 6.6 | 2.7 | 9.3 | 18.0 | 5.0 | 3.6 |
| | Human | 20 | 0-48 | 16.1 | NA | 1.38 | NA | 38.4 | NA | NA | 4.36 | 5.77 | 0.43 |
| Bile | Monkey | 10 | 0-24 | 0.21 | NA | 6.28 | NA | 0.77 | 1.40 | 2.00 | NA | 0.37 | NA |
| Feces | Rat | 1 | 0-24 | 11.7 | NA | NA | NA | NA | NA | NA | 29.8 | 50.8 | NA |
| | Monkey | 10.8 | 0-168 | 22.3 | - | - | - | 52.1 | - | - | 15.0 | 9.3 | 1.4 |
| | Human | 20 | 0-72 | 0.87 | NA | NA | NA | 15.4 | NA | NA | 1.82 | 1.8 | 0.18 |

Vehicle: 0.2 w/v% HCO-60 solution containing 1 v/v% ethanol and 0.5 w/v% CMC.  M1: CH523447.  M2, M3: CH5098293.  M4: CH5108987.  M5: CH5098291.

Table 13  *In Vitro* Metabolism of Metabolite M4 (CH5108987) in Incubation with Human Liver S9, Microsomes and Cytosol under Different Conditions[8]

| Cofactor | ADH Inhibitor | Metabolic Rate (pmol/mg protein/h) | | |
|----------|---------------|------|------------|---------|
| | | S9 | Microsomes | Cytosol |
| Cofactor (-) | - | <4.8 | <4.8 | <4.8 |
| NADPH gen. | - | 7.5 | 6.7 | NT |
| NADP+ | - | NT | 27.0 | NT |
| NAD+ | - | 91.5 | 52.6 | 71.4 |
| NAD+ | 4-Methylpyrazole | NT | NT | 23.2 |

NADPH gen.: NADPH regeneration system.  NT: Not tested.  ADH: Alcohol dehydrogenase.

Table 14  *In Vitro* Metabolism of [$^{14}$C]Tofogliflozin in Recombinant CYP Enzymes[8]

| Test System | Incubation | Conc. (μM) | Analyte | Radioactivity (%) | | | | | | | | | | | | | |
|-------------|-----------|-----------|---------|------|------|------|------|------|------|------|------|------|------|------|------|------|------|
| | | | | 1A2 | 2A6 | 2B6 | 2C8 | 2C9 | 2C18 | 2C19 | 2D6 | 2E1 | 3A4 | 3A5 | 4A11 | 4F2 | 4F3B |
| rhCYP, NADPH | 1 h | 1 | Tofogliflozin | 98.6 | 98.8 | 99.1 | 98.5 | 98.9 | 74.4 | 98.7 | 97.8 | 99.1 | 84.8 | 85.8 | 97.6 | 99.1 | 97.7 |
| | | | M2, M3 | ND | ND | ND | 0.2 | ND | 8.2 | 0.2 | 1.0 | ND | 13.0 | 12.6 | ND | ND | ND |
| | | | M4 | ND | 0.3 | 0.3 | 0.3 | ND | 8.4 | ND | 0.3 | ND | ND | ND | 1.8 | ND | 1.6 |
| rhCYP, NADPH | 15 min | 50 | Tofogliflozin | 99.1 | 99.3 | ND | 99.3 | 99.1 | ND | 99.1 | 98.9 | 99.3 | 89.0 | 91.7 | ND | ND | ND |
| | | | Hydroxylated tofogliflozin | 0.1 | 0 | ND | 0 | 0.1 | ND | 0 | 0.5 | 0 | 7.6 | 6.9 | ND | ND | ND |

M2, M3 (CH5098293): Secondary hydroxylated metabolite.  M4 (CH5108987): First hydroxylated metabolite.

Table 15  *In Vitro* Inhibitory Effect of Chemicals on the Metabolism of [$^{14}$C]Tofogliflozin in Human Hepatocytes Incubations[8]

| CYP | Conc. (μM) | Incubate Time (h) | Inhibitor | Inhibition of Formation (%) | | | |
|-----|-----------|-------------------|-----------|--------|------|------|------|
| | | | | M2, M3 | M4 | M5 | M1 |
| CYP | 1 | 5 | 1-Aminobenzotriazole | 100 | 60 | 67.9 | 70.4 |
| 3A | 1 | 5 | Ketoconazole | 66.7 | 37.3 | 67.6 | 23.1 |
| 4A | 1 | 5 | 10-Undecynoic acid | 21.6 | 100 | 47.8 | 96.7 |

M1: CH523447.  M2, M3: CH5098293.  M4: CH5108987.  M5: CH5098291.

[8]  PMDA Database.   http://www.pmda.go.jp/drugs/2014/P201400036/index.html (Accessed Mar 2016).

Table 16    Inhibitory Effect of Each Inhibitor on the Metabolism of [$^{14}$C]Tofogliflozin for
Each CYP Isoform in Human Liver Microsomes[8]

| CYP | Conc. (μM) | Inhibitor | %Inhibition |
|---|---|---|---|
| 1A2 | 50 | Furafylline | 8.1 |
| 2A6 | 50 | 8-Methoxypsoralen | -17.6 |
| 2C9 | 50 | Sulfaphenazole | -5.9 |
| 2C19 | 50 | S-(+)-N-3-Benzylnirvanol | 18.9 |
| 2D6 | 50 | Quinidine | 13.5 |
| 2E1 | 50 | Diethyldithiocarbamate | 9.1 |
| 3A4 | 50 | Ketoconazole | 73.0 |

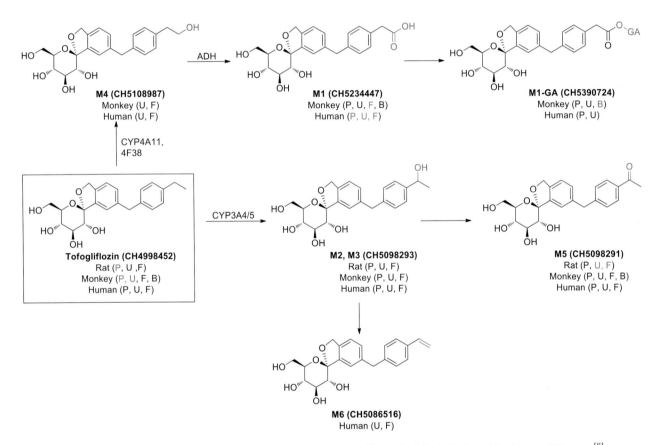

Figure C    Proposed Pathways for *In Vivo* Biotransformation of [$^{14}$C]Tofogliflozin in Rats, Monkeys and Humans[8]
The red labels represent the main components in the matrices.    F = Feces, P = Plasma, U = Urine, B = Bile and GA = Glucuronic acid.

[8]  PMDA Database.    http://www.pmda.go.jp/drugs/2014/P201400036/index.html (accessed Mar 2016).

# Excretion

Table 17    Excretion Profiles in Male Rats, Monkeys and Healthy Humans after Oral or Intravenous Dose of [$^{14}$C]Tofogliflozin[8, 15]

| Species | Dose (mg/kg) | Route | Time (h) | Urine (% of dose) | Feces (% of dose) | Bile (% of dose) | Other[a] (% of dose) | Recovery (% of dose) |
|---|---|---|---|---|---|---|---|---|
| SD rat | 1 | i.v.[b] | 0-168 | 54.9 ± 2.5 | NA | NA | NA | 54.9 ± 2.5 |
| SD rat | 1 | p.o.[c] | 0-168 | 44.6 ± 9.0 | 52.7 ± 7.5 | NA | NA | 97.4 ± 1.9 |
| Cynomolgus monkey | 1 | i.v.[b] | 0-168 | 42.9 ± 5.13 | 44.7 ± 4.11 | NA | 6.45 ± 2.77 | 94.1 ± 5.94 |
| Cynomolgus monkey | 10 | p.o.[c] | 0-168 | 33.0 ± 8.09 | 44.9 ± 7.67 | NA | 11.6 ± 7.74 | 89.7 ± 7.58 |
| Cynomolgus monkey | 10 | p.o.[c] | 0-24 | NA | NA | 28.2 | NA | 28.2 |
| Healthy human | 20 mg | p.o.[c] | 0-72 | 77 | 21.7 | NA | - | 98.7 |

[a] Others contained cage wash, cage debris and so on.    [b] The vehicle for i.v. administration was 20% PEG400 in solution.    [c] The vehicle for p.o. administration was 0.2 w/v% HCO-60 solution containing 1 v/v% ethanol and 0.5 w/v% CMC.

# Drug-Drug Interaction

Table 18    *In Vitro* Evaluation of Tofogliflozin and Metabolite M1 (CH5234447) as Inhibitors and Inductors of CYP Enzymes[8]

| Isoforms | Tofogliflozin and Metabolite as Inhibitors | | Tofogliflozin as a Inducer | | | |
|---|---|---|---|---|---|---|
| | IC$_{50}$ (µM) | | Isoform | Conc. (µM) | Fold Induction[a] | % of Positive Control[a] |
| | Tofogliflozin | M1 (CH5234447) | | | | |
| CYP1A2 | >50 | >50 | CYP1A2[b] | 0.5 | 1.07 | 0.07 |
| CYP2B6 | >50 | >50 | | 5 | 1.03 | 0.03 |
| CYP2C8 | >50 | >50 | | 50 | 1.13 | 0.07 |
| CYP2C9 | >50 | >50 | CYP3A4[b] | 0.5 | 1.17 | 2.23 |
| CYP2C19 | >50 | 27.1 ± 6.5 | | 5 | 1.03 | 2.57 |
| CYP2D6 | >50 | >50 | | 50 | 0.8 | -6.17 |
| CYP3A4/5 | >50 | >50 | CYP2B6[c] | 0.5, 5, 50 | 1.0 | NA |

[a] The value represented mean of 3 determinations.    [b] Analytical method: HPLC.    [c] Analytical method: RTqPCR.

Table 19    *In Vitro* Evaluation of Tofogliflozin and Metabolite as Substrates and Inhibitors of Transporters[8]

| Transporter | Tofogliflozin and Metabolite as Substrates | | | | | Tofogliflozin and Metabolite as Inhibitors | |
|---|---|---|---|---|---|---|---|
| | Inhibitor | Transport Ratios in Apical Direction | | | | IC$_{50}$ (µM) | |
| | | Tofogliflozin | | M1 | | | |
| | | LLC-PK1 | LMDR1 | LLC-PK1 | LMDR1 | Tofogliflozin | M1 |
| P-gp | No | 0.92 | 8.87 | 1.16 | 0.57 | >500 | No |
| | Elacridar (0.5 µM) | 0.91 | 1.07 | 1.22 | 0.72 | | |
| OCT2 | - | No | | NT | | No inhibitory effect | No inhibitory effect |
| OAT1 | - | No | | NT | | No inhibitory effect | No inhibitory effect |
| OATP1B1 | - | No | | NT | | >370[a] | >500[a] |
| OATP1B3 | - | No | | NT | | NT | NT |
| OAT3 | - | No | | NT | | NT | NT |

NT: Not tested.    [a] The substrates of the inhibition study were simvastatin (1 µM) and fluvastatin (1 µM).

[8]  PMDA Database.  http://www.pmda.go.jp/drugs/2014/P201400036/index.html (accessed Mar 2016).
[15]  Nagata, T.; Fukuzawa, T.; Takeda, M., et al. *Br. J. Pharmacol.* **2013**, *170*, 519-531.

# 6　Non-Clinical Toxicology

## Summary

Single-Dose Toxicity
- ❖ Acute toxicity by the oral route in rodents:
  - • Rat ALD: 1000 mg/kg.

Repeated-Dose Toxicity
- ❖ Sub- and chronic toxicity for up to 3 months in mice, 6 months in rats and 12 months in monkeys:
  - • By the longest studies employed, the average exposure at NOAELs was approximate 5-7 folds in mice, 2-4 folds in rats, and 36 folds in monkeys, respectively, compared to that of MRHD (20 mg/day).
  - • Most lethality derived from the pharmacology of tofogliflozin, i.e., promotion of glucose excretion and reduction of energy supply in turn.　Meanwhile, increases of AST, ALT, BUN and T-KB reflected enhancements of gluconeogenesis, protein catabolism and lipid metabolism, which was consistent with the pathological finding of elevated glycogen in liver cells.[8]
  - • As kidneys were the major pharmaceutical target organs, renal lesions were verified, e.g., mineral deposition in the renal cortex and medulla, and proliferation of renal tubular epithelium.　Other toxicities, as increases in trabecular (femur and sternum) and reductions of RBCs, were considered species-specific.

Safety Pharmacology
- ❖ Safety pharmacology was illustrated by core battery of studies on tofogliflozin, as well as M2, M3 (CH5098293, hydroxide) and M1 (CH5234447, carboxylic), which raised no concern on CNS, CVS and RS.

Genotoxicity
- ❖ Tofogliflozin, and its primary human metabolite M1, got least potential for genotoxicity, based on the negative results in the standard battery of *in vitro/in vivo* mutagenicity and clastogenicity studies.

Reproductive and Developmental Toxicity
- ❖ Fertility and early embryonic development in rats:
  - • NOAELs were 320 mg/kg/day for fertility and early embryonic development.
- ❖ Embryo-fetal development in rats and rabbits:
  - • Maternal (malnutrition, premature delivery and abortion) and fetal (slight developmental retardation and anomalies) effects occurred at HD (320 mg/kg/day for rats and 200 mg/kg/day for rabbits) in both species, which was considered to be hypoglycaemia-mediated.　NOAELs for embryo-fetal development and dams were 80 and 60 mg/kg/day in rats and rabbits, respectively, approximately 50-fold clinical exposure.
- ❖ Pre- and postnatal development in rats:
  - • Similar effects to EFD studies occurred in $F_0$ dams and $F_1$ fetus, but no effect emerged on $F_1$ physiological behavior and sexual maturity.　NOAELs were 200 and 80 mg/kg/day for maternal and offspring, respectively.
- ❖ Tofogliflozin distributed to fetal tissues in pregnant rats, including membrane, fetus, brain, liver, kidneys, and gastrointestinal tract, the ratio of concentration relative to plasma was below 5.48.[8]
- ❖ Milk excretion of tofogliflozin was also found in lactating rats and excretion ration was: milk/plasma = 0.28-1.84.[8]

Carcinogenicity
- ❖ For mice, NOAELs were 11 × and 38 × MRHD for males and females respectively.
- ❖ For rats, NOAELs were 37 × and 76 × MRHD for males and females respectively.
- ❖ No increase in incidence of neoplasm.

Special toxicity
- ❖ Tofogliflozin showed no absorption at 290-700 nm, which determined no concern about phototoxicity.[8]

## Single-Dose Toxicity

Table 20　Single-Dose Toxicity Studies of Tofogliflozin by Oral Administration[8]

| Species | Dose (mg/kg) | ALD | | Finding |
| --- | --- | --- | --- | --- |
| | | Dose (mg/kg) | AUC$_{0-24}$ (μg·h/mL) | |
| SD rat | 1000, 2000 | 1000 | Male, 632; Female, 888 | 1000 mg/kg: 1/5 male and 1/5 female died at 3 days post-dose. 2000 mg/kg: 4/5 males died, 1/5 female died at 2-5 days post-dose. |

Vehicle: 0.5% (w/v) CMC-Na containing 0.2% (w/v) PEG60 hydrogenated castor oil.

[8] PMDA Database.　http://www.pmda.go.jp/drugs/2014/P201400036/index.html (accessed Mar 2016).

## Repeated-Dose Toxicity

Table 21    Repeated-Dose Toxicity Studies of Tofoglilozin by Oral Administration[8]

| Species | Duration (Month) | Dose (mg/kg/day) | NOAEL | | | Finding |
|---|---|---|---|---|---|---|
| | | | Dose (mg/kg/day) | $AUC_{0-24}$ (μg·h/mL) | Safety Margin (× MRHD)[a] | |
| ICR mouse | 3 | 0, 20, 80, 320, 640 | 20 | Male: 14.9; Female: 9.94 | Male: 7; Female: 5 | ↑ Food consumption; ↑ AST, LDH and CK ; ↑ Kidney and liver weights, hypertrophy of renal tubular epithelial cells. |
| SD rat | 1 | 0, 10, 40, 160, 640/480[b] | 40 | Male: 31.7; Female: 53.0 | Male: 15; Female: 25 | Change in serum globulin, ↑ adrenal glands weight, anemia (↓ RBC, Ht and Hb). |
| | 6 | 0, 5, 40, 320 | 5 | Male: 4.84; Female: 9.13 | Male: 2; Female: 4 | ↑ Lipid metabolism, protein catabolism and gluconeogenesis ; Mild anemia (↓ RBC, Hb, MCHC), ↑ adrenal glands, liver and kidney weights, ↑ trabecular bone (femur, sternum). |
| Cynomolgus monkey | 1 | 30, 100, 300 | 100 | Male: 464; Female: 419 | Male: 217; Female: 196 | ↑ Glucose excretion at all doses, ↑ BUN and TG in HD males, ↑ liver and kidney weights at HD. |
| | 3 | 30, 100, 300/200[c] | 30 | Male: 82.5; Female: 74.1 | Male: 38; Female: 35 | ↓ Body weight in HD females, ↑ glucose excretion at all doses, ↓ RBC, lymphocyte, neutrophil, Ht and Hb in MD and HD males, ↑ liver weights at HD, ↑ kidney weights and ↓ thymus weights at MD and HD. |
| | 12 | 10, 30, 100 | 30 | Male: 76.7; Female: 76.4 | Male: 36; Female: 36 | ↑ Glucose excretion at all doses, significant ↑ TK-B at Week 8, ↑ renal weights yet not dose-proportional. Pathologically visible lesions limited to HD, including atrophy of lymph node, acinar (parotid gland, lower jaw gland, pancreas, lacrimal gland, mammary gland), mucosa (stomach, intestine), liver, epithelium (uterus, vagina); Dilation of the distal tubule, adrenal cortex hypertrophy, ↓ fat droplets, bone marrow hypoplasia. |

Vehicle: 0.5% (w/v) CMC-Na containing 0.2% (w/v) PEG60 hydrogenated castor oil.    [a] Calculated based on MRHD exposure estimates for 20 mg ($AUC_{0-24}$ = 2.14 μg·h/mL).    [b] The dose reduced to 480 from 640 mg/kg/day after 7-day administration in order to avoid death.    [c] The dose reduced to 200 from 300 mg/kg/day after 31-day administration in order to avoid death.

## Safety Pharmacology

Table 22    Overall Safety Pharmacological Evaluation of Tofogliflozin and Metabolites[8]

| Study | Test System | Dose | NOAEL | | | Finding |
|---|---|---|---|---|---|---|
| | | | Dose | $C_{max}$ (μg/mL) | Safety Margin[a] (× MRHD) | |
| Central nervous effect | SD Rat | 10, 80, 640 mg/kg | NA | NA | NA | 10, 80 mg/kg: ↑ Urinary excretion; 640 mg/kg ($C_{max}$ = 50.2 μg/mL, 100 × MRHD): ↑ Urinary excretion, ↓ body temperature, eyelid closure. |
| Cardiovascular effect | HEK293 cell expressing hERG channel | 10, 30, 100, 300, 1000 μM | 100 μM | - | 450 | $IC_{20}$ = 554 μM. |
| | | M1: 100, 300, 1000 μM | 1000 μM | - | 5700[b] | No inhibition. |
| | | M2, M3: 30, 100, 300, 1000 μM | 300 μM | - | 11500[c] | 8.7% inhibition at 1000 μM. |
| | Cynomolgus monkey | 10, 30, 100 mg/kg | 100 mg/kg | 22.8[d] | 45 | No effect on BP, HR, ECG or body temperature. |
| Respiratory effect | SD rat | 10, 80, 640 mg/kg | 640 mg/kg | 50.2[e] | 100 | No effect. |

Vehicle: 0.5% (w/v) CMC-Na containing 0.2 % (w/v) PEG60 hydrogenated castor oil.    M1 (CH5234447): Carboxylic tofogliflozin.    M2, M3 (CH5098293): Hydroxide tofogliflozin.    [a] Calculated based on MRHD exposure estimates for 20 mg QD ($C_{max}$ = 0.509 μg/mL).    [b] Derived from clinical trial CSG0101JP, $C_{max}$ (free form) = 0.175 μM.    [c] Derived from clinical trial BP22320 $C_{max}$ (free from) = 0.026 μM.    [d] Plasma concentration at 4 h post-dose.    [e] Derived from the first day TK on 1 month repeated dose toxicity in male rats.

[8]  PMDA Database.    http://www.pmda.go.jp/drugs/2014/P201400036/index.html (accessed Mar 2016).

## Genotoxicity

Table 23    Genotoxicity Studies of Tofogliflozin and Metabolite (M1)[8]

| Assay | Species/System | Test Article | Dose | Finding |
|---|---|---|---|---|
| *In vitro* Ames assay | *S. typhimurium* TA100, TA1535, TA98, TA1537; *E. coli* WP2*uvr*A | Tofogliflozin | 78.1-5000 μg/plate | Negative. |
| | | M1 | 313-5000 μg/plate | Negative. |
| *In vitro* chromosome aberration test | CHL cell | Tofogliflozin | -S9: 200-400 μg/mL +S9: 400-600 μg/mL | Negative. |
| | | M1 | 1.05-4.2 mg/mL | Negative. |
| *In vivo* micronucleus test | SD rat (male) | Tofogliflozin | 250, 500, 1000 mg/kg/day | Negative. |

Vehicle: DMSO for *in vitro* assays, saline for metabolite; 0.5% (w/v) CMC-Na containing 0.2% (w/v) PEG60 hydrogenated castor oil for *in vivo* tests.    M1: CH5234447.

## Reproductive and Developmental Toxicity

Table 24    Reproductive and Developmental Toxicity Studies of Tofogliflozin[8]

| Study | Species | Dose (mg/kg/day) | NOAEL | | |
|---|---|---|---|---|---|
| | | | Dose (mg/kg/day) | AUC$_{0-24}$ (μg·h/mL) | Safety Margin[a] (× MRHD) |
| Fertility and early embryonic development | SD rat | 20, 80, 320 | 320 | NA | NA |
| Embryo-fetal development | SD rat | 20, 80, 320 | 80 | 125 | 58 |
| | NZW rabbit | 20, 60, 200 | 60 | 111 | 52 |
| Pre- and postnatal development | SD rat | 20, 80, 200 | F$_0$: 200; F$_1$: 80 | NA | NA |

Vehicle: 0.5% (w/v) CMC-Na containing 0.2% (w/v) PEG60 hydrogenated castor oil.    [a] Calculated based on MRHD exposure estimates for 20 mg (AUC$_{0-24}$ = 2.14 μg·h/mL).

## Carcinogenicity

Table 25    Carcinogenic Toxicity Studies of Tofogliflozin[8]

| **104-Week Carcinogenic Study in ICR Mouse** | | | | | | |
|---|---|---|---|---|---|---|
| Dose (mg/kg/day) | | 0 (Water) | 0 (Vehicle) | 10 | 30/40[a] | 80/125[b] | NOAEL (mg/kg/day)[c] |
| Survival Rate (%) | Male | 53.3 | 55.0 | 48.3 | 40.0 | NA | 30:125 |
| | Female | 43.3 | 38.3 | 48.3 | 33.3 | 43.3 | (11:38 × MRHD) |
| **104-Week Carcinogenic Study in SD Rat** | | | | | | |
| Dose (mg/kg/day) | | 0 (Water) | 0 (Vehicle) | 15 | 35 | 100 | NOAEL (mg/kg/day)[d] |
| Survival Rate (%) | Male | 43.6 | 50.9 | 45.5 | 54.5 | 69.1 | 100 |
| | Female | 34.5 | 47.3 | 50.9 | 38.2 | 43.6 | (MRHD) |
| Finding | Increased incidence of tumors related to drug administration was not observed. | | | | | |

n = 55 for each dose and each gender in both mice and rat studies; Calculated based on MRHD exposure estimates for 20 mg (AUC$_{0-24}$ = 2.14 μg·h/mL).    [a] In male mice, after 39 weeks administration, administration was stopped, then resumed on week 41, the dose reduced to 30 mg/kg/day.    [b] In male mice 80 mg/kg/day, in female mice 125 mg/kg/day.    [c] The AUC$_{0-24}$ ratio of male and female was 23.9:82.    [d] The ratio of AUC$_{0-24}$ of male and female was 78.7:163.

[8]  PMDA Database.   http://www.pmda.go.jp/drugs/2014/P201400036/index.html (accessed Mar 2016).

# CHAPTER

## 28

## Umeclidinium Bromide

# Umeclidinium Bromide

(Incruse®/Incruse Ellipta®/Encruse®)

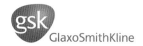

Research code: GSK-573719

## 1   General Information

❖ Umeclidinium bromide is an inhaled long-acting muscarinic antagonist (LAMA), which was first approved in Apr 2014 by EMA.

❖ Umeclidinium bromide was discovered and marketed by GlaxoSmithKline Plc.

❖ Umeclidinium bromide, an inhaled LAMA, competitively inhibits the binding of acetylcholine (ACh) with muscarinic receptors on airway smooth muscle, resulting in bronchodilation.

❖ Umeclidimium bromide is indicated for the treatment of patients with chronic obstructive pulmonary disease (COPD).

❖ Available as inhalation powder, with strength of 62.5 μg umeclidimium bromide, and the recommended dose is 62.5 μg once daily.

❖ The 2015 sale of Incruse Ellipta® was 21.4 million US$, referring to the financial reports of GlaxoSmithKline.

### Key Approvals around the World

|  | EU (EMA) | US (FDA) | Japan (PMDA) |
|---|---|---|---|
| First approval date | 04/28/2014 | 04/30/2014 | 03/26/2015 |
| Application or approval No. | EMA/H/C/002809 | 205382 | 22700AMX00633 22700AMX00634 |
| Brand name | Incruse® | Incruse Ellipta® | Encruse® |
| Indication | Chronic obstructive pulmonary disease (COPD) | | |
| Authorisation holder | GSK | GSK | GSK |

* Till Mar 2016, it had not been approved by CFDA (China).

## Active Ingredient

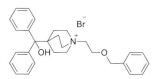

*Molecular formula*:   $C_{29}H_{34}NO_2 \cdot Br$
*Molecular weight*:   508.49
*CAS No.*:   869113-09-7 (Umeclidinium bromide)
*Chemical name*:   1-[2-(Benzyloxy)ethyl]-4-(hydroxydi-phenylmethyl)-1-azoniabicyclo[2.2.2]octane bromide

*No Parameters of Lipinski's "Rule of 5"*

## Drug Product*

*Dosage route*:   Oral inhalation
*Strength*:   55 μg (Umeclidinium)
     62.5 μg (Umeclidinium bromide)
*Dosage form*:   Powder
*Inactive ingredient*: Lactose monohydrate and magnesium stearate.
*Recommended dose*: The recommended starting dose is one inhalation once daily.

* Sourced from EMA drug label information

## 2   Key Patents Information

### Summary

❖ Incruse®/Ellipta® (Umeclidinium bromide) was initially approved by EMA on Apr 28, 2014.

❖ Umeclidinium was originally discovered by GSK, and its compound patent application was filed as PCT application by GSK in 2005.

❖ The compound patent will expire in 2025 foremost, which has been granted in the United States, Europe and Japan successively.

Table 1   Umeclidinium's Compound Patent Protection in Drug-Mainstream Country

| Country | Publication/Patent NO. | Application Date | Granted Date | Estimated Expiry Date |
|---------|------------------------|------------------|--------------|------------------------|
| WO | WO2005104745A2 | 04/27/2005 | / | / |
| US | US7488827B2 | 04/27/2005 | 02/10/2009 | 04/27/2025 |
| | US7498440B2 | 04/27/2005 | 03/03/2009 | 04/27/2025 |
| EP | EP1740177B1 | 04/27/2005 | 08/08/2012 | 04/27/2025 |
| JP | JP5014121B2 | 04/27/2005 | 08/29/2012 | 02/06/2028ᵃ |
| CN | CN102040602A | 04/27/2005 | Examination | / |

ᵃ The term of this patent is extended by 1015 days.

Table 2   Originator's International Patent Application List (Patent Family)

| Publication NO. | Title | Applicant/Assignee/Owner | Publication Date |
|-----------------|-------|--------------------------|------------------|
| **Technical Subjects** | **Active Ingredient (Free Base)'s Formula or Structure and Preparation** | | |
| WO2005104745A2 | Muscarinic acetylcholine receptor antagonists | GSK | 11/10/2005 |
| **Technical Subjects** | **Formulation and Preparation** | | |
| WO2013153146A1 | Aggregate particles | GSK | 10/17/2013 |
| WO2014027045A1 | Chemical process | GSK | 02/20/2014 |
| **Technical Subjects** | **Indication or Methods for Medical Needs** | | |
| WO2015015446A1 | Topical compositions for treatment of excessive sweating and methods of use thereof | GSK | 02/05/2015 |
| **Technical Subjects** | **Combination Including at Least Two Active Ingredients** | | |
| WO2011067212A1 | Combinations of a muscarinic receptor antagonist and a beta-2 adrenoreceptor agonist | GSK | 06/09/2011 |
| WO2012168160A1 | Dry powder inhaler compositions comprising umeclidinium | GSK | 12/13/2012 |
| WO2012168161A1 | Combination comprising umeclidinium and a corticosteroid | GSK | 12/13/2012 |
| WO2014095924A1 | Combination of umeclidinium, fluticasone propionate and salmeterol xinafoate for use in the treatment of inflammatory or respiratory tract diseases | GSK | 06/26/2014 |
| WO2015181262A1 | Fluticasone furoate in the treatment of COPD | GSK | 12/03/2015 |

The data was updated until Jan 2016.

# 3 Chemistry

## Route 1: Original Discovery Route

**Synthetic Route:** Commercially available ethyl isonipecotate **1** was alkylated with 2-chloroethanol **2** in the presence of DBU in hot toluene and then chlorinated with sulfurous dichloride to give ethyl 1-(2-chloroethyl)piperidine-4-carboxylate **3**. This material was then treated with KHMDS in toluene to affect a transannular substitution reaction resulting in the cyclized quinuclidine **4**. Excess of phenyllithium was added to ester **4** in dibutyl ether to give tertiary alcohol **5** in 50% yield over three steps. Amine **5** was finally alkylated with benzyl 2-bromoethyl ether **6** in refluxing IPA to afford the umeclidinium bromide in 87% yield and with 44% overall yield.[1-4]

# 4 Pharmacology

## Summary

### Mechanism of Action

❖ Umeclidinium bromide is a novel inhaled LAMA, which exerts bronchodilatory activity by competitively inhibiting the binding of ACh to muscarinic cholinergic receptors subtypes on airway smooth muscle.

❖ Umeclidinium bromide appeared to show competitive kinetics in both target binding and calcium mobilization. The compound competes with [$^3$H]-$N$-methyl-scopolamine binding for human M1-M5 mAChRs ($K_i$ = 0.05-0.16 nM).

❖ The major metabolite M33 was a functional inhibitor of mAChR-1 and mAChR-3 *in vitro*, about 10-fold less potent than umeclidinium bromide.

❖ Umeclidinium bromide showed no significant radio-ligand binding inhibition for a panel of 50 receptors, ion channels, enzymes and transporters, except κ-opioid receptors, σ-receptors, Ca$^{2+}$ channels, Na$^+$ channels and dopamine transporters ($K_i$ = 69-780 nM).

### In Vitro Efficacy

❖ Muscarinic antagonist activity in CHO cells containing mAChRs:
- Human M1 AChR: pA$_2$ = 9.6.
- Human M2 AChR: pA$_2$ = 10.1.
- Human M3 AChR: pA$_2$ = 10.6.

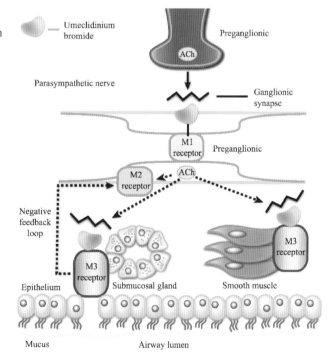

[1] Hossner, F.; Strachan, J. B. WO2014027045A1, **2014**.
[2] Laine, D. I.; McCleland, B.; Thomas, S., et al. *J. Med. Chem.* **2009**, *52*, 2493-2505.
[3] Laine, D. I.; Palovich, M. R.; McCleland, B. W., et al. WO2005104745A2, **2005**.
[4] Laine, D. I.; Palovich, M. R.; McCleland, B. W., et al. US20070185155A1, **2007**.

❖ Muscarinic antagonist reversibility:
- In CHO cells transfected with the human recombinant M3 mAChRs:
  ◆ The rightward shift of Ach concentration-response curves (CRC): washing < absence of washing.
- In human bronchus:
  ◆ On $T_{1/2}$ = 63-14 min (1-100 nM).
  ◆ Off $T_{1/2}$ = 119-299 min (1-100 nM).
  ◆ Induced rightward shift of the carbochol response curve: $EC_{50}$ = 11.5 µM and maximum contraction = 73.4%.

*In Vivo* Efficacy
❖ Methacholine-induced bronchoconstriction in mouse models:
- $ED_{50}$ = 0.02 µg/mouse, 5 h post instillation.
- Maximum inhibition: 80% at 0.05 µg/mouse, 30 min post instillation.
❖ Acetylcholine-induced bronchoconstriction in Dunkin-Hartley guinea pig models:
- Significant inhibition (74.4%) at 4 h after 0.25 µg/guinea pig.
- ≥50% inhibition at 2.5 (for >48 h) and 25 (for >5 days) µg/guinea pig.

# Mechanism of Action

Table 3    Receptor Binding Activity of Umeclidinium Bromide and Its Metabolites in CHO Cells[5-7]

| Compound | Test | mAChR Subtype | | | | |
|---|---|---|---|---|---|---|
| | | M1 | M2 | M3 | M4 | M5 |
| Umeclidinium bromide | $K_i$ (nM) | 0.16 ± 0.01 | 0.15 ± 0.01 | 0.06 ± 0.01 | 0.05 ± 0.01 | 0.13 ± 0.003 |
| | $K_d$ (nM) | NA | 0.16 | 0.03 | NA | NA |
| | $K_{on}$ ($M^{-1} \cdot min^{-1}$) | NA | $(2.22 ± 0.11) × 10^9$ | $(5.676 ± 0.45) × 10^8$ | NA | NA |
| | $K_{off}$ ($min^{-1}$) | NA | 0.074 ± 0.004 | 0.0089 ± 0.0012 | NA | NA |
| M33 | $IC_{50}$ (nM) | <10 | NA | <10 | NA | NA |
| M14 | $IC_{50}$ (nM) | 1202 | 1660 | 562 | NA | NA |

$K_i$: Inhibition constant.   CHO: Chinese hamster ovary.   M1-M5, muscarinic subtype 1-5.   $pK_i$: Corresponding negative log value.   Ligand binding assays with umeclidinium bromide and [$^3$H]-*N*-methyl scopolamine (0.5 nM) were performed using a scintillation proximity assay for M1, M2, and M3 mAChRs and a filtration assay for M4 and M5 mAChRs.   The presence of vehicle [1% dimethylsulfoxide (DMSO)], the concentration of umeclidinium bromide (0.01-300 nM).   The $K_i$ for umeclidinium bromide was calculated according to Cheng and Prusoff (1973), where $K_i = IC_{50}/([L]/K_d + 1)$, $K_d$ = 0.17, 0.28, 0.16, 0.07 and 0.2 nM for M1-M5 mAChRs, respectively, and [L] is the assay concentration of radioligand.

Table 4    The Off-Target Activity of Umeclidinium Bromide against Other Receptors and Ion Channels[5, 6]

| Test | κ-Opioid Receptor | σ-Receptor | $Ca^{2+}$ Channel | $Na^+$ Channel | Dopamine Transporter |
|---|---|---|---|---|---|
| $K_i$ (nM) | 69 | 220 | 330 | 170 | 780 |

Umeclidinium bromide (1 µM) inhibited radioligand binding by less than 50% at 41 of the 50 receptors, ion channels and transporters screened.   Those targets that were not muscarinic receptors were greater than 50% inhibition of radioligand binding, and a further concentration response study was performed to determine the $IC_{50}$ and $K_i$.

[5]   European Medicines Agency (EMA) Database.   http://www.ema.europa.eu/docs/en_GB/document_library/EPAR_-_Public_assessment_report/human/002809/WC500167431.pdf (accessed Mar 2016).
[6]   Japan Pharmaceuticals and Medical Devices Agency (PMDA) Database.   http://www.pmda.go.jp/drugs/2014/P201400076/index.html (accessed Mar 2016).
[7]   Michael S.; Luttmann M. A.; Foley J. J., et al. *J. Pharmacol. Exp. Ther.* **2013**, *345*, 260-270.

## *In Vitro* Efficacy

Table 5　Reversibility of Antagonism at M3 ACh Receptor in CHO Cell[5-8]

| Umeclidinium Bromide (nM) | Ach Effect, EC$_{50}$ (nM) | | Tiotropium (nM) | Ach Effect, EC$_{50}$ (nM) | |
|---|---|---|---|---|---|
| | 180 min Washout | No Washout | | 90 min Washout | No Washout |
| 0 | 0.22 | 0.24 | 0 | 0.27 | 0.26 |
| 3.3 | 0.94 | 26.9 | 3.3 | 2.93 | 110 |
| 33 | 1.98 | 243 | 10 | 3.87 | 1170 |
| 330 | 4.23 | 1486 | 33 | 4.37 | 2726 |

EC$_{50}$: 50% effective concentration, blockade of Ach-induced calcium mobilization.　M3 ACh receptors were pretreated with umeclidinium bromide or tiotropium for 30 min and then washed for 180 or 90 min before Ach challenge in CHO cells containing M3 mAChRs.

Table 6　Muscarinic Antagonism Activity and Reversibility of Umeclidinium Bromide[5-8]

| Drug | Muscarinic Antagonism (pA$_2$)[a] | | | Muscarinic Antagonist Reversibility Profile[b] | | | | | | | |
|---|---|---|---|---|---|---|---|---|---|---|---|
| | | | | On T$_{1/2}$ (min) | | | Off T$_{1/2}$ (min) | | | EC$_{50}$ (μM) | Maximum Contraction (%) |
| | hM1 | hM2 | hM3 | 1 nM | 10 nM | 100 nM | 1 nM | 10 nM | 100 nM | | |
| Umeclidinium bromide | 9.6 | 10.1 | 10.6 | 63 | 27 | 14 | 119 | 145 | 299 | 11.5 | 73.4 |
| Ipratropium bromide | NA | NA | NA | 29 | 10 | 4 | 20 | 29 | 86 | 0.3 | 99.2 |
| Tiotropium bromide | NA | NA | NA | 17 | 8 | 2 | 106 | 167 | 435 | 4.6 | 63.1 |

[a] Muscarinic antagonism activity in CHO cell containing human mAChR.　pA$_2$ = -log[I].　[b] Carbachol-induced contraction of isolated strips of human bronchus. Bronchial strips were isolated from human airway and suspended in static tissue baths.　Cumulative carbachol concentration-response curves were obtained in the presence and absence of umeclidinium bromide, besides ipratropium, tiotropium, and atropine were also tested as comparators.　Tiotropium had no effect at 0.1 nM, yet suppressed the maximal carbachol response by 68% and 66% at 1 and 10 nM, respectively.　Atropine (10 nM) induced a parallel-shift of the carbachol response, yielding a pK$_B$ of 9.6.　On T$_{1/2}$: Onset halftime.　Off T$_{1/2}$: Offset halftime.　EC$_{50}$: 50% effective concentration.

## *In Vivo* Efficacy

Table 7　*In Vivo* Effects of Umeclidinium Bromide in Animal Models[5-8]

| Animal Model | | | Dose (μg/instillation) | Route & Duration (Day) | Effect | |
|---|---|---|---|---|---|---|
| Study | Animal | Test | | | ED$_{50}$ (μg) | Finding |
| Methacholine-induced bronchoconstriction | Balb/c mouse | Bronchocon-striction | 0.005-5 | Intranasal, single dose | 0.02 (5 h) | Maximum inhibition: 80% at 30 min post-dose of 0.05 μg. |
| | | | 0.025 | Intranasal, QD × 5 | NA | Significant inhibition from Day 1 (35%) to Day 5 (60%). |
| Acetylcholine-induced bronchoconstriction[a] | Dunkin-Hartley guinea pig | Penh elicited | 0.25, 2.5, 25 | Intranasal, single dose | NA | Dose-dependent inhibition. ≥50% Inhibition for >48 h at 2.5 μg/guinea pig, and >5 days at 25 μg/guinea pig. |
| | | Airway tone and heart rate | 0.025, 0.25, 2.5 | Intranasal, single dose | NA | Significant inhibition (74.4%, $P$ <0.05) at 4 h after 0.25 μg/guinea pig. Dose-related decrease in heart rate after administration of ACh. |

[a] 4, 24, 48, 72, 96 and 120 h after drug or vehicle administration, guinea pigs were placed into a whole body plethysmograph box.　Animals were exposed to an aerosol of acetylcholine (ACh) produced by an ultrasonic nebulizer.　Collected values were retained and Penh (enhanced pause) was calculated.

[5]　EMA Database.　http://www.ema.europa.eu/docs/en_GB/document_library/EPAR_-_Public_assessment_report/human/002809/WC500167431.pdf (accessed Mar 2016).
[6]　PMDA Database.　http://www.pmda.go.jp/drugs/2014/P201400076/index.html (accessed Mar 2016).
[7]　Michael S.; Luttmann M. A.; Foley J. J., et al. *J. Pharmacol. Exp. Ther.* **2013**, *345*, 260-270.
[8]　U.S. Food and Drug Adiminstration (FDA) Database.　http://www.accessdata.fda.gov/drugsatfda_docs/nda/2014/205382Orig1s000ClinPharmR.pdf (accessed Mar 2016).

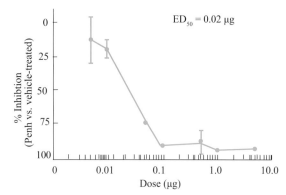

**Study:** Effects of umeclidinium bromide on methacholine-induced bronchocon-striction in Balb/c mouse.

**Animal:** Balb/c mouse.

**Administration:** Single dose intratracheally. Umeclidinium bromide: 0.005-5 µg/mouse; Vehicle control: 0.5% Tween 80.

**Test:** Bronchoconstriction (Standard plethysmograph, Penh) Penh = [(expiratory time/relaxation time)-1] × (peak expiratory flow/peak inspiratory flow).

**Results:** $ED_{50}$ was 0.02 µg/mouse at 4 h after instillation.

Figure A    Effects of Intratracheal Umeclidinium Bromide on Methacholine-induced Bronchoconstriction in Mice[6, 7]

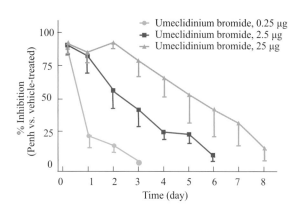

**Study:** Effects of intratracheal umeclidinium bromide on acetylcholine-induced bronchoconstriction in guinea pig.

**Animal:** Guinea pig (Dunkin-Hartley).

**Administration:** Single dose intratracheally. Umeclidinium bromide: 0.25, 2.5, 25 µg/guinea pig; Vehicle control: 0.5% Tween 80.

**Test:** Standard plethysmograph (Penh served as a surrogate measure of changes in airway tone). Penh = [(expiratory time/relaxation time)-1] × (peak expiratory flow/peak inspiratory flow).

**Results:** Umeclidinium bromide showed dose-dependently inhibition effect, ≥50% inhibition for >2 days at 0.25 µg/guinea pig and for >5 days at 2.5 µg/guinea pig.

Figure B    Effects of Intratracheal Umeclidinium Bromide on Acetylcholine-Induced Bronchoconstriction in Guinea Pigs[6, 7]

# 5   ADME & Drug-Drug Interaction

## Summary

### Absorption of Umeclidinium

❖ Exhibited a non-linear pharmacokinetics in humans following intravenous dosing. The increases in $C_{max}$ and AUC were not dose-proportional in the dose range of 20 to 65 µg umeclidinium.

❖ Had low inhaled bioavailability (12.8%) in humans.

❖ Was absorbed moderately ($T_{max}$ = 0.083 h) in humans after inhalation administration.

❖ Showed a half-life of 3.35 h in rats, much shorter than that in dogs (11.6 h), after infusion administrations.

❖ Had high clearance in humans (151 L/h), dogs (32.5 mL/min/kg) and rats (328 mL/min/kg), in contrast to liver blood flow, after intravenous administrations.

❖ Exhibited an extensive tissue distribution in humans, rats and dogs, with apparent volumes of distribution at 86.2 L, 14.6 and 4.67 L/kg, respectively, after intravenous administrations.

❖ Showed a low permeability in MDCK cell monolayer model.

### Distribution of Umeclidinium

❖ Exhibited moderate plasma protein binding in mice (86.7%-88.8%), rats (84.3%-86.9%), rabbits (74.8%-78.8%), dogs (77.2%-83.0%) and humans (87.1%-88.9%). Note that umeclidinium was mainly bound to AGP.

❖ Had a $C_b$:$C_p$ ratio of 0.541-0.560 in humans, suggesting rare penetration into red blood cells.

❖ Lister hooded-pigmented rats after single intravenous administration:

[6]  PMDA Database.   http://www.pmda.go.jp/drugs/2014/P201400076/index.html (accessed Mar 2016).
[7]  Michael S.; Luttmann M. A.; Foley J. J., et al. *J. Pharmacol. Exp. Ther.* **2013**, *345*, 260-270.

- Umeclidinium was rapidly and well distributed into most tissues, except for the central nervous system (CNS), with rare or no radioactivity in the brain.
- Relatively higher concentration levels were observed in kidneys, liver, pituitary, small intestine wall, thyroid and pancreas.
- The radioactivity could be detected in all of the high concentration tissues by 72 h post-dose.
- Some accumulations in the uveal tract and retina were detected.

## Metabolism of Umeclidinium

- ❖ Showed moderate stability in human liver microsomes and hepatocytes, but high stability in rat and dog hepatocytes.
- ❖ CYP2D6 was the major metabolizing enzyme in human liver microsomes, and CYP3A4 and CYP1A1 were playing minor roles.
- ❖ Overall, the parent drug represented the most abundant component in rat and dog plasma.
- ❖ The main routes of metabolism in humans were likely to be *via* O-dealkylation to M14 and hydroxylation to M33. Other routes were conjugation with glutathione and methylation and/or glucuronidation of the hydroxylated metabolites.
- ❖ All the metabolites in human were also observed in at least one of other species used for nonclinical toxicology assay.

## Excretion of Umeclidinium

- ❖ Was predominantly excreted in feces in humans and tested animals, with the parent drug as the most significant component in rat feces and M14 in dog feces.
- ❖ About 0.17% and 55.6% of [$^{14}$C]umeclidinium were recovered *via* biliary excretion in bile duct-cannulated (BDC) rats and dogs, respectively.

## Drug-Drug Interaction

- ❖ Umeclidinium had strong inhibition for CYP2D6 (IC$_{50}$ = 0.1 μM) and moderate inhibition for CYP3A4 (1.0 μM for diethoxyfluorescein, and 8.0 μM for 7-benzyloxyguinoline).
- ❖ Umeclidinium had no induction for any CYPs.
- ❖ Umeclidinium was a substrate of P-gp, but had no inhibition for P-gp.
- ❖ Umeclidinium was a subatrate of OCT1 and OCT2, but not for OCT3, OCTN1 or OCTN2, and had inhibition for OCT2 (IC$_{50}$ = 1.4 μM).

# Absorption

Table 8　*In Vivo* Pharmacokinetic Parameters of Umeclidinium in Rats and Dogs after Intravenous Infusion Dose of Umeclidinium Bromide[6]

| Species | Route | Dose (mg/kg) | Vehicle | $T_{max}$ (h) | $C_{max}$ (ng/mL) | $AUC_{inf}$ (ng·h/mL) | $T_{1/2}$ (h) | Cl (mL/min/kg) | $V_{ss}$ (L/kg) |
|---|---|---|---|---|---|---|---|---|---|
| Rat (male) | i.v. (1 h infusion) | 0.5 | Saline/solution | 0.33-0.67 | 30.3±1.56 | 25.2±1.59 | 3.35±0.998 | 328±22.5 | 14.6±6.59 |
| Dog (male) | i.v. (1 h infusion) | 1 | 20% aqueous cavitron and <1% DMSO/solution | 0.75-1.0 | 651±194 | 502±74 | 11.6±1.7 | 32.5±4.53 | 4.67±1.73 |

Table 9　*In Vivo* Pharmacokinetic Parameters of Umeclidinium in Humans after Intravenous and Oral Dose of Umeclidinium Bromide[6]

| Species | Route | Analyte | Dose (μg) | $T_{max}$ (h) | $C_{max}$ (ng/mL) | $AUC_{inf}$ (ng·h/mL) | Cl/F (L/h) | $V_{ss}$ (L) | F (%) |
|---|---|---|---|---|---|---|---|---|---|
| Healthy human (male) | i.v. | Umeclidinium | 65 | 0.53 | 0.906 | 0.268 | 151 | 86.2 | - |
| | i.v. | [$^{14}$C]Umeclidinium | 65 | 0.5 | 1.39 | 1.04 | 46.5 | 1801 | - |
| | p.o. | [$^{14}$C]Umeclidinium | 1000 | 4 | 0.07 | 0.796 | 988 | 66958 | 5.4 |
| | i.v. | Umeclidinium | 20 | 0.483 | 0.376 | 0.132 | 108 | 12.8 | - |
| | i.v | | 50 | 0.483 | 1.14 | 0.525 | 95.3 | 16.2 | - |
| | i.v. | | 65 | 0.483 | 1.55 | 0.543 | 90.9 | 14.5 | - |
| | i.h. | | 1000 | 0.083 | 1.66 | 1.33 | 752 | 2717 | 12.8 |

[6] PMDA Database. http://www.pmda.go.jp/drugs/2014/P201400076/index.html (accessed Mar 2016).

Table 10    *In Vitro* Permeability of Umeclidinium Bromide in MDCK II-MDR1 Cell Monolayer Model[6]

| Test Article | Rate A→B (nM/h/cm²) | Rate B→A (nM/h/cm²) | Efflux Ratio | P-gp Substrate | Recovery A→B (%) | Recovery B→A (%) | Papp (1 × 10⁻⁶ cm/s) | Permeability Class |
|---|---|---|---|---|---|---|---|---|
| [¹⁴C]Umeclidinium | 0.0010 ± 0.000 | 0.015 ± 0.0070 | 7-17 | Y | 88 ± 1.6 | 75 ± 3.0 | - | - |
| [¹⁴C]Umeclidinium + GF120918A | 0.0020 ± 0.0010 | 0.0020 ± 0.0010 | 0.8 | - | 89 ± 0.6 | 82 ± 4.9 | 0.24 | Low |
| [³H]Amprenavir | 0.0010 ± 0.000 | 0.32 ± 0.14 | 53 | Y | 87 ± 1.7 | 92 ± 1.1 | - | - |
| [³H]Amprenavir + GF120918A | 0.26 ± 0.017 | 0.30 ± 0.11 | 1.2 | - | 97 ± 1.0 | 100 ± 2.2 | 280 | High |

[¹⁴C]Umeclidinium concentration: 3 µM.    P-glycoprotein inhibitor: GF120918A (2 µM).    Positive control: [³H]amprenavir (3 µM).    Values were the mean ± SD of 3 monolayers.    A compound was classified as a P-gp substrate if the apical efflux ratio in the absence of inhibitor GF120918A was 2 and this efflux collapsed to about 1 in the presence of inhibitor.    Passive membrane permeabilities were classed as low (<10 nm/s), moderate (10 to 100 nm/s) or high (>100 nm/s).

## Distribution

Table 11    *In Vitro* Plasma Protein Binding of [¹⁴C]Umeclidinium and Metabolites in Several Species[6]

| Plasma Protein Binding | | | Isolated Human Protein Binding[c] | | Blood Cell Partition | | | |
|---|---|---|---|---|---|---|---|---|
| Species | Conc. (ng/mL) | %Bound | Protein | %Bound | Species | Conc. (ng/mL) | Cb:Cp[b] | Blood Cell Association (%) |
| Mouse (male)[a] | 5-200 | 86.7-88.8 | HSA | 67.2 | Mouse | 50-500 | 0.732-0.778 | 26.2-30.5 |
| Rat (male)[a] | 5-200 | 84.3-86.9 | | | Rat | 50-500 | 0.670-0.691 | 25.4-27.6 |
| Rabbit (female)[a] | 5-200 | 74.8-78.8 | AGP | 84.9 | Rabbit | 50-500 | 0.729-0.747 | 6.70-9.01 |
| Dog (male)[a] | 5-200 | 77.2-83.0 | | | Dog | 50-500 | 0.520-0.533 | 2.00-4.40 |
| Human (female)[a] | 2 | 88.9 | γ-globulin | 64.6 | Human | 50-500[c] | 0.541-0.560 | 6.35-7.62 |
| Human (male)[b] | 2-200 | 87.1-88.8 | | | | | | |

[a] Incubation of umeclidinium bromide salt with plasma at 37 °C for 8 h.    [b] Incubation of [¹⁴C]umeclidinium with blood at 37 °C for 30 min.    [c] Values were mean ± SD of 3 individuals.    Incubation of umeclidinium (1 ng/mL) in PBS solutions containing HSA (40 mg/mL), AGP (0.8 mg/mL) and γ-globulin (7 mg/mL) at 37 °C for 6 h.

Table 12    *In Vivo* Tissue Distribution of [¹⁴C]Umeclidinium in Rats (Lister Hooded-Pigmented) after Single Intravenous Dose of 1 mg/kg [¹⁴C]Umeclidinium Bromide[6]

| Tissues | Radioactivity (µg eq./mL or µg eq./g) | | | | | | Tissue/Blood AUC₀₋₈₄₀ Ratio |
|---|---|---|---|---|---|---|---|
| | 0.5 h | 1.5 h | 24 h | 72 h | 240 h | 840 h | |
| Blood | 0.348 | 0.050 | BLQ | BLQ | BLQ | BLQ | 1.0 |
| Kidney cortex | >ULQ | 4.37 | 1.18 | 0.551 | 0.122 | BLQ | >241 |
| Kidney medulla | >ULQ | 2.28 | 2.96 | 0.922 | 0.026 | 0.008 | >293 |
| Liver | 6.94 | 1.22 | 0.071 | 0.014 | BLQ | BLQ | 27.8 |
| Brain | 0.008 | BLQ | BLQ | BLQ | BLQ | BLQ | - |
| Pituitary | 3.83 | 1.78 | 0.914 | 0.532 | 0.282 | BLQ | 261 |
| Thyroid | 2.13 | 2.76 | 1.11 | 0.465 | 0.169 | BLQ | 19.2 |
| Salivary gland | 1.87 | 2.30 | 1.43 | 0.174 | 0.017 | BLQ | 123 |
| Preputial gland | 1.41 | 2.05 | 1.34 | 0.459 | 0.029 | BLQ | 13.6 |
| Pancreas | 2.07 | 2.90 | 2.12 | 0.726 | 0.019 | BLQ | 20.0 |
| Stomach wall | 1.89 | 1.69 | 1.56 | 0.290 | 0.040 | BLQ | 145 |
| Small intestine wall | 3.76 | 3.02 | 0.182 | 0.022 | 0.010 | BLQ | 60.0 |
| Large intestine wall | 1.46 | 1.45 | 1.81 | 0.146 | 0.023 | BLQ | 126 |
| Uveal tract/ retina | 0.653 | 0.757 | 0.289 | 0.586 | 0.499 | 0.371 | 455 |

Vehicle: 0.9% (w/v) aqueous sodium chloride.    Upper limit of quantification = 7.03 µg equivalents umeclidinium free base/g of tissue.    Lower limit of quantification = 0.007 µg equivalents umeclidinium free base/g of tissue.    NS: Not sectioned.

[6]  PMDA Database.    http://www.pmda.go.jp/drugs/2014/P201400076/index.html (accessed Mar 2016).

# Metabolism

Table 13    *In Vitro* Metabolic Stability of [$^{14}$C]Umeclidinium in Hepatocytes and Liver Microsomes[6]

| %Remaining of Parent and %Formation of Metabolites | | | | | |
|---|---|---|---|---|---|
| Analyte | Liver Microsomes[a] (% of total radioactivity) | | Hepatocytes[b] (%Remaining or % of Total Metabolism) | | |
| Species | Human | Species | Human | Rat | Dog |
| Umeclidinium | 48.5 | Umeclidinium[c] | 57 | 74 | 72 |
| M14 | 19.3 | M14[d] | 22.9 | 37.9 | 25.9 |
| M33 | 20.0 | M33/M34[d] | 18.4 | BLQ | 18.0 |
| M56 | 4.51 | M52[d] | 3.5 | ND | BLQ |
| M61 | 3.82 | M45/M59[d] | 5.2 | BLQ | BLQ |

The turnovers of umeclidinium in 24 h in human, rat and dog hepatocytes were 43%, 26% and 28%, respectively.    [$^{14}$C] Umeclidinium (0.075 μM) was incubated with human liver microsomal preparations (0.25 mg/mL) containing CYP inhibitor for 30 min.    BLQ: Peak detected by MS and radio detection but below quantitation limit.
[a] [$^{14}$C]umeclidinium (0.075 μM) was incubated with human liver microsomes at 37 °C for 30 min.    [b] [$^{14}$C]Umeclidinium (10, 50 μM) was incubated with hepatocytes for up to 24 h.    [c] % Remaining.    [d] % of total metabolism.

Table 14    *In Vitro* Metabolic Phenotype of Umeclidinium in Human Liver Microsomes and Recombinant CYPs[6]

| Hunan Liver Microsomes[a] | | | Recombinant CYP Enzyme[b] | | | | | |
|---|---|---|---|---|---|---|---|---|
| CYPs (inhibitor) | %Inhibition | | CYPs | % of Total Radioactivity | | | | |
| | M14 | M33 | | Umeclidinium | M14 | M33 | M56 | M61 |
| CYP1A2 (Furafylline) | 8.0 | 0.0 | CYP1A1 | 71.4 | 21.8 | ND | ND | ND |
| CYP2C8 (Montalukast) | 9.7 | 15 | CYP1A2 | 93.9 | ND | ND | ND | ND |
| CYP2C9 (Sulphaphenazole) | 0.0 | 6.3 | CYP2A13 | 93.9 | ND | ND | ND | ND |
| | | | CYP2C8 | 96.9 | ND | ND | ND | ND |
| CYP2C19 (Benzylnirvanol) | 27 | 16 | CYP2C9 | 96.2 | ND | ND | ND | ND |
| | | | CYP2C19 | 98.7 | ND | ND | ND | ND |
| CYP2D6 (Quinidine) | 90 | 100 | CYP2D6 | 45.9 | 11.7 | 22.2 | 7.10 | 4.30[a] |
| | | | CYP2E1 | 96.6 | √ | ND | ND | ND |
| CYP3A4 (Azamulin) | 52 | 0.0 | CYP3A4 | 95.8 | 3.64[a] | ND | ND | ND |
| | | | CYP3A5 | 98.1 | ND | ND | ND | ND |

ND: Not detected.    √: Peak detected by MS but not quantifiable form radiochromatogram.    Peak identified by retention time only.    [a] Incubation of [$^{14}$C] umeclidinium (0.075 μM) with human liver microsomal preparations (0.25 mg/mL) containing CYP inhibitor for 30 min.    [b] Incubation of umeclidinium (0.075 μM) with bactosomes expressing individual CYPs at 37 °C for 30 min (or 5 min for CYP2D6).

Table 15    Metabolites in Plasma, Urine, Bile and Feces in Humans and Non-clinical Test Species after Single Dose of Umeclidinium[6]

| Matrix | Species | Route | Dose (mg/kg) | Time (h) | % of Radioactivity (% of dose) | | | | | | | | | |
|---|---|---|---|---|---|---|---|---|---|---|---|---|---|---|
| | | | | | Parent | M14 | M33 | M34 | M37 | M51 | M58 | M63 | M65 | M66 |
| Plasma | Rat | i.v. | 1 | 0-2 | 98 | - | - | - | - | - | - | - | - | - |
| | Dog | i.v. | 1 | 0-3 | 94.7 | BLQ | BLQ | BLQ | - | BLQ | - | - | - | - |
| | Human | i.h. | 1 mg | 0.083 | √ | 4[c] | - | - | - | - | - | - | - | - |
| | | | | 1 | √ | 10[c] | - | - | - | - | - | - | - | - |
| Urine | Rat | i.v. | 1 | 0-24 | 90.2 (13.7) | 3.5 (0.5) | BLQ | ND | ND | NA | NA | NA | NA | NA |
| | Dog | i.v. | 1 | 0-48 | 18.6 (1.8) | 11.8 (1.1) | 29.8 (2.9) | 1.0 (0.1) | ND | 11.8 (1.1) | ND | NA | NA | NA |

[6]  PMDA Database.    http://www.pmda.go.jp/drugs/2014/P201400076/index.html (accessed Mar 2016).

*Continued*

| Matrix | Species | Route | Dose (mg/kg) | Time (h) | % of Radioactivity(% of dose) | | | | | | | | | |
|--------|---------|-------|--------------|----------|--------|-----|-----|-----|-----|-----|-----|-----|-----|-----|
| | | | | | Parent | M14 | M33 | M34 | M37 | M51 | M58 | M63 | M65 | M66 |
| Urine | BDC dog | i.v. (10 min infusion) | 0.2 | 0-48 | 24.9 (1.7) | 9.1 (0.6) | 22.9 (1.6) | 2.6 (0.2) | ND | 10.2 (0.7) | ND | ND | ND | ND |
| Bile | BDC dog | i.v. (10 min infusion) | 0.2 | - | 7.5 (4.3) | 16.3 (9.4) | 8.7 (5.0)[a] | NA[a] | 7.4 (4.3)[b] | ND | 2.2 (1.3) | 6.0 (3.4) | 7.2 (4.2) | 6.6 (3.8) |
| Feces | Dog | i.v. | 1 | 0-72 | 21.9 (12.0) | 25.9 (14.2) | 4.4 (2.4) | 4.9 (2.7) | 4.7 (2.6) | 6.0 (3.3) | BLQ | NA | NA | NA |
| | Rat | i.v. | 1 | 0-48 | 85.7 (53.2) | 3.2 (2.0) | BLQ | BLQ | 3.1 (1.9) | NA | NA | NA | NA | NA |

M14 (*O*-dealkylation product), M33 (hydroxy), M34 (methyl catecol), M37 (hydroxylation), M51 (dihydrodiol), M58 (hydroxylation), M63 (dihydrodiol), M65 (dihydration, glycylcysteine conjugation) and M65 (dihydration, oxygenation, glycylcysteine conjugation).   √: Presence.   BLQ: Below limit of quantification.   ND: Not detected.   NA: Not applicable.   BDC: Bile duct-cannulated.   [a] Co-elution M33/M34.   [b] Co-elution M37/M54.   [c] % of Umeclidinium.

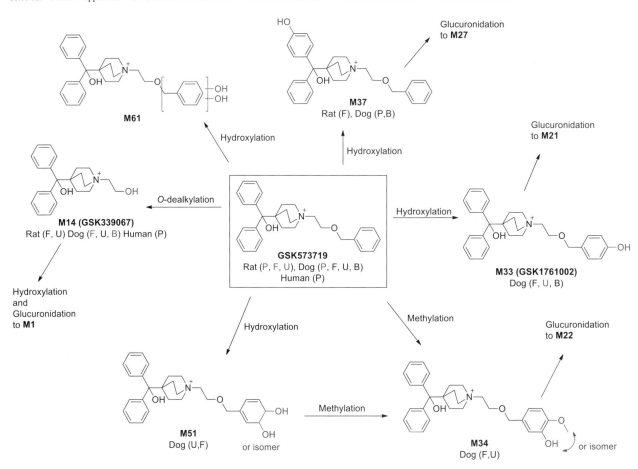

Figure C    Proposed Pathways for *In Vivo* Biotransformation of Umeclidinium in Rats, Dogs and Humans[6]

The red labels represent the major components in the matrices.    P = Plasma, U = Urine, F = Feces and B = Bile.

[6]  PMDA Database.  http://www.pmda.go.jp/drugs/2014/P201400076/index.html (accessed Mar 2016).

# Excretion

Table 16 Excretion Profiles of [$^{14}$C]Umeclidinium in Rats and Humans after Single Intravenous and Oral Dose of [$^{14}$C]Umeclidinium Bromide[6, 8]

| Species | State | Route | Dose (mg/kg) | Time (h) | Bile (% of dose) | Urine (% of dose) | Feces (% of dose) | Recovery (% of dose) |
|---|---|---|---|---|---|---|---|---|
| Rat (male) | Intact | i.v.(30 min infusion) | 1 | 0-96 | ND | 16.9 ± 1.43 | 65.3 ± 1.87 | 93.9 ± 1.16[a] |
| | | p.o. | 1 | 0-96 | ND | 0.10 ± 0.00 | 96.4 ± 1.91 | 96.5 ± 1.91[a] |
| Rat (male) | BDC | p.o. | 1 | 0-48 | 0.17 ± 0.06 | 0.13 ± 0.06 | 92.9 ± 3.19 | 93.8 ± 2.29[a] |
| Dog (male) | Intact | i.v. (1 h infusion) | 1 | 0-168 | ND | 11.9 ± 1.50 | 61.8 ± 0.78 | 74.5 ± 0.84[a] |
| | | p.o. | 1 | 0-168 | ND | 0.43 ± 0.31 | 95.2 ± 8.00 | 96.5 ± 8.26[a] |
| Dog (male) | BDC | i.v. (slow bolus) | 0.01 | 0-48 | 55.6 | 14.2 | 3.30 | 73.8[a] |
| Human (male & female) | Intact | i.v. | 0.065 mg | NA | - | 22 | 58 | ~81 |
| | | p.o. | 1 mg | NA | - | <1 | 92 | <93 |

Vehicle: 0.9% (w/v) aqueous sodium chloride. BDC: Bile duct-cannulated. ND: Not detected. [a] Containing excretion in other tissues, such as liver, lungs, gastrointestinal tract and carcass.

# Drug-Drug Interaction

Table 17 Evaluation of Umeclidinium as an Inhibitor and an Inducer of Enzymes[6]

| Umeclidinium as an Inhibitor[a] | | Umeclidinium as an Inducer[c] | | | | | | |
|---|---|---|---|---|---|---|---|---|
| | | | Fold Induction (male) | | | Fold Induction (female) | | |
| CYPs | IC$_{50}$ (µM) | CYPs | 30 µg/kg/d | 200 µg/kg/d | 2000 µg/kg/d | 30 µg/kg/d | 200 µg/kg/d | 2000 µg/kg/d |
| CYP1A2 | >33 | CYP1A1 | 0.13 ± 0.19 | 1.1 ± 1.3 | 0.24 ± 0.14 | 0.62 ± 0.23 | 0.44 ± 0.22 | 7.7 ± 11 |
| CYP2C9 | >33 | CYP1A2 | 0.92 ± 0.079 | 1.0 ± 0.056 | 0.00096 ± 0.00035 | 1.0 ± 0.18 | 0.51 ± 0.45 | 0.72 ± 0.23 |
| CYP2C19 | 14 | CYP2B1 | 1.1 ± 0.52 | 2.4 ± 1.4 | 0.14 ± 0.0087 | 0.77 ± 0.24 | 4.2 ± 2.6 | 1.6 ± 0.89 |
| CYP2D6 | 0.1 | CYP2B2 | 0.34 ± 0.25 | 0.62 ± 0.72 | 0.15 ± 0..042 | 0.52 ± 0.26 | 1.2 ± 0.79 | 0.29 ± 0.21 |
| CYP3A4 | 1.0[b] | CYP2E1 | 0.74 ± 0.15 | 1.2 ± 0.24 | 0.000042 ± 0.000022 | 1.2 ± 0.19 | 0.87 ± 0.77 | 1.1 ± 0.27 |
| CYP3A4 | 8.0[b] | CYP3A2 | 1.6 ± 0.53 | 1.6 ± 0.58 | 0.000088 ± 0.000039 | NA | NA | NA |
| | | CYP3A23 | 0.86 ± 0.24 | 1.6 ± 0.59 | 0.032 ± 0.016 | 1.3 ± 0.094 | 1.5 ± 1.2 | 1.1 ± 0.56 |
| | | CYP4A1 | 2.3 ± 0.73 | 3.6 ± 0.27 | 0.0076 ± 0.0056 | 1.1 ± 0.26 | 0.76 ± 0.66 | 0.91 ± 0.22 |

[a] Incubation of umeclidinium with bulk mixture containing microsomes and probe substrate for 15 min at 42°C Umeclidinium 0.03-33 µM (*in vitro*). [b] 1.0 for substrate diethoxyfluorescein, and 8.0 for substrate 7-benzyloxyguinoline. [c] 1 h inhalation (dry powder) for 4 weeks on rats (*in vivo*).

Table 18 *In Vitro* Evaluation of Umeclidinium as a Substrate of Human Organic Cation Transporters[6]

| Transporter | Uptake (µL/mg protein) | | | | | | |
|---|---|---|---|---|---|---|---|
| | 0.5 min | 1 min | 3 min | 5 min | 10 min | 30 min | 60 min |
| Mock[a] | 4.0 | 6.5 | 10.4 | 12.9 | 18.4 | 40.9 | 73.7 |
| OCT1 | 15.7 | 28.4 | 78.2 | 117 | 202 | 415 | 516 |
| OCT2 | 9.6 | 12.7 | 20.3 | 31.9 | 48.5 | 125 | 200 |
| OCT3 | 8.6 | 12.1 | 14.6 | 15.5 | 19.1 | 40.3 | 61.8 |
| Mock[b] | 9.8 | 6.0 | 9.8 | 11.6 | 14.0 | 28.5 | 49.5 |
| OCTN1[c] | 5.8 | 6.9 | 7.1 | 10.2 | 19.8 | 32.6 | 28.2 |
| OCTN2[c] | 5.8 | 10.4 | 10.3 | 13.3 | 14.0 | 23.4 | 53.9 |

The uptake time course of [$^{14}$C]umeclidinium (1.8 µM) was assessed by HEK293 cells expressing human OCT1, OCT2, OCT3, OCTN1, OCTN2 and Mock at 37 °C for up to 60 min. [a] For OCT1, OCT2 and OCT3. [b] For OCTN1 and OCTN2. [c] Positive control: [$^3$H]Ergothioneine (5.0 nM) per 3 min = 36.6 ± 4.1 µL/mg protein (OCTN1, n = 3) versus 2.3 ± 0.3 µL/mg protein (Mock, n = 3). [$^3$H]Carnitine (5.9 nM) per 3 min = 179.2 ± 7.3 µL/mg protein (OCTN2, n = 3) versus 9.0 ± 0.6 µL/mg protein (Mock, n = 3).

[6] PMDA Database. http://www.pmda.go.jp/drugs/2014/P201400076/index.html (accessed Mar 2016).
[8] FDA Database. http://www.accessdata.fda.gov/drugsatfda_docs/nda/2014/205382Orig1s000ClinPharmR.pdf (accessed Mar 2016).

Table 19  *In Vitro* Evaluation of Umeclidinium as an Inhibitor of P-gp[6]

| Compound | Conc. (μM) | Digoxin Transport Rate (pM/cm²/h) | Digoxin Transport Rate (% of Control) |
|---|---|---|---|
| Umeclidinium | 0.1 | 2.5 ± 0.17 | 100 ± 7.1 |
| | 0.3 | 2.6 ± 0.25 | 100 ± 10 |
| | 1 | 2.1 ± 0.19 | 85 ± 7.6 |
| | 3 | 2.3 ± 0.20 | 96 ± 8.1 |
| | 10 | 2.3 ± 0.14 | 94 ± 5.8 |
| | 30 | 2.5 ± 0.15 | 100 ± 6.0 |
| | 100 | 2.2 ± 0.046 | 91 ± 1.9 |
| [³H]Digoxin only | 0.03 | 2.5 ± 0.092 | 100 ± 3.7 |
| GF120918A | 2 | 0.59 ± 0.046 | 24 ± 1.9 |

Test system: MDCKII-MDR1 cells.  MDCKII-MDR1 cells were preincubated (37 °C) for 30 min with receiver working solutions with and without GF120918A (2 μM).  Concentration (μM): 0.1, 0.3, 1, 3, 10, 30 and 100.  P-glycoprotein inhibitor: GF120918A (2 μM).

# 6  Non-Clinical Toxicology

## Summary

### Single-Dose Toxicity
❖ No specific single-dose toxicity study was reviewed.

### Repeated-Dose Toxicity
❖ Repeated-dose toxicity studies by inhalation administration for up to 26 weeks in rats and up to 39 weeks in dogs:
  • By the longest studies employed, the NOAEL in rats was 87.1 μg/kg/day (23.9/27.2 × MRHD), and that in dogs was 109 μg/kg/day (12.5/19.2 × MRHD).
  • The main target organs of toxicity in both species were respiratory tract and lungs.  Besides, the heart was identified as a target organ in the dog.

### Safety Pharmacology
❖ Safety pharmacology studies with umeclidinium bromide, including inhalation studies on CNS, *in vitro* and intravenous studies on CVS, as well as inhalation studies on RS:
  • Moderately dilated pupil was observed for rats at 322 and 1994 μg/kg, which was an expected pharmacological effect, but no other change in CNS was observed.[8]
  • Umeclidinium bromide was a weak hERG blocker with a low potential to induce QT prolongation, besides, it increased heart rate, decreased RR interval, and blocked AV, which could be attributed to the antimuscarinic effects.
  • Single inhaled doses of umeclidinium bromide at 215 and 2260 mg/kg administered to rats generated increases in respiratory rate (18% to 45%) and decreases in tidal volume (3% to 17%).

### Genotoxicity
❖ Umeclidinium bromide was negative in genetic toxicology testing based on results from the *in vitro* bacterial reverse mutation assay, *in vitro* mouse lymphoma assay, and *in vivo* rat micronucleus test.

### Reproductive and Developmental Toxicity
❖ Fertility and early embryonic development in rats:
  • Fertility and reproductive performance were not affected in males and females, with exposure margin of 84 and 44 on AUC basis, respectively.
❖ Embryo-fetal development in rats and rabbits:
  • No adverse effect was seen on embryo-fetal survival and development in either species, following up to 44- and 165-fold clinical AUC expousure, respectively.
❖ Pre- and postnatal development in rats:
  • Umeclidinium provided an overall safety margin of 22 × MRHD on AUC basis, but was detected in pups, reflecting potential excretion in breast milk.
❖ It is unknown whether umeclidinium bromide was excreted in human breast milk.

[6]  PMDA Database.  http://www.pmda.go.jp/drugs/2014/P201400076/index.html (accessed Mar 2016).
[8]  FDA Database.  http://www.accessdata.fda.gov/drugsatfda_docs/nda/2014/205382Orig1s000ClinPharmR.pdf (accessed Mar 2016).

Carcinogenicity
- ❖ Traditional 2-year carcinogenicity studies of umeclidinium bromide by the inhalation route were conducted in mice and rats.
  - No tumor was considered test-article related.
  - Non-neoplastic finding was found, including upper respiratory tract irritancy, accumulation of eosinophilic inclusions, accumulation of alveolar macrophages, and effect on the eyes and harderian glands.

## Repeated-Dose Toxicity

Table 20 Repeated-Dose Toxicity Studies of Umeclidinium by Inhalation Administration[5, 6, 8]

| Species | Duration (Week) | Dose (µg/kg/day) | NOAEL Dose (µg/kg/day) | AUC$_{0-t}$[a] (ng·h/mL) | Mean Safety margin[b] (× MRHD) | Finding |
|---|---|---|---|---|---|---|
| SD rat | 13 | 0, 38, 102, 288, 924 | 288 | 21.1/16.0 | 56.8/43.1 | Tolerated at all doses up to 924 µg/kg/day. Target organ of toxicity: Lungs and tracheal bifurcation. 924 µg/kg/day: In the nasal cavity, degeneration/regeneration of the respiratory epithelium graded moderate in severity. |
| | 26 | 0, 87.1, 289, 987 | 87.1 | 8.88/10.1 | 23.9/27.2 | Tolerated at all doses up to 987 µg/kg/day. Umeclidinium-induced toxicity was primarily seen in animals given ≥289 µg/kg/day. Target organ of toxicity: The nasal cavity/sinus, nasopharynx, larynx, tracheal bifurcation and the lungs. Minimal increases in neutrophil count (males only) and reduced body weight gain, microscopic changes seen in the nasal cavity/sinus, nasopharynx, larynx and tracheal bifurcation. |
| Beagle dog | 13 | 0, 40.7, 187, 1070 | 1070 | 26.5/24.3 | 71.3/65.4 | Tolerated at all doses up to 1070 µg/kg/day. None of the changes were considered to be adverse. |
| | 39 | 0, 109, 421, 1002 | 109 | 4.64/7.13 | 12.5/19.2 | Tolerated at all doses up to 1002 mg/kg/day. Umeclidinium-induced toxicity was primarily seen in dogs given 421 or 1002 µg/kg/day. Target organ of toxicity: The heart, lungs, larynx and nasal turbinates. |

Vehicle: Lactose with 1% w/w magnesium stearate. [a] Male/Female. [b] Calculated with clinical AUC$_{ss}$ (0.3716 ng·h/mL) at proposed umeclidinium dose of 62.5 µg/day from a 24-week study in COPD patients.

## Safety Pharmacology

Table 21 Safety Pharmacology Studies of Umeclidinium Bromide by Inhalation or Injection Administration[9]

| Study | System | Dose | Vehicle | Finding |
|---|---|---|---|---|
| Cardiovascular effect | HEK293 cell expressing hERG channel | Up to 48.997 µM | 0.1% DMSO in extracellular solution | A weak hERG blocker (IC$_{50}$ = 9.41 µM) without significant potential to induce QT prolongation. |
| | Conscious Beagle dog (M) | 0.3, 3, 10 µg/kg, i.v. for over 1 min | 0.9% (w/v) NaCl | At 10 µg/kg: Heart rate increased with a maximum change of 49 bpm (from predose average of 65 bpm), RR interval decreased to 0.545 sec, pulse pressure reduced of 7 mmHg, PR interval increased to 0.118 sec, AV block was observed in 3 out of 4 animals with an incidence ranging between 7-93. At 0.3 µg/kg: Arrhythmias (ventricular ectopic beats) were observed. |
| Respiratory effect | Conscious CD rat (M) | 36, 215, 2660 µg/kg inhalation | 0.8% w/w in Lactose | At 215 or 2660 µg/kg: Increased respiratory rate of 18%-45%, decreased tidal volume of 3%-17%. |
| Neurological effect | Conscious CD rat (M) | 36, 322, 1994 µg/kg inhalation | 8% w/w in Lactose | No toxicologically significant adverse effect on neurological function. |

[5] EMA Database. http://www.ema.europa.eu/docs/en_GB/document_library/EPAR_-_Public_assessment_report/human/002809/WC500167431.pdf (accessed Mar 2016).
[6] PMDA Database. http://www.pmda.go.jp/drugs/2014/P201400076/index.html (accessed Mar 2016).
[8] FDA Database. http://www.accessdata.fda.gov/drugsatfda_docs/nda/2014/205382Orig1s000ClinPharmR.pdf (accessed Mar 2016).
[9] FDA Database. http://www.accessdata.fda.gov/drugsatfda_docs/nda/2014/205382Orig1s000PharmR.pdf (accessed Mar 2016).

# Genotoxicity

Table 22    Genotoxicity Studies of Umeclidinium Bromide[9]

| Assay | Species/ System | Metabolism | Dose | Finding |
|---|---|---|---|---|
| *In vitro* bacterial reverse mutation assay | *S. typhimurium* TA98, TA100, TA1535, and TA1537 *E. coli* WP2 uvrA pKM101 | ±S9 | 5, 15, 50, 150, 500, 1500 and 2500 μg/plate (±S9) for *S. typhimurium* 5, 15, 150, 500, 1500, 2500 and 5000 μg/plate for WP2 uvrA pKM101 | Negative. |
| *In vitro* mouse lymphoma mutation assay | L5178Y t/k$^{+/-}$ cell | ±S9 | 25, 50, 75, 100, 125, 150, 175, 200, 225 and 250 μg/mL (-S9, 3 h) 20, 40, 60, 80,100, 125, 150, 175, 200, 250 and 300 μg/mL (+S9, 3 h) 10, 20, 40, 60, 80, 90, 100, 110, 125 and 150 μg/mL (-S9, 24 h) | Negative. |
| *In vivo* rat bone marrow micronucleus assay | SD rat | + | Single, p.o., 0, 10, or 20 mg/kg/day | Negative. |

Vehicle: DMSO for *in vitro* study, 0.9% NaCl for *in vivo* study.

# Reproductive and Developmental Toxicity

Table 23    Reproductive and Developmental Toxicology Studies of Umeclidinium Bromide by Inhalation or Injection Administration[6, 9]

| Study | Species | Estimated Achieved Dose (μg/kg/day) | NOAEL Dose (μg/kg/day) | NOAEL AUC (ng·h/mL) | NOAEL Safety Margin[a] (× MRHD) | Finding |
|---|---|---|---|---|---|---|
| Fertility and early embryonic development | SD rat | 0, 30, 60, 180 s.c. (M); 3.37, 29.1, 100, 294 inhalation (F) | s.c., 180 inhalation, 294 | 31.1[b]/16.2[c] | 84/44 | Tolerated at all doses for male and female rats. No toxicologically significant adverse effect in the fertility and early embryonic development. |
| Embryo-fetal development | SD rat | 0, 31.7, 96.9, 278, inhalation for 1 h | 278 | 16.2[c] | 44 | Tolerated at all doses. No toxicologically significant adverse effect on embryo-fetal development. |
| | NZW rabbit | 40, 100, 180 s.c. | 180 | 61.4 | 165 | Tolerated at all doses. In all treated groups: Slightly low overall mean food consumption during the treatment period. No toxicologically significant adverse effect of treatment on embryo-fetal survival, growth or development. |
| Pre- and postnatal development | Wistar rat | 10, 60, 180 s.c. | Materal:180 | 24.9 | 67 | Tolerated at all doses for male and female rats. At 180 μg/kg/day: Slight reductions in $F_0$ body weight gains, food consumption and preweaning pup body weight. |
| | | | $F_1$: 60[d] | 8.07 | 22 | No toxicologically significant adverse effect in the fertility and early embryonic development. |

Vehicle: 1% (w/w) magnesium stearate in lactose for inhalation; 0.9% Sodium chloride for subcutaneous injection.    [a] Calculated with clinical AUC$_{ss}$ (0.3716 ng·h/mL) at proposed umeclidinum dose of 62.5 μg/day from a 24-week study in COPD patients.    [b] Extrapolated from study 14-day s.c. toxicity & TK study in rats.    [c] Extrapolated from 13-week rat inhalation study.    [d] Detected in pups, reflecting potential excretion in breast milk.

[6]  PMDA Database.   http://www.pmda.go.jp/drugs/2014/P201400076/index.html (accessed Mar 2016).
[9]  FDA Database.   http://www.accessdata.fda.gov/drugsatfda_docs/nda/2014/205382Orig1s000PharmR.pdf (accessed Mar 2016).

# Carcinogenicity

Table 24    Carcinogenicity Studies of Umeclidinium Bromide by Inhalation Administration[6, 9]

| Species | Estimated Achieved Dose (μg/kg/day) | Duration | NOAEL | | | Finding |
|---|---|---|---|---|---|---|
| | | | Dose (μg/kg/day) | Mean $AUC_{0-t}$ (ng·h/mL) | Safety Margin[a] (× MRHD) | |
| CD-1 mouse | Male: 58.6, 188, 533 Reduced to 32.7, 102, 295 from Week 67 | 60 min/day, reduced to 30 min/day from Week 67, 104 weeks in total | 295 | 8.21 | 22 | No effect of the test article on the factors contributory to death. Reduced body weight gain over Week 0-72, accompanied by minimally lower food consumption. |
| | Female: 20.8, 63.7, 200 | 60 min/day for 104 Weeks | 200 | 6.87 | 18 | Local irritation in the larynx and nasal turbinates, a small increase in foamy alveolar macrophages in the lungs and an increase in porphyrin concretions in the harderian glands. No test article-related neoplastic change. |
| SD rat | Male & Female: 30.1, 101, 267 Reduced to 14.7, 45.0, 137 from Week 73 | 60 min/day, reduced to 30 min/day from Week 73, 104 weeks in total | 137 | 6.75 | 18 | No adverse effect on survival of either sex. Local irritation in the larynx, tracheal bifurcation and nasal cavity. Lower body weight gain of males over Week 1-66 with slightly lower food consumption, except for at HD throughout the study. No test article-related neoplastic change. |

Vehicle: Lactose with 1% (w/w) magnesium stearate.    [a] Calculated with clinical $AUC_{ss}$ (0.3716 ng·h/mL) at proposed umeclidinium dose of 62.5 μg/day from a 24-week study in COPD patients.

[6]  PMDA Database.   http://www.pmda.go.jp/drugs/2014/P201400076/index.html (accessed Mar 2016).

[9]  FDA Database.   http://www.accessdata.fda.gov/drugsatfda_docs/nda/2014/205382Orig1s000PharmR.pdf (accessed Mar 2016).

# CHAPTER

## 29

## Vaniprevir

# Vaniprevir

## (Vanihep®)

Research code: MK-7009

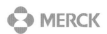

---

## 1 General Information

❖ Vaniprevir is a hepatitis C virus (HCV) non-structural 3/4A protease inhibitor, which was approved in Sep 2014 by PMDA of Japan.

❖ Vaniprevir was discovered and marketed by Merck & Co.

❖ Vaniprevir is an HCV NS3/4A protease inhibitor. Inhibition of HCV NS3/4A protease prevents the proteolytic processing of the HCV nonstructural polyprotein, which is essential for viral replication.

❖ Vaniprevir is indicated for the treatment of patients with HCV infection.

❖ Available as oral capsule, with each containing 150 mg of vaniprevir and the recommended dose is 300 mg twice daily taken with or without food last for 12 weeks.

❖ The sale of Vanihep® was not available up to Mar 2016.

### Key Approvals around the World*

|  | Japan (PMDA) |
|---|---|
| First approval date | 09/26/2014 |
| Application or approval No. | 22600AMX01313000 |
| Brand name | Vanihep®/バニヘップ® |
| Indication | HCV infection |
| Authorisation holder | Merck & Co. |

* Till Mar 2016, it had not been approved by FDA (US), EMA (EU) and CFDA (China).

## Active Ingredient

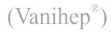

*Molecular formula*: $C_{38}H_{55}N_5O_9S$
*Molecular weight*: 757.94
*CAS No.*: 923590-37-8 (Vaniprevir)
*Chemical name*: (5R,7S,10S)-10-(1,1-dimethylethyl)-N-{(1R,2R)-1-[N-(cyclopropanesulfonyl)carbamoyl]-2-ethylcyclopropyl}-15,15-dimethyl-3,9,12-trioxo-2,3,5,6,7,8,9,10,11,12,14,15,16,17,18,19-hexadecahydro-2,23:5,8-dimethano-1H-benzo[n][1,10,3,6,12] dioxatriaza-cyclohenicosine-7-carboxamide

*Parameters of Lipinski's "Rule of 5"*

| MW | $H_D$ | $H_A$ | FRB[a] | PSA[a] | cLogP[a] |
|---|---|---|---|---|---|
| 757.94 | 3 | 14 | 6 | 189Å² | 3.90 ± 1.02 |

[a] Calculated by ACD/Labs software V11.02.

## Drug Product*

*Dosage route*: Oral
*Strength*: 150 mg (Vaniprevir)
*Dosage form*: Capsule
*Inactive ingredient*: Glycerin fatty acid ester, polysorbate 80, polyoxyl 35 castor oil, butylhydroxyanisol, dibutylhydroxytoluene, medium-chain fatty acid triglyceride, lecithin, gelatin, sorbitol sorbitan solution, glycerin, titanium oxide, ferric oxide and yellow ferric oxide.
*Recommended dose*: The recommended starting dose is 300 mg twice daily taken with or without food last for 12 weeks.

* Sourced from Japan PMDA drug label information

## 2  Key Patents Information

### Summary

❖ Vanihep® (Vaniprevir) was approved by PMDA of Japan on Sep 26, 2014.
❖ Vaniprevir was originally developed by Merck & Co., and its compound patent application was filed as PCT application by Merck & Co. in 2006.
❖ The compound patent will expire in 2026 foremost, which has been granted in the United States, Europe, Japan and China successively.

Table 1    Vaniprevir's Compound Patent Protection in Drug-Mainstream Country

| Country | Publication/Patent NO. | Application Date | Granted Date | Estimated Expiry Date |
|---|---|---|---|---|
| WO | WO2007015787A1 | 07/14/2006 | / | / |
| US | US7470664B2 | 07/12/2006 | 12/30/2008 | 01/26/2027[a] |
|  | US8216999B2 | 07/12/2006 | 07/10/2012 | 01/26/2027[b] |
| EP | EP1910404B1 | 07/14/2006 | 11/27/2013 | 07/14/2026 |
|  | EP1924593B1 | 07/14/2006 | 09/16/2009 | 07/14/2026 |
| JP | JP4621282B2 | 07/14/2006 | 01/26/2011 | 06/03/2030[c] |
|  | JP5345117B2 | 07/14/2006 | 11/20/2013 | 07/14/2026 |
| CN | CN101228181B | 07/14/2006 | 09/18/2013 | 07/14/2026 |

[a] The term of this patent is extended by 196 days.    [b] The term of this patent is extended by 416 days (TD).    [c] The term of this patent is extended by 1420 days.

Table 2    Originator's International Patent Application List (Patent Family)

| Publication NO. | Title | Applicant/Assignee/Owner | Publication Date |
|---|---|---|---|
| Technical Subjects | Active Ingredient (Free Base)'s Formula or Structure and Preparation | | |
| WO2007015787A1 | HCV NS3 protease inhibitors | Merck & Co. | 02/08/2007 |
| Technical Subjects | Salt, Crystal, Polymorphic, Solvate (Hydrate), Isomer, Derivative Etc. and Preparation | | |
| WO2011025849A1 | Processes for preparing protease inhibitors of hepatitis C virus | Merck & Co. | 03/03/2011 |
| WO2012082672A2 | Process and intermediates for preparing macrolactams | Merck & Co. | 06/21/2012 |
| Technical Subjects | Formulation and Preparation | | |
| WO2015120014A1 | Novel disintegration systems for pharmaceutical dosage forms | Merck & Co. | 08/13/2015 |
| Technical Subjects | Combination Including at Least Two Active Ingredients | | |
| WO2013033901A1 | Heterocyclic-substituted benzofuran derivatives and methods of use thereof for the treatment of viral diseases | Merck & Co. | 03/14/2013 |
| WO2013033899A1 | Substituted benzofuran compounds and methods of use thereof for the treatment of viral diseases | Merck & Co. | 03/14/2013 |
| WO2013034047A1 | Heterocyclic-substitued benzofuran derivatives and methods of use thereof for the treatment of viral diseases | Merck & Co. | 03/14/2013 |
| WO2013034048A1 | Substituted benzofuran compounds and methods of use thereof for the treatment of viral diseases | Merck & Co. | 03/14/2013 |
| WO2013033971A1 | Tetracyclic heterocycle compounds and methods of use thereof for the treatment of viral diseases | Merck & Co. | 03/14/2013 |
| WO2013066753A1 | Compositions useful for the treatment of viral diseases | Merck & Co. | 05/10/2013 |
| Technical Subjects | Others | | |
| WO2008112108A1 | In vivo HCV resistance to anti-viral inhibitors | Merck & Co. | 09/18/2008 |

The data was updated until Jan 2016.

# 3 Chemistry

## Route 1: Original Discovery Route

BPO: Benzoyl peroxide
MS: Molecular sieves
Zhan 1B catalyst: 1,3-Bis(2,4,6-trimethylphenyl)-4,5-dihydroimidazol-2-ylidene[2-(*i*-propoxy)-5-(*N*,*N*-dimethylaminosulfonyl)phenyl]
    methyleneruthenium(II) dichloride

*Synthetic Route*:    The original synthesis started with 3-bromo-*o*-xylene **1**, which was dibrominated with *N*-bromosuccinimde (NBS) and benzoyl peroxide, to afford dibenzylbromide **2** in 95% yield.    Displacement of the bromines with benzylamine **3** with concomitant ring closure gave 2-benzyl-4-bromoisoindoline **4**.    Removal of the benzyl protective group with 1-chloro-ethyl chloroformate **5** and the following CDI-promoted carbamate formation afforded **8** in excellent yield.    Installation of the vinyl group using potassium vinyltrifluoroborate under Pd(II)-catalyzed cross-coupling and then acidic removal of Boc group gave key intermediate **11** as the hydrochloride salt in 90% yield across a two-step sequence.    Compound **11**, as a stable white powder, was then coupled to linker acid **12** to form bis-olefins **13**.    Macrocyclization *via* olefin metathesis catalyzed by Zhan 1B catalyst, selectively generated **14** as *trans*-isomer.    This key intermediate was transformed into the ultimate target by hydrogenation, hydrolysis and amide formation with **17** in 68% yield over three steps, and with the overall yield of 12%.[1-3]

[1]   Holloway, M. K.; Liverton, N. J.; Ludmerer, S. W., et al. WO2007015855A1, **2007**.
[2]   Holloway, M. K.; Liverton, N. J.; Ludmerer, S. W., et al. US7470664B2, **2008**.
[3]   McCauley, J. A.; McIntyre, C. J.; Rudd, M. T., et al. *J. Med. Chem.* **2010**, *53*, 2443-2463.

## Route 2

**20** + **21** (·HCl) → TEA, MeCN, 21 to 38 °C, 97% → **22**

**22** → i. **22**, **23**, t-BuOLi, Toluene, 10 °C; ii. 3M HCl, 15 to 30 °C; iii. 50% NaOH, r.t. 65% → **24**

Br⌐⌐⌐Br **23**

**24** → Boc₂O, IPAc, 35 °C, 85% → **25**

**25** → i. **25**, Alcalase, 0.1M K₂HPO₄, DMSO, 40 °C; ii. 5N NaOH, 47% → **26** (>99% ee)

**26** → i. 50% NaOH, MeOH, 40 °C; ii. 12M HCl, IPAc → **27**

H₂N–SO₂–cyclopropane **28**

**27** → i. **27**, CDI, IPAc, 40 °C; ii. **28**, DBU, 15 to 40 °C, 92% → **29**

**29** → Ru/C, H₂, MeOH, 50 psi, 90% → **30** (99.0% ee)

**30** → TsOH, n-PrOH, 60 °C, 74% → **14** (·TsOH)

IPAc: Isopropyl acetate
BPO: Dibenzoyl peroxide
DMPU: 1,3-Dimethyl-3,4,5,6-tetrahydro-2(1H)-pyrimidinone or N,N'-dimethyl-N,N'-trimethylene urea
DCHA: Dicyclohexylamine
MCy: Methylcyclohexane

*Synthetic Route*: Beginning with bis-benzylbromide **2**, which was prepared by bromination of commercially available 3-bromo-o-xylene **1** and then was subjected to benzylamine **3** under basic conditions followed by acidification afforded the isoindoline **4** as toluene sulfonic acid salt in 90% yield. This salt was then treated with base and acylative removal of the benzyl protecting group took place through the use of acetyl chloride **5**. Hydrochloric acid in refluxing methanol liberated indoline **6** which was isolated as the HCl salt with 88% yield. Next, exposure of **6** to alcohol **7** in the presence of CDI and warm DMF gave rise to carbamate **8** in 91% yield. Palladium-catalyzed Heck installation of n-hexenyl fragment **9** and subsequent hydrogenation of the olefin with concomitant removal of the Boc protecting group delivered macrocycle precursor **11** with 96% yield across three steps. Next, an intramolecular lactamization reaction furnished the macrocyclic system **12** in 57% yield. Saponification of the prolinate ester gave **13** in excellent yield. This acid was then coupled with cyclopropylamine **14** under standard coupling conditions to achieve vaniprevir in 87% yield.

The preparation of hexenyl fragment **9** started with the lithiation of commercially available ethyl isobutyrate **16** and homoallylative quench with 1-bromo-4-butene **15** to provide hexenyl ester **17** in 88% yield. Next, DIBAL-H reduction followed by CDI-mediated carbamate formation with L-t-leucine **19** and subsequent treatment with DCHA furnished the key hexenyl fragment **9** with 85% yield over two steps.

The assembly of cyclopropylamine **14** began with condensation of the HCl salt of glycine ethyl ester **21** with benzaldehyde **20** to furnish imine **22** in 97% yield, which then underwent a well-designed bis-alkylation reaction whereby lithiation of the glycine derivative followed by an S_N2 reaction afforded vinyl cyclopropane **24** in 65% yield after acid-base workup. Boc-protection and enzymatic resolution with alcalase gave a 47% yield of enantiopure **26** in >99% ee. Saponification of the ester and CDI-promoted amide bond formation provided **29** in 92% yield. Finally, catalytic hydrogenation of the olefin and TsOH salt formation gave key fragment **14** in 67% yield over two steps and 3% overall yield.[4-6]

[4] Song, Z. J.; Wang, Y.; Artino, L. M., et al. WO2011025849A1, **2011**.
[5] Song, Z. J.; Wang, Y.; Artino, L. M., et al. US8637449B2, **2014**.
[6] Song, Z. J.; Tellers, D. M.; Journet, M., et al. *J. Org. Chem.* **2011**, *76*, 7804-7815.

# Route 3

Hex-Li: Hexyllithium
DMPU: 1,3-Dimethyl-3,4,5,6-tetrahydro-2(1*H*)-pyrimidinone
DCHA: Dicyclohexylamine
HOPO: 2-Hydroxypyridine-*N*-oxide

*Synthetic Route:*    To deliver an alternative coupling process to avoid the key Heck reaction, which resulted in a 13% yield loss due to regioisomer formation, the use of a Sonogashira-type coupling was also disclosed in the same reference[4-6], which diminish the regioisomer issue.    The preparation of the alkyne linker relied upon a key "zipper" reaction to convert an internal alkyne **4** to the required terminal alkyne **6** in 80% yield.    Subsequent carbamate formation with CDI and tert-butylglycine **7** followed by treatment with DCHA yielded the salt of alkyne linker **8** with 72% yield over two steps.    The Sonogashira reaction of **8** and aryl bromide **9** was mediated by the X-Phos/Pd(II) catalyst.    In contrast to the Heck reaction, this Sonogashira coupling step proceeded in a near quantitative yield without production of multiple isomers.    Subsequent hydrogenation of this coupling product **10** yielded precursor **11** in excellent yield across two steps.    The overall yield of this Sonogashira amendment was 37%, ~10%-15% higher than the original Heck route due to the absence of regioisomers generated.[4-6]

[4]   Song, Z. J.; Wang, Y.; Artino, L. M., et al. WO2011025849A1, **2011**.
[5]   Song, Z. J.; Wang, Y.; Artino, L. M., et al. US8637449B2, **2014**.
[6]   Song, Z. J.; Tellers, D. M.; Journet, M., et al. *J. Org. Chem.* **2011**, *76*, 7804-7815.

# 4 Pharmacology

## Summary

Mechanism of Action

❖ Vaniprevir is a reversible, macrocyclic inhibitor of HCV NS3/4A protease which is essential for HCV replication. HCV NS3/4A protease is involved in proteolytic processing of the HCV nonstructural polyprotein by cleaving four known sites along the virally encoded polyprotein.

❖ In a biochemical assay, vaniprevir inhibited the proteolytic activity of recombinant HCV NS3/4A proteases from all 6 HCV genotypes.
- Genotype 1a/1b, 2a, 4a, 5a, 6a: $IC_{50}$ = 0.016-0.54 nM.
- Genotype 2b: $IC_{50}$ = 1.4 nM.
- Genotype 3a: $IC_{50}$ = 53 nM.
- Mutant genotype 1b: $IC_{50}$ = 6-101 nM.

❖ Vaniprevir showed high selectivities (>10000 folds) for a panel of 169 receptors, ion channels and enzymes.

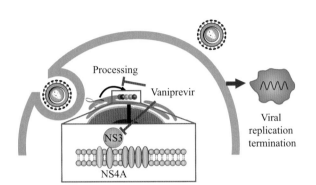

*In Vitro* Efficacy

❖ Anti-HCV replicons in HCV replicon cells:
- GT 1a/1b: $EC_{50}$ = 1-3 nM, $EC_{90}$ = 3.9-4 nM.
- GT 2a: $EC_{50}$ = 2.7-7 nM, $EC_{90}$ = 35.5 nM.
- GT 2b/5a: $EC_{50}$ = 1.8-61 nM, $EC_{90}$ = 5.9-157 nM.
- GT 3a: $EC_{50}$ = 70 nM, $EC_{90}$ = 337 nM.

❖ Inhibitions of vaniprevir in the presence of human serum proteins in Con1 cell line:
- GT 1b 50% NHS: 5.7 folds increase in $EC_{50}$.
- GT 1b 40% NHS: 3.1 folds increase in $EC_{50}$.

❖ Substitution changes during vaniprevir selection:
- GT 1a/1b mutation in NS3/4A: A156 and D168.

❖ Anti-HCV activities against HCV containing NS3/4A substitutions in cell culture:
- GT 1a in replicon assays:
  ◆ V36, Q41, T54, V55, Q80, V107: $EC_{50}$ = 0.5-2.1 nM (0.6-2.3 folds change).
  ◆ R155, D168A/E: $EC_{50}$ = 39.9->1000 nM (44.3->1000 folds change).
  ◆ A156S, V158I, D168N: $EC_{50}$ = 1.0-6.3 nM (1.1-7 folds change).
- GT 1b in replicon assays:
  ◆ V36, Q41, T54, V55, Q80: $EC_{50}$ = 0.7-14.6 nM (0.4-7.7 folds).
  ◆ R155, A156, D168: $EC_{50}$ = 29->2000 nM (15.3->1000 folds).
  ◆ A156S, D168N, V170: $EC_{50}$ = 5.0-9.7 nM (2.6-5.1 folds).
- GT 1a in transient assays: R155, A156, D168: 21.5-346 folds.
- GT 1b in transient assays:
  ◆ V36, Q41, F43, T54, T55, Y56, R109, I153: 0.3-9.9 folds.
  ◆ R155, A156, D168, V170: 32-463 folds.
  ◆ A156S, V163I, V170I: 0.4-3.7 folds.
- HCV from clinical:
  ◆ GT 1a/1b mutation: $EC_{50}$ = 2.9-27 nM.

*In Vivo* Efficacy

❖ The effects of vaniprevir on HCV-infected chimpanzee:
- HCV genotype 1a infection.
  ◆ Decrease 5 Log IU/mL in plasma at 5 mg/kg BID and 2-3 Log at 1 mg/kg BID.
- HCV genotype 1b infection:
  ◆ Reduced viral load for 2-3 Log IU/mL at 1 mg/kg BID.

❖ HCV genotype 3a infection: The viral load was reduced to 10% at 5 mg/kg.

# Mechanism of Action

Table 3    The Activity and Selectivity of Vaniprevir against NS3/4A Proteases in Wild Type and Mutant HCV Genotypes[7, 8]

| NS3/4A Proteases Genotype | IC$_{50}$ ± SD (nM) | NS3/4A Proteases Genotype/Mutation | $K_i$ ± SD (nM) | Fold Change |
|---|---|---|---|---|
| GT 1a | 0.028 ± 0.003 | GT 1b (BK) Wild type | 0.079 | 1 |
| GT 1b | 0.016 ± 0.004 | GT 1b V36A/L/M | 0.08-0.16 | 1.0-2.1 |
| GT 2a | 0.540 ± 0.016 | GT 1b R155K/Q | 18.9/47 | 239/595 |
| GT 2b | 1.4 ± 0.10 | GT 1b A156S | 0.200 | 2.5 |
| GT 3a | 53 ± 5 | GT 1b A156T/V | 15.7/88.1 | 199/>1000 |
| GT 4a | 0.10 ± 0.02 | GT 1b D168E | 0.544 | 6.9 |
| GT 5a | 0.160 ± 0.07 | GT 1b D168V/Y | 82/120 | >1000 |
| GT 6a | 0.07 ± 0.02 | GT 1b V170A | 0.061 | 0.8 |
| GT 1b R155K | 9 ± 4 | GT 1a Wild type | 0.074 | 1 |
| GT 1b A156T | 6 ± 1 | GT 1a R155K | 34 | 459 |
| GT 1b A156V | 57 ± 5 | GT 2a (JFH) Wild type | 0.904 | 2 |
| GT 1b D168Y | 101 ± 15 | GT 2a D168A/E | 150/2.8 | 166/3.1 |

GT: Genotype.    IC$_{50}$: 50% inhibitory concentration.    SD: The detected of enzyme inhibition of protease using Time-Resolved Fluorescence assay (TRF) to measure the IC$_{50}$ value of the compound.

Table 4    Off-Target Activity of Vaniprevir and Telaprevir[7, 9]

| Protease | IC$_{50}$ (nM) | |
|---|---|---|
| | Vaniprevir | Telaprevir |
| Chymotrypsin | 520 | 3000 |
| Trypsin | >10000 | >10000 |
| Cathepsin B | >10000 | 4400 |
| Cathepsin F | >10000 | >10000 |
| Cathepsin K | >10000 | 630 |
| Cathepsin L | >10000 | 3500 |
| Cathepsin S | >10000 | 300 |
| Cathepsin V | >10000 | 1350 |
| Chymase | >10000 | 30 |
| Pancreatic elastase 1 | >10000 | 30 |
| Neutrophil elastase 2 | >10000 | 8000 |

The selectivities of vaniprevir in non-target molecules were better than telaprevir.    In a broader MDS Pharma Services (Panlabs) screen performed to assess potential off-target activities, >10000-fold selectivity was observed against 169 receptors, enzymes and ion channels tested.

[7]    Japan Pharmaceuticals and Medical Devices Agency (PMDA) Database.    http://www.pmda.go.jp/drugs/2014/P201400135/index.html (accessed Mar 2016).
[8]    Kinoshita, K.; Iwasa, T.; Takase, A., et al. *Nihon Yakurigaku Zasshi.* **2015**, *146*, 159-170.
[9]    Liverton, N. J.; Carroll, S. S.; Dimuzio, J., et al. *Antimicrob. Agents Chemother.* **2010**, *54*, 305-311.

## *In Vitro* Efficacy

Table 5    Anti-HCV Activity of Vaniprevir in HCV Replication Cells[7, 8]

| HCV Genotype | NS3/4A | Replicon Strain | Assay | Efficacy (Mean ± SD, nM) | |
|---|---|---|---|---|---|
| | | | | EC$_{50}$ | EC$_{90}$ |
| GT 1b | Wild type | Con1 | HEPREP | 3 ± 1 | NA |
| | | | TaqMan | 1.9 ± 0.8 | 3.9 ± 2.1 |
| GT 2a | Wild type | JFH | HEPREP | 7 ± 2 | NA |
| | | | TaqMan | 2.7 ± 2.8 | 35.3 ± 11.5 |
| GT 1a | Wild type | H77 | TaqMan | 1 ± 0.7 | 4 ± 2.8 |
| GT 2b:2a | NS3/4A AY232740[a] | JFH | TaqMan | 31 ± 11 | 45 ± 9 |
| GT 2b:2a | NS3/4A AY232732[a] | JFH | TaqMan | 11.5 ± 0.7 | 40 ± 3 |
| GT 3a:2a | NS3/4A GU045445.1[a] | JFH | TaqMan | 70 ± 28 | 337 ± 68.8 |
| GT 5a:2a | NS3/4A AF 064490[a] | JFH | TaqMan | 1.8 ± 0.6 | 5.9 ± 0.6 |
| GT 5a:2a | NS3/4A GU 945429[a] | JFH | TaqMan | 61 ± 20 | 157 ± 10 |

Huh-7 cell with G T1b replicon (HB1): CC$_{50}$ = 58 nM

HEPREP: Hepatitis C replication.    NHS: Normal human serum.    NA: Not available.    [a] Genbank accession numbers, NS3/4A from genotype 2b/3a/5a expressed in genotype 2a HCV replicons.

Table 6    Inhibition of Vaniprevir in the Presence of Human Serum Proteins in Con1 Cell Line[7]

| HCV Genotype | Assay | Serum/Protein | Efficacy Mean ± SD (nM) | |
|---|---|---|---|---|
| | | | EC$_{50}$ | EC$_{90}$ |
| GT 1b | HEPREP | 10% FBS | 3 ± 1 | NA |
| | | 50% NHS | 17 ± 5 | NA |
| | TaqMan | 10% FBS | 1.9 ± 0.8 | 3.9 ± 2.1 |
| | | 40% NHS | 5.9 ± 1.4 | 25.0 ± 6.1 |

The effect of vaniprevir on HCV replication (HEPREP) was evaluated by RT-PCR (TaqMan) assay.    HEPREP: Hepatitis C replication.    NHS: Normal human serum. NA: Not available.

Table 7    Substitution Change During Vaniprevir Selection[7, 8]

| HCV Replicon Genotype | Vaniprevir (nM) | Mutant Strain (the number of colonies) |
|---|---|---|
| GT 1b | 20 | A156T (2), D168E/V/Y (8) |
| | 30 | D168H/V/Y (11) |
| | 40 | D168E/G/V/Y (10) |
| | 80 | D168V/Y (11) |
| GT 2a | 65 | D168E/Y (2) |
| | 325 | A156S (2), D168E (1) |

[7]  PMDA Database.    http://www.pmda.go.jp/drugs/2014/P201400135/index.html (accessed Mar 2016).
[8]  Kinoshita, K.; Iwasa, T.; Takase, A., et al. *Nihon yakurigaku zasshi.* **2015**, *146*, 159-170.

Table 8    Anti-HCV Activity of Vaniprevir against HCV Replicon Carrying NS3/4A Substitutions in Replicon Assays[7]

| NS3/4A Wild type and Mutation | Genotype 1a | | | | NS3/4A Wild type and Mutation | Genotype 1b | | | |
|---|---|---|---|---|---|---|---|---|---|
| | EC$_{50}$ (nM) | Fold | EC$_{90}$ (nM) | Fold | | EC$_{50}$ (nM) | Fold | EC$_{90}$ (nM) | Fold |
| Wild type (H77) | 0.9 ± 0.6 | 1 | 3.3 ± 2.4 | 1 | Wild type (con1) | 1.9 ± 0.8 | 1 | 3.9 ± 2.1 | 1 |
| V36A | 2.1 ± 1.3 | 2.3 | 7.0 ± 5.3 | 2.1 | V36A | 9.3 ± 7.3 | 4.9 | 16.6 ± 9.2 | 4.3 |
| V36L | 1.3 ± 0.4 | 1.4 | 4.7 ± 1.8 | 1.4 | V36L | 1.0 ± 0.7 | 0.5 | 2.8 ± 1.0 | 0.7 |
| V36M | 1.3 ± 0.9 | 1.4 | 4.5 ± 2.3 | 1.4 | V36M | 2.7 ± 1.4 | 1.4 | 8.5 ± 3.1 | 2.2 |
| Q41R | 1.6 ± 0.6 | 1.8 | 4.7 ± 1.9 | 1.4 | Q41L | 0.7 ± 0.5 | 0.4 | 2.2 ± 1.4 | 0.6 |
| T54A | 1.0 ± 0.7 | 1.1 | 2.5 ± 1.9 | 0.8 | Q41R | 2.1 ± 0.9 | 1.1 | 5.1 ± 2.0 | 1.3 |
| T54S | 1.4 ± 1.0 | 1.6 | 4.7 ± 3.6 | 1.4 | F43S | 14.6 ± 8.7 | 7.7 | 57.7 ± 33.4 | 14.8 |
| V55A | 1.6 ± 0.5 | 1.8 | 5.0 ± 0.3 | 1.5 | T54C | 6.0 ± 5.6 | 3.2 | 12.4 ± 8.0 | 3.2 |
| V55I | 0.5 ± 0.2 | 0.6 | 1.4 ± 0.5 | 0.4 | T54G | 5.6 ± 4.2 | 2.9 | 18.6 ± 12.5 | 4.8 |
| Q80K | 1.4 ± 0.8 | 1.6 | 4.5 ± 2.2 | 1.4 | V55A | 2.1 ± 1.1 | 1.1 | 4.8 ± 2.1 | 1.2 |
| Q80R | 1.6 ± 0.7 | 1.8 | 6.4 ± 2.6 | 1.9 | V55I | 1.7 ± 0.6 | 0.9 | 6.8 ± 2.8 | 1.7 |
| V107I | 0.7 ± 0.4 | 0.8 | 2.2 ± 1.1 | 0.7 | Y56F | 0.8 ± 0.3 | 0.4 | 3.9 ± 1.8 | 1.0 |
| R155K | >1000 | >1000 | >1000 | >250 | Y56H | 2.0 ± 0.8 | 1.1 | 5.5 ± 1.4 | 1.4 |
| R155T | 389 ± 115 | 432 | 933 ± 138 | 283 | Q80R | 1.1 ± 0.4 | 0.6 | 4.2 ± 1.4 | 1.1 |
| A156S | 5.1 ± 3.7 | 5.7 | 17.0 ± 9.1 | 5.2 | Q86R | 0.8 ± 0.5 | 0.4 | 3.2 ± 2.0 | 0.8 |
| V158I | 1.0 ± 0.4 | 1.1 | 4.1 ± 1.7 | 1.2 | V107I | 5.9 ± 5.4 | 3.1 | 14.9 ± 12.7 | 3.8 |
| D168A | >500 | >500 | >500 | >125 | R155G | 267 ± 204 | 142 | 586 ± 360 | 150 |
| D168E | 39.9 ± 32.1 | 44.3 | 193 ± 213 | 58 | R155K | 402 ± 194 | 212 | 945 ± 228 | 242 |
| D168N | 6.3 ± 4.0 | 7 | 27 ± 19 | 8.2 | R155Q | 240 ± 153 | 126 | 649 ± 214 | 166 |
| | | | | | R155W | 363 ± 154 | 191 | 707 ± 187 | 181 |
| | | | | | A156G | 29 ± 16 | 15.3 | 54 ± 11 | 13.8 |
| | | | | | A156S | 9.7 ± 3.1 | 5.1 | 50.0 ± 12.8 | 12.8 |
| | | | | | A156T | 95.8 ± 33.7 | 50 | 400 ± 164 | 103 |
| | | | | | A156V | 588 ± 163 | 309 | 4247 ± 123 | 1089 |
| | | | | | D168A | 277 ± 157 | 146 | >500 | >125 |
| | | | | | D168E | 37.0 ± 6.0 | 19.5 | 193 ± 82 | 49.5 |
| | | | | | D168G | 1093 ± 408 | 575 | 1715 ± 361 | 440 |
| | | | | | D168K | >2000 | >1000 | >2000 | >250 |
| | | | | | D168N | 5.0 ± 2.8 | 2.6 | 18.0 ± 12 | 4.6 |
| | | | | | D168T | >2000 | >1000 | >2000 | >250 |
| | | | | | D168V | 1160 ± 800 | 610 | >2000 | >500 |
| | | | | | D168Y | 491 ± 100 | 258 | 1262 ± 186 | 324 |
| | | | | | V170A | 5.4 ± 2.9 | 2.8 | 28.5 ± 11.5 | 7.3 |
| | | | | | V170T | 8.3 ± 6.1 | 4.5 | 16.2 ± 11.1 | 4.2 |

Fold: Compared to Wild type.

[7]  PMDA Database.   http://www.pmda.go.jp/drugs/2014/P201400135/index.html (accessed Mar 2016).

Table 9    Anti-HCV Activity of Vaniprevir against HCV Replicons Containing NS3/4A Substitutions in Transient Assay[7]

| Mutation | GT 1a (H77) | | GT 1b (con1) | |
|---|---|---|---|---|
| | EC$_{50}$ (nM) | Fold | EC$_{50}$ (nM) | Fold |
| Wild type | $4.5 \pm 1.8$ | 1 | $4.1 \pm 3.9$ | 1.0 |
| V36A | $15.7 \pm 7.5$ | 3.5 | $4.2 \pm 1.0$ | 1.0 |
| V36L | ND | – | $8.9 \pm 9.7$ | 2.2 |
| V36M | ND | – | $14.8 \pm 10.3$ | 3.6 |
| Q41R | ND | – | $3.7 \pm 0.6$ | 0.9 |
| F43S | ND | – | $40.5 \pm 6.4$ | 9.9 |
| T54A | ND | – | $4.7 \pm 2.7$ | 1.1 |
| T55S | ND | – | $1.5 \pm 0.5$ | 0.3 |
| Y56H | ND | – | $2.9 \pm 0.7$ | 0.7 |
| R109K | ND | – | $4.2 \pm 2.1$ | 1.0 |
| I153V | ND | – | $3.7 \pm 4.2$ | 0.9 |
| R155G | $1517 \pm 171$ | 337 | $1543 \pm 386$ | 376 |
| R155K | $422 \pm 101$ | 93.8 | $450 \pm 392$ | 110 |
| R155M | $149 \pm 102$ | 33.1 | $130 \pm 87.8$ | 32 |
| R155N | $262 \pm 91$ | 58.2 | $380 \pm 181$ | 93 |
| R155Q | $450 \pm 533$ | 100 | $600 \pm 278$ | 146 |
| R155S | $760 \pm 104$ | 169 | $320 \pm 185$ | 78 |
| R155T | $290 \pm 121$ | 64.4 | $420 \pm 216$ | 102 |
| A156N | $430 \pm 244$ | 95.6 | $300 \pm 91.7$ | 73 |
| A156S | ND | – | $15.0 \pm 17.1$ | 3.7 |
| A156T | $301 \pm 232$ | 66.9 | $440 \pm 191$ | 107 |
| A156V | $1555 \pm 744$ | 346 | $690 \pm 200$ | 161 |
| V163I | ND | – | $6.1 \pm 7.7$ | 1.5 |
| D168A | $798 \pm 390$ | 177 | $830 \pm 340$ | 202 |
| D168E | $96.7 \pm 89.6$ | 21.5 | $150 \pm 79.7$ | 36 |
| D168G | $790 \pm 95.4$ | 176 | $660 \pm 495$ | 161 |
| D168H | $1260 \pm 607$ | 280 | $550 \pm 455$ | 134 |
| D168V | $1473 \pm 1120$ | 327 | $450 \pm 331$ | 110 |
| D168Y | $1277 \pm 375$ | 284 | $1900 \pm 303$ | 463 |
| V170I | ND | – | $1.6 \pm 0.6$ | 0.4 |

Fold: Compared to wild type.    NS3/4A cloned expression transiently in cell culture.

[7] PMDA Database.    http://www.pmda.go.jp/drugs/2014/P201400135/index.html (accessed Mar 2016).

Table 10    The Inhibition of Vaniprevir on NS3/4A Proteases in Wild Type and Mutant HCV
Genotypes from Clinical Patient Isolates[7, 9]

| NS3/4A Origin | HCV Genotype | EC$_{50}$ (nM) |
|---|---|---|
| Con1 | 1b | 4.1 ± 3.9 |
| H77 | 1a | 4.5 ± 1.8 |
| Ps20 | 1b | 2.9 ± 1.1 |
| Ps30 | 1b | 27 ± 1.1 |
| Ps31 | 1b | 3.4 ± 4.0 |
| Ps32 | 1b | 3.8 ± 1.8 |
| Ps33 | 1b | 9.5 ± 0.3 |
| Ps36 | 1a | 4.9 ± 1.4 |
| Ps37 | 1a | 6.5 ± 1.9 |
| Ps38 | 1a | 6.0 ± 2.0 |
| Ps40 | 1a | 2.9 ± 1.2 |
| Ps41 | 1a | 19 ± 1.6 |

Data were the geometric averages of three or more determinations.

## *In Vivo* Efficacy

Table 11    The Effect of Vaniprevir in HCV-Infected Chimpanzees[7, 8]

| Infected HCV Genotype | Administration | | Finding |
|---|---|---|---|
| | Drug (mg/kg, p.o.) | Duration (Day) | |
| 1a | Vaniprevir: 5 | BID × 7 | Decreased 5 Log IU/mL in plasma. |
| | Vaniprevir: 1 | BID × 7, from Week 3 | The viral load has been reduced by 2-3 Log IU/mL. |
| | Vaniprevir: 1/Ribavirin: 4 g | BID × 7, from Week 3/QD × 28 | Ribavirin alone didn't suppress the growth of virus. No combination effect was observed in the two drugs. |
| | Vaniprevir: 5/MK-0608: 2 | BID × 84/QD × 47 | Suppressed the virus to the low limit of quantification. |
| | Vaniprevir: 1/MK-3281: 4 | BID × 7 | Decreased the viral load by 2-3 Log IU/mL in the HCV genotype 1a infection animal. |
| | | BID × 7 | |
| 1b | Vaniprevir: 1 | BID × 7, from Week 3 | Reduced 2-3 Log IU/mL viral load. |
| | Vaniprevir: 1/Ribavirin: 4 g | BID × 7, from Week 3/QD × 28 | No combination effect was observed in the two drugs. |
| | Vaniprevir: 1/MK-3281: 4 | BID × 7/BID × 7 | Reduced the viral load by 3-4 Log IU/mL in the HCV genotype 1b infection animal. |
| 3a | Vaniprevir: 5 | BID × 3 | The viral load was reduced to 10%. |

Using TaqMan HCV viral load assays for quantification of plasma viral load as RNA levels.

[7]  PMDA Database.   http://www.pmda.go.jp/drugs/2014/P201400135/index.html (accessed Mar 2016).
[8]  Kinoshita, K.; Iwasa, T.; Takase, A., et al. *Nihon Yakurigaku Zasshi.* **2015**, *146*, 159-170.
[9]  Liverton, N. J.; Carroll, S. S.; Dimuzio, J., et al. *Antimicrob. Agents Chemother.* **2010**, *54*, 305-311.

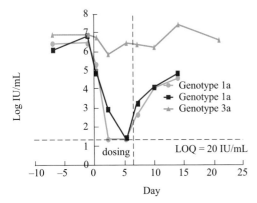

**Study:** HCV infection of chimpanzees.

**Animal:** Chimpanzee.

**Administration:** Vaniprevir, p.o., 5 mg/kg, genotype 1a BID × 7 days; genotype 3a, BID × 3 days.   Vehicle control: NA.

**Test:** Measured by RT-PCR (TaqMan) assay.

**Results**: Two cases of HCV genotype 1a infected chimpanzee showed a decrease of 5 Log IU/mL in plasma.   Viral load was observed in the second day and the fifth day after administration of the drug.   A decrease of about 1 Log IU / mL of plasma viral load was observed in HCV genotype 3a infected chimpanzee.

Figure A    The Infection of HCV Genotype 1a and 3a in Pan Troglodytes[7, 8]

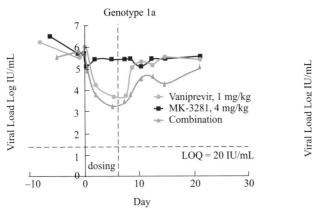 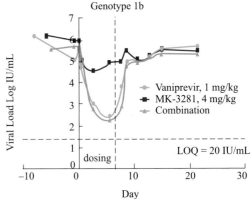

Figure B    The Combination of Vaniprevir with MK-3281 in HCV-infected Chimpanzees[7]

**Study:** The infection of HCV genotype 1a and 1b in chimpanzee.

**Animal:** Chimpanzee.

**Administration:** Vaniprevir, p.o., 1 mg/kg, BID × 7 days.   MK-3281, p.o., 4 mg/kg, BID × 7 days.   Vehicle control: NA.

**Test:** Measured by RT-PCR (TaqMan) assay.

**Results**: The combination of the two drugs decreased the virus in 2-3 Log IU/mL in the HCV genotype 1a infected animal.   The combination of the two drugs decreased the virus in 3-4 Log IU/mL in the HCV genotype 1b infected animal.   There were no synergy effect of the two drugs.

## 5   ADME & Drug-Drug Interaction

## Summary

Absorption of Vaniprevir

* Exhibited a non-linear pharmacokinetics in rats, dogs, monkeys and humans following oral dosing.   The increases in $C_{max}$ and AUC appeared to be more than dose-proportional in the dose range of 5 to 500 mg/kg (rats), 5-30 mg/kg (dogs), 5-100 mg/kg (monkeys), and 40-1000 mg (humans) of vaniprevir.
* Had low oral bioavailability in rats (0-5%), dogs (12%) and monkeys (2%).
* Was absorbed rapidly with the $T_{max}$ occurring 0.5 to 1.3 h in rats, dogs and monkeys after 5 mg/kg oral administration, and $T_{max}$ increased as the dose increased.   $T_{max}$ in humans was 1.01-4.0 h after oral administration.
* Showed a half-life ranging between 0.9-1.3 h in non-clinical species after intravenous administration, and the half-life in humans was 4.13-6.89 h after oral administration.
* Had high clearance in rats (74 mL/min/kg), but moderate in dogs (11 mL/min/kg) and monkeys (18 mL/min/kg), in contrast to liver blood flow, after intravenous administrations.   The clearance in humans was 45.3 L/h after 1000 mg oral administration.

[7]  PMDA Database.   http://www.pmda.go.jp/drugs/2014/P201400135/index.html (accessed Mar 2016).
[8]  Kinoshita, K.; Iwasa, T.; Takase, A., et al. *Nihon yakurigaku zasshi.* **2015**, *146*, 159-170.

❖ Exhibited a confined tissue distribution in rats, dogs and monkeys, with apparent volumes of distribution at 1.9, 0.3 and.0.4 L/kg, respectively, after intravenous administration.

## Distribution of Vaniprevir

❖ Exhibited very high plasma protein binding in mice (99.0%), rats (99.5%), rabbits (99.0%) and dogs (99.3%), and high in humans (97.7%-98.8%) and monkeys (98.2%-98.7%).　Note that vaniprevir mainly bound to HSA.

❖ Had a $C_b:C_p$ ratio of 0.8 in humans, suggesting little penetration into red blood cells.

❖ SD and Long-Evans male rats after a single oral administration:
  - Concentrations of radioactivity were measurable in the medulla of the brain at one sampling time, 4 h post-dose, all other lobes of the brain had no quantifiable radioactivity, suggesting that [$^{14}$C]vaniprevir has limited penetration of the blood brain barrier.
  - Relatively higher concentration levels were observed in GI tract contents, kidneys, stomach, small intestine and liver. Vaniprevir was not measurable at any collection time point in cerebellum, cerebrum, eye lens, olfactory lobe, and spinal cord.
  - Elimination of radioactivity from tissues was complete in the majority of tissues by 24 h post-dose.
  - The amount of radioactive equivalents was similar and low in both pigmented and non-pigmented rats indicating that vaniprevir did not bind to melanin.

❖ Vaniprevir exhibited good liver exposure in rats, dogs, and monkeys after oral administration.　The AUC ratios of vaniprevir in liver and plasma of rats, dogs, and monkeys after a 5 mg/kg oral dose were >874, 102 and 455, respectively. In rats, the liver exposure increased more than dose proportionally between 5 and 30 mg/kg, but less than dose proportionally between 30 and 300 mg/kg.　Liver exposure in dogs was more than dose proportional between 2 and 5 mg/kg.

## Metabolism of Vaniprevir

❖ Several metabolites of vaniprevir (M6, M7, M8, M9 and M10) were observed in liver microsomes or S9 and hepatocytes of humans, rats, dogs and mice.

❖ Overall, the parent drug represented the most abundant component in human and non-clinical species plasma, and metabolites were trace or below the limit of quantitation.

❖ Vaniprevir was mainly metabolized by CYP3A.

## Excretion of Vaniprevir

❖ Was predominantly excreted in feces in humans, with parent as the major component in human feces.

❖ About 52.1% and 53.0% of radioactivities were recovered *via* biliary excretion in bile duct-cannulated (BDC) rats and dogs.

## Drug-Drug Interaction

❖ Vaniprevir was an inhibitor of CYP3A ($IC_{50}$ = 18.8 μM) and UGT1A1 ($IC_{50}$ = 19 μM).

❖ Vaniprevir was not an inducer of CYP450 (CYP3A4, 2B6 or 1A2).

❖ Vaniprevir was a substrate of P-gp, OATP1B1 and OATP1B3, but not of BCRP.

❖ Vaniprevir had inhibition for P-gp ($IC_{50}$ = 38 μM), OATP1B1 ($IC_{50}$ = 0.3 μM), OATP1B3 ($IC_{50}$ = 0.3 μM), BESP ($IC_{50}$ = 1.3 μM), BCRP ($IC_{50}$ = 13 μM), MRP2 ($IC_{50}$ = 42.2 μM), MRP3 ($IC_{50}$ = 9.9 μM) and MRP4 ($IC_{50}$ = 8.0 μM).

## Absorption

Table 12　*In Vivo* Pharmacokinetic Parameters of Vaniprevir in Rats, Dogs, Monkeys and Chimpanzee after Single Intravenous and Oral Dose of Vaniprevir[7]

| Species | Route | Dose (mg/kg) | Vehicle | $T_{max}$ (h) | $C_{max}$ (μM) | $AUC_{0-24}$ (μM·h) | $T_{1/2}$ (h) | Cl (mL/min/kg) | $V_{ss}$ (L/kg) | F (%) |
|---|---|---|---|---|---|---|---|---|---|---|
| Rat (male) | i.v. | 2 | DMSO | NA | NA | 0.6 ± 0.1 | 0.9 ± 0.7 | 74 ± 9 | 1.9 ± 1.6 | - |
| | p.o. | 5 | PEG400 | 0.5 | 0-0.1 | 0.0-0.1 | NA | NA | NA | 0-5 |
| Rat (male) | p.o. | 30 | 10% Tween 80 | 1.0 ± 0.0 | 1.7 ± 1.0 | 3.4 ± 1.6 | NA | NA | NA | NA |
| | | 100 | | 4.7 ± 2.3 | 6.2 ± 3.4 | 30 ± 9 | NA | NA | NA | NA |
| | | 300 | | 24 ± 0 | 18.5 ± 14.0 | 217 ± 143 | NA | NA | NA | NA |
| | | 500 | | 18 ± 10 | 41.2 ± 23.7 | 604 ± 379 | NA | NA | NA | NA |
| Dog (male) | i.v. | 2 | DMSO | NA | NA | 4.1 ± 0.7 | 1.2 ± 0.0 | 11 ± 2 | 0.3 ± 0.1 | - |
| | p.o. | 5 | PEG400 | 1.3 ± 0.6 | 0.5 ± 0.2 | 1.2 ± 0.4 | NA | NA | NA | 12 ± 2 |

[7] PMDA Database.　http://www.pmda.go.jp/drugs/2014/P201400135/index.html (accessed Mar 2016).

*Continued*

| Species | Route | Dose (mg/kg) | Vehicle | $T_{max}$ (h) | $C_{max}$ ($\mu$M) | $AUC_{0-24}$ ($\mu$M·h) | $T_{1/2}$ (h) | Cl (mL/min/kg) | $V_{ss}$ (L/kg) | F (%) |
|---|---|---|---|---|---|---|---|---|---|---|
| Dog (male) | p.o. | 10 | 10% Tween 80 | 1 | 0.7 | 1.5 | NA | NA | NA | NA |
| | | 15 | | 1.0 ± 0.0 | 13 ± 12 | 19 ± 16 | NA | NA | NA | NA |
| | | 30 | | 6 | 14 | 93 | NA | NA | NA | NA |
| Monkey (male) | i.v. | 2 | DMSO | NA | NA | 2.5 ± 0.3 | 1.3 ± 0.2 | 18 ± 2.0 | 0.4 ± 0.1 | - |
| | p.o. | 5 | PEG400 | 1.3 ± 0.6 | 0.01-0.18 | 0.05-0.24 | NA | NA | NA | 2 ± 1 |
| Monkey (male) | p.o. | 50 | PEG400 | 4 | 0.8 | 3.1 | NA | NA | NA | NA |
| | p.o. | 100 | 10% Tween 80 | 3 | 26 | 126 | NA | NA | NA | NA |
| Chimpanzee (male & female[a]) | p.o. | 10 | Chocolate milk | 2, 4 | 0.7, 1.1 | 3.8, 6.5 | NA | NA | NA | NA |
| Rabbit (female) | p.o. | 240 | 10% Tween 80 | 1.3 ± 0.6 | 1.7 ± 0.2 | 7.5 ± 1.6 | NA | NA | NA | NA |

F% (0-5) for rats were calculated using mean i.v. $AUC_{0-2}$ and the lowest and mean p.o. $AUC_{0-2}$.   [a] The values were from one male chimpanzee and one female chimpanzee.   PEG: Polyethyleneglycol.

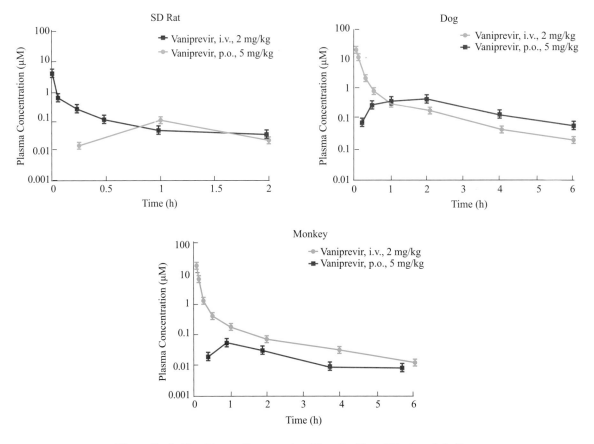

Figure C   *In Vivo* Plasma Concentration-Time Profiles of Vaniprevir in Rats, Dogs and Monkeys after Single Oral and Intravenous Dose of Vaniprevir[7]

[7]  PMDA Database.   http://www.pmda.go.jp/drugs/2014/P201400135/index.

Table 13    *In Vivo* Pharmacokinetic Parameters of Vaniprevir in Healthy Male Japanese after Single Oral Dose of Vaniprevir[7]

| Species | Route | Dose (mg) | $T_{max}$ (h) | $C_{max}$ (μM) | $AUC_{inf}$ (μM·h) | $AUC_{0-24}$ (μM·h) | $T_{1/2}$ (h) | Cl/F (L/h) | F (%) |
|---|---|---|---|---|---|---|---|---|---|
| | p.o. | 40 | 1.5 (1.0-2.02) | 0.02 (0.015-0.028) | 0.071 (0.055-0.091) | 0.055 (0.042-0.072) | 5.89 (18) | NA | NA |
| | p.o. | 75 | 1.01 (0.50-2.00) | 0.083 (0.059-0.116) | 0.174 (0.135-0.225) | 0.162 (0.124-0.212) | 6.89 (47) | NA | NA |
| | p.o. | 200 | 1.75 (1.50-3.00) | 0.319 (0.229-0.444) | 0.933 (0.724-1.20) | 0.918 (0.703-1.20) | 5.96 (22) | NA | NA |
| Healthy Japanese | p.o. | 400 | 2.0 (1.50-3.00) | 1.59 (1.14-2.22) | 3.15 (2.44-4.06) | 3.09 (2.36-4.04) | 4.59 (25) | NA | NA |
| | p.o. | 600 | 3.0 (2.00-4.00) | 3.74 (2.69-5.20) | 8.82 (6.85-11.4) | 8.71 (6.67-11.4) | 4.13 (6) | NA | NA |
| | p.o. | 800 | 3.02 (3.00-6.00) | 6.35 (4.55-8.87) | 16.6 (12.9-21.5) | 16.4 (12.6-21.5) | 4.14 (20) | NA | NA |
| | p.o. | 1000 | 4.00 (3.00-4.00) | 9.44 (6.79-13.1) | 30.5 (23.7-39.3) | 30.2 (23.2-39.5) | 4.27 (40) | 45.3 (49) | 0.175 (44) |

The values of $T_{1/2}$ and Cl/F were geometric mean (CV%), others were median (minimal-maximum).

## Distribution

Table 14    *In Vitro* Plasma Protein Binding and Blood Partitioning of Vaniprevir in Several Species[7]

| | Plasma Protein Binding% | | | | | Blood Partitioning | | |
|---|---|---|---|---|---|---|---|---|
| Species | Conc. (μM)[a] | %Bound | Species | Category | %Bound[b] | Species | Conc. (μM)[c] | $C_b$:$C_p$ |
| Mouse | 10 | 99.0 ± 0.0 | Humans | HSA (40 mg/mL) | 95.3 ± 0.9 | Rat | 0.1 | 0.7 ± 0.1 |
| Rat | 1-10 | 99.5 ± 0.1 | | | | | 1 | 0.7 ± 0.0 |
| Rabbit | 10 | 99.0 ± 0.2 | Humans | AGP (1 mg/mL) | 60.9 ± 7.3 | | 10 | 0.8 ± 0.3 |
| Dog | 1-10 | 99.3 ± 0.0 | | | | | 0.1 | 0.8 ± 0.4 |
| Monkey | 0.1-10 | 98.2 ± 0.1-98.7 ± 0.1 | Hepatic insufficient humans[d] | Mild | 97.0 ± 0.7 | Dog | 1 | 0.7 ± 0.1 |
| Chimpanzee | 10 | 98.9 ± 0.1 | | Moderate | 97.3 ± 0.6 | | 10 | 0.7 ± 0.3 |
| Human | 0.1-10 | 97.7 ± 0.3-98.8 ± 0.5 | | Severe | 97.5 | Human | 0.1-10 | 0.8 ± 0.0 |

$C_b$:$C_p$ = Blood to plasma concentration ratio.    [a] [³H]/[¹⁴C]Vaniprevir.    [b] Vaniprevir.    [c] [³H]Vaniprevir.    [d] The concentration of vaniprevir was 10 μM.

Table 15    *In Vivo* Tissue Distribution of [¹⁴C]Vaniprevir in Rats after Single Oral Dose of 60 mg/kg Vaniprevir[7]

| Tissues | SD Rat/Male | | | | | Long-Evans Rat/Male | | | |
|---|---|---|---|---|---|---|---|---|---|
| | Radioactivity (ng eq./g) | | | | | Radioactivity (ng eq./g) | | | |
| | 2 h | 4 h | 24 h | 72 h | 168 h | 4 h | 24 h | 168 h | 672 h |
| Blood | 5730 | 8910 | ND | ND | ND | 9400 | ND | ND | ND |
| Kidneys | 9060 | 10600 | ND | ND | ND | 3770 | ND | ND | ND |
| Liver | 145000 | 126000 | 1850 | 263 | BLQ | 140000 | 2070 | BLQ | ND |
| Adrenal gland | 6480 | 8360 | ND | ND | ND | 2830 | ND | ND | ND |
| Lungs | 4720 | 4870 | ND | ND | ND | 1950 | ND | ND | ND |
| Fat (brown) | 6730 | 9230 | ND | ND | ND | 2040 | ND | ND | ND |
| Large intestine contents | 1340 | 1100000 | 83200 | 279 | ND | 44800 | 126000 | 331 | ND |
| Large intestine | 1680 | 4730 | 397 | ND | ND | 1470 | 576 | ND | ND |
| Small intestine contents | 907000 | 2600000 | 26100 | ND | ND | 190000 | 4680 | ND | ND |
| Stomach contents | 1590000 | 1940000 | 275000 | ND | ND | 910000 | 1450 | ND | ND |

BLQ: Below the limit of quantitation (<244 ng equivalents [¹⁴C]vaniprevir/g).

[7]  PMDA Database.    http://www.pmda.go.jp/drugs/2014/P201400135/index.html (accessed Mar 2016).

Table 16   *In Vivo* Liver and Plasma Exposure in Rats, Dogs and
Monkeys after Single Oral Dose of Vaniprevir[7]

| Species | Route | Dose (mg/kg) | Plasma AUC (μM·h) | Liver AUC (μM·h) | Liver/Plasma AUC Ratio |
|---------|-------|--------------|-------------------|------------------|------------------------|
| Rat | p.o. | 5 | <0.1 | 87.4 | >874 |
|  | p.o. | 30 | 0.952 | 1597 | 1678 |
|  | p.o. | 300 | 183 | 6728 | 37 |
| Dog | p.o. | 2 | 0.22 ± 0.13 | 21.2 ± 8.1 | 96 |
|  | p.o. | 2 | 7.2 ± 1.1 | 406 ± 94 | 56 |
|  | p.o. | 5 | 2.238 | 228 | 102 |
| Monkey | p.o. | 5 | 0.062 | 28.2 | 455 |

## Metabolism

### Key Findings:[7]

❖  Vaniprevir was mainly metabolized by CYP3A.

Table 17   Metabolites in *In Vitro* S9, Hepatocytes and *In Vivo* Plasma, Bile and Feces in Humans and Non-clinical Test Species
after Single Intravenous and Oral Dose of Vaniprevir[7]

| Matrix | Species | Route | Dose (mg/kg) | Time (h) | % of Radioactivity | | | | | | | | | | | |
|--------|---------|-------|--------------|----------|-----|-----|-----|-----|-----|-----|-----|-----|-----|-----|-----|-----|
| | | | | | M0 | M1 | M3 | M4 | M5 | M6 | M7 | M8 | M9 | M10 | M13 | M14 |
| S9 | Rat | *In vitro* | 10 μM | 4 | NA | - | - | - | - | - | - | - | - | √ | NA | NA |
| | Dog | | | | NA | - | - | - | - | - | - | - | - | - | NA | NA |
| | Rabbit | | | | NA | - | √ | - | - | √ | √ | √ | √ | √ | NA | NA |
| | Mouse | | | | NA | - | √ | - | - | √ | √ | √ | √ | √ | NA | NA |
| | Human | | | | NA | - | - | - | - | - | √ | √ | √ | √ | NA | NA |
| Hepatocytes | Rat | *In vitro* | 10 μM | 4 | NA | - | - | - | - | - | - | - | - | - | NA | NA |
| | Dog | | | 4 | NA | - | - | - | - | - | - | √ | - | - | NA | NA |
| | Mouse | | | 4 | NA | - | √ | - | - | √ | √ | √ | √ | √ | NA | NA |
| | Human | | | 4 | NA | - | - | - | - | - | - | - | √ | √ | NA | NA |
| Plasma | Mouse | p.o. | 300 | NA | √ | NA | NA | NA | NA | √ | √ | √ | √ | √ | NA | NA |
| | Rat | p.o. | 114 | NA | √ | - | - | - | - | trace | trace | trace | trace | trace | - | - |
| | Dog | p.o. | 5 | NA | √ | - | - | - | - | - | - | - | - | - | - | - |
| | Human | p.o. | 575 mg | 2 | √ | - | - | - | - | - | - | - | - | - | - | - |
| Urine | Dog | p.o. | 5 | 0-172 | The amount of radioactivity recovered in urine was too low to profile. | | | | | | | | | | | |
| | Rat | i.v. | 2 | 0-72 | 33 | Oxidative metabolites : 67 (M6, M7, M8, M9, M10) | | | | | | | | | | |
| Bile | Rat | i.v. | 2 | 0-72 | NA | - | √ | - | - | √ | √ | √ | √ | - | - | - |
| | Dog | p.o. | 5 | 0-72 | 30 | Oxidative metabolites : 70 (M6, M7, M8, M9, M10) | | | | | | | | | | |
| Feces | Mouse | p.o. | 300 | NA | √ | - | - | - | - | √ | √ | √ | √ | √ | NA | NA |
| | Rat | p.o. | 60 | 0-24 | 37.9 | - | - | - | - | 3.1 | 2.2 | 2.3 | 1.4 | 24.3 | 2.4 | - |
| | Dog | p.o. | 5 | 0-24 | 18.4 | 1.6 | 1.6 | 3.4 | 4.7 | 10.1 | 17.2 | 6.0 | 1.0 | 8.6 | - | 1.1 |
| | Rabbit | p.o. | 240 | 0-72 | √ | NA | NA | NA | NA | √ | √ | √ | √ | √ | NA | NA |
| | Human | p.o. | 575 mg | 0-96 | 23.1 | 4.9 | 2.9 | 2.2 | 6.1 | 5.3 | 6.3 | 1.5 | 3.1 | 19.7 | - | 6.2 |
| | Mouse | p.o. | 300 | NA | √ | - | - | - | - | √ | √ | √ | √ | √ | NA | NA |

√: Detected.   -: Not observed.   NA: Not available.

---

[7]  PMDA Database.   http://www.pmda.go.jp/drugs/2014/P201400135/index.html (accessed Mar 2016).

Figure D    Proposed Pathways for *In Vivo* Biotransformation of Vaniprevir in Mice, Rats, Dogs and Humans after Single Oral Dose of Vaniprevir[7]

The red labels represent the major components in matrices.    P = Plasma, U = Urine, B = Bile and F = Feces.

[7]  PMDA Database.    http://www.pmda.go.jp/drugs/2014/P201400135/index.html (accessed Mar 2016).

## Excretion

Table 18    Excretion Profiles of [$^{14}$C or $^3$H]Vaniprevir in Various Species after Single Intravenous
and Oral Dose of Vaniprevir[7]

| Species | State | Route | Dose (mg/kg) | Time (h) | Bile (% of dose) | Urine (% of dose) | Feces (% of dose) | Recovery (% of dose) |
|---------|-------|-------|--------------|----------|------------------|-------------------|-------------------|----------------------|
| Rat | BDC | i.v. | 2 | 0-72 | 52.1 | 15.6 | 4.2 | 71.7 |
| Rat | Intact | p.o. | 60 | 0-240 | NS | 0.5 ± 0.5 | 81.3 ± 6.7 | 81.8 ± 6.3 |
| Dog | BDC | i.v. | 2 | 0-72 | 53.0 ± 3.3 | 3.5 ± 2.9 | 12.0 ± 4.8 | 68.5 ± 6.3 |
| Dog | Intact | p.o. | 5 | 0-172 | NS | 0.78 ± 0.4 | 87.3 ± 6.43 | 91.5 ± 4.26 |
| Rabbit | Intact | p.o. | 240 | 0-72 | NS | 0.5 ± 0.1 | 66.9 ± 14.1 | 67.3 ± 14.1 |
| Human | Intact | p.o. | 575 mg | 0-168 | NS | 0.4 ± 0.2 | 95.5 ± 1.2 | 96.0 ± 1.1 |

NS: Not studied.

## Drug-Drug Interaction

Table 19    *In Vitro* Evaluation of Vaniprevir as an Inhibitor and an Inducer of Enzymes[7]

| Vaniprevir as an Inhibitor | | Vaniprevir as an Inducer | | |
|---------|-----------|--------|------------|---------------------|
| Enzyme | IC$_{50}$ (µM) | Enzyme | Conc.(µM) | % of Positive Control |
| CYP1A2 | >50 | | | |
| CYP2C8 | >50 | CYP3A | 20 | 18 |
| CYP2C9 | 26.4 | | | |
| CYP2C19 | >50 | | | |
| CYP2B6 | 50.6 | CYP2B6 | 20 | No |
| CYP3A[a] | 18.8 | | | |
| CYP3A[b] | 28.4 | CYP1A2 | 20 | No |
| UGT1A1 | 19 | | | |

[a] Midazolam 1'-hydroxylation.    [b] Testosterone 6β-hydroxylation.

Table 20    *In Vitro* Evaluation of Vaniprevir as an Inhibitor and a Substrate of Transporters[7]

| Transporter | Vaniprevir as a Substrate | | | | Vaniprevir as an Inhibitor, IC$_{50}$ (µM) | | | | | | | |
|-------------|------|------|---------|---------|------|---------|---------|------|------|------|------|------|
| | P-gp | BCRP | OATP1B1 | OATP1B3 | P-gp | OATP1B1 | OATP1B3 | BESP | BCRP | MRP2 | MRP3 | MRP4 |
| Results | Yes | No | Yes | Yes | 38 | 0.30 | 0.30 | 1.3 | 13 | 42.2 | 9.9 | 8.0 |

## 6    Non-Clinical Toxicology

### Summary

Single-Dose Toxicity
❖ Acute toxicity by the oral route in rodents:
  • Mouse MTD: 2000 mg/kg.

Repeated-Dose Toxicity
❖ Sub- and chronic toxicological potential by the oral route in rats (up to 6 months) and dogs (up to 9 months):
  • As the longest studies employed, the NOAEL in rats was 120 mg/kg/day (8.3 × MRHD), while that in dogs was 15 mg/kg/day (2.9 × MRHD).
  • The cross-species adverse effects concentrated on liver and biliary system disorders which can be monitored clinically. Furthermore, all lesions were identified mild, and given that both liver and gall bladder epithelium were regenerative. Hypernomic concern should not be required.

[7]  PMDA Database.   http://www.pmda.go.jp/drugs/2014/P201400135/index.html (accessed Mar 2016).

Safety Pharmacology

❖ No apparent toxicity was observed in the core battery of safety pharmacology studies.

Genotoxicity

❖ No genetic risk was verified by the standard battery of genotoxicity assays.

Reproductive and Developmental Toxicity

❖ Fertility and early embryonic development in rats:
  • The NOAEL was 250 mg/kg/day (HD) for both males and females.
❖ Embryo-fetal development in rats and rabbits:
  • The maternal NOAEL was 120 mg/kg/day (3.8 × MRHD) in rats and 120 mg/kg/day (0.37 × MRHD) in rabbits. The NOAEL for fetus was 120 mg/kg/day (3.8 × MRHD) in rats and 240 mg/kg/day (2.0 × MRHD) in rabbits.
❖ Pre- and postnatal development in rats:
  • The NOAEL was determined as 120 and 180 mg/kg/day for $F_0$ and $F_1$ in rats.
❖ Vaniprevir can be transferred through placenta and excreted through milk.

Carcinogenicity

❖ There was non-neoplastic findings up to 26 weeks in transgenic mice or up to 104 weeks in rats.

Special toxicity

❖ Vaniprevir had no absorption within the range of natural light (290-700 nm), and distributed rarely to light-exposed tissues (e.g., skin, eyes), so it would hardly cause phototoxicity.[7]

## Single-Dose Toxicity

Table 21　Single-Dose Toxicity Studies of Vaniprevir by Oral Administration[7]

| Species | Dose (mg/kg) | MTD (mg/kg) | Finding |
|---------|--------------|-------------|---------|
| ICR mouse | 2000 | 2000 | Eyelid ptosis, loose stools, decreased locomotor activity. |

Vehicle: 10% (w/v) Tween 80.

## Repeated-Dose Toxicity

Table 22　Repeated-Dose Toxicity Studies of Vaniprevir by Oral Administration[7]

| Species | Duration | Dose (mg/kg/day) | NOAEL Dose (mg/kg/day) | NOAEL $AUC_{0-24}$[a] (µM·h) | NOAEL Safety Margin[b] (× MRHD) | Finding |
|---------|----------|------------------|------|------|------|---------|
| SD rat | 5 weeks | 40, 100, 250 | 100 | 52.7 | 2.1 | Salivation, loose stools, slight increase of total bilirubin and white blood cells (2-fold in males), loss of body weight in one case and reduction of reticulocytes and mucous stool were observed at 250 mg/kg/day. A dose-dependent increase in relative histopathological changes. |
| | 6 months | 60, 120, 360 | 120 | 209 | 8.3 | Mortality, severe weight loss, deteriorated physiological condition, serum biochemical changes indicated liver toxicity, and centrilobular hepatocellular hypertrophies with an increase in liver weight were observed at 360 mg/kg/day. |
| Beagle dog | 5 weeks | 0, 15, 30, 250 | 30 | 83.3 | 3.3 | One female was dead in 250 mg/kg/day group. Salivation, liquid stool, vomiting, reduction of body weight and food consumption were observed at 250 mg/kg/day. A dose-dependent increase in relative histopathological changes. |
| | 9 months | 5/10, 15, 45/30, 150/75[c] | 15 | 72.3 | 2.9 | Mortality and deteriorated physiological condition were observed at 75 mg/kg/day. Necrosis of liver cell with an increase of liver enzyme levels (8-fold) and vacuolization of gallbladder epithelium were observed at 45/30 mg/kg/day. |

Vehicle: 10% (w/v) Tween 80.　[a] Male/Female.　[b] Calculated with MRHD exposure of 300 mg (BID), i.e., 25.3 µM·h.　[c] Dose shift during the study.

[7] PMDA Database.　http://www.pmda.go.jp/drugs/2014/P201400135/index.html (accessed Mar 2016).

## Safety Pharmacology

Table 23　Safety Pharmacology Studies of Vaniprevir[7]

| Study | System | Dose | Finding |
|---|---|---|---|
| Neurobehavioral effect | FOB in SD rats (male and female) | 40, 100, 250 mg/kg/day, p.o. for 5 weeks | No observed baneful effect on neurological function, i.e., general behavior, spontaneous action, nervous reflex and thermoregulation. |
| | FOB in conscious CD-1 mice | 100 mg/kg, p.o. | |
| Cardiovascular function | CHO-K1 cell expressing hERG channel | 3, 10, 30 μM | The inhibition of hERG was 36% at 30 μM. |
| | Unanesthetized Beagle dog | 15, 30, 250 mg/kg, p.o. | No effect on the monitored parameters, i.e., HR, artery pressure (SBP, DBP and MAP), ECG (PR, QRS, QT and QTcf intervals). |
| | Hybrid dog (Anesthesia, vagotomy, artificial respiration) | 1, 3, 10 mg/kg, i.v. | |
| Respiratory function | Unanesthetized SD rat | 40, 100, 250 mg/kg, p.o. | No anomaly on respiratory rate, tidal volume, min ventilation and PenH (airway resistance index). |

## Genotoxicity

Table 24　Genotoxicity Studies of Vaniprevir[7]

| Assay | Species/System | Metabolism | Dose | Finding |
|---|---|---|---|---|
| In vitro bacterial reverse mutation assay (Ames) | S. typhimurium TA1535, TA97a, TA98, TA100; E. coli WP2uvrA pKM101 | ±S9 | 30-6000 μg/plate | Negative. |
| In vitro mammalian cell chromosomal aberration study | CHO | ±S9 | 5-100 μM | Negative. |
| In vivo bone marrow micronucleus test | ICR mouse | + | 500, 1000, 2000 mg/kg, p.o. | Negative. |

Vehicle: 10% (w/v) Tween 80 for in vivo tests, DMSO for in vitro tests.

## Reproductive and Developmental Toxicity

Table 25　Embryonic and Developmental Toxicology Studies of Vaniprevir by Oral Administration[7]

| Study | Species | Dose (mg/kg/day) | NOAEL | | | | Finding |
|---|---|---|---|---|---|---|---|
| | | | Endpoint | Dose (mg/kg/day) | $AUC_{0-24}$ (μM·h) | Safety Margin[a] (× MRHD) | |
| Fertility and early embryonic development | SD rat | 60, 120, 250 | Male fertility | 250 | 818 | 32.3 | No drug-related adverse effect on mating performance, fertility and embryo/fetal survival rate, and no harm to male/female reproductive organ. |
| | | | Female fertility | 250 | 378 | 14.9 | |
| Embryo-fetal development | SD rat | 60, 80, 120 | Maternal | 120 | 95 | 3.8 | No drug-related toxicological effect at either endpoint. |
| | | | Fetal development | 120 | 95 | 3.8 | |
| | Dutch Belted rabbit | 60, 120, 240 | Maternal | 120 | 9.42 | 0.37 | No drug-related toxicity except for excessive maternal weight loss at HD. |
| | | | Fetal development | 240 | 49.9 | 2.0 | |
| Pre- and postnatal development | SD rat | 80, 120, 180 | $F_0$ | 120 | 95.9 | 3.8 | Other than slight decrease of maternal body weight at HD, no observed anomaly at either endpoint. |
| | | | $F_1$ | 180 | 414 | 16.4 | |

Vehicle: 10% (w/v) Tween 80.　Safety margin was calculated with MRHD of 300 mg (BID) was 25.3 μM·h.

[7]　PMDA Database.　http://www.pmda.go.jp/drugs/2014/P201400135/index.html (accessed Mar 2016).

# Carcinogenicity

Table 26 Carcinogenicity Toxicity Studies of Vaniprevir by Oral Administration[7]

| Species | Duration (Week) | Dose (mg/kg/day) | $AUC_{0-24}$ at HD ($\mu M \cdot h$)[a] | Safety Margin[a] ($\times$ MRHD)[b] | Finding |
|---|---|---|---|---|---|
| CB6F1-non TgrasH2 mouse | 4 | 0, 75, 150, 300, 450, 900 | 278/290 | 11.0/11.5 | NOAEL: 300 mg/kg/day. Mice were found be dead at 900 and 450 mg/kg/day respectively. No explainable cause of death from the pathological findings. |
| B6F1-TgrasH2 mouse | 26 | 0, 75, 150, 300 | 278/290 | 11.0/11.5 | Negative. |
| SD rat | 104 | 0, 30, 60, 120 | 354/186 | 10.7 | Negative. |

Vehicle: 10% (w/v) Tween 80. [a] Male/Female. [b] Calculated with MRHD exposure of 300 mg (BID) , i.e., 25.3 $\mu M \cdot h$.

[7] PMDA Database. http://www.pmda.go.jp/drugs/2014/P201400135/index.html (accessed Mar 2016).

# CHAPTER

30

## Vonoprazan Fumarate

# Vonoprazan Fumarate

## (Takecab®)

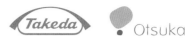

## 1  General Information

- ❖ Vonoprazan fumarate is a proton pump inhibitor (PPI), which was first approved in Dec 2014 by PMDA of Japan.

- ❖ Vonoprazan fumarate was discovered by Takeda, co-developed and co-marketed by Takeda and Otsuka.

- ❖ Vonoprazan fumarate belongs to potassium-competitive acid blockers (P-CAB), inhibiting $H^+$, $K^+$-ATPase (proton pump) which is the final step of acid secretion in the gastric parietal cells.

- ❖ Vonoprazan fumarate is indicated for gastric ulcer, duodenal ulcer and reflux esophagitis.

- ❖ Available as tablet, with each containing 10 mg or 20 mg of vonoprazan fumarate and the recommended dose is 20 mg orally once daily until disease progression or unacceptable toxicity.

- ❖ The sale of Takecab® was not available up to Mar 2016.

### Key Approvals around the World*

| | Japan (PMDA) |
|---|---|
| First approval date | 12/26/2014 |
| Application or approval No. | 22600AMX01389; 22600AMX01390 |
| Brand name | Takecab® |
| Indication | Gastric ulcer, Duodenal ulcer and Reflux esophagitis |
| Authorisation holder | Takeda; Otsuka |

* Till Mar 2016, it had not been approved by FDA (US), EMA (EU) and CFDA (China).

## Active Ingredient

*Molecular formula*: $C_{17}H_{16}FN_3O_2S \cdot C_4H_4O_4$
*Molecular weight*: 461.46
*CAS No.*: 881681-00-1 (Vonoprazan)
  1260141-27-2 (Vonoprazan fumarate)
*Chemical name*: 1-[5-(2-Fluorophenyl)-1-(pyridin-3-ylsulfonyl)-1H-pyrrol-3-yl]-N-methylmethanamine monofumarate

*Parameters of Lipinski's "Rule of 5"*

| MWᵃ | H_D | H_A | FRBᵇ | PSAᵇ | cLogPᵇ |
|---|---|---|---|---|---|
| 345.39 | 1 | 5 | 5 | 72.4Å² | 2.36 ± 0.56 |

ᵃ Molecular weight of vonoprazan.  ᵇ Calculated by ACD/Labs software V11.02.

## Drug Product*

*Dosage route*: Oral
*Strength*: 10 mg/20 mg (Vonoprazan)
*Dosage form*: Tablet
*Inactive ingredient*: D-mannitol, crystalline cellulose, croscarmellose sodium, hydroxypropyl cellulose, fumaric acid, magnesium stearate, hypromellose, macrogol 6000, titanium oxide (all tablets), yellow ferric oxide (10 mg tablets) and ferric oxide (20 mg tablets).
*Recommended dose*: The recommended starting dose is 20 mg orally once daily for adults (gastric ulcer, duodenal ulcer and reflux esophagitis).
  The recommended starting dose is 10 mg orally once daily for adults (gastric ulcer or duodenal ulcer at the time of low-dose aspirin administration; Gastric ulcer or duodenal ulcer at the time of non-steroidal anti-inflammatory drugs administration).

* Sourced from Japan PMDA drug label information

## 2 Key Patents Information

### Summary

❖ Takecab® (Vonoprazan fumarate) was approved by PMDA of Japan on Dec 26, 2014.

❖ Vonoprazan was originally discovered by Takeda and then co-developed by Otsuka, and its compound patent application was filed as PCT application by Takeda in 2006.

❖ The compound patent will expire in 2026 foremost, which has been granted in Japan, Europe, the United States and China successively.

Table 1    Vonoprazan's Compound Patent Protection in Drug-Mainstream Country

| Country | Publication/Patent NO. | Application Date | Granted Date | Estimated Expiry Date |
|---------|------------------------|------------------|--------------|------------------------|
| WO | WO2007026916A1 | 08/29/2006 | / | / |
| US | US7977488B2 | 08/29/2006 | 07/12/2011 | 08/11/2028[a] |
| | US8338461B2 | 08/29/2006 | 12/25/2012 | 08/29/2026 |
| EP | EP1919865B1 | 08/29/2006 | 04/06/2011 | 08/29/2026 |
| | EP2327692B1 | 08/29/2006 | 07/18/2012 | 08/29/2026 |
| JP | JP4035559B1 | 08/29/2006 | 01/23/2008 | 08/29/2031[b] |
| | JP5204426B2 | 08/29/2006 | 06/05/2013 | 08/29/2026 |
| CN | CN101300229B | 08/29/2006 | 10/05/2011 | 08/29/2026 |

[a] The term of this patent is extended by 713 days.    [b] The term of this patent is extended by 5 years.

Table 2    Originator's International Patent Application List (Patent Family)

| Publication NO. | Title | Applicant/Assignee/Owner | Publication Date |
|-----------------|-------|--------------------------|------------------|
| **Technical Subjects** | **Active Ingredient (Free Base)'s Formula or Structure and Preparation** | | |
| WO2007026916A1 | 1-Heterocyclylsulfonyl, 2-aminomethyl, 5-(hetero-) aryl substituted 1H-pyrrole derivatives as acid secretion inhibitors | Takeda | 03/08/2007 |
| **Technical Subjects** | **Salt, Crystal, Polymorphic, Solvate (Hydrate), Isomer, Derivative Etc. and Preparation** | | |
| WO2006036024A1 | Proton pump inhibitors | Takeda | 04/06/2006 |
| WO2010098351A1 | Process for producing pyrrole compound | Takeda | 09/02/2010 |
| WO2014133059A1 | Method for producing sulfonyl chloride compound | Takeda | 09/04/2014 |
| **Technical Subjects** | **Formulation and Preparation** | | |
| WO2010013823A2 | Pharmaceutical composition | Takeda | 02/04/2010 |
| WO2014003199A1 | Liquid preparations of amines and organic acids stabilized by salts | Takeda | 01/03/2014 |

The data was updated until Jan 2016.

# 3   Chemistry

## Route 1:   Original Discovery Route

TPAP: *Tetra-n*-propylammonium perruthenate
NMMO: *N*-methylmorpholine *N*-oxide

*Synthetic Route*:   Commercially available 2-fluoroacetophenone **1** was brominated to yield α-bromo-acetophenone derivative **2**, and this compound was treated with ethyl 2-cyanoacetate **3** under basic conditions to provide ketoester **4** in essentially quantitative yield.   Next, intermolecular condensation of **4** upon treatment of 4 M HCl furnished the *tri*-substituted pyrrole **5** in 53% yield.   Next, reduction of the chloride under hydrogenolytic conditions facilitated arrival at pyrrole **6**, albeit in merely 18% yield.   Subsequent DIBAL-H reduction, followed by the oxidation with TPAP and NMMO afforded the corresponding aldehyde **8** in 60% yield across the two steps.   Next, *N*-pyrrole substitution with pyridine-3-sulfonyl chloride **9** gave rise to *N*-sulfonylpyrrole **10** in 82% yield.   The reductive amination of **10** afforded vonoprazan, which was treated with fumaric acid *via* co-crystallization provided vonoprazan fumarate in 74% for two steps.   The overall yield was 3%.[1-5]

[1]   Kajino, M.; Hasuoka, A.; Nishida, H. WO2007026916A1, **2007**.
[2]   Kajino, M.; Hasuoka, A.; Nishida, H. US7498337B2, **2009**.
[3]   Kajino, M.; Hasuoka, A.; Tarui, N., et al. WO2006036024A1, **2006**.
[4]   Kajino, M.; Hasuoka, A.; Takagi, T. US8048909B2, **2011**.
[5]   Sun, P.; Lv, X.; Wu, C., et al. CN104327051A, **2015**.

## Route 2

*Synthetic Route:* The 10 g scaled-up synthetic route was initiated by reductive amination of 5-(2-fluorophenyl)-1*H*-pyrrole-3-carbaldehyde **1** and the following conversion to *N*-Boc-protected methylaminomethyl derivative **3** prior to sulfonylation. Sulfonylation of pyrrole **3** was performed in the same manner as previously described in route **1** to yield the 1-arylsulfonylated pyrroles **5**. The vonoprazan precursor **5** was finally deprotected by treatment with TFA and successive salification with fumaric acid to obtain the titled compound with the yield of 90%. The overall yield was 66%.[6]

## 4  Pharmacology

### Summary

Mechanism of Action

❖ Vonoprazan fumarate is P-CAB, which inhibits $H^+$, $K^+$-ATPase ($IC_{50}$ = 19.3 nM, pH = 6.5), the final step of acid secretion ($IC_{50}$ = 300 nM) in the gastric parietal cells.

❖ Vonoprazan fumarate did not show the anti-microbial activity for *H. pylori* (MIC >277 µg/mL), nor affected the anti-*H. pylori* activity of AMPC, CAM and MNZ.

❖ Vonoprazan fumarate had no significant inhibition in the off-target activity assays for a panel of 133 functional proteins including receptors, ion channels, transporters and enzymes at 10 µM, except L-type calcium channels, muscarinic M1, M2 and M3 receptors, 5-HT₂ receptor, σ receptor and sodium channel.[7]

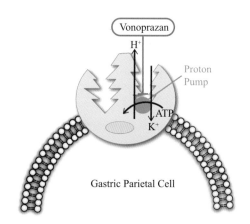

*In Vivo* Efficacy

❖ Upper gastrointestinal tract lesion formation:
  - Reflux esophagitis in SD rat: $ID_{50}$ = 1.27 mg/kg.
  - Aspirin-induced gastric mucosal damage in SD rat: $ID_{50}$ = 0.73 mg/kg.
  - Indomethacin-induced gastric mucosal damage in Lewis rat: $ID_{50}$ = 1.65 mg/kg.

[6] Lu, X.; Zhang, Y.; Huo, L., et al. CN105085484A, **2015**.
[7] Japan Pharmaceuticals and Medical Devices Agency (PMDA) Database. http://www.pmda.go.jp/drugs/2014/P201400173/index.html (accessed Mar 2016).

❖ Gastric acid secretion:
- Basal acid secretion in SD rat: $ID_{50}$ = 1.26 mg/kg.
- Histamine-stimulated acid secretion in SD rat: $ID_{50}$ = 0.86 mg/kg.
- 2-Deoxy-D-glucose-stimulated acid secretion in SD rat: $ID_{50}$ = 0.83 mg/kg.
- Histamine-stimulated acid secretion in beagle dog: $ID_{50}$ = 0.21 mg/kg.

## Mechanism of Action

Table 3    Efficacy of Vonoprazan Fumarate and Metabolites on Porcine $H^+$, $K^+$-ATPase and Acid Production[7, 8]

| Compound | $H^+$, $K^+$-ATPase (pig gastric mucosa) | | Acid Production (rabbit gastric mucosa) |
| --- | --- | --- | --- |
| | $IC_{50}$ (nM, pH = 6.5) | $IC_{50}$ (nM, pH = 7.5) | $IC_{50}$ (nM) |
| Vonoprazan fumarate | 19.3 | 28 | 300 |
| SCH28080 | 140 | 2500 | NA |
| Lansoprazole | 7600 | 66000 | NA |
| M- I | >10000 | | NA |
| M- II | >10000 | | NA |
| M-III | >10000 | | 3000 |
| M-IV-Sul | 4120 | 4610 | 3000 |

The $H^+$, $K^+$-ATPase inhibition was 3.03% at 10 μM vonoprazan fumarate.    ATPase activity was determined by measuring the inorganic phosphate amount generated by ATP degradation and the $H^+$, $K^+$-ATPase activity was determined by subtracting the activity of the absence of activity in the presence of potassium ions.    SCH28080: A potassium-competitive acid blocker.

Table 4    *In Vitro* Efficacy of Compounds against *H. pylori*[7]

| Strain | MIC (μM) | | | | |
| --- | --- | --- | --- | --- | --- |
| | Vonoprazan Fumarate | Lansoprazol | AMPC | CAM | MNZ |
| ATCC43504 | >277 | 86.6 | 0.0855 | 0.0836 | 748 |
| ATCC43579 | >277 | 21.7 | 0.342 | 0.0418 | 23.4 |
| ATCC43629 | >277 | 21.7 | 0.0855 | 0.167 | 23.4 |
| ATCC43526 | >277 | 43.3 | 0.171 | 0.0836 | 748 |
| ATCC700392 | >277 | 43.3 | 0.171 | 0.0836 | 11.7 |
| ATCC43503 | >277 | 21.7 | 0.171 | 0.0418 | 5.84 |

AMPC: Amoxicilin.    CAM: Clarithromycin.    MV2: Metronidazole.

Table 5    *In Vitro* Off-Target of Vonoprazan Fumarate in Different Functional Protein[7]

| Target | $IC_{50}$ (nM) | Effect | |
| --- | --- | --- | --- |
| | | Conc. (μM) | %Inhibition |
| L-type calcium channel | 2270 | 10 | >80 |
| Muscarinic M1 receptor | 1490 | 10 | >80 |
| Muscarinic M3 receptor | 800 | 10 | >80 |
| 5-HT$_2$ receptor | 1430 | 10 | >80 |

The off-target activity was studied from 133 kinds of functional protein; Table 5 showed the channels and receptors inhibition >80%.

[7]  PMDA Database.   http://www.pmda.go.jp/drugs/2014/P201400173/index.html (accessed Mar 2016).
[8]  Hori, Y.; Imanishi, A.; Matsukawa, J., et al. *J Pharmacol. Exp. Ther.* **2010**, *335*, 231-238.

## *In Vivo* Efficacy

Table 6    *In Vivo* Efficacy of Vonoprazan Fumarate in Animal Models[7-9]

| Animal Model | | | Dose (mg/kg) | Route (single dose) | Effect | | |
|---|---|---|---|---|---|---|---|
| Study | Model | Animal | | | ED (mg/kg) | ID50 (mg/kg) | Finding |
| Upper gastrointestinal tract lesion formation inhibitory effect | Reflux esophagitis | Fasting SD rat (male) | 0.5, 1, 2, 4 | p.o., 1 h | 2 | 1.27 | Inhibited reflux esophagitis. |
| | Aspirin-induced gastric mucosal damage | Fasting SD rat (male) | 0.5, 1, 2, 4 | p.o., 1 h | 1 | 0.73 | Inhibited aspirin-induced gastric mucosal injury. |
| | Indomethacin-induced gastric mucosal damage | Fasting Lewis rat (male) | 0.5, 1, 2, 4 | p.o., 1 h | 2 | 1.65 | Inhibited indomethacin-induced gastric mucosal damage. |
| Gastric acid secretion inhibitory action | Basal acid secretion | Fasting SD rat (male) | 0.5, 1, 2, 4 | p.o., 1 h | 2 | 1.26 | Inhibited basal acid secretion. The effect: Vonoprazan fumarate > Lansoprazole. |
| | Histamine-stimulated acid secretion | Fasting SD rat (male) | 0.5, 1, 2, 4 | p.o., 1 h | 1 | 0.86 | Inhibited histamine-stimulated acid secretion. Higher stomach perfusate pH compared with the lansoprazole. |
| | 2-Deoxy-D-glucose-stimulated acid secretion | Fasting SD rat (male) | 0.5, 1, 2, 4 | p.o., 1 h | 1 | 0.83 | Inhibited 2-deoxy-D-glucose-stimulated acid secretion. |
| | pH of stomach perfusate | Fasting SD rat (male) | 2 | i.v., 1 h | NA | NA | Raised the pH of stomach perfusate more than lansoprazole. |
| | Histamine-stimulated acid secretion | Fasting Beagle dog (male) | 0.1-1 | p.o. | NA | 0.21 | Dose-dependently inhibited histamine-stimulated acid secretion lasting for more than 48 h. |

ID50: 50% inhibitory dose.

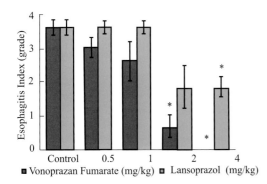

**Study:** Esophagitis in reflux esophagitis model.

**Animal:** SD rat.

**Model:** Under ether anesthesia, an abdominal incision was made in the midline of the SD rat.    Ligated pylorus and boundary portion of anterior stomach and gastric body, after then, sutured the abdominal incision.

**Administration:** Treated blindedly, p.o., after fasting for 24 h; 0.5-4 mg/kg vonoprazan fumarate.

**Test:** The damage of the esophageal portion from excised gastroesophageal portion. Esophagitis index: 0, lesion area for 0%; 1, lesion area for 1%-25%; 2, lesion area for 26%-50%; 3, lesion area for 51%-75%; 4, lesion area for >75% or perforation.

**Result:** Vonoprazan fumarate had significant inhibition of esophagitis at 2 mg/kg, and complete inhibition at 4 mg/kg.    $^*P \leq 0.025$.

Figure A    The Inhibitory Effect of Vonoprazan Fumarate and Lansoprazole on Reflux Esophagitis Model[7]

[7]  PMDA Database.   http://www.pmda.go.jp/drugs/2014/P201400173/index.html (accessed Mar 2016).
[8]  Hori, Y.; Imanishi, A.; Matsukawa, J., et al. *J. Pharmacol. Exp. Ther.* **2010**, *335*, 231-238.
[9]  Hori, Y.; Matsukawa, J.; Takeuchi, T., et al. *J. Pharmacol. Exp. Ther.* **2011**, *337*, 797-804.

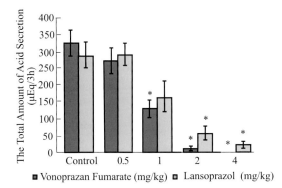

**Study:** Histamine-stimulated acid secretion rat model.

**Animal:** SD rat.

**Model:** Histamine dihydrochloride 30 mg/kg was administered subcutaneously into SD rat.

**Administration:** Treated blindedly, p.o., after fasting for 24 h.    Vonoprazan fumarate: 0.5, 1, 2, 4 mg/kg.

**Test:** The amount of gastric acid secretion from excised gastroesophageal portion.

**Result:** Vonoprazan fumarate had significant inhibition of acid secretion at 1 mg/kg, and complete inhibition at 4 mg/kg.    $^*P \leq 0.025$.

Figure B    The Inhibitory Effect of Vonoprazan Fumarate and Lansoprazole on Histamine-Stimulated Acid Secretion in Rat Model[7]

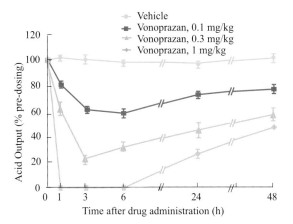

**Study:** Histamine-stimulated acid secretion in Heidenhain pouch dogs.

**Animal:** Male Beagle dog.

**Model:** Histamine dihydrochloride 30 μg/kg was administered subcutaneously one day before (acid output as 100%) and 1, 3, 6, 24 and 48 h after drug or vehicle administration.

**Administration:** Treated blindedly, p.o., after fasting for 24 h.    Vonoprazan fumarate: 0.1, 0.3 and 1 mg/kg.

**Test:** The total acid output during the 90-min period after each time point was calculated and expressed as a percentage of the pre-dosing value measured one day before the administration.

**Result:** Vonoprazan fumarate inhibited histamine-stimulated acid secretion in a dose-dependent manner and the inhibitory effect lasted for more than 48 h.

Figure C    The Inhibitory Effect of Vonoprazan Fumarate and Lansoprazole on Histamine-Stimulated Acid Secretion in Heidenhain Pouch Dog[7]

# 5    ADME & Drug-Drug Interaction

## Summary

### Absorption of Vonoprazan

❖  Had low oral bioavailability in rats (10.3%), but high in dogs (52.4%).

❖  Was absorbed rapidly in rats and dogs ($T_{max}$ = 0.3-1 h), but rapidly to moderately in humans (1.0-1.75 h).

❖  Showed a half-life ranging between 5.11-8.66 h in humans, much longer than that in rats (1.3-1.8 h) and dogs (1.1-1.9 h), after oral administrations.

❖  Showed a high permeability, with a $Papp_{(A \to B)}$ 17.8 × 10⁻⁶ cm/s in Caco-2 cell monolayer model.

### Distribution of Vonoprazan

❖  Exhibited moderate serum protein binding in humans (85.2%-88.0%), rats (67.3%-69.5%) and dogs (71.7%-83.3%).

❖  Had blood cell partitions in rats (60.3%-62.9%), dogs (30.0%-40.6%) and humans (43.7%-46%).

❖  In rats after single oral administration:

•  Tissue concentration of total radioactivity showed a maximum at 1 h post-dose in most tissues.

•  The total radioactivity was distributed throughout the body, particularly high radioactivity in the liver and stomach wall. Radioactivity in each tissue was nearly lost until 168 h post-dose, the residual of the vonoprazan and derived components were not observed.

•  In melanin affinity study, the intraocular plasma concentration of the colored rats was higher than that of the white rats.

[7]  PMDA Database.    http://www.pmda.go.jp/drugs/2014/P201400173/index.html (accessed Mar 2016).

Metabolism of Vonoprazan

❖ Could be metabolized in human, rat, dog and monkey liver microsomes and hepatocytes.

❖ The M-I , M-III and vonoprazan $N$-demethylation were mainly metabolized by CYP3A4 isoenzymes in humans, and some were metabolized by CYP2B6, CYP2C19 and CYP2D6.

❖ Overall, the major components in human plasma were M-IV-sul, M-I-G and parent.

❖ The test using a variety of animal liver cytosol and human sulfotransferase (SULT) expression cytosol, [$^{14}$C]vonoprazan was metabolized to vonoprazan $N$-sulfate by SULT2A1.

Excretion of Vonoprazan

❖ Was predominantly excreted in feces in rats and in urine in dogs after oral administrations.

❖ About 88.0% of [$^{14}$C]vonoprazan was recovered *via* biliary excretion in bile duct-cannulated (BDC) rats.

Drug-Drug Interaction

❖ Vonoprazan was an inhibitor of CYP3A4/5 ($IC_{50}$ = 29 μM) and CYP2B6 ($IC_{50}$ = 16 μM).

❖ Vonoprazan was not an inducer of CYP1A2, 2B6 or 3A4.

❖ Vonoprazan was not a substrate of P-gp, but had inhibition for P-gp, $IC_{50}$ of 50.3 μM.

❖ Vonoprazan was not a substrate of OATP1Bl or OATP1B3.

❖ Vonoprazan showed weak inhibitory effects against OAT3 and OCT2.

# Absorption

Table 7    *In Vivo* Pharmacokinetic Parameters of Vonoprazan and Metabolites in Rats and Dogs after Single Intravenous and Oral Dose of Vonoprazan[7]

| Species | Route | Dose (mg/kg) | Analyte | $T_{max}$ (h) | $C_{max}$ (ng/mL) | $AUC_{inf}$ (ng·h/mL) | $T_{1/2}$ (h) | F (%) |
|---|---|---|---|---|---|---|---|---|
| Rat (male) | i.v. | 0.75 | Vonoprazan | - | - | 99.2 ± 7.1 | 1.2 ± 0.1 | - |
| | | 2.25 | Vonoprazan | - | - | 384 ± 44.9 | 1.3 ± 0.0 | - |
| | p.o. | 2 | Vonoprazan | 0.3 ± 0.0 | 17.4 ± 4.3 | 27.2 ± 5.0 | 1.3 ± 0.1 | 10.3 ± 2.0 |
| | | 6 | Vonoprazan | 0.4 ± 0.1 | 195 ± 78.2 | 417 ± 110 | 1.3 ± 0.1 | - |
| | | 18 | Vonoprazan | 0.5 ± 0.0 | 953 ±184 | 2629 ± 500 | 1.8 ± 0.2 | - |
| Dog (male) | i.v | 0.1 | Vonoprazan | - | - | 44 ± 4 | 1.2 ± 0.2 | - |
| | p.o. | 0.3 | Vonoprazan | 1.0 ± 0.0 | 29.5 ± 12.5 | 68 ± 32 | 1.1 ± 0.2 | 52.4 ± 24.8 |
| | p.o. | 0.1 | Vonoprazan | 0.8 | 5.3 | 13.9 | 1.1 | - |
| | | | M1 | 1.0 | 40.5 | 138 | 2.5 | - |
| | | | M2 | 6.0 | 4.0 | 60.4 | 10.4 | - |
| | p.o. | 0.3 | Vonoprazan | 0.6 | 29.9 | 80.4 | 1.3 | - |
| | | | M1 | 1.3 | 88.4 | 409 | 3.0 | - |
| | | | M2 | 7.0 | 10.3 | 167 | 11.3 | - |
| | p.o. | 1 | Vonoprazan | 0.6 | 149 | 601 | 1.9 | - |
| | | | M1 | 1.5 | 169.4 | 1352 | 3.5 | - |
| | | | M2 | 8.0 | 29.2 | 518 | 31.5 | - |

Vehicle: Physiological saline solution for i.v. and 5% MC for p.o..

[7]  PMDA Database.   http://www.pmda.go.jp/drugs/2014/P201400173/index.html (accessed Mar 2016).

Table 8 *In Vivo* Pharmacokinetic Parameters of Vonoprazan and Metabolites in Rats by Portal Vein Absorption after Single Dose of Vonoprazan[7]

| Tissue | Dose (mg/kg) | Route | Time (h) | Conc. (ng/mL) | | | | | |
| --- | --- | --- | --- | --- | --- | --- | --- | --- | --- |
| | | | | Vonoprazan | M1 | M1-G | M2 | M2-G | Other |
| Portal plasma | 2 | Jejunum | 0-0.5 | 1035 | 30 | 7 | 4 | 1 | 76 |
| | | | 0.5-1 | 1340 | 33 | 11 | 4 | 1 | 105 |
| | | | 1-1.5 | 928 | 18 | 6 | 1 | 0 | 58 |
| | | | 1.5-2 | 541 | 13 | 4 | 1 | 0 | 48 |
| | 18 | Jejunum | 0-0.5 | 5357 | 111 | 39 | 13 | 5 | 342 |
| | | | 0.5-1 | 10195 | 194 | 21 | 34 | 2 | 616 |
| | | | 1-1.5 | 9103 | 193 | 16 | 41 | 6 | 766 |
| | | | 1.5-2 | 7710 | 128 | 9 | 15 | 2 | 449 |

Table 9 *In Vivo* Pharmacokinetic Parameters of Vonoprazan in Rats by Lymph Absorption after Single Dose of Vonoprazan[7]

| Dose (mg/kg) | Route | Time (h) | Cumulative Recovery Rate (% of Dose) | | | |
| --- | --- | --- | --- | --- | --- | --- |
| | | | Lymph | Urine | Feces | The Total Recovery Rate |
| 2 | p.o. | 2 | 0.2 | - | - | - |
| | | 4 | 0.3 | 10.8 | - | - |
| | | 8 | 0.4 | 13.6 | - | - |
| | | 24 | 0.6 | 17.1 | 79 | 96.6 |

Table 10 *In Vivo* Pharmacokinetic Parameters of Vonoprazan in Humans after Single Oral Dose of Vonoprazan[7]

| Species | Dose (mg) | $T_{max}$ (h) | $C_{max}$ (ng/mL) | $AUC_{inf}$ (ng·h/mL) | $T_{1/2}$ (h) |
| --- | --- | --- | --- | --- | --- |
| Healthy human (male) | 1 | 1.5 | 0.692 | 4.27 | 5.11 |
| | 5 | 1.5 | 4.25 | 31.6 | 7.62 |
| | 10 | 1.75 | 9.69 | 60.8 | 6.95 |
| | 20 | 1.5 | 25.0 | 162 | 6.85 |
| | 40 | 1.5 | 71.9 | 475 | 7.09 |
| | 80 | 1.5 | 130 | 911 | 8.66 |
| | 120 | 1.0 | 304 | 1985 | 6.58 |

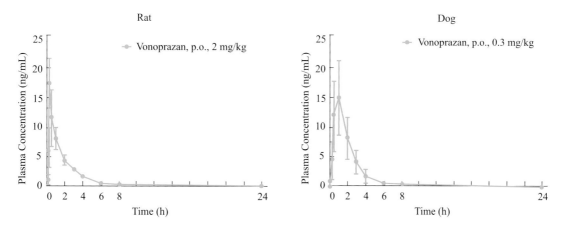

Figure D *In Vivo* Plasma Concentration-Time Profiles of Vonoprazan in Rats and Dogs after Single Oral Dose of Vonoprazan[7]

[7] PMDA Database. http://www.pmda.go.jp/drugs/2014/P201400173/index.html (accessed Mar 2016).

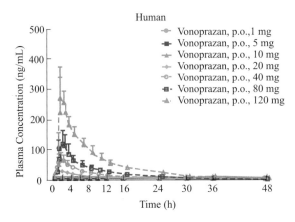

Figure E   *In Vivo* Plasma Concentration-Time Profiles of Vonoprazan in Humans after Single Oral Dose of Vonoprazan[7]

Table 11   *In Vitro* Permeability of Vonoprazan in Caco-2 Cell Monolayer Model[7]

| Test Article | Conc.( μM) | Papp$_{(A \to B)}$ (1 × 10$^{-6}$cm/s) | Papp$_{(B \to A)}$ (1 × 10$^{-6}$cm/s) | Efflux Ratio | Permeability Class |
|---|---|---|---|---|---|
| [14C]Vonoprazan | 3 | 17.8 | 21.3 | 1.2 | High |
| [3H]Digoxin | 3 | 2.01 | 9.44 | 4.7 | Moderate |
| [3H]Estrone-3-sulfate | 0.1 | 2.76 | 17.7 | 6.4 | Moderate |
| [14C]Antipyrine | 10 | 42.1 | 42.4 | 1.0 | High |
| [14C]Mannitol | 10 | 0.735 | 0.641 | 0.9 | Low |

## Distribution

Table 12   *In Vitro* Plasma Protein Binding and Blood Partitioning of Vonoprazan in Several Species[7]

| Plasma Protein Binding (%) | | | Human Isolated Protein Binding (%) | | | Blood Partitioning | | |
|---|---|---|---|---|---|---|---|---|
| Species | Conc. (ng/mL) | %Bound | Protein | Conc. (ng/mL) | %Bound | Species | Conc. (ng/mL) | Blood Cell Association (%) |
| Rat | 100-10000 | 67.3-69.5 | 4% HSA | 100-10000 | 43.0-44.6 | Rat | 100-10000 | 60.3-62.9 |
| Dog | 100-10000 | 71.7-83.3 | 0.05% AGP | 100-10000 | 21.4-45.7 | Dog | 100-10000 | 30.0-40.6 |
| Human | 100-10000 | 85.2-88.0 | 4% HSA/0.05% AGP | 100-10000 | 51.1-60.1 | Human | 100-10000 | 43.7-46 |

Table 13   *In Vivo* Plasma Protein Binding of Vonoprazan in Several Species[7]

| Species | Dose (mg/kg) | Plasma Protein Binding (%) | | | | | | |
|---|---|---|---|---|---|---|---|---|
| | | 0.25 h | 0.5 h | 1 h | 2 h | 4 h | 8 h | 24 h |
| Rat | 2 | 94.1 | - | 95.1 | 94.9 | - | - | 82.8 |
| Dog | 0.3 | - | 94.0 | - | 92.0 | 90.7 | 88.5 | 88.9 |

[7]  PMDA Database.   http://www.pmda.go.jp/drugs/2014/P201400173/index.html (accessed Mar 2016).

Table 14   *In Vivo* Tissue Distribution of [$^{14}$C]Vonoprazan in Rats after Single Oral Dose of 2 mg/kg [$^{14}$C]Vonoprazan[7]

| Tissue | Species | Radioactivity (ng eq./g) | | | | | | Tissue/Plasma AUC$_{0-168}$ Ratio |
|---|---|---|---|---|---|---|---|---|
| | | 0.25 h | 1 h | 2 h | 24 h | 48 h | 168 h | |
| Blood | White rat | 397 | 710 | 368 | 23 | 13 | 5 | 1.0 |
| Plasma | White rat | 436 | 1045 | 611 | 27 | 14 | 3 | 1.48 |
| | Pigmented rat | 687 | 1196 | 427 | 29 | 12 | 2 | 1.42 |
| Brain | White rat | 31 | 47 | 31 | 2 | 2 | 1 | 0.08 |
| Spinal cord | White rat | 31 | 46 | 33 | 2 | 2 | 1 | 0.08 |
| Pituitary gland | White rat | 271 | 858 | 1067 | 13 | <LOQ | <LOQ | 1.73 |
| Eyes | White rat | 47 | 93 | 55 | 4 | 2 | 1 | 0.14 |
| | Pigmented rat | 147 | 557 | 444 | 320 | 266 | 135 | 2.55 |
| Submandibular gland | White rat | 329 | 687 | 504 | 9 | 6 | 2 | 1.06 |
| Thyroid | White rat | 588 | 511 | 279 | 18 | | <LOQ | 0.81 |
| Thymus | White rat | 134 | 268 | 219 | 8 | 7 | 2 | 0.46 |
| Heart | White rat | 474 | 568 | 313 | 8 | 5 | 2 | 0.81 |
| Lungs | White rat | 1204 | 1846 | 1379 | 149 | 82 | 35 | 3.45 |
| Liver | White rat | 14754 | 9646 | 6021 | 735 | 435 | 69 | 18.3 |
| Spleen | White rat | 304 | 746 | 381 | 13 | 9 | 4 | 0.98 |
| Pancreas | White rat | 492 | 572 | 344 | 9 | 6 | 2 | 0.86 |
| Kidneys | White rat | 2884 | 5718 | 3854 | 265 | 163 | 63 | 9.31 |
| Skin | White rat | 85 | 290 | 208 | 18 | 13 | 6 | 0.5 |
| Marrow | White rat | 190 | 560 | 328 | 19 | 12 | 3 | 0.81 |
| Stomach | White rat | 3074 | 1759 | 1402 | 103 | 26 | 3 | 3.49 |
| Intestinal | White rat | 4174 | 2689 | 2666 | 45 | 6 | 2 | 5.45 |

LOQ: Limit of quantitation.

## Metabolism

Table 15   *In Vitro* Metabolism of Vonoprazan in Hepatocytes and Liver Microsomes[7]

| Study | Species | Gender | Metabolism of Vonoprazan or the Formation of Metabolites (nM) | | | | | |
|---|---|---|---|---|---|---|---|---|
| | | | Vonoprazan | M-I | M-II | M-III | M-IV-Sul | Vonoprazan N-Demethylation |
| Hepatocyte | Rat | NA | 3180 | 996 | 8 | 45 | 71 | 961 |
| | Dog | NA | 1324 | 241 | 5 | 13 | 25 | 595 |
| | Monkey | NA | 5560 | 2118 | 25 | 301 | 54 | 1585 |
| | Human | Female | 1593 | 399 | 5 | 101 | 298 | 521 |
| | | Male | 1496 | 192 | 6 | 46 | 469 | 473 |
| Liver microsomes | Mouse | NA | 1249 | 132 | 11 | 130 | - | 383 |
| | Rat | Male | 1440 | 387 | 14 | 89 | - | 595 |
| | | Female | 1192 | 62 | 14 | 19 | - | 758 |
| | Dog | NA | 695 | 154 | 0 | 19 | - | 314 |
| | Monkey | NA | 1916 | 562 | 10 | 170 | - | 798 |
| | Human | NA | 1135 | 314 | 0 | 166 | - | 466 |

[7]   PMDA Database.   http://www.pmda.go.jp/drugs/2014/P201400173/index.html (accessed Mar 2016).

Table 16    *In Vitro* Metabolic Phenotype of Vonoprazan in Human Liver Microsomes[7]

| CYP | Human Liver Microsomes | | | | CYP | Human Liver Microsomes | | | | |
| | Correlation (r) | | | | | Metabolism/Generation Rate (pmol/h/pmol P450) | | | | |
| | Vonoprazan | M-I | M-III | Vonoprazan N-Demethylation | | Vonoprazan | M-I | M-II | M-III | Vonoprazan N-Demethylation |
|---|---|---|---|---|---|---|---|---|---|---|
| 1A2 | 0.114 | 0.158 | 0.162 | 0.176 | 1A1 | 2.4 | 0.1 | 0.0 | 0.2 | 2.3 |
| 2A6 | 0.136 | 0.120 | 0.087 | 0.139 | 1A2 | 0.3 | 0.2 | 0.0 | 0.1 | 0.2 |
| 2B6 | 0.410 | 0.348 | 0.377 | 0.337 | 2A6 | 0.0 | 0.1 | 0.3 | 0.1 | 0.3 |
| 2C8 | 0.495 | 0.465 | 0.398 | 0.528 | 2B6 | 9.8 | 4.0 | 0.0 | 1.1 | 5.0 |
| 2C9 | 0.0437 | 0.118 | 0.0307 | -0.0217 | 2C8 | 1.4 | 0.2 | 0.0 | 0.0 | 0.9 |
| 2C19 | 0.487 | 0.530 | 0.299 | 0.590 | 2C9 | 0.2 | 0.1 | 0.3 | 0.0 | 0.7 |
| 2D6 | 0.209 | 0.166 | 0.252 | 0.0561 | 2C19 | 24.7 | 2.2 | 0.1 | 0.5 | 17.6 |
| 2E1 | 0.237 | 0.292 | 0.257 | 0.335 | 2D6 | 26.5 | 0.1 | 0.4 | 1.1 | 20.3 |
| 3A4/5 | 0.916 | 0.902 | 0.940 | 0.862 | 2E1 | 0.0 | 0.1 | 0.1 | 0.1 | 0.2 |
| 4A11 | 0.0788 | 0.113 | 0.0372 | 0.156 | 3A4 | 16.9 | 3.0 | 0.2 | 2.7 | 3.6 |

Table 17    *In Vitro* Metabolism of Vonoprazan in Liver Cytosol and Human SULT Expression Cytosol[7]

| PAPS | Human Liver Cytosol | | | | Human SULT Expression Cytosol | | |
| | Percentage of Total Radioactivity (%) | | | | Metabolism/Generation Speed (pmol/h/mg protein) | | |
| | Species | Vonoprazan | Vonoprazan N-Demethylation | Others | SULTs | Vonoprazan | Vonoprazan N-Demethylation |
|---|---|---|---|---|---|---|---|
| + | Rat | 93.0 | 0.2 | 6.8 | 1A1 | 36.5 | <LOQ |
| | Dog | 92.9 | <LOD | 7.1 | 1A3 | 52.5 | <LOQ |
| | Human | 90.2 | 3.2 | 6.6 | 1B1 | 70.5 | <LOD |
| - | Rat | 93.2 | <LOD | 6.8 | 1E1 | 21.5 | <LOQ |
| | Dog | 92.6 | <LOQ | 7.4 | 2A1 | 13276 | 13508 |
| | Human | 92.6 | <LOD | 7.4 | | | |

At 10 μM/L vonoprazan.    PAPS: 3'-Phosphodiester adenosine-5'-phospho-sulfate.    LOD: Limit of detection.    LOQ: Limit of quantitation.    SULT: Sulfotransferase.

[7]  PMDA Database.  http://www.pmda.go.jp/drugs/2014/P201400173/index.html (accessed Mar 2016).

Table 18 Metabolites in Tissues, Plasma, Urine, Bile and Feces in Humans and Non-clinical Species after Single Oral Dose of Vonoprazan[7]

| Matrix | Species | Dose (mg/kg) | Time (h) | Gender | % of Radioactivity or % of Dose | | | | | | |
|---|---|---|---|---|---|---|---|---|---|---|---|
| | | | | | M0 | M-I | M-I-G | M-II | M-II-G | M-III | M-IV-Sul |
| Liver | Rat | 2 | 0-24 | Male | 4.3 | 19.8 | 3.23 | 2.75 | 0.45 | NA | NA |
| Kidneys | Rat | 2 | 0-24 | Male | 5.8 | 55.3 | 6.24 | 0.78 | 0.65 | NA | NA |
| Stomach | Rat | 2 | 0-24 | Male | 64.4 | 4.5 | 1.75 | 1.18 | 0.36 | NA | NA |
| Intestinal | Rat | 2 | 0-24 | Male | 13.1 | 4.79 | 7.10 | 0.8 | 0.60 | NA | NA |
| Plasma | Rat | 2 | 0-24 | Male & female | 0.9 | 51.9 | 11.8 | 7.4 | 4.5 | NA | NA |
| | Dog | 0.3 | 0-24 | Male | 1.9 | 8.8 | 14.0 | 5.2 | 39.4 | NA | NA |
| | Human | 15 mg | 0-24 | Male | 13.9 | 8.2 | 19.2 | 6.8 | NA | 4.3 | 16.9 |
| Urine | Rat | 2 | 0-24 | Male & female | 13.3 | 0.6 | 8.2 | 4.4 | 8.9 | NA | NA |
| | Dog | 0.3 | 0-24 | Male | 0.9 | 1.0 | 1.4 | 1.7 | 72.4 | NA | NA |
| | Human | 15 mg | 0-24 | Male | 12.0 | 2.8 | 20.6 | 0.1 | NA | 1.1 | 11.4 |
| Bile | Rat | 2 | 0-24 | Male & female | 0.1 | 1.8 | 34.2 | 0.3 | 2.5 | NA | NA |
| Feces | Rat | 2 | 0-48 | Male & female | 1.0 | 2.1 | 11.1 | 0.5 | 0.8 | NA | NA |
| | Dog | 0.3 | 0-168 | Male | 1.6 | 2.2 | 1.9 | 1.6 | 0.3 | NA | NA |
| | Human | 15 mg | 0-336 | Male | 4.4 | 1.0 | ND | 0.2 | NA | 2.4 | 15.9 |

% of Radioactivity for tissues and plasma.   % of dose for urine, feces and bile.

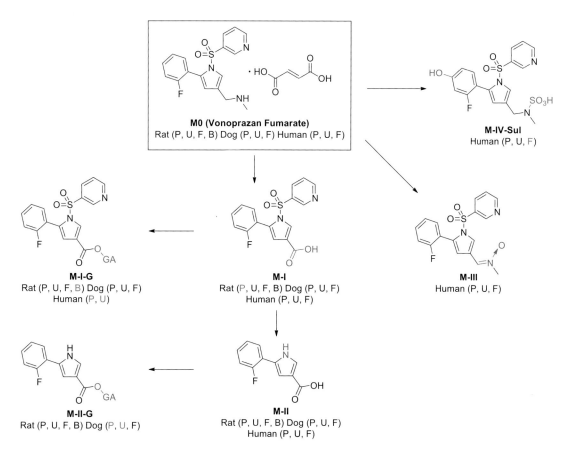

Figure F    Proposed Pathways for *In Vivo* Biotransformation of Vonoprazan in Rats, Dogs and Humans[7]
The red labels represent the main components in the matrices.    P = Plasma, U = Urine, F = Feces, B = Bile and GA = Glucuronic acid.

[7]  PMDA Database.   http://www.pmda.go.jp/drugs/2014/P201400173/index.html (accessed Mar 2016).

## Excretion

Table 19    Excretion Profiles of [$^{14}$C]Vonoprazan in Rats and Dogs after Single Dose of Vonoprazan[7]

| Species | State | Route | Dose (mg/kg) | Time (h) | Bile (% of dose) | Urine (% of dose) | Feces (% of dose) | Recovery (% of dose) |
|---|---|---|---|---|---|---|---|---|
| Rat (male) | Intact | p.o. | 2 | 0-168 | - | 16.8 | 80.3 | 97.7 |
| Dog (male) | Intact | p.o. | 0.3 | 0-168 | - | 64.4 | 34.3 | 98.7 |
| Rat (male) | BDC | i.d. | 2 | 0-24 | 88.0 | 8.7 | 2.1 | 98.8 |

i.d.: Intraduodenum.

## Drug-Drug Interaction

Table 20    *In Vitro* Evaluation of Vonoprazan as an Inhibitor and an Inducer of Enzymes[7]

| | Vonoprazan as an Inhibitor | | | | | Vonoprazan as an Inducer | | | |
|---|---|---|---|---|---|---|---|---|---|
| | Direct Inhibition | | Time-Dependent Inhibition | | | | | % of Positive Control | |
| CYPs | IC$_{50}$ (µM) | % Remaining Activity | IC$_{50}$ (µM) | % Remaining Activity | Compound | Con. (µM) | CYP1A2[c] | CYP2B6[d] | CYP3A4/5[e] |
| 1A2 | >30 | 88.3 | >30 | 89.0 | Omeprazole | 50 | 100 | - | - |
| 2B6 | 16 | 37.9 | 2.6 | 16.8 | Phenobarbital | 1000 | - | 100 | - |
| 2C8 | >30 | 70.7 | >30 | 72.3 | Rifampicin | 10 | - | - | 100 |
| 2C9 | >30 | 87.7 | >30 | 76.2 | | 0 | 3.4 ± 1.1 | 10.5 ± 2.7 | 1.1 ± 0.6 |
| 2C19 | >30 | 64.3 | 13 | 34.0 | | 1 | 3.6 ± 1.1 | 11.8 ± 3.1 | 0.9 ± 0.5 |
| 2D6 | >30 | 61.3 | >30 | 64.3 | Vonoprazan | 3 | 3.9 ± 1.1 | 12.4 ± 3.3 | 0.8 ± 0.4 |
| 3A4/5[a] | 29 | 49.9 | 10 | 32.6 | | 10 | 5.4 ± 2.2 | 13.9 ± 2.8 | 0.7 ± 0.4 |
| 3A4/5[b] | >30 | 61.3 | 9.8 | 32.4 | | 30 | 7.3 ± 1.7 | 12.4 ± 2.1 | 0.6 ± 0.3 |

[a] The index activity was midazolam 1'-hydroxylation.    [b] The index activity was testosterone 6β-hydroxylation.    [c] The induction period was 2 days.    [d] The induction period was 3 days.    [e] The induction period was 4 days.

Table 21    *In Vitro* Effect of Incorporated Drug on Human Plasma Protein Binding of Vonoprazan[7]

| Incorporated Drug | Conc. (µg/mL) | Unbound (ng/mL) Vonoprazan | Relative (%) | Incorporated Drug | Conc. (µg/mL) | Unbound (ng/mL) Control | Unbound (ng/mL) Incorporated Drug | Relative (%) |
|---|---|---|---|---|---|---|---|---|
| Control | 0 | 19.9 | 100 | [$^3$H]Warfarin | 1 | 6.1 | 6.1 | 100 |
| Warfarin | 1 | 18.4 | 92.5 | [$^3$H]Ibuprofen | 20 | 80.4 | 82.1 | 102 |
| Ibuprofen | 20 | 22.1 | 111 | [$^3$H]Diazepam | 0.3 | 2.6 | 2.6 | 100 |
| Diazepam | 0.3 | 19.3 | 97.0 | [$^{14}$C]Phenytoin | 2 | 66.6 | 64.9 | 97.4 |
| Phenytoin | 2 | 20.0 | 100 | [$^3$H]Propranolol | 0.1 | 2.2 | 2.3 | 104 |
| Propranolol | 0.1 | 20.0 | 100 | [$^3$H]Digoxin | 0.01 | 7.9 | 7.5 | 94.9 |
| Diclofenac | 1 | 19.5 | 98.0 | [$^{14}$C]Diclofenac | 1 | 2.7 | 2.5 | 92.6 |
| Loxoprofen | 5.5 | 21.6 | 108 | Loxoprofen | 5.5 | 168.1 | 167.5 | 99.6 |
| Meloxicam | 1 | 20.8 | 104 | Meloxicam | 1 | 1.0 | 1.0 | 100 |
| Celecoxib | 1.5 | 21.2 | 106 | Celecoxib | 1.5 | <1.0 | <1.0 | 100 |
| SR26334 | 2.5 | 20.3 | 102 | SR26334 | 2.5 | 64.4 | 63.6 | 98.8 |

Control: No vonoprazan.    Vonoprazan conc.: 100 ng/mL (salt).

[7]  PMDA Database.    http://www.pmda.go.jp/drugs/2014/P201400173/index.html (accessed Mar 2016).

Table 22    *In Vitro* Evaluation of Vonoprazan as an Inhibitor and a Substrate of Transporters[7]

| As a Substrate of OATP1B1 and OATP1B3[a] | | | | | | As an Inhibitor[b] | | | | |
| Compound | Inhibitor | Time (min) | Uptake (µL/mg protein) | | | Transporter | Substrate | Conc. (µM) | IC$_{50}$ (µM) | Residual Activity (%) |
| | | | Control | OATP1B1 | OATPAB3 | | | | | |
| Vonoprazan | - | 0.5 | 107 | 113 | 107 | P-gp | [$^3$H]Digoxin | 3 | 50.3 | 39.7 |
| | | 1 | 163 | 174 | 164 | BCRP | Prazosin | 0.01 | - | 97.6 |
| | | 2 | 281 | 333 | 278 | OATP1B1 | [$^3$H]E$_2$17$\beta$G | 0.05 | - | 95.7 |
| | | 5 | 447 | 450 | 453 | OATP1B3 | [$^3$H]E$_2$17$\beta$G | 0.05 | - | 81.7 |
| | Rifampicin | 2 | 228 | 230 | 230 | OAT1 | *p*-Aminohippuric acid | 1 | - | 84.2 |
| [$^3$H]E$_2$17$\beta$G | - | 2 | 0.526 | 149 | 16.1 | OAT3 | Estrone-3-sulfate | 0.05 | - | 58.1 |
| | | | | | | OCT2 | Metformin | 10 | - | 76.0 |

[a] At 10 µM rifampicin and 0.05 µM [$^3$H]E$_2$17$\beta$G.    [b] Vonoprazan conc.: 30 µM for all except 100 µm for P-gp and BCRP.

# 5   Non-Clinical Toxicology

## Summary

### Single-Dose Toxicity

❖ Single-dose oral administration of vonoprazan in rodent and non-rodent species:
  • Rat MNLD: 200 mg/kg.
  • Dog MNLD: 10 mg/kg.

### Repeated-Dose Toxicity

❖ Repeated-dose oral administration of vonoprazan in rats (up to 26 weeks) and dogs (up to 39 weeks):
  • For rats: The NOAEL was 5 mg/kg/day (0.46 and 0.43 × MRHD for Japanese and British, respectively) in males and 10 mg/kg/day (3.5 and 3.3 × MRHD for Japanese and British, respectively) in females, determined by the 26-week study, and the observations resulted from pharmacological action of vonoprazan.
  • For dogs: The NOAEL was 0.6 mg/kg/day (0.91 and 0.85 × MRHD for Japanese and British, respectively) in males and 0.6 mg/kg/day (0.75 and 0.71 × MRHD for Japanese and British, respectively) in females, determined by the 39-week study, and the observation resulted from pharmacological action of vonoprazan.

### Safety Pharmacology

❖ Safety pharmacology studies were not conducted or required to support the proposed indication.

### Genotoxicity

❖ No genetic risk was found in a standard battery of genotoxicity studies.

### Reproductive and Developmental Toxicity

❖ Fertility and early embryonic development in rats:
  • The NOAEL was ≥300 mg/kg/day for both males and females.
❖ Embryo-fetal development in rats and rabbits:
  • The NOAELs for maternal were 30 mg/kg/day in rats and 3 mg/kg/day in rabbits.   The NOAELs for fetus were 100 mg/kg/day in rats and >30 mg/kg/day in rabbits.
❖ Pre- and postnatal developments in rats:
  • The NOAEL was determined as 10 mg/kg/day for F$_0$ and F$_1$ in rats.

### Carcinogenicity

❖ Increased incidence of tumor was found in liver and stomach in 2-year mouse and rat tests.

### Special toxicity

❖ Only minor irritation of function was found in paravenous tolerance study.

[7]  PMDA Database.   http://www.pmda.go.jp/drugs/2014/P201400173/index.html (accessed Mar 2016).

## Single-Dose Toxicity

Table 23    Single-Dose Toxicity Studies of Vonoprazan by Oral Administration[7]

| Species | Dose (mg/kg) | MNLD (mg/kg) | Finding |
|---|---|---|---|
| SD rat | 0, 600, 2000 | 600 | 600 mg/kg: Salivation, mydriasis, decreased stools and body weight gain.<br>2000 mg/kg: Salivation, mydriasis, decreased locomotor activity, action tremor, all died rats with a prone position. |
|  | 0, 200, 600, 2000 | 200 | ≥200 mg/kg: Salivation, mydriasis.<br>600 mg/kg: One female: died; others: decreased activity, action tremor.<br>2000 mg/kg: Decreased locomotor activity, tonic convulsions, then died. |
| Beagle dog | 10, 60<br>(Single ascending dose) | 60 | 60 mg/kg: Vomiting, ↑ ALT. |
|  | 0.6, 20<br>(Single ascending dose) | 20 | 20 mg/kg: Vomiting. |
|  | 0, 2, 10, 60<br>(Single ascending dose) | 10 | >10 mg/kg: Vomiting.<br>60 mg/kg: ↑ ALT and AST, ↓ body temperature, one male and one female died. |

Vehicle: 0.5% (w/v) MC.

## Repeated-Dose Toxicity

Table 24    Repeated-Dose Toxicity Studies of Vonoprazan by Oral Administration[7]

| Species | Duration (Week) | Dose (mg/kg/day) | NOAEL Dose (mg/kg/day) | AUC$_{0-24}$ (ng·h/mL) | Safety Margin (× MRHD) Japanese[a] | Safety Margin (× MRHD) British[b] | Finding |
|---|---|---|---|---|---|---|---|
| SD rat | 4 | 1, 3, 10, 30, 100 | 30/>100[a] | 2239/13375 | 4.9/29.2 | 4.6/27.4 | 1 mg/kg: No observed effect.<br>3 mg/kg: ↑ Stomach weight, gastric parietal cells vacuolation, squamous cell hyperplasia of the forestomach boundary edge, cervical mucus cell hyperplasia, globule leukocyte infiltration, eosinophilic infiltration.<br>≥10 mg/kg: ↑ Stomach weight, gastric parietal cells vacuolation, squamous cell hyperplasia of the forestomach boundary edge, cervical mucus cell hyperplasia, globule leukocyte infiltration, eosinophilic infiltration.<br>≥30 mg/kg: Parietal cell atrophy, ↑ gastrin.<br>100 mg/kg (male): ↓ Hb, MCV, MCH and MCHC, ↓ fibrinogen, ↑ ALT, AST and ALP, hepatocyte vacuolization, thyroid follicular epithelial cell hypertrophy. |
|  | 13 | 1, 10, 100, 300 | 10 | 989/1343 | 2.2/2.9 | 2.0/2.7 | ≥10 mg/kg: ↑ Stomach weight, gastric parietal cells vacuolation and atrophy, stomach chief cells acidification, squamous cell hyperplasia of the forestomach boundary edge, globule leukocyte infiltration, ↑ gastrin.<br>≥100 mg/kg: Urine increased, ↑ ALP and TChol, ↓ TG and glucose, gastric chief cell hyperplasia, inflammatory cell infiltration, pyloric growth band expansion, centrilobular hepatocellular hypertrophy, liver cell vacuolization, adrenal clear cell hypertrophy.<br>300 mg/kg: ↓ MCV and MCH, ↓ fibrinogen, gastric mucous metaplasia, thyroid follicular epithelial cell hypertrophy. |

[7]  PMDA Database.    http://www.pmda.go.jp/drugs/2014/P201400173/index.html (accessed Mar 2016).

*Continued*

| Species | Duration (Week) | Dose (mg/kg/day) | NOAEL Dose (mg/kg/day) | NOAEL AUC$_{0-24}$ (ng·h/mL) | NOAEL Safety Margin (× MRHD) Japanese[a] | NOAEL Safety Margin (× MRHD) British[b] | Finding |
|---|---|---|---|---|---|---|---|
| SD rat | 26 | 1, 5, 10, 30 | 5/10 | 210/1615 | 0.46/3.5 | 0.43/3.3 | ≥5 mg/kg: ↑ Stomach weight, stomach chief cells acidification, squamous cell hyperplasia of the forestomach boundary edge, globule leukocyte infiltration. ≥10 mg/kg: ↑ Gastrin, gastric parietal cell vacuolization and atrophy, gastric mucosa fibrosis (male). 30 mg/kg: Urine increased, ↑ CK, gastric mucosa fibrosis, gastric inflammatory cell infiltration and vasodilatation, centrilobular hepatocellular hypertrophy, liver cell vacuolization, adrenal clear cell hypertrophy. |
| Beagle dog | 4 | 0.6, 2, 6, 20 | 0.6 | 491/493 | 1.1/1.1 | 1.0/1.0 | ≥2 mg/kg: Vomiting, gastric parietal cells atrophy and vacuolation, single cell necrosis, fundic gland mucosa inflammatory cell infiltration. ≥6 mg/kg: Salivation, ↓ chloride. 20 mg/kg (female): Loose stool. |
| Beagle dog | 13 | 1, 1.3, 1.6, 2 | <1 | Not established | NA | NA | ≥1 mg/kg: ↑ ALT, single cell necrosis of gastric bottom gland cells, fundic gland mucosa inflammatory cell infiltration, stomach muscle layer degeneration, fundic gland mucosa hyperplasia, gastric parietal cells vacuolization. ≥1.6 mg/kg: Vomiting. |
| Beagle dog | 39 | 0.3, 0.6, 2 | 0.6 | 415/346 | 0.91/0.75 | 0.85/0.71 | ≥0.3 mg/kg: Gastric parietal cells vacuolization. ≥0.6 mg/kg: ↑ Gastrin. 2 mg/kg: ↑ Eosinophil, ↑ reticulocyte, ↑ ALT, gastric wall thickening, stomach muscle layer degeneration (male). |

Vehicle: 0.5% (w/v) MC. Values XXX/XXX represented male/female. [a] Exposure multiples based on multiple 40 mg doses in a 7-day multiple rising dose study (TAK-438/CPH-002 Japan study) that resulted in AUC$_{0-24}$ values of 485.5 ng·h/mL. [b] Exposure multiple based on multiple 40 mg doses in male subjects in a 7-day multiple rising dose study (TAK-483_107 UK study) that resulted in AUC$_{0-24}$ values of 488.4 ng·h/mL.

# Genotoxicity

Table 25    Genotoxicity Studies of Vonoprazan[7]

| Assay | Species/System | Metabolism | Dose | Finding |
|---|---|---|---|---|
| *In vitro* bacterial reverse mutation assay (Ames) | *S. typhimurium* TA100, TA1535, TA 98, TA1537; *E. coli* WP2uvrA | ±S9 | 1.5-5000 µg/plate | Negative. |
| *In vitro* chromosomal aberration study in cultured mammalian cell | CHL cell | ±S9 | 25-300 µg/mL | Negative. |
| *In vivo* bone marrow micronucleus test | SD rat | - | 62.5, 125, 250 mg/kg/day, p.o. | Negative. |

Vehicle: 0.5% (w/v) MC for *in vivo* tests, DMSO for *in vitro* tests.

[7]  PMDA Database.    http://www.pmda.go.jp/drugs/2014/P201400173/index.html (accessed Mar 2016).

# Reproductive and Developmental Toxicity

Table 26   Embryonic and Developmental Toxicology Studies of Vonoprazan by Oral Administration[7]

| Study | Species | Dose (mg/kg/day) | NOAEL | | Finding |
| | | | Endpoint | Dose (mg/kg/day) | |
|---|---|---|---|---|---|
| Fertility and early embryonic development | SD rat | 0, 30, 100, 300 | Male fertility | ≥300 | 100 mg/kg: Mydriasis.<br>300 mg kg: Mortality (male), tremor, prone position, vulva fur contamination by urine, ↓ body weight, BWG, food consumption. |
| | | | Female fertility | ≥300 | |
| | | | Embryo | ≥300 | |
| Embryo-fetal development | SD rat | 0, 30, 100, 300 | Maternal | 30 | 100 mg/kg: Dams, ↓ BWG, food consumption. Fetus, ↓ BW, placental weight and ossification sacro-coccygeal vertebral number, ↑ tail anomaly, anal stenosis, membranous part ventricular septal defect, subclavian artery origin anomaly. |
| | | | Fetal development | 100 | |
| | Rabbit | 0, 3, 10, 30 | Maternal | 3 | 10 mg/kg: Dams, ↓ feces amount, ↓ food consumption, ↓ body weight.<br>30 mg/kg: Dams, abortion. |
| | | | Fetal development | >30 | |
| Pre- and postnatal development | SD rat | 0, 1, 3, 10, 100 | $F_0/F_1$ | 10 | 100 mg/kg: $F_0$, ↓ BWG, ↓ food consumption. $F_1$ at four days after birth, adjustment excluded children liver caudate lobe discoloration nest (white and black), low birth weight. |

Vehicle: 0.5% (w/v) MC solution.

# Carcinogenicity

Table 27   2-Year Carcinogenicity Studies of Vonoprazan by Oral Administration[7]

| Species | Dose (mg/kg/day) | Finding |
|---|---|---|
| B6C3F1 mouse | 0, 6, 20, 60, 200 | ≥6 mg/kg: Gastric neuroendocrine cell tumors (male), gastric neuroendocrine cell hyperplasia (male).<br>≥20 mg/kg: Hepatocellular adenoma.<br>≥60 mg/kg: Gastric neuroendocrine cell tumors (female), gastric neuroendocrine cell hyperplasia (female), hepacellular adenoma (female), hepatocellular carcinoma (male).<br>200 mg/kg: ↓ Survival, ↓ BWG (male), hepatocellular carcinoma (female), gastric adenoma. |
| SD rat | 0, 5, 15, 50, 150 | ≥5 mg/kg: ↑ Gastrin, gastric neuroendocrine cell tumors, gastric neuroendocrine cell hyperplasia, hyperplastic gastric disease, centrilobular hepatocellular hypertrophy.<br>≥15 mg/kg: Gastric mucosa atrophy, localized tegmental epithelium cell hyperplasia.<br>≥50 mg/kg: Pyloric gland intestinal metaplasia, liver cell adenoma, hepatocellular carcinoma, hepatocellular and bile duct cell adenoma (male: 50 mg/kg only).<br>150 mg/kg: ↓ BWG, hepatocellular carcinoma (female), hepatocellular and bile duct cell adenoma (male). |

Vehicle: 0.5 % (w/v) MC.

# Special Toxicity

Table 28   Special Toxicity Studies of Vonoprazan[7]

| Study | Species | Dose | Finding |
|---|---|---|---|
| Venous irritation test | Rabbit | 3 mg/site | None. |
| Paravenous tolerance study | Rabbit | 0.3 mg/site | Minor reversible changes. |
| *In vivo* phototoxicity assay | Mouse | 0, 20, 60, 200 mg/kg | Negative. |

Vehicle: 0.5% (w/v) MC.

[7]  PMDA Database.   http://www.pmda.go.jp/drugs/2014/P201400173/index.html (accessed Mar 2016).

# CHAPTER

31

## Vorapaxar Sulfate

# Vorapaxar Sulfate

## (Zontivity®)

Research code: SCH-530348

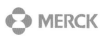

## 1 General Information

- ❖ Vorapaxar sulfate is a protease-activated receptor-1 (PAR-1) antagonist, which was first approved in May 2014 by US FDA.

- ❖ Vorapaxar sulfate was discovered and marketed by Merck & Co.

- ❖ Vorapaxar sulfate is a PAR-1 antagonist, which is critical in primate and human platelet aggregation and smooth muscle cell proliferation induced by thrombin.

- ❖ Vorapaxar sulfate is indicated for the reduction of thrombotic cardiovascular events in patients with a history of myocardial infarction (MI) or with peripheral arterial disease (PAD).

- ❖ Available as tablet, with each containing 2.08 mg of vorapaxar and the recommended dose is 2.08 mg orally once daily until disease progression or unacceptable toxicity.

- ❖ The sale of Zontivity® was not available up to Mar 2016.

### Key Approvals around the World*

|  | US (FDA) | EU (EMA) |
|---|---|---|
| First approval date | 05/08/2014 | 01/19/2014 |
| Application or approval No. | NDA 204886 | EMEA/H/C/002814 |
| Brand name | Zontivity® | Zontivity® |
| Indication | The reduction of thrombotic cardiovascular events in patients with a history of MI or with PAD. | The reduction of thrombotic cardiovascular events in patients with a history of MI or with PAD |
| Authorisation holder | Merck & Co. | Merck & Co. |

* Till Mar 2016, it has not been approved by PMDA (Japan) and CFDA (China).

## Active Ingredient

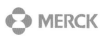

*Molecular formula*: $C_{29}H_{33}FN_2O_4 \cdot H_2SO_4$
*Molecular weight*: 590.70
*CAS No.*: 618385-01-6 (Vorapaxar)
705260-08-8 (Vorapaxar sulfate)
*Chemical name*: Ethyl (1R,3aR,4aR,6R,8aR,9S,9aS)-9-{(1E)-2-[5-(3-fluorophenyl)pyridin-2-yl]ethen-1-yl}-1-methyl-3-oxododecahydronaphtho[2,3-c]furan-6-yl] carbamate sulfate

*Parameters of Lipinski's "Rule of 5"*

| MW[a] | $H_D$ | $H_A$ | FRB[b] | PSA[b] | cLogP[b] |
|---|---|---|---|---|---|
| 492.58 | 1 | 6 | 6 | 77.5Å$^2$ | 5.39 ± 0.55 |

[a] Molecular weight of vorapaxar. [b] Calculated by ACD/Labs software V11.02.

## Drug Product*

*Dosage route*: Oral
*Strength*: 2.08 mg (Vorapaxar)
*Dosage form*: Tablet
*Inactive ingredient*: Lactose monohydrate, microcrystalline cellulose, croscarmellose sodium, povidone, magnesium stearate, lactose monohydrate, hypromellose, titanium dioxide, triacetin (glycerol triacetate) and iron oxide yellow.
*Recommended dose*: The recommended dose is 2.08 mg once daily, used with aspirin and/or clopidogrel according to their indications or standard of care.
There is limited clinical experience with other antiplatelet drugs or with vorapaxar sulfate as the only antiplatelet agent.

* Sourced from US FDA drug label information

# 2 Key Patents Information

## Summary

❖ Zontivity® (Vorapaxar sulfate) has got five-year NCE market exclusivity protection after it was initially approved by US FDA on May 08, 2014.

❖ Vorapaxar was originally discovered by Schering Plough (now a subsidiary of Merck & Co.), and its compound patent application was filed as PCT application by Schering Plough in 2003.

❖ The compound patent will expire in 2023 foremost, which has been granted in Europe, the United States, Japan and China successively.

Table 1    Vorapaxar's Compound Patent Protection in Drug-Mainstream Country

| Country | Publication/Patent NO. | Application Date | Granted Date | Estimated Expiry Date |
|---------|------------------------|------------------|--------------|------------------------|
| WO | WO03089428A1 | 04/14/2003 | / | / |
| US | US7304078B2 | 04/14/2003 | 12/04/2007 | 04/06/2024[a] |
| EP | EP1495018B1 | 04/14/2003 | 11/14/2007 | 04/14/2023 |
| JP | JP4558331B2 | 04/14/2003 | 10/06/2010 | 04/14/2023 |
| CN | CN1659162B | 04/14/2003 | 08/31/2011 | 04/14/2023 |

[a] The term of this patent is extended by 358 days.

Table 2    Originator's International Patent Application List (Patent Family)

| Publication NO. | Title | Applicant/Assignee/ Owner | Publication Date |
|-----------------|-------|---------------------------|------------------|
| **Technical Subjects** | **Active Ingredient (Free Base)'s Formula or Structure and Preparation** | | |
| WO03089428A1 | Tricyclic thrombin receptor antagonists | Schering Plough | 10/30/2003 |
| **Technical Subjects** | **Salt, Crystal, Polymorphic, Solvate (Hydrate), Isomer, Derivative Etc. and Preparation** | | |
| WO0196330A2 | Thrombin receptor antagonists | Schering Plough | 12/20/2001 |
| WO2006076415A2 | Exo- and diastereo-selective syntheses of himbacine analogs | Schering Plough | 07/20/2006 |
| WO2006076452A2 | An exo-selective synthesis of himbacine analogs | Schering Plough | 07/20/2006 |
| WO2006076564A1 | Synthesis of himbacine analogs | Schering Plough | 07/20/2006 |
| WO2006076565A2 | Preparation of chiral propargylic alcohol and ester intermediates of himbacine analogs | Schering Plough | 07/20/2006 |
| WO2008005348A1 | Synthesis of diethyl{[5-(3-fluorophenyl)-pyridine-2-yl]methyl} phosphonate used in the synthesis of himbacine analogs | Schering Plough | 01/10/2008 |
| WO2015013083A1 | Co-crystal of the PAR-1 receptor antagonist vorapaxar and aspirin | Merck & Co. | 01/29/2015 |
| WO2010141525A1 | Active metabolite of a thrombin receptor antagonist | Schering Plough | 12/09/2010 |
| **Technical Subjects** | **Formulation and Preparation** | | |
| WO2008005352A2 | Solid dose formulations of a thrombin receptor antagonist | Schering Plough | 01/10/2008 |
| WO2008005353A2 | Immediate-release tablet formulations of a thrombin receptor antagonist | Schering Plough | 01/10/2008 |
| WO2008039406A2 | Rapidly disintegrating lyophilized oral formulations of a thrombin receptor antagonist | Schering Plough | 04/03/2008 |
| WO2008079260A2 | Disintegration promoters in solid dose wet granulation formulations | Schering Plough | 07/03/2008 |
| **Technical Subjects** | **Indication or Methods for Medical Needs** | | |
| WO2007075808A2 | Methods for preventing and/or treating a cell proliferative disorder | Schering Plough | 07/05/2007 |
| WO2007075964A2 | Thrombin receptor antagonists as phophylaxis to complications from cardiopulmonary surgery | Schering Plough | 07/05/2007 |
| WO2008118320A1 | Reduction of adverse events.after percutaneous intervention by use of a thrombin receptor antagonist | Schering Plough | 10/02/2008 |
| WO2010057066A1 | Pharmacokinetically-based dosing regimens of a thrombin receptor antagonist | Schering Plough | 05/20/2010 |

*Continued*

| Publication NO. | Title | Applicant/Assignee/ Owner | Publication Date |
|---|---|---|---|
| WO2010093629A1 | PAR-1 antagonism in fed or antacid-dosed patients | Schering Plough | 08/19/2010 |
| WO2011041217A1 | The use of a PAR-1 antagonist in combination with a P2Y12 ADP receptor antagonist for inhibition of thrombosis | Schering Plough | 04/07/2011 |
| **Technical Subjects** | **Combination Including at Least Two Active Ingredients** | | |
| WO2007117621A1 | Use of combination preparations containing thrombin receptor antagonists for treating cardiovascular disorders | Schering Plough | 10/18/2007 |
| WO2009124103A2 | Combination therapies comprising PAR1 antagonists with PAR4 antagonists | Schering Plough | 10/08/2009 |
| WO2010144339A2 | A thrombin receptor antagonist and clopidogrel fixed dose tablet | Schering Plough | 12/16/2010 |

The data was updated until Jan 2016.

# 3   Chemistry

## Route 1:   Original Discovery Route

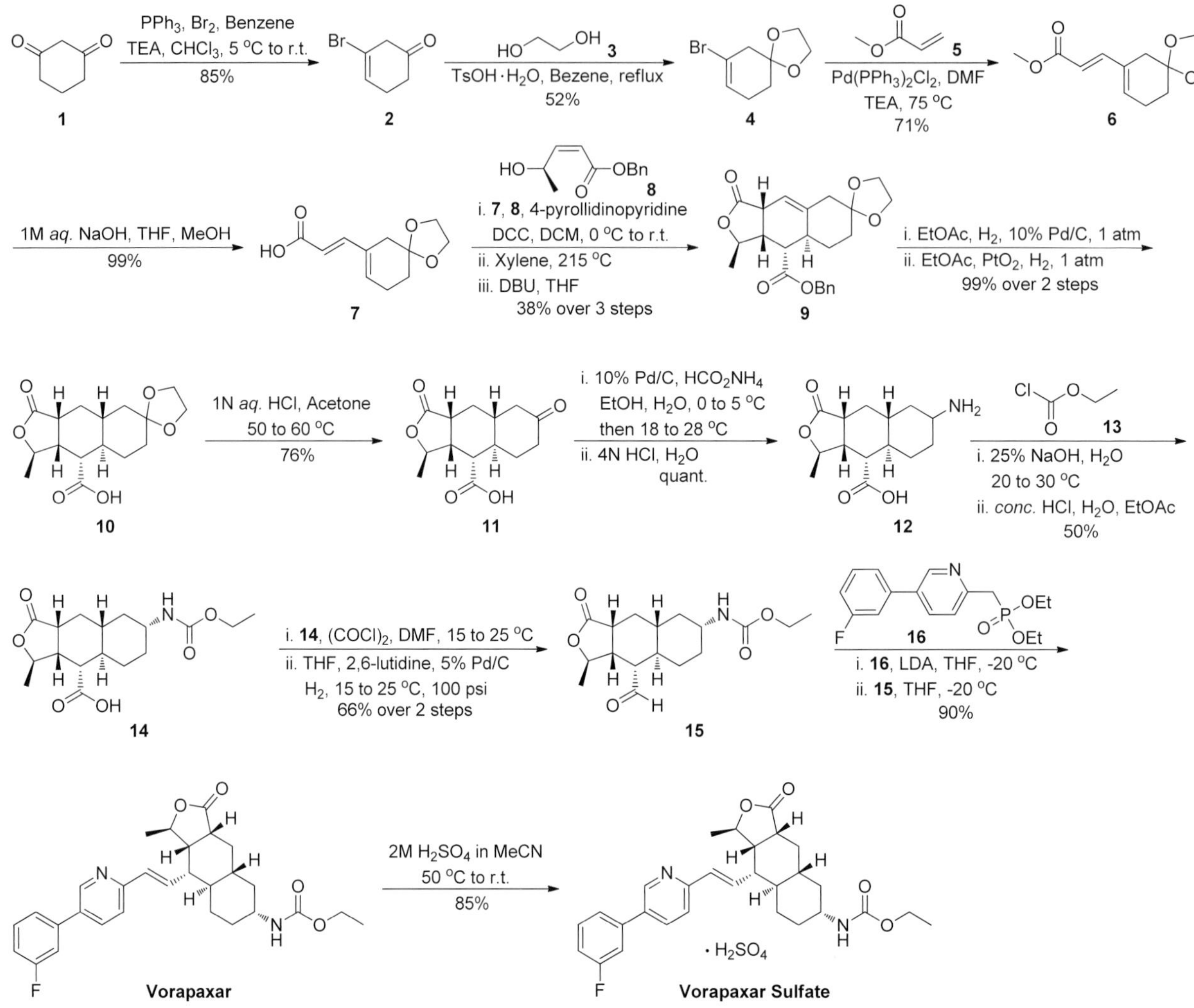

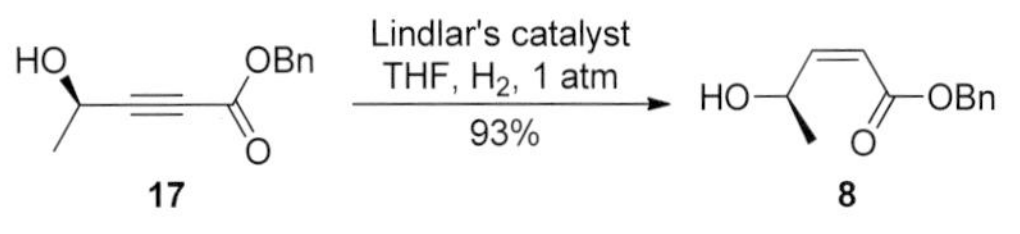

PPh$_3$, Br$_2$, Benzene
TEA, CHCl$_3$, 5 °C to r.t.
85%

**1**   **2**

HO᠆OH  **3**
TsOH·H$_2$O, Bezene, reflux
52%

**4**

**5**
Pd(PPh$_3$)$_2$Cl$_2$, DMF
TEA, 75 °C
71%

**6**

HO᠆OBn
**8**
i. **7**, **8**, 4-pyrollidinopyridine
DCC, DCM, 0 °C to r.t.
ii. Xylene, 215 °C
iii. DBU, THF
38% over 3 steps

1M aq. NaOH, THF, MeOH
99%

**7**

**9**

i. EtOAc, H$_2$, 10% Pd/C, 1 atm
ii. EtOAc, PtO$_2$, H$_2$, 1 atm
99% over 2 steps

1N aq. HCl, Acetone
50 to 60 °C
76%

**10**   **11**

i. 10% Pd/C, HCO$_2$NH$_4$
EtOH, H$_2$O, 0 to 5 °C
then 18 to 28 °C
ii. 4N HCl, H$_2$O
quant.

**12**

**13**
i. 25% NaOH, H$_2$O
20 to 30 °C
ii. conc. HCl, H$_2$O, EtOAc
50%

**14**

i. **14**, (COCl)$_2$, DMF, 15 to 25 °C
ii. THF, 2,6-lutidine, 5% Pd/C
H$_2$, 15 to 25 °C, 100 psi
66% over 2 steps

**15**

**16**
i. **16**, LDA, THF, -20 °C
ii. **15**, THF, -20 °C
90%

**Vorapaxar**

2M H$_2$SO$_4$ in MeCN
50 °C to r.t.
85%

· H$_2$SO$_4$

**Vorapaxar Sulfate**

Lindlar's catalyst
THF, H$_2$, 1 atm
93%

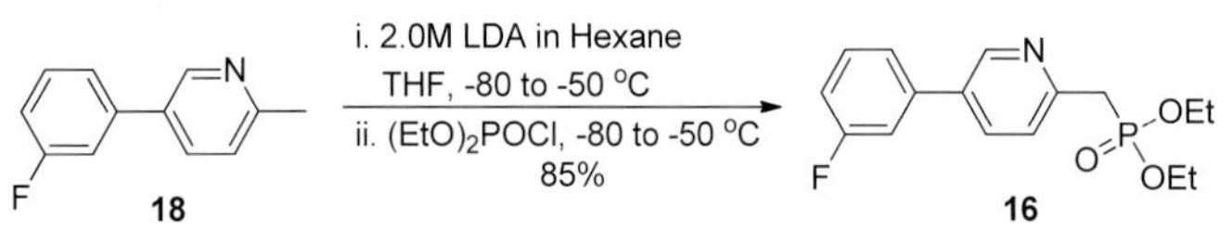

**17**   **8**

i. 2.0M LDA in Hexane
THF, -80 to -50 °C
ii. (EtO)$_2$POCl, -80 to -50 °C
85%

**18**   **16**

*Synthetic Route*:   Lactone **15** was derived from synthons **7** and **8**, which were readily prepared from commercial starting materials.    Acid **7** was constructed in four steps starting from enolation and bromination of cyclohexane-1,3-dione **1** and protection of resultant vinyl bromide **2** produced vinyl bromide **4** which first underwent a Heck reaction with methacrylate **5** followed by saponification of the ester **6** to afford the desired acid **7** in 31% over four steps.    Acid **7** was then esterified with *cis*-allylic alcohol **8** (prepared by hydrogenation of the alkyne **17** with Lindlar's catalyst in 93% yield) by way of a DCC coupling, and upon heating in refluxing xylenes, an intramolecular Diels-Alder reaction occurred and upon subsequent subjection to DBU, the tricyclic system **9** was secured in 38% over three steps as a single enantiomer.    Diastereoselective hydrogenation reduced the olefin with concomitant benzyl removal to generate key fragment **10**.    Next, acidic ketone revelation followed by reductive amination with ammonium formate delivered primary amines **12** as a mixture of diastereomers in 76% yield over two steps.   These amines were then converted to the corresponding carbamates, and resolution by means of recrystallization yielded 50% of **14** as the desired diastereomer.   Next, oxidation state adjustment of acid **14** to aldehyde **15** proceeded in 66% yield over two steps.   Finally, deprotonation of phosphonate **16** followed by careful addition of **15** and subsequent acidic quench delivered vorapaxar sulfate by the two-step protocol in 90% and 85% yield, respectively.   Thus, the overall yield was about 2%.[1-5]

# Route 2

TMAC: Trimethyacetyl chloride

[1]  Chackalamannil, S.; Clasby, M. C.; Greenlee, W. J., et al. WO03089428A1, **2003**.
[2]  Chackalamannil, S.; Greenlee, W. J.; Wang, Y., et al. US7304078B2, **2007**.
[3]  Thiruvengadam, T. K.; Wang, T.; Liao, J., et al. WO2006076564A1, **2006**.
[4]  Chackalamannil, S.; Asberom, T.; Xia, Y., et al. US6063847A, **2000**.
[5]  Lambert, J. B.; Liu, X. *J. Organomet. Chem.* **1996**, *521*, 203-210.

*Synthetic Route*:  In this strategy, conjugate addition of acrolein **1** to nitromethane in the presence of KOH, followed by treatment with sodium pyrosulfite gave nitro disulfonate **2** in 83% yield, which underwent hydrolysis with glyoxylic acid yielded 4-nitroheptanedial **3** in 86% yield.  The further cyclization in the presence of pyrrolidine and benzoic acid provided cyclo-hexenecarbaldehyde **4** in 75% yield, which went through Knoevenagel condensation with malonic acid **5** to lead to conjugated acid **6** in 60% yield.  Future esterification with propargyl alcohol **7** furnished the corresponding amide **8**, whose alkyne group was hydrogenatively reduced over Lindlar's catalyst to yield the olefin **9** in 74% yield over two steps.  Thermal Diels-Alder cyclization of triene **9** along with the sequential treatment with DBU furnished *cis*-lactone **10**, which was finally reduced to give primary amines **11**, coupled with **12** as illustrated in the first route to provide amide **13** in 85% yield over two steps. Finally, saponification of **13** in 5% aqueous NaOH and workup with diluted HCl provided **14** in 99% yield.[6-8]

Hereof, protection of 3-butyn-2(*R*)-ol **15** with HMDS in the presence of concentrated $H_2SO_4$ in refluxing THF yielded the corresponding silyl ether, which, after deprotonation with hexyllithium, underwent carbamoylation with 1-(diphenylcarbamoyl)imidazole **16** in THF/toluene to provide propargyl alcohol **7** in 84% yield.[6-8]  TFAA-induced rearrangement of 5-bromo-2-methylpyridine-1-oxide **17** secured the trifluoroacetate, without isolation, which was hydrolyzed in MeOH solution to yield (5-bromopyridin-2-yl)methanol trifluoroacetate salt **18** in 63% yield.  Basification of **18** followed by chlorination with $SOCl_2$ furnished 5-bromo-2-(chloromethyl)pyridine **19**, which was subsequently condensed with diethyl phosphite in the presence of LiHMDS to afford phosphonate **20**.  Suzuki coupling of bromopyridine derivative **20** with 3-fluorophenylboronic acid **21** actually afforded the desired phenylpyridine **22** in 75% yield over three steps.  Moreover, the entire way involving fifteen steps achieved in 6% overall yield.[6-8]

## 4  Pharmacology

## Summary

### Mechanism of Action

- ❖ Vorapaxar sulfate is a slowly reversible inhibitor of PAR-1 ($K_d$ = 1.2 nM), a thrombin receptor, which is critical in primate and human platelet aggregation and smooth muscle cell proliferation induced by thrombin.
- ❖ Vorapaxar sulfate inhibited thrombin-induced ($IC_{50}$ = 47 nM) and thrombin receptor agonist peptide (TRAP)-induced ($IC_{50}$ = 76 nM) platelet aggregation.
- ❖ The metabolite M20 inhibited thrombin-induced $\beta$-arrestin association with PAR-1 ($IC_{50}$ = 11.2 nM) for 15 min, and inhibited thrombin-induced calcium flux ($IC_{50}$ = 12.1 nM) in washed human platelets after 1 h pre-incubation.
- ❖ Vorapaxar sulfate showed no significant radioligand binding inhibition on a panel of 65 physiologically important receptors and a panel of 38 G-protein coupled receptors at 6 μM, except rat chloride channel.[9]
- ❖ Binding affinity:
  - PAR-1: $K_d$ = 1.2 nM (M20: $K_d$ = 1.6 nM).
  - Washed human platelet: $K_d$ = 1.08-1.2 nM.
- ❖ *In vitro* efficacy:
  - Stimulated human platelet aggregation: $IC_{50}$ = 15-76 nM.
  - Stimulated $Ca^{2+}$ transient in human CASMC and rat ASMC: $K_b$ = 0.63-2.9 nM.

### Ex Vivo Efficacy

- ❖ *Ex vivo* inhibition of aggregation of platelets derived from cynomolgus monkey.
  - haTRAP-induced aggregation in whole blood:
    - ♦ MED = 0.05 mg/kg (60% inhibition).
    - ♦ Complete inhibition at 0.1 mg/kg from 2 to 5 h after dosing and >90% inhibition at 24 h after dosing.

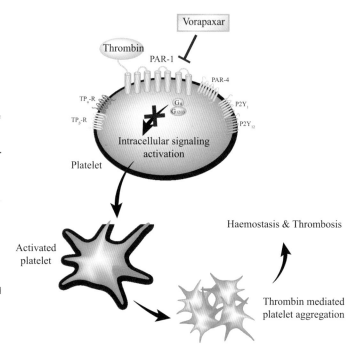

[6]  Wu, G. G.; Sudhakar, A.; Wang, T., et al. WO2006076415A2, **2006**.

[7]  Sudhakar, A.; Kwok, D-L.; Wu, G. G., et al. WO2006076452A2, **2006**.

[8]  Yong, K. H.; Zavialov, I. A.; Yin, J., et al. US20080004449A1, **2008**.

[9]  U.S. Food and Drug Administration (FDA) Database.  http://www.accessdata.fda.gov/drugsatfda_docs/nda/2014/204886Orig1s000PharmR.pdf (accessed Mar 2016).

- Folts thrombosis model:
  - SCH602539: MED = 0.1 mg/kg.　Inhibited haTRAP-induced platelet aggregation at 0.1 mg/kg (>70% inhibition), but not ADP-induced at 1 mg/kg.
  - Cangrelor: MED = 0.1 μg/kg/min.　Inhibited ADP-induced platelet aggregation, but not haTRAP or collagen-induced aggregation.

## Mechanism of Action

Table 3　Binding and Inhibition Efficacy of Vorapaxar Sulfate and Its Metabolites[9-11]

| Study | Target | Condition | Effect | |
|---|---|---|---|---|
| | | | Vorapaxar Sulfate | M20 |
| Binding affinity | PAR | NA | $K_d = 1.5$ nM | NA |
| | PAR-1 | Washed human platelet | $K_d = 1.2 \pm 0.3$ nM, $T_{1/2} = 190 \pm 50$ min | $K_d = 1.6 \pm 0.5$ nM; $T_{1/2} = 206$ min |
| | Human platelet membrane | haTRAP-induced | $K_i = 8.5$ nM | NA |
| | Washed human platelet | Saturation binding | $K_d = 1.2$ nM | $K_d = 1.6$ nM |
| | Washed human platelet | Competition binding | $K_i = 1.0$ nM | $K_i = 1.0$ nM |
| | Washed human platelet | Association binding | $K_{on} = 0.00406$ nM$^{-1}$min$^{-1}$, $K_{off} = 0.00440$ min$^{-1}$, $K_d = 1.08$ nM, $T_{1/2} = 158$ min | $K_{on} = 0.00369$ nM$^{-1}$min$^{-1}$, $K_{off} = 0.00842$ min$^{-1}$, $K_d = 1.14$ nM, $T_{1/2} = 82$ min |
| | Washed human platelet | Dissociation | $K_{off} = 0.003731$ min$^{-1}$, $T_{1/2} = 186$ min | $K_{off} = 0.003332$ min$^{-1}$, $T_{1/2} = 208$ min |
| Inhibition of Ca$^{2+}$ efflux | Human CASMC | TK agonist-induced | $EC_{50} = 4.5$ nM | NA |
| | Washed human platelets | Thrombin-induced[b] | $IC_{50} = 13.1$ and 6.7 nM, | $IC_{50} = 12.1$ and 5.0 nM, |
| Inhibition of Ca$^{2+}$ transient | Human CASMC | TK agonist-induced | $K_b = 0.63$ nM | $K_b = 13.1$ nM |
| | Rat ASMC | TK agonist-induced | $K_b = 1.3$ nM | $K_b = 3.9$ nM |
| | Human CASMC | Thrombin-induced | $K_b = 1.1$ nM | $K_b = 3.9$ nM |
| | Rat ASMC | Thrombin-induced | $K_b = 2.9$ nM | NA |
| Thymidine incorporation | Human CASMC | Thrombin-induced | $K_b = 1.1$ | NA |
| | Human CASMC | Factor Xa-stimulated | $K_i = 9.6$ | NA |
| Inhibition of human platelet aggregation | Aggregation | Thrombin-induced | $IC_{50} = 47$ nM | NA |
| | | TRAP-induced | $IC_{50} = 76$ nM | NA |
| | | SFLLRN-induced[a] | $IC_{50} = 41.0$ and 106 nM | $IC_{50} = 42.9$ and 120 nM |
| | | PAR-1-induced | <5% (1 μM) | <10% (1 μM) |
| | | PAR-4-induced | <80% (1 μM) | <80% (1 μM) |
| | | ADP-induced | <80% (1 μM) | <80% (1 μM) |
| | | haTRAP-induced | $IC_{50} = 15$ nM | NA |
| Inhibition of β-arrestin association with PAR-1 | β-arrestin association | Thrombin-induced[c] | $IC_{50} = 12.1$, 9.92 and 9.97 nM | $IC_{50} = 11.2$, 11.1 and 9.37 nM |

Vorapaxar sulfate inhibition of haTRAP-stimulated P-selectin expression in washed human platelets.　[a] Inhibition of TRAP peptide (SFLLRN) induced platelet aggregation in human PRP after 1 and 2 h pre-incubation.　The inhibition of SFLLRN-induced platelet aggregation was >75% at 300 nM vorapaxar sulfate.　[b] Inhibition of thrombin induced calcium flux in washed human platelets after 1 and 2 h pre-incubation.　[c] Inhibition of β-arrestin association with PAR-1 induced by thrombin for 15, 90 or 180 min.　haTRAP: High affinity thrombin receptor activating peptide.　TK: TFLLRNPNDK-NH2 (a PAR-1 selective agonist).　CASMC: Coronary aortic smooth muscle cells.　ASMC: Aortic smooth muscle cells.　$K_b$: Antagonist dissociation constant.　The antagonist dissociation constant, $K_b$, using Gaddum analysis.　SFLLRN: TRAP peptide.　$K_d = K_{off}/K_{on}$.　$T_{1/2} = 0.693/K_{off}$.

[9] FDA Database.　http://www.accessdata.fda.gov/drugsatfda_docs/nda/2014/204886Orig1s000PharmR.pdf (accessed Mar 2016).
[10] European Medicines Agency (EMA) Database.　http://www.ema.europa.eu/docs/en_GB/document_library/EPAR_Public_assessment_report/human/002814/WC500183331.pdf (accessed Mar 2016).
[11] Hawes, B. E.; Zhai, Y.; Hesk, D., et al. *Eur. J. Pharmacol.* **2015**, 762, 221-228.

Table 4    The Off Target Activity of Vorapaxar Sulfate[9]

| Receptor | Species | Conc. (µM) | %Inhibition | Selectivity |
|---|---|---|---|---|
| P2X | Rat | 6 | 40 | >600 |
| 5-HT$_{2B}$ | Human | 6 | 43 | >66 |
| L-calcium channel | Rat | 6 | 35 | >5000 |
| Chloride channel | Rat | 6 | 58 | <6.5 |
| ADO transporter | Guinea pig | 6 | 53 | ~30000 |
| 5-HT transporter | Human | 6 | 31 | <984 |

## *Ex Vivo* Efficacy

Table 5    *Ex Vivo* the Platelet Aggregation Effect of Vorapaxar Sulfate[9]

| Animal Model | | Compound | Dose (mg/kg) | Route & Duration | Effect | |
|---|---|---|---|---|---|---|
| Study/Model | Animal | | | | MED (mg/kg) | Finding |
| haTRAP stimulated in whole blood | Cynomolgus monkey | Vorapaxar sulfate | 0.05, 0.1, 0.3, 1, 3 | p.o., single dose (1-24 h) | 0.05 | 0.05 mg/kg: 60% inhibition of *ex vivo* platelet aggregation at 3 h after dosing. 0.1 mg/kg: Complete inhibition of *ex vivo* haTRAP-induced platelet aggregation from 2 to 5 h after dosing and >90% inhibition at 24 h after dosing. |
| | | SCH602539 | 0.1, 0.3, 1 | p.o., single dose (1-24 h) | 0.1 | 0.1 mg/kg: Resulted in complete inhibition of *ex vivo* platelet aggregation from 3 to 6 h after dosing and >60% inhibition of *ex vivo* haTRAP-induced platelet aggregation at 24 h after dosing. |
| Folts thrombosis model | Cynomolgus monkey | SCH602539 | 0.1, 0.3, 1 | i.v., single dose (30 min) | 0.1 | Reduced the frequency of CFRs by 50% at 0.1 mg/kg. Inhibited *ex vivo* platelet aggregation in response to the PAR-1 selective agonist peptide haTRAP by more than 70%, but did not inhibit platelet aggregation induced by ADP at two highest doses. |
| | | Cangrelor | 0.1, 0.2, 0.3 (µg/kg) | i.v., infusion × 30 min | 0.1 (µg/kg/min) | Reduced the frequency of CFRs by 40% at 0.1 µg/kg/min. Inhibited *ex vivo* platelet aggregation induced by ADP, but did not inhibit platelet aggregation induced by haTRAP or collagen at two highest doses. |
| | | Combination of SCH 602539 and cangrelor | NA | NA | NA | Inhibited the aggregation induced by haTRAP and ADP in a dose-related manner with the level of inhibition similar to that for each drug alone. |

SCH602539: Structurally similar analog of vorapaxar sulfate.    CFRS: Cyclic flow reductions.    MED: Minimum effective dose.

[9]  FDA Database.    http://www.accessdata.fda.gov/drugsatfda_docs/nda/2014/204886Orig1s000PharmR.pdf (accessed Mar 2016).

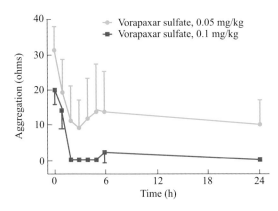

**Study:** Platelet aggregation in response to 1 μM haTRAP in whole blood from cynomolgus monkey model.

**Animal:** Cynomolgus monkey.

**Model:** haTRAP-induced platelet aggregation was evaluated in whole blood collected from cynomolgus monkey.

**Administration:** Treated for 1-24 h, p.o., vorapaxar sulfate: 0.05 and 0.1 mg/kg.

**Test:** Platelet aggregation.

**Result:** Treatment with 0.1 mg/kg vorapaxar sulfate resulted in a complete inhibition effect.

**Figure A** *Ex Vivo* Platelet Aggregation of Vorapaxar Sulfate in Whole Blood from Cynomolgus Monkey Models after a Single Administration[9]

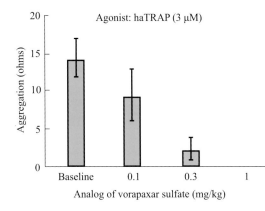

**Study:** Platelet aggregation of analog of vorapaxar.

**Animal:** Cynomolgus monkey.

**Model:** Folts thrombosis model.

**Administration:** Treated for 30 min, i.v., analog of vorapaxar sulfate: 0.1, 0.3 and 1 mg/kg.

**Starting:** After stable CFRs were achieved.

**Test:** Platelet aggregation.

**Result:** Treatment with 0.1 mg/kg analog of vorapaxar sulfate reduced the frequency of CFRs by 50%.

**Figure B** *Ex Vivo* Platelet Aggregation of Analog of Vorapaxar Sulfate in Monkeys Subjected to Folts Thrombosis Models after a Single Administration[9]

# 5  ADME & Drug-Drug Interaction

## Summary

### Absorption of Vorapaxar

❖ Exhibited a linear pharmacokinetics in humans following oral dosing.　The increases in $C_{max}$ and AUC appeared to be dose-proportional in the dose range of 1 to 20 mg vorapaxar.

❖ Had moderate oral bioavailability in rats (33%), high in monkeys (86%) and humans (88.7%).

❖ Was absorbed slowly in rats ($T_{max}$ = 3.3 h), but rapidly in monkeys ($T_{max}$ = 1 h) and humans ($T_{max}$ = 1-1.5 h).

❖ Showed a half-life of 159 h in humans, much longer than that in non-clinical species (5.1-13 h), after intravenous administrations.

❖ Had moderate clearance in rats (21 mL/min/kg), but low in monkeys (3 mL/min/kg), in contrast to liver blood flow, after intravenous administrations.

❖ Showed an extensive tissue distribution in rats and monkeys, with apparent volumes of distribution at 4.6 and 2.2 L/kg, respectively, after intravenous administrations.

❖ Had a high permeability, with the $P_{app(A→B)}$ = 27.9-34.0 × 10$^{-6}$ cm/s in Caco-2 cell monolayer model.

### Distribution of Vorapaxar

❖ Exhibited very high plasma protein binding in humans (99.82%-99.84%), mice (99.7%-99.8%), rats (99.6%-99.7%), rabbits (99.8%) and monkeys (99.8%).　Note that the drug was highly bound to human serum albumin compared to $α_1$-acid glycoprotein at physiological concentrations.

❖ Had a $C_b$:$C_p$ ratio of 0.56-0.60 in humans, suggesting the drug did not preferentially distribute into red blood cells.

❖ SD and Long-Evans male rats after single oral administration:

---

[9] FDA Database.　http://www.accessdata.fda.gov/drugsatfda_docs/nda/2014/204886Orig1s000PharmR.pdf (accessed Mar 2016).

- The drug was widely distributed to all tissues, except for the lens of eyes.
- Concentrations of radioactivity were measurable in the brain at two sampling times, 2 & 8 h post-dose, suggesting that [$^{14}$C]vorapaxar had limited penetration of the blood brain barrier.
- Other than the gastrointestinal tract, the higher concentration levels were observed in liver, spleen, adrenal gland, pituitary, thyroid gland, kidneys and brown fat.
- Elimination of radioactivity from tissues was complete in the majority of tissues at 168 h post-dose, but the levels of radioactivity in pituitary and testes were still detected.
- The pigmented rats at 168 h post-dose had concentrations in pigmented region of skin and eyes with the half-life much great than 168 h.

## Metabolism of Vorapaxar

❖ Overall, the parent drug represented the most abundant component, with M20 (mono-hydroxy metabolite) as the major metabolite in human plasma.

❖ Several metabolites of vorapaxar (M5, M7a, M8, M16, M17, M19, M19a, M20, M20b, M21 and M24) were observed in plasma of humans, rabbits, monkeys, rats and mice.

❖ CYP3A4 was the major metabolizing enzyme, with CYP2C19, 1A1, 1A2 involved.

## Excretion of Vorapaxar

❖ Was predominantly excreted in feces of humans and animal species, with the M19 as the major component in feces.

❖ Vorapaxar was eliminated primarily in the form of metabolites, with no parent drug detected in urine.

❖ About 27%-31% of radioactivity was recovered *via* biliary excretion in bile duct-cannulated (BDC) rats after oral administrations.

## Drug-Drug Interaction

❖ Vorapaxar was an inhibitor of CYP2C8 ($IC_{50}$ = 1.5 μM), CYP2A6, CYP2C19, CYP2D6 and CYP2C9 ($IC_{50} \geq 30$ μM).

❖ Vorapaxar had a low potential induction to CYPs. 10 and 30 μM Vorapaxar resulted in an increase in CYP1A2 activity of 2.66- and 2.97-fold, respectively, and in CYP2B6 activity of 3.91- and 4.66-fold, respectively.

❖ Vorapaxar had weak inhibition for OATP1B1, OATP1B3, OAT1 and OCT2 ($IC_{50}$ >10 μM), but had strong inhibition for OAT3 ($IC_{50}$ = 2.2 μM) and BCRP ($IC_{50}$ = 2.5 μM).

❖ Vorapaxar was not a substrate, but a strong inhibitor of P-gp ($IC_{50}$ = 1.2 μM).

# Absorption

Table 6 *In Vivo* Pharmacokinetic Parameters of Vorapaxar in Rats and Monkeys after Single Oral and Intravenous Dose of Vorapaxar[9, 10]

| Species | Route | Dose (mg/kg) | $T_{max}$ (h) | $C_{max}$ (μg/mL) | $AUC_{0-48}$ (μg·h/mL) | $T_{1/2}$ (h) | Cl (mL/min/kg) | $V_{ss}$ (L/kg) | F (%) |
|---|---|---|---|---|---|---|---|---|---|
| Rat | i.v. | 10 | NA | NA | 7.9 | 5.1 | 21 | 4.6 | - |
| | p.o. | 10 | 3.3 | 0.33 | 2.6 | NA | NA | NA | 33 |
| Monkey | i.v. | 1 | NA | NA | 5.6 | 13 | 3.0 | 2.2 | - |
| | p.o. | 1 | 1.0 | 0.65 | 4.8 | NA | NA | NA | 86 |

Table 7 *In Vivo* Pharmacokinetic Parameters of Vorapaxar in Healthy Adult Volunteers after Single Oral and Intravenous Dose of Vorapaxar[12]

| Species | Route | Dose (mg) | $T_{max}$ (h) | $C_{max}$ (ng/mL) | $AUC_{0-24}$ (ng·h/mL) | $T_{1/2}$ (h) | F (%) |
|---|---|---|---|---|---|---|---|
| Human | i.v. | 73.7 μg | 0.30 (0.25-0.50) | 1.17 (11) | 43.2$^b$ (25) | 159 (22) | - |
| | p.o. | 2.5 | 1.25 (1.00-2.00) | 27.0 (14) | 1300$^a$ (19) | 196 (35) | 88.7 |
| | p.o. | 1 | 1.00 (0.5-4.0) | 9.78 (31) | 58.5 (24) | NA | NA |
| | p.o. | 3 | 1.00 (0.5-1.0) | 38.2 (25) | 225 (15) | NA | NA |
| | p.o. | 5 | 1.00 (0.5-2.0) | 56.4 (25) | 315 (21) | NA | NA |
| | p.o. | 10 | 1.00 (1.0-2.0) | 85.4 (24) | 592 (14) | NA | NA |
| | p.o. | 20 | 1.5 (1.0-4.0) | 188 (32) | 1280 (23) | NA | NA |

The values of $C_{max}$ and $AUC_{0-24}$ were geometric mean (CV%).  $^a$ $AUC_{0-t}$.  $^b$ $AUC_{0-t}$ and first sample collected were at 0.25 h post i.v. bolus administration.

[9] FDA Database. http://www.accessdata.fda.gov/drugsatfda_docs/nda/2014/204886Orig1s000PharmR.pdf (accessed Mar 2016).
[10] EMA Database. http://www.ema.europa.eu/docs/en_GB/document_library/EPAR_Public_assessment_report/human/002814/WC500183331.pdf (accessed Mar 2016).
[12] FDA Database. http://www.accessdata.fda.gov/drugsatfda_docs/nda/2014/204886Orig1s000ClinPharmR.pdf (accessed Mar 2016).

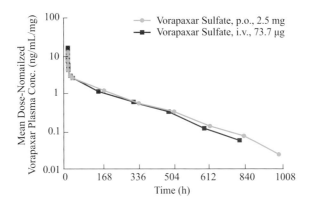

Figure C   *In Vivo* Plasma Concentration-Time Profiles after Single Oral Dose of Unlabeled Vorapaxar Sulfate and Intravenous [[14]C]Vorapaxar Sulfate[12]

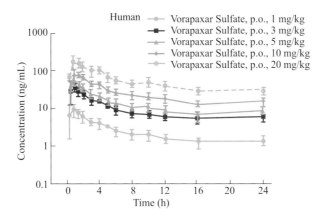

Figure D   *In Vivo* Plasma Concentration-Time Profiles of Vorapaxar in Humans after Single Oral Dose of Vorapaxar Sulfate[12]

Table 8   *In Vitro* Permeability of Vorapaxar and M20 in Caco-2 and LLC-PK1 Cell Monolayer Model[9, 10]

| Drug | Cell Type | Conc. (μM) | Papp (1 × 10⁻⁶ cm/s) | Efflux Ratio | Permeability Class |
|------|-----------|------------|----------------------|--------------|--------------------|
| Vorapaxar | Caco-2 | NA | 27.9-34.0 | NA | High |
| M20 | LLC-PK1 cell | 1 | 25.4 | 0.9 | High |
| Verapamil | LLC-PK1 cell | 1 | 31.9 | 1.4 | High |
| Metoprolol | LLC-PK1 cell | 1 | 31.3 | 1.1 | High |
| Mannitol | LLC-PK1 cell | 1 | 3.4 | 0.9 | Moderate |

[9]   FDA Database.   http://www.accessdata.fda.gov/drugsatfda_docs/nda/2014/204886Orig1s000PharmR.pdf (accessed Mar 2016).
[10]  EMA Database.   http://www.ema.europa.eu/docs/en_GB/document_library/EPAR_Public_assessment_report/human/002814/WC500183331.pdf (accessed Mar 2016).
[12]  FDA Database.   http://www.accessdata.fda.gov/drugsatfda_docs/nda/2014/204886Orig1s000ClinPharmR.pdf (accessed Mar 2016).

# Distribution

Table 9    *In Vitro* Plasma Protein Binding and Blood Partitioning of Vorapaxar and Metabolites[9]

| Binding of [¹⁴C]Vorapaxar or M20 to Plasma Protein of Different Species | | | | | Binding of Vorapaxar to Isolated Human Plasma Protein | | |
|---|---|---|---|---|---|---|---|
| | M20 | | Vorapaxar | | Study | Conc. (µg/mL) | %Bound |
| Species | Conc. (µg/mL) | %Bound | Conc. (µg/mL) | %Bound | | | |
| CD1 mouse | 0.19 | 98.86 | 0.0353-9.02 | 99.7-99.8 | HSA 4% | 0.05, 0.5 | 99.1, 99.2 |
| SD rat | NA | NA | 0.0353-9.02 | 99.6-99.7 | HSA 3% | 0.05, 0.5 | 99.0, 99.0 |
| Pregnant NZW-rabbit | 0.54 | 99.4 | 0.0353-9.02 | 99.8 | HSA 2% | 0.05, 0.5 | 98.6, 98.7 |
| Cynomolgus monkey | 0.83 | 97.9 | 0.0353-9.02 | 99.8 | 1% $\alpha_1$-acid glycoprotein + HSA, 4% | 0.05, 0.5 | 99.2, 99.3 |
| Human | 0.03-0.05 | 99.0-99.2 | 0.0353-9.02 | 99.9 | 1% $\alpha_1$-acid glycoprotein + HSA, 3% | 0.05, 0.5 | 99.2, 99.1 |
| | | | 0.02-0.04 | 99.8 | 1% $\alpha_1$-acid glycoprotein + HSA, 2% | 0.05, 0.5 | 98.8, 99.0 |

The report stated that in the concentration range of 50-500 ng/mL, ≤11.1% and 1% of [¹⁴C]vorapaxar partitioned to blood cellular components and to platelets, respectively.    HSA: Human serum albumin.

## Other Findings:[12]

❖  The mean blood-to-plasma radioactivity ratio ranged from 0.56-0.60 over 120 h in humans.

Table 10    Tissue Distribution and Excretion Pattern of [¹⁴C]Vorapaxar-Derived Radiocarbon in Sprague Dawley and Long-Evans Rats after Single Oral Dose of [¹⁴C]Vorapaxar[9, 10]

| Species | SD Rat | | | | | | | | Long-Evans Rat | | | | | | | |
|---|---|---|---|---|---|---|---|---|---|---|---|---|---|---|---|---|
| | Radioactivity (ng eq./g) | | | | | | | | Radioactivity (ng eq./g) | | | | | | | |
| Tissues | 0.25 h | 2 h | 8 h | 24 h | 48 h | 72 h | 168 h | Tissue/Blood AUC$_{0-168}$ Ratio | 0.25 h | 2 h | 8 h | 24 h | 48 h | 72 h | 168 h | Tissue/Blood AUC$_{0-168}$ Ratio |
| Blood | 47.7 | 239 | 232 | BLQ | BLQ | BLQ | BLQ | 1.00 | BLQ | 259 | 251 | 91.3 | BLQ | BLQ | BLQ | 1.00 |
| Brain | BLQ | 149 | 163 | BLQ | BLQ | BLQ | BLQ | 0.68 | BLQ | 266 | 174 | BLQ | BLQ | BLQ | BLQ | 0.53 |
| Kidneys | 154 | 1440 | 1600 | 416 | 91.8 | BLQ | BLQ | 9.86 | 145 | 1580 | 1930 | 607 | 55.6 | BLQ | BLQ | 7.44 |
| Pituitary gland | BLQ | 846 | 2240 | 4010 | 908 | 618 | 555 | 55.0 | BLQ | 987 | 2930 | 1550 | 952 | 955 | 424 | 30.7 |
| Spleen | 177 | 2280 | 2320 | 910 | 300 | BLQ | BLQ | 17.9 | BLQ | 1660 | 3030 | 1920 | 223 | 99.7 | BLQ | 16.4 |
| Thyroid gland | 66.1 | 1420 | 2130 | 567 | 92.0 | BLQ | BLQ | 12.4 | 228 | 2160 | 5860 | 1170 | 170 | 25.9 | BLQ | 18.7 |
| Liver | 967 | 3110 | 1910 | 314 | 83.0 | BLQ | BLQ | 12.1 | 791 | 4080 | 3880 | 596 | 71.1 | BLQ | BLQ | 13.2 |
| Adrenal gland | 155 | 2010 | 3130 | 2160 | 314 | BLQ | BLQ | 27.2 | 146 | 2100 | 4100 | 2680 | 182 | 89.0 | BLQ | 21.1 |
| Lungs | 113 | 949 | 1190 | 354 | 75.3 | BLQ | BLQ | 7.52 | 90.3 | 1180 | 2100 | 554 | 41.1 | BLQ | BLQ | 7.23 |
| Fat (brown) | 115 | 941 | 1570 | 174 | 28.8 | BLQ | BLQ | 7.26 | 118 | 1750 | 1760 | 310 | BLQ | BLQ | BLQ | 5.82 |
| Large intestine | 70.3 | 511 | 2130 | 331 | 122 | 22.6 | BLQ | 10.8 | 1020 | 5000 | 3020 | 763 | 63.4 | 29.4 | BLQ | 12.9 |
| Stomach | 1420 | 1340 | 767 | 496 | 144 | 47.9 | BLQ | 9.04 | 2190 | 1660 | 1060 | 545 | 51.4 | BLQ | BLQ | 5.68 |
| Testis | BLQ | 154 | 214 | 67.0 | 20.4 | BLQ | 72.5 | 1.35 | BLQ | 258 | 252 | 91.8 | BLQ | 63.9 | BLQ | 1.67 |
| Eyeballs | BLQ | 36.0 | 130 | 197 | BLQ | BLQ | BLQ | 0.98 | BLQ | 409 | 858 | 1040 | 1040 | 989 | 1040 | 29.1 |
| Skin | BLQ | 251 | 460 | 184 | BLQ | BLQ | BLQ | 1.74 | BLQ | 438 | 553 | 412 | 71.9 | 217 | 126 | 6.38 |

BLQ: Below quantifiable limit of 56.6 ng vorapaxar eq./g.

[9]   FDA Database.    http://www.accessdata.fda.gov/drugsatfda_docs/nda/2014/204886Orig1s000PharmR.pdf (accessed Mar 2016).
[10]  EMA Database.    http://www.ema.europa.eu/docs/en_GB/document_library/EPAR_Public_assessment_report/human/002814/WC500183331.pdf (accessed Mar 2016).
[12]  FDA Database.    http://www.accessdata.fda.gov/drugsatfda_docs/nda/2014/204886Orig1s000ClinPharmR.pdf (accessed Mar 2016).

# Metabolism

Table 11   *In Vitro* Identification of Human CYP450 Enzymes Responsible for the Metabolism of Vorapaxar[9, 10, 13]

| Parameter | HLM with High CYP3A4 Activity | CYP3A4 | Recombinant CYP450 Enzymes | | | |
|---|---|---|---|---|---|---|
| | | | Inhibitor | Enzyme | Inhibitor Conc. (μM) | %Inhibition |
| Vorapaxar Conc. (μM) | 10 | 10 | Ketoconazole | CYP3A4/5 | 2 | 89 |
| % Formation of M19 | 11.5 | - | | | | |
| $K_m$ (μM) | 23.5 | 22.9 | Tranylcypromine | CYP2C19 | 100 | 34 |
| $V_{max}$ (pM/nM P450/min) | 57.9 | 166 | | | | |
| $V_{max}/K_m$ (μL/nM P450/min) | 2.46 | 7.25 | Ticlopidine | CYP2C19/CYP2B16 | 20 | 5 |

The metabolism of [$^{14}$C]vorapaxar was evaluated using human liver microsomes from a single donor with high CYP3A4 activity and 19 recombinant CYP450 enzymes in incubations for 30-120 min at 37 ℃ in the presence of an NADPH generating system.

Table 12   Correlation (r) Value Between M19 Formation Rates from Vorapaxar and CYP450 Enzyme Specific Activities[9, 10, 13]

| P450 Enzyme Specific Reaction | CYP450 Involved | M19 (r value) |
|---|---|---|
| Phenacetin *O*-Deethylation | CYP1A2 | 0.22 |
| Coumarin 7-Hydroxylation | CYP2A6 | 0.38 |
| Bupropion Hydroxylation | CYP2B6 | 0.14 |
| Paclitaxel 6α-Hydroxylation | CYP2C8 | 0.13 |
| Diclofenac 4'-Hydroxylation | CYP2C9 | 0.11 |
| *S*-Mephenytoin 4'-Hydroxylation | CYP2C19 | 0.22 |
| Dextromethorphan *O*-Demethylation | CYP2D6 | 0.68 |
| Chlorzoxazone 6-Hydroxylation | CYP2E1 | 0.44 |
| Midazolam 1'-Hydroxylation | CYP3A4/5 | 0.75 |
| Testosterone 6β-Hydroxylation | CYP3A4/5 | 0.92 |
| Lauric Acid 12-Hydroxylation | CYP4A11 | 0.10 |

Table 13   Metabolites formed after Incubation of [$^{14}$C]Vorapaxar (10 μM) with HLM, HLS9 and CYP450 Enzymes[13]

| Matrix | % of Radioactivity | | | | | | |
|---|---|---|---|---|---|---|---|
| | Parent | M18 | M19 | M20a | M22 | M23 | M24 |
| HLM | 92.7 | - | 5.12 | - | - | - | - |
| S9 | 95.7 | - | 3.42 | - | - | - | - |
| CYP1A1 | 96.3 | - | 1.96[a] | 1.73[a] | - | BIT | BIT |
| CYP1A2 | 98.3 | - | 0.23[a] | 0.78[a] | - | BIT | - |
| CYP2B6 | 97.7 | - | - | 0.44 | - | BIT | - |
| CYP2C9 | 98.8 | - | BIT | - | - | - | - |
| CYP2C19 | 94.1 | - | 5.91 | - | - | BIT | - |
| CYP2D6 | 98.1 | - | - | 0.48 | - | - | - |
| CYP3A4 | 72.5 | 0.63 | 22.1[a] | 0.68[a] | 1.0 | - | BIT |
| CYP3A5 | 93.9 | - | 0.15[a] | 3.65[a] | - | - | - |
| Control microsomes | 98.7 | - | - | - | - | - | - |

BIT: Below integration threshold of flow scintillation analyzer detected by MS.   [a] M19 and M20a were not separated in the radiochromatogram.

[9]   FDA Database.   http://www.accessdata.fda.gov/drugsatfda_docs/nda/2014/204886Orig1s000PharmR.pdf (accessed Mar 2016).
[10]   EMA Database.   http://www.ema.europa.eu/docs/en_GB/document_library/EPAR_Public_assessment_report/human/ 002814/WC500183331.pdf (accessed Mar 2016).
[13]   Ghosal, A.; Lu, X.; Penner, N., et al. *Drug Metab. Dispos*. **2011**, *39*, 30-38.

Table 14    Metabolites in Plasma, Urine and Feces in Humans and Non-clinical Species after Single Oral Dose of Vorapaxar[9, 12]

| Matrix | Species | Gender | Route | Dose (mg/kg) | Time (h) | % of Radioactivity or % of Dose | | | | | | | | | | | |
|---|---|---|---|---|---|---|---|---|---|---|---|---|---|---|---|---|---|
| | | | | | | M0 | M5 | M7a | M8 | M16 | M17 | M19 | M19a | M20 | M20b | M21 | M24 |
| Plasma | Mouse | Male | p.o. | 75 | 6 | 80.7 | NA | NA | NA | BIT | NA | 15.0 | BIT | 2.2 | NA | NA | NA |
| | Rat | Male | p.o. | 3 | 4 | 67.7 | NA | 1.5 | ND | NA | 1.6 | 23.5 | 4.3 | BIT | ND | ND | 1.5 |
| | | Female | p.o. | 3 | 4 | 73.4 | NA | 1.8 | 0.8 | NA | 2.3 | 10.6 | 3.5 | ND | BIT | 3.9 | BIT |
| | Rabbit[c] | Female | p.o. | 20 | 24 | 100 | ND | 4.94 | NA | NA | NA | 4.11 | ND | 16.7 | NA | NA | NA |
| | Monkey | Male | p.o. | 0.5 | 8 | 53.5 | ND | NA | ND | 2.3 | BIT | 2.2 | BIT | 38.2 | NA | 3.8 | NA |
| | | Female | p.o. | 0.5 | 8 | 46.5 | BIT | NA | BIT | 3.6 | BIT | 2.1 | BIT | 43.2 | NA | 4.7 | NA |
| | Human | M & F | p.o. | 2.5 mg | 0-24 | 181[a] | NA | NA | NA | NA | NA | NA | NA | 32.2[a] | NA | NA | NA |
| Urine[b] | Mouse | M & F | p.o. | 75 | NA | 0.3 | NA | NA | NA | 0.02 | NA | 2.0 | NA | 0 | NA | BLQ | NA |
| | Rat (BDC) | Male | p.o. | 3 | NA | 0 | NA | NA | NA | ND | NA | 0.87 | NA | ND | NA | ND | NA |
| | | Female | p.o. | 3 | NA | 0 | NA | NA | NA | ND | NA | 0.54 | NA | ND | NA | 0 | NA |
| | Rabbit | M & F | p.o. | 20 | 7 days | 2 | NA | 38.2 | NA | 18 | NA | 14 | NA | NA | NA | NA | NA |
| | Monkey (BDC) | M & F | p.o. | 0.5 | NA | 0 | NA | NA | NA | 0.7 | NA | 0.05 | NA | 0 | NA | 0 | NA |
| | Human[d] | M & F | p.o. | 9.3 mg | 0-168 | ND | NA | NA | 0.42 | 0.41 | 1.40 | 1.21 | ND | ND | ND | ND | NA |
| Feces[b] | Mouse | M & F | p.o. | 75 | NA | 36.1 | NA | NA | NA | 2.7 | NA | 56.7 | NA | 0.63 | NA | BLQ | NA |
| | Rat (BDC) | Male | p.o. | 3 | NA | 15 | NA | NA | NA | ND | NA | 83.7 | NA | ND | NA | ND | NA |
| | | Female | p.o. | 3 | NA | 9.2 | NA | NA | NA | ND | NA | 50.6 | NA | ND | NA | 8.3 | NA |
| | Monkey (BDC) | M & F | p.o. | 0.5 | NA | 5.9 | NA | NA | NA | 33.7 | NA | 9.35 | NA | 4.4 | NA | 6.5 | NA |
| | Human[d] | M & F | p.o. | 9.3 mg | 0-168 | 1.59 | NA | NA | ND | 2.30 | 0.87 | 18.4 | 3.51 | 0.68 | 2.44 | 6.96 | NA |

% of radioactivity for plasma, urine and feces in non-clinical test species.    % of dose for urine and feces in humans.    M5 = Monohydroxy-vorapaxar-gluc.    M7a = Monohydroxy-vorapaxar-gluc.    M8 = Monohydroxy-vorapaxar-gluc.    M16 = Carboxylic acid metabolite (SCH 609528).    M17 = M + 34.    M19 = Amine metabolite (SCH 540679).    M15, M19a, M20, M20b, M21, M24 = Monohydroxy-vorapaxar (M20 = SCH 2046273).    ND: Not detected.    BIT: Detection by LC-MS only.    BLQ: Below quantifiable limits.    M & F: Male & female.    [a] AUC$_{0-24}$ (ng·h/mL).    [b] Retention time was obtained from LC-MS experiments.    [c] Percent relative to parent.    [d] % of dose.

[9]  FDA Database.  http://www.accessdata.fda.gov/drugsatfda_docs/nda/2014/204886Orig1s000PharmR.pdf (accessed Mar 2016).
[12]  FDA Database.  http://www.accessdata.fda.gov/drugsatfda_docs/nda/2014/204886Orig1s000ClinPharmR.pdf (accessed Mar 2016).

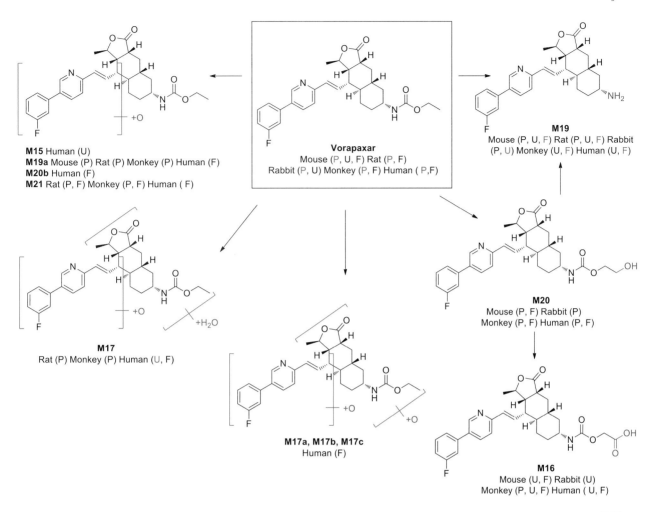

**Figure E**  Proposed Pathways for *In Vivo* Biotransformation of Vorapaxar in Mice, Rats, Rabbits, Monkeys and Humans[9, 12]

The red labels represent the main components in matrices.  P = Plasma, U = Urine and F = Feces.

## Excretion

Table 15  Excretion Profiles of [14C]Vorapaxar in Various Species after Single Intravenous and Oral Dose of [14C]Vorapaxar[9, 12]

| Species | State | Route | Dose (mg/kg) | Time (h) | Bile (% of dose) | Urine (% of dose) | Feces (% of dose) | Recovery (% of dose) |
|---|---|---|---|---|---|---|---|---|
| Mouse (male) | Intact | p.o. | 75 | NA | - | 2 | 87 | 89 |
| Rat (male & female) | BDC | p.o | 10 | NA | 27-31 | 2.2 | 46-49 | 75.2-82.2 |
| | | i.d. | NA[b] | NA | 3.3-4.5 | 0.13-0.14 | 83-86 | ~90.6 |
| Rat (male) | Intact | i.v. | NA | 0-96 | - | 3.0 | NA | >90 |
| Rat (female) | Intact | i.v. | NA | 0-96 | - | 2.6 | NA | >90 |
| Rat (male & female)[a] | Intact | p.o. | 3 | 72 | - | <1 | >82 | >83 |
| Monkey (male) | Intact | i.v. | NA | 0-120 | - | 5.0 | NA | >90 |
| Monkey (female) | Intact | i.v. | NA | 0-120 | - | 6.0 | NA | >90 |
| Human | Intact | p.o. | 9.3 mg | 0-168 | - | 4.23 | 42.2 | 46.43 |

[a] 15% of the dose was not excreted at 168 h after dosing and presumably remained in the carcass tissue.   [b] Following a single oral dose of 10 mg/kg [14C]vorapaxar to rats, bile collected post-dose was administered intraduodenally to a different set of rats.

[9]  FDA Database.   http://www.accessdata.fda.gov/drugsatfda_docs/nda/2014/204886Orig1s000PharmR.pdf (accessed Mar 2016).
[12]  FDA Database.   http://www.accessdata.fda.gov/drugsatfda_docs/nda/2014/204886Orig1s000ClinPharmR.pdf (accessed Mar 2016).

## Drug-Drug Interaction

Table 16    *In Vitro* Evaluation of Vorapaxar and Metabolite as Inhibitors of Enzymes[9, 14]

| Vorapaxar | | M20 | | | |
| --- | --- | --- | --- | --- | --- |
| | | | Control Inhibitor | | |
| Enzyme | IC$_{50}$ (µM) | Enzyme | Compound | IC$_{50}$ (µM) | IC$_{50}$ (µM) |
| CYP1A2 | No | CYP2B6 | Ticlopidine | 0.43 | >1.0 |
| CYP3A4/5 | No | | | | |
| CYP2A6 | ≥30 | CYP2C19 | Benzylnirvanol | 0.19 | >1.0 |
| CYP2B6 | No | | | | |
| CYP2C8 | 1.5 | CYP2D6 | Quinidine | 0.17 | >1.0 |
| CYP2C9 | ≥30 | | | | |
| CYP2C19 | ≥30 | CYP3A4[a] | Ketoconazole | 0.023 | >1.0 |
| CYP2D6 | ≥30 | CYP3A4[b] | Ketoconazole | 0.030 | >1.0 |

Using pooled human liver microsomes with P450 marker substrates to detect the effect of vorapaxar on CYP.    [a] Midazolam 1'-hydroxylation.    [b] Testosterone 6$\beta$-hydroxylation.

Table 17    *In Vitro* Evaluation of Vorapaxar as an Inducer of CYP450 Enzymes Expression in Cultured Human Hepatocytes[9]

| Treatment | Conc. (µM) | CYP1A2 | | CYP2B6 | | CYP2C8 | | CYP2C9 | | CYP2C19 | | CYP3A4/5 | |
| --- | --- | --- | --- | --- | --- | --- | --- | --- | --- | --- | --- | --- | --- |
| | | Enzyme Activity[a] | Fold | Enzyme Activity[a] | Fold | Enzyme Activity[a] | Fold | Enzyme Activity[a] | Fold | Enzyme Activity[a] | Fold | Enzyme Activity[a] | Fold |
| Dimethyl sulfoxide | 0.1% | 87.4 ± 82.6 | 1.00 ± 0.94 | 41.2 ± 9.7 | 1.00 ± 0.24 | 683 ± 314 | 1.00 ± 0.46 | 1340 ± 420 | 1.00 ± 0.31 | 7.20 ± 7.80 | 1.00 ± 1.08 | 2280 ± 1770 | 1.00 ± 0.78 |
| Vorapaxar | 1 | 99.7 ± 102 | 1.08 ± 0.10 | 50.6 ± 10.4 | 1.24 ± 0.09 | 764 ± 367 | 1.11 ± 0.15 | 1420 ± 330 | 1.08 ± 0.10 | 7.3 ± 7.71 | 1.04 ± 0.06 | 2360 ± 1740 | 1.07 ± 0.06 |
| | 10 | 237 ± 213 | 2.66 ± 0.57 | 151 ± 36 | 3.91 ± 1.80 | 1170 ± 410 | 1.80 ± 0.29 | 1630 ± 230 | 1.27 ± 0.32 | 12.3 ± 14.2 | 1.63 ± 0.22 | 3300 ± 2690 | 1.44 ± 0.10 |
| | 30 | 266 ± 297 | 2.97 ± 0.96 | 173 ± 84 | 4.66 ± 3.00 | 1030 ± 210 | 1.82 ± 1.12 | 1590 ± 300 | 1.27 ± 0.49 | 9.02 ± 8.67 | 1.39 ± 0.23 | 2490 ± 2630 | 1.11 ± 0.49 |
| Omeprazole | 100 | 1790 ± 1370 | 27.0 ± 15.2 | 454 ± 267 | 11.5 ± 6.8 | 2770 ± 1300 | 4.09 ± 0.44 | 2250 ± 1000 | 1.68 ± 0.47 | 8.87 ± 5.04 | 1.87 ± 1.25 | 6920 ± 4340 | 3.76 ± 1.62 |
| Phenobarbital | 750 | 175 ± 43 | 2.24 ± 0.38 | 519 ± 76 | 12.8 ± 1.8 | 2670 ± 1290 | 3.86 ± 0.14 | 2590 ± 680 | 2.01 ± 0.52 | 22.5 ± 26.7 | 2.86 ± 0.39 | 10400 ± 5200 | 6.11 ± 3.15 |
| Rifampin | 10 | 139 ± 83 | 2.16 ± 0.97 | 336 ± 51 | 8.38 ± 1.72 | 3200 ± 990 | 5.09 ± 1.44 | 3090 ± 310 | 2.47 ± 0.87 | 58.3 ± 80.1 | 6.08 ± 2.80 | 11000 ± 2900 | 8.09 ± 6.96 |

Three preparations of human hepatocytes from three separate human livers were treated once daily for three consecutive days with vehicle (0.1% dimethyl sulfoxide), one of three concentrations of vorapaxar (1, 10, and 30 µM) or one of three known human CYP inducers (100 µM omeprazole, 750 µM phenobarbital or 10 µM rifampin). After treatment, cells were harvested to prepare microsomes for the analysis of phenacetin *O*-dealkylase (marker for CYP1A2), bupropion hydroxylase (marker for CYP2B6), amodiaquine *N*-dealkylase (marker for CYP2C8), diclofenac 4′-hydroxylase (marker for CYP2C9), *S*-mephenytoin 4′-hydroxylase (marker for CYP2C19) and testosterone 6$\beta$-hydroxylase (marker for CYP3A4/5) activity.    [a] Enzyme activity: pmol/mg protein/min.    Values were the mean ± SD of three determinations (human hepatocyte preparations H749, H753 and H754) rounded to three significant figures.

**Key Findings:**[9]
❖  Vorapaxar was not a substrate of P-gp.

[9]  FDA Database.  http://www.accessdata.fda.gov/drugsatfda_docs/nda/2014/204886Orig1s000PharmR.pdf (accessed Mar 2016).
[14]  Xia, Y.; Chackalamannil, S.; Greenlee, W. J., et al. *Bioorg. Med. Chem. Lett.* **2010**, *20*, 6676-6679.

Table 18  *In Vitro* Evaluation of Vorapaxar as an Inhibitor of Transporters[9, 10]

| Transporter | Cell Type | Substrate | IC$_{50}$ (µM) | |
|---|---|---|---|---|
| | | | Vorapaxar | M20 |
| OATP1B1 | MDCKII | [$^3$H]Pitavastatin | >10 | >10 |
| OATP1B3 | MDCKII | [$^3$H]BSP | >10 | >10 |
| OAT1 | MDCKII | [$^3$H]Cidofovir | >10 | >10 |
| OAT3 | MDCKII | [$^3$H]Estrone Sulfate | 2.2 ± 0.5 | 0.6 ± 0.1 |
| OCT2 | CHO-K1 | [$^{14}$C]Metformin | >10 | >10 |
| BCRP | Membrane vesicles from baculovirus infected *spodoptera frugiperda* cells containing human BCRP | [$^3$H]Methotrexate | 2.5 ± 0.3 | 1.6 ± 0.2 |
| P-gp | Caco-2 | [$^3$H]Digoxin | 1.2 | NA |

The IC$_{50}$ value for cyclosporine A was 0.8 µM.   BCRP: Breast cancer resistance protein.   OATP: Organic anion transporting polypeptide.   OAT: Organic anion transporter.   OCT: Organic cation transporter.

# 6  Non-Clinical Toxicology

## Summary

### Single-Dose Toxicity

❖ Acute toxicity studies by the oral route in rats and monkeys:[9]
  • Rat LD$_{50}$: >2000 mg/kg.
  • Monkey LD$_{50}$: >800 mg/kg.

### Repeated-Dose Toxicity

❖ Sub- and chronic toxicity studies by the oral route in mice (up to 3 months), rats (up to 6 months) and monkeys (up to 12 months):
  • Findings generally occurred at high animal-to-human exposures and with the exception of phospholipidosis (all species), and seemed to be species specific (rat retinal vacuolation) and reversible.
  • The principal treatment-related findings were urinary bladder and ureter hyperplasia in mice, hepatic vascular thrombi, lymphoid necrosis and retinal vacuolation in rats and phospholipidosis in all species.

### Safety Pharmacology

❖ The core battery of ancillary safety pharmacology studies:
  • Single doses up to 100 mg/kg did not significantly affect central neurological or respiratory function in rats.
  • Single doses up to 20 mg/kg did not significantly alter HR, blood pressures, ECG interval duration (RR, QT, PR and QRS) or ECG morphology in cynomolgus monkeys; inhibited hERG current in mouse L cells with a nominal IC$_{50}$ of 341 nM.   Did not significantly affect action potential parameters in dog Purkinje fibers up to a maximum measured concentration of 200 nM.   Since vorapaxar was >99% bound to protein, the concentration of 200 nM was 38 times higher than the expected unbound plasma concentration (5.3 nM) following administration of the 40 mg loading dose in humans.[9]
  • Single doses up to 3 mg/kg did not significantly affect GI and renal parameters in rats.

### Genotoxicity

❖ Vorapaxar presented no mutagenic or clastogenic potential in a battery of *in vitro* and *in vivo* studies.

### Reproductive and Developmental Toxicity

❖ Fertility and early embryonic development in rats:
  • Reproductive parameters, mating and fertility indices were not affected.
❖ Embryo-fetal development in rats and rabbits:
  • Slight delays in development and decreased fetal body weights were observed at MD (25 mg/kg/day for rats, 10 mg/kg/day for rabbits) and HD (75 mg/kg/day for rats, 20 mg/kg/day for rabbits) in both species, and limited maternal toxicity was observed at HD in the dams and does.

[9]  FDA Database.   http://www.accessdata.fda.gov/drugsatfda_docs/nda/2014/204886Orig1s000PharmR.pdf (accessed Mar 2016).
[10]  EMA Database.   http://www.ema.europa.eu/docs/en_GB/document_library/EPAR_Public_assessment_report/human/002814/WC500183331.pdf (accessed Mar 2016).

❖ Pre- and postnatal development in rats:
- The overall NOAEL was 5 mg/kg/day (3.8 × MRHD). Limited $F_0$ maternal toxicity was identified; Clear toxicities demonstrated in the $F_1$ generation, particularly developmental delays and a reduced growth rate from postpartum into adulthood. In the adult female $F_1$s, there were some evidences for maternal toxicities and reductions in fertility at HD (50 mg/kg/day).
- Vorapaxar, as well as M9, M12 and M14, were excreted through milk.[9]

## Carcinogenicity
❖ Two-year carcinogenicity bioassays in mice and rats:
- No vorapaxar-related tumor.
- Exposure (AUC) margin was estimated to be 28 and 34 times in mice, and to be 10 and 29 times in rats, compared to the human exposure ($AUC_{0-24}$ of 1320 ng·h/mL) at the RHD of 2.5 mg QD.

## Special Toxicity
❖ Phototoxicity: No drug-related cutaneous erythema or corneal epithelial indicative of photoallergy.[9]

# Repeated-Dose Toxicity

Table 19　Repeated-Dose Toxicity Studies of Vorapaxar by the Oral Route[9]

| Species | Duration | Dose (mg/kg/day) | NOAEL Dose (mg/kg/day) | NOAEL $AUC_{0-24}$ (ng·h/mL) | NOAEL Safety Margin[a] (× MRHD) | Finding |
|---|---|---|---|---|---|---|
| Mouse | 3 months | 0, 25, 75, 150 | Male: <25 Female: 25 | Male: 61000 Female: 75800 | Male: 46.2 Female: 57.4 | Mortality at HD. Epithelial hyperplasia in the kidney, ureters, and urinary bladder. Vacuolation in epididymides, kidneys, testes, urinary bladder, ureters and small intestine shown to be phospholipidosis by EM. |
| SD rat | 2 weeks | 0, 30, 75 | 75 | Male: 98200 Female: 192000 | Male: 7.4 Female: 14.5 | Retinal vacuolation in the eyes fixed immediately in Davidson's fixative or in Davidson's fixative after 6 h refrigeration in situ, but not in Carnoy's fixative or in Davidson fixative after 24 h refrigeration in situ. |
| | 1 month | 0, 3, 30, 50, 100 | 3 | Male: 1182 Female: 1785 | Male: 0.9 Female: 1.4 | Vacuolation in the bile duct, in macrophages in liver, spleen, lymph nodes, small intestine and inner nuclear layer of retina. |
| | 3 months | 0, 50, 100, 200 | <50 | Male: 22500 Female: 51900 | Male: 17.0 Female: 39.3 | Mortality and morbidity at MD and HD. Phospholipidosis, confirmed by EM, in all drug-treated groups in bile ducts, seminal vesicles and macrophages in liver, spleen, lungs, lymph nodes and SI. Retinal vacuolation at 50 mg/kg. |
| | 6 months | 0, 3, 10, 30 | M: 3 F: 10 | Male: 2250 Female: 9310 | Male: 1.7 Female: 7.0 | Vacuolation of bile duct epithelium and seminal vesicles. Retinal vacuolation at 30 mg/kg and two animals at 10 mg/kg. |
| Cynomolgus monkey | 1 month | 0, 0.5, 5, 20 | 20 | Male: 45016 Female: 55426 | Male: 34.1 Female: 42.0 | BUN values exceeded the normal range and were increased compared to predose at MD and HD, but which were not considered adverse. |
| | 3 months | 0, 30, 60, 90 | 30 | Male: 121000 Female: 112000 | Male: 91.7 Female: 84.8 | Vacuolated macrophages in the spleen, and lymph nodes at MD and HD; Vacuolated macrophages in adrenal gland, spleen, bone marrow, SI, thymus and vacuolation of liver Kupffer cells with Kupffer cell hyperplasia in HDF. |
| | 6 months | 0, 0.5, 5, 20 | 20 | Male: 155250 Female: 162500 | Male: 117.6 Female: 123.1 | None drug-related. |
| | 12 months | 0, 0.5, 5, 20 | 5 | Male: 27900 Female: 27800 | Male: 21 Female: 21 | Adrenal weights relative to body weight increased in 2 HD. |

Vehicle: PEG400. 　[a] Calculated with human $AUC_{0-24}$ of 1320 ng·h/mL at 2.5 mg/day.

[9] FDA Database.　http://www.accessdata.fda.gov/drugsatfda_docs/nda/2014/204886Orig1s000PharmR.pdf (accessed Mar 2016).

# Safety Pharmacology

Table 20 Safety Pharmacological Studies of Vorapaxar[9]

| Study | Species/Strain | Treatment | Finding |
|---|---|---|---|
| CNS | SD rat | Up to 100 mg/kg, p.o. | No adverse effect. |
| Cardiovascular effect | Male cynomolgus monkey | Up to 20 mg/kg, p.o. | No significant alteration on heart rate, blood pressures (systolic, diastolic and mean), ECG interval duration (RR, QT, PR and QRS) or ECG morphology. |
| | Mouse L cell expressing hERG channel | NA | Nominal $IC_{50}$: 341 nM. |
| | Dog Purkinje fiber | Up to 200 nM | No effect on action potential. |
| Respiratory effect | SD rat | Up to 100 mg/kg, p.o. | No effect on respiratory function. |
| Renal and GI function | SD rat | Up to 3 mg/kg | No noticeable effect. |

# Genotoxicity

Table 21 Genotoxicity Studies of Vorapaxar[9]

| Assay | Species/Strain | Metabolism Activity | Treatment | Finding |
|---|---|---|---|---|
| In vitro microbial reverse mutation assay | S. typhimurium/TA98, TA100, TA1535, TA1537; E. coli/WP2 uvrA | ±S9 | 0-5000 µg/plate | Negative. |
| In vitro chromosome aberration assay in mammalian cells | HPBL | ±S9 | 0-1200 µg/mL | Negative. |
| In vivo mouse bone marrow erythrocyte micronucleus assay | NA | + | Two doses of 250 mg/kg/day | Negative. |

Vehicle: DMSO for in vitro studies, 0.04% MC for in vivo studies.

[9] FDA Database. http://www.accessdata.fda.gov/drugsatfda_docs/nda/2014/204886Orig1s000PharmR.pdf (accessed Mar 2016).

## Reproductive and Developmental Toxicity

Table 22    Reproductive and Developmental Toxicology Studies of Vorapaxar by Oral Administration[9]

| Studies | Species | Dose (mg/kg/day) | NOAEL | | | | Finding |
|---------|---------|------------------|-------|-------|-------|-------|---------|
| | | | Endpoint | Dose (mg/kg/day) | AUC (ng·h/mL) | Safety Margin[a] (× MRHD) | |
| Fertility and early embryonic development | SD rat | 0, 5, 25, 50 | Parental | 25 | Male: 23460 Female: 41460 | Male: 18 Female: 31 | No mortality; ↓ food consumption in HDM; ↑ Mating duration (30%) but within concurrent and historical range; ↑ Testis weight (6%) in HD males. |
| | | | Embryo/fertility | 50 | Male: 52700 Female: 88300 | Male: 40 Female: 67 | No drug-related embryo/fetal/offspring effects. |
| Embryo-fetal development | SD rat | 0, 5, 25, 75 | Mater | 25 | 73500 | 56 | No mortality; No remarkable necropsy or unusual placental findings; ↑ Mean post-implantation loss in MD and HD but within historical range. |
| | | | Fetal malformation | 25 | 73500 | 56 | ↓ Mean fetal weight at HD; Rare malformations in ventricular chamber in hearts and higher incidence of skeletal abnormality at HD. |
| | NZW rabbit | 0, 2, 10, 20 | Mater | 20 | 117000 | 89 | No remarkable necropsy or unusual placental findings; 1 Absorption at MD; 2 Mortality at LD and MD. |
| | | | Fetal toxicity | 20 | 117000 | 89 | |
| | | | Malformation | 10 | 34600 | 26 | Dose-related ↑ litter# and fetus# with any malformation but most in one litter. |
| Pre- and postnatal development | SD rat | 0, 5, 25, 50 | $F_0$ | 50 | 88300 | 67 | $F_0$ dams: No drug-related toxicity. $F_1$: Similar litter size across all group; ↑ incidence of dead or missing pups (primarily PND1~3, 5-fold) at HD; ↓ $F_1$ BW and BWGs at HD; No malformation and delay of sexual maturation in any group; ↑ Mean $T_{max}$ of response to the auditory startle stimulus, and ↓ ambulatory locomotor activity at HD. |
| | | | $F_1$ | 5 | 5025 | 3.8 | |
| | | | $F_2$ | 25 | 41460 | 31 | |
| | | 0, 50 (Cross-fostering) | NA | NA | NA | NA | ↑ $F_1$ deaths/litter (≥ 2-fold) and ↓ physical development in Groups ($F_{0 (50)}$/$F_{1 (50)}$) and ($F_{0 (50)}$ × $F_{1 (0)}$); No effects on $F_1$ sexual maturation and fertility. ↓ $F_2$ birth and survival. |

Vehicle: 0.4% (w/v) MC.    [a] Calculated with human $AUC_{0-24}$ of 1320 ng·h/mL at 2.5 mg/day.

## Carcinogenicity

Table 23    104-Week Carcinogenicity Studies of Vorapaxar by Oral Administration[9]

| Species | Dose (mg/kg/day) | NOAEL | | | Finding |
|---------|------------------|-------|-------|-------|---------|
| | | Dose (mg/kg/day) | AUC (ng·h/mL) | Safety Margin[a] (× MRHD) | |
| SD rat | 0, 3, 10, 30 | 30 | Male, 13100 Female, 37900 | Male: 10 Female 29 | ↑ Basal cell tumor of the skin and histiocytic sarcoma in HD males, but not significant. ↑ Hepatocellular adenoma (not significant) and uterine adenoma (4-fold above the max historical data) in HD females. |
| CD-1 mouse | 0, 1, 5, 15 | 15 | Male, 36600 Female, 45480 | Male: 28 Female: 34 | ↑ Bronchiolo-alveolar adenoma at HD, but not significant. |

Vehicle: 0.4% (w/v) MC.    [a] Calculated with human $AUC_{0-24}$ of 1320 ng·h/mL at 2.5mg/day.

[9]   FDA Database.   http://www.accessdata.fda.gov/drugsatfda_docs/nda/2014/204886Orig1s000PharmR.pdf (accessed Mar 2016).

# Appendix

## I

## Abbreviation

# Abbreviation

| | | | |
|---|---|---|---|
| (+)-DAA | (+)-dehydroabietylamine | $AUC_{tot}$ | area under the plasma concentration-time |
| 2-MeTHF | 2-methyltetrahydrofuran | | curve appears in this category |
| 2-NsCl | 2-nitrobenzencsulfonyl chloride | Ba/F3 | murine pro-B cell line |
| 2-PrOH | 2-propanol | BALF | broncho alveolar lavage fluid |
| 3,4-DHP | 3,4-dihydropyran | $BBr_3$ | boron tribromide |
| 5-FU | 5-fluorouracil | BCG | bacillus Calmette-Guérin |
| 5-HT | serotonin | Bcl-2 | B-cell lymphoma-2 |
| A→B | apical to basal | BCR | B cell receptor |
| A2780 | human ovarian cancinoma cell line | BCRP | breast cancer resistance protein |
| A375 | human melanoma cell line | BDC | bile duct-cannulated |
| A549 | human non-small cell lung cancer cell line | bFGF | basic fibroblast growth factor |
| AAG | $\alpha$1-acid glycoprotein | BID | twice daily |
| AARS | aminoacyl-tRNA synthetases | $B(i\text{-}PrO)_3$ | triisopropyl borate |
| ABCB1 | P-gp coding gene | BLQ | below the lower limit of quantification |
| ABCG2 | BCRP coding gene | Bn | benzyl |
| ABSSSI | acute bacterial skin and skin structure | BnBr | benzyl bromide |
| | infections | Boc | *tert*-butoxycarbonyl |
| Ac | acetyl | $Boc_2O$ | *di-tert*-butyl dicarbonate |
| AcCl | acetyl chloride | $B(OMe)_3$ | trimethyl borate |
| ACh | acetylcholine | BPO | benzoyl peroxide |
| $(Ac)_2O$ | acetic anhydride | BRCA1 | breast cancer susceptibility gene 1 |
| ADDP | 1,1'-(azodicarbonyl)dipiperidine | BrCN | bromine cyanide |
| AIDS | acquired immune deficiency syndrome | BSEP | bile salt export pump |
| Akt | serine/threonine-specific protein kinases | BT-549 | breast carcinoma cell line |
| ALCL | anaplastic large-cell lymphoma | BTBSC | $(R,R)$-(-)-$N,N'$-bis(3,5-*di-tert*-butylsali- |
| ALD | aproximate letal dose | | cylidene)-1,2-cyclohexanediamine |
| ALK | anaplastic lymphoma kinase | BTPHNP | $(11R,13S)$-11-(1H-benzo[*d*][1,2,3]tria- |
| ALP | alkaline phosphatase | | zol-1-yl)-13-phenyl-7a,8,9,10,11,13-he- |
| ALT | alanine aminotransferase | | xahydronaphtho[1,2-*e*]pyrido[2,1-*b*][1,3] |
| AMG | alpha-methyl-D-glucopyranoside | | oxazine |
| AOE | acute otitis externa | $Bu_3P$ | tributylphosphane |
| APD | action potential duration | BuLi | butyllithium |
| APPE-19 | retinal epithelial cells | BUN | blood urea nitrogen |
| APTT | activated partial thromboplastin time | BuOEt | butyl ethyl ether |
| ASMC | aortic smooth muscle cells | $(Bu_3Sn)_2$ | hexabutylditin |
| AST | aspartate aminotransferase | BVDV | bovine viral diarrhea virus |
| ATP | adenosine triphosphate | BW | body weight |
| AUC | area under the curve | BWG | body weight gain |
| $AUC_{0-24}$ | area under the plasma concentration-time | BxPC-3 | human pancreatic cancer cell line |
| | curve from time 0 to 24 hours | Caco-2 | colon adenocarcinoma-2 cell |
| $AUC_{inf}$ | area under the plasma concentration-time | CAL-51 | basal-like breast cancer cell |
| | curve from 0 to infinity | $CaMK2\alpha$ | calmodulin-dependent protein kinase $2\alpha$ |

| | | | |
|---|---|---|---|
| cAMP | cyclic-3',5'-adenosine monophosphate | DCHA | dicyclohexylamine |
| CASMC | coronary artery smooth muscle cells | DCM | dichloromethane |
| $C_b$:$C_p$ | blood-to-plasma concentration ratio | DEA | diethylamine |
| CbzCl | benzyl carbonochloridate | (DHQ)$_2$PHAL | hydroquinine 1,4-phthalazinediyl diether |
| $CC_{50}$ | 50% cytotoxic concentration | DIAD | diisopropyl azodicarboxylate |
| CCD1070sk | skin fibroblasts | DIBAL-H | diisobutylaluminium hydride |
| CDI | $N,N'$-carbonyldiimdazole | DIO | diet induced obesity |
| CFDA | China Food and Drug Administration | DIPA | diisopropylamine |
| CFRs | cyclic flow reductions | DIPEA | diisopropylethylamine |
| CFU | colony-forming units | DLBCL | diffuse large B-cell lymphoma |
| CHL | chinese hamster lung cell line | DMA | dimethylacetamide |
| CHMP | committee for human medicinal products | DMAP | 4-dimethylaminopyridine |
| CHO | chinese hamster ovary | DMD | duchenne muscular dystrophy |
| CHP | cumene hydroperoxide | DME | dimethoxyethane |
| CI | combination index | DMEAD | bis(2-methoxyethyl)azodicarboxylate |
| CK | creatine kinase | DMF | $N,N$-dimethylformamide |
| Cl/F | apparent total body clearance | DMPU | 1,3-dimethyl-3,4,5,6-tetrahydro- |
| $CL_{50}$ | defined as the concentration that induces 50% maximum cleavage | | 2($1H$)-pyrimidinone; $N,N'$-dimethyl-$N,N'$-trimethylene urea |
| $Cl_{int}$ | intrinsic clearance | DMSO | dimethyl sulfoxide |
| CLL | chronic lymphoid leukemia | DNA | deoxyribonucleic acid |
| CLN1 | the gene encoding palmitoyl-protein thioesterase-1 (PPT1) | DPDPE | a selective δ-opioid receptor agonist |
| | | DPP-4 | dipeptidyl peptidase-4 |
| cLogP | calculated partition coefficient | DPPA | diphenylphosphoryl azide |
| $C_{max}$ | maximum drug concentration in the plasma after dosing | DU145 | human prostate cancer cell lines |
| | | DYSF | dysferlin |
| CMC | carboxy methylated cellulose | EB | ethambutol |
| CNS | central nervous system | $EC_{50}$ | 50% effective concentration |
| COPD | chronic obstructive pulmonary disease | ECG | electrocardiogram |
| CPIV | canine parainfluenza virus | ED | effect dose |
| CPT1A | carnitine palmitoyltransferase 1A | EDC | $N$-(3-dimethylaminopropyl)-$N'$-ethyl-carbodiimide |
| CRC | concentration-response curves | | |
| CSF | cerebrospinal fluid | EDCI | $N$-(3-dimethylaminopropyl)-$N'$-ethyl-carbodiimide hydrochloride |
| CV | coefficient of variation | | |
| CVS | cardiovascular system | EEG | electroencephalography |
| CXCL9 | C-X-C motif chemokine 9 | EFD | embryo-fetal development |
| Cy | cyclohexyl | EG | ethylene glycol |
| CYP | cytochrome P450 enzymes | EGFR | epidermal growth factor receptor |
| D2 receptor | dopamine D2 receptor | ELISA | enzyme-linked immunosorbent assay |
| DABCO | 1,4-diazabicyclo(2.2.2)octane | EM | electron microscope |
| DAMGO | [D-Ala2, NMe-Phe4, Gly-ol5]-enkephalin | EMA | European Medicines Agency |
| | | EML4 | echinoderm microtubule associated protein like 4 |
| DBP | diastolic blood pressure | | |
| DBU | 1,8-diazabicyclo[5,4,0]undec-7-ene | EMS | ethyl methanesulfonate |
| DCC | 1,3-dicyclohexylcarbodiimde | EMs | extensive metabolizers |
| DCE | 1,2-dichloroethane | EQ | equivalent |

| | | | |
|---|---|---|---|
| ERK | extracellular signal-regulated kinase | HCl | hydrochloric acid |
| Et | ethyl | Hct | hematocrit |
| Et$_2$O | diethyl ether | HCT-116 | human colon carcinoma cell line |
| EtOAc | ethyl acetate | HCT-8 | human colon carcinoma cell line |
| EtOH | ethanol | HCV | hepatitis C virus |
| (EtO)$_2$POCl | diethyl chlorophosphate | HD | high dose |
| EU | European Union | H$_D$ | hydrogen bond donor |
| F% | percentage of bioavailability | HDAC | histone deacetylase |
| FACS | fluorescence activated cell sorting | HEC | hydroxyethylcellulose |
| FBS | fetal bovine serum | HED | human equivalent dose |
| FCS | fetal calf serum | HEK | human embryonic kidney |
| FDA | Food and Drug Administration | HeLa | human cervical cancer cell line |
| FEED | fertility and early embryonic development | HepG2 | human liver hepatocellular carcinoma |
| FFA | free fatty acid | HEPREP | hepatitis C replication |
| FITC | fluorescein isothiocyanate | hERG | human ether-a-go-go related gene |
| FL | follicular lymphoma | HexLi; Hex-Li | hexyllithium |
| FLIPR | fluorometric imaging plate reader | HIV | human immunodeficiency virus |
| FLT3 | Fms-like tyrosine kinase-3 | HL60 | human promyelocytic leukemia cells |
| fMLP | $N$-formyl-methionyl-leucyl-phenylalanine | HLM | human liver microsomes |
| FOB | functional observation battery | HMDS | hexamethyldisilazane |
| FQ-R | fluoroquinolone-resistant | HMG-CoA | 3-hydroxy-3-methylglutaryl-coenzyme A |
| FRB | freely rotatable bonds | HMPA | hexamethylphosphoramide |
| FREC | fluorquinolone-resistant E. coli | HOAc | acetic acid |
| FRET | fluorescence resonance energy transfer | HOAt | 1-hydroxy-7-azabenzotriazole |
| G- | gram-negative | HOBt | 1-hydroxybenzotriazole hydrate |
| G+ | gram-positive | HOPO | 2-hydroxypyridine-$N$-oxide |
| GA | glucuronic acid | HPBL | human peripheral blood lymphocyte |
| GCS | glucosylceramide synthase | HPBMC | peripheral blood mononuclear cell |
| GD | gestation day | HPMC | hydroxypropyl methylcellulose |
| GGT | $\gamma$-glutamyl transpeptidase | HP$\beta$CD | hydroxypropyl-$\beta$-cyclodextrin |
| GI tract | gastrointestinal tract | HR | heart rate |
| GLP | good laboratory practice | HRE | human primary renal epithelial cells |
| GPCRs | G-protein-coupled receptors | HSA | human serum albumin |
| GSK | GlaxoSmithKline | HSV-1, 2 | herpes simplex virus type 1, 2 |
| GT | genotype | HT29 | human colon carcinoma |
| GTP | guanosine triphosphates | HuH-7 | human hepatoma cell line |
| h | hour | HUVEC | human umbilical vein endothelial cell |
| H$_A$ | hydrogen bond acceptors | hv | light source |
| HATU | $O$-(7-azabenzotriazol-1-yl)-$N,N,N',N'$-tetramethyluronium hexafluorophosphate | i.d. | intraduodenal |
| | | i.p. | Intraperitoneal injection |
| | | i.t. | intratracheally |
| | | i.v. | intravenous |
| HBCx | human breast cancer xenografts | IC$_{50}$ | 50% inhibitory concentration |
| HBTU | $N,N,N',N'$-tetramethyl-$O$-(1H-benzotriazol-1-yl)uronium hexafluorophosphate | IC$_{90}$ | 90% inhibitory concentration |
| | | ID$_{50}$ | 50% inhibitory does |
| HCC827 | human lung cancer cell line | IGF-1R | insulin-like growth factor 1 receptor |

| | |
|---|---|
| IL | interleukin |
| IMS | industrial methylated spirits |
| IMs | intermediate metabolizers |
| INCL | infantile neuronal ceroid lipofuscinosis |
| INH | isoniazid |
| iNHL | indolent non-Hodgkin lymphoma |
| INSR | insulin receptor |
| IOP | intraocular pressure |
| IPA | isopropanol |
| IPAc | isopropyl acetate |
| IPF | idiopathic pulmonary fibrosis |
| $i$-Pr | isopropyl |
| $i$-Pr$_2$O | isopropyl ether |
| $i$-PrMgCl | isopropylmagnesium chloride |
| $i$-PrOH | isopropanol |
| ($i$-PrO)$_3$La | triisopropoxylanthanum |
| J82 | human bladder carcinoma |
| Jurkat | human T-lymphoma cell line |
| K562 | human chronic myelogenous leukemia |
| Karpas299 cells | human non-hodgkin's Ki-positive cell line |
| KB-3-1 | human cervical carcinoma cell |
| $K_d$ | equilibrium dissociation constant |
| Kg | kilogram |
| KHMDS | potassium hexamethyldisilazide |
| $K_i$ | inhibition constant |
| kinact | theoretical maximum enzyme inactivation rate |
| KKAy mice | type 2 diabetes mice |
| $K_m$ | Michaelis-Menten enzyme affinity constant |
| KOAc | potassium acetate |
| $K_{off}$ | dissociation rate constant |
| $K_{on}$ | association rate constant |
| KRAS | v-Ki-ras2 Kirsten rat sarcoma viral oncogene homolog |
| LAH | lithium aluminium hydride |
| LAMA | long-acting muscarinic antagonist |
| LC/MS | liquid chromatography and mass spectrometry |
| LC$_{50}$ | lethal concentration, 50% |
| LD | low dose |
| LD$_{50}$ | lethal dose, 50% |
| LDA | lithium diisopropylamide |
| LDH | lactate dehydrogenase |
| D-DIPT | D-(-)-diisopropyl tartrate |
| LiAlH$_4$ | lithium aluminium hydride |

| | |
|---|---|
| LiHMDS | lithium hexamethyldisilazide |
| Lindlar's catalyst | palladium on calcium carbonate |
| LLC-PK1 | pig porcine kidney cell line |
| LLOQ | lower limit of quantification |
| LN | lymph node |
| LNCaP | lymph node carcinoma of prostate |
| LOEL | lowest observed effect level |
| LOK | lymphocyte-oriented kinase |
| LOQ | limit of quantitation |
| LPA | lysophosphatidic acid |
| LPS | lipopolysaccharide |
| LS174T | human colon cancer cell |
| LSC | liquid scintillation counting |
| mAb | monoclonal antibody |
| MABP | mean arterial blood pressure |
| MAO | monoamine oxidase |
| Max | maximum |
| MBC | minimum bactericidal concentration |
| MC | methylcellulose |
| MC3 receptor | melanocortin 3 receptor |
| MCF-7 | human breast cancer cell line |
| MCH(C) | mean corpuscular hemoglobin (contentration) |
| Mcl-1 | myeloid cell leukemia-1 |
| $m$-CPBA | 3-chloroperbenzoic acid |
| MCV | mean corpuscular volume |
| Mcy | methylcyclohexane |
| MD | medium dose |
| MDA-MB-231 | human breast adenocarcinoma |
| MDBK | the Madin-Darby bovine kidney cells |
| MDCK | Madin-Darby canine kidney cell line |
| MDICB | (-)-B-methoxydiisopinocampheylborane |
| MDR | multi-drug resistance |
| MDR1 | multidrug resistance protein 1, also known as P-glycoprotein 1 |
| MDR-TB | multidrug-resistant tuberculosis |
| Me | methyl |
| Me$_2$SO$_2$ | dimethylsulfone |
| Me$_3$Al | trimethylaluminium |
| MeCN | acetonitrile |
| MED | minimum effective dose |
| mED | maximal effect dose |
| MeI | iodomethane |
| MEK | methylethyl ketone |
| MEMCl | 2-methoxyethoxymethyl chloride |
| MeMgCl | methylmagnesium chloride |

| | | | |
|---|---|---|---|
| MeNH$_2$ | methylamine | MsOH | methanesulfonic acid |
| MeOH | methanol | MSSA | methicillin-susceptible S. aureus |
| MeONa | sodium methoxide | MSSE | methicillin-susceptible S. epidermidis |
| MFC | minimal fungicidal concentration | MT2 | human T cell line |
| MFC$_{50}$ | minimum fungicidal concentration required to kill (defined at a >99.9% reduction in colony count from the original inoculum) 50% of the strains tested | MTBE | tert-butylmethyl ether |
| | | MTD | maximum tolerated dose |
| | | MW | molecular weight |
| | | NA | not available |
| MFC$_{90}$ | minimum fungicidal concentration required to kill (defined at a >99.9% reduction in colony count from the original inoculum) 90% of the strains tested | NA/STZ mice | nicotinamide/streptozotocin-induced diabetic mice |
| | | NaBH(OAc)$_3$ | sodium triacetoxyborohydride |
| | | NaBH$_3$CN | sodium cyanoborohydride |
| | | NaBH$_4$ | sodium borohydride |
| mg | milligram | NADPH | nicotinamide adenine dinucleotide phosphate |
| MI | myocardial infarction | NAG | N-acetyl-$\beta$-D-glucosaminidase |
| MiaPaca-2 | human pancreatic cancer cell | NaHMDS | sodium hexamethyldisilazide |
| MIBK | methylisobutyl ketone | NaN$_3$ | sodium azide |
| MIC | minimum inhibitory concentration | NBS | N-bromosuccinimide |
| MIC$_{50}$ | minimum inhibitory concentration required to inhibit the growth of 50% of isolates tested | n-BuLi | n-butyllithium |
| | | (n-Bu)$_3$P | tri-n-butylphosphine |
| | | NC | not calculated |
| MIC$_{90}$ | minimum inhibitory concentration required to inhibit the growth of 90% of isolates tested | NCI-H2228 cell | human non-small cell lung cancer cell line |
| | | NCI-H460 | human non-small cell lung cancer cell line |
| Min | minimum | ND | not detected |
| MIP-1$\alpha$ | macrophage inflammatory protein-1$\alpha$ | NDA | new drug application |
| mL | milliliter | (NHC)Pd- | |
| MLA | mouse lymphoma assay | (allyl)Cl | allyl[1,3-bis(2,6-diisopropylphenyl) imidazol-2-ylidene]chloropalladium(II) |
| MLD | minimal lethal dose | | |
| MMS | methyl methanesulfonate | NHLF | normal human lung fibroblast |
| MN | micronucleus | NH$_4$OAc | ammonium acetate |
| MNLD | maximum non-lethal dose | NHS | normal human serum |
| MNNG | 1-methyl-3-nitro-1-nitrosoguanidine | NIH-3T3 | mouse embryonic fibroblast cell line |
| Mo7e | human megakaryocytic leukemic cell line | NIS | N-iodosuccinimide |
| | | NK1 | neurokinin 1 receptor |
| MOPS | 3-(N-morpholino)propanesulfonic acid | nM | nanomolar |
| MRC5 | human fetal lung fibroblast cell line | NMM | N-methylmorpholine |
| (M)RHD | (maximum) recommended human dose | NMMO | N-methylmorpholine N-oxide |
| MRSA | methicillin-resistant S. aureus | NMP | N-methyl-2-pyrrolidone |
| MRSE | methicillin-resistant S. epidermidis | NMRI | nuclear magnetic resonance imaging |
| MS | molecular sieves | NO(A)EL | no observed (adverse) effect level |
| Ms | methanesulfonyl | NOD | non-obese diabetic |
| MsCl | methanesulfonyl chloride | NOMO-1 | human promonocytic leukemia cell line |
| MSCoNS | methicillin-susceptible coagulase-negative staphylococci | NP | normal phenotype |

| | | | |
|---|---|---|---|
| *n*-PrOH | 1-propanol | | dichloropalladium(II), complex with |
| nRTKs | non-receptor tyrosine kinases | | dichloromethane |
| NRU | neutral red uptake | Pd(MeCN)$_2$Cl$_2$ | bis(acetonitrile)dichloropalladium(II) |
| NS3/4A | HCV protease | Pd(OAc)$_2$ | palladium(II) acetate |
| NSCLC | non-small cell lung cancer | Pd(PPh$_3$)$_2$Cl$_2$ | bis(triphenylphosphine)palladium(II) |
| NT | not tested | | chloride |
| O.D. | *oculus dexter* | Pd(PPh$_3$)$_4$ | terakis(triphenylphosphine)palladium(0) |
| O.L. | *oculus laevus* | Pd(*t*-Bu$_3$P)$_2$ | bis(*tri-t*-butylphosphine)palladium(0) |
| OAT | organic anion transporter | Pd$_2$(dba)$_3$ | tris(dibenzylideneacetone)dipalladium(0) |
| OATP | organic anion-transporting polypeptide | PDE4 | phosphodieasterase 4 |
| OCT | organic cation transporter | PDGF | platelet-derived growth factor |
| OCTN1 | organic cation transporter N1 | PDGFR | platelet derived growth factor receptor |
| Off t$_{1/2}$ | offset half-time | PEG 400 | polyethylene glycol 400 |
| OGTT | oral glucose tolerance test | PEG-IFN$\alpha$ | polyethylene glycol interferon alpha |
| OIC | opioid-induced constipation | PF50 | potentiation factor at 50% cell viability |
| On t$_{1/2}$ | onset half-time | PG | propylene glycol; plasma glucose |
| OVA | ovalbumin | P-gP | P-glycoprotein |
| OX1R | orexin receptor 1 | PH | pulmonary hypertension |
| OX2R | orexin receptor 2 | Ph$_2$CH$_2$ | diphenylmethane |
| p.c. | post challenge | PhCl | chlorobenzene |
| p.i. | post infectious | PhCO$_2$H | benzoic acid |
| p.o. | *per os*, oral administration | PhLi | phenyllithium |
| p.s. | post surgery | PhSH | phenthiol |
| PAA | phenylacetic acid | PI3K$\delta$ | phosphatidylinositol 3-kinase p110$\delta$ |
| PAD | peripheral arterial disease | | isoform |
| PAG | phenylacetylglycine | PISP | penicillin-intermediate S. pneumoniae |
| PAGN | phenylacetylglutamine | PKAC$\alpha$ | protein kinase A catalytic $\alpha$ |
| PAI | pharmacological activity index | PKC | protein kinase C |
| PANC-1 | human pancreatic cancer cell line | pKi | corresponding negative logarithmic value |
| Papp | apparent permeability coefficients | PLT | blood platelet |
| PAR-1 | protease-activated receptor-1 | PMDA | Pharmaceuticals and Medical Devices |
| PARP | poly(ADP-ribose) polymerase | | Agency |
| PAS | pituitary-adrenocortical system | PMs | poor metabolizers |
| PaTu8988 | human pancteatic cancer cell line | PND | postnatal day |
| PBMC | peripheral blood mononuclear cell | PO(OEt)$_2$H | diethyl phosphite |
| PC-3 | human prostate cancer cell line | PO(OEt)$_3$ | triethyl phosphate |
| P-CAB | potassium-competitive acid blocker | POCl$_3$ | phosphorus oxychloride |
| PCE | polychromatic erythrocyte | P(OPh)$_3$ | triphenyl phosphite |
| PCR | polymerase chain reaction | P(*o*-tol)$_3$ | *tri-o*-tolylphosphine |
| PCV | packed cell volume | PPE | porcine pancreatic elastase |
| PCy$_3$ | tricyclohexylphospine | PPh$_3$ | triphenylphosphine |
| [Pd(allyl)Cl]$_2$ | allylpalladium chloride dimer | PPI | proton pump inhibitor |
| Pd(dppf)Cl$_2$ | [1,1'-bis(diphenylphosphino) | PPND | pre- and postnatal development |
| | ferrocene]dichloropalladium(II) | PPTS | pyridinium *p*-toluenesulfonate |
| Pd(dppf)Cl$_2$ | | PRSP | penicillin-resistant S. pneumoniae |
| • CH$_2$Cl$_2$ | [1,1'-bis(diphenylphosphino)ferrocene] | PSSP | penicillin-susceptible S. pneumoniae |

| | | | |
|---|---|---|---|
| PT | prothrombin time | SD rat | Sprague-Dawley rat |
| P(*t*-Bu)$_3$ • HBF$_4$ | *tri-tert*-butylphosphine tetrafluoroborate | SDH | succinate dehydrogenase |
| PTCL | peripheral T-cell lymphoma | SFLLRN | TRAP peptide |
| PTT | partial thromboplastin time | SGC-7901 | human gastric cancer cell line |
| PTX | patient-derived tumor xenograft | SGLT2 | sodium-glucose co-transporter-2 |
| PZA | pyrazinamide | SLK | ste2-like kinase |
| Q4D | once a day for four days | SM | sreptomycin |
| QD | once daily | SPhos | 2-dicyclohexylphosphine-2',6'-dimethoxybiphenyl |
| QID | quater in die | | |
| QSAR | quantitative structure-activity relationship | SRB | sulforhodamine B |
| | | Src | non-receptor tyrosine kinases homologous to the Rous sarcoma virus oncogene v-src |
| QTc | corrected QT interval | | |
| r.t. | room tempreture | | |
| *rac*-BINAP | racemic-2,2'-bis(diphenylphosphino)-1,1'-binaphthyl | (*S,R*)-*t*-Bu-Josiphos | bis(1,5-cyclooctadiene)rhodium(I) trifluoromethanesulfonate |
| Raji | human Burkitt B-cell lymphoma cell line | | |
| RBC | red blood cell | STAT3 | signal transducer and activator of transcription 3 |
| REM | rapid eye movement | | |
| RET | rearranged during transfection | STZ | streptozotocin |
| RFP | rifampicin | SULT | sulfotransferase |
| Rh(COD)$_2$OTf | bis(1,5-cyclooctadiene) rhodium(I) trifluoromethanesulfonate | SW-620 | human colon carcinoma cell line |
| | | SWS | slow-wave sleep |
| RNA | ribonucleic acid | T$_{1/2}$ | half-life time |
| ROCK | Rho-associated coiled-coil containing protein kinase | t$_{1/2}$ | terminal elimination half-life |
| | | T24 | urinary bladder cancer cell |
| RPMI | roswell park memorial institute | T2DM | type 2 diabetes mellitus |
| RS | respiratory system | TB | tubercle bacillus |
| RT4 | rat schwannoma cell | TBAB | tetrabutylammonium bromide |
| RTKs | receptor tyrosine kinase | TBAF | tetrabutylammonium fluoride |
| RuCl(*p*-cymene)[(*S,S*)-Ts-DPEN] | [*N*-[(1*S*,2*S*)-2-(amino-κ*N*)-1,2-diphenyl-ethyl]-4-methylbenzenesulfonamidato-κ*N*]chloro[(1,2,3,4,5,6-η)-1-methyl-4-(1-methylethyl)benzene]-ruthenium | TBAH | tetrabutylammonium hydroxide |
| | | TBAHS | tetrabutylammonium hydrogen sulfate |
| | | TBDMS | *tert*-butyldimethylsilane; *tert*-butyldimethylsilyl |
| | | | |
| | | TBDMSCl | *tert*-butyldimethylsilyl chloride |
| s.c. | subcutaneous | TBME | *tert*-butylmethyl ether |
| S/T PKs | serine/threonine-specific protein kinases | *t*-BuNO$_2$ | *tert*-butyl nitrite |
| S6RP | S6 ribosomal protein | *t*-BuOH | *tert*-butyl alcohol |
| S9 | liver S9 fraction | *t*-BuOK | potassium *tert*-butoxide |
| SBP | systolic blood pressure | *t*-BuONa | sodium *tert*-butoxide |
| SCE | monkey Schlemm's canal endothelial cells | *t*-Butyl Xphos | 2-*di-tert*-butylphosphino-2',4',6'-triisopropyl-1,1'-biphenyl |
| | | | |
| SCID mice | severe combined immunodeficient mice | TCT | cyanuric chloride |
| | | TEA | triethylamine |
| SCN | suprachiasmatic nucleus | TEER | trans-epithelial electrical resistance |
| SCV | s colony variant | Tf$_2$O | trifluoromethanesulfonic anhydride |
| SD | standard deviation | TFA | trifluoroacetic acid |

| | | | |
|---|---|---|---|
| TFAA | trifluoroacetic anhydride | US / U.S. | United States |
| TFE | trifluoroethanol | USH1 | one of usher syndrome type I gene |
| TfOH | trifluoromethanesulfonic acid | UVA | ultraviolet A-rays |
| TG | transport glucose; triglyceride | UVR | ultraviolet radiation |
| TGI | tumor growth inhibition | $V_d$ | volume of distribution |
| THF | tetrahydrofuran | $V_d/F$ | apparent distribution volume |
| THP-1 | human acute monocytic leukemia cell line | VEGF | vascular endothelial growth factor |
| Ti($i$-PrO)$_4$ | titanium tetraisopropanolate | Vero | monkey kidney epithelial cell line |
| Ti(OEt)$_4$ | titanium ethoxide | VMAT2 | vesicular monoamine transporter 2 |
| TID | 3 times a day | VR | vancomycin-resistant |
| TIPSCl | triisopropylsilyl chloride | VS | vancomycin-susceptible |
| TK | toxicokinetics | VSEfa | vancomycin-susceptible E. faecalis |
| TLR9 | toll-like receptor 9 | $V_{ss}$ | apparent volume of distribution at steady |
| TM cells | monkey trabecular meshwork cells | | state |
| TMAC | trimethyacetyl chloride | WBC | white blood cell |
| $T_{max}$ | time to maximum plasma concentration | WT | wild type |
| TMDS | 1,1,3,3-tetramethyldisiloxane | Xantphos | 4,5-bis(diphenylphosphino)-9,9- |
| TMOA | trimethyl orthoacetate | | dimethylxanthene |
| TMSCl | trimethylsilyl chloride | XDR | extensively-drug resistant |
| TNBC | triple negative breast cancer | XPhos | 2-dicyclohexylphosphino-2',4',6'- |
| TNF-$\alpha$ | tumor necrosis factor $\alpha$ | | triisopropylbiphenyl |
| TPAP | *tetra-n*-propylammonium perruthenate | Y | tyrosine-specific protein kinases |
| TRAP | thrombin receptor agonist peptide | ZDF rat | Zucker diabetic fatty rat |
| tRNA | aminoacyl-transfer ribonucleic acid | Zhan 1B | |
| TsCl | 4-toluensulfonyl chloride | catalyst | 1,3-bis(2,4,6-trimethylphenyl)-4,5-dihy- |
| TsNH$_2$ | 4-toluenesulfonamide | | droimidazol-2-ylidene[2-($i$-propoxy)-5- |
| TsOH | 4-toluenesulfonic acid | | ($N,N$-dimethylaminosulfonyl)phenyl] |
| TsOH · H$_2$O | 4-toluenesulfonic acid monohydrate | | methyleneruthenium(II) dichloride |
| U2OS | human osteosarcoma cancer cell | ZO-1 | zonula occludens-1 |
| UDS | unscheduled DNA synthesis | $\gamma$-GLB | $\gamma$-globulin |
| UGE | urinary glucose excretion | $\mu$g | microgram |
| UGT | uridine diphosphate glucuronosyl-transferase | $\mu$M | micromolar |

# Appendix

## Sales Worldwide (2014-2015)

# Sales Worldwide (2014-2015)

| Active ingredient | Trade name | 2014-sale ($Million, Fiscal Year) | 2015-sale ($Million, Fiscal Year) |
|---|---|---|---|
| Alectinib Hydrochloride | Alecensa® | 13.2 | 71.3 |
| Apatinib | 艾坦® | N/A | N/A |
| Apremilast | Otezla® | 69.8 | 471.7 |
| Asunaprevir | Sunvepra® | 55 | 288 |
| Ataluren | Translarna® | 1.4 | 33.7 |
| Belinostat | Beleodaq® | 4.9 | 10.1 |
| Ceritinib | Zykadia® | 31 | 79 |
| Chidamide | Epidaza®/爱谱沙® | N/A | N/A |
| Daclatasvir Dihydrochloride | Daklinza® | 201 | 1315 |
| Delamanid | Deltyba® | N/A | N/A |
| Eliglustat Tartrate | Cerdelga® | 5.3 | 73.3 |
| Empagliflozin | Jardiance® | 10.1 | N/A |
| Finafloxacin | Xtoro® | N/A | N/A |
| Idelalisib | Zydelig® | 23 | 132 |
| Ipragliflozin L-Proline | Suglat® | 30.8 | 51.6 |
| Luseogliflozin Hydrate | Lusefi® | 22.4 | 5.7 |
| Naloxegol Oxalate | Movantik®/Moventig® | N/A | 39 |
| Nintedanib Esylate | Ofev®/ Vargatef® | N/A | N/A |
| Olaparib | Lynparza® | N/A | 94 |
| Oritavancin Diphosphate | Orbactiv® | 0.8 | 9.1 |
| Phenothrin | Sumithrin® | N/A | N/A |
| Ripasudil Hydrochloride Hydrate | Glanatec® | N/A | N/A |
| Suvorexant | Belsomra® | N/A | N/A |
| Tasimelteon | Hetlioz® | 12.8 | 44.3 |
| Tavaborole | Kerydin® | N/A | N/A |
| Tedizolid Phosphate | Sivextro® | N/A | N/A |
| Tofogliflozin Hydrate | Deberza®/Apleway® | N/A | N/A |
| Umeclidinium Bromide | Incruse® | N/A | 21.4 |
| Vaniprevir | Vanihep® | N/A | N/A |
| Vonoprazan Fumarate | Takecab® | N/A | N/A |
| Vorapaxar Sulfate | Zontivity® | N/A | N/A |

Note: All the sales data come from the financial reports of the marketing-authorisation holder.

# Appendix

# III

# Worldwide Approved NCEs
# (2001-2015)

# Worldwide Approved NCEs (2001-2015)

| | | | |
|---|---|---|---|
| **Year 2001** | **Bimatoprost** Lumigan®/Latisse® 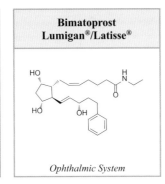 *Ophthalmic System* | **Bosentan Hydrate** Tracleer® 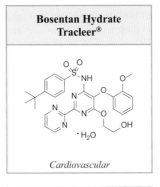 *Cardiovascular* | **Caspofungin Acetate** Cancidas® 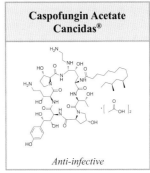 *Anti-infective* |
| **Desloratadine** Aerius®/Clarinex®/ Neoclarityn® <br> *Respiratory* | **Dexmethylphenidate Hydrochloride** Focalin®/Attenade® <br> *Central Nervous System* | **Dutasteride** Avodart®/Avolve® 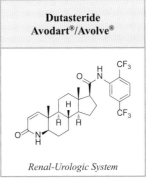 *Renal-Urologic System* | **Edaravone** Radicut®/Arone® 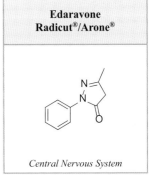 *Central Nervous System* |
| **Eletriptan Hydrobromide** Relpax®/Relert® 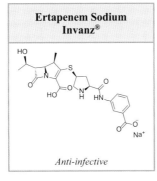 *Central Nervous System* | **Ertapenem Sodium** Invanz® 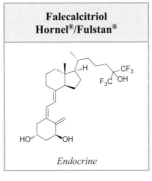 *Anti-infective* | **Falecalcitriol** Hornel®/Fulstan® 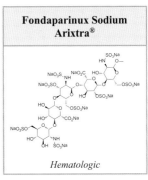 *Endocrine* | **Fondaparinux Sodium** Arixtra® <br> *Hematologic* |
| **Frovatriptan Succinate Hydrate** Frova®/Migard® <br> *Central Nervous System* | **Fudosteine** Cleanal®/Spelear® <br> *Respiratory* | **Imatinib Mesylate** Gleevec®/Glivec® 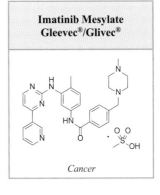 *Cancer* | **Levocetirizine Dihydrochloride** Xyzal®/Xusal® 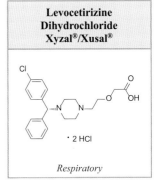 *Respiratory* |

## Methyl Aminolevulinate Hydrochloride
### Metvix®/Metvixia®

*Cancer*

## Pimecrolimus
### Elidel®

*Dermatologic System*

## Tegaserod Maleate
### Zelmac®/Zelnorm®

*Gastrointestinal System*

## Telithromycin
### Ketek®

*Anti-infective*

## Tenofovir Disoproxil Fumarate Spiriva®

*Anti-infective*

## Tiotropium Bromide Hydrate Spiriva®

*Respiratory*

## Travoprost Travatan®/ Travatan Z®

*Ophthalmic System*

## Valganciclovir Hydrochloride Valcyte®/ Valixa®

*Anti-infective*

## Ziprasidone
### Geodon®/Zeldox®

*Central Nervous System*

# Year 2002

## Adefovir Dipivoxil
### Hepsera®

*Anti-infective*

## Amrubicin Hydrochloride
### Calsed®

*Cancer*

## Aripiprazole
### Abilify®

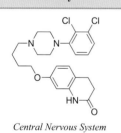

*Central Nervous System*

## Atomoxetine Hydrochloride
### Strattera®

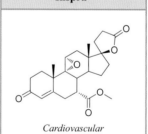

*Central Nervous System*

## Eplerenone
### Inspra®

*Cardiovascular*

## Escitalopram Oxalate
### Lexapro®/Cipralex®

*Central Nervous System*

## Etoricoxib
### Arcoxia®

*Anti-arthritic*

## Ezetimibe
### Zetia®/Ezetrol®

*Cardiovascular*

## Fulvestrant
### Faslodex®

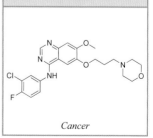

*Cancer*

## Gefitinib
### Iressa®

*Cancer*

**Landiolol Hydrochloride**
**Onoact®**

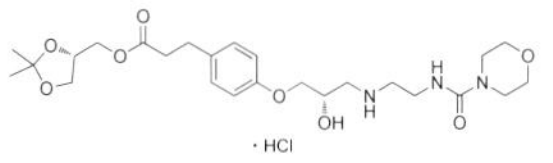

*Cardiovascular*

**Memantine Hydrochloride**
**Namenda®/Axura®/Ebixa®**

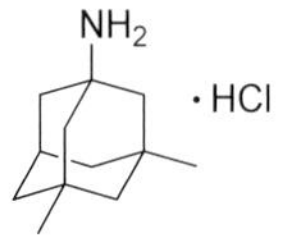

*Central Nervous System*

**Micafungin Sodium**
**Funguard®/Mycamine®**

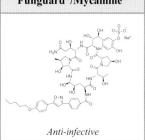

*Anti-infective*

**Miglustat**
**Zavesca®**

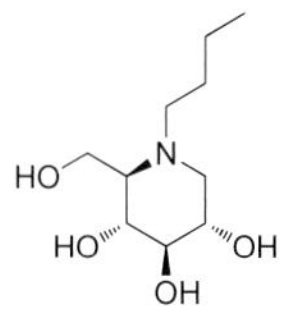

*Metabolic*

**Mycophenolate Sodium**
**Myfortic®**

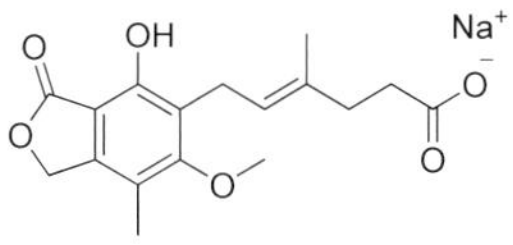

*Immunologic*

**Neridronate Sodium**
**Nerixia®**

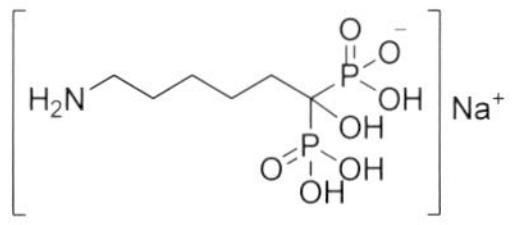

*Metabolic*

**Nitazoxanide**
**Alinia®**

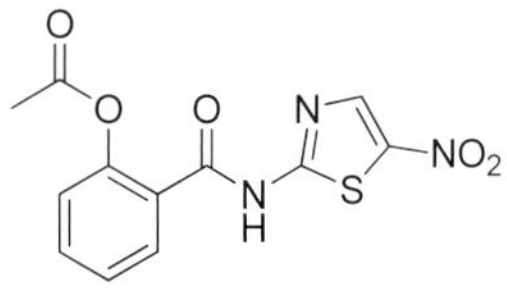

*Cryptosporidium*

**Nitisinone**
**Orfadin®**

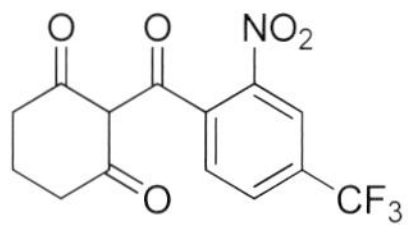

*Metabolic*

**Olmesartan Medoxomil**
**Benicar®/Olmetec®**

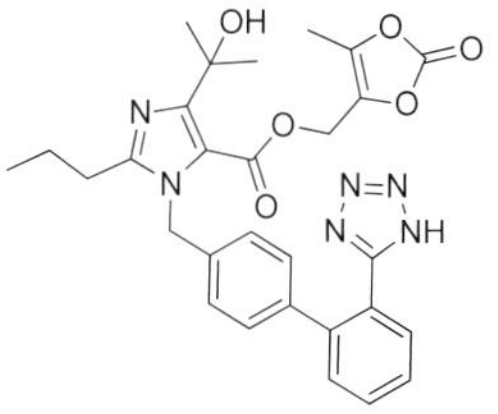

*Cardiovascular*

**Parecoxib Sodium**
**Dynastat®**

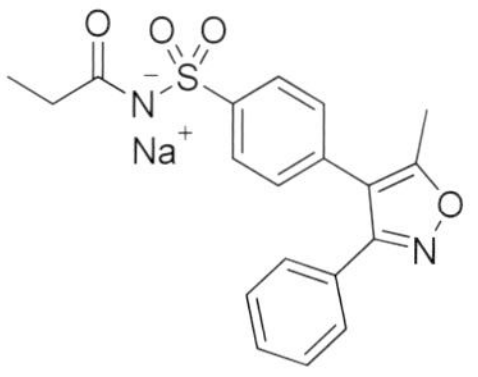

*Anti-arthritic*

**Pazufloxacin Mesylate**
**Pazucross®/Pasil®**

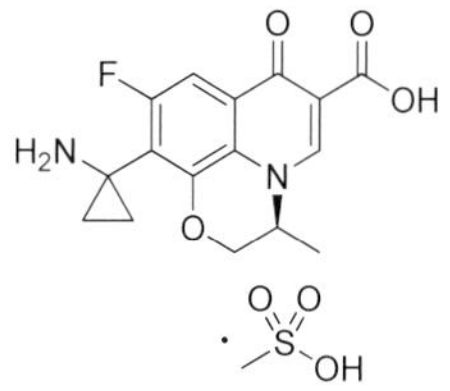

*Anti-infective*

**Prulifloxacin**
**Sword®**

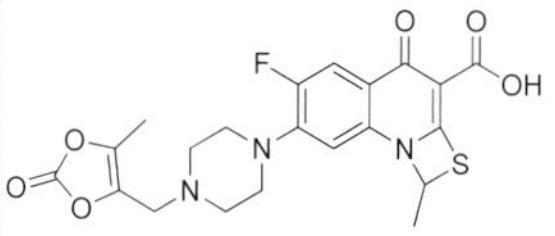

*Anti-infective*

**Rosuvastatin Calcium**
**Crestor®**

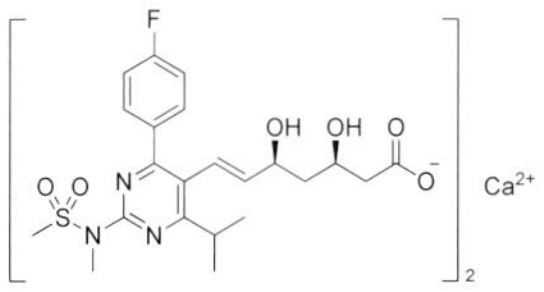

*Cardiovascular*

**Sivelestat Sodium Hydrate**
**Elaspol®**

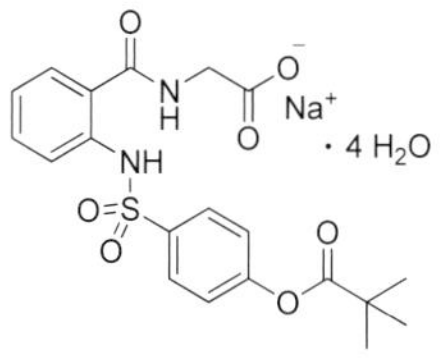

*Respiratory*

**Sodium Oxybate**
**Xyrem®**

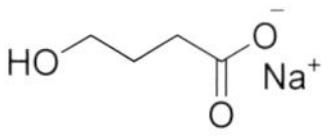

*Central Nervous System*

**Tadalafil**
**Cialis®/Adcirca®**

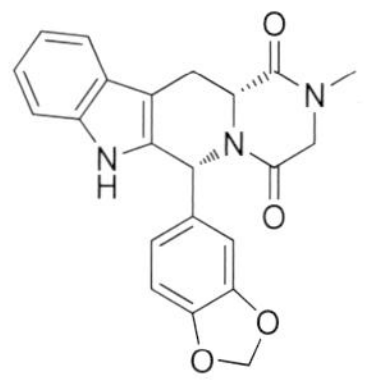

*Renal-Urologic System*

**Treprostinil Sodium**
**Remodulin®/**
**Orenitram®/Tyvaso®**

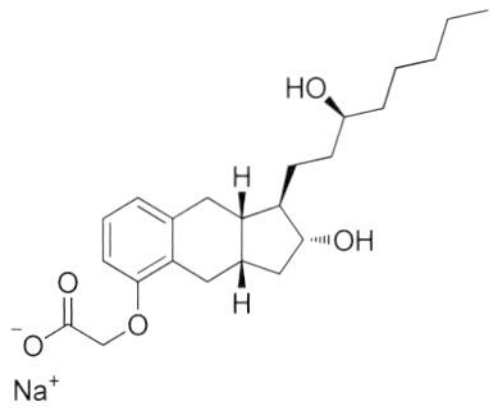

*Cardiovascular*

**Voriconazole**
**Vfend®**

*Anti-infective*

# Year
# 2003

**Abarelix**
**Plenaxis®**

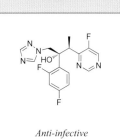

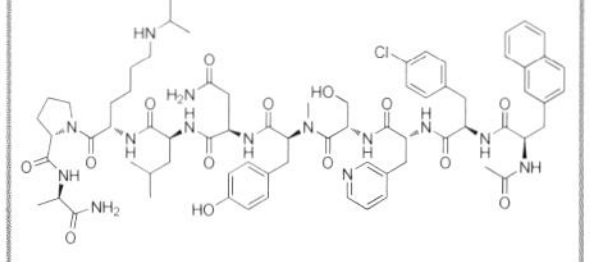

*Cancer*

**Alfuzosin Hydrochloride**
**Uroxatral®/Xatral®**

*Renal-Urologic System*

**Aprepitant**
**Emend®**

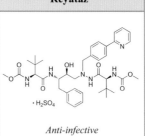

*Gastrointestinal System*

**Atazanavir Sulfate**
**Reyataz®**

*Anti-infective*

**Azelnidipine**
**Calblock®**

*Cardiovascular*

**Belotecan Hydrochloride**
**Camtobell®**

*Cancer*

**Bortezomib**
**Velcade®**

*Cancer*

**Carglumic Acid**
**Carbaglu®**

*Metabolic*

**Daptomycin**
**Cubicin®**

*Anti-infective*

**Emtricitabine**
**Emtriva®**

*Anti-infective*

**Esomeprazole Sodium**
**Nexium IV®**

*Gastrointestinal System*

**Everolimus Certican®/**
**Zortress®/Afinitor®**

*Cancer*

**Fosamprenavir Calcium**
**Lexiva®/Telzir®**

*Anti-infective*

**Fosfluconazole**
**Prodif®**

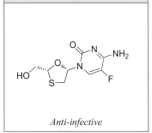

*Anti-infective*

**Gemifloxacin Mesylate**
**Factive®**

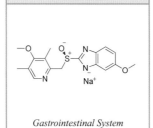

*Anti-infective*

**Ibandronate Sodium**
**Hydrate Boniva®/**
**Bondronat®/Bonviva®**

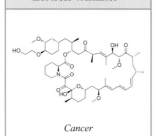

*Metabolic*

**Palonosetron Hydrochloride**
**Aloxi®**

*Gastrointestinal System*

**Pitavastatin Calcium**
**Livalo®**

*Cardiovascular*

**Rupatadine Fumarate**
**Rupafin®**

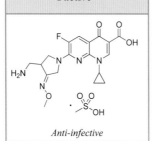

*Respiratory*

**Sertaconazole Nitrate**
**Ertaczo®/Dermofix®/**
**Zalain®**

*Anti-infective*

**Talaporfin Sodium**
**Laserphyrin®**

*Cancer*

**Vardenafil Hydrochloride**
**Levitra®/Vivanza®/Staxyn®**

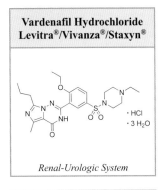

*Renal-Urologic System*

**Ximelagatran**
**Exanta®**

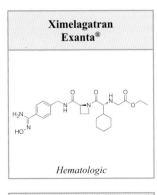

*Hematologic*

**Year
2004**

**Azacitidine**
**Vidaza®**

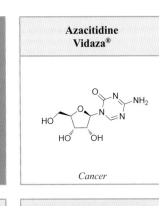

*Cancer*

**Ciclesonide Alvesco®/**
**Omnaris®**

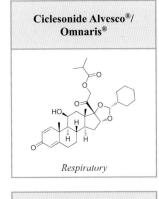

*Respiratory*

**Cinacalcet Hydrochloride**
**Sensipar®/Mimpara®/**
**Regpara®**

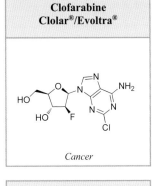

*Metabolic*

**Clofarabine**
**Clolar®/Evoltra®**

*Cancer*

**Darifenacin Hydrobromide**
**Emselex®/Enablex®/**
**Xelena®**

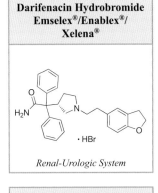

*Renal-Urologic System*

**Duloxetine Hydrochloride**
**Cymbalta®/Ariclaim®**

*Central Nervous System*

**Erlotinib Hydrochloride**
**Tarceva®**

*Cancer*

**Eszopiclone**
**Lunesta®**

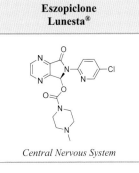

*Central Nervous System*

**Indisetron Dihydrochloride**
**Sinseron®**

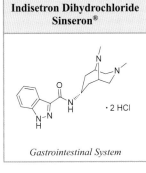

*Gastrointestinal System*

**Mitiglinide Calcium**
**Hydrate Glufast®**

*Metabolic*

**Pemetrexed Disodium**
**Hydrate Alimta®**

*Cancer*

**Pregabalin**
**Lyrica®**

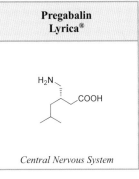

*Central Nervous System*

**Solifenacin Succinate**
**Vesicare®**

*Renal-Urologic System*

**Strontium Ranelate**
**Osseor®/Protelos®/Protos®**

*Metabolic*

**Trospium Chloride**
**Sanctura®**

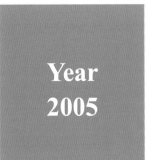

*Renal-Urologic System*

**Year
2005**

**Anecortave Acetate**
**Retaane®**

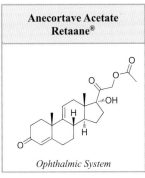

*Ophthalmic System*

| | |
|---|---|
| **Conivaptan Hydrochloride**<br>**Vaprisol®**<br>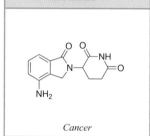<br>· HCl<br>*Cardiovascular* | **Deferasirox**<br>**Exjade®**<br><br>*Iron chelator* |

| | |
|---|---|
| **Doripenem Hydrate**<br>**Finibax®/Doribax®**<br>· H₂O<br>*Anti-infective* | **Eberconazole Nitrate**<br>**Ebernet®**<br>· HNO₃<br>*Dermatologic System* |

**Conivaptan Hydrochloride**
**Vaprisol®**

· HCl

*Cardiovascular*

**Deferasirox**
**Exjade®**

*Iron chelator*

**Doripenem Hydrate**
**Finibax®/Doribax®**

· H₂O

*Anti-infective*

**Eberconazole Nitrate**
**Ebernet®**

· HNO₃

*Dermatologic System*

**Entecavir Hydrate**
**Baraclude®**

· H₂O

*Anti-infective*

**Ivabradine Hydrochloride**
**Procoralan®/Corlentor®**

· HCl

*Cardiovascular*

**Lenalidomide**
**Revlimid®**

*Cancer*

**Luliconazole**
**Lulicon®/Luzu®**

*Anti-infective*

**Lumiracoxib**
**Prexige®**

*Anti-arthritic*

**Magnesium**
**Isoglycyrrhizinate**
**天晴甘美®**

· 4 H₂O

Mg²⁺

*Anti-infective*

**Nelarabine**
**Arranon®/Atriance®**

*Cancer*

**Nepafenac**
**Nevanac®**

*Ophthalmic System*

**Posaconazole**
**Noxafil®**

*Anti-infective*

**Ramelteon**
**Rozerem®**

*Central Nervous System*

**Rasagiline Mesylate**
**Azilect®**

*Central Nervous System*

**Revaprazan Hydrochloride**
**Revanex®**

· HCl

*Gastrointestinal System*

**Sorafenib Tosylate**
**Nexavar®**

*Cancer*

**Tamibarotene**
**Amnolake®**

*Cancer*

**Tigecycline**
**Tygacil®**

*Anti-infective*

**Tipranavir**
**Aptivus®**

*Anti-infective*

**Udenafil**
**Zydena®**

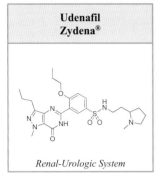

*Renal-Urologic System*

**Year**
**2006**

**Anidulafungin**
**Eraxis®/Ecalta®**

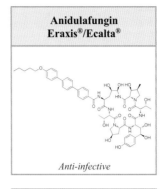

*Anti-infective*

**Arformoterol Tartrate**
**Brovana®**

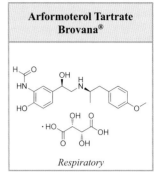

*Respiratory*

**Clevudine**
**Levovir®/Revovir®**

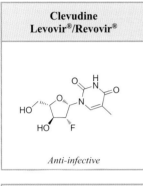

*Anti-infective*

**Darunavir Ethanolate**
**Prezista®**

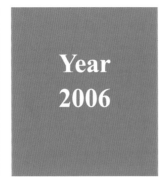

*Anti-infective*

**Dasatinib Hydrate**
**Sprycel®**

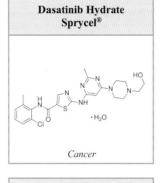

*Cancer*

**Decitabine**
**Dacogen®**

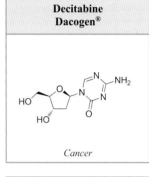

*Cancer*

**Etonogestrel**
**Implanon®/Nexplanon®**

*Endocrine*

**Lubiprostone**
**Amitiza®**

*Gastrointestinal System*

**Mozavaptan Hydrochloride**
**Physuline®**

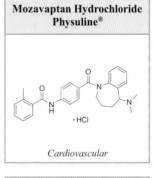

*Cardiovascular*

**Paliperidone**
**Invega®**

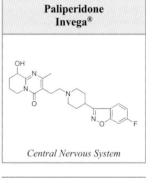

*Central Nervous System*

**Ranolazine**
**Ranexa®**

*Cardiovascular*

**Rimonabant**
**Acomplia®/Zimulti®**

*Metabolic*

**Rotigotine**
**Neupro®/Leganto®**

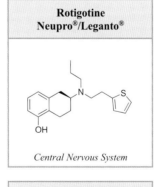

*Central Nervous System*

**Silodosin**
**Urief®/Rapaflo®/Silodyx®**

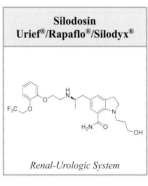

*Renal-Urologic System*

**Sitagliptin Phosphate**
**Monohydrate Januvia®/**
**Glactiv®**

*Metabolic*

**Sitaxentan Sodium**
**Thelin®**

*Cardiovascular*

**Sunitinib Malate**
**Sutent®**

*Cancer*

**Telbivudine**
**Tyzeka®/Sebivo®**

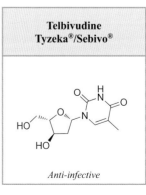

*Anti-infective*

| Varenicline Tartrate Chantix®/Champix® | Vorinostat Zolinza® | **Year 2007** | Aliskiren Hemifumarate Tekturna®/Rasilez® |
|---|---|---|---|
| *Central Nervous System* | *Cancer* | | *Cardiovascular* |

| Ambrisentan Letairis®/Volibris® | Armodafinil Nuvigil® | Fesoterodine Fumarate Toviaz® | Fluticasone Furoate Veramyst®/Avamys®/ Allermist® |
|---|---|---|---|
| *Cardiovascular* | *Central Nervous System* | *Renal-Urologic System* | *Respiratory* |

| Fosaprepitant Dimeglumine Emend®/Ivemend®/ Proemend® | Garenoxacin Mesylate Hydrate Geninax® | Imidafenacin Uritos®/Staybla® | Ixabepilone Ixempra® |
|---|---|---|---|
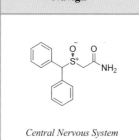
| *Gastrointestinal System* | *Anti-infective* | *Renal-Urologic System* | *Cancer* |

| Lapatinib Ditosylate Hydrate Tykerb®/ Tyverb® | Lisdexamfetamine Dimesylate Vyvanse®/ Elvanse®/Venvanse® | Maraviroc Selzentry®/Celsentri® | Nilotinib Hydrochloride Hydrate Tasigna® |
|---|---|---|---|
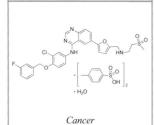
| *Cancer* | *Central Nervous System* | *Anti-infective* | *Cancer* |

| Raltegravir Potassium Isentress® | Retapamulin Altabax®/Altargo® | Rufinamide Inovelon®/Banzel® | Sevelamer Carbonate Renvela® |
|---|---|---|---|
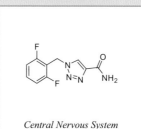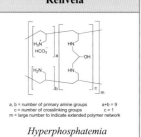
| *Anti-infective* | *Dermatologic System* | *Central Nervous System* | *Hyperphosphatemia* |

| Temsirolimus Torisel® | Trabectedin Yondelis® | Vildagliptin Galvus®/ Jalra®/Xiliarx®/Equa® | **Year 2008** |
|---|---|---|---|
| 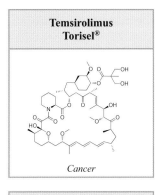 | 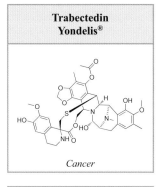 | 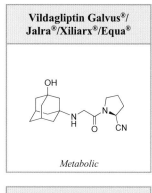 | 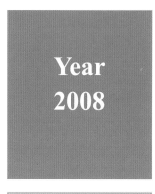 |
| *Cancer* | *Cancer* | *Metabolic* | |

| Alvimopan Hydrate Entereg® | Blonanserin Lonasen® | Ceftobiprole Medocaril Sodium Zeftera®/Zevtera® | Choline Fenofibrate Trilipix® |
|---|---|---|---|
| 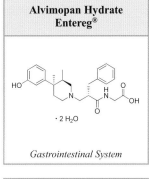 | 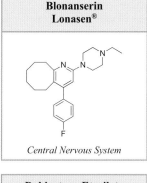 | 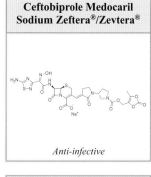 | 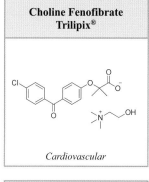 |
| *Gastrointestinal System* | *Central Nervous System* | *Anti-infective* | *Cardiovascular* |

| Clevidipine Butyrate Cleviprex® | Dabigatran Etexilate Mesylate Pradaxa®/ Prazaxa® | Degarelix Acetate Firmagon®/Gonax® | Desvenlafaxine Succinate Hydrate Pristiq® |
|---|---|---|---|
| 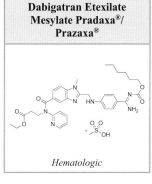 | | 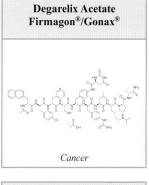 | 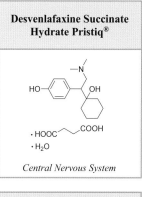 |
| *Cardiovascular* | *Hematologic* | *Cancer* | *Central Nervous System* |

| Eltrombopag Olamine Promacta®/Revolade® | Etravirine Intelence® | Febuxostat Uloric®/ Adenuric®/Febutaz® | Fospropofol Disodium Lusedra® |
|---|---|---|---|
| | | 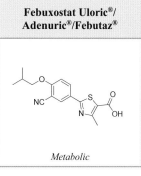 | |
| *Hematologic* | *Anti-infective* | *Metabolic* | *Central Nervous System* |

| Lacosamide Vimpat® | Methylnaltrexone Bromide Relistor® | Pirfenidone Pirespa®/Esbriet® | Plerixafor Mozobil® |
|---|---|---|---|
| | | 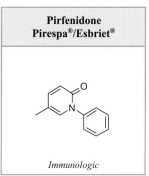 | 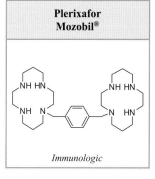 |
| *Central Nervous System* | *Gastrointestinal System* | *Immunologic* | *Immunologic* |

| | | | |
|---|---|---|---|
| **Regadenoson Hydrate**<br>**Lexiscan®/Rapiscan®** | **Rivaroxaban**<br>**Xarelto®** | **Sitafloxacin Hydrate**<br>**Gracevit®** | **Sugammadex Sodium**<br>**Bridion®** |

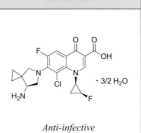

· 3/2 H₂O → · 3/2 $H_2O$

*Cardiovascular* — *Hematologic* — *Anti-infective* — *Muscle Relaxants*

| | | | |
|---|---|---|---|
| **Tafluprost Taflotan®/**<br>**Tapros®/Zioptan®** | **Tapentadol Hydrochloride**<br>**Nucynta®/Palexia®** | **Tetrabenazine**<br>**Xenazine®/Choreazine®** | |

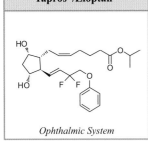

**Year 2009**

*Ophthalmic System* — *Central Nervous System* — *Central Nervous System*

| | | | |
|---|---|---|---|
| **Agomelatine**<br>**Thymanax®/Valdoxan®** | **Amifampridine Phosphate**<br>**Firdapse®/Zenas®** | **Antofloxacin Hydrochloride**<br>**优朋®** | **Asenapine Maleate**<br>**Saphris®/Sycrest®** |

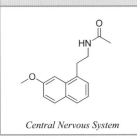

*Central Nervous System* — *Central Nervous System* — *Anti-infective* — *Central Nervous System*

| | | | |
|---|---|---|---|
| **Bazedoxifene Acetate**<br>**Conbriza®/Viviant®** | **Besifloxacin Hydrochloride**<br>**Besivance®** | **Capsaicin**<br>**Qutenza®** | **Dapoxetine Hydrochloride**<br>**Priligy®** |

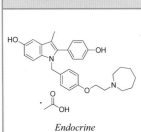

*Endocrine* — *Ophthalmic System* — *Central Nervous System* — *Renal-Urologic System*

| | | | |
|---|---|---|---|
| **Dexamethasone Cipecilate**<br>**Erizas®** | **Dexlansoprazole**<br>**Dexilant®/Kapidex®** | **Dronedarone Hydrochloride**<br>**Multaq®** | **Eslicarbazepine Acetate**<br>**Exelief®/Zebinix®/Stedesa®** |

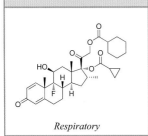

*Respiratory* — *Gastrointestinal System* — *Cardiovascular* — *Central Nervous System*

## Iloperidone
### Fanapt®

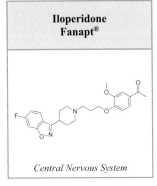

*Central Nervous System*

## Indacaterol Maleate
### Onbrez®/Arcapta®/ Hirobriz®

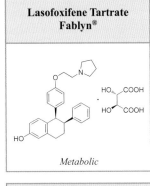

*Respiratory*

## Lasofoxifene Tartrate
### Fablyn®

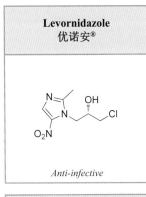

*Metabolic*

## Levornidazole
### 优诺安®

*Anti-infective*

## Mifamurtide Sodium Hydrate Mepact®

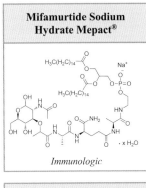

*Immunologic*

## Minodronic Acid Hydrate
### Bonoteo®/Recalbon®

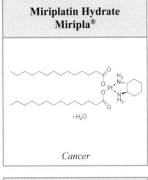

*Metabolic*

## Miriplatin Hydrate
### Miripla®

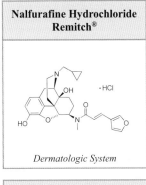

*Cancer*

## Nalfurafine Hydrochloride
### Remitch®

*Dermatologic System*

## Pazopanib Hydrochloride
### Votrient®

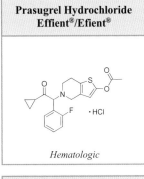

*Cancer*

## Pralatrexate
### Folotyn®

*Cancer*

## Prasugrel Hydrochloride
### Effient®/Efient®

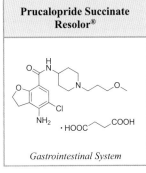

*Hematologic*

## Prucalopride Succinate
### Resolor®

*Gastrointestinal System*

## Romidepsin
### Istodax®

*Cancer*

## Saxagliptin Hydrate
### Onglyza®

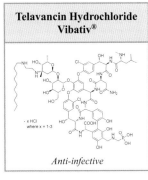

*Metabolic*

## Telavancin Hydrochloride
### Vibativ®

*Anti-infective*

## Tolvaptan
### Samsca®

*Cardiovascular*

## Ulipristal Acetate
### EllaOne®/Ella®/Esmya®

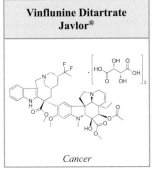

*Endocrine*

## Vinflunine Ditartrate
### Javlor®

*Cancer*

## Year 2010

## Alcaftadine
### Lastacaft®

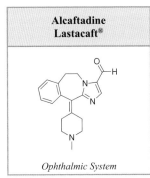

*Ophthalmic System*

## Alogliptin Benzoate
### Nesina®/Vipidia®

*Metabolic*

## Bilastine
### Bilaxten®

*Respiratory*

## Cabazitaxel
### Jevtana®

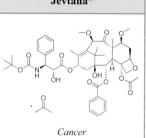

*Cancer*

## Ceftaroline Fosamil Acetate
### Teflaro®/Zinforo®

*Anti-infective*

## Dalfampridine/Fampridine
### Ampyra®/Fampyra®

*Central Nervous System*

## Diquafosol Tetrasodium
### Diquas®

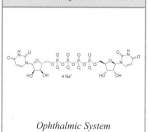

*Ophthalmic System*

## Eribulin Mesylate
### Halaven®

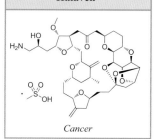

*Cancer*

## Fimasartan Potassium
### Trihydrate Kanarb®

*Cardiovascular*

## Fingolimod Hydrochloride
### Gilenya®/Imusera®

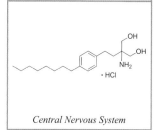

*Central Nervous System*

## Laninamivir Octanoate
### Hydrate Inavir®

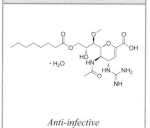

*Anti-infective*

## Lurasidone Hydrochloride
### Latuda®

*Central Nervous System*

## Peramivir Hydrate
### Rapiacta®/Peramiflu®

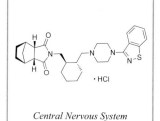

*Anti-infective*

## Roflumilast Daxas®/
### Daliresp®/Libertek®

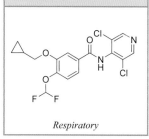

*Respiratory*

## Ticagrelor
### Brilinta®/Brilique®/Possia®

*Hematologic*

## Vernakalant Hydrochloride
### Brinavess®/Kynapid®

*Cardiovascular*

## Zucapsaicin
### Zuacta®/Civanex®

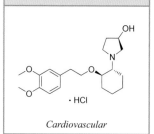

*Anti-arthritic*

## Year 2011

## Abiraterone Acetate
### Zytiga®

*Cancer*

## Apixaban
### Eliquis®

*Hematologic*

## Avanafil Zepeed®/
### Stendra®/Spedra®

*Renal-Urologic System*

**Azilsartan Medoxomil Potassium Edarbi®/Ipreziv®**

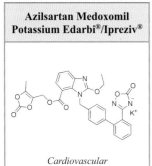

*Cardiovascular*

**Boceprevir Victrelis®**

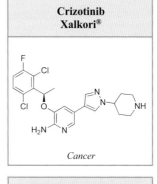

*Anti-infective*

**Crizotinib Xalkori®**

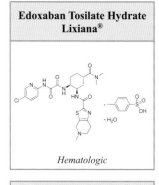

*Cancer*

**Edoxaban Tosilate Hydrate Lixiana®**

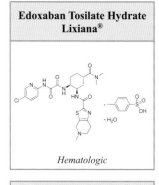

*Hematologic*

**Eldecalcitol Edirol®**

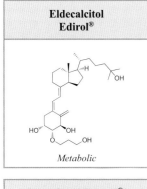

*Metabolic*

**Fidaxomicin Dificid®/Dificlir®**

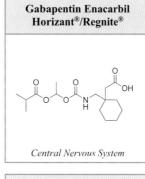

*Anti-infective*

**Gabapentin Enacarbil Horizant®/Regnite®**

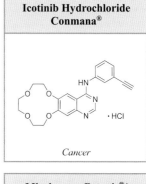

*Central Nervous System*

**Icotinib Hydrochloride Conmana®**

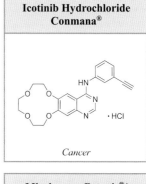

*Cancer*

**Iguratimod Iremod®/ Kolbet®/Careram®**

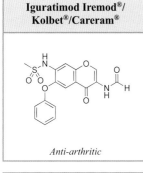

*Anti-arthritic*

**Imrecoxib Hengyang®**

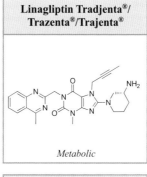

*Anti-arthritic*

**Linagliptin Tradjenta®/ Trazenta®/Trajenta®**

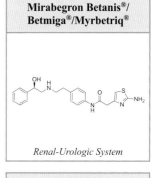

*Metabolic*

**Mirabegron Betanis®/ Betmiga®/Myrbetriq®**

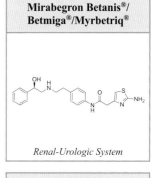

*Renal-Urologic System*

**Retigabine/Ezogabine Trobalt®/Potiga®**

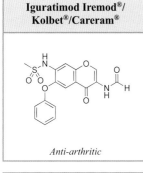

*Central Nervous System*

**Rilpivirine Hydrochloride Edurant®**

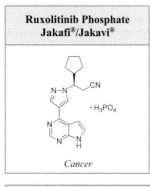

*Anti-infective*

**Ruxolitinib Phosphate Jakafi®/Jakavi®**

*Cancer*

**Tafamidis Meglumine Vyndaqel®**

*Central Nervous System*

**Telaprevir Incivek®/ Incivo®/Telavic®**

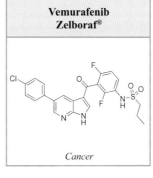

*Anti-infective*

**Vandetanib Caprelsa®**

*Cancer*

**Vemurafenib Zelboraf®**

*Cancer*

**Vilazodone Hydrochloride Viibryd®**

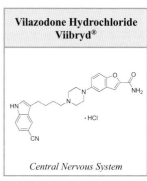

*Central Nervous System*

# Year 2012

## Aclidinium Bromide
### Bretaris Genuair®/ Eklira Genuair®/Tudorza Pressair®

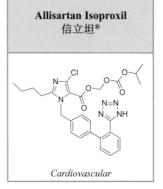

*Respiratory*

## Allisartan Isoproxil
### 信立坦®

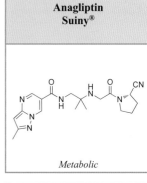

*Cardiovascular*

## Anagliptin
### Suiny®

*Metabolic*

## Axitinib
### Inlyta®

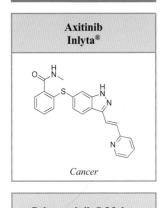

*Cancer*

## Azilsartan
### Azilva®

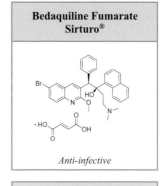

*Cardiovascular*

## Bedaquiline Fumarate
### Sirturo®

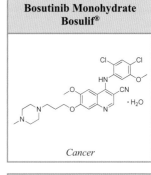

*Anti-infective*

## Bosutinib Monohydrate
### Bosulif®

*Cancer*

## Cabozantinib S-Malate
### Cometriq®

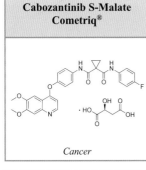

*Cancer*

## Carfilzomib
### Kyprolis®

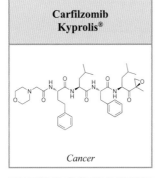

*Cancer*

## Dapagliflozin Propanediol Monohydrate
### Forxiga®/Farxiga®

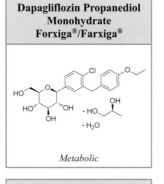

*Metabolic*

## Enzalutamide
### Xtandi®

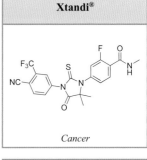

*Cancer*

## Gemigliptin L-tartrate Sesquihydrate
### Zemiglo®

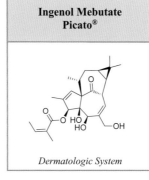

*Metabolic*

## Glycopyrronium Bromide
### Enurev®/Seebri®/Robinul®

*Respiratory*

## Ingenol Mebutate
### Picato®

*Dermatologic System*

## Ivacaftor
### Kalydeco®

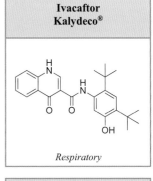

*Respiratory*

## Linaclotide
### Linzess®/Constella®

*Gastrointestinal System*

## Lomitapide Mesylate
### Juxtapid®/Lojuxta®

*Cardiovascular*

## Lorcaserin Hydrochloride Hemihydrate Belviq®

*Metabolic*

## Omacetaxine Mepesuccinate
### Synribo®

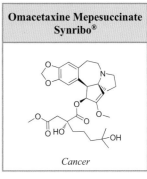

*Cancer*

| | | | |
|---|---|---|---|
| **Pasireotide Diaspartate**<br>**Signifor®** | **Perampanel Hydrate**<br>**Fycompa®** | **Pixantrone Dimaleate**<br>**Pixuvri®** | **Ponatinib Hydrochloride**<br>**Iclusig®** |

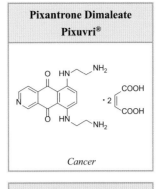

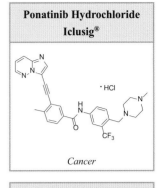

| | | | |
|---|---|---|---|
| *Endocrine* | *Central Nervous System* | *Cancer* | *Cancer* |

| | | | |
|---|---|---|---|
| **Radotinib Dihydrochloride**<br>**Supect®** | **Regorafenib Monohydrate**<br>**Stivarga®** | **Teneligliptin Hydrobromide**<br>**Hydrate Tenelia®** | **Teriflunomide**<br>**Aubagio®** |

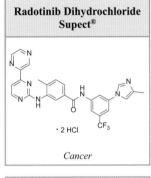

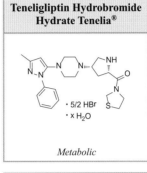

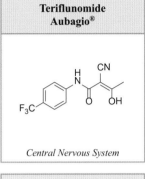

| | | | |
|---|---|---|---|
| *Cancer* | *Cancer* | *Metabolic* | *Central Nervous System* |

| | | | |
|---|---|---|---|
| **Tofacitinib Citrate**<br>**Xeljanz®/Jakvinus®** | **Vismodegib**<br>**Erivedge®** | | **Acotiamide Hydrochloride**<br>**Acofide®** |

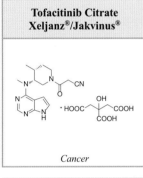

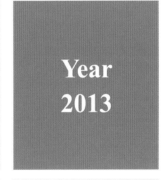

**Year 2013**

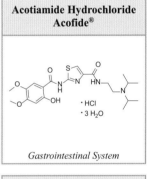

| | | | |
|---|---|---|---|
| *Cancer* | *Cancer* | | *Gastrointestinal System* |

| | | | |
|---|---|---|---|
| **Afatinib Dimaleate**<br>**Gilotrif®/Giotrif®** | **Canagliflozin Hemihydrate**<br>**Invokana®/Canaglu®** | **Cetilistat**<br>**Oblean®** | **Cholic Acid**<br>**Orphacol®** |

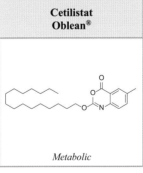

| | | | |
|---|---|---|---|
| *Cancer* | *Metabolic* | *Metabolic* | *Metabolic* |

| | | | |
|---|---|---|---|
| **Cobicistat**<br>**Tybost®** | **Dabrafenib Mesylate**<br>**Tafinlar®** | **Dimethyl Fumarate**<br>**Tecfidera®** | **Dolutegravir Sodium**<br>**Tivicay®** |

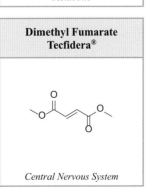

| | | | |
|---|---|---|---|
| *Anti-infective* | *Cancer* | *Central Nervous System* | *Anti-infective* |

| | | | |
|---|---|---|---|
| **Efinaconazole**<br>**Jublia®** | **Elvitegravir**<br>**Vitekta®** | **Esomeprazole Strontium**<br>**Esomezol®** | **Glycerol Phenylbutyrate**<br>**Ravicti®** |
| 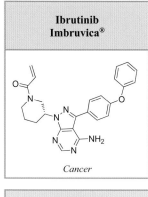 | 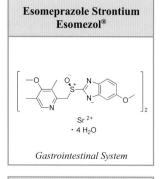 | 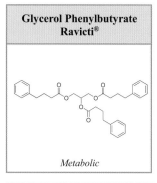 | |
| *Dermatologic System* | *Anti-infective* | *Gastrointestinal System* | *Metabolic* |

| | | | |
|---|---|---|---|
| **Ibrutinib**<br>**Imbruvica®** | **Istradefylline**<br>**Nouriast®** | **Levomilnacipran**<br>**Hydrochloride**<br>**Fetzima®** | **Lobeglitazone Sulfate**<br>**Duvie®** |
| | 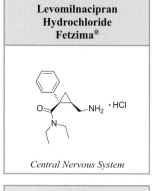 | 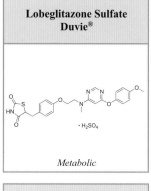 | |
| *Cancer* | *Central Nervous System* | *Central Nervous System* | *Metabolic* |

| | | | |
|---|---|---|---|
| **Macitentan**<br>**Opsumit®** | **Olodaterol Hydrochloride**<br>**Striverdi Respimat®** | **Ospemifene**<br>**Osphena®** | **Pomalidomide**<br>**Pomalyst®/Imnovid®** |
| 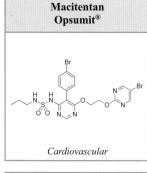 | 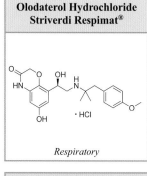 | 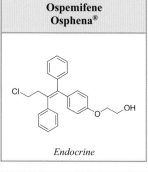 | 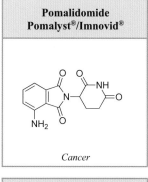 |
| *Cardiovascular* | *Respiratory* | *Endocrine* | *Cancer* |

| | | | |
|---|---|---|---|
| **Riociguat**<br>**Adempas®** | **Saroglitazar**<br>**Lipaglyn®** | **Simeprevir Sodium**<br>**Olysio®/Sovriad®** | **Sofosbuvir**<br>**Sovaldi®** |
| | | 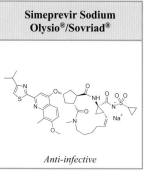 | 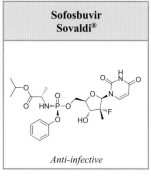 |
| *Cardiovascular* | *Metabolic* | *Anti-infective* | *Anti-infective* |

| | | | |
|---|---|---|---|
| **Topiroxostat**<br>**Uriadec®/Topiloric®** | **Trametinib Dimethyl**<br>**Sulfoxide Mekinist®** | **Vortioxetine Hydrobromide**<br>**Brintellix®** | |
| | 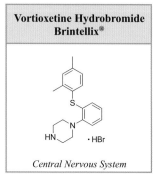 | | **Year**<br>**2014** |
| *Metabolic* | *Cancer* | *Central Nervous System* | |

| | | | |
|---|---|---|---|
| **Alectinib Hydrochloride**<br>**Alecensa®** | **Apatinib Mesylate**<br>艾坦® | **Apremilast**<br>**Otezla®** | **Asunaprevir**<br>**Sunvepra®** |
| *Cancer* | *Cancer* | *Anti-arthritic* | *Anti-infective* |
| **Ataluren**<br>**Translarna®** | **Belinostat**<br>**Beleodaq®** | **Ceritinib**<br>**Zykadia®** | **Chidamide**<br>**Epidaza®/爱谱沙®** |
| *Cancer* | *Cancer* | *Cancer* | *Cancer* |
| **Daclatasvir Dihydrochloride**<br>**Daklinza®** | **Delamanid**<br>**Deltyba®** | **Eliglustat Tartrate**<br>**Cerdelga®** | **Empagliflozin**<br>**Jardiance®** |
| *Anti-infective* | *Anti-infective* | *Metabolic* | *Metabolic* |
| **Finafloxacin**<br>**Xtoro®** | **Idelalisib**<br>**Zydelig®** | **Ipragliflozin L-Proline**<br>**Suglat®** | **Luseogliflozin Hydrate**<br>**Lusefi®** |
| *Anti-infective* | *Cancer* | *Metabolic* | *Metabolic* |
| **Morinidazole**<br>迈灵达® | **Naloxegol Oxalate**<br>**Movantik®** | **Nintedanib Esylate**<br>**Ofev®** | **Olaparib**<br>**Lynparza®** |
| *Anti-infective* | *Gastrointestinal System* | *Cancer* | *Cancer* |

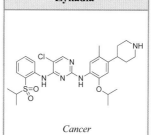
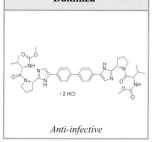
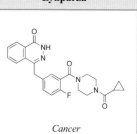

| | | | |
|---|---|---|---|
| **Oritavancin Diphosphate**<br>**Orbactiv®** | **Phenothrin**<br>**Sumithrin®** | **Ripasudil Hydrochloride**<br>**Hydrate Glanatec®** | **Suvorexant**<br>**Belsomra®** |
| *Anti-infective* | *Dermatologic System* | *Ophthalmic System* | *Central Nervous System* |
| **Tasimelteon**<br>**Hetlioz®** | **Tavaborole**<br>**Kerydin®** | **Tedizolid Phosphate**<br>**Sivextro®** | **Tofogliflozin Hydrate**<br>**Deberza®/Apleway®** |
| *Central Nervous System* | *Anti-infective* | *Anti-infective* | *Metabolic* |
| **Umeclidinium Bromide**<br>**Incruse®/Ellipta®** | **Vaniprevir**<br>**Vanihep®** | **Vonoprazan Fumarate**<br>**Takecab®** | **Vorapaxar Sulfate**<br>**Zontivity®** |
| *Respiratory* | *Anti-infective* | *Gastrointestinal System* | *Hematologic* |
| **Year**<br>**2015** | **Aripiprazole Lauroxil**<br>**Aristada®** | **Brexpiprazole**<br>**Rexulti®** | **Cangrelor Tetrasodium**<br>**Kengrexal®/Kengreal®** |
| | *Central Nervous System* | *Central Nervous System* | *Hematologic* |
| **Cariprazine Hydrochloride**<br>**Vraylar®** | **Cobimetinib Fumarate**<br>**Cotellic®** | **Dasabuvir Sodium Hydrate**<br>**Exviera®** | **Deoxycholic Acid**<br>**Kybella®** |
| *Central Nervous System* | *Cancer* | *Anti-infective* | *Dermatologic System* |

| **Eluxadoline** **Viberzi®** | **Esflurbiprofen** **Loqoa®** | **Flibanserin** **Addyi®** | **Isavuconazonium Sulfate** **Cresemba®** |
|---|---|---|---|
| 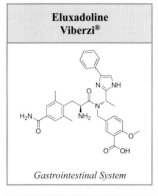 | 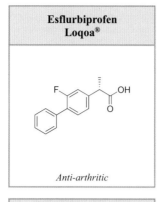 | 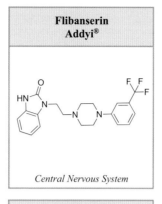 | 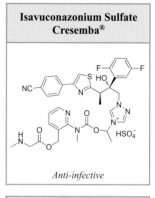 |
| *Gastrointestinal System* | *Anti-arthritic* | *Central Nervous System* | *Anti-infective* |

| **Ixazomib Citrate** **Ninlaro®** | **Lenvatinib Mesylate** **Lenvima®** | **Lesinurad** **Zurampic®** | **Omarigliptin** **Marizev®** |
|---|---|---|---|
| 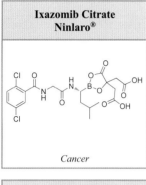 | 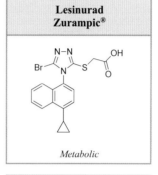 | 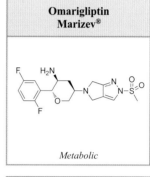 | |
| *Cancer* | *Cancer* | *Metabolic* | *Metabolic* |

| **Osimertinib Mesylate** **Tagrisso®** | **Palbociclib** **Ibrance®** | **Panobinostat Lactate** **Farydak®** | **Rolapitant Hydrochloride** **Hydrate Varubi®** |
|---|---|---|---|
| | | 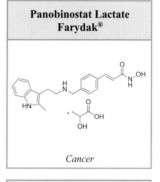 | 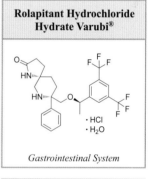 |
| *Cancer* | *Cancer* | *Cancer* | *Gastrointestinal System* |

| **Safinamide** **Methanesulfonate** **Xadago®** | **Selexipag** **Uptravi®** | **Sonidegib Phosphate** **Odomzo®** | **Trelagliptin Succinate** **Zafatek®** |
|---|---|---|---|
| | | 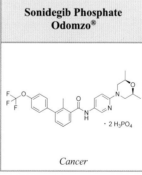 | 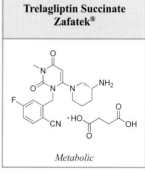 |
| *Central Nervous System* | *Cardiovascular* | *Cancer* | *Metabolic* |

| **Uridine Triacetate** **Xuriden®** | | | |
|---|---|---|---|
|  | | | |
| *Metabolic* | | | |

# Appendix

# IV

# Worldwide Approved NCEs (Sorted by Indication 2001-2015)

# Worldwide Approved NCEs
## (Sorted by Indication 2001-2015)

| | | |
|---|---|---|
| **Anti-Infectives** | **Ertapenem Sodium**<br>**Invanz®** *2001*<br>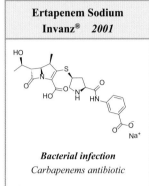<br>***Bacterial infection***<br>*Carbapenems antibiotic* | **Prulifloxacin**<br>**Sword®** *2002*<br>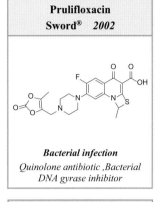<br>***Bacterial infection***<br>*Quinolone antibiotic ,Bacterial*<br>*DNA gyrase inhibitor* |

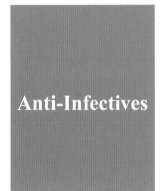

**Daptomycin**
**Cubicin®** *2003*

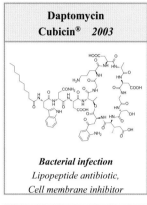

***Bacterial infection***
*Lipopeptide antibiotic,*
*Cell membrane inhibitor*

---

**Gemifloxacin Mesylate**
**Factive®** *2003*

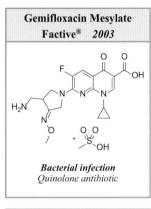

***Bacterial infection***
*Quinolone antibiotic*

**Doripenem Hydrate**
**Finibax®/Doribax®** *2005*

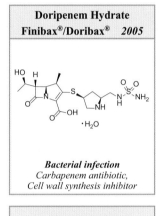

***Bacterial infection***
*Carbapenem antibiotic,*
*Cell wall synthesis inhibitor*

**Tigecycline**
**Tygacil®** *2005*

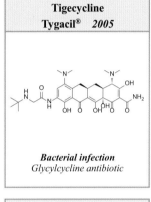

***Bacterial infection***
*Glycylcycline antibiotic*

**Retapamulin**
**Altabax®/Altargo®** *2007*

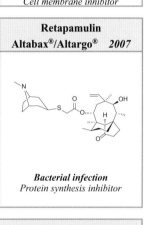

***Bacterial infection***
*Protein synthesis inhibitor*

---

**Ceftobiprole Medocaril**
**Sodium Zeftera®/**
**Zevtera®** *2008*

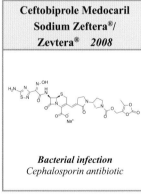

***Bacterial infection***
*Cephalosporin antibiotic*

**Sitafloxacin Hydrate**
**Gracevit®** *2008*

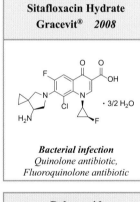

***Bacterial infection***
*Quinolone antibiotic,*
*Fluoroquinolone antibiotic*

**Levornidazole**
优诺安® *2009*

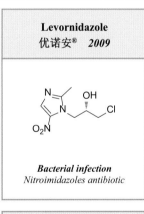

***Bacterial infection***
*Nitroimidazoles antibiotic*

**Ceftaroline Fosamil Acetate**
**Teflaro®/Zinforo®** *2010*

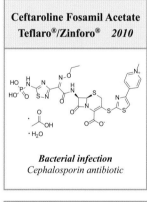

***Bacterial infection***
*Cephalosporin antibiotic*

---

**Bedaquiline Fumarate**
**Sirturo®·** *2012*

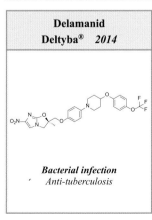

***Bacterial infection***
*Anti-Tuberculosis, Proton-*
*translocating ATP synthetase*
*inhibitor*

**Delamanid**
**Deltyba®** *2014*

***Bacterial infection***
·  *Anti-tuberculosis*

**Morinidazole**
迈灵达® *2014*

***Bacterial infection***
*Nitroimidazoles antibiotic*

**Oritavancin Diphosphate**
**Orbactiv®** *2014*

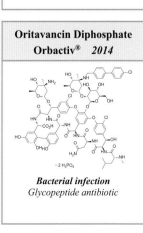

***Bacterial infection***
*Glycopeptide antibiotic*

### Voriconazole
### Vfend® *2002*

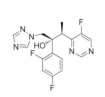

**Bacterial infection, Fungal infection**
Azole antifungal, Triazole antifungal agent

### Caspofungin Acetate
### Cancidas® *2001*

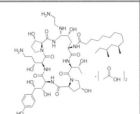

**Fungal infection**
Echinocandin antifungal, Glucan synthesis inhibitor

### Micafungin Sodium
### Funguard®/
### Mycamine® *2002*

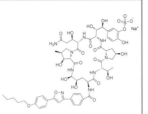

**Fungal infection**
Echinocandin antifungal , Fungal cell walls synthesis inhibitor

### Fosfluconazole
### Prodif® *2003*

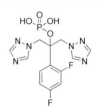

**Fungal infection**
Azole antifungal, Prodrug of fluconazole

### Sertaconazole Nitrate
### Ertaczo®/Dermofix®/
### Zalain® *2003*

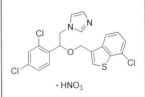

**Fungal infection**
Imidazole antifungal

### Eberconazole Nitrate
### Ebernet® *2005*

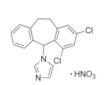

**Fungal infection**
Azole antifungal agent

### Luliconazole
### Lulicon®/Luzu® *2005*

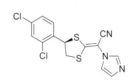

**Fungal infection**
Imidazole antifungal, Lanosterol demethylase inhibitor

### Posaconazole
### Noxafil® *2005*

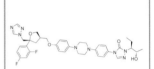

**Fungal infection**
Azole antifungal, Blocker of the synthesis of ergosterol

### Anidulafungin
### Eraxis®/Ecalta® *2006*

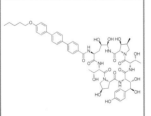

**Fungal infection**
Echinocandin antifungal

### Efinaconazole
### Jublia® *2013*

**Fungal infection**
14α-demethylase inhibitor

### Tavaborole
### Kerydin® *2014*

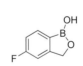

**Fungal infection**
Oxaborole antifungal

### Isavuconazonium Sulfate
### Cresemba® *2015*

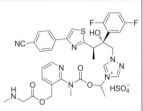

**Fungal infection**
Azole antifungal

### Adefovir Dipivoxil
### Hepsera® *2002*

**HBV infection**
Nucleotide analog reverse transcriptase

### Entecavir Hydrate
### Baraclude® *2005*

**HBV infection**
Hepatitis B virus nucleoside analog reverse transcriptase inhibitor

### Clevudine
### Levovir®/Revovir® *2006*

**HBV infection**
DNA polymerase inhibitor

### Telbivudine
### Tyzeka®/Sebivo® *2006*

**HBV infection**
HBV nucleoside analogue reverse transcriptase inhibitor

### Tenofovir Disoproxil Fumarate Viread® 2001

**HBV infection, HIV infection**
*Reverse transcriptase inhibitor*

### Boceprevir Victrelis® 2011

**HCV infection**
*HCV NS3/4A protease inhibitor*

### Telaprevir Incivek®/ Incivo®/Telavic® 2011

**HCV infection**
*HCV NS3/4A protease inhibitor*

### Simeprevir Sodium Olysio®/Sovriad® 2013

**HCV infection**
*NS3/4A protease inhibitor*

### Sofosbuvir Sovaldi® 2013

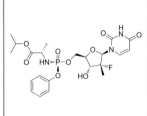

**HCV infection**
*HCV NS5B polymerase inhibitor, Nucleotide analogue*

### Asunaprevir Sunvepra® 2014

**HCV infection**
*HCV NS3/4A protease inhibitor*

### Daclatasvir Dihydrochloride Daklinza® 2014

**HCV infection**
*HCV NS5A inhibitor*

### Vaniprevir Vanihep® 2014

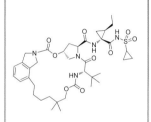

**HCV infection**
*HCV NS3/4A protease inhibitor*

### Dasabuvir Sodium Hydrate Exviera® 2015

**HCV infection**
*HCV NS5B RNA polymerase inhibitor*

### Atazanavir Sulfate Reyataz® 2003

**HIV infection**
*Protease inhibitor*

### Emtricitabine Emtriva® 2003

**HIV infection**
*Nucleoside reverse transcriptase inhibitor (NRTI)*

### Fosamprenavir Calcium Lexiva®/Telzir® 2003

**HIV infection**
*Protease inhibitor, Prodrug of amprenavir*

### Tipranavir Aptivus® 2005

**HIV infection**
*Nonpeptidic protease inhibitor (PI)*

### Darunavir Ethanolate Prezista® 2006

**HIV infection**
*Protease inhibitor*

### Maraviroc Selzentry®/ Celsentri® 2007

**HIV infection**
*CCR5 co-receptor antagonist*

### Raltegravir Potassium Isentress® 2007

**HIV infection**
*HIV-1 integrase inhibitor*

**Etravirine**
**Intelence®** *2008*

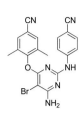

***HIV infection***
*Non-nucleoside reverse transcriptase inhibitor (NNRTI)*

**Rilpivirine Hydrochloride**
**Edurant®** *2011*

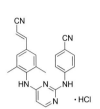

***HIV infection***
*Non-nucleoside reverse transcriptase inhibitor (NNRTI)*

**Cobicistat**
**Tybost®** *2013*

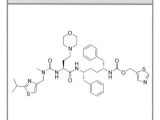

***HIV infection***
*CYP3A inhibitor*

**Dolutegravir Sodium**
**Tivicay®** *2013*

***HIV infection***
*Integrase inhibitor*

**Elvitegravir**
**Vitekta®** *2013*

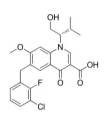

***HIV infection***
*HIV-1 integrase strand transfer inhibitor*

**Pazufloxacin Mesylate**
**Pazucross®/Pasil®** *2002*

***Others***
*Quinolone antibiotic*

**Nitazoxanide**
**Alinia®** *2002*

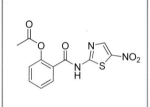

***Parasitic infection***
*Pyruvate: ferredoxin oxidoreductase (PFOR)*

**Laninamivir Octanoate Hydrate**
**Inavir®** *2010*

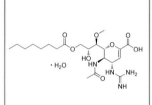

***Viral infection***
*Neuraminidase inhibitor*

**Peramivir Hydrate**
**Rapiacta®/**
**Peramiflu®** *2010*

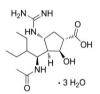

***Viral infection***
*Neuraminidase inhibitor*

**Cardiovascular and Hematological System**

**Ranolazine**
**Ranexa®** *2006*

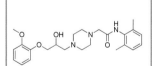

***Angina pectoris***
*Sodium channel modulator, Partial fatty acid oxidation inhibitor*

**Landiolol Hydrochloride**
**Onoact®** *2002*

***Arrhythmia***
*Adrenergic receptor antagonist, Ultra short-acting beta blocker , Cardio-selective beta blocker*

**Dronedarone Hydrochloride**
**Multaq®** *2009*

***Arrhythmia***
*Atrial potassium channel blocker, Class III antiarrhythmic agent, Benzofuran derivative*

**Vernakalant Hydrochloride**
**Brinavess®/Kynapid®**
*2010*

***Arrhythmia***
*Atrial potassium channel blocker, Class III antiarrhythmic agent*

**Eltrombopag Diolamine**
**Promacta®/Revolade®**
*2008*

***Bleeding and blood coagulation disorders***
*Thrombopoietin receptor agonist*

**Edaravone**
**Radicut®/Arone®** *2001*

***Cerebral vascular disease***
*Neuroprotective agent as a potent antioxidant*

| | | | |
|---|---|---|---|
| **Dabigatran Etexilate Mesylate Pradaxa®/ Prazaxa®** *2008* | **Apixaban Eliquis®** *2011* | **Edoxaban Tosilate Hydrate Lixiana®** *2011* | **Rivaroxaban Xarelto®** *2008* |

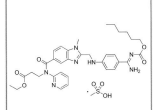

***Thrombosis, Cerebral vascular disease***
*Direct thrombin inhibitor*

***Thrombosis, Cerebral vascular disease***
*Direct factor Xa inhibitor*

***Thrombosis, Cerebral vascular disease***
*Direct factor Xa inhibitor*

***Cerebral vascular disease, Thrombosis***
*Factor Xa inhibitor*

| | | | |
|---|---|---|---|
| **Ticagrelor Brilinta®/ Brilique®/Possia®** *2010* | **Ivabradine Hydrochloride Procoralan®/ Corlentor®** *2005* | **Cangrelor Tetrasodium Kengrexal®/ Kengreal®** *2015* | **Prasugrel Hydrochloride Effient®/Efient®** *2009* |

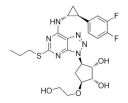

***Coronary heart disease***
*P2Y12 platelet inhibitor*

***Heart failure, Coronary heart disease***
*Selective and specific cardiac pacemaker If inhibitor*

***Thrombosis, Coronary heart disease, Miocardial infarction***
*P2Y12 platelet receptor inhibitor*

***Coronary heart disease, Thrombosis***
*P2Y12 platelet inhibitor*

| | | | |
|---|---|---|---|
| **Tolvaptan Samsca®** *2009* | **Eplerenone Inspra®** *2002* | **Sacubitril/Valsartan Entresto®** *2015* | **Ezetimibe Zetia®/ Ezetrol®** *2002* |

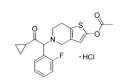

***Heart failure***
*Selective vasopressin V2-receptor antagonist*

***Hypertension, Heart failure***
*Aldosterone antagonist*

***Hypertension, Heart failure, Miocardial infarction***
*Angiotensin II receptor antagonist, Angiotensin II receptor blocker (ARB)*

***Hyperlipemia***
*Cholesterol absorption blocker*

| | | | |
|---|---|---|---|
| **Rosuvastatin Calcium Crestor®** *2002* | **Pitavastatin Calcium Livalo®** *2003* | **Choline Fenofibrate Trilipix®** *2008* | **Lomitapide Mesylate Juxtapid®/Lojuxta®** *2012* |

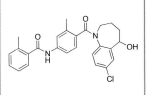 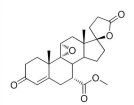 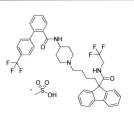

***Hyperlipemia***
*HMG-CoA reductase inhibitor*

***Hyperlipemia***
*HMG-CoA reductase inhibitor*

***Hyperlipemia***
*PPAR-α receptor agonist*

***Hyperlipemia***
*Microsomal triglyceride transfer protein (MTP or MTTP) inhibitor*

**Saroglitazar**
**Lipaglyn®  2013**

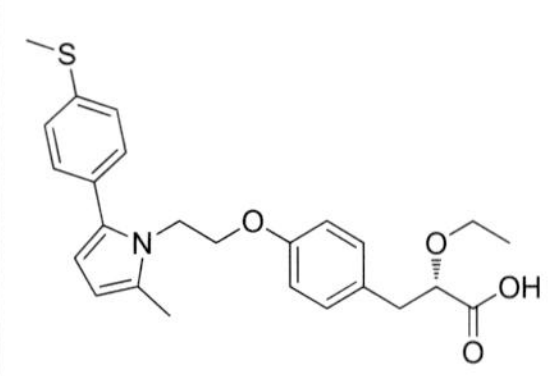

*Hyperlipemia*
*PPAR agonist, PPAR agonist*

**Bosentan Hydrate**
**Tracleer®  2001**

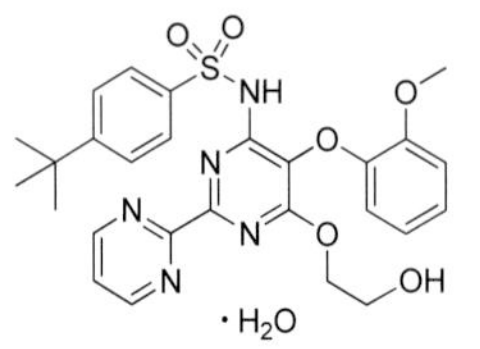

· H₂O

*Hypertension*
*Dual endothelin receptor*
*antagonist*

**Olmesartan Medoxomil**
**Benicar®/Olmetec®  2002**

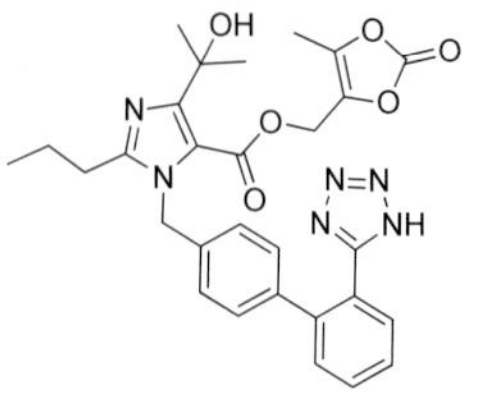

*Hypertension*
*Angiotensin II receptor*
*antagonist*

**Treprostinil Sodium**
**Remodulin®/Orenitram®/**
**Tyvaso®  2002**

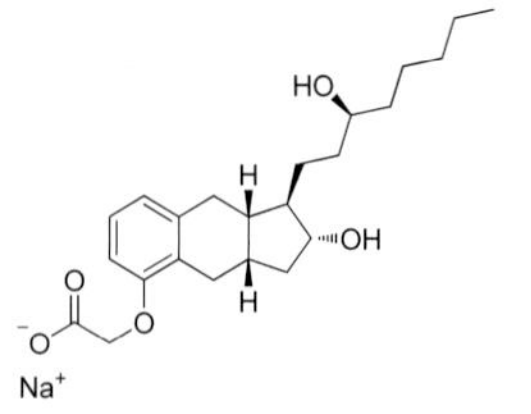

Na⁺

*Hypertension*
*Prostacyclin vasodilator, Platelet*
*aggregation inhibitors*

**Azelnidipine**
**Calblock®  2003**

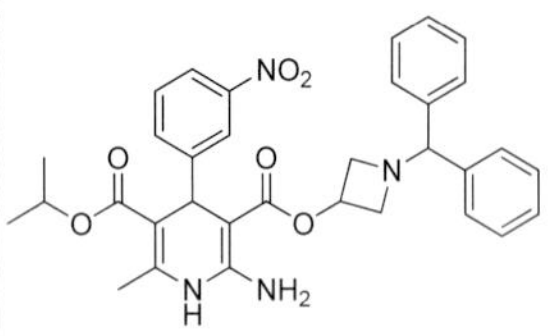

*Hypertension*
*Dihydropyridine calcium*
*channel blocker*

**Silodosin Urief®/Rapaflo®/**
**Silodyx®  2006**

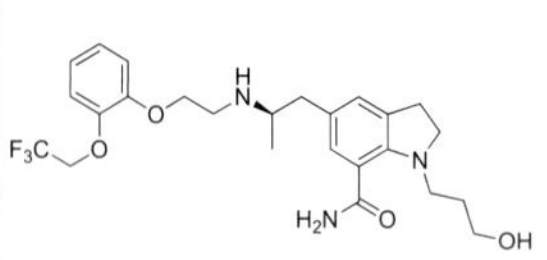

*Hypertension*
*α-1 adrenergic receptor*
*antagonist*

**Aliskiren Hemifumarate**
**Tekturna®/Rasilez®  2007**

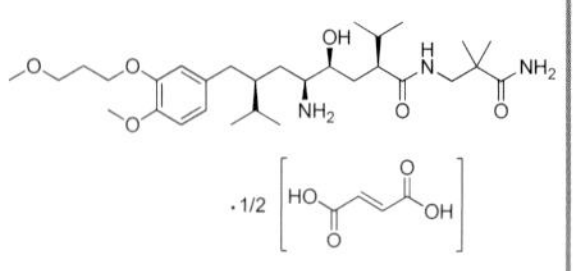

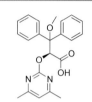

*Hypertension*
*Renin inhibitor (RI)*

**Ambrisentan Letairis®/**
**Volibris®  2007**

*Hypertension*
*Type A endothelin receptor (ETA)*
*antagonist*

**Clevidipine Butyrate**
**Cleviprex®  2008**

*Hypertension*
*Dihydropyridine calcium*
*channel blocker*

**Fimasartan Potassium**
**Trihydrate**
**Kanarb®  2010**

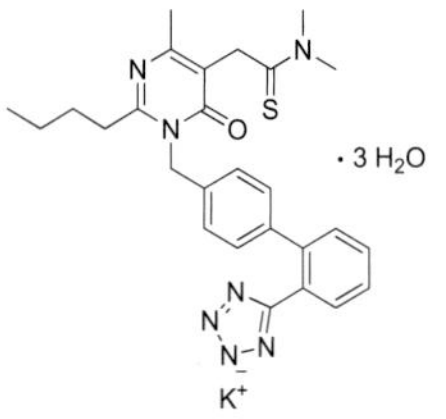

· 3 H₂O

K⁺

*Hypertension*
*Angiotensin II receptor*
*antagonist*

**Azilsartan Medoxomil**
**Potassium Edarbi®/**
**Ipreziv®  2011**

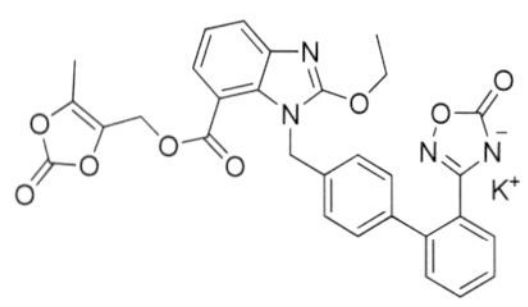

K⁺

*Hypertension*
*Angiotensin II receptor*
*antagonist*

**Allisartan Isoproxil**
**信立坦®  2012**

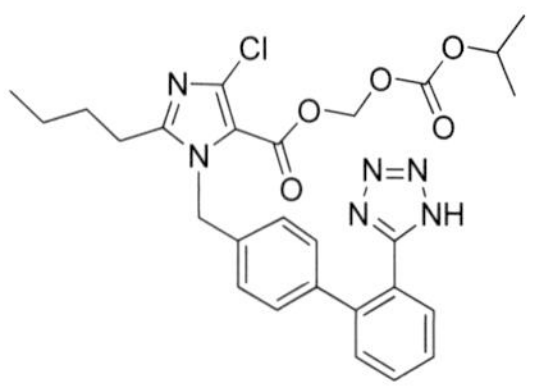

*Hypertension*
*Angiotensin II receptor*
*antagonist, Angiotensin II*
*receptor blocker (ARB)*

**Azilsartan**
**Azilva®  2012**

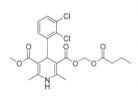

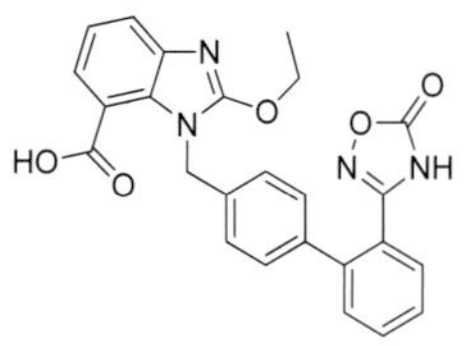

*Hypertension*
*Angiotensin II receptor*
*antagonist*

**Macitentan**
**Opsumit®  2013**

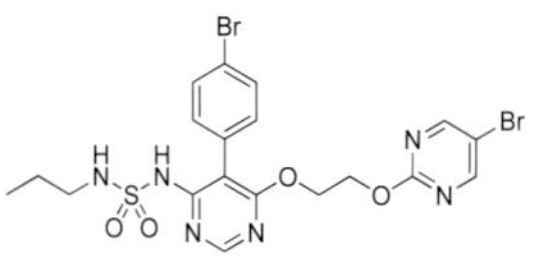

*Hypertension*
*Endothelin receptor antagonist*
*(ERA)*

**Riociguat**
**Adempas®  2013**

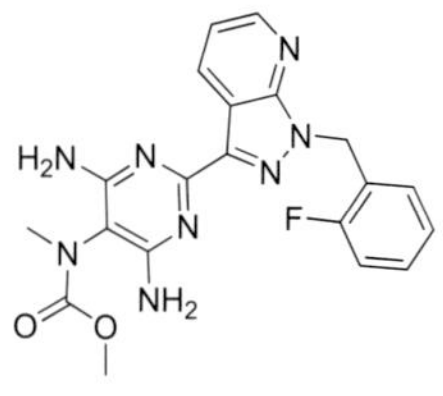

*Hypertension*
*Soluble guanylate cyclase (sGC)*
*stimulator*

**Selexipag**
**Uptravi®  2015**

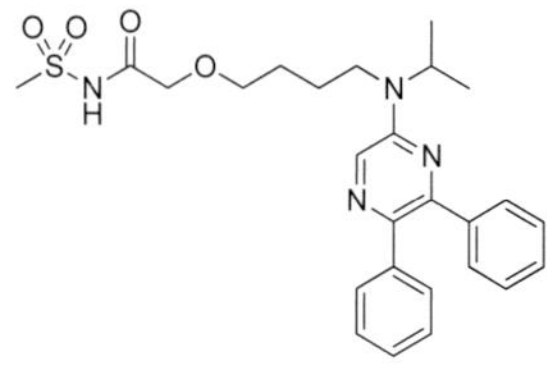

*Hypertension*
*Prostacyclin receptor*
*(prostaglandin I2 receptor)*
*agonist*

### Vorapaxar Sulfate
### Zontivity® 2014

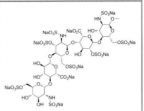

· H₂SO₄

***Miocardial infarction,***
***Thrombosis***
*PAR-1 antagonist*

### Pazufloxacin Mesylate
### Pazucross®/Pasil® 2002

***Anti-infectives***
*Quinolone antibiotic*

### Fondaparinux Sodium
### Arixtra® 2001

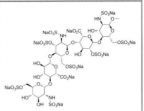

***Thrombosis, Pulmonary***
***vascular disease***
*Factor Xa inhibitor*

# Dermatologic

### Desloratadine
### Aerius®/Clarinex®/
### Neoclarityn® 2001

***Allergic diseases***
*Histamine H1 receptor*
*antagonist*

### Pimecrolimus
### Elidel® 2001

***Allergic diseases***
*Calcineurin inhibitor*

### Rupatadine Fumarate
### Rupafin® 2003

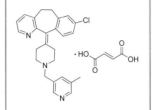

***Allergic diseases***
*(PAF antagonist, Histamine H1*
*antagonist*

### Bilastine
### Bilaxten® 2010

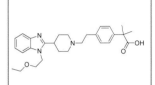

***Allergic diseases***
*Histamine H1 receptor*
*antagonist*

### Levocetirizine
### Dihydrochloride
### Xyzal®/Xusal® 2001

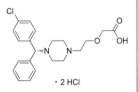

· 2 HCl

***Allergic diseases, Cutaneous***
***and subcutaneous infection***
*Histamine H1 receptor*
*antagonist*

### Ertapenem Sodium
### Invanz® 2001

***Cutaneous and subcutaneous***
***infection***
*Carbapenems antibiotic*

### Daptomycin
### Cubicin® 2003

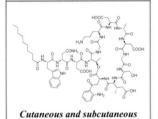

***Cutaneous and subcutaneous***
***infection***
*Lipopeptide antibiotic, Cell*
*membrane inhibitor*

### Sertaconazole Nitrate
### Ertaczo®/Dermofix®/
### Zalain® 2003

· HNO₃

***Cutaneous and subcutaneous***
***infection***
*Imidazole antifungal*

### Eberconazole Nitrate
### Ebernet® 2005

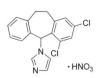

· HNO₃

***Cutaneous and subcutaneous***
***infection***
*Azole antifungal agent*

### Tigecycline
### Tygacil® 2005

***Cutaneous and subcutaneous***
***infection***
*Glycylcycline antibiotic*

### Ceftobiprole Medocaril
### Sodium Zeftera®/
### Zevtera® 2008

***Cutaneous and subcutaneous***
***infection***
*Cephalosporin antibiotic*

### Telavancin Hydrochloride
### Vibativ® 2009

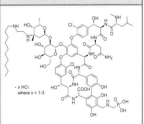

· x HCl
where x = 1-3

***Cutaneous and subcutaneous***
***infection***
*Glycopeptide antibiotic*

## Ceftaroline Fosamil Acetate Teflaro®/Zinforo® 2010

*Cutaneous and subcutaneous infection*
Cephalosporin antibiotic

## Apremilast Otezla® 2014

*Cutaneous and subcutaneous infection*
PDE4 inhibitor

## Oritavancin Diphosphate Orbactiv® 2014

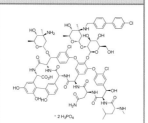

· 2 H₃PO₄

*Cutaneous and subcutaneous infection*
Glycopeptide antibiotic

## Phenothrin Sumithrin® 2014

*Cutaneous and subcutaneous infection*
Synthetic pyrethroid, Voltage-gated sodium channels opener

## Tedizolid Phosphate Sivextro® 2014

*Cutaneous and subcutaneous infection*
Oxazolidinone antibiotic

## Methyl Aminolevulinate HCl Metvix®/Metvixia® 2001

· HCl

*Skin cancer*
Protoporphyrin IX (sensitizer)

## Nalfurafine Hydrochloride Remitch® 2009

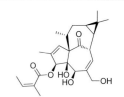

· HCl

*Others*
κ -opioid receptor agonist

## Ingenol Mebutate Picato® 2012

*Others*
Cell death inducer

## Digestive System

## Esomeprazole Sodium Nexium IV® 2003

*Antiacid and antiulcer*
PPI

## Revaprazan Hydrochloride Revanex® 2005

· HCl

*Antiacid and antiulcer*
PPI, Reversible H+/K+-ATPase inhibitor

## Dexlansoprazole Dexilant®/Kapidex® 2009

*Antiacid and antiulcer*
PPI

## Esomeprazole Strontium Esomezol® 2013

Sr²⁺
· 4 H₂O

*Antiacid and antiulcer*
PPI

## Vonoprazan Fumarate Takecab® 2014

*Antiacid and antiulcer*
P-CAB

## Aprepitant Emend® 2003

*Antiemetic*
Substance P/NK1 receptor antagonist

## Indisetron Dihydrochloride Sinseron® 2004

· 2 HCl

*Antiemetic*
Serotonin (5-HT3/5-HT4) receptor antagonist

**Fosaprepitant Dimeglumine Emend®/Ivemend®/ Proemend®** *2007*

***Antiemetic***
*NK1, Substance P receptor antagonist*

**Acotiamide Hydrochloride Hydrate Acofide®** *2013*

***Dyspepsia and gastric motility***
*Peripheral AChE inhibitor*

**Fidaxomicin Dificid®/Dificlir®** *2011*

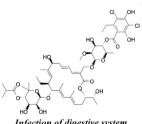

***Infection of digestive system***
*Bacterial RNA polymerase inhibitor, Macrolides antibiotic*

**Lubiprostone Amitiza®** *2006*

***Intestinal function disorder***
*Chloride channel activator*

**Prucalopride Succinate Resolor®** *2009*

***Intestinal function disorder***
*Serotonin (5-HT4) receptor agonist*

**Linaclotide Linzess®/ Constella®** *2012*

***Intestinal function disorder***
*Guanylate cyclase-C agonist*

**Eluxadoline Viberzi®** *2015*

***Intestinal function disorder***
*μ-opioid receptor agonist*

**Methylnaltrexone Bromide Relistor®** *2008*

***Poisoning***
*μ-opioid receptor antagonist*

**Naloxegol Oxalate Movantik®** *2014*

***Poisoning***
*Opioid receptor*

## Endocrine and Metabolic System

**Neridronate Sodium Nerixia®** *2002*

***Bone metabolism***
*Bisphosphonate*

**Mitiglinide Calcium Hydrate Glufast®** *2004*

***Diabetes and complications***
*K+(ATP) channels blocker*

**Pregabalin Lyrica®** *2004*

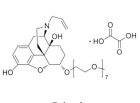

***Diabetes and complications***
*GABA receptor inhibitor*

**Sitagliptin Phosphate Hydrate Januvia®/ Glactiv®** *2006*

***Diabetes and complications***
*DPP-4 inhibitor*

**Vildagliptin Galvus®/ Jalra®/Xiliarx®/ Equa®** *2007*

***Diabetes and complications***
*DPP-4 inhibitor*

**Saxagliptin Hydrate Onglyza®** *2009*

***Diabetes and complications***
*DPP-4 inhibitor*

**Alogliptin Benzoate**
**Nesina®/Vipidia®**   *2010*

*Diabetes and complications*
*DPP-4 inhibitor*

**Linagliptin Tradjenta®/**
**Trazenta®/Trajenta®**   *2011*

*Diabetes and complications*
*DPP-4 inhibitor*

**Anagliptin**
**Suiny®**   *2012*

*Diabetes and complications*
*DPP-4 inhibitor*

**Dapagliflozin Propanediol**
**Monohydrate**
**Forxiga®/Farxiga®**   *2012*

*Diabetes and complications*
*SGLT2 inhibitor*

**Gemigliptin L-tartrate**
**Sesquihydrate**
**Zemiglo®**   *2012*

*Diabetes and complications*
*DPP-4 inhibitor*

**Teneligliptin**
**Hydrobromide Hydrate**
**Tenelia®**   *2012*

*Diabetes and complications*
*DPP-4 inhibitor*

**Canagliflozin Hemihydrate**
**Invokana®/Canaglu®**
*2013*

*Diabetes and complications*
*SGLT2 inhibitor*

**Lobeglitazone Sulfate**
**Duvie®**   *2013*

*Diabetes and complications*
*PPAR agonist*

**Saroglitazar**
**Lipaglyn®**   *2013*

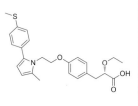

*Diabetes and complications*
*PPAR agonist*

**Empagliflozin**
**Jardiance®**   *2014*

*Diabetes and complications*
*SGLT2 inhibitor*

**Ipragliflozin L-Proline**
**Suglat®**   *2014*

*Diabetes and complications*
*SGLT2 inhibitor*

**Luseogliflozin Hydrate**
**Lusefi®**   *2014*

*Diabetes and complications*
*SGLT2 inhibitor*

**Tofogliflozin Hydrate**
**Deberza®/Apleway®**   *2014*

*Diabetes and complications*
*SGLT2 inhibitor*

**Omarigliptin**
**Marizev®**   *2015*

*Diabetes and complications*
*DPP-4 inhibitor*

**Trelagliptin Succinate**
**Zafatek®**   *2015*

*Diabetes and complications*
*DPP-4 inhibitor*

**Falecalcitriol**
**Hornel®/Fulstan®**   *2001*

*Metabolic disorder*
*Active vitamin D3 derivative*

**Miglustat**
**Zavesca®   2002**

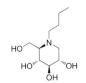

*Metabolic disorder*
*Glucosylceramide synthase*
*inhibitor*

**Carglumic Acid**
**Carbaglu®   2003**

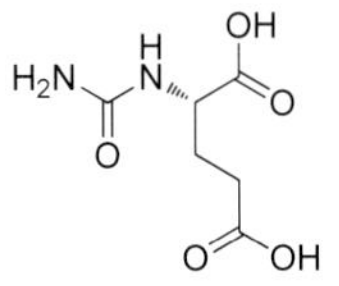

*Metabolic disorder*
*CPS1 activator*

**Ibandronate Sodium**
**Hydrate Boniva®/**
**Bondronat®/**
**Bonviva®   2003**

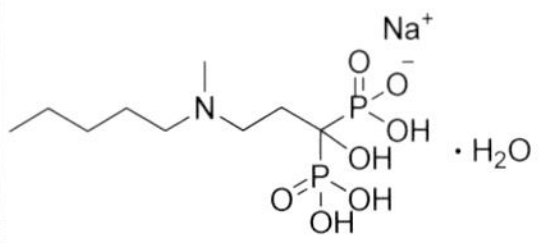

*Metabolic disorder*
*Bisphosphonate*

**Cinacalcet Hydrochloride**
**Sensipar®/Mimpara®/**
**Regpara®   2004**

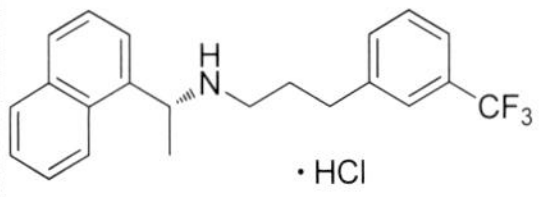

*Metabolic disorder*
*Calcium-sensing receptor*
*agonist*

**Conivaptan Hydrochloride**
**Vaprisol®   2005**

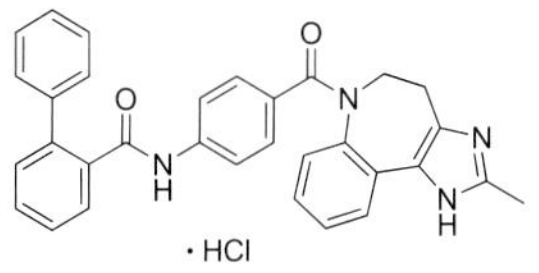

Metabolic disorder
*Vasopressin receptor antagonist*

**Mozavaptan Hydrochloride**
**Physuline®   2006**

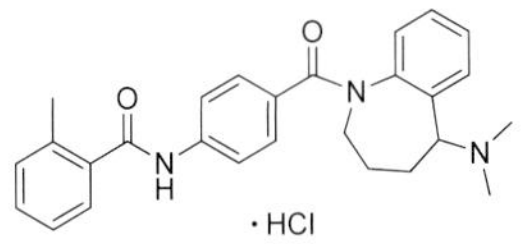

*Metabolic disorder*
*Vasopressin receptor antagonist*

**Febuxostat Uloric®/**
**Adenuric®/Febutaz®   2008**

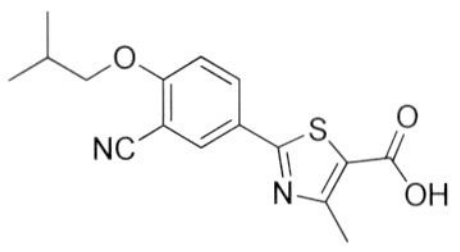

*Metabolic disorder*
*Xanthine oxidase inhibitor*

**Tafamidis Meglumine**
**Vyndaqel®   2011**

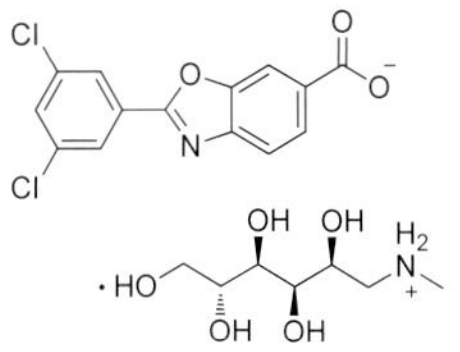

*Metabolic disorder*
*Transthyretin stabilizer*

**Pasireotide Diaspartate**
**Signifor®   2012**

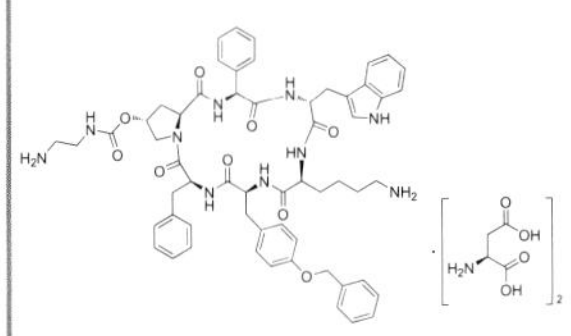

*Metabolic disorder*
*Cyclohexapeptide somatostatin*
*analogue, Somatostatin receptor 5*

**Cholic Acid**
**Orphacol®   2013**

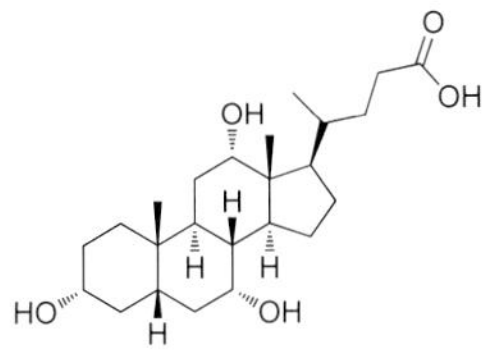

*Metabolic disorder*
*Bile acid*

**Glycerol Phenylbutyrate**
**Ravicti®   2013**

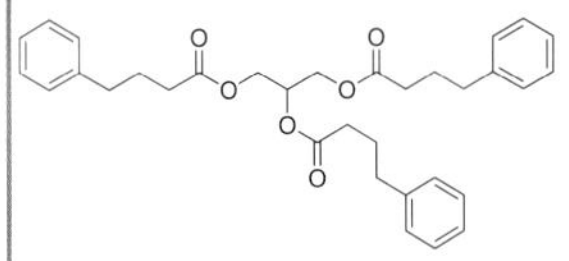

*Metabolic disorder*
*Nitrogen-binding agent*

**Topiroxostat Uriadec®/**
**Topiloric®   2013**

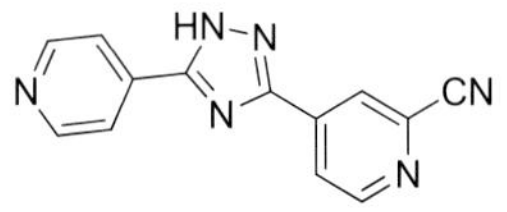

*Metabolic disorder*
*Xanthine oxidase inhibitor*

**Eliglustat Tartrate**
**Cerdelga®   2014**

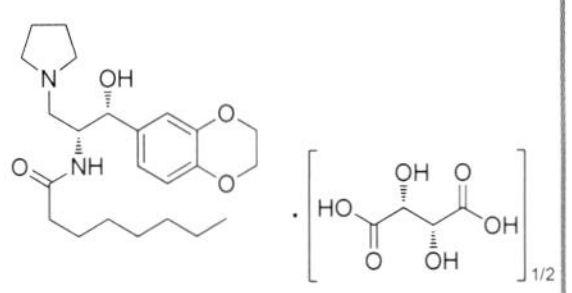

*Metabolic disorder*
*Glucosylceramide synthase*
*inhibitor*

**Uridine Triacetate**
**Xuriden®   2015**

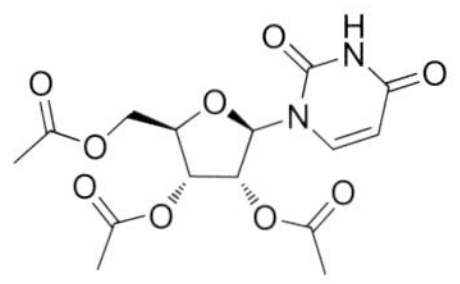

*Metabolic disorder*
*Pyrimidine analog*

**Tolvaptan**
**Samsca®   2009**

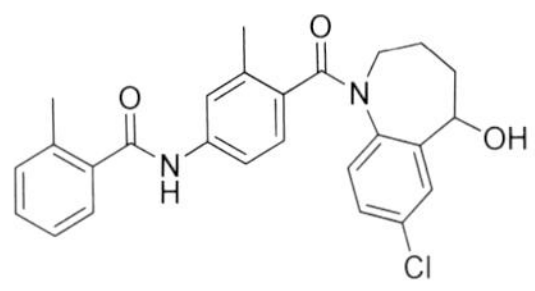

*Metabolic disorder*
*Selective vasopressin V2-*
*receptor antagonist*

**Lorcaserin Hydrochloride**
**Hemihydrate**
**Belviq®   2012**

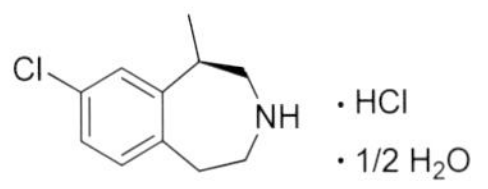

*Obesity*
*Selective 5-HT2C receptor*
*agonist, Serotonin receptor*
*agonist*

## Cetilistat
### Oblean®  *2013*

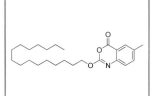

***Obesity***
*Pancreatic lipase inhibitor*

## Deoxycholic Acid
### Kybella®  *2015*

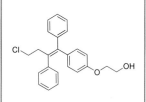

***Obesity***
*GPCR*

# Genitourinary System

## Ulipristal Acetate
### EllaOne®/Ella®/
### Esmya®  *2009*

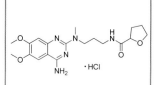

***Acyeterion***
*Progesterone agonist/antagonist*

## Ospemifene
### Osphena®  *2013*

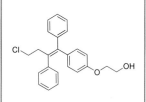

***Gynecological diseases***
*Estrogen agonist/antagonist*

## Dutasteride
### Avodart®/Avolve®  *2001*

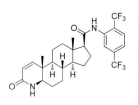

***Prostate drug***
*5-α-reductase inhibitor*

## Alfuzosin Hydrochloride
### Uroxatral®/Xatral®  *2003*

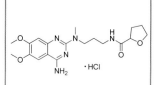

***Prostate drug***
*α1 adrenergic antagonist*

## Silodosin
### Urief®/Rapaflo®/
### Silodyx®  *2006*

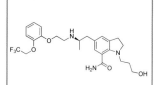

***Prostate drug***
*α1 adrenergic antagonist*

## Vardenafil Hydrochloride
### Levitra®/Vivanza®/
### Staxyn®  *2003*

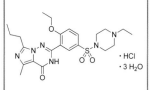

***Sexual dysfunction***
*PDE-5 inhibitor*

## Udenafil
### Zydena®  *2005*

***Sexual dysfunction***
*PDE-5 inhibitor*

## Dapoxetine Hydrochloride
### Priligy®  *2009*

***Sexual dysfunction***
*Serotonin transporter inhibitor, SSRI*

## Avanafil
### Zepeed®/Stendra®/
### Spedra®  *2011*

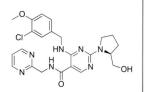

***Sexual dysfunction***
*PDE5 inhibitor*

## Flibanserin
### Addyi®  *2015*

***Sexual dysfunction***
*5HT1A receptor agonist, 5HT2A receptor antagonist*

## Darifenacin Hydrobromide
### Emselex®/Enablex®/
### Xelena®  *2004*

***Urethral disease***
*M3 muscarinic acetylcholine receptor antagonist*

## Solifenacin Succinate
### Vesicare®  *2004*

***Urethral disease***
*Competitive muscarinic acetylcholine receptor antagonist*

## Trospium Chloride
### Sanctura®  *2004*

***Urethral disease***
*Muscarinic antagonist*

**Fesoterodine Fumarate**
**Toviaz®** *2007*

**Urethral disease**
*Competitive muscarinic receptor antagonist, Specific muscarinic receptor antagonist*

**Imidafenacin**
**Uritos®/Staybla®** *2007*

**Urethral disease**
*Muscarinic acetylcholine receptor antagonist, M3 and M1 receptors antagonist*

**Mirabegron**
**Betanis®/Betmiga®/**
**Myrbetriq®** *2011*

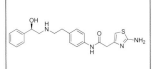

**Urethral disease**
*β3 adrenergic agonist*

## Musculoskeletal System

**Etoricoxib**
**Arcoxia®** *2002*

**Arthritis**
*COX-2 selective inhibitor*

**Zucapsaicin Zuacta®/**
**Civanex®** *2010*

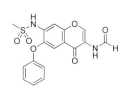

**Arthritis**
*TRPV1 channel agonist, TRPV1 (vanilloid VR1 receptor)*

**Iguratimod Iremod®/**
**Kolbet®/Careram®** *2011*

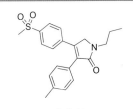

**Arthritis**
*NF-κB activation inhibitor*

**Imrecoxib**
**Hengyang®** *2011*

**Arthritis**
*Selective COX-2 inhibitor*

**Esflurbiprofen**
**Loqoa®** *2015*

**Arthritis**
*COX inhibitor*

**Polmacoxib**
**Acelex®** *2015*

**Arthritis**
*COX-2 inhibitor*

**Falecalcitriol Hornel®/**
**Fulstan®** *2001*

**Bone metabolism**
*Active vitamin D3 derivative*

**Neridronate Sodium**
**Nerixia®** *2002*

**Bone metabolism**
*Bisphosphonate*

**Strontium Ranelate**
**Osseor®/Protelos®/**
**Protos®** *2004*

**Bone metabolism**
*Calcium sensing receptor stimulator*

**Bazedoxifene Acetate**
**Conbriza®/Viviant®** *2009*

**Bone metabolism**
*SERM*

**Minodronic Acid Hydrate**
**Bonoteo®/Recalbon®** *2009*

**Bone metabolism**
*Bisphosphonate*

**Eldecalcitol**
**Edirol®** *2011*

**Bone metabolism**
*Orally active vitamin D analogue*

### Ibandronate Sodium Hydrate Boniva®/ Bondronat®/Bonviva®  *2003*

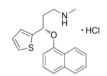

**Bone metabolism, Sports injury**
*Bisphosphonate*

### Pregabalin Lyrica®  *2004*

**Muscular disease**
*GABA receptor inhibitor*

### Amifampridine Phosphate Firdapse®/Zenas®  *2009*

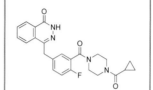

**Muscular disease**
*Potassium channel blocker*

### Ataluren Translarna®  *2014*

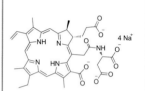

**Muscular disease**
*Nonsense mutations regulator*

### Duloxetine Hydrochloride Cymbalta®/Ariclaim® *2004*

**Muscular disease, Sports injury**
*SNRI*

### Neoplasm

### Olaparib Lynparza®  *2014*

**Brain tumor, Cancer of the female reproductive system**
*PARP inhibitor*

### Talaporfin Sodium Laserphyrin®  *2003*

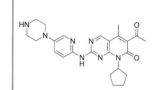

**Brain tumor, Lung Cancer**
*Photosensitizer*

### Fulvestrant Faslodex®  *2002*

**Breast cancer**
*Estrogen receptor antagonist*

### Ixabepilone Ixempra®  *2007*

**Breast cancer**
*Microtubule inhibitor*

### Lapatinib Ditosylate Hydrate Tykerb®/ Tyverb®  *2007*

**Breast cancer**
*HER2/EGFR tyrosine kinase inhibitor*

### Palbociclib Ibrance®  *2015*

**Breast cancer**
*CDK4/CDK6 inhibitor*

### Belotecan Hydrochloride Camtobell®  *2003*

**Cancer of the female reproductive system, Lung Cancer**
*Topoisomerase I inhibitor*

### Trabectedin Yondelis®  *2007*

**Cancer of the female reproductive system, Sarcoma Plant alkaloids, Cell apoptosis induction agent**

### Regorafenib Monohydrate Stivarga®  *2012*

**Colorectal cancer**
*Tyrosine kinase inhibitor*

### Apatinib Mesylate 艾坦®  *2014*

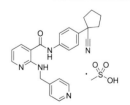

**Gastric and esophageal cancer**
*VEGFR2 tyrosine kinase inhibitor*

| | | | |
|---|---|---|---|
| **Vandetanib**<br>**Caprelsa®** *2011* | **Cabozantinib *S*-Malate**<br>**Cometriq®** *2012* | **Lenvatinib Mesylate**<br>**Lenvima®** *2015* | **Sorafenib Tosylate**<br>**Nexavar®** *2005* |
| 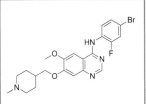<br><br>***Head and neck cancer***<br>*Multi-targeted RTKs inhibitor,*<br>*Tyrosine Kinase inhibitor* | ***Head and neck cancer***<br>*Multi-targeted RTKs inhibitor* | ***Head and neck cancer***<br>*VEGFR2/VEGFR3 kinase*<br>*inhibitor* | ***Head and neck cancer, Kidney***<br>***cancer, Liver and gallbladder***<br>***cancer***<br>*Multi-targeted kinase inhibitor* |

| | | | |
|---|---|---|---|
| **Sunitinib Malate**<br>**Sutent®** *2006* | **Axitinib**<br>**Inlyta®** *2012* | **Temsirolimus**<br>**Torisel®** *2007* | **Pazopanib Hydrochloride**<br>**Votrient®** *2009* |
| 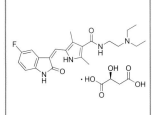<br><br>***Kidney cancer***<br>*Tyrosine kinase inhibitor* | 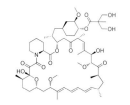<br><br>***Kidney cancer***<br>*VEGFR and PDGF tyrosine*<br>*kinase inhibitor* | ***Kidney cancer, Lymphoma***<br>*mTOR inhibitor* | 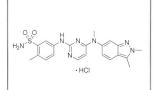<br><br>***Kidney cancer, Sarcoma***<br>*Multi-targeted RTKs inhibitor* |

| | | | |
|---|---|---|---|
| **Imatinib Mesylate**<br>**Gleevec®/Glivec®** *2001* | **Clofarabine**<br>**Clolar®/Evoltra®** *2004* | **Tamibarotene**<br>**Amnolake®** *2005* | **Dasatinib Hydrate**<br>**Sprycel®** *2006* |
| ***Leukemia***<br>*Tyrosine kinase inhibitor* | ***Leukemia***<br>*Purine nucleoside metabolic*<br>*inhibitor* | ***Leukemia***<br>*RARα agonist* | ***Leukemia***<br>*Multi-targeted inhibitor* |

| | | | |
|---|---|---|---|
| **Decitabine**<br>**Dacogen®** *2006* | **Nilotinib Hydrochloride**<br>**Hydrate Tasigna®** *2007* | **Bosutinib Monohydrate**<br>**Bosulif®** *2012* | **Omacetaxine**<br>**Mepesuccinate**<br>**Synribo®** *2012* |
| ***Leukemia***<br>*Nucleoside metabolic inhibitor* | ***Leukemia***<br>*Bcr-Abl kinase inhibitor* | ***Leukemia***<br>*Kinase inhibitor* | ***Leukemia***<br>*Protein translation inhibitor* |

**Ponatinib Hydrochloride**
**Iclusig®  2012**

*Leukemia*
*Multi-targeted tyrosine kinase inhibitor*

**Radotinib Dihydrochloride**
**Supect®  2012**

*Leukemia*
*Bcr-Abl tyrosine kinase inhibitor, PDGFR inhibitor*

**Nelarabine Arranon®/**
**Atriance®  2005**

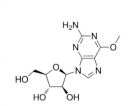

*Leukemia, Lymphoma*
*Nucleoside metabolic inhibitor*

**Ibrutinib**
**Imbruvica®  2013**

*Leukemia, Lymphoma*
*BTK inhibitor*

**Idelalisib**
**Zydelig®  2014**

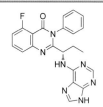

*Leukemia, Lymphoma*
*PI3Kδ kinase inhibitor*

**Bortezomib**
**Velcade®  2003**

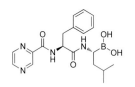

*Leukemia, Lymphoma,*
*Myeloma*
*Proteasome inhibitor*

**Miriplatin Hydrate**
**Miripla®  2009**

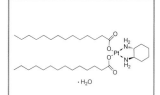

*Liver and gallbladder cancer*
*Lipophilic platinum complex*

**Amrubicin Hydrochloride**
**Calsed®  2002**

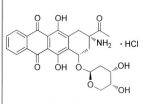

*Lung Cancer*
*Topoisomerase inhibitor*

**Gefitinib**
**Iressa®  2002**

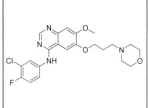

*Lung Cancer*
*EGFR tyrosine kinase inhibitor*

**Pemetrexed Disodium**
**Hydrate**
**Alimta®  2004**

*Lung Cancer*
*Folate analog metabolic inhibitor*

**Crizotinib**
**Xalkori®  2011**

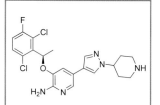

*Lung Cancer*
*ALK inhibitor, c-Met inhibitor,*
*ROS1 RTKs inhibitor*

**Icotinib Hydrochloride**
**Conmana®  2011**

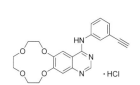

*Lung Cancer*
*EGFR tyrosine kinase inhibitor*

**Afatinib Dimaleate**
**Gilotrif®/Giotrif®  2013**

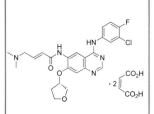

*Lung Cancer*
*Kinase inhibitor*

**Alectinib Hydrochloride**
**Alecensa®  2014**

*Lung Cancer*
*ALK inhibitor*

**Ceritinib**
**Zykadia®  2014**

*Lung Cancer*
*ALK inhibitor*

**Nintedanib Esylate**
**Ofev®  2014**

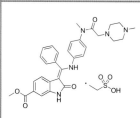

*Lung Cancer*
*Tyrosine kinase inhibitor*

**Osimertinib Mesylate**
**Tagrisso®** *2015*

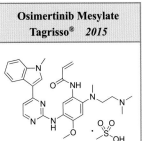

*Lung Cancer*
*EGFR inhibitor,Thr790met*
*mutant inhibitor*

**Erlotinib Hydrochloride**
**Tarceva®** *2004*

*Lung Cancer, Pancreatic cancer*
*EGFR tyrosine kinase inhibitor*

**Vorinostat**
**Zolinza®** *2006*

*Lymphoma*
*HDAC inhibitor*

**Pralatrexate**
**Folotyn®** *2009*

*Lymphoma*
*Folate analog metabolic*
*inhibitor*

**Romidepsin**
**Istodax®** *2009*

*Lymphoma*
*HDAC inhibitor*

**Pixantrone Dimaleate**
**Pixuvri®** *2012*

*Lymphoma*
*DNA intercalating agent,*
*Cytotoxic antibiotics*

**Belinostat**
**Beleodaq®** *2014*

*Lymphoma*
*HDAC inhibitor*

**Chidamide**
**Epidaza®/爱谱沙®** *2014*

*Lymphoma*
*HDAC inhibitor*

**Lenalidomide**
**Revlimid®** *2005*

*Lymphoma, Myeloma*
*Angiogenesis inhibitor*

**Plerixafor**
**Mozobil®** *2008*

*Lymphoma, Myeloma*
*CXCR4 inhibitor*

**Vemurafenib**
**Zelboraf®** *2011*

*Melanoma*
*B-Raf kinase inhibitor*

**Dabrafenib Mesylate**
**Tafinlar®** *2013*

*Melanoma*
*B-Raf kinase inhibitor*

**Trametinib Dimethyl**
**Sulfoxide**
**Mekinist®** *2013*

*Melanoma*
*MEK inhibitor*

**Cobimetinib Fumarate**
**Cotellic®** *2015*

*Melanoma*
*MEK inhibitor*

**Carfilzomib**
**Kyprolis®** *2012*

*Myeloma*
*Proteasome inhibitor*

**Pomalidomide**
**Pomalyst®/Imnovid®** *2013*

*Myeloma*
*Immunomodulators*

**Ixazomib Citrate**
**Ninlaro® 2015**

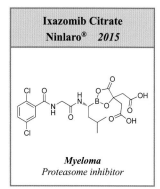

*Myeloma*
*Proteasome inhibitor*

**Panobinostat Lactate**
**Farydak® 2015**

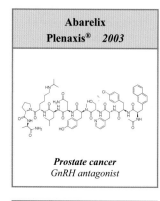

*Myeloma*
*HDAC inhibitor*

**Abarelix**
**Plenaxis® 2003**

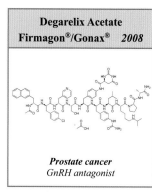

*Prostate cancer*
*GnRH antagonist*

**Degarelix Acetate**
**Firmagon®/Gonax® 2008**

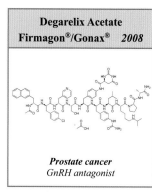

*Prostate cancer*
*GnRH antagonist*

**Cabazitaxel**
**Jevtana® 2010**

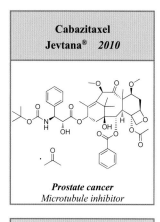

*Prostate cancer*
*Microtubule inhibitor*

**Abiraterone Acetate**
**Zytiga® 2011**

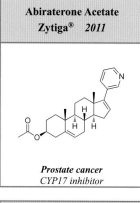

*Prostate cancer*
*CYP17 inhibitor*

**Enzalutamide**
**Xtandi® 2012**

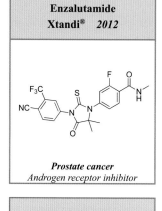

*Prostate cancer*
*Androgen receptor inhibitor*

**Mifamurtide Sodium**
**Hydrate**
**Mepact® 2009**

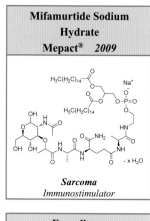

*Sarcoma*
*Immunostimulator*

**Methyl Aminolevulinate**
**HCl Metvix®/**
**Metvixia® 2001**

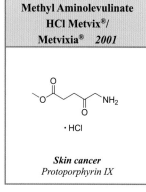

*Skin cancer*
*Protoporphyrin IX*

**Vismodegib**
**Erivedge® 2012**

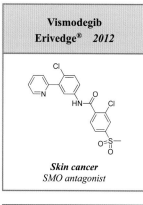

*Skin cancer*
*SMO antagonist*

**Sonidegib Phosphate**
**Odomzo® 2015**

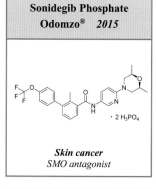

*Skin cancer*
*SMO antagonist*

**Everolimus**
**Certican®/Zortress®/**
**Afinitor® 2003**

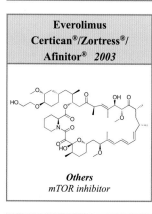

*Others*
*mTOR inhibitor*

**Azacitidine**
**Vidaza® 2004**

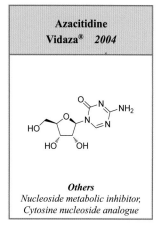

*Others*
*Nucleoside metabolic inhibitor,*
*Cytosine nucleoside analogue*

**Ulipristal Acetate**
**EllaOne®/Ella®/**
**Esmya® 2009**

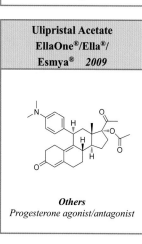

*Others*
*Progesterone agonist/antagonist*

**Vinflunine Ditartrate**
**Javlor® 2009**

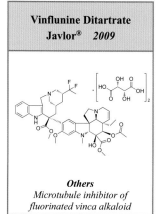

*Others*
*Microtubule inhibitor of*
*fluorinated vinca alkaloid*

**Ruxolitinib Phosphate**
**Jakafi®/Jakavi® 2011**

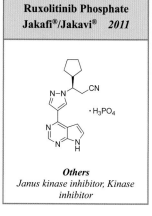

*Others*
*Janus kinase inhibitor, Kinase*
*inhibitor*

## Nervous System

### Varenicline Tartrate
Chantix®/Champix®   *2006*

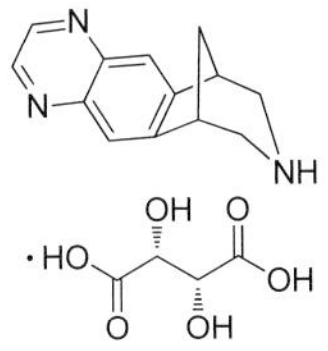

**Addiction**
*Nicotinic receptor partial agonist*

### Memantine Hydrochloride
Namenda®/Axura®/
Ebixa®   *2002*

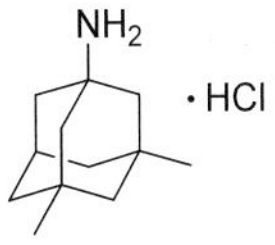

**Alzheimer's disease**
*NMDA-receptor antagonist*

### Frovatriptan Succinate
Hydrate Frova®/
Migard®   *2001*

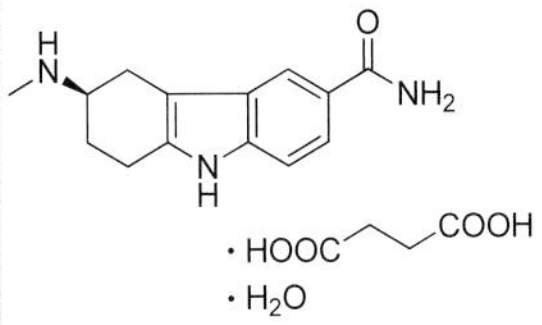

**Analgesic**
*5-HT1B/1D serotonin receptor
agonist, Serotonin receptor
agonist*

### Tapentadol Hydrochloride
Nucynta®/Palexia®   *2008*

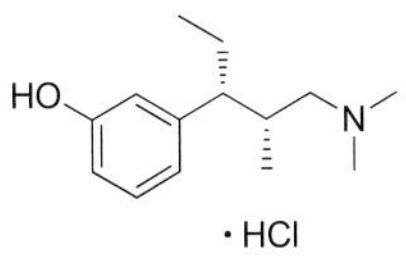

**Analgesic**
*μ-opioid receptor agonist and
norepinephrine reuptake
inhibitor*

### Capsaicin
Qutenza®   *2009*

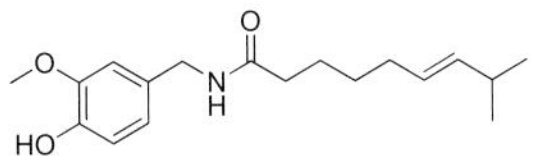

**Analgesic**
*TRPV1 channel agonist,
Vanilloid receptor agonist*

### Pregabalin
Lyrica®   *2004*

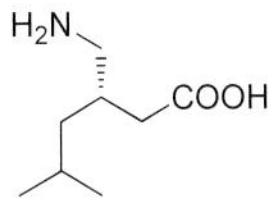

**Analgesic**
*GABA receptor inhibitor*

### Fospropofol Disodium
Lusedra®   *2008*

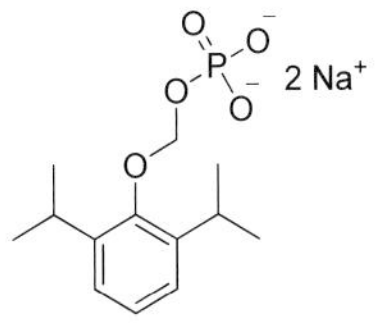

**Anesthetic**
*GABA receptor enhance*

### Escitalopram Oxalate
Lexapro®/Cipralex®   *2002*

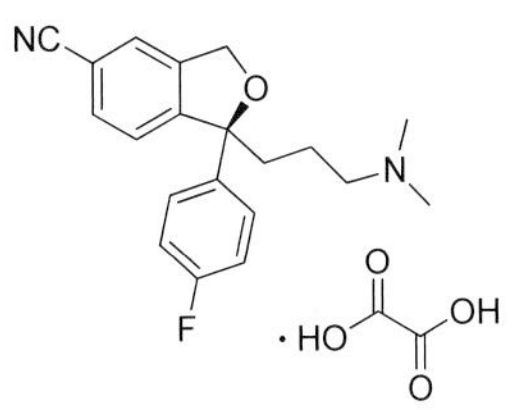

**Antidepressants or anti-anxiety**
*Selective serotonin reuptake
inhibitor*

### Desvenlafaxine
Succinate Hydrate
Pristiq®   *2008*

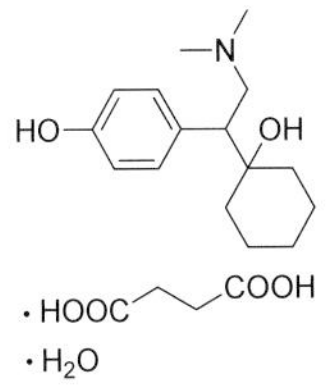

**Antidepressants or anti-anxiety**
*SNRI*

### Agomelatine
Thymanax®/
Valdoxan®   *2009*

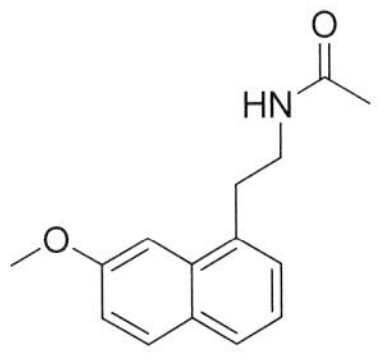

**Antidepressants or anti-anxiety**
*5-HT2C/5-HT2B antagnist,
MT1/MT2 agonist*

### Vilazodone Hydrochloride
Viibryd®   *2011*

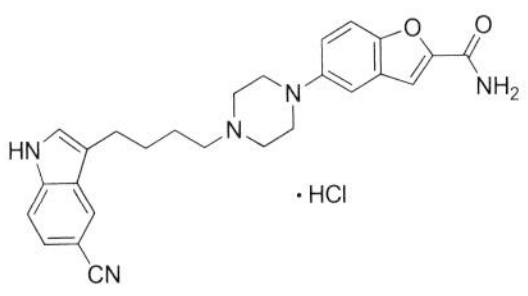

**Antidepressants or anti-anxiety**
*5-HT1A receptor partial agonist*

### Levomilnacipran
Hydrochloride
Fetzima®   *2013*

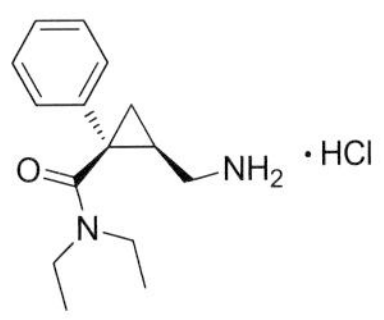

**Antidepressants or anti-anxiety**
*SNRI*

### Vortioxetine Hydrobromide
Brintellix®   *2013*

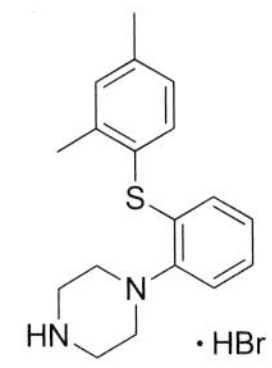

**Antidepressants or anti-anxiety**
*5-HT modulator and stimulator*

### Duloxetine Hydrochloride
Cymbalta®/Ariclaim®
*2004*

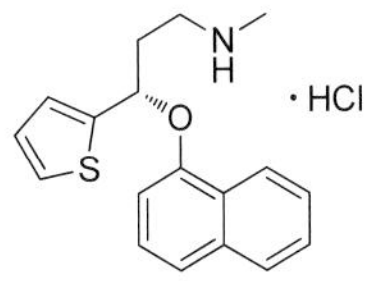

**Antidepressants or anti-anxiety**
*SNRI*

### Ziprasidone
Geodon®/Zeldox®   *2001*

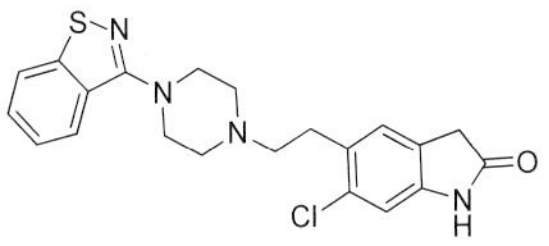

**Antipsychotics**
*Dopamine D2 and 5HT2
antagonist*

| **Paliperidone**<br>**Invega® 2006** | **Blonanserin**<br>**Lonasen® 2008** | **Asenapine Maleate**<br>**Saphris®/Sycrest® 2009** | **Iloperidone**<br>**Fanapt® 2009** |
|---|---|---|---|
| | | 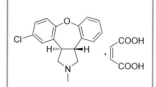 | |
| ***Antipsychotics***<br>*D2 dopamine receptor antagonist; 5HT2A serotonin receptor antagonist* | ***Antipsychotics***<br>*Serotonin receptor antagonist, Dopamine receptor antagonist* | ***Antipsychotics***<br>*5-HT2A serotonin receptor antagonist, Dopamine D2 receptor antagonist* | ***Antipsychotics***<br>*5-HT2 serotonin receptor antagonist, Dopamine receptor antagonist* |

| **Lurasidone Hydrochloride**<br>**Latuda® 2010** | **Aripiprazole lauroxil**<br>**Aristada® 2015** | **Cariprazine Hydrochloride**<br>**Vraylar® 2015** | **Brexpiprazole**<br>**Rexulti® 2015** |
|---|---|---|---|
| 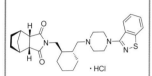 | 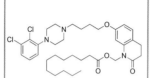 | 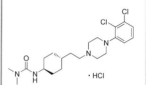 | 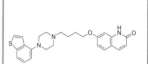 |
| ***Antipsychotics***<br>*5HT2A receptor, D2 dopamine receptor antagonist* | ***Antipsychotics***<br>*5-HT1A receptor agonist, 5-HT2A antagonist, Dopamine D2 receptor agonist* | ***Antipsychotics***<br>*5-HT1A receptor agonist, 5-HT2A antagonist, Dopamine D2 receptor agonist* | ***Antipsychotics***<br>*5-HT1A receptor agonist, 5-HT2A antagonist, Dopamine D2 receptor agonist* |

| **Aripiprazole**<br>**Abilify® 2002** | **Rufinamide Inovelon®/**<br>**Banzel® 2007** | **Lacosamide**<br>**Vimpat® 2008** | **Eslicarbazepine Acetate**<br>**Exelief®/Zebinix®/**<br>**Stedesa® 2009** |
|---|---|---|---|
| 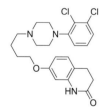 | 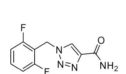 | 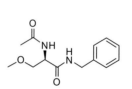 | 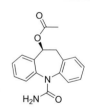 |
| ***Antipsychotics***<br>*5-HT1A receptor agonist, 5-HT2A antagonist, Dopamine D2 receptor agonist* | ***Epilepsy***<br>*Voltage-gated sodium channel modulator* | ***Epilepsy***<br>*Sodium channel enhancer* | ***Epilepsy***<br>*Voltage-gated sodium channels inhibitor* |

| **Retigabine/Ezogabine**<br>**Trobalt®/Potiga® 2011** | **Dalfampridine/Fampridine**<br>**Ampyra®/Fampyra® 2010** | **Fingolimod Hydrochloride**<br>**Gilenya®/Imusera® 2010** | **Teriflunomide**<br>**Aubagio® 2012** |
|---|---|---|---|
| | | | |
| ***Epilepsy***<br>*Potassium channel opener* | ***Multiple sclerosis***<br>*Potassium channel blocker* | ***Multiple sclerosis***<br>*Sphingosine 1-phosphate receptor modulator* | ***Multiple sclerosis***<br>*Pyrimidine synthesis inhibitor, Dihydroorotate dehydrogenase blocker* |

**Dimethyl Fumarate**
**Tecfidera®** *2013*

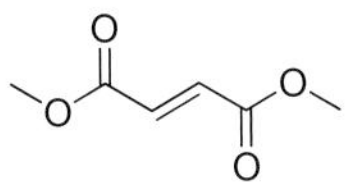

***Multiple sclerosis***
*Hypoxic cell radiosensitizer,*
*Nicotinic receptor agonist*

**Rasagiline Mesylate**
**Azilect®** *2005*

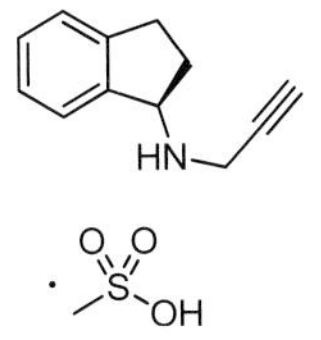

***Parkinson's disease***
*Irreversible MAO-B inhibitor*

**Istradefylline**
**Nouriast®** *2013*

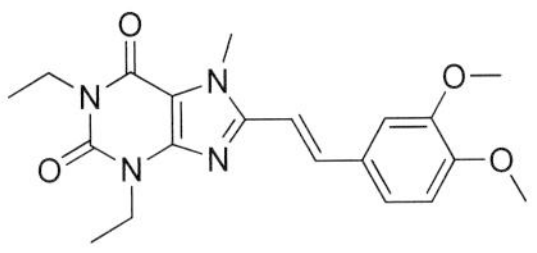

***Parkinson's disease***
*Adenosine A2A receptor*
*antagonist*

**Safinamide**
**Methanesulfonate**
**Xadago®** *2015*

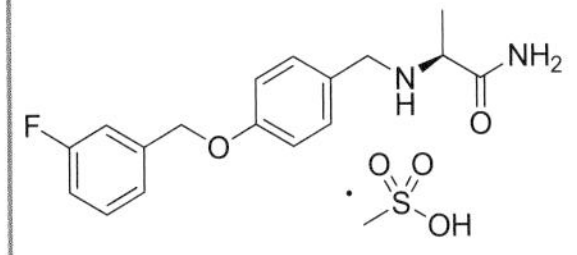

***Parkinson's disease***
*MAO-B inhibitor, Sodium*
*channel blocker, Glutamate*
*release inhibitor, Dopamine*
*receptor*

**Sodium Oxybate**
**Xyrem®** *2002*

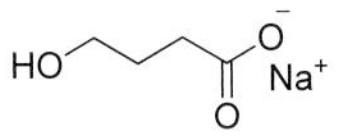

***Sleep disorder***
*CNS depressant, Central nervous*
*system depressant*

**Eszopiclone**
**Lunesta®** *2004*

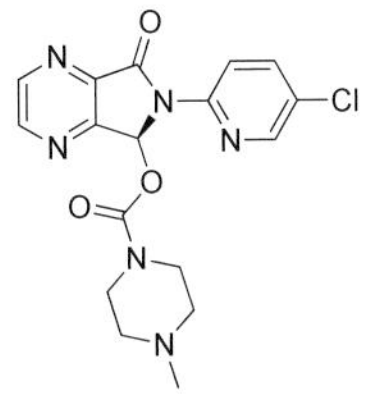

***Sleep disorder***
*Gamma aminobutyric acid*
*receptor*

**Ramelteon**
**Rozerem®** *2005*

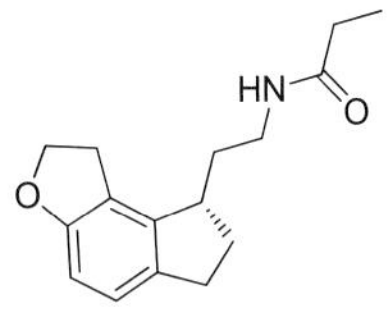

***Sleep disorder***
*Melatonin receptor agonist*

**Armodafinil**
**Nuvigil®** *2007*

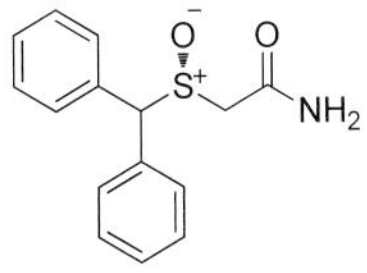

***Sleep disorder***
*Indirect dopamine receptor*
*agonist, Dopamine reuptake*
*inhibitor*

**Suvorexant**
**Belsomra®** *2014*

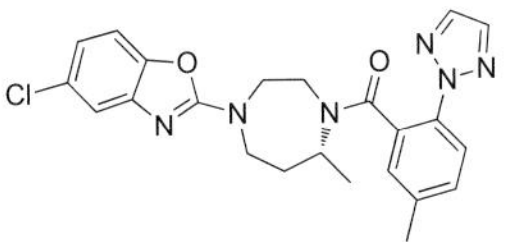

***Sleep disorder***
*Orexin receptor antagonist*

**Tasimelteon**
**Hetlioz®** *2014*

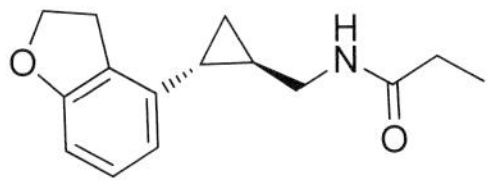

***Sleep disorder***
*Melatonin receptor agonist*

**Dexmethylphenidate HCl**
**Focalin®/Attenade®** *2001*

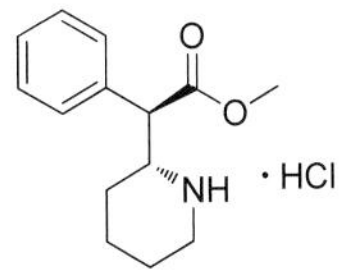

***Others***
*Norepinephrine-dopamine*
*reuptake inhibitor*

**Edaravone**
**Radicut®/Arone®** *2001*

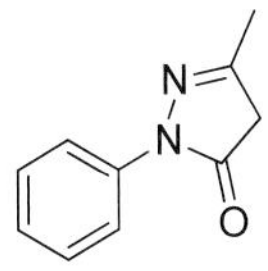

***Others***
*Neural protective agent*

**Atomoxetine Hydrochloride**
**Strattera®** *2002*

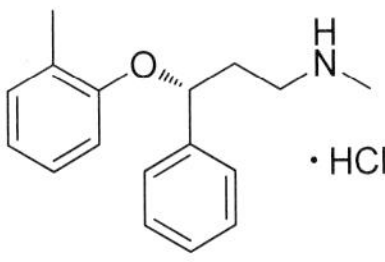

***Others***
*Norepinephrine reuptake*
*inhibitor*

**Rotigotine**
**Neupro®/Leganto®** *2006*

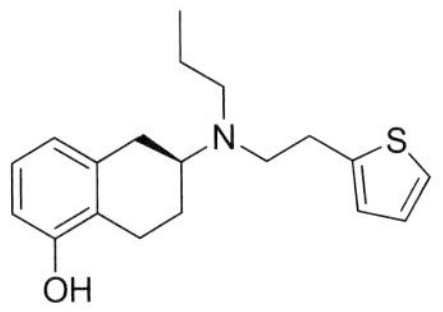

***Others***
*Non-ergoline dopamine agonist*

**Lisdexamfetamine**
**Dimesylate Vyvanse®/**
**Elvanse®/Venvanse®** *2007*

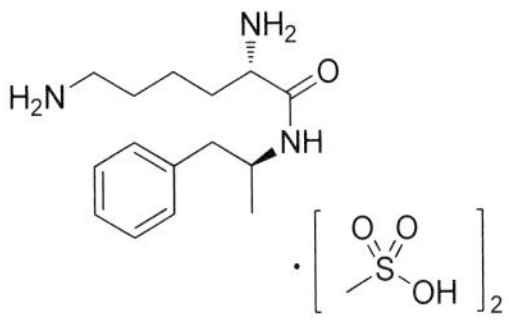

***Others***
*CNS stimulant*

**Sugammadex Sodium**
**Bridion®** *2008*

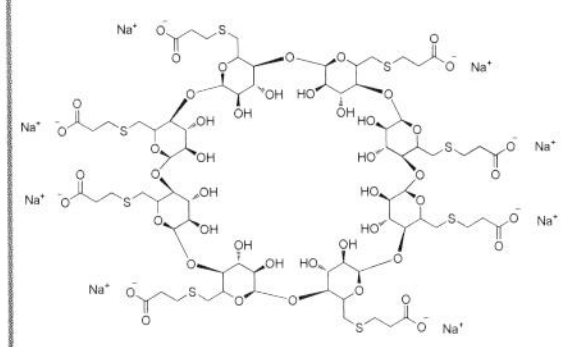

***Others***
*SRBA*

## Tetrabenazine Xenazine®/Choreazine® *2008*

**Others**
*VMAT2 inhibitor*

## Gabapentin Enacarbil Horizant®/Regnite® *2011*

**Others**
*GABA receptor agonist*

## Ophthalmic and ENT

## Levocetirizine Dihydrochloride Xyzal®/Xusal® *2001*

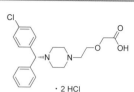

· 2 HCl

**Ear infection, Rhinitis**
*Histamine H1 receptor antagonist*

## Finafloxacin Xtoro® *2014*

**Ear infection**
*Quinolone antibiotic*

## Valganciclovir Hydrochloride Valcyte®/Valixa® *2001*

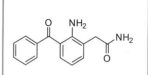

· HCl

**Ear infection**
*CMV nucleoside analogue DNA polymerase inhibitor*

## Nepafenac Nevanac® *2005*

**Ear infection**
*Prostaglandin H synthase (cyclooxygenase) inhibitor*

## Besifloxacin Hydrochloride Besivance® *2009*

· HCl

**Ear infection**
*Fluoroquinolone antibiotic*

## Bimatoprost Lumigan®/Latisse® *2001*

**Glaucoma**
*Prostaglandin analog*

## Travoprost Travatan®/Travatan Z® *2001*

**Glaucoma**
*Selective FP prostanoid receptor agonist*

## Tafluprost Taflotan®/Tapros®/Zioptan® *2008*

**Glaucoma**
*Selective FP prostanoid receptor agonist*

## Ripasudil Hydrochloride Hydrate Glanatec® *2014*

· HCl
· 2 H₂O

**Glaucoma**
*Rho kinase inhibitor*

## Fluticasone Furoate Veramyst®/Avamys®/Allermist® *2007*

**Rhinitis**
*GR, Anti-inflammitory corticosteroid*

## Dexamethasone Cipecilate Erizas® *2009*

**Rhinitis**
*Glucocorticoid class steroid drug, GR*

## Desloratadine Aerius®/Clarinex®/Neoclarityn® *2001*

**Rhinitis**
*Histamine H1 receptor antagonist*

## Garenoxacin Mesilate Hydrate Geninax® *2007*

· H₂O

**Others**
*Quinolone antibiotic, DNA topoisomerase inhibitor*

**Sitafloxacin Hydrate**
**Gracevit®  2008**

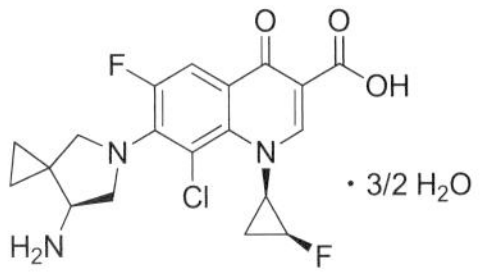

*Others*
*Quinolone antibiotic*

**Alcaftadine**
**Lastacaft®  2010**

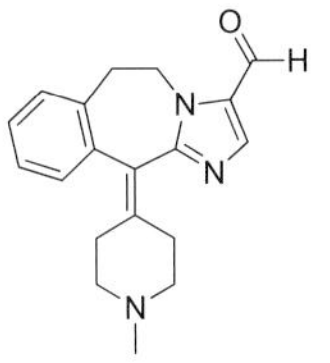

*Others*
*H1 histamine receptor antagonist*

**Diquafosol Tetrasodium**
**Diquas®  2010**

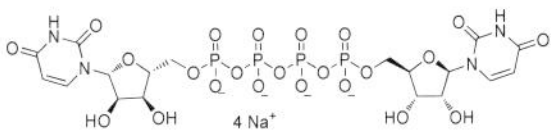

*Others*
*P2Y2 purinoceptor receptor*
*agonist*

**Respiratory**

**Ciclesonide**
**Alvesco®/Omnaris®  2004**

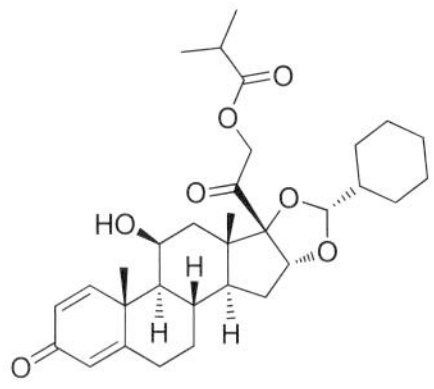

*Asthma*
*GR*

**Tiotropium Bromide**
**Hydrate Spiriva®  2001**

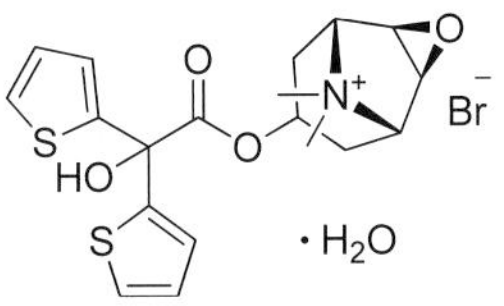

*Chronic obstructive pulmonary*
*disease*
*Muscarinic acetylcholine*
*receptor antagonist*

**Arformoterol Tartrate**
**Brovana®  2006**

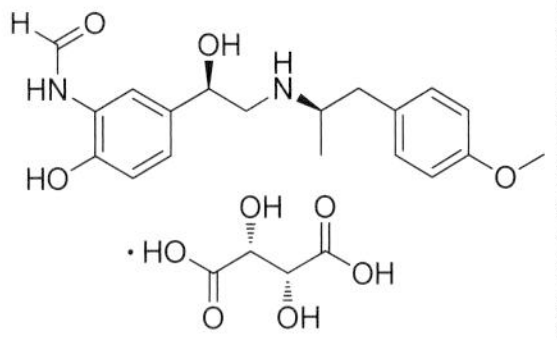

*Chronic obstructive pulmonary*
*disease*
*Long acting β-adrenoceptor*
*agonist*

**Indacaterol Maleate**
**Onbrez®/Arcapta®/**
**Hirobriz® 2009**

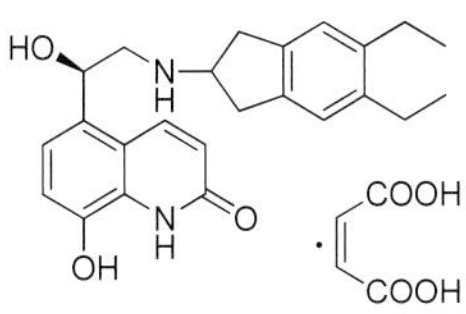

*Chronic obstructive pulmonary*
*disease*
*Long-acting β2-adrenergic*
*agonist*

**Roflumilast**
**Daxas®/Daliresp®/Libertek®**
**2010**

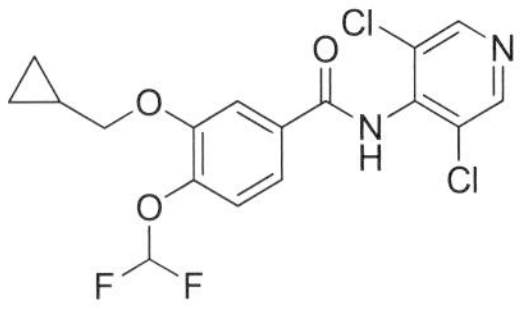

*Chronic obstructive pulmonary*
*disease*
*PDE-4 inhibitor*

**Aclidinium Bromide**
**Bretaris Genuair®/Eklira**
**Genuair®/Tudorza**
**Pressair®  2012**

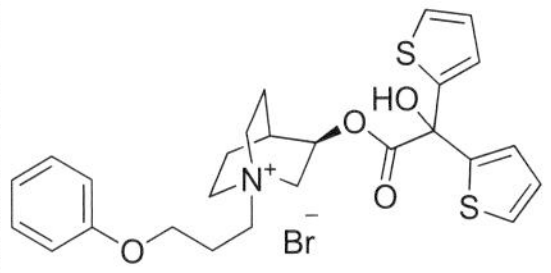

*Chronic obstructive pulmonary*
*disease*
*Muscarinic M3 receptor*
*antagonist*

**Glycopyrronium Bromide**
**Enurev®/Seebri®/Robinul®**
**2012**

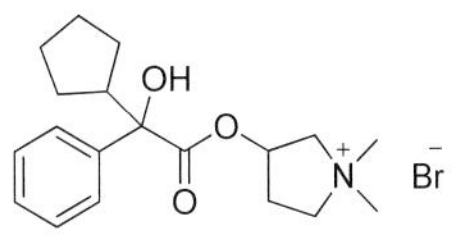

*Chronic obstructive pulmonary*
*disease*
*Muscarinic antagonist*

**Olodaterol Hydrochloride**
**Striverdi Respimat®  2013**

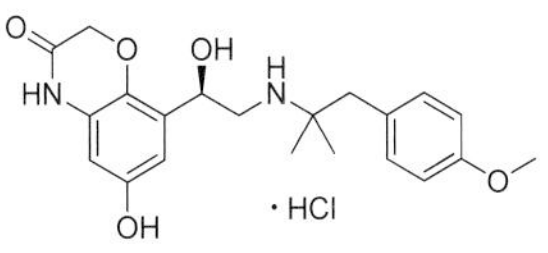

*Chronic obstructive pulmonary*
*disease*
*LABA*

**Umeclidinium Bromide**
**Incruse®/Ellipta®  2014**

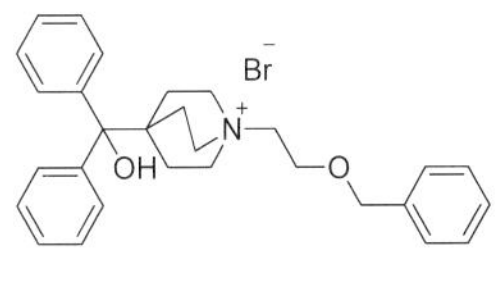

*Chronic obstructive pulmonary*
*disease*
*LAMA*

**Nintedanib Esylate**
**Ofev®  2014**

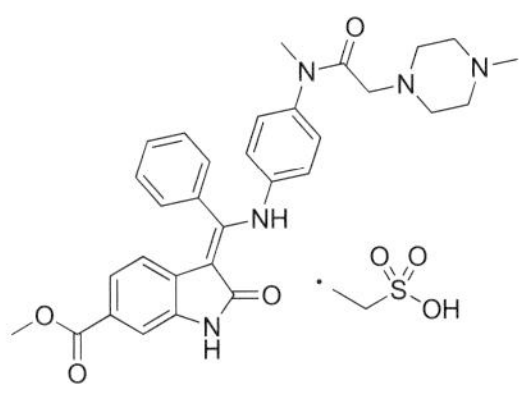

*Lung Cancer*
*Tyrosine kinase inhibitor*

**Telithromycin**
**Ketek®  2001**

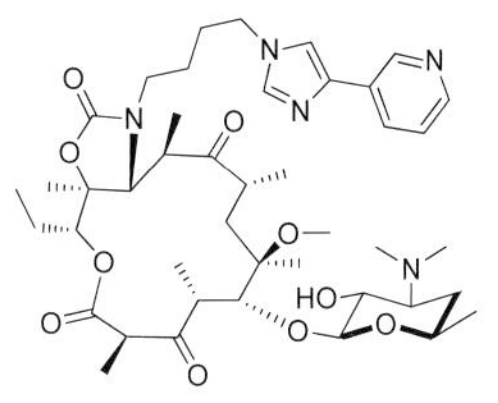

*Respiratory tract infection*
*Macrolides antibiotic*

**Sitafloxacin Hydrate**
**Gracevit®  2008**

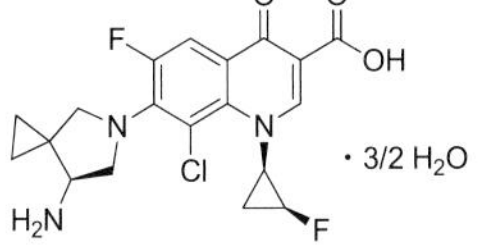

*Respiratory tract infection*
*Quinolone antibiotic,*
*Fluoroquinolone antibiotic*

| **Antofloxacin Hydrochloride**<br>优朋® *2009* | **Telavancin Hydrochloride**<br>Vibativ® *2009* | **Ceftaroline Fosamil Acetate**<br>Teflaro®/Zinforo® *2010* | **Fudosteine**<br>Cleanal®/Spelear® *2001* |
|---|---|---|---|
| | | | |
| ***Respiratory tract infection***<br>*Quinolone antibiotic* | ***Respiratory tract infection***<br>*Glycopeptide antibiotic* | ***Respiratory tract infection***<br>*Cephalosporin antibiotic* | ***Others***<br>*MUC5AC mucin hypersecretion inhibitor* |

| **Sivelestat Sodium Hydrate**<br>Elaspol® *2002* | **Pirfenidone**<br>Pirespa®/Esbriet® *2008* | **Ivacaftor**<br>Kalydeco® *2012* | |
|---|---|---|---|
| | | | |
| ***Others***<br>*Neutrophil elastase inhibitor* | ***Others***<br>*TGF-β1 inhibitor, Collagen inhibitor* | ***Others***<br>*CFTR potentiator* | |

# 客户反馈表

**1、工作类别、领域**

A. 立项人员　　B. 研发人员　　C. 管理人员　　D. 科研人员　　E. 其他

**2、您所关注的板块**

A. 药物基本信息（结构、适应症、用法用量、杂质辅料）

B. 药物的市场信息：批准与销售　　C. 专利信息　　D. 化学合成信息

E. 药理药效信息　　F. 药代信息　　G. 毒理信息

**3、该书是否能帮助到您**

A. 非常有帮助，解决了手边棘手问题　　B. 很有帮助，能查询不少想知道的数据

C. 有帮助，可以学习不少知识　　D. 根本没帮助

**4、对该书内容数据详细程度的意见**

A. 数据太多，不能突出核心数据　　B. 数据全面　　C. 数据太少，部分内容缺失

缺失内容请填写

**5、总结单页是否能涵盖您所关心的问题**

A. 是，非常全面　　　B. 否，内容太简单。需要丰富的方面：

C. 否，缺少部分内容。缺少部分：

**6、专利内容是否足够**

A. 是　　B. 否，缺少

**7、化学合成路线内容是否足够**

A. 是　　B. 否，缺少

**8、药理药效内容是否足够**

A. 是　　B. 否，缺少

**9、药代内容是否足够**

A. 是　　B. 否，缺少

**10、毒理内容是否足够**

A. 是　　B. 否，缺少

**11、何种渠道得知此书？若经推荐购买，推荐人为：**

**12、您希望下一卷做哪些内容、形式的改进：**

以上内容您可拍照发送至bookstore@pharmacodia.com或上传至药渡官方微信公众号；

感谢您在百忙之中的帮忙，请留下联系方式，您会及时了解药渡的最新资讯！

联系人：　　　　　　电话：　　　　　　微信：

邮箱：　　　　　　　联系地址：

微信公众号

购书详询：400-851-9921